Fundamental Mathematics for Computer Applications

Fundamental Mathematics for Computer Applications

Useful for

- Bachelor of Computer Application (BCA) and B.Sc. (IT)
- Foundation of Mathematics for Computer Science and I.T. related Courses

Dr. SUDHIR KUMAR PUNDIR
M.Sc., M.Phil, NET (C.S.I.R.), Ph.D.
Head, Department of Mathematics
S.D. (P.G.) College,
Muzaffarnagar (U.P.)

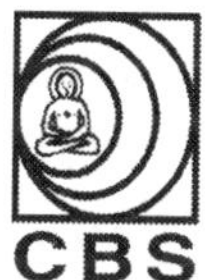

CBS Publishers & Distributors Pvt Ltd
New Delhi • Bengaluru • Chennai • Kochi • Kolkata • Mumbai
Hyderabad • Nagpur • Patna • Pune • Jharkhand • Uttarakhand

Disclaimer
Science and technology are constantly changing fields. New research and experience broaden the scope of information and knowledge. The author has tried his best in giving information available to him while preparing the material for this book. Although, all efforts have been made to ensure optimum accuracy of the material, yet It is quite possible some errors might have been left uncorrected, The publisher, printer and author will not be held responsible for any inadvertent errors or inaccuracies.

Fundamental Mathematics for Computer Applications

ISBN: 978-93-88527-66-8

First Edition: 2019

Published by **Satish Kumar Jain** and produced by **Varun Jain** for
CBS Publishers & Distributors Pvt. Ltd.,
4819/XI Prahlad Street, 24 Ansari Road, Daryaganj, New Delhi - 110002
delhi@cbspd.com, cbspubs@airtelmail.in • www.cbspd.com
Ph.: 23289259, 23266861, 23266867 • Fax: 011-23243014
Corporate Office: 204 FIE, Industrial Area, Patparganj, Delhi - 110 092
Ph: 49344934 • Fax: 011-49344935
E-mail: publishing@cbspd.com • publicity@cbspd.com
Branches:
- ***Bengaluru:*** 2975, 17th Cross, K.R. Road, Bansankari 2nd Stage, Bengaluru - 70 • Ph: +91-80-26771678/79 • Fax: +91-80-26771680 E-mail: cbsbng@gmail.com, bangalore@cbspd.com
- ***Chennai:*** No. 7, Subbaraya Street, Shenoy Nagar, Chennai - 600030 Ph: +91-44-26681266, 26680620 • Fax: +91-44-42032115 E-mail: chennai@cbspd.com
- ***Kochi:*** Ashana House, 39/1904, A.M. Thomas Road, Valanjambalam, Ernakulum, Kochi • Ph: +91-484-4059061-65 Fax: +91-484-4059065 • E-mail: cochin@cbspd.com
- ***Kolkata:*** 6-B, Ground Floor, Rameshwar Shaw Road, Kolkata - 700014 Ph: +91-33-22891126/7/8 • E-mail: kolkata@cbspd.com
- ***Mumbai:*** 83-C, Dr. E. Moses Road, Worli, Mumbai - 400018 Ph: +91-9833017933, 022-24902340/41 • E-mail: mumbai@cbspd.com

Representatives:
- Hyderabad: 0-9885175004
- Patna: 0-9334159340
- Jharkhand: 0-9811541605
- Nagpur: 0-9021734563
- Pune: 0-9623451994
- Uttarakhand: 0-9716462459

Printed at:
India Binding House, Noida, UP (India)

Preface

In the absence of good and comprehensives text book of Mathematics in single unit, for the bachelor student of computer applications (BCA) and many other fields, students have to read a number of books, which quite often are not easily available. They have to purchase several books on a single subject of mathematics otherwise they are forced to seek the help of tution. To overcome this difficulty the book has been written to cover the core courses of mathematics in computer application and many other computer and IT related professional course.

This book provide theoretical background of the subject with well graded set of detailed solved examples. It is a collection and compilation work from vanrus sources and has been endeavored to include as much as information could be possible. There is a plenty of slope in the form of exercise for the reader to try and solve the problem on his own.

I express my gratitude to the authors and publishers of various books I consulted.

I wish to sincerely thank Sh S.K. Jain and Sh Varun Jain,Managing Director, CBS Publishers and Distributors, New Delhi for his encouragement and help in bringing out this publication in a present nice form.

My special thanks to Sh. B.M. Singh, Sh. Sunil Dutt, Sh. Puneet Verma and entire team of CBS Publishers and Distributors, New Delhi whose encouragement and unstinted support enabled me to complete my book. Mr. Peeyush Goel, M/s Dreamshapers also deserve special mention for nice type setting.

I must also record my appreciation due to my wife Dr. Rimple, daughter Rijuta and son Shrish for their understanding and love during the long period that I have taken to complete this book.

Above all I am thankful to The Almighty God, without whose grace nothing is possible for any one.

Readers are welcomed to point out errors, if any and send their valuable suggestions for improving the quality of the book.

Dr. SUDHIR KUMAR PUNDIR

email : skpundir05@yahoo.co.in

CONTENTS

Ch 9. Indeterminate Forms 279-292

Ch 10. Maxima and Minima 293-320

Ch 11. Partial Differentiation and Change of Variables 321-352

Ch 12. Tangent and Normal 353-364

Ch 13. Curvature 365-382

Ch 17. Multiple Integrals 483-510

Ch 18. Rectification of Curves 511-524

Ch 19. Area of Bounded Curves 525-536

Ch 20. Surface and Volume of Solid of Revolutions 537-556

Ch 21. Sequences 557-580

Ch 22. Infinite Series 581-618

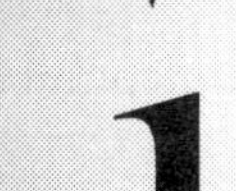

1 Sets, Relation and Functions

1.1 INTRODUCTION

The concept of set is fundamental in all branches of mathematics. It was developed by German mathematician George Cantor. Classical set theory, also termed as crisp set theory, is fundamental to the study of pure mathematics. This chapter introduces the notations and terminology of set theory.

1.2 NUMBER SYSTEM

The number system plays a key role in mathematics. The real number system **R** is one of the most important and beautiful mathematical system. There are different ways of introducing the real number system, but the most common way is to start with Peano's Axioms for the natural numbers. The axioms for natural numbers, discovered by the Italian Mathematician Peano are:

(i) 1 is a natural number

(ii) Each natural number n has a successor $(n+1)$.

(iii) Two natural numbers are equal if their successors are equal.

(iv) Except 1, each natural number is a successor of natural number.

(v) Any set of natural numbers which contains 1 and the successor of every natural number $(k+1)$ whenever it contains k in the set **N** of natural numbers.

- Axiom (v) is commonly known as the axiom of induction or principle of finite induction.
- The above axioms completely define the set of natural numbers.

DEFINITION. *The numbers* 1, 2, 3, ... *are called natural numbers*. We represent the set of natural numbers by **N**.

i.e., $\mathbf{N} = \{1,2,3, \ldots\}$

The Peano's axioms can be used to extend the set **N** of natural numbers to another large system, known as the set of integers.

DEFINITION. *The numbers* ... , –3, –2, –1, 0, 1, 2, 3... *are called integers.* We represent the set of integers by **Z**.

i.e., $\mathbf{Z} = \{ \ldots -3, -2, -1, 0,1,2,3,.. \}$

Integers can be used to define the rational numbers.

DEFINITION. *Any number of the form p/q, where* $p,q \in \mathbf{Z}$, $q \neq 0$ *and* p,q *have no common factor (except* ± 1) *is called a rational number.*

The set of rational numbers is denoted by **Q**.

$$\mathbf{Q} = \left\{\frac{p}{q};\ p,q \in \mathbf{Z}, q \neq 0\right\}$$

- The set of rational numbers consists of integers and fractions.

Definition. *Any number which is not rational, is called an irrational number.*

e.g., $\sqrt{2}$, $\sqrt{3}$ etc. It should be noted that every rational number can be expressed as a terminating or recurring decimal whereas every irrational number can be expressed as a non-terminating infinite decimal.

1.2.1 Real Number

A number which is either rational or irrational is called a real number. The set of real numbers is denoted by **R.**

1.2.2 Integral Powers of a Real Number

Let $a \in \boldsymbol{R}$, and n be any positive integer then we can define $a^n = a.a.a...n$ times.

In particular

$$a = a$$
$$a^2 = a.a$$
$$a^3 = a.a.a = a^2.a \text{ and so on.}$$

Also, if n is any negative integer, then we have $x^{-n} = (x^n)^{-1} = (x^{-1})^n$

1.3 INTERVAL

A subset S of **R** *is called an interval if a, b* $\in$ *S, x* $\in$ **R** *such that a < x < b implies x* $\in$ *S.* There are following four type of intervals.

(i) a ○———○ $b \Rightarrow\ ]a, b[\ = \{x : a < x < b\}$

(ii) a ●———● $b \Rightarrow [a, b] = \{x : a \le x \le b\}$

(iii) a ○———● $b \Rightarrow\ ]a, b] = \{x : a < x \le b\}$

(iv) a ●———○ $b \Rightarrow [a, b[\ = \{x : a \le x < b\}$

- The set $]a, b[$ in which the end points are not included, is called an open interval.
- The set $[a, b]$ also contains both its end points, is called a closed interval.
- The sets $[a, b[$ and $]a, b]$ are called half open (or half closed) intervals or semi-open (or semi-closed) as they contain only one end point.

Apart from the four types of intervals listed above; there are a few more types: These are

(i) $]a, \infty[\ = \{x : a < x\}$ (open right ray)

(ii) $[a, \infty[\ = \{x : a \le x\}$ (closed right ray)

(iii) $]-\infty, b[\ = \{x : x < b\}$ (open left ray)

(iv) $]\ \infty, b] = \{x : x \le b\}$ (closed left ray)

(v) $]-\infty, \infty[\ =$ (open interval)

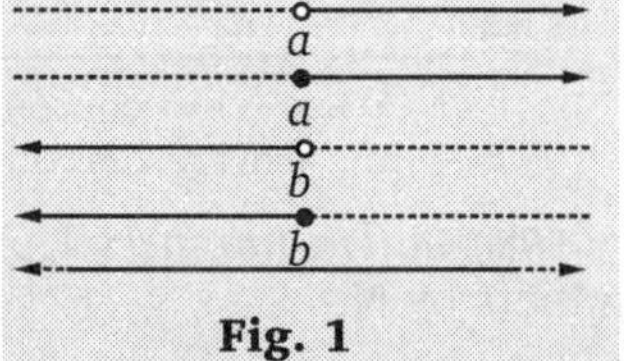

Fig. 1

- If S is any interval and if c and d are two elements of S, then all numbers lying between c and d are also elements of S.

1.3.1 Length of an Interval

The number b – a is called length of the intervals $]a, b[$, $[a, b[$, $]a, b]$ *and* $[a, b]$. If the length of the interval is finite, the interval is said to be finite and if the length is infinite, then it is known as infinite interval.

1.3.2 Absolute Value of a Real Number

The absolute value of a real number a denoted by $|a|$ *is the real number a, – a or 0 according as a is positive, negative or zero, i.e.,* $|a| = \begin{cases} a & \text{if} \quad a \ge 0 \\ -a & \text{if} \quad a < 0 \end{cases}$

From the above definition, it is clear that

(i) $|a| = \max.\{a - a\}$ (ii) $-|a| = \min.\{a - a\}$ (iii) $|a| \ge a \ge -|a|$

1.3.3 Some Useful Results

(i) $|xy| = |x|.|y|$ (ii) $|x+y| \leq |x|+|y|$

(iii) $|x-y| \geq ||x| - |y||$ (iv) $|x-y| \leq |x| + |y|$

(v) $\left|\frac{x}{y}\right| = \frac{|x|}{|y|}$ (vi) If $\in > 0$, then $|x-y| < \varepsilon \Leftrightarrow y - \in < x < y + \in$

1.4 CONCEPT OF SETS

The theory of sets is one of the most important tools of pure mathematics. Pure mathematics is the study of sets equipped with assigned structures, known as mathematical systems. In this section, we shall study some fundamental concept of set theory.

Definition: *'A set is a well defined collection of objects'.*

The objects of a set are called the elements or members of that set and their membership is defined by certain conditions.

The sets are usually denoted by the capital letters of English alphabets: Say $A, B, C, \ldots, X, Y, Z$.

For example :

(i) The collection of the letters *a, b, c, d,..*

(ii) The collection of all natural numbers denoted by **N**.

(iii) The students of M.Sc., Mathematics in C.C.S. University, Meerut.

(iv) The collection of vowels in English alphabet. This set containing only five elements, namely *a, e, i, o, u*.

(v) The collection of all states in Indian union.

If S is a set, an object a in the collection S is called an element of S. This fact is expressed in symbol as $a \in S$ (read as a is in S or a belongs to S). If a is not in S, we write $a \notin S$. For example, $4 \in \mathbf{R}$, the set of real numbers, but $\sqrt{-2} \notin \mathbf{R}$.

Here, Greek letter $\in$ denotes 'belongs to'. It is the abbreviation of the Greek word meaning 'is'.

- By the term 'well defined' we mean that we are given a collection of objects, with certain definite property, so that we are able to determine whether a given object belongs to our collection or not. Thus, every collection of objects is not a set.
- Set and aggregate both have the same meaning.
- The elements of a set must be distinguished from one another. The collection of sand particles does not form a set.
- The collection of rich persons of a city is not a set. However the collection of those persons of city whose wealth exceeds, a fixed amount, say rupees fifty thousands, is a set.
- The order is not preserved in case of a set, whereas order is necessarily preserved in case of sequence. That is to say, each of the sets {1,2,3}, {3,2,1}, {1,3,2} denotes the same sets.
- The repetition of an element does not change the nature of a set, *i.e.*, each of the sets {1,2,3}, {1,2,2,3}, {1,3,3,2} denotes the same sets.

1.4.1. Representation of a Set

There are two ways of representing a set:

(i) Roster or tabulation method

(ii) Set-builder or rule method

Roster Method: In this method, the elements of the set are listed within braces, and separated by comma.

For example:

(i) A= {1,2,3,4,5,6}

(ii) The set of vowels of English alphabet may be represent as {a, e, i, o, u}.

(iii) The set of natural numbers from 1 to 100 may be written as **N**= {1,2,3, ..., 100}. We use three dots in the middle to include the missing elements.

(iv) The set of positive integers, which is a non-ending set may be written as $\mathbf{Z}^+ = \{1,2,3,...\}$. The three dots in the end means that the elements continue in the same manner.

(v) The set of prime numbers is written as P = {2, 3, 5, 7, 11, 13, 17, 19, ...}

Set-Builder Method: In this method, we first try to find a property which characterizes the elements of a set, that is, a property P, in which all the elements of the set possess and in which no other objects possess. Then, we describe the set as $\{x : x \text{ has property } P\}$.

This is to be read as "the set of all x such that x has property P".

For example:

(i) The set of all integers can be written as $\mathbf{Z} = \{x : x \text{ is an integer}\}$

(ii) The set $A = \{1, 2, 3,4, 5\}$ can be written as $\mathbf{A} = \{x \in \mathbf{N} : x \leq 5\}$.

(iii) The set of complex numbers can be written as $\mathbf{C} = \{a+ib : a, b \in \mathbf{R}\}$

(iv) The set A = {1,8,27, ...} can be written as $A = \{x^3 : x \in \mathbf{Z}^+\}$.

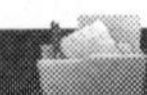

Solved Examples

1. *Use the Roster method to identify each set:*

(a) *The set of possible integers greater than 8 and less than 14.*

(b) *The set of numbers whose elements are the first five positive odd integers.*

(c) *The set of even positive integers.*

(d) *The set of even positive integers that are divisible by 10.*

(e) *The set of all vowels in English alphabets which precedes r.*

SOLUTION. (a) {9, 10, 11, 12, 13}

(b) {1,3,5,7,9}

(c) {2, 4, 6, 8, 10 ...}

(d) {10,20,30,40,50 ...}

(e) $\{a, e, i, o\}$

2. *Use the set-builder method, to identify the following sets :*

(a) $A = \{1,3,5,7,9,...\}$

(b) $B = \left\{1, \frac{1}{4}, \frac{1}{9}, \frac{1}{16}, \frac{1}{25}, ...\right\}$

(c) $C = \{0,1, 2, 3, ...\}$

(d) $D = \left\{\frac{1}{2}, \frac{2}{3}, \frac{3}{4}, \frac{4}{5}, ...\right\}$

SOLUTION. (a) The set of odd positive integers.

(b) Here, elements of the set B are the reciprocals of the squares of the natural numbers.

So, the set $B = \left\{\frac{1}{n^2} : n \in \mathbf{N}\right\}$

(c) The set of whole numbers.

(d) Here, each element in the given set has the denominator one more than the numerator. Hence,

$$D = \left\{x : x = \frac{n}{n+1} : n \in \mathbf{N}\right\}$$

3. *Write the set* $\left\{\frac{1}{2}, \frac{2}{5}, \frac{3}{10}, \frac{5}{26}, ...\right\}$ *in the set-builder form.*

SOLUTION. We observe that each element in the given set has the denominator one more than the square of the numerator. Also, the numerator begins with 1. Hence, in the set builder form, the given set can be written as

$$\left\{x : x = \frac{n}{n^2+1} : n \in \mathbf{N}\right\}$$

Exercise- 1.1

1. Which of the following collections are sets?

(i) All Mathematics students in your college.

(ii) All poor hockey players in the college.

(iii) All odd numbers less than 20.

(iv) The collection of good teachers in your college.

(v) All successful and rich people in your city.

(vi) The people in your immediate family (father, mother, sister, brother).

2. Write the members of each of following sets by the Roster method.

(i) {x : x is odd whole number less than 14}

(ii) $\{x : x^2 < 36 \text{ and } x \in \mathbf{N}\}$

(iii) {x : squares of all whole numbers less than 8}
(iv) {$x : x$ is a prime number, $10 < x < 20$}
(v) {x: x is a composite number less than 20}
(vi) {$x : x < x$ }

3. Rewrite the following sets using set-builder method.
(i) $A = \{2,4,6,8, \ldots\}$
(ii) $B = \left\{1, \frac{1}{2}, \frac{1}{3}, \frac{1}{4}, \ldots\right\}$
(iii) $C = \{0, 3, 6, 9, 12, \ldots\}$
(iv) $D = \{0, 4, 6, 8, 10, \ldots\}$

4. List the elements of the following sets.
(i) $A = \{x : x^2 \leq 16 : x \in \mathbf{Z}\}$
(ii) $B = \{x : 1 \leq x \leq 5$ and $x \in \mathbf{N}\}$
(iii) $C = \{x : x \in \mathbf{N}$ and x is a factor of 15}
(iv) $D = \{x : x$ is a month of year having 31 days}
(v) $E = \{x : x \in \mathbf{Z}$ and $3x - 2 = 3\}$
(vi) $E = \{x : x$ is an integer lying between $-1/2$ and $1/2$ }

5. Use the appropriate symbols $\in$ or $\notin$ to fill in the blanks below:
(i) 12 … the set of all numbers dividing 84.
(ii) K … the set of all vowels of the English alphabets.
(iii) $\frac{1}{2}$ ... the set of natural number.
(iv) India … the set of members of UNO.
(v) $\sqrt{2}$ … The set of rational number
(vi) 15 … the set of multiples of 3.

ANSWERS

1. (i), (iii), (vi)

2. (i) {1, 3, 5, 7, 9, 11, 13} (ii) {1, 2, 3, 4, 5} (iii) {0, 1, 4, 9, 16, 25, 36, 49}
(iv) {11, 13, 17, 19} (v) {1, 4, 6, 8, 9, 10, 12, 14, 15, 16, 18} (vi) ϕ

3. (i) $A = \{x : x = 2n : n \in \mathbf{N}\}$ (ii) $\{1/n : n \in \mathbf{N}\}$
(iii) $\{x : x = 3n$, n is the whole number (iv) $\{x : x = 2n$, n is the whole number}

4. (i) {–4, –3, –2, –1, 0, 1, 2, 3, 4} (ii) {1, 2, 3, 4, 5} (iii) {3, 5}
(iv) {Jan, March, May, July, August, October, December}

5. (i) $\in$ (ii) $\notin$ (iii) $\notin$ (iv) $\in$ (v) $\notin$ (vi) $\in$

1.5 TYPE OF SETS

(i) Empty Set: *A set containing no elements is called empty set and is denoted by the symbol* ϕ.

For example:
(i) $\phi = \{x : x$ is a negative integer whose square is $-1\}$
(ii) $\phi = \{x : x$ is a natural number lying between 2 and 3}
(iii) ϕ = {the set of such persons, who never die}
(iv) $\phi = \{x : x$ is a real numbers, $x^2 < 0\}$
(v) $\phi = \{x : x$ is an even prime number greater than 5}
(vi) ϕ = {the set of real solutions of equation $x^2 + 1 = 0$ }
(vii) $\phi = \{x : x$ is a straight ling passing through three distinct points on a circle}

- The empty set is also known as null set or void set.
- In the Roster method, the empty set is denoted by {}.
- To describe the null set, we can use any property, which is not true for any element.
- It is wrong to use the expression 'an empty' or 'a null set' as there is one and only one empty set through, it may have many-many descriptions. We shall always call 'The empty or the null set.'
- A set consisting of at least one element is called a non-empty or non-void set.
- { ϕ } is not a null set.

(ii) Singleton Set: *Set containing only one element is a singleton set*. The set {a} is a singleton set.

- {0} is not a null set, since it contains 0 as its member. It is a singleton set.
- A room containing only one man is not same thing as a man. In a similar way, the singleton set {a} is not the same thing as the element a.

(iii) Finite Set: *A set is said to be finite if it consists of only finite number of elements.* Here, the process of counting the different elements comes to an end.

For example:

(i) Set of natural numbers less than 50.
(ii) Set of all persons in a city.
(iii) Set of English alphabets.
(iv) Set of all persons on the earth.

(iv) Infinite Set: *A set which is not finite is said to be an infinite set, i.e.*, it contains infinite number of elements. Here, process of counting the different elements never comes to an end.

For example:

(i) Set of natural numbers $\mathbf{N} = \{1,2,3, \ldots\}$
(ii) Set of all points of plane.
(iii) Set of all even integers.
(iv) Set of rational numbers lying between two integers.

(v) Equal Sets: *Two sets are said to be equal if they contain exactly the same elements.*

For example:

$A = \{x : x$ is a letter in the word 'Area'$\}$, *i.e.*, $A = \{a, r, e\}$

And $B = \{y : y$ is a letter in the word 'ear'$\}$, *i.e.*, $B = \{a, r, e\}$

Here A and B are equal sets.

1.5.1 Cardinal Number of a Set

The number of distinct elements contained in a finite set A is called cardinal number of A and is denoted by $n(A)$.

1.5.2 Equivalent Sets

Two finite sets are said to be equivalent if they have the same cardinal number.

- Equivalent sets are not always equal but equal sets are always equivalent.
- The number of distinct elements in a finite set is also called the order of the set.
- If the order of a set is zero, the set is empty.
- If the order of a set is one, the set is singleton.
- The order of an infinite set is never defined.

1.6 SUBSET

Let A and B be two sets. *The set A is said to be a subset of the set B if every element of A is also an element of B.* Symbolically, we write $A \subseteq B$.

When A is subset of B, it means that 'A is contained in B' or 'B contains A'. Here B is called superset of A and is written as $B \supseteq A$.

- Every set is a subset of itself.
- Empty set is a subset of every set.
- If A is not a subset of B, we write $A \not\subseteq B$.
- An element cannot be a subset of a set, only a set can be subset of a set.

1.6.1 Proper Subset

We know that for A to be a subset of B all that is needed is that every element of A is in B. It is possible that every element of B may or may not be in A. If it so happens that every element of B is also in A, then we will have $B \subset A$. Obviously, then A and B are the same set, so that we have $A \subset B$ and $B \subset A \Leftrightarrow A = B$.

If every element of A is in B, but every element of B is not in A , *i.e.*, if $A \subset B$ and $B \not\subset A$, then A is said to be a proper subset of B.

For example:

(i) $\{a, b\}$ is a proper subset of $\{a, b, c\}$.

(ii) Set of natural numbers **N** is a proper subset of set **Z** of integers.

- Here, it follows that every element of A is an element of B and B contains at least one element which does not belong to A.
- If the subset is not proper, it is called **improper subset.** $A \subseteq A$ and $\phi \subseteq A$ are improper subsets.

1.6.2 NUMBER OF SUBSETS OF A SET

If A is a set contains n distinct elements. Let $0 < r \leq n$. If we consider those subsets of A that have r elements each, then we know that the number of ways in which r elements can be choose out of n elements is ${}^nC_r$. Therefore, the number of subsets of A having r elements each is ${}^nC_r$.

Hence, the total number of subsets of A is equal to

$$^nC_0 + {}^nC_1 + {}^nC_2 + ... + {}^nC_n = (1+1)^n = 2^n$$

For example:

(i) If a set A has one element, then it has $2^1 = 2$ subsets.

(ii) If a set A has two elements, then it has $2^2 = 4$ subsets.

- The number of proper subsets of a set with n elements is 2^{n-1}.
- The collection of all possible subsets of a given set A is called power set. It is denoted by $P(A)$. For example : If A = {1,2,3} then the power set $P(A)$ = {ϕ, {1}, {2}, {3}, {1,2}, {1,3}, {2,3}, {1,2,3}}.
- $P(\phi) = \{\phi\}$
- The power set of any given set is always non-empty.

1.7 UNIVERSAL SET

In any discussion , we are given particular set and we consider different subsets of the given set. This given set is called Universal Set. Generally, it is denoted by U.

For Example:

(i) The universal set is of real numbers **R**, while considering the set of natural numbers, whole numbers, integers and rational numbers.

(ii) The set of alphabets is the universal set from which the letters of any word may be chosen to form a set.

(iii) In geometry, we discuss set of lines, triangles and circles, then the universal set is the plane, in which the lines, triangles and circles lie.

- Universal set is a superset of each of the given sets.
- The universal set is not unique.

1.7.1 COMPLEMENT OF A SET

Let U be the universal set and the set $A \subseteq U$. Complement of set A with respect to the universal set U is the set of all those elements of U which are not the elements of A and is denoted by A' or A^c,

$$A' = \{x : x \in \text{U and } x \notin A\}$$

For example:

(i) If U= {1, 2, 3, 4, 5, 6, 7, 8, 9, 11} and A= {1, 2, 3} then A'= {4, 5, 6, 7, 8, 9, 11}.

- Complement of the universal set is the null set and *vice-versa*.
- $(A')' = A$
- If $A \subseteq B$, then $B' \subseteq A'$.
- $x \in A' \Leftrightarrow x \notin A$

RECAPITULATIONS

- A set containing no element is called empty set.
- Set containing finite number of elements is called finite otherwise infinite.
- The number of distinct elements contained in a finite set is called its cardinality.
- Two finite sets are said to be equivalent if they have same cardinality.
- A set A is said to be subset of a set B if every elements of A belongs to B.
- Total number of subsets of a set A of n elements is 2^n.
- $A' = \{x : x \in A' \text{ and } x \notin A\}$

Solved Examples

1. *Let $A = \{1,2,3\}$, then find $P(A)$.*

SOLUTION. Since $A = \{1, 2, 3\}$ then,

$P(A) = \{\phi, \{1\}, \{2\}, \{3\}, \{1,2\}, \{1,3\}, \{2,3\}, \{1,2,3\}\}$

2. *Let $A = \{a,b,c,d\}$, $B = \{a,b,c\}$ and $C = \{b,d\}$, find all sets X such that*

(i) $X \subset B$ and $X \subset C$

(ii) $X \subset A$ and $X \not\subset B$

SOLUTION. (i) Here, we have

$P(B) = \{\phi, \{a\}, \{b\}, \{c\}, \{a, b\}, \{a,c\}, \{b,c\}, \{a,b,c\}\}$.

And $P(C) = \{\phi, \{b\}, \{d\}, \{b, d\}\}$, then $X \subset B$ and $X \subset C$ implies

$X \in P(B)$ and $X \in P(C)$

$X = \{\phi, \{b\}\}$

(ii) Here, we have, $X \subset A$ and $X \not\subset B$, which implies that

$X \in P(A)$ and $X \notin P(B)$

Therefore

$X = \{\{d\}, \{a,b,d\}, \{b,c,d\}, \{a,c,d\}, \{a,d\}, \{b,d\}, \{c,d\}, \{a,b,c,d\}\}$

3. *Write down all the subsets of the following sets.*

(i) $\{a\}$ (ii) $\{a,b\}$

(iii) $\{a,b,c\}$ (iv) ϕ

SOLUTION. (i) Let $A = \{a\}$. Since A contains only one element, therefore, the total number of subsets is $2^1 = 2$, which are given by ϕ and $\{a\}$.

(ii) Here, total number of subsets, $= 2^2 = 4$, which are given by ϕ, $\{a\}$, $\{b\}$, $\{a, b\}$

(iii) Here, total number of subsets $= 2^3 = 8$, given by

$\phi, \{a\}, \{b\}, \{c\}, \{a,b\}, \{a,c\}, \{b,c\}, \{a,b,c\}$

(iv) since ϕ contains no element therefore the number of subsets $= 2^0 = 1$. The only subset is ϕ.

4. *Which of the following sets are empty. Also, give the reason.*

(i) $A = \{x : x \neq x$, is a real number$\}$.

(ii) $B = \{x : x + 4 = 4\}$

(iii) $C = \{x : x^3 - 3 = 0$ and x is rational number$\}$

SOLUTION. (i) Here, $A = \{x : x \neq x, x$ is a real number$\}$. Since $x \neq x$ is not true $\Rightarrow$ $A = \phi$

(ii) $B = \{x : x + 4 = 4\}$

$= \{x : x = 0\} = \{0\}$

$\Rightarrow B$ has one element 0, therefore $B \neq \phi$.

(iii) Since there is no rational number whose square is 3, so $x^3 - 3 = 0$ is not satisfied for any rational number. Therefore, C is an empty set.

5. *Which of the following sets are finite and which are infinite.*

(i) The set of natural numbers divisible by 2.

(ii) The set of natural numbers less then 8.

(iii) The set of integers whose square is even.

(iv) The set of integers greater than −18.

(v) The set of lines passing through a point.

(vi) The set of points of a plane at a fixed distance from a given point in the plane.

(vii) The set of points common to two given parallel lines.

(viii) *The set of the roots of a polynomial of n degree.*

SOLUTION. (i) The given set is {2, 4, 6, 8, ...}. It has an infinite number of elements, therefore it is an infinite set.

(ii) The given set is {1,2,3,4,5,6,7}. It has seven elements, *i.e.*, finite number of elements. Hence, it is a finite set.

(iii) The given set is {..., – 8, – 6, – 4, – 2, 0, 2, 4, 6, 8,...}. It has infinite number of elements, therefore it is an infinite set.

(iv) Here, the given set is {–17, –16, ... , 0, 1, 2 ...}. It has infinite number of elements therefore, it is an infinite set.

(v) Since infinite number of lines can pass through a fixed point, therefore the given set is an infinite set.

(vi) Since the points in a plane at a fixed distance from a given point in the plane lie on a circle with the given point as centre and the number of points on a circle is infinite. Therefore, the given set is an infinite set.

(vii) Since two parallel lines cannot meet anywhere, therefore, the set of points common to two given parallel lines is empty, therefore the given set cannot be infinite. Hence, it is a finite set.

(viii) Since, a polynomial of n degree always have atmost n roots.

Therefore, the given set is always a finite set.

6. *Which of the following sets are equivalent* ϕ *,{0} and* $\{\phi\}$.

SOLUTION. Since ϕ has no element. Also, {0} and $\{\phi\}$, each contains one element namely 0 and ϕ respectively. Hence, {0} and $\{\phi\}$ are equivalent.

7. *Which of the following sets are equal ?*

$A = \{1,2,3\}$, $B = \{2,3,4\}$,

$C = \{3,2,1\}$, $D = \{2,3,5\}$

SOLUTION. Since $1 \in A$ but $1 \notin B$, therefore $A \neq B$. A and C have exactly the same element, therefore $A = C$.

Also, $1 \in C$ but $1 \notin D \Rightarrow C \neq D$

$4 \in B$ but $4 \notin C \Rightarrow B \neq C$

$1 \in A$ but $1 \notin D \Rightarrow A \neq D$

Hence, only A and C are equal sets.

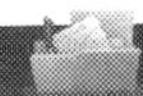

Exercise-1.2

1. Fill in the blanks:

(i) A set which contains no element is called ... set.

(ii) If $A = \{1,2,3\}$ and $B = \{3,2,1\}$ then they are said to be ...

(iii) If $A = \{a, b, c\}$ and $B = \{c, d, e\}$ then they are said to be ...

(iv) If every element of a set B is also an element of A, then B is said to be ... of A.

(v) The empty set is a ... of every set.

(vi) Every set is a .... of itself.

(vii) The set **Z** of integers is a ... of set of natural numbers **N**.

2. Which of the followings sets are equal?

(i) $A = \{1,2,3\}$

(ii) $B = \{1,2,2,3\}$

(iii) $C = (x \in \mathbf{R} : x^3 - 6x^2 + 11x - 6 = 0)$

3. Which of the following sets are equivalent to the set {4,7,11,17,20}?

(i) {5,1,2,3,4}

(ii) {all odd numbers less then 10}

(iii) {the months of a year of 30 days}

(iv) {all the prime numbers which lie between 10 and 25}.

4. Which of the following sets are finite and which are infinite ?

(i) $\{x \in \mathbf{N} : x > 10\}$

(ii) $\{x \in \mathbf{N} : x < 100\}$

(iii) $\{x \in \mathbf{R} : 1 \le x \le 2\}$

(iv) Set of vowels in English alphabets.

(v) The set of prime numbers less than 100.

(vi) The set of multiple of 8.

5. Which of the following statements are true? Give the reason.

(i) For any two sets A and B either $A \subseteq B$ or $B \subseteq A$

(ii) Every subset of a finite set is finite.

(iii) A subset of an infinite set may be finite.

(iv) Every set has a proper subset.

(v) A set containing n elements have 2^n subsets.

(vi) If $A = \{1,2,3,4,5,6\}$ and B = {whole numbers less than 6}, then $A = B$.

(vii) The empty set has no proper subset.

6. Examine which of the following sets are empty?

(i) The set of tigers in your class.

(ii) The set of triangles having three equal sides.

(iii) The set of all numbers which, when added to zero, yield sum greater than the original.

(iv) The set of odd numbers which are divisible by 2.

7. Which of the following statements are true?

(i) If $x \in A$ and $A \subset B$, then $x \in B$

(ii) If $A \subset B$ and $B \subset C$, then $A \subset C$

(iii) If $A \not\subset B$ and $B \not\subset C$, then $A \not\subset C$

(iv) If $x \in A$ and $A \not\subset B$, then $x \in B$

(v) If $A \subset B$ and $x \notin B$, then $x \notin A$

8. Are the following sets, *i.e.*, (A and B) are equal.

(i) $A = \{x : x$ is a letter of the word 'LITTLE'$\}$
$B = \{x : x$ is a letter in the word 'TITLE'$\}$

(ii) $A = \{x : x$ is a letter in the word 'FOLLOW'$\}$
$B = \{x : x$ is a letter in the word 'WOLF'$\}$

(iii) $A = \{x : x$ is a letter in the word 'LOYAL'$\}$
$B = \{x : x$ is a letter In the word 'ALLOY'$\}$

9. Write down all possible subsets of each of the following sets.

(i) $\{a\}$ (ii) $\{0,1\}$ (iii) $\{a, b, c\}$

(iv) $\{1, \{1\}\}$ (v) ϕ

10. Which of the following statements are true?

(i) $\{a, \phi\} \in \{a, \{a, \phi\}\}$

(ii) If $A \subseteq B$ and $B \subseteq C$, then $A \subseteq C$

(iii) If $A \in B$ and $B \subseteq C$, then $A \in C$

(iv) If $A \subset B$ and $B \in C$, then $A \in C$

(v) If $A \subseteq B$ and $B \in C$, then $A \subseteq C$

ANSWERS

1. (i) empty (ii) equal (iii) equivalent (iv) subset (v) subset (vi) subset (vii) super set.

2. $A = B = C$ **3.** (i), (ii), (iv) **4.** (ii), (iv), (v) are finite sets and (i), (iii), (vi) are infinite.

5. (i) F (ii) T (iii) T (iv) F (v) T (vi) F (vii) T **6.** (i), (iii), (iv),

7. (i), (ii), (v) **8.** (i) Equal, (ii) Equal, (iii) Equal

9. (i) ϕ, {a};(ii) ϕ ,{0},{1},{0,1}; (iii) ϕ ,{a},{b},{c}, {a, b},{b,c},{a,c}, {a,b,c}(iv) {1}; {1}, {{1}}, {1,{1}};

10. (i) , (ii), (iii), (iv), (v)

1.8 VENN DIAGRAMS

A set can be represented by closed figures like circles, triangles, rectangles, etc. The point in the interior of the figure represents the elements of the set. Such a representations is called a Venn diagram. In Venn diagram, the universal set is usually represented by a rectangular region and its subset by closed bounded regions inside the rectangular region. For example, if A is a subset of B, *i.e.*, $A \subset B$. This is shown in figure 2.

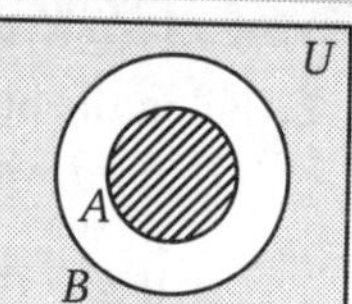

Fig. 2

- The diagrams drawn to represent sets are called Venn diagram or Venn-Euler diagrams, after the name of British mathematician **Venn.**
- If A and B are two sets, which are not equal, but have common elements, then to represent A and B, We draw two intersecting circles.
- Two disjoint sets are represented by two-intersecting circles.
- Venn diagrams are to be used for clarity and are no substitute for precise proof.

1.9 OPERATIONS ON SETS

1.9.1 UNION AND INTERSECTION OPERATIONS

(i) Union of Two sets

Let A and B be two sets. Then union of A and B, denoted by $A \cup B$ is the set of all those elements, which either belongs to A or B or to both A and B.

It should be noted that the common elements are to be taken only once.

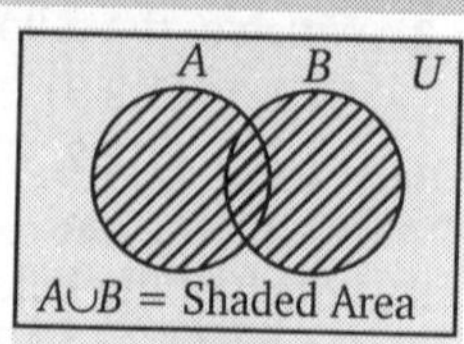

Fig. 3

Symbolically: $A \cup B = \{x : x \in A \text{ or } x \in B\}$ It is shown in the adjoining figure 3.

For example:

(i) Let $A = \{3,4,5,6,7\}$ and $B = \{5,6,7,8,9\}$
Then $A \cup B = \{3, 4, 5, 6, 7, 8, 9\}$

(ii) Let $A = \{x : x = 2n, n = 1, 2, 3, ...\} = \{2, 4, 6, 8, ...\}$
$B = \{x : x = 3n, n = 1, 2, 3, ...\} = \{3, 6, 9, 12, ...\}$
Then $A \cup B = \{x : x$ is multiple of 2 or a multiple of 3$\}$
$= \{2, 3, 4, 6, 8, 10, 12, ...\}$

(iii) Let A = set of even natural numbers $= \{2, 4, 6, 8,...\}$
and B = set of natural numbers $= \{1, 2, 3, 4, 5,...\}$
Then $A \cup B = \{1, 2, 3, 4,...\}$

- $x \in (A \cup B) \Leftrightarrow x \in A$ or $x \in B$.
- $x \notin (A \cup B) \Leftrightarrow x \notin A$ and $x \notin B$
- $A \cup B = B \cup A$, *i.e.*, union of sets is commutative.
- $A \cup A' = U$ and $A \cup U = U$
- $A \cup \phi = A$
- If *A, B, C, D, ..., Z* is a finite family of sets, then their union is denoted by $A \cup B \cup C \cup D ... \cup Z$.
- $(A \cup B) \cup C = A \cup (B \cup C)$, *i.e.*, a union of sets is associative.

(ii) Intersection of Two sets

Let A and B be two sets. Then intersection of A and B, denoted by $A \cap B$ is the set of all those elements, which belongs to both A and B.

Symbolically: $A \cap B = \{x : x \in A$ and $x \in B\}$ It is shown in the adjoining figure 4.

For example:

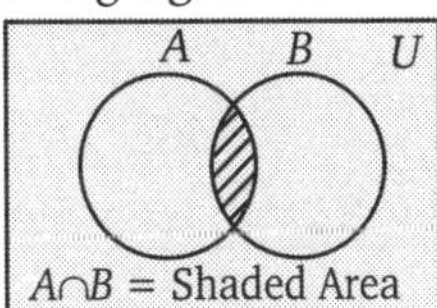

$A \cap B$ = Shaded Area

Fig. 4

(i) Let $A = \{2, 4, 6, 8, 10\}$ and $B = \{1, 2, 3, 4, 5\}$
Then $A \cap B = \{2, 4\}$

(ii) If $A = \{x : x = 3n, n \in \mathbf{Z}\}$
$B = \{x : x = 4n, n \in \mathbf{Z}\}$
Then $A \cap B = \{x : x$ is multiple of 3 and x is a multiple of 4$\}$
$= \{x : x$ is multiple of 3 and 4 both$\}$
$= \{x : x = 12n, n \in \mathbf{Z}\}$

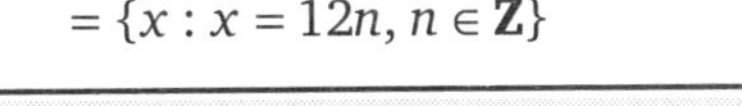

- $x \in (A \cap B) \Leftrightarrow x \in A$ and $x \in B$.
- $x \notin (A \cap B) \Leftrightarrow x \notin A$ or $x \notin B$
- $A = A \cap A$, *i.e.*, intersection of sets is idempotent.
- $A \cap \phi = \phi$
- $A \cap U = A$, where U is a universal set.
- $A \cap B = B \cap A$, *i.e.*, intersection of sets is commutative.
- $(A \cap B) \cap C = A \cap (B \cap C)$ intersection of sets is associative.
- If *A,B,C,D, ...,Z* is a finite family of sets, then their intersection is denoted by $A \cap B \cap C ... \cap Z$.

(iii) Distributive Property of Union and Intersection

(i) $A \cup (B \cap C) = (A \cup B) \cap (A \cup C)$ (ii) $A \cap (B \cup C) = (A \cap B) \cup (A \cap C)$

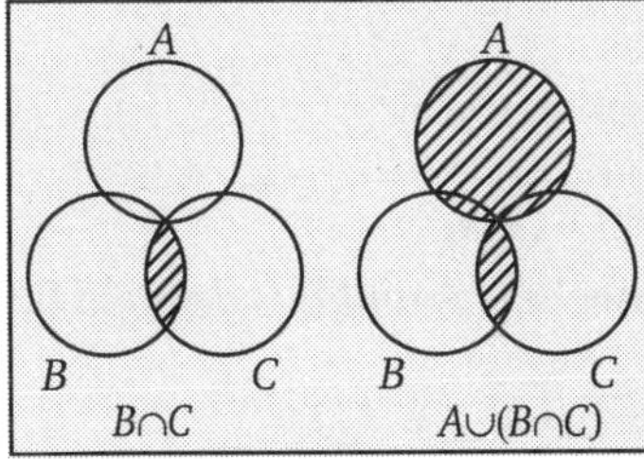

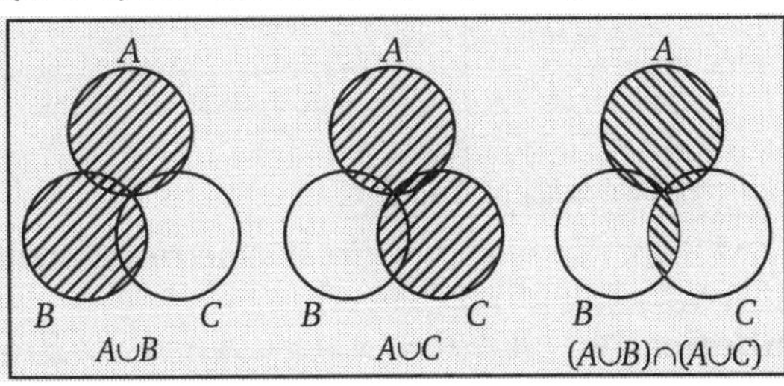

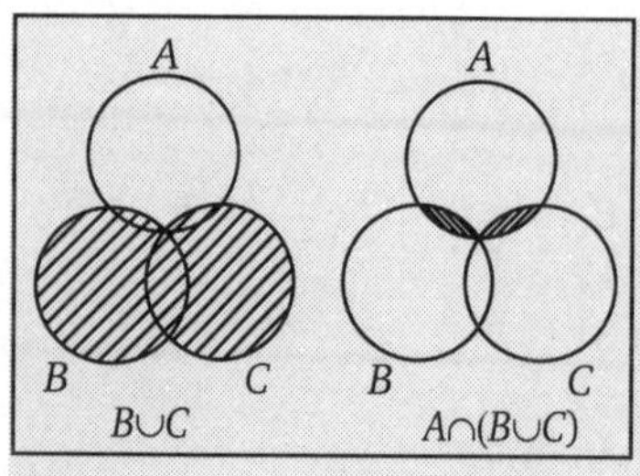

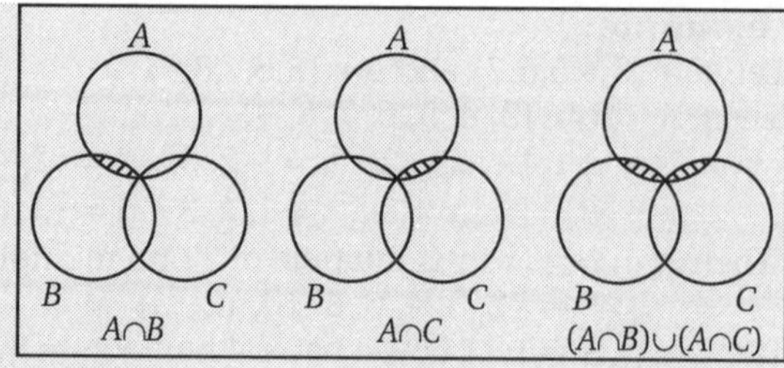

Fig. 5

1.9.2. Disjoint Sets

When two sets have no common elements, they are called disjoint sets. Thus, if $A \cap B = \phi$, then A and B are disjoint. It is shown in the adjoining figure 6.

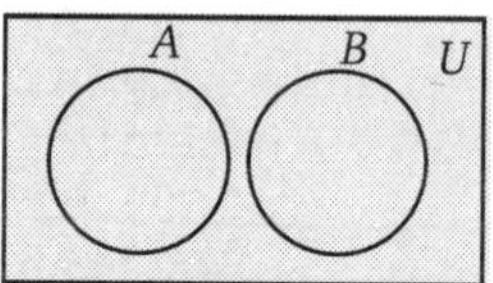

Fig. 6

For example:

(i) If $A = \{2, 4, 6, 8\}$ and $B = \{1, 3, 5, 7, 9\}$

Then, $A \cap B = \phi$

(ii) If A = Boys in school , B = Girls in school

Then, $A \cap B = \phi$

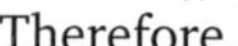

- If $A \cap B \neq \phi$, , then A and B are said to be intersecting or overlapping sets.
- A family of sets is said to be pair-wise disjoint family of sets if and only if any two sets of this family are disjoint. For example, classes of A_2, A_3, A_5 and A_7 defined as $A_2 = \{2, 2^2, 2^3, ...\}$; $A_3 = \{3, 3^2, 3^3, ...\}$; $A_5 = \{5, 5^2, 5^3, ...\}$ and $A_7 = \{7, 7^2, 7^3, ...\}$ are pair-wise disjoint.
- $\phi \cap A = \phi$, *i.e.*, null set is disjoint from every subset.

1.9.3 Difference of Two Sets

If A and B are two sets, then the set of all elements which belong to A but do not belong to B is called the difference of sets A and B and is denoted by A ~ B. The set of all elements which belong to B but do not belong to A is called the difference of sets B and A and is denoted by B ~ A.

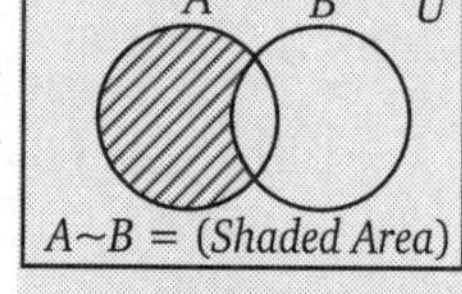

Fig. 7

Therefore,

$$A \sim B = \{x : x \in A \text{ and } x \notin B\} = A \cap B'$$

And $$B \sim A = \{x : x \notin A \text{ and } x \in B\} = B \cap A'$$

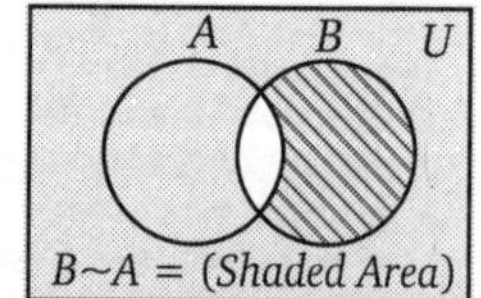

Fig. 8

For example:

(i) Let $A = \{1, 2, 3, 4, 5\}$ and $B = \{-1, 0, 1, 2\}$

Then, $A \sim B = \{3, 4, 5\}$ and $B \sim A = \{-1, 0\}$

- $x \in (A - B) \Leftrightarrow x \in A$ and $x \notin B$.
- $x \notin (A - B) \Rightarrow x \in A$ and $x \in B$
- $x \notin A$ and $x \in B \Rightarrow x \notin (A - B)$
- $A \sim B \neq B \sim A$, *i.e.*, difference of two sets is not commutative.
- $A \subset B$ then $A \sim B = \phi$
- The sets $A \sim B$, $A \cap B$ and $B \sim A$ are mutually disjoint.
- Difference of a set with the universal set is known as complementation.
- $A \sim B$ is a subset of A and $B \sim A$ is a subset of B.

1.9.4 Symmetric Difference of Two Sets

If A and B are two sets, then the symmetric difference of two sets A and B is denoted by AΔB is given by $A \Delta B = (A \sim B) \cup (B \sim A)$

Symbolically: $A \Delta B = \{x : (x \in A \text{ and } x \notin B) \text{ or } (x \in B \text{ and } x \notin A)\}$

For example:

(i) If $A = \{1,2,3,4,5,6,7,8\}$ and $B = \{1,3,5,6,7,8,9\}$

Then $A \sim B = \{2, 4\}$ and $B \sim A = \{9\}$

and $A \Delta B = \{2, 4, 9\}$

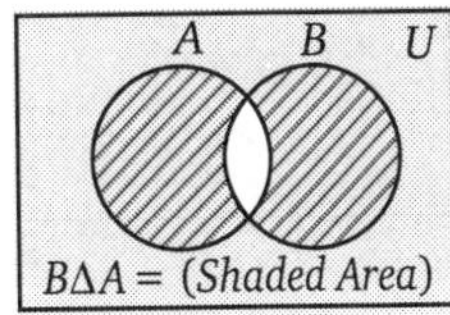

$B\Delta A$ = (Shaded Area)

Fig. 9

1.9.5 EQUIVALENT SETS

Two finite sets A and B are equivalent if their cardinal numbers are same , *i.e.*, $n(A) = n(B)$.

1.9.6 LAW OF EXCLUDED MIDDLE AND LAW OF CONTRADICTION

Two special properties of set operations are known as the excluded middle axioms and law of contradiction. The excluded middle axioms are very important because they are the only set operations described here that are not valid for both classical sets and fuzzy sets. Let A be any subset of universal set X. Then , we define.

(i) Axiom of the excluded middle: $A \cup \overline{A} = X$

(ii) Axiom of the contradiction: $A \cap \overline{A} = \phi$

THEOREM 1. (i) $A \cup \phi = A$ (ii) $A \cap \phi = \phi$ (iii) $A \cup A = A$

(iv) $A \cap A = A$ (v) $A \cup B = B \cup A$ (vi) $A \cap B = B \cap A$

PROOF. (i) Let x be an arbitrary element of $A \cup B$.

i.e., $x \in A \cup \phi$

Then, by definition $x \in A \cup B \Leftrightarrow x \in A$ or $x \in B$

i.e., $x \in A \cup \phi \Rightarrow x \in A$ or $x \in \phi$

$\Leftrightarrow x \in A$ ($\because \phi$ is a null set $\Rightarrow x \notin \phi$)

Therefore, $A \cup \phi = A$

(ii) Let x be an arbitrary element of $A \cap \phi$.

$x \in A \cap \phi \Leftrightarrow x \in A$ and $x \in \phi$ ($\because \phi$ is a null set)

Therefore, $A \cap \phi = \phi$

(iii) Let x be an arbitrary element of $A \cup A$,

$x \in A \cup A \Leftrightarrow x \in A$ or $x \in A$ (Repeated statement)

$\Leftrightarrow x \in A$

Therefore, $A \cup A = A$

(iv) Let x be an arbitrary element of $A \cap A$,

$x \in A \cap A \Leftrightarrow x \in A$ and $x \in A$ (Repeated statement)

$\Leftrightarrow x \in A$

Therefore, $A \cap A = A$

(v) Let x be an arbitrary element of $A \cup B$,

$x \in A \cup B \Leftrightarrow x \in A$ or $x \in B$ (Writing in reverse order)

$\Leftrightarrow x \in B$ or $x \in A \Leftrightarrow x \in B \cup A$

Therefore, $A \cup B = B \cup A$

(vi) Let x be an arbitrary element of $A \cap B$

$x \in A \cap B \Leftrightarrow x \in A$ and $x \in B$ (Writing in reverse order)

$\Leftrightarrow x \in B$ and $x \in A \Leftrightarrow x \in B \cap A$

Therefore, $A \cap B = B \cap A$

THEOREM 2. *For any three sets A, B and C*

(i) $A \cup (B \cup C) = (A \cup B) \cup C$ (ii) $A \cap (B \cap C) = (A \cap B) \cap C$

(iii) $A \cup (B \cap C) = (A \cup B) \cap (A \cup C)$ (iv) $A \cap (B \cup C) = (A \cap B) \cup (A \cap C)$

[MEERUT(BCA)–2001, 07,12, 14; DELHI(BCA)–2010]

PROOF. (i) Let x be an arbitrary element of $A \cup (B \cup C)$, then

$x \in A \cup (B \cup C)$

$\Leftrightarrow$ $x \in A$ or $x \in (B \cup C) \Leftrightarrow x \in A$ or ($x \in B$ or $x \in C$)

$\Leftrightarrow$ ($x \in A$ or $x \in B$) or $x \in C$ (By associativity)

$\Leftrightarrow$ $x \in (A \cup B)$ or $x \in C \Leftrightarrow x \in (A \cup B) \cup C$

Therefore, $A \cup (B \cup C) = (A \cup B) \cup C$

(ii) Let x be an arbitrary element of $A \cap (B \cap C)$, then

$x \in A \cap (B \cap C)$

$\Leftrightarrow$ $x \in A$ and $x \in (B \cap C) \Leftrightarrow x \in A$ and ($x \in B$ and $x \in C$)

$\Leftrightarrow$ ($x \in A$ and $x \in B$) and $x \in C$ (By associativity)

$\Leftrightarrow$ $x \in (A \cap B)$ and $x \in C \Leftrightarrow x \in (A \cap B) \cap C$

Therefore, $A \cap (B \cap C) = (A \cap B) \cap C$

(iii) Let x be an arbitrary element of $A \cup (B \cap C)$, then

$x \in A \cup (B \cap C)$

$\Leftrightarrow$ $x \in A$ or $x \in (B \cap C) \Leftrightarrow x \in A$ or ($x \in B$ and $x \in C$)

$\Leftrightarrow$ ($x \in A$ or $x \in B$) and ($x \in A$ or $x \in C$) $\Leftrightarrow x \in (A \cup B)$ and $x \in (A \cup C)$

$\Leftrightarrow$ $x \in (A \cup B) \cap (A \cup C)$

Therefore, $A \cup (B \cap C) = (A \cup B) \cap (A \cup C)$

(iv) Let x be an arbitrary element of $A \cap (B \cup C)$, then

$x \in A \cap (B \cup C)$

$\Leftrightarrow$ $x \in A$ and $x \in (B \cup C) \Leftrightarrow x \in A$ and ($x \in B$ or $x \in C$)

$\Leftrightarrow$ ($x \in A$ and $x \in B$) or ($x \in A$ and $x \in C$) $\Leftrightarrow x \in (A \cap B)$ or $x \in (A \cap C)$

Therefore, $A \cap (B \cup C) = (A \cap B) \cup (A \cap C)$

THEOREM 3. *(i)* $(A')' = A$ *(ii)* $A \cup A' = U$, *where U is the universal set.*

(iii) $A \cap A' = \phi$ *(iv)* $(A \cup B)' = A' \cap B'$ *(De' Morgan's Law)*

(v) $(A \cap B)' = A' \cup B'$ *(De' Morgan's Law)*

[MEERUT(BCA)–2001, 02, 03, 04, 08, 09, 10, 14; DELHI(BCA)–2009; KANPUR(BCA)–2013]

PROOF. (i) Let x be an arbitrary element of $(A')'$,

$x \in (A')' \Leftrightarrow x \notin A' \Leftrightarrow x \in A$

Therefore, $(A')' = A$

(ii) Let x be an arbitrary element of $(A \cup A')$,

$x \in (A \cup A') \Leftrightarrow x \in A$ or $x \in A' \Leftrightarrow x \in A$ or $x \in U - A$

$\Leftrightarrow$ $x \in A$ or ($x \in U, x \notin A$) $\Leftrightarrow x \in U$

Therefore, $A \cup A' = U$

(iii) Let x be an arbitrary element of $(A \cap A')$,

$x \in (A \cap A') \Leftrightarrow x \in A$ and $x \in A'$ but if $x \in A$ then $x \notin A'$

Therefore, $A \cap A' = \phi$

(iv) Let x be an arbitrary element of $(A \cup B)'$,

$x \in (A \cup B)' \Leftrightarrow x \notin (A \cup B) \Leftrightarrow x \notin A$ and $x \notin B$

$\Leftrightarrow$ $x \in A'$ and $x \in B' \Leftrightarrow x \in A' \cap B'$

Therefore, $(A \cup B)' = A' \cap B'$

(v) Let x be an arbitrary element of $(A \cap B)'$,

$x \in (A \cap B)' \Leftrightarrow x \notin (A \cap B) \Leftrightarrow x \notin A$ or $x \notin B$

$\Leftrightarrow \quad x \in A'$ or $x \in B' \quad \Leftrightarrow x \in A' \cup B'$

Therefore, $\quad (A \cap B)' = A' \cup B'$

RECAPITULATIONS

- $A \cup B = \{x : x \in A$ or $x \in B)$
- $x \notin A \cup B \Leftrightarrow x \notin A$ and $x \notin B$
- $x \in A - B \Leftrightarrow x \in A$ and $x \notin B$
- $A \cup \phi = A$
- $(A')' = A$
- $A \cap A' = \phi$
- $(A \cap B)' = A' \cup B'$
- $A \cap B = \{x : x \in A$ and $x \in B)$
- $x \notin A \cap B \Leftrightarrow x \notin A$ or $x \notin B$
- $A \Delta B = (A \sim B) \cup (B \sim A)$
- $A \cap \phi = \phi$
- $A \cup A' = U$
- $(A \cup B)' = (A' \cap B')$

Solved Examples

1. *Show that (i) $A \subset (A \cup B)$,*
(ii) $(A \cap B) \subset A$.

SOLUTION. (i) Let $x \in A$ be arbitrary then $x \in A$ certainly but may or may not belong to B.

$\Rightarrow \quad x \in A \cup B$

Therefore, $x \in A$

$\Rightarrow x \in A \cup B$ gives $A \subset A \cup B$

(ii) Let $x \in A \cap B$ where x is arbitrary

$x \in A \cap B$

$\Rightarrow x \in A$ and $x \in B$

In particular,

$x \in A \cap B$

$\Rightarrow \quad x \in A$

Therefore, $(A \cap B) \subset A$

- In a similar manner we can show that (i) $B \subset (A \cup B)$ and (ii) $A \cap B \subset B$.

2. *Let A and B be two sets, if $A \cap X = B \cap X = \phi$ and $A \cup X = B \cup X$ for some set X, prove that $A = B$.*

SOLUTION. Given that $A \cup X = B \cup X$

$\Rightarrow A \cap (A \cup X) = A \cap (B \cup X)$

(taking intersection by A on both sides)

$\Rightarrow \quad A = A \cap (B \cup X)$

$(\because A \cap (A \cup X) = A)$

$\Rightarrow \quad A = (A \cap B) \cup (A \cap X)$

(By distributive law)

$\Rightarrow \quad A = (A \cap B) \cup \phi$

$\Rightarrow \quad A = A \cap B$

$\Rightarrow \quad A \subset (A \cap B)$

$\Rightarrow \quad A \subset B \quad \ldots(1)$

Again consider, $A \cup X = B \cup X$

$\Rightarrow B \cap (A \cup X) = B \cap (B \cup X)$

(taking intersection with B)

$\Rightarrow \quad B \cap (A \cup X) = B$

$\Rightarrow \quad (B \cap A) \cup (B \cap X) = B$

(By distributive law)

$\Rightarrow \quad (B \cap A) \cup \phi = B$

(Given $B \cap X = \phi$)

$\Rightarrow \quad (B \cap A) = B$

$(\therefore A \cap B = B \cap A)$

$\Rightarrow \quad A \cap B = B$

$\Rightarrow \quad B \subset A \cap B$

$\Rightarrow \quad B \subset A \quad \ldots(2)$

Hence, (1) and (2) gives $A \subset B$ and $B \subset A$.

$\Rightarrow \quad A = B$

3. *For any two sets A and B, show that*
(i) $P(A \cap B) = P(A) \cap P(B)$,
(ii) $P(A) \cup P(B) \subset P(A \cup B)$

SOLUTION. (i) Let $X \in P(A \cap B)$

$\Rightarrow X \subset A \cap B$

$\Rightarrow X \subset A$ and $X \subset B$

$\Rightarrow X \in P(A)$ and $X \in P(B)$

$\Rightarrow X \in P(A) \cap P(B)$

Therefore,

$P(A \cap B) \subset P(A) \cap P(B) \quad \ldots(1)$

Now, let $X \in P(A) \cap P(B)$

$\Rightarrow X \in P(A)$ and $X \in P(B)$

$\Rightarrow X \subset A$ and $X \subset B$

$\Rightarrow X \subset A \cap B$

$\Rightarrow X \in P(A \cap B)$

Therefore,

$P(A) \cap P(B) \subset P(A \cap B) \quad \ldots(2)$

From (1) and (2), we conclude that

$P(A \cap B) \subset P(A) \cap P(B)$

and $P(A) \cap P(B) \subset P(A \cap B)$ which

gives

$P(A \cap B) = P(A) \cap P(B)$

(ii) Let $X \in P(A) \cup P(B)$

$\Rightarrow X \in P(A)$ or $X \in P(B)$

$\Rightarrow X \subset A$ or $X \subset B$

$\Rightarrow X \subset A \cup B$

$\Rightarrow X \in P(A \cup B)$

Therefore,

$P(A) \cup P(B) \subset P(A \cup B)$

1.9.6 Some More Results

1. If A and B are any two sets, then

(i) $A - B = A \cap B'$

(ii) $A - B = A \Leftrightarrow A \cap B = \phi$

(iii) $(A - B) \cup B = A \cup B$

(iv) $A \subset B \Leftrightarrow B' \subset A'$

(v) $(A - B) \cup (B - A) = (A \cup B) - (A \cap B)$

2. If A and B are any two sets, then

(i) $A - (B \cap C) = (A - B) \cup (A - C)$

(ii) $A - (B \cup C) = (A - B) \cap (A - C)$

(iii) $A \cap (B - C) = (A \cap B) - (A \cap C)$

Exercise-1.3

1. Let $A = \{a, b\}$, $B = \{a, b, c\}$. Is $A \subset B$? Find $A \cup B$ and $A \cap B$.

2. If $A = \{1,2,3,4\}$, $B = \{2,4,6,8\}$, $C = \{3,4,5,6\}$ and universal set $U = \{1,2,3,4,...9\}$. Verify that $A \cap (B \cup C) = (A \cap B) \cup (A \cap C)$.

3. If A, B , C are subsets of a set X, then show that $A \subseteq B$ and $B \subseteq C \Rightarrow A \subseteq C$.

4. Find the union of the following sets:

(i) $A = \{x : x \text{ is an even integer}\}$, $B = \{x : x \text{ is an odd integer}\}$.

(ii) $A = \{x : x \text{ is a multiple of } 2\}$, $B = \{x : x \text{ is a multiple of } 3\}$.

(iii) $A = \{x : x \text{ is a rational number }\}$, $B = \{x : x \text{ is an irrational number}\}$.

(iv) $A = \{x : x \text{ is a negative integer}\}$, $B = \{x : x \text{ is a non-negative integer}\}$

5. Find the intersection of the following sets.

(i) $A = \{x : x \text{ is an even integer}\}$, $B = \{x : x \text{ is an odd integer}\}$

(ii) $A = \{x : x \text{ is a rational number }\}$, $B = \{x : x \text{ is an irrational number}\}$.

(iii) $A = \{x : x \text{ is a multiple of } 5\}$, $B = \{x : x \text{ is a multiple of } 2\}$

(iv) $A = \{x : x \text{ is a rational number }\}$, $B = \{x : x \text{ is a real number}\}$

6. If $A = \{1,2,3,4\}$, $B = \{2,4,6,8\}$ and $C = \{3,4,5,6\}$, find

(i) $(A \cup B) \cap C$ (ii) $A \cup (B \cap C)$

7. Write T for true and F for false statement.

(i) $A \in (A \cup B)$ (T/F)

(ii) $(A \cup B) \in B$ (T/F)

(iii) $(A \cap B) \in A$ (T/F)

(iv) $A \cup A = A$ and $A \cap A = A$ (T/F)

(v) If $A \cap B = \phi$, then $A \cap \phi = B$ (T/F)

(vii) If A and B are disjoint sets, then intersection of their union and intersection is the null set. (T/F)

(viii) If A is the proper subset of U, then the union of A and A' is U. (T/F)

(ix) $U' = \phi$ and $\phi' = U$ (T/F)

(x) $(A \cup B)' = A' \cap B'$ (T/F)

(xi) $A \cap A'$ is always empty (T/F)

(xii) $(A \cap B)' = A' \cup B'$ (T/F)

8. If $A = \{1, 2, 3, 4, 5, 6, 7, 8\}$ and $B = \{1, 3, 5, 6, 7, 8, 9\}$, then show that

$A \Delta B = \{2, 4, 9\}$

9. Let $A = \{x : x \in \mathbf{N}\}$,

$B = \{x : x = 2n : n \in \mathbf{N}\}$,

$C = \{x : x = 2n\text{–}1 : n \in \mathbf{N}\}$

and $D = \{x : x \text{ is a prime natural number}\}$. Find

(i) $A \cap B$ (ii) $A \cap C$

(iii) $A \cap D$ (iv) $B \cap C$

(v) $B \cap D$ (vi) $C \cap D$

10. For any two sets A and B, prove that $P(A) = P(B)$ implies that $A = B$

11. For any two sets A and B, show that

(i) $A \cup (A \cap B) = A$

(ii) $A \cap (A \cup B) = A$

(iii) $(A \cup B) \cap (A \cap B') = A$

(iv) $A' \cup B = U \Rightarrow A \subset B$

(v) $A \subset B \Leftrightarrow B' \subset A'$

(vi) $B \subset A \Leftrightarrow A \cap B = B$ [MEERUT(BCA)–2007]

12. Let $A = \{1, 2, 3, 4\}$, $B = \{2, 3, 4, 5\}$ and $C = \{4, 5, 6, 7\}$. Verify that
   (i) $A \cup (B \cap C) = (A \cup B) \cap (A \cup C)$
   (ii) $A \cap (B \cup C) = (A \cap B) \cup (A \cap C)$
   (iii) $A \cap (B - C) = (A \cap B) - (A \cap C)$
   (iv) $A - (B \cup C) = (A - B) \cap (A - C)$
   (v) $A - (B \cap C) = (A - B) \cup (A - C)$

13. Show that
   (i) If a set has only even element, then it has 2 subsets.
   (ii) If $B \subset A$ and B has one element less than that of A, show that A has twice as many subset as B has.
   (iii) A set with 2 elements has 2^2 subsets, a set with 3 elements has 2^3 subsets and so on.

14. If $X = \{4^n - 3n - 1 : n \in \mathbf{N}\}$ and $Y = \{9(n-1) : n \in \mathbf{N}\}$, show that $X \subset Y$.

15. Show that $A - B$, $A \cap B$ and $B - A$ are pairwise disjoint.

16. Show that $A \cup B \subseteq A \cap B$ implies that $A = B$.

17. If $A_i = \{0, i\}$, $i \in \mathbf{Z}$, show that
   (i) $A_1 \cup A_2 = \{0, 1, 2\}$
   (ii) $A_3 \cap A_4 = \{0\}$
   (iii) $\sum_{i=5}^{10} A_i = \{0,5,6,7,8,9,10\}$

[MEERUT(BCA)–2002; BHOPAL(BCA)–2006]

18. IF $A = \{2, 4, 6, 8, 10, 12\}$, $B = \{3, 4, 5, 6, 7, 8, 10\}$, then show that $(A - B) \cup (B - A) = \{2, 3, 4, 5, 7\}$.

[MEERUT(BCA)–2012; RAJ–2006; NAGPUR–2004]

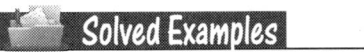

ANSWERS

1. (i) Yes. $\{a, b, c\}$, $\{a, b\}$;

4. (i) $A \cup B = \{x : x$ is non-zero integer$\}$ (ii) $A \cup B = \{x : x$ is a multiple of 2 or 3$\}$
(iii) $A \cup B = \{x : x$ is a real number$\}$ (iv) $A \cup B = \{x : x$ is an integer$\}$

5. (i) ϕ (ii) ϕ (iii) 10 (iv) $\{x : x$ is a rational number$\}$

6. (i) $\{3, 4, 6\}$, (ii) $\{1, 2, 3, 4, 6\}$

7. (i) T (ii) F (iii) T (iv) T (v) F (vi) T (vii) T
(viii) T (ix) T (x) T (xi) T (xii) T

9. (i) B (ii) C (iii) D (iv) ϕ (v) 2 (vi) $D - \{2\}$

1.10 SOME RESULTS ON VENN DIAGRAMS

If A is a finite set, and $n(A)$ = No. of elements in the set A.

The following results may be remembered for direct application :

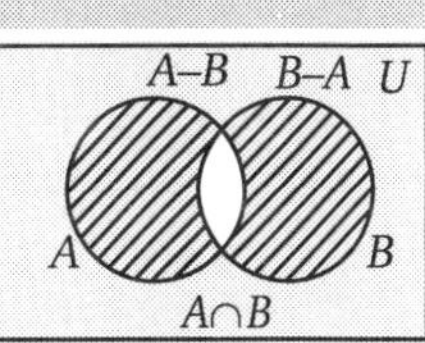

Fig. 10

(i) $n(A \cup B) = n(A) + n(B) - n(A \cap B)$
(ii) $n(A \cup B) = n(A) + n(B)$, provided A and B are disjoints
(iii) $n(A \cap B') = n(A) - n(A \cap B)$
(iv) $n(B \cap A') = n(B) - n(A \cap B)$
(v) $n(A \cup B) = n(A \cap B') + n(B \cap A') + n(A \cap B)$
(vi) $n(A \Delta B) = n(A) + n(B) - 2n(A \cap B)$
(vii) $n(A' \cup B') = n[(A \cap B)'] = n(U) - n(A \cap B)$
(viii) $n(A' \cap B') = n[(A \cup B)'] = n(U) - n(A \cup B)$
(ix) $n(A - B) = n(A) - n(A \cap B) \Rightarrow n(A - B) + n(A \cap B) = n(A)$
(x) $n(A \cup B \cup C) = n(A) + n(B) + n(C) - n(A \cap B) - n(B \cap C) - n(A \cap C) + n(A \cap B \cap C)$

1. *In a group of athletic teams in a school, 21 are in the basket ball, 26 in the hockey team and 29 in the football team. If 14 play hockey and basket ball, 12 play football and basket ball, 15 play hockey and football and 8 play all the three games. Find*
(i) how many players are there in all
(ii) how many play football only.

SOLUTION. Let A, B and C denote the set of players, who play basket ball, hockey and football respectively. Then, according to question, we have $n(A) = 21$, $n(B) = 26$, $n(C) = 29$, $n(A \cap B) = 14$, $n(A \cap C) = 12$, $n(B \cap C) = 15$ and $n(A \cap B \cap C) = 8$

Therefore, $n(A \cup B \cup C)$

$= [n(A) + n(B) + n(C) + n(A \cap B \cap C)] - [n(A \cap B) + n(A \cap C) + n(B \cap C)]$

$= [21 + 26 + 29 + 8] - [14 + 12 + 15] = 43$

Hence, the total number of players is 43. Now, the number of players playing football only is $[29 - (7+8+4)] = 10$.

2. *In a canteen, out of 123 students, 42 students buy ice-cream, 36 buy burst and 10 buy cakes, 15 students buy ice-cream and 11 buy ice-cream and buns but no cakes. Draw Venn diagram to illustrate the above information and find (i) how many students buy nothing at all (ii) how many students buy at least two items. (iii) how many students buy all three items.*

SOLUTION. Define the sets A, B and C such that

A = Set of students who buy cakes

B = Set of students who buy ice-cream

C = Set of students who buy buns

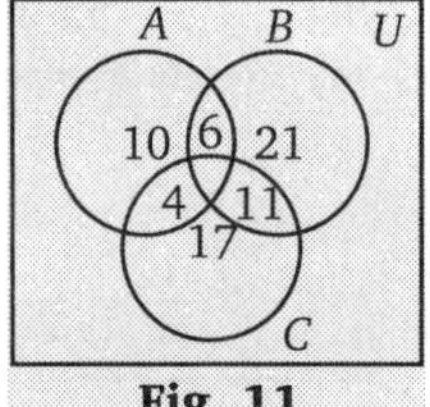

Fig. 11

According to question, we have,

$n(A) = 10$; $n(B) = 42$; $n(C) = 36$;

$n(B \cap C) = 15$; $n(A \cap B) = 10$;

$n[(A \cap C) - B] = 4$;

$n[(B \cap C) - A] = 11$

and $n[A - B \cup C] = 10$

Now we have

$n(B \cup C) = n(B) + n(C) - n(B \cap C)$

$= 42 + 36 - 15 = 63$

$n(B \cup C) - n(B) = 63 - 42 = 21$

and $n(B \cup C) - n(C) = 63 - 36 = 27$

The above distribution of the students can be illustrated by Venn diagram (Figure 11). Now, total number of students buying something.

$= 10 + 6 + 21 + 4 + 4 + 11 + 17 = 73$

(i) Number of students who did not buy anything

$= 123 - 73 = 50$

(ii) Number of students buying at least two items

$= 6+4+4+11 = 25$

And

(iii) Number of students buying all three items = 4

3. *In a group of 50 people, 35 speak Hindi, 25 speak both English and Hindi and all people speak at least one of the two language. How many people speak only English and not Hindi. How many speak English.*

[MEERUT(BCA)–2003, 07, 15; DELHI–2009, 14 AMRITSAR–2010]

SOLUTION. Given: $n(H) = 35$, $n(H \cap E) = 25$, $n(H \cup E) = 50$

Using $n(H \cup E) = n(H) + n(E) - n(H \cap E)$

$\Rightarrow n(E) = n(H \cap E) + n(H \cup E) - n(H)$

$= 50 + 25 - 35 = 40$

4. *In a city of 1000 families, it was found that 40% families buy newspaper A, 20% families buy newspaper B, and 10% buy C. Only 5% families buy A and B, 3% buy B and C and 4% buy A and C and 2% family buy all the three newspapers. Find the number of families which buy:*

(i) A only *(ii) B only*

(iii) none of A, B and C

[DELHI(BCA)–2005]

SOLUTION. Let P, Q and R respectively denote the set of families buy newspaper A, B and C. Then, for the universal set is

$n(P) = 40\%$ of $1000 = 400$,

$n(R) = 100$, $n(Q) = 200$,

$n(P \cap Q) = 50$, $n(Q \cap R) = 30$, $n(R \cap P) = 40$, $n(P \cap Q \cap R) = 20$ and $n(U) = 1000$

(i) Number of families which buy newspaper A only

$= n(P \cap Q' \cap R')$

$= n[P \cap (Q \cup R)']$

$= n(P) - n[(P \cap Q) \cup (P \cap R)]$

$= n(P) - n(P \cap Q) + n(P \cap R) - n[(P \cap Q) \cap (P \cap R)]$

$= n(P) - \{n(P \cap Q) + n(P \cap R) - n(P \cap Q \cap R)\}$

$= 400 - (50 + 40 - 20)$

$= 330$

(ii) Number of families which buy newspaper B

$= n(P' \cap Q \cap R')$
$= n(Q \cap P' \cap R')$
$= n[Q \cap (P \cup R)']$
$= n(Q) - n[Q \cap (P \cup R)]$
$= n(Q) - n[(Q \cap P) \cup (Q \cap R)]$
$= n(Q) - \{n(Q \cap P) + n(Q \cap R) - n(Q \cap P) \cap n(Q \cap R)\}$
$= n(Q) - \{n(P \cap Q) + n(Q \cap R) - n(P \cap Q \cap R)\}$
$= 200 - (50 + 30 - 20)$
$= 140$

(iii) The number of families which buy none of A, B and C

$= n(P' \cap Q' \cap R')$
$= n[P \cup Q \cup R]'$ (By Demorgan's law)
$= n(U) - [n(P) + n(Q) + n(R) - n(P \cap Q) - n(Q \cap R) - n(R \cap P) + n(P \cap Q \cap R)]$
$= 1000 - (400 + 200 + 100 - 50 - 30 - 40 + 20)$
$= 400$

5. *A computer company must hire 20 programmer to handle system programming jobs and 30 programmers for application programming. Of these, hired 5 are expected to perform jobs of both types. How many programmers must be hired.*

[MEERUT–2002; ROHILKHAND(BCA)–2008; BIKANER–2010]

SOLUTION. Let A denote the programmers to handle system programming and B denote the programmers for application programming. Then,

$n(A) = 20, n(B) = 30, n(A \cap B) = 5$

Now, using

$n(A \cup B) = n(A) + n(B) - n(A \cap B)$
$= 20 + 30 - 5 = 45$

6. *In a class of 25 students, 12 have taken Mathematics, 8 have taken Mathematics but not Biology. Find the number of students who have taken Mathematics and Biology and those who have taken Biology but not Mathematics.*

[MEERUT(BCA)–2006, 08; BIKANER–2010; BHOPAL–2010]

SOLUTION. Here, total no. of students = 25

No. of students taken Mathematics only = 8

No. of students taken Mathematics and Biology = 4

Hence, no. of students taken Biology only = 25 – (8 + 4) = 13

Exercise-1.4

1. Out of 80 students who secured first class marks in Mathematics or in Physics, 50 obtained first class marks in Mathematics, 10 in both Physics and Mathematics. How many students secured first class marks in Physics only?
2. The Mathematics club in a school held an open house on three afternoons. 115, 110 and 135 students attended both the first, second and third afternoons respectively. 25 attended just the first, 30 attended both the first and second days, 80 attended both the first and third days, and 60 attended both the second and third days. How many attended (i) all three days (ii) just the second day (iii) just the third day?
3. In a school of 250 pupils, 100 are girls, and 200 pupils stay at school for lunch. If 40 girls go home for lunch. Find the number of boys who go home for lunch.
4. In a class of 150 students, the following results were obtained in a certain examination. 45 students failed in Maths; 50 students failed in Physics, 48 students failed in Chemistry, 35 failed in both Maths and Chemistry, 25 failed in the three subject. Find the number of students who have failed in at least one subject.

ANSWERS

1. 30 **2.** 20, 30, 15 **3.** 10 **4.** 71

1.11 ORDERED PAIR

Sometimes, there are situations in which order is very important. Some results may be affected by order and other are not.

Definition: *An ordered pair is a pair of entries whose components occur in a specific order.* It is written by listing the two components in the specific order, separating them by a comma and enclosing the pair in parentheses.

Symbolically: If A and B are two sets, then by ordered pair of elements, we must mean a pair (a,b): $a \in A$, $b \in B$ in that order.

- It may be noted that (a, b) is not the same as $\{a, b\}$. The former denotes an ordered pair whereas the latter denotes a set.
- $(a, b) \neq (b, a)$ unless $a = b$.
- Ordered pair may have the same first and second components, *i.e.*, two elements of an ordered pair need not be distinct.
- Two ordered pairs are said to be equal when both the first components are equal and their second components are also equal.

1.11.1 CARTESIAN PRODUCT OF TWO SETS

The set of all ordered pairs of elements (a,b), $a \in A$, $b \in B$ is called the cartesian product of two sets A and B. It is denoted by $A \times B$.

Symbolically: $A \times B = \{(a, b) : a \in A, b \in B\}$

For example :

If $A = \{2, 3\}$ *and* $B = \{4,5,6\}$, then $A \times B = \{(2, 4), (2, 5), (2, 6), (3, 4), (3, 5), (3, 6)\}$

- $A \times B = \phi \Leftrightarrow A = \phi$ or $B = \phi$
- If A and B are finite sets, then $n(A \times B) = n(A). n(B)$
- If either A or B are infinite sets, then $A \times B$ is an infinite set.

1.11.2 ORDERED TRIPLET

If A, B, C are three sets, then by ordered triple product of elements, we mean a triplet $(a, b, c) : a \in A, b \in B, c \in C$ in that order.

This is also called ordered 3-tuple.

The set of all ordered triplets (a, b, c): $a \in A$, $b \in B$, $c \in C$ is also called the cartesian triple product of three sets A, B and C and is denoted by $(A \times B \times C)$

Symbolically: $A \times B \times C = \{(a, b, c): a \in A, b \in B, c \in C\}$

- In general, the cartesian product on n sets $A_1, A_2, \ldots, A_n$ is a ordered n-tuples $(a_1, a_2, \ldots, a_n)$, where $a_1 \in A_1$, $a_2 \in A_2$, ..., $a_n \in A_n$. It is denoted by $A_1 \times A_2 \ldots \times A_n$ or briefly by $\prod_{i=1}^{n} A_i$ where Π stands for the product.

Solved Examples

1. *If $A = \{1, 2\}$ and $B = \{a, b, c\}$, find the value of $A \times B$, $B \times A$, $A \times A$, $B \times B$.*

SOLUTION. We have $A = \{1, 2\}$ and $B = \{a, b, c\}$.

Therefore,

$A \times B = \{(1, a), (1, b), (1, c), (2, a), (2, b), (2, c)\}$

$B \times A = \{(a, 1), (a, 2), (b, 1), (b, 2), (c, 1), (c, 2),\}$

$A \times A = \{(1, 1), (1, 2), (2, 1), (2, 2)\}$

$B \times B = \{(a, a), (a, b), (a, c), (b, a), (b, b), (b, c), (c, a), (c, b), (c, c)\}$

2. *If $A = \{1, 2, 3\}$, $B = \{a, b, c, d\}$ and $C = \{-1, -2\}$, find $A \times B$, $B \times A$ and $C \times (B \cup C)$.*

SOLUTION. Given that $A = \{1, 2, 3\}$, $B = \{a, b, c, d\}$ and $C = \{-1, -2\}$.

Therefore,

$A \times B = \{(1, a), (1, b), (1, c), (1, d), (2,a),(2,b),(2,c),(2,d),(3,a), (3, b), (3, c), (3, d)\}$

$B \times A = \{(a, 1), (b, 1), (c, 1), (d, 1), (a, 2), (b, 2), (c, 2), (d, 2), (a, 3), (b, 3), (c, 3), (d, 3)\}$

Also, $B \cup C = \{a, b, c, d, -1, -2\}$

Therefore,

$C \times (B \cup C) = \{(-1, a), (-1,b), (-1, c), (-1,d), (-1,-1), (-1,-2), (-2, a), (-2, b), (-2, c), (-2, d), (-2, -1), (-2, -2)\}$

3. *Find the values of a and b if* $(4a-2, b+4) = (2a, 4)$.

SOLUTION. Since we know that two ordered pairs (a_1, b_1) and (a_2, b_2) are said to be equal if $a_1 = a_2$ and $b_1 = b_2$. Therefore, for the equality of two given ordered pairs, we have $4a - 2 = 2a$ and $b + 4 = 4$

Therefore, $4a - 2a = 2$

$\Rightarrow a=1$ and $b + 4 = 4 \Rightarrow b = 0$

4. *If* $A = \{1,2,3, 4\}$ *and* $B = \{4, 5\}$, *represent* $A \times B$, $B \times A$ *and* $B \times B$ *pictorially and find their values.*

SOLUTION. Given $A= \{1, 2, 3, 4\}$ and $B = \{4, 5\}$

$A \times B = \{(1, 4), (1, 5), (2,4), (2, 5), (3, 4), (3, 5),(4,4), (4,5)\}$

$B \times A = \{(4, 1), (5, 1), (4, 2), (5, 2), (4, 3), (5, 3), (4, 4), (5,4)\}$

And $B \times B = \{(4, 4), (4, 5), (5,4), (5, 5)\}$

Pictorially, $A \times B$, $B \times B$ and $B \times A$ can be represented as shown in figure 12.

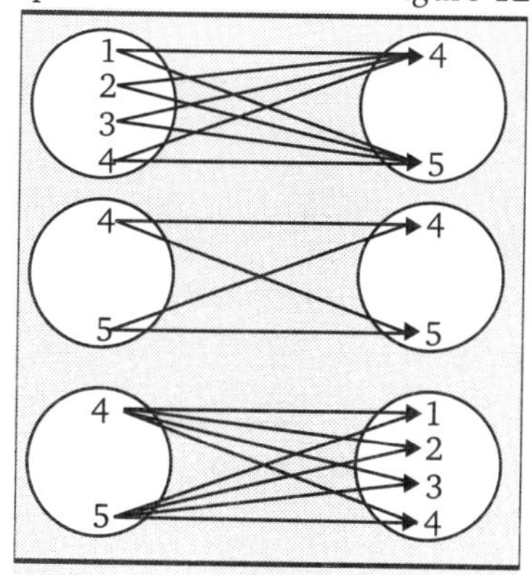

Fig. 12

EXAMPLE 5. *Let* $A = \{1, 2, 3, 4\}$ *and* $B = \{5, 7, 9\}$.

Determine (i) $A \times B$, *(ii)* $B \times A$. *Also represent* $A \times B$ *and* $B \times A$ *graphically.*

SOLUTION. (i) Given $A = \{1, 2, 3, 4\}$ and $B = \{5, 7, 9\}$. Then,

$A \times B = \{(1, 5), (1, 7), (1,9), (2, 5), (2, 7), (2, 9) (3, 5), (3, 7), (3, 9), (4, 5), (4, 7), (4, 9)\}$

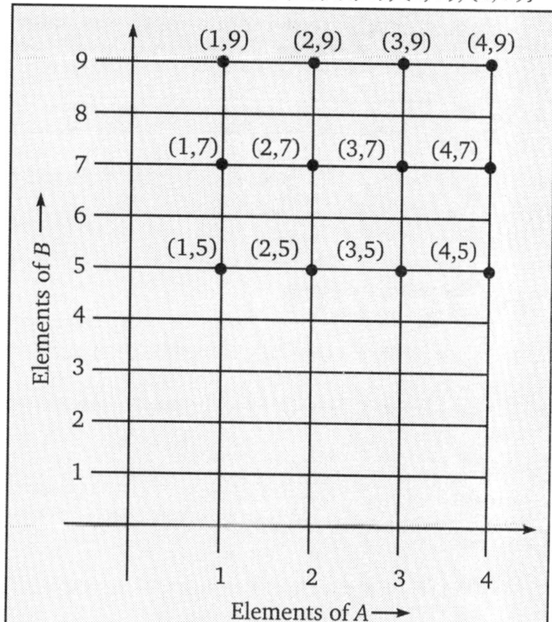

Fig. 13 $A \times B$

Now, $B \times A = \{(5, 1), (5,2), (5, 3) (5, 4) (7, 1), (7, 2), (7, 3) (7, 4) (9,1),(9,2), (9 3) (9, 4)\}$

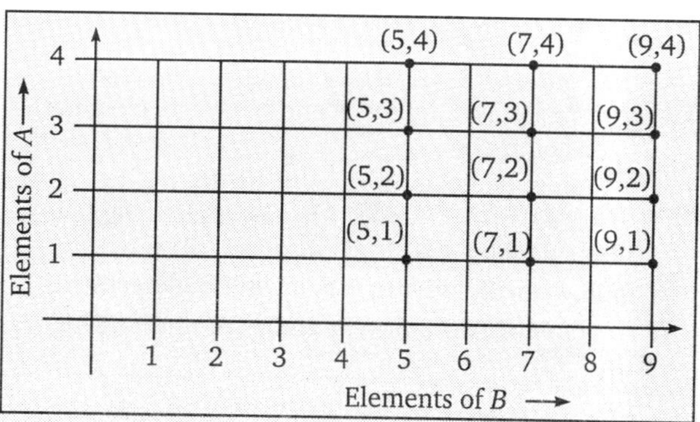

Fig. 14 $B \times A$

SOME RESULTS

1. For any three subsets A, B and C , we have.

(i) $A \times (B \cap C) = (A \times B) \cap (A \times C)$

(ii) $A \times (B \cup C) = (A \times B) \cup (A \times C)$

2. For any sets A, B, C, D we have $(A \times B) \cap (C \times D) = (A \cap C) \times (B \cap D)$

- $(A\times B) \cap (B\times A) = (A \cap B)\times (B \cap A)$
- $A \times (B' \cup C')' = A \times (B \cap C) = (A \times B) \cap (A\times C)$
- $A \times (B' \cap C')' = A \times (B \cup C) = (A \times B) \cup (A \times C)$

3. If A and B are two non-empty sets having n elements in common, then $A \times B$ and $B \times A$ have n^2 elements in common.

- For any three sets, A, B, C, we have $A \times (B - C) = (A \times B) - (A \times C)$
- If A and B are any two non-empty sets, then $A \times B = B \times A$ iff $A = B$.
- If $A \subseteq B$, then $A \times A \subseteq (A \times B) \cap (B \times A)$
- If $A \subseteq B$, then $A \times C \subseteq B \times C$ for any set C.
- If $A \subseteq B$ and $C \subseteq D$, then $A \times C \subseteq B \times D$.
- $A \times B = A \times C \Rightarrow B = C$

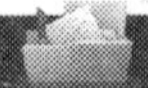

Exercise-1.5

1. If $A = \{a, b, c\}$, $B = \{d\}$, $C = \{2\}$, then verify
(i) $A\times(B \cup C) = (A\times B) \cup (A\times C)$
(ii) $A\times (B \cap C) = (A\times B) \cap (A\times C)$
(iii) $A \times (B - C) = (A \times B) - (A \times C)$
(iv) $(A \cap B)\times C = (A\times C) \cap (B\times C)$

2. If $A = \{2, 3\}$, $B = \{1, 2, 3\}$, $C = \{2, 3, 4\}$, show that $A\times A = (B \times B) \cap (C \times C)$.

3. If $A = \{1, 2, 3\}$, $B = \{4, 5\}$ and $C = \{1, 2, 3, 4, 5\}$, then show that $(C\times B) - (A\times B) = B\times B$.

4. The ordered pairs (2,7), (4, 8) and (5, 9) and among nine elements of the set $A \times B$. Determine the other six elements of $A \times B$.

5. Let $A = \{2, 3, 5, 7\}$, $B = \{1, 12, 13, 15\}$. How many elements are there in $A \times B$? In $B \times A$? Is $A \times B = B \times A$? Is $n(A \times B) = n(B \times A)$?

6. Let A and B be two sets. Show that the sets $A \times B$ and $B \times A$ have an element in common if and only if the sets A and B have an element in common.

7. Some elements of $A \times B$ are (a, x), (a, y), (d, z). If $A : \{a, b, c\ d\}$, find the remaining elements of $A\times B$ such that $n(A\times B)$ is least.

8. If A and B are two sets having 3 elements in common. If $n(A) = 5$, $n(B) = 4$, find $n(A\times B)$ and $n\{(A\times B) \cap (B\times A)\}$.

9. The ordered pairs (1, 1), (2, 2) and (3, 3) are among the elements in the set $A\times B$. If A and B have elements each, how many elements in all does the set $A\times B$ have? Also find the remaining elements.

10. If A and B are two sets such that $n(A) = 3$ and $n(B) = 2$. If $(x, 1)$, $(y, 2)$, $(z, 1)$ are in $A\times B$, find A and B, where x, y, z are distinct.

11. Write 'T' for true and 'F' for false statement:

(a) If $A = (a, b)$ and $B = (b, a)$, then $A \times B = \{(a, b)\ (b, a)\}$ (T/F)

(b) $\{(a, x), (a, y), (b, x), (b, y)\}$ is product set. (T/F)

(c) If $n(A) = x$ and $n(B) = y$ and $A \cap B = \phi$, then $n\ (A\times B) = xy$ (T/F)

(d) If A and B are non-empty sets, then $A\times B$ is a non-empty set of ordered pairs (x, y) such that $x \in A$ and $y \in A$. (T/F)

12. (a) If $A = \{1, 2, 3\}$, $B = \{4, 5\}$ and $C = \{1, 2, 3, 4, 5\}$. Find
(i) $A\times B$, (ii) $C\times B$, (iii) $B\times B$

(b) If $A = \{1, 2, 3, 4\}$ and $B = \{5, 7, 9\}$, find $(A\times B) \cap (A \cap B)$.

ANSWERS

4. (2, 8), (2, 9), (4, 7), (4, 9), (5, 7), (5, 8)
5. 16, 16, No, yes
7. (a, y), $(a, 2)$, (b, x), (b, y), (b, z), (c, x), (c, z), (d, x), (d, y)
8. 20, 9
9. 9, (1, 2), (1, 3), (2, 1), (2, 3), (3, 1), (3, 2)
10. $A = \{x, y, z\}$, $B = \{1, 2\}$,
11. (a) F (b) T (c) T (d) F

12. (a) (i) $A\times B$ = (1, 4), (1, 5), (2, 4), (2, 5), (3, 4), (3, 5)
(ii) $C\times B$ = {(1, 4), (1, 5), (2, 4), (2, 5), (3, 4), (3, 5), (4, 4), (4, 5), (5, 4), (5, 5), }
(iii) $B\times B$ = {(4, 4), (4, 5), (5, 5)} (b) ϕ

1.12 RELATION

Let us take two sets of natural numbers N_1 and N_2. We define R as a relation between them such that N_1 is a square of N_2. Then we can write $1R1$, $2R4$, $3R9$, ...

In terms of ordered pair, we can write

$$R = \{(1, 1), (2, 4), (3, 9), (4, 16), ...\} = \{(x, y : x, y \in \mathbf{N} \text{ and } y = x^2\}$$

The relation from set **N** to **N** is a subset of **N**×**N** such that $y = x^2$.

DEFINITION: *Let A and B be two sets. Then a relation R from A to B is a subset of A×B.*

Symbolically: R is a relation from A to $B \Leftrightarrow R \subseteq A\times B$.

- If R is a relation from A to B, then A is called the domain and B the range of R.
- If R is a relation from a non-empty set A to a non-empty set B and if $(a, b) \in R$, then we write aRb, read as "a is related to b by the relation R." On the other hand, if $(a, b) \notin R$, we write $a\not{R}b$ and say that 'a is not related to b by the relation R'.
- In particular, any subset $A \times A$ defined a relation in A, known as **Binary relation.**

☛ ILLUSTRATIONS

(i) If $a, b \in \mathbf{N}$ and R is defined as "a is divisor of b" then R is relation on **N**.
The subset N×N, which corresponds to the relation R is $S = \{(n, r): n \in \mathbf{N}, r \in \mathbf{N}\}$
Here, it is clear that (1, 3), (2, 4), (3, 9) (4, 8), (4, 4), are in S, whereas (2, 3), (4, 5), (5, 6) are not in S.

(ii) If R is a relation from set $A = \{1,2,3\}$ to the set $B = \{-1, -2\}$ defined by $x + y = 0$, then $R = \{(1, -1), (2, -2)\}$. Here, domain of R is {1, 2} and Range = {–1, –2}.

(iii) If $A = \{a, b, c, d, e\}$ and $B = \{f, g, h, i\}$ and let $R = \{(a, g), (a, i), (d, h), (e, f)\}$ by a relation from A to B then Domain of $R = \{a, d, e\}$ and Range of $R = \{g, i, h, f\}$

(iv) If $a, b \in \mathbf{R}$, the set of real numbers and R is "$|a - b|$ is a rational number" then R is a relation on **R**. The subset S of **R** × **R** which corresponds to the relation is

$$S = \{(a, b + a): a \in \mathbf{R}, b \in \mathbf{Q}\}$$

It is observed that $\left(1, 2\frac{1}{2}\right), \left(\pi, 1-\frac{1}{2}\right)$ belongs to S, while $(\sqrt{2}, \pi+\sqrt{2}) \notin$ S.

(v) If $A = \{2, 3, 4\}$and $B = \{a, b, c\}$, then $R = \{(2, b), (3, c), (2, a), (4, a)\}$ being a subset of $A\times B$, is a relation from $A\times B$. Here $(2, b), (3, c), (2, a), (4, a) \in R$, so we may write $2Rb$, $3Rc$, $2Ra$, $4Ra$. But $(3, b) \notin R$ therefore, $3 \not{R}\ b$.

(vi) If $a, b \in \mathbf{N}$ and R is defined by "$a - b$ is divisible by a number $n \in \mathbf{N}$", then R is a relation on **N**. The subset S of **N** × **N** corresponding to the relation by

$$S = \{n, n + rm : n \in \mathbf{N}, r \in \mathbf{N}\}$$

Here, $m = 3$, $(2, 8), (5, 11) \in S$ [$\because 2 - 8 = 6$, which is divisible by 3]
While $(3, 8) \in S$ [$\because 3 - 8 = 5$, which is not divisible by 3]

1.12.1 TOTAL NUMBER OF RELATIONS

Let A and B be two non-empty finite sets consisting p and q elements respectively, then $A \times B$ consists of $p\,q$ ordered pairs. Therefore, total number of subset of $A \times B$ is 2^{pq}.

- For a non-empty set A, $\phi \in A \times A$, therefore it is a relation on A, called **void** or **empty** relation on A.
- The void relation ϕ and the universal relation $A \times B$ are called trivial relation from A to B.
- The void and universal relation on set A respectively the smallest and the largest relation on A.

1.12.2 IDENTITY RELATION

Let A be a set. The identity relation on A is the relation $I_A = \{(x, x) : x \in A\}$ on A.

For example : If $A = \{a, b, c\}$ then the relation $I_A = \{(a, a), (b, b), (c, c)\}$is the identity relation. $R=\{(a, a), (b, b)\}$ is not an identity relation as $(c, c) \notin R$.

1.12.3 INVERSE OF A RELATION

Let A, B be two non-empty sets and R be a relation from a set A to B and let (x,y), number of the subset D of $A \times B$ corresponding to the relation R from A to B.

For the relation R from the set A to the set B, there corresponds a relation from the set B to the set A called the inverse of the relation, denoted by R^{-1} such that the subset $B \times A$ corresponding to the relation R^{-1} is $= \{(y, x): (x, y) \in D\}$.

i.e., $$yR^{-1}x \Leftrightarrow xRy$$

For example:

(i) Let $A = \{a, b, c\}$ and $B = \{1,2,3\}$ be two sets and let $R = \{(a, 1), (a, 2), (b, 1), (b, 2)\}$ be a relation from A to B then $R^{-1} = \{(1, a), (2, a), (1, b), (2, b)\}$

(ii) If $A = \{1, 2, 3\}$, $B = \{5, 6, 7\}$ and let $R = \{(1, 5), (2, 5), (2, 7)\}$ be a relation from A to B.
Then $R^{-1} = \{(5, 1), (5, 2), (7, 2)\}$ which is a relation from B to A.
Also, Domain $(R) = \{1, 2\} =$ Range (R^{-1})
And, Range $(R) = \{5, 7\} =$ Domain (R^{-1})

(iii) The inverse of the relation "*is less than*" in **R** "*is greater than*".

- It may be noted that sometimes, the inverse of a relation coincides with the relation itself.
  For example, the inverse of the relation "perpendicular to" in the set of straight lines coincides with itself.

1.13 CLASSIFICATION OF RELATIONS

(a) Reflexive Relation: Let R be a relation on a set A.

"*A relation R is said to be reflexive if* $(x, x) \in R\ \forall\ x \in A$" *i.e.,* $x\,R\,x\ \forall\ x \in A$

ILLUSTRATIONS

(i) In a set of integers, a relation R defined by $x\,R\,y$ iff $x - y$ is divisible by 4, then R is a reflexive relation because $x - x = 0$ which is divisible by 4.

(ii) The universal relation on a non-empty set A is reflexive.

(iii) The relation "is less than," *i.e.*, '<' in the set of rational number is not reflexive, because no member have the relation is less than to itself.

(iv) The relation "is a factor of" in the set of rational number is reflexive, since every rational number is a factor of itself.

(v) The relation "is less than or equal to." *i.e.*, $\leq$ is in the set of natural number is reflexive.

$$n \leq n\ \forall\ n \in \mathbf{N}$$

(b) Symmetric Relation. *A relation R on a set A is said to be symmetric if*

$$(y, x) \in R \text{ whenever } (x, y) \in R\ \forall\ x, y \in R$$

i.e., $$x\,R\,y \Leftrightarrow y\,R\,x\ \forall\ x, y \in R$$

ILLUSTRATIONS

(i) Let l_1, l_2 be two lines such that l_1 is perpendicular to l_2, *i.e.*, $l_1 \perp l_2$. Then $l_1 \perp l_2 \Rightarrow l_2 \perp l_1$. Therefore the relation $\perp$ is symmetric.

(ii) The identity and the universal relation on a non-empty set are symmetric relations.

(iii) Consider the set **N** of natural numbers and the relation 'is less than'. This relation is not symmetric. Since if $2 < 3$ then $3 \nless 2$.

Let $A = \{1, 2, 3\}$ and relations R_1 and R_2 defined by

$R_1 = \{(1, 2), (1, 3), (3, 1), (2, 1)\}$ and $R_2 = \{(1, 2), (2, 3), (3, 1)\}$

Then R_1 is a symmetric relation, but R_2 is not symmetric.

(c) Transitive Relation: *A relation R on a set A is said to be transitive iff* $(x,y) \in R$ *and* $(y, z) \in R \Rightarrow (x, z) \in R \;\forall\; x, y, z \in A$, *i.e.*, $x R y, y R z \Rightarrow xRz$.

ILLUSTRATIONS

(i) Let a, b, c be three numbers such that a is a factor of b and b is a factor of c, then obviously a is a factor of c. Therefore, 'is a factor of' is a transitive relation.

(ii) If l_1, l_2, l_3 are three lines such that $l_1 \perp l_2$ and $l_2 \perp l_3$ then it is obvious that l_1 is parallel to l_3. Therefore the relation "$\perp$" is not transitive.

(iii) The identity and universal relation on a non-empty set are transitive.

(iv) Let l_1, l_2, l_3 be three straight lines, such that l_1 is parallel to l_2 and l_2 is parallel to l_3 then it is clear that l_1 is parallel to l_3. Therefore, 'is parallel to' is a transitive relation.

(d) Anti-symmetric Relation. *A relation R on a non-empty set A is said to be an anti-symmetric relation iff* $(x, y) \in R$ *and* $(y, x) \in R \Rightarrow x = y \;\forall\; x, y \in R$

- The identity relation R on a set A is an anti – symmetric relation.
- If $(x, y) \in R$ and $(y, x) \notin R$, then it may be noted that $x = y$.
- The universal relation on a set A containing at least two elements is not anti – symmetric.

1.13.1 EQUIVALENCE RELATIONS

A relation R on a set E is said to be equivalence if it is

(i) Reflexive, (ii) Symmetric and (iii) Transitive

ILLUSTRATIONS

(i) In a set of integers, a relation R is defined by $x R y$ if and only if $x - y$ is divisible by 4. Then R is an equivalence relation. Since

(a) For $x R x$, $x - x = 0$ is divisible by 4. Therefore, it is reflexive.

(b) For $x R y$. Let $x - y = 4m$ so $y - x = 4m$, which is also divisible by 4. Therefore, it is symmetric.

(c) For $x R y$, let $x - y = 4m$; for $y R z$, let $y - z = 4n$. By adding these two equations, we get $x - z = 4(m + n)$,
which is divisible by 4. Therefore it is transitive.

(ii) Let R be a relation on the set of all lines in a plane L defined by $(l_1, l_2) \in R$ if and only if line l_1 is parallel to l_2, then R is an equivalence relation because

(a) For each line $l \in L$, we have l is parallel to $l \Rightarrow lRl \Rightarrow R$ is reflexive.

(b) Let $l_1, l_2 \in L$ such that $(l_1, l_2) \in R$, then
$\Rightarrow (l_1, l_2) \in R \Rightarrow l_1$ is parallel to $l_2 \Rightarrow l$ is symmetric.

(c) Let $l_1, l_2, l_3 \in L$ such that (l_1, l_2) and $(l_2, l_3) \in R$, then obviously $(l_1, l_3) \in R$ because if l_1 is parallel to l_2 and l_2 is parallel to l_3, then l_3 should be parallel to l_1.

1.13.2 CONGRUENCE MODULO 'm'

Let m be an arbitrary but fixed integer. If $x - y$ is divisible by m, then two integers x and y are said to be congruence modulo m of one another.

Symbolically: $x \equiv y \pmod{m}$ is $x - y$ divisible by m.
For example: $32 \equiv 2$ (mol 3), as $32 - 2 = 30$ which is divisible by 3.

1.13.3 COMPOSITION OF RELATIONS

Let R_1 and R_2 be two relations from set A to B and B to C respectively, then we can define a relation $R_1 \, o \, R_2$ from A to C, such that $(x, z) \in R_1 \, o \, R_2$ if and only if there exist $y \in Y$ such that $(x, y) \in R_1$ and $(y, z) \in R_2$.

This relation is called composition of R_1 and R_2.

- $R_1 o R_2 \neq R_2 o R_1$
- $(R_2 o R_1)^{-1} = R_1^{-1} o R_2^{-1}$

For example : Let A, B, C be three sets such that $A = \{-1, -2\}$, $B = \{p, q, r\}$ and $C = \{\alpha, \beta, \gamma\}$

Also, $R_1 = \{(-1, p), (-1, r), (-2, q)\}$ is a relation from A and B *and*

$R_2 = \{(p, \alpha), (q, \beta), (r, \gamma)\}$ is a relation from set to B to C.

Then $R_2 o R_1$ is a relation from A to C given by

$$R_2 o R_1 = \{(-1, \alpha), (-1, \gamma), (-2, \beta)\}$$

THEOREM 4. *The intersection of two equivalence relations on a set is an equivalence relation.*

PROOF. Let R_1, R_2 be two equivalence relation on a set A. To show $(R_1 \cap R_2)$ also an equivalence relation.

(i) Let $a \in A$ and a is arbitrary.
Since R_1 and R_2 both are reflexive on A.
$\therefore$ $(a, a) \in R_1$ and $(a, a) \in R_2$
$\Rightarrow$ $(a, a) \in R_1 \cap R_2$
Therefore, $(R_1 \cap R_2)$ is reflexive.

(ii) Let $a, b \in A$ such that $(a, b) \in R_1 \cap R_2$
$(a, b) \in R_1 \cap R_2 \Rightarrow (a, b) \in R_1$ and $(a, b) \in R_2$
Also, R_1 and R_2 both are symmetric on A.
Therefore, $(b, a) \in R_1$ and $(b, a) \in R_2 \Rightarrow (b, a) \in R_1 \cap R_2 \Rightarrow (R_1 \cap R_2)$ is symmetric on A.

(iii) Let $a, b, c \in$ A such that $(a, b) \in R_1 \cap R_2$, $(b, c) \in R_1 \cap R_2$
Then, $(a, b) \in R_1 \cap R_2$ and $(b, c) \in R_1 \cap R_2$
$\Rightarrow$ $\{(a, b\} \in R_1$ and $(a, b) \in R_2$ and $\{(b, c) \in R_1$ and $(b, c) \in R_2\}$
$\Rightarrow$ $\{(a, b) \in R_1, (b, c) \in R_1\}$ and $\{(a, b) \in R_2, (b, c) \in R_2\}$
$\Rightarrow$ $(a, c) \in R_1$ and $(a, c) \in R_2$ [$\because R_1$ and R_2 both are transitive.]
$\Rightarrow$ $(a, c) \in R_1 \cap R_2$
Therefore, $(R_1 \cap R_2)$ is transitive on A.

From (i), (ii) and (iii), we conclude that $R_1 \cap R_2$ is reflexive, symmetric and transitive, and hence $R_1 \cap R_2$ is an equivalence relation.

- The union of two equivalence relations on a set is not necessarily an equivalence relation.

THEOREM 5. *If R is an equivalence relation, then R^{-1} is also an equivalence relation.*

PROOF. Let R be an equivalence relation on a set A. Then by definition of relation on a set, we have

$$R \subseteq A \times A \Rightarrow R^{-1} \subseteq A \times A$$

Therefore, R^{-1} is a relation on A.

Now, to show R^{-1} is an equivalence relation.

(i) Let $a \in$ A, then $(a, a) \in R$
($\because$ R is an equivalence relation and hence reflexive)
$\Rightarrow$ $(a, a) \in R^{-1}$
Thus, $(a, a) \in R^{-1} \; \forall \; a \in R \Rightarrow R^{-1}$ is reflexive on A.

(ii) Let $(a, b) \in R^{-1}$, then $(a, b) \in R^{-1} \Rightarrow (b, a) \in R$
$\Rightarrow$ $(a, b) \in R$ ($\because$ R is symmetric)
$\Rightarrow$ $(b, a) \in R^{-1}$
Therefore R^{-1} is symmetric .

(iii) Let $(a, b) \in R^{-1}$ and $(b, c) \in R^{-1}$ then $(a, b) \in R^{-1} \Rightarrow (b, a) \in R$
and $(b, c) \in R^{-1} \Rightarrow (c, b) \in R$
Now, $(c, b) \in R$ and $(b, a) \in R$
$(c, a) \in R$ ($\because$ R is transitive)
$(a, c) \in R^{-1}$
Therefore R^{-1} is transitive .
From (i), (ii) and (iii), we conclude that R^{-1} is an equivalence relation.

RECAPITULATIONS

- If $n(A) = p$, $n(B) = q$ then total number of subsets of $A \times B = 2^{pq}$.
- **Reflexive Relation:** xRx, $\forall\, x \in A$
- **Symmetric relation:** $xRy \Leftrightarrow yRx\ \forall\, x, y \in R$
- **Transitive relation:** $xRy, yRz \Rightarrow xRz$
- **Anti-symmetric relation:** $xRy \Rightarrow yRx \Leftrightarrow x = y$
- **Equivalence relation:** Reflexive, symmetric and transitive **(RST).**
- **Partial ordered relation:** Reflexive, anti-symmetric and transitive **(RAT)**
- R is equivalence $\Rightarrow R^{-1}$ is equivalence.
- Intersection of two equivalence relations on a set is again equivalence.

Solved Examples

1. *Let* **Z** *be the set of integers. Define a relation R on* **Z** *such that $x\,R\,y$ holds if and only if $x - y$ is divisible by 5, $x \in$* **Z**, *$y \in$* **Z**. *Show that it is an equivalence relation.*

SOLUTION. (i) For each $x \in$ **Z**, $x - x$ i.e., 0 is divisible by 5.
Therefore, for all $x \in$ **Z** , $x\,R\,x \Rightarrow$ x is reflexive.

(ii) Let $x\,R\,y$
$\Rightarrow x - y$ is divisible by 5.
$\Rightarrow y - x$ is divisible by 5.
Thus $xRy = yRx$
Therefore R is symmetric.

(iii) Let us suppose xRy and yRz, then $(x - y)$ and $(y - z)$ are both divisible by 5. Hence, 5 is also a divisor of $(x - y) + (y - z)$.
5 is a divisor of $(x - z)$.
Therefore, $xRy, yRz \Rightarrow xRz \Rightarrow R$ is transitive.
From (i), (ii) and (iii), we conclude that R is an equivalence relation.

2. *Let* **N×N** *be the set of ordered pairs of natural numbers. Also, let R be the relation in* **N×N**, *defined by $(a, b)\ R\ (c, d)$ if and only if $a+d = b+c$. Show that R is an equivalence relation.*

SOLUTION. (i) For all $(a, b) \in$ **N×N**, we have $a+b = b+a$, i.e., $(a, b)\ R\ (b, a)$.
Therefore, R is reflexive.

(ii) Let $(a, b)\ R\ (c, d)$, then, by definition of R
$(a+d) = (b+c)$
or $(c+b) = (d+a)$
$(c, d)\ R\ (a, b)$
$\Rightarrow R$ is symmetric.

(iii) Let us suppose $(a, b)\ R\ (c, d)$ and $(c, d)\ R\ (e, f)$, then
$a + d = b+c$ and $c+f = d+e$
$\Rightarrow (a + d)+(c+f) = (b + c) + (d + e)$
$\Rightarrow\ a + f = b + e$
$\Rightarrow (a, b)R(e, f)$
Therefore, R is transitive.
Hence, from (i), (ii) and (iii), we conclude that R is an equivalence relation.

3. *If R is the relation on natural number defined by $x+4y = 20$. Find the domain and range of the relation R.*

SOLUTION. Let $x + 4y = 20$

$$\Rightarrow \quad y = \frac{20 - x}{4}$$

For $x = 4, y = 4$ and for $x = 8, y = 3$.
For $x = 16, y = 1$ and for $x = 12, y = 2$
Therefore, Domain = {4, 8, 12, 16}
and range = {4, 3, 2, 1}

4. *A relation R defined on the set of integers* **Z**, *as follows*

$(x, y) \in R \Rightarrow x^2 + y^2 = 25$

Express R and R^{-1} as the sets of ordered pairs and hence find their respective domains.

SOLUTION. Since $(x, y) \in R \Leftrightarrow x^2 + y^2 = 25$

$\Rightarrow \quad y = \pm\sqrt{25 - x^2}$

If $x = 0 \quad \Rightarrow \quad y = 5$.

Therefore, $(0,5) \in R$ and $(0,-5) \in R$

Now, $x = 3 \quad \Rightarrow \quad y = \sqrt{25-9} = \pm 4$

$(3, 4) \in R$, $(-3, 4) \in R$, $(3, -4) \in R$ and $(-3, -4) \in R$

$x = \pm 4 \quad \Rightarrow y = \pm 3$

Therefore, $(4, 3) \in R$, $(-4, 3) \in R$, $(4, -3) \in R$ and $(-4, -3) \in R$

$x = \pm 5 \quad \Rightarrow y = \sqrt{25-25} = 0$

$\therefore$ $(5, 0) \in R$ and $(-5, 0) \in R$

Here, it is clear that for any other integral value of x, y is not an integer. Therefore,

$R = \{(0, 5), (0, -5), (3, 4), (-3, 4), (3, -4), (-3, -4), (4, 3), (-4, 3), (4, -3), (-4, -3), (5, 0), (-5, 0)\}$

and $R^{-1} = \{(5, 0), (-5, 0), (4, 3), (4, -3), (-4, 3), (-4, -3), (3, 4), (3, -4), (-3, 4), (-3, -4), (0, 5), (0, -5)\}$

Also, Domain $(R) = \{(0, 3, -3, 4, -4, 5, -5\}$ = domain of (R^{-1}).

5. *Consider the set $A = \{a, b, c\}$. Give an example of a relation R on A which is*

(i) reflexive and symmetric but not transitive.

(ii) symmetric and transitive, but not reflexive.

(iii) reflexive and transitive, but not symmetric.

SOLUTION. (i) Given $A = \{a, b, c\}$

Let $R = \{(a, a), (a, b), (b, a), (b, c), (c, b), (b, b), (c, c)\}$ on A.

Clearly, R is reflexive and symmetric but not transitive.

(ii) Let $R = \{(a, a), (a, b), (b, a), (b, b)\}$ on A.

Here, R is symmetric and transitive but not reflexive.

(iii) Let $R = \{(a, a), (b, b), (c,c), (a, b)\}$ on A.

Here, R is reflexive, transitive but not symmetric.

6. *If R is a relation in* **N**×**N**, *show that the relation* **R** *defined by (a, b) R (c, d) if and only if ad = bc is an equivalence relation.*

SOLUTION. (i) Since $ab = ba \ \forall \ a, b \in$ **N**.

Therefore, $(a, b) \ R \ (a, b) \forall \ a, b \in$ **N** $\Rightarrow R$ is reflexive.

(ii) We have $(a, b) \ R \ (c, d)$ iff $ad = bc$ $\forall \ a, b, c, d \in$ **N**

Now, $(c, d) \ R \ (a, b)$ iff $cb = da \ \forall \ a, b, c, d \in$ **N** $\Rightarrow R$ is symmetric.

(iii) We have $(a, b) \ R \ (c, d)$ iff $ad = bc$ $\forall \ a, b, c, d \in$ **N**

Therefore, $(a, b) \ R \ (c, d)$, $(c, d) \ R \ (e, f) \Rightarrow (a, b) \ R \ (e, f) \ \forall \ a, b, c, d \in$ **N**

Using $(a, d), (c, f) = (b, c)(d, e)$

$\Rightarrow \qquad (a, f) = (b, e)$

$\Rightarrow$ R is transitive

Hence, from (i), (ii) and (iii), we conclude that R is an equivalence relation.

7. *If* **Z** *be a set of non-zero integers and a relation R defined by $xRy \Rightarrow x^y = y^x$ $\forall \ x, y \in$* **Z**, *then show that R is not an equivalence relation on* **Z**.

SOLUTION. (i) Let $x \in$ **Z**, then $x^x = x^x$, $\forall \ x \in$ **Z**

$\Rightarrow \quad xRx$, $\forall \ x \in$ **Z**

Therefore, R is reflexive.

(ii) Let $x, y \in$ **Z**, such that xRy, *i.e.*, $x^y = y^x$

$\Rightarrow x^y = y^x \Rightarrow y^x = x^y$

Therefore, $xRy \Rightarrow yRx$, $\forall \ x, y \in$ **Z**

$\Rightarrow$ R is symmetric.

(iii) Let $x, y, z \in$ **Z** such that xRy and yRz

i.e., $x^y = y^x$ and $y^z = z^y$ which does not give $x^z = z^x$

$\Rightarrow R$ is not transitive.

Hence, we conclude that R is not an equivalence relation.

8. *Let A* = **R**×**R** (**R** *is the set of real numbers) and define the following relation on A : (a, b) R (c, d) iff $a^2 + b^2 = c^2 + d^2$*

(i) Verify that (A, R) is an equivalence relation.

(ii) *Describe geometrically what the equivalence classes are for this reason.*

SOLUTION. (i) we have $(a, b)R(c, d)$

$\Rightarrow a^2 + b^2 = c^2 + d^2$

$\Rightarrow c^2 + d^2 = a^2 + b^2$

$\Rightarrow (c, d)R(a, b)$ ...(1)

$\Rightarrow$ R is symmetric.

Now, $(a, b)R(c, d)$ and

$(c, d)R(x, y) \Rightarrow a^2 + b^2 = c^2 + d^2$

and $c^2 + d^2 = x^2 + y^2$

$\Rightarrow a^2 + b^2 = x^2 + y^2$

$\Rightarrow (a, b)R(x, y)$ ...(2)

$\Rightarrow$ R is transitive.

Again $(a, b)R(a, b)$

$\Leftrightarrow a^2 + b^2 = a^2 + b^2$ ...(3)

$\Rightarrow$ R is reflexive.

Hence, from (1), (2) and (3), we conclude that R is an equivalence relation.

(ii) For any point (a, b), the sum $a^2 + b^2$ is the square of the distance from the origin. The equivalence classes are, therefore, the set of points in the place which have the same distance from the origin. Hence, the equivalence classes are concentric circles centered on the origin.

9. *Let R be the binary relation defined as* $R = \{(a, b) \in R^2 : a - b \le 3\}$. Determine whether R is reflexive, symmetric, anti symmetric and transitive.

SOLUTION. We have $(a, b) \in R^2 : a - b \le 3$.

$\Rightarrow (a, a) \in R^2 : a - a \le 3$ *i.e.,* $0 \le 3$, which is true. So, R is reflexive.

In a similar way, we can easily show that R is neither symmetric, anti symmetric nor transitive.

Exercise-1.6

1. If R is the relation 'is less than' from $A = \{1, 2, 3, 4, 5\}$ to $B = \{1, 4, 5\}$, find the set of ordered pairs corresponding to R. Also find R^{-1}.
2. A relation R defined from a set $A = \{2, 3, 4, 5\}$ to a set $B = \{3, 6, 7, 10\}$ as follows : $(x, y) \in R \Rightarrow x$ divides y. Write R as a set of ordered pairs and determine the domain and range of R. Also find R^{-1}.
3. Find the domain and range of $A = \{1, 2, 3, 4, 5, 6\}$ when the relation are defined as
   (i) xR_1y if and only if $x - y > 0$
   (ii) xR_2y if and only if $x + y < 0$
4. Two sets A and B are given by $A = \{1, 2, 8, 9\}$ and $B = \{2, 3, 4, 6, 7\}$ and if R is the relation form A to B given by $\{(1,2), (1,3), (2,4), (2,6)\}$, then which of the following statement is true?
   (i) Domain (R) = Range (R^{-1}) and Range (R) = Domain (R^{-1})
   (ii) Domain (R) = Domain (R^{-1}) and Range (R) = Range (R^{-1})
   (iii) Domain (R) = Range (R^{-1}) and Range (R) = Domain (R^{-1})
   (iv) Domain (R) = Range (R)
5. If R is a relation on a set A, then which of the following statement is not true?
   (i) If R is reflexive then R^{-1} is reflexive.
   (ii) If R is symmetric then R^{-1} is symmetric.
   (iii) If R is transitive, then R^{-1} is transitive.
   (iv) None of these
6. Find the domain and range of the following relations:
   (i) $R = \{(x + 1, x + 5)\} : x \in \{0, 1, 2, 3, 4, 5\}$
   (ii) $R = \{(x, x^3) : x$ is a prime number, less than $10\}$
   (iii) $R = \{(a, b) : a \in \mathbf{N}, a < 5, b = 4\}$
   (iv) $R = \{(a, b) : b = |a - l|, a \in \mathbf{Z}$, and $|a| \le 3\}$
7. Let R_1 be the relation defined on the set of reals $\mathbf{R}$ such as $(a, b) \in R_1$ if and only if $1 + ab > 0$ for all $a, b \in \mathbf{R}$. Show that R_1 is reflexive, symmetric but not transitive.
8. Let R be relation on $\mathbf{N} \times \mathbf{N}$, defined by $(a,b) R (c,d)$ if and only if ad $(b+c) = bc(a+d)$. Show that R is an equivalence relation.
9. Show that the relation 'congruence modulo m' on the set of integers is an equivalence relation.
10. Let R_1 be a relation on the set of reals defined by $R_1 = \{(a, b) \in R \times R : a^2 + b^2 = 1\}$ Show that R_1 is not an equivalence relation on R.
11. In a set L of all straight lines in a plane, discuss which of the following two relations are equivalence relations on L.
    (i) $R_1 = \{(x, y): x, y \in L$ and x is parallel to $y\}$
    (ii) $R_2 = \{(x, y): x, y \in L$ and x is perpendicular to $y\}$.

12. Show that the relation
$R = \{(a, b): a-b = \text{even integer} \ \forall \ a, b \in \mathbf{Z}\}$, *i.e.*, $aRb \Leftrightarrow a-b$ = even integer, is an equivalence relation.

13. Show that the relation R in **N**, the set of natural numbers, defined by xRy if $x^2 - 4xy + 3y^2 = 0$, (x, $y \in \mathbf{N}$) is reflexive, not symmetric and not transitive.

14. For the given relation R on a set S, determine which are equivalence relations:

(i) S is the set of all rational numbers, aRb if and only if $a = b$

(ii) S is the set of all real numbers iff

(a) $|a| = |b|$ (b) $a \geq b$

(iii) S is the set of all triangles in a plane, aRb iff a is congruent to b.

(iv) S is the set of all triangles in a plane, aRb iff a and b have equal perimeters.

15. An integer m is said to be related to another integer n if m is a multiple of n. Show that this relation is reflexive and transitive but not symmetric.

16. Let R be a relation defined on the set of natural number **N** as $R = \{(x, y): x, y \in \mathbf{N}, 2x + y = 41\}$. Find the domain and range of R.

17. Let O be the origin. Define a relation between two points P and Q in a plane if $PO = OQ$. Show that the relation is an equivalence relation.

18. Given the relation $R = \{(1, 2), (2, 3)\}$ on the set of natural number **N**, add a minimum of ordered pairs so that the enlarged relation is symmetric, transitive and reflexive.

19. Let **N** denote the set of all natural numbers and R be the relation on $\mathbf{N} \times \mathbf{N}$ defined by $(a, b) R (c, d) \Leftrightarrow ad(b + c) = bc(a + d)$. Show that R is an equivalence relation.

20. Show that the relation, which is symmetric and transitive, is not necessarily reflexive.

ANSWERS

1. $aRb = \{(1, 4), (1, 5), (2, 4), (3,4), (2, 5), (3, 5), (4, 5)\}$,
$R^{-1} = \{(4, 1), (5, 1), (4, 2), (5, 2), (4, 3), (5, 3), (5, 4)\}$

2. Domain $(R) = \{2, 3, 5\}$, Range $(R) = \{3, 6, 10\}$, $R^{-1} = \{(6, 2), (10, 2), (3, 3), (6, 3), (10, 5)\}$

3. (i) $\{2, 3, 4, 5, 6\}$, $\{1, 2, 3, 4, 5\}$, (ii) ϕ, ϕ **4.** (iii) **5.** (iv) **6.** (i) Domain $(R) = \{1, 2, 3, 4, 5, 6\}$, Range $(R) = \{5, 6, 7, 8, 9, 10\}$ (ii) Domain $(R) = \{2, 3, 5, 7\}$, Range $(R) = \{8, 27, 125, 243\}$ (iii) Domain $(R) = \{1,2,3,4\}$, Range $(R) = \{4\}$ (iv) Domain $(R) = \{0, -1, -2, -3, 1, 2, 3\}$, Range $(R) = \{1, 2, 3, 4, 0, 1, 2\}$ **11.** R_1 = Equivalence relation, R_2 = Not equivalence **14.** (i), (ii)

16. Domain $(R) = \{1, 2, ..., 19, 20\}$, Range $(R) = \{39, 37, 35, ..., 5, 3, 1\}$ **18.** $\{(1, 2), (2, 1), (2, 3), (3, 2), (1, 3), (3, 1), (1, 1), (2, 2), (3, 3), (4, 4), ...\}$

1.14 FUNCTIONS

DEFINITION: *Let A and B be two sets, then the rule or correspondance, which associates each element of A to a unique element of B, is called a function from set A to set B.*

[MEERUT(BCA)–2002, 03, 04, 06, 08, 14, 15, 16, 17; DELHI–2014]

If a general element of set A is denoted by x, and of set B is denoted by y, then we say that y is a function of x if, for every $x \in A$, one and only one value of $y \in B$ can be determined.

Symbolically: If f is a function from a set A to a set B, then we write $f : A \to B$, read as f is a function from A to B or f maps A to B.

1.14.1 RANGE AND DOMAIN OF A FUNCTION

Let an element $y \in B$ be corresponded by an element $x \in A$, then y is called the image of x and is denoted by $f(x)$. Here, x is defined as the pre-image of y.

The set A is called the domain and the set B is called the co-domain of the function f.

The set of all f-images of the elements of A, is called image set or the range of f and is denoted by

$$f(A) \quad \text{or} \quad \{f(x) : x \in A\}$$

Evidently, $f(A) \subseteq B$.

Thus, a mapping $f : A \to B$ is the set of ordered pairs $\{(a, b) : a \in A, b \in B\}$, so that no two ordered pairs have the same finite element.

$$f = \{(a, b): a \in A, b \in B, b = f(a) \ \forall \ a \in A\}$$

For example: Let $A = \{-2, -1, 0, 1, 2\}$ and B is the set of whole numbers for every $x \in A$, $f(x) \in B$ and $f(x) = x^2$.

Here, A is the domain and B is the co-domain.

$f(a)$ is the value of the function $f(x)$, when x takes the value a, *i.e.*, when x is replaced by a.

The elements of the co-domain which is equal to $f(x)$ form the range.

When $x = -2, f(-2) = (-2)^2 = 4$

When $x = -1, f(-1) = 1$

When $x = 0, f(0) = 0$

When $x = 1, f(1) = 1$

When $x = 2, f(2) = 4$.

Which can be illustrated in the figure (15).

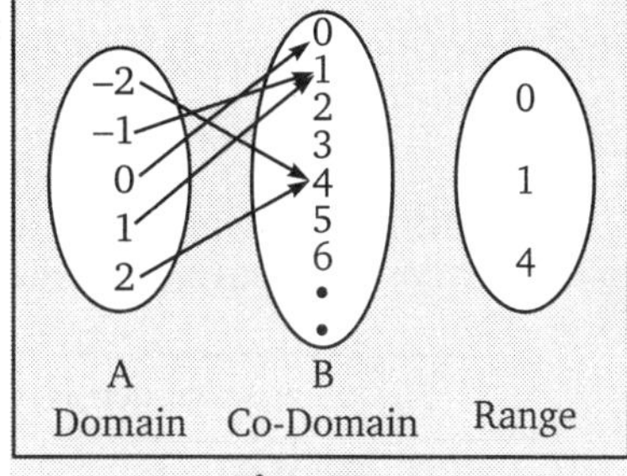

Fig. 15

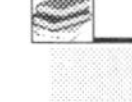

- If $f : A \to B$ then a single element in A cannot have more than one image in B. However, two or more elements in A may have the same images in B.
- Every element in A must have its image in B, but every element in B may not have its pre-image in A.
- To each element x in A, there exists a unique element y in B such that $y = f(x)$.
- The unique element y of B is called the value of f at x (the image of f under x), and written as $y = f(x)$.
- The range of f consist of those elements in B which appear as the image of at least one element in A.
- Range of a function is the image of its domain.
- Range is a subset of co-domain.

1.15 TYPE OF FUNCTIONS

(a) One-One Function: *A function f from A to B, i.e., $f : A \to B$ is said to be one-one (or injective) iff distinct elements of A have distinct images.*

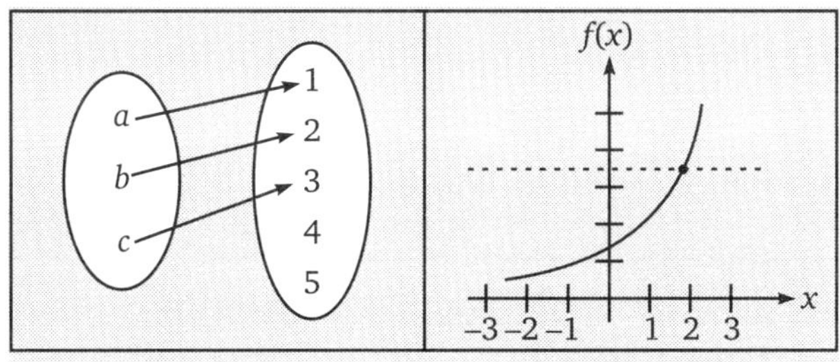

Fig. 16 **Fig. 17**

Symbolically: f is one-one if for $x_1, x_2 \in A$, we have

$$x_1 \neq x_2 \quad \Rightarrow f(x_1) \neq f(x_2) \ \forall \ x_1, x_2 \in A$$

or $f(x_1) = f(x_2) \Rightarrow \quad x_1 = x_2 \ \forall \ x_1, x_2 \in A$

It is also called Univalent function.

Graphically, a function is one-one if and only if no line parallel to x-axis meets the graph of the function in more than one point.

(b) Many-One Function: *A function $f : A \to B$ is called many-one, if at least one element of co-domain B has two or more than two pre-images in domain A.*

Symbolically: f is many-one if for $x_1, x_2 \in A$, we have $x_1 \neq x_2 \Rightarrow f(x_1) = f(x_2)$
This can be illustrated in the following figures.

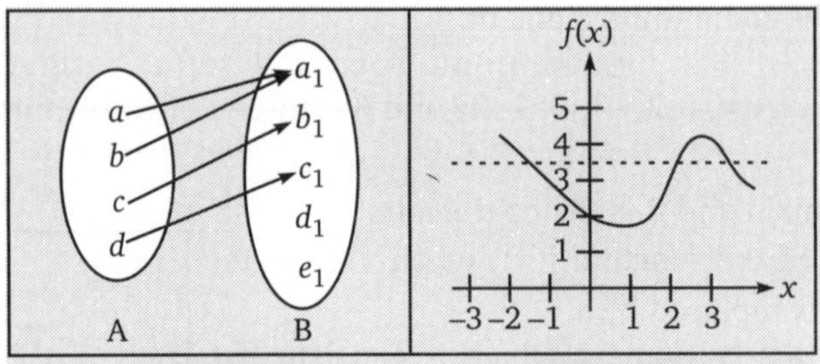

Fig. 18 **Fig. 19**

Graphically, a function is many-one if and only if a line parallel to x-axis meets the graph of the function in more than one point.

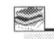

- One-many function does not exist.

(c) Onto Function: *A function $f : A \rightarrow B$ is called an onto function, if there is no element of B which is not an image of some element of A, i.e.,* every element of B appears as the image of at least one element of A. This is illustrated in Figure 20.

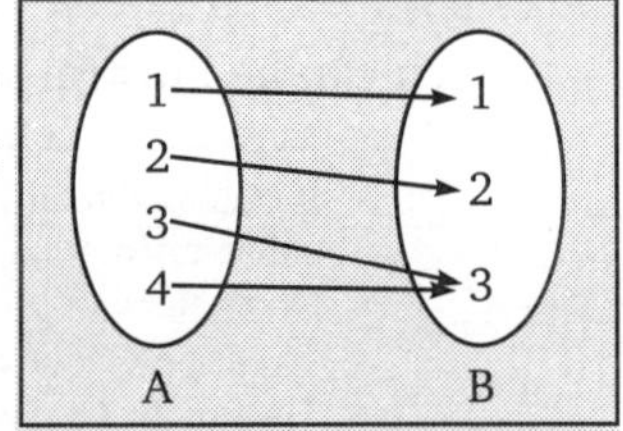

Fig. 20 Onto Function

- In an onto function, Range = Co-domain
- Onto function is also called surjective.

(d) Into Function: *A function $f : A \rightarrow B$ is called an into function, if there is at least one element of set B which has no pre-image in the set A. This is illustrated in Figure* 21.

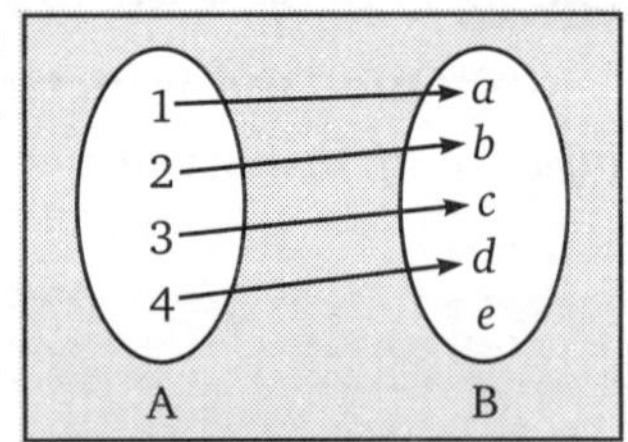

Fig. 21 Into Function

- In an into function, Range $\subset$ Co-domain.

(e) One-One Into Function: *A function $f : A \rightarrow B$ is called a one-one into function, if it is both one-one and into, i.e., the different points in A are joined to different points in B and there are some points in B which are not joined to any point in A.* This is illustrated in Figure 22.

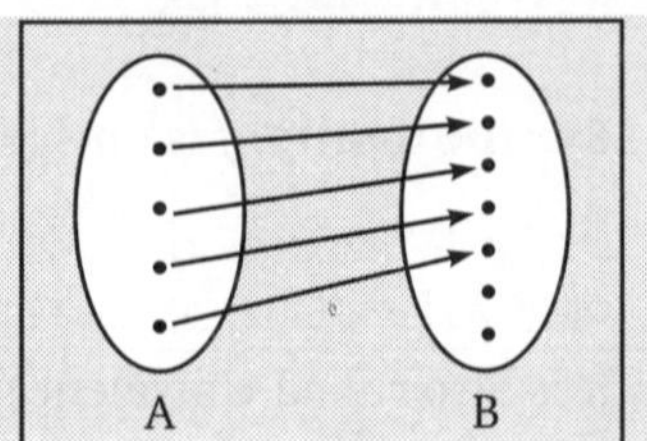

Fig. 22 One-One Into Function

Symbolically : For One-one into function
(i) Range $\subset$ Co-domain.
(ii) $f(x_1) \neq f(x_2) \Rightarrow x_1 \neq x_2.$

(f) One-One Onto Function: *A function $f : A \to B$ is both one-one and onto, if the different points in A are joined to different points in B and no point in B is left vacant.* This is illustrated in Figure 23.

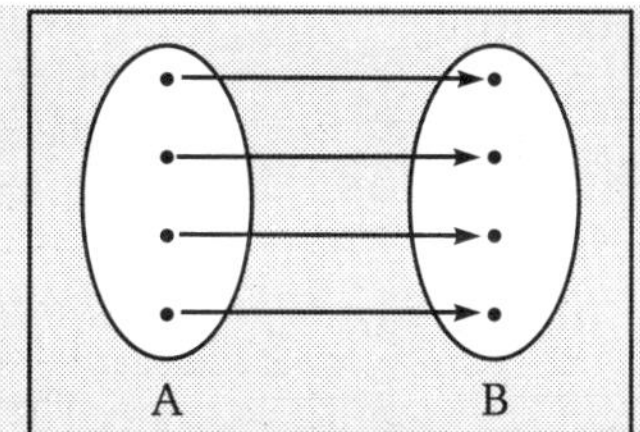

Fig. 23 One-One Onto Function

- One-one onto mapping is also known as bijective.
- For a one-to-one onto function,
  Range = Co-domain, and $x_1 \neq x_2 \Rightarrow f(x_1) \neq f(x_2)$ or $f(x_1) = f(x_2) \Rightarrow x_1 = x_2$

(g) Many-One Into Function: *A function $f : A \to B$ which is both many-one and into function is called a many-one into function, i.e., two or more points in A are joined to some points in B and there are some point in B which are not joined to any point in A.* Therefore, for many-one into function.

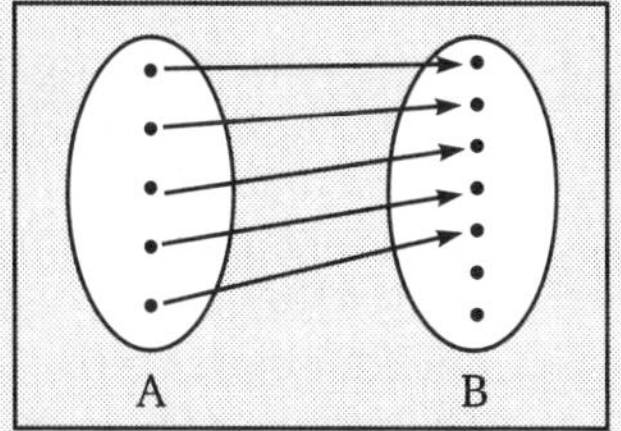

Fig. 24 Many-One Into Function

(i) Range $\subset$ Co-domain.

(ii) $x_1 \neq x_2 \Rightarrow f(x_1) = f(x_2)$

(h) Many-One Onto Function: *A function $f : A \to B$ which is both many-one and onto function is called a many one onto function, i.e., in B one point is joined to at least one point in A and two or more points in A are joined to some points in B.* Therefore, for many-one onto function.

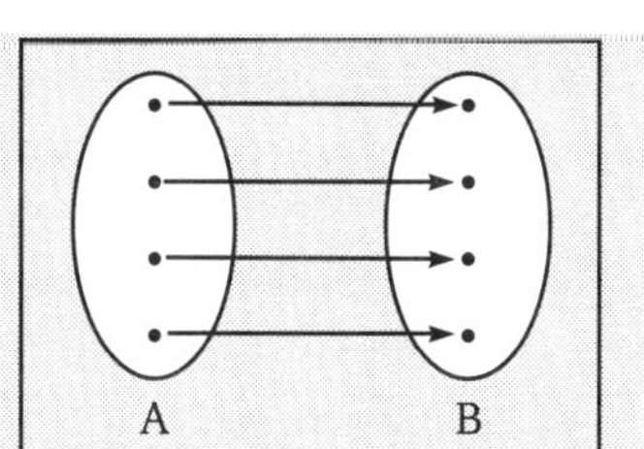

Fig. 25 Many-One Onto Function

(i) Range = Co-domain.

(ii) $x_1 \neq x_2 \Rightarrow f(x_1) = f(x_2)$

RECAPITULATIONS

- For a function $f : A \to B$, A = domain, B = co-domain.
- **For one-one function:** $x_1 \neq x_2 \Rightarrow f(x_1) \neq f(x_2)\ \forall\ x_1, x_2 \in A$ or $f(x_1) = f(x_2) \Rightarrow x_1 = x_2\ \forall\ x_1, x_2 \in A$
- **For many-one function:** $x_1 \neq x_2 \Rightarrow f(x_1) = f(x_2),\ \forall\ x_1, x_2 \in A$
- **For onto function:** Range = co-domain
- **For into function:** Range $\subset$ co-domain
- **For one-one into function:**
  (i) Range $\subset$ co-domain
  (ii) $f(x_1) \neq f(x_2) \Rightarrow x_1 \neq x_2$
- **For one-one onto function:**
  (i) Range = codomain
  (ii) $x_1 \neq x_2 \Rightarrow f(x_1) \neq f(x_2)$ or $f(x_1) = f(x_2) \Rightarrow x_1 = x_2$
- **For many-one into function:**
  (i) Range $\subset$ co-domain
  (ii) $x_1 \neq x_2 \Rightarrow f(x_1) = f(x_2)$
- **For many-one onto function:** (i) Range = co-domain (ii) $x_1 \neq x_2 \Rightarrow f(x_1) = f(x_2)$

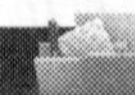

Solved Examples

1. *Let $f : \mathbf{R} \rightarrow \mathbf{R}$ be a function defined by*

$$f(x) = \begin{cases} 3x - 1 \text{ when } & x > 3 \\ x^2 - 2 \text{ when } & -2 \leq x \leq 3 \\ 2x + 3 \text{ when } & x < -2 \end{cases}$$

Find (i) f(2), (ii) f(4), (iii) f(–1), (iv) f(–3)

SOLUTION. (i) $f(2) = (2)^2 - 2 = 4 - 2 = 2$

(ii) $f(4) = 3(4) - 1 = 12 - 1 = 11$

(iii) $f(-1) = (-1)^2 - 2 = 1 - 2 = -1$

(iv) $f(-3) = 2(-3) + 3 = -6 + 3 = -3$

2. *For $y = +\sqrt{x}$, say whether it is a function or not. If it is a function, find its domain and range.*

SOLUTION. Here we have $y = +\sqrt{x}$ ...(1)

Since y is real if $x \geq 0$ and is unique and finite for each $x \geq 0$.

Therefore, (1) is a function with domain $[0, \infty[$.

Again from (1), $y \geq 0 \ \forall \ x \geq 0$

Hence, range = $[0, \infty[$

3. *Find the domain of*

$$f(x) = \frac{x^3 - x^2 + 4x + 2}{3x + 11}$$

SOLUTION. Since f is defined for all real values of x except when $3x + 11 = 0$

i.e., when, $x = -\frac{11}{3}$

Hence, domain of $f = \mathbf{R} - \left\{-\frac{11}{3}\right\}$

4. *Let $f : \mathbf{N} - \{1\} \rightarrow \mathbf{N}$ be defined by f(n) = the highest prime factor of n. Show that f is neither one-one nor onto. Also, find the range f.*

SOLUTION. Since we have

$f(6)$ = the highest prime factor of 6 = 3

$f(9)$ = the highest prime factor of 9 = 3

$f(12)$ = the highest prime factor of 12 = 3

Therefore, f is a many-one function.

Clearly, image of any $n \in \mathbf{N} - \{1\}$ is the largest prime number that divides n. So the range of f consists of prime numbers only. Consequently, range of $f \neq \mathbf{N}$ (Co-domain)

$\Rightarrow f$ is not onto function.

Hence, f is neither one-one nor onto. The range of f is the set of all prime numbers.

5. *Let A = {1, 2}. Find all one-to-one function from A to A.*

SOLUTION. Let $f : A \rightarrow A$ be a one-one function.

Then, for $f(1)$, there are two choices, *i.e.,* 1 or 2.

Let us first suppose $f(1) = 1$.

As $f : A \rightarrow A$ is one-one, $f(2) = 2$

Therefore, we have

$$f(1) = 1, f(2) = 2$$

Now, let $f(1) = 2$

Since, $f : A \rightarrow A$ is one-one, therefore $f(2) = 1$.

Therefore, we have $f(1) = 2$ and $f(2) = 1$.

Hence, we have two one-one function say f and g form A and A given by $f(1) = 1, f(2) = 2$ and $f(2) = 1$ and $f(1) = 2$.

6. *Let $\{x \in \mathbf{R} : -1 \leq x \leq 1\} = B$. Show that $f : A \rightarrow B$ given by $f(x) = x\,|x|$ is one-one and onto.*

SOLUTION. Let x, y be any two elements in A, then $x \neq y \Rightarrow x|x| \neq y|y| \Rightarrow f(x) \neq f(y)$.

Therefore, f is one-one.

Since, range of $f = f(A) = B$ so $f : A \rightarrow B$ is onto mapping. Hence f is one-one and onto.

7. *Find the domain and range of the function.*

$$f(x) = -\sqrt{-5 - 6x - x^2}$$

SOLUTION. Given that,

$$f(x) = -\sqrt{-5 - 6x - x^2}$$

For f to be real, $-5 - 6x - x^2 \geq 0$

$$\begin{aligned} \Rightarrow \quad & x^2 + 6x + 5 \leq 0 \\ \Rightarrow \quad & x^2 + 6x \leq -5 \\ \Rightarrow \quad & x^2 + 6x + 9 \leq -5 + 9 \\ \Rightarrow \quad & (x + 3)^2 \leq 4 \\ \Rightarrow \quad & |x + 3|^2 \leq 4 \\ \Rightarrow \quad & |x + 3| \leq 2 \\ \Rightarrow \quad & -2 \leq x + 3 \leq 2 \\ \Rightarrow \quad & -2 - 3 \leq x \leq 2 - 3 \\ \Rightarrow \quad & -5 \leq x \leq -1 \end{aligned}$$

Therefore, domain of $f(x) = [-5, -1]$

To find the range of $f(x)$, put $y = f(x)$

Therefore,

$$f(x) = -\sqrt{-5 - 6x - x^2}, \ y \leq 0$$

$\Rightarrow \quad y^2 = -5 - 6x - x^2$

$\Rightarrow \quad x^2 + 6x + (y^2 + 5) = 0$

For real x, discriminant ≥ 0,

i.e., $(6)^2 - 4 \times 1 \times (y^2 + 5) \geq 0$

$\Rightarrow \quad 36 - 4y^2 - 20 \geq 0$

$\Rightarrow \quad -4y^2 \geq -16$

$\Rightarrow \quad y^2 \leq 4$

$\Rightarrow \quad |y|^2 \leq 4$

$\Rightarrow \quad |y| \leq 2$

i.e., $\quad -2 \leq y \leq 2$

But $y \leq 0$ therefore, $-2 \leq y \leq 0$.

Hence, Range of $f = [-2, 0]$

- For a finite set A, if $f : A \to A$ is onto function, then f is one-one.
- For a finite set A, if $f : A \to A$ is a one-one, then f is onto.

8. *If $f : \mathbf{R} \to \mathbf{R}$ be a function defined by $f(x) = 4x^3 - 7$, show that the function f is bijective.*

SOLUTION. Given that $f(x) = 4x^3 - 7$; $x \in \mathbf{R}$

***f* is one-one :** Let $x_1, x_2 \in \mathbf{R}$

Now, $\quad f(x_1) = f(x_2)$

$\Rightarrow \quad 4x_1^3 - 7 = 4x_2^3 - 7$

$\Rightarrow \quad 4x_1^3 = 4x_2^3$

$\Rightarrow \quad x_1^3 = x_2^3$

$\Rightarrow \quad x_1^3 - x_2^3 = 0$

$\Rightarrow (x_1 - x_2)(x_1^2 + x_1x_2 + x_2^2) = 0$

$$\Rightarrow (x_1 - x_2)\left[\left(x_1 + \frac{x_2}{2}\right)^2 + \frac{3x_2^2}{4}\right]$$

$$\left\{\because \left[\left(x_1 + \frac{x_2}{2}\right)^2 + \frac{3x_2^2}{4} \neq 0\right]\right\}$$

$\Rightarrow \quad (x_1 - x_2) = 0$

$\Rightarrow \quad x_1 = x_2$

Therefore, f is one-one.

***f* is one-one :** Let $c \in \mathbf{R}$

$f(x) = c \Rightarrow 4x^3 - 7 = c$

$$\Rightarrow x = \left(\frac{c+7}{4}\right)^{1/3}$$

Now, $\left(\frac{c+7}{4}\right)^{1/3} \in \mathbf{R}$ and

$$f\left\{\left(\frac{c+7}{4}\right)^{1/3}\right\}$$

$$= 4\left[\left(\frac{c+7}{4}\right)^{1/3}\right]^3 - 7$$

$$= c + 7 - 7 = c$$

Which implies that c is the image of $\left(\frac{c+7}{4}\right)^{1/3}$

Therefore, f is onto. Hence, f is objective function.

10. *Find the domain and range of the function* $f(x) = \dfrac{1}{2 - \cos 3x}$

[MEERUT(BCA)–2001, 12; ROHILKHAND–2005, 14]

SOLUTION. We have $f(x) = \dfrac{1}{2 - \cos 3x}$

We know that the value of cos $3x$ lies between -1 and 1 for all $x \in \mathbf{R}$.

i.e., $-1 \leq \cos 3x \leq 1 \; \forall \; x \in \mathbf{R}$ and $2 - \cos 3x \neq 0 \; \forall \; x \in \mathbf{R}$.

$\Rightarrow f(x)$ is defined for all $x \in \mathbf{R}$. Hence, domain of $f(x)$ is $\mathbf{R}$.

Further, the maximum value of cos $3x = 1$

$\Rightarrow$ max. value of $f(x) = \dfrac{1}{2-1} = 1$.

Similarly, the minimum value of cos $3x = -1$

$\Rightarrow$ min. value of $f(x) = \dfrac{1}{2-(-1)} = \dfrac{1}{3}$.

$\Rightarrow$ Range of $f = \left[\dfrac{1}{3}, 1\right]$.

10. *Find the domain and range of the following functions:*

(i) $f(x) = \sin x - \cos x$

(ii) $f(x) = |\sin x|$

[MEERUT(BCA)–2004, 08; KANPUR–2010; ROHILKHAND–2011; BUNDELKHAND–2012]

SOLUTION. (i) $f(x) = \sin x - \cos x$

$$= \sqrt{2}\left(\frac{1}{\sqrt{2}}\sin x - \frac{1}{\sqrt{2}}\cos x\right)$$

$$= \sqrt{2}\sin x\left(x - \frac{\pi}{4}\right)$$

Now, domain of $\sin x\left(x - \frac{\pi}{4}\right)$ is

R, so domain of $f(x)$ is **R**. Also,

range of $\sin x\left(x-\frac{\pi}{4}\right)$ is [–1, 1]

so range of $f(x)$ is $[-\sqrt{2},\sqrt{2}]$.

(ii) $f(x) = |\sin x|$

Clearly, domain of sin x is the set of real numbers, **R**

$\Rightarrow$ domain($|\sin x|$) = **R**.

Also, range of sin x is [–1, 1].

Hence, Range($|\sin x|$) = [0,1].

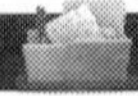

Exercise-1.7

1. Let A = {–2, –1, 0, 1, 2} and $f : A \to \mathbf{Z}$ be given by $f(x) = x^2 - 2x - 3$. Find :
   (i) the range of f,
   (ii) pre-image of 6, –3 and 5.
2. Find the domain and range of the following function
   $$f(x)=\sqrt{(x-1)(3-x)}$$
3. Find the range of the following function
   $$f(x)=\frac{1}{(2x-3)(x+1)}$$
4. Find the domain and range of the following functions :
   (i) $f(x)=\frac{x^2-1}{x-1}$ (ii) $y = -|x|$
   (iii) $f(x)=\frac{|x-1|}{x-1}$ (iv) $y=\sqrt{x-3}$
5. If A = {–1, 0, 2, 5, 6, 11},
   B = {–2, –1, 0, 18, 25, 108}
   and $f(x) = x^2 - x - 2$, find $f(A)$.
6. Let A be the set of two positive integers. Let $f : A \to \mathbf{Z}^+$, set of positive integers be defined by $f(n) = p$, where p is the highest prime factor of n. If range of f = {3}, find A.
7. Find the domain for which the function $f(x) = 2x^2 - 1$ and $g(x) = 1 - 3x$ are equal.
8. Let $f_1 : \mathbf{R} \to \mathbf{R}$ and $f_2 : \mathbf{C} \to \mathbf{C}$ be two functions defined as $f_1(x) = x^3$ and $f_2(x) = x^3$. Show that they are not equal.
9. Let A = {p, q, r, s} and B = {1, 2, 3}. Which of the following relations from A to B not a function?
   (i) R_1 = {(p, 1), (q, 2), (r, 1), (s, 2)}
   (ii) R_2 = {(p, 1), (q, 1), (r, 1), (s, 1)}
   (iii) R_3 = {(p, 1), (q, 2), (r, 2), (s, 3)}
   (iv) R_4 = {(p, 2), (q, 3), (r, 2), (s, 2)}
10. Write the following relations as sets of ordered pairs and find which of them are functions :
    (i) {(x, y) : $y = 3x$, $x \in$ (1, 2, 3), $y \in$ (3, 6, 9, 12)}
    (ii) {(x, y) : $y > x + 1$, x = 1, 2 and y = 2, 4, 6}
    (iii) {(x, y) : $x + y = 3$ $x, y \in$ (0, 1, 2, 3)}
11. Express the following functions as sets of ordered pairs, and find their range :
    (i) $f_1 : A \to \mathbf{R} : f_1(x) = x^2 + 1$ where A = {–1, 0, 2, 4}
    (ii) $f_2 : A \to \mathbf{N} : f_2(x) = 2x$ where $A = \{x : x \in \mathbf{N}, x \le 10\}$
12. Let $f : \mathbf{R} \to \mathbf{R}$ be a function such that $f(x) = 2^x$. Determine :
    (i) range of f
    (ii) {$x : f(x) = 1$}
    (iii) whether $f(x + y) = f(x)\cdot f(y)$ holds
13. Let $f : \mathbf{R}^+ \to \mathbf{R}$, be a function such that $f(x) = \log x$. Determine :
    (i) the image set of domain of f
    (ii) {$x : f(x) = -2$}
    (iii) whether $f(xy) = f(x) + f(y)$ holds
14. Give an example of a map which is :
    (i) one-to-one but not onto
    (ii) not one to one, but onto
    (iii) neither one-to-one nor onto

ANSWERS

1. (i) $f(A)$ = {– 4, –3, 0, 5}, (ii) ϕ, {1, 2}, –2 **2.** Domain = [1, 3], Range = [–1, 1] **3.** $\left]-\infty \frac{-8}{25}\right] \cup [0, \infty[$

4. (i) **R** – {1}, **R** – {2}, (ii) **R** : **R** – **R**$^+$, (iii) **R** – {1}, {–1, 1}, (iv) [3, ∞[, [0, ∞] **5.** $f(A)$ = {1, –2, 18, 28, 108} **6.** A = {3, 6} or (3, 9) or [3, 12] etc. **7.** (–2, 1/2) **9.** (iii) **10.** (i) {(1, 3), (2, 6), (3, 9)}, function, (ii) {(1, 4), (1, 6), (3, 4), (3, 6)}, not function (iii) {(0, 3), (1, 2), (2, 1), (3, 0)}, function **11.** (i) $f_1 = \{x, f(x) : x \in A\}$ = {(–1, 2), (0, 1), (2, 5), (4, 17)} (ii) $f_2 = \{(x, g(x)) : x \in A\}$= {(1,2),(2,4), (3, 6), ..., (10, 20)} **12.** (i) Range of f = **R**$^+$, the set of positive real numbers, (ii) ($x : f(x) = 1$) = {0}, (iii) $f(x+y) = f(x).f(y)$ holds for all $x, y \in \mathbf{R}$

14. (i) $n \to n^2 : \mathbf{N} \to \mathbf{N}$ (ii) $n \to |n| : \mathbf{Z} \to \mathbf{N} \cup \{0\}$ (iii) $n \to |n|^2 : \mathbf{Z} \to \mathbf{N} \cup \{0\}$

❑❑❑❑❑❑

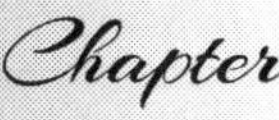

2

Determinants

2.1 INTRODUCTION

A determinant is an arrangement of numbers in rows and columns but it always has a square form and can be reduced to a single value. Therefore, a determinant is distinct from matrix in the sense that the determinant is always in square shape and it has a numerical value. The arrangement of the numbers of a determinant is enclosed within two vertical parallel lines.

Consider two homogeneous linear equations

$$a_1x + b_1y = 0$$
$$a_2x + b_2y = 0;$$

Multiplying the first equation by b_2 and second by b_1 and then subtracting and dividing by x, we obtained

$$a_1b_2 - a_2b_1 = 0$$

This result is sometimes written as

$$\begin{vmatrix} a_1 & b_1 \\ a_2 & b_2 \end{vmatrix} = 0$$

and the expression on the left is called determinant.

2.1.1 Order of a Determinant

The determinant of a square matrix of order n is known as determinant of order n.

2.2 DETERMINANT OF ORDER TWO

Let $a_{11}, a_{12}, a_{21}, a_{22}$ be any four number (real or complex). Then

$$|A| = \begin{vmatrix} a_{11} & b_{12} \\ a_{21} & b_{22} \end{vmatrix}$$

represent the number $a_{11}a_{22} - a_{21}a_{12}$ and is called a determinant of order two.

For Example $\quad |A| = \begin{vmatrix} 5 & 2 \\ 3 & -7 \end{vmatrix} = (5)(-7) - (3)(2) = -35 - 6 = -41$

2.3 DETERMINANT OF ORDER THREE

Let $\quad |A| = \begin{vmatrix} a_{11} & a_{12} & a_{13} \\ a_{21} & a_{22} & a_{23} \\ a_{31} & a_{32} & a_{33} \end{vmatrix}$

is called a determinant of order 3 and its value can be obtained as follows:

$$|A| = a_{11}\begin{vmatrix} a_{22} & a_{23} \\ a_{32} & a_{33} \end{vmatrix} - a_{12}\begin{vmatrix} a_{21} & a_{23} \\ a_{31} & a_{33} \end{vmatrix} + a_{13}\begin{vmatrix} a_{21} & a_{22} \\ a_{31} & a_{32} \end{vmatrix}$$
$$= a_{11}(a_{22}a_{33} - a_{32}a_{23}) - a_{12}(a_{21}a_{33} - a_{31}a_{23}) + a_{13}(a_{21}a_{32} - a_{31}a_{22})$$

For Example, $|A| = \begin{vmatrix} 2 & 3 & 4 \\ -1 & 2 & 3 \\ 4 & -2 & 1 \end{vmatrix} = 2\begin{vmatrix} 2 & 3 \\ -2 & 1 \end{vmatrix} - 3\begin{vmatrix} -1 & 3 \\ 4 & 1 \end{vmatrix} + 4\begin{vmatrix} -1 & 2 \\ 4 & -2 \end{vmatrix}$

$= 2(2 + 6) - 3(-1 -12) + 4(2 - 8) = 16 + 39 - 24 = 31$

- The value of a determinant is not changed if it is expanded along any row or column.
- When no reference of the corresponding matrix is needed, we may denote a determinant by D.
- The determinant of a square zero matrix is zero.

Solved Examples

1. *Find the value of* $\begin{vmatrix} \cos\alpha & -\sin\alpha \\ \sin\alpha & \cos\alpha \end{vmatrix}$.

SOLUTION. We have $|A| = \begin{vmatrix} \cos\alpha & -\sin\alpha \\ \sin\alpha & \cos\alpha \end{vmatrix}$

$= \cos^2\alpha - (-\sin^2\alpha)$

$= \cos^2\alpha + \sin^2\alpha = 1$

2. *Find the value of* $\begin{vmatrix} 1 & \omega \\ \omega & -\omega \end{vmatrix}$.

SOLUTION. We have

$|A| = \begin{vmatrix} 1 & \omega \\ \omega & -\omega \end{vmatrix}$

$= -\omega - \omega^2 = -(\omega + \omega^2) = -(-1) = 1.$

3. *Solve for x.*

$\begin{vmatrix} x & 3 \\ 5 & 2x \end{vmatrix} = \begin{vmatrix} 5 & -4 \\ 5 & 3 \end{vmatrix}$

SOLUTION. We have $\begin{vmatrix} x & 3 \\ 5 & 2x \end{vmatrix} = \begin{vmatrix} 5 & -4 \\ 5 & 3 \end{vmatrix}$

$\Rightarrow \quad 2x^2 - 15 = 15 + 20$

$\Rightarrow \quad 2x^2 = 50$

$\Rightarrow \quad x^2 = 25$

$\Rightarrow \quad x = \pm 5$

4. *Find the value of* $\begin{vmatrix} a & h & g \\ h & b & f \\ g & f & c \end{vmatrix}$.

SOLUTION. Let $\Delta = \begin{vmatrix} a & h & g \\ h & b & f \\ g & f & c \end{vmatrix}$

Then

$\Delta = a(bc - f^2) - h(hc - fg) + g(hf - bg)$

$= abc - af^2 - ch^2 + fgh + fgh - bg^2$

$= abc + 2fgh - af^2 - bg^2 - ch^2$

5. *Find the value of* $\begin{vmatrix} 0 & 1 & \sec\theta \\ \tan\theta & -\sec\theta & \tan\theta \\ 1 & 0 & 1 \end{vmatrix}$.

SOLUTION. Let $\Delta = \begin{vmatrix} 0 & 1 & \sec\theta \\ \tan\theta & -\sec\theta & \tan\theta \\ 1 & 0 & 1 \end{vmatrix}$

Expand along R_1

$\Delta = 0 + 1(-1)^3 \begin{vmatrix} \tan\theta & \tan\theta \\ 1 & 1 \end{vmatrix}$

$+ \sec\theta(-1)^4 \begin{vmatrix} \tan\theta & -\sec\theta \\ 1 & 0 \end{vmatrix}$

$= -(\tan\theta - \tan\theta) + \sec\theta(0 + \sec\theta)$

$= \sec\theta(0 + \sec\theta) = \sec^2\theta.$

2.4 CO-FACTORS AND MINORS OF AN ELEMENT

If in the expansion of a determinant $|a_{ij}|$, all the factor containing a_{ij}, are collected and their sum is denoted by $a_{ij} A_{ij}$ then the factor A_{ij} is called the co-factor of the element a_{ij}. Hence, in a determinant of order n

$$|a_{ij}| = a_{i1}A_{i1} + a_{i2}A_{i2} + \ldots + a_{in}A_{in} = \sum_{j=1}^{n} a_{ij}A_{ij}$$

Now, let M_{ij} be the $(n - 1) \times (n - 1)$ sub-matrix of $|a_{ij}|_{n \times n}$ obtained by deleting the ith row and j^{th} column. Then $|M_{ij}|$ is called the minor of the element a_{ij} the determinant $|a_{ij}|$ of order n. Thus, we can express the determinant as a linear combination of the minors of the elements of any row or any column.

- $(-1)^{i+j}$ is 1 or –1 according as $i + j$ is even or odd.
  $\therefore A_{ij}$ and M_{ij} coincides if $i + j$ is even and if $i + j$ is odd then we have $A_{ij} = -M_{ij}$.

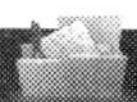

Solved Examples

1. *Find the minors and cofactors of elements of the determinant* $\begin{vmatrix} 5 & -2 \\ 3 & 7 \end{vmatrix}$.

SOLUTION. Minor of the element a_{11} is $M_{11} = |7| = 7$

Minor of the element a_{12} is $M_{12} = 3$

Minor of the element a_{21} is $M_{21} = -2$

Minor of the element a_{22} is $M_{22} = 5$

Hence, $A_{11} = (-1)^{1+1}M_{11} = 7$

$A_{12} = (-1)^{1+2}M_{12} = -3$

$A_{21} = (-1)^{2+1}M_{21} = 2$

$A_{22} = (-1)^{2+2}M_{22} = 5$

2. *Find all the minors and cofactors of the elements in following determinants*

$$\begin{vmatrix} 4 & 3 & 1 \\ 1 & 3 & 2 \\ 2 & 1 & 5 \end{vmatrix}$$

SOLUTION. Here, $a_{11} = 4, a_{12} = 3, a_{13} = 1$

$a_{21} = 1, a_{22} = 3, a_{23} = 2$

$a_{31} = 2, a_{32} = 1, a_{33} = 5$

$$M_{11} = \begin{vmatrix} 3 & 2 \\ 1 & 5 \end{vmatrix} = 15 - 2 = 13$$

$$M_{12} = \begin{vmatrix} 1 & 2 \\ 2 & 5 \end{vmatrix} = 5 - 4 = 1$$

$$M_{13} = \begin{vmatrix} 1 & 3 \\ 2 & 1 \end{vmatrix} = 1 - 6 = -5$$

$$M_{21} = \begin{vmatrix} 3 & 1 \\ 1 & 5 \end{vmatrix} = 15 - 1 = 14$$

$$M_{22} = \begin{vmatrix} 4 & 1 \\ 2 & 5 \end{vmatrix} = 20 - 2 = 18$$

$$M_{23} = \begin{vmatrix} 4 & 3 \\ 2 & 1 \end{vmatrix} = 4 - 6 = -2$$

$$M_{31} = \begin{vmatrix} 3 & 1 \\ 3 & 2 \end{vmatrix} = 6 - 3 = 3$$

$$M_{32} = \begin{vmatrix} 4 & 1 \\ 1 & 2 \end{vmatrix} = 8 - 1 = 7$$

$$M_{33} = \begin{vmatrix} 4 & 3 \\ 1 & 3 \end{vmatrix} = 12 - 3 = 9.$$

The co–factors are

$A_{11} = (-1)^{1+1}M_{11} = 1 \times 13 = 13$

$A_{12} = (-1)^{1+2}M_{12} = -1 \times 1 = -1$

$A_{13} = (-1)^{1+3}M_{13} = 1 \times (-5) = -5$

$A_{21} = (-1)^{2+1}M_{21} = -1 \times 14 = -14$

$A_{22} = (-1)^{2+2}M_{22} = 1 \times 18 = 18$

$A_{23} = (-1)^{2+3}M_{23} = -1 \times (-2) = 2$

$A_{31} = (-1)^{3+1}M_{31} = 1 \times 3 = 3$

$A_{32} = (-1)^{3+2}M_{32} = -1 \times 7 = -7$

$A_{33} = (-1)^{3+3}M_{33} = 1 \times 9 = 9.$

3. *Find the minor and co-factors of elements of the following determinant*

$$\begin{vmatrix} 2 & -3 & 5 \\ 6 & 0 & 4 \\ 1 & 5 & -7 \end{vmatrix}.$$

SOLUTION. We have

$$M_{11} = \begin{vmatrix} 0 & 4 \\ 5 & -7 \end{vmatrix} = 0 - 20 = -20$$

$A_{11} = -20$

$$M_{12} = \begin{vmatrix} 6 & 4 \\ 1 & -7 \end{vmatrix} = -42 - 4 = -46$$

$A_{12} = 46$

$$M_{13} = \begin{vmatrix} 6 & 0 \\ 1 & 5 \end{vmatrix} = 30 - 0 = 30$$

$A_{13} = 30$

$$M_{21} = \begin{vmatrix} -3 & 5 \\ 5 & -7 \end{vmatrix} = 21 - 25 = -4$$

$A_{21} = 4$

$$M_{22} = \begin{vmatrix} 2 & 5 \\ 1 & -7 \end{vmatrix} = -14 - 5 = -19$$

$A_{22} = -19$

$$M_{23} = \begin{vmatrix} 2 & -3 \\ 1 & 5 \end{vmatrix} = 10 + 3 = 13$$

$A_{23} = -13$

$$M_{31} = \begin{vmatrix} -3 & 5 \\ 0 & 4 \end{vmatrix} = -12 - 0 = -12$$

$A_{31} = -12$

$$M_{32} = \begin{vmatrix} 2 & 5 \\ 6 & 4 \end{vmatrix} = 8 - 30 = -22 \qquad M_{33} = \begin{vmatrix} 2 & -3 \\ 6 & 0 \end{vmatrix} = 0 + 18 = 18$$

$$A_{32} = 22 \qquad A_{33} = 18.$$

2.5 PROPERTIES OF DETERMINANTS

THEOREM 1. *The value of a determinant does not change when rows and columns are interchanged.*

PROOF. Let $|A| = \begin{vmatrix} a_1 & b_1 & c_1 \\ a_2 & b_2 & c_2 \\ a_3 & b_3 & c_3 \end{vmatrix}$ be a determinant of order three.

Expanding $|A|$ along the first row, we get

$$|A| = a_1(b_2c_3 - b_3c_2) - b_1(a_2c_3 - a_3c_2) + c_1(a_2b_3 - a_3b_2)$$

$$= a_1(b_2c_3 - b_3c_2) - a_2(b_1c_3 - b_3c_1) + a_3(b_1c_2 - b_2c_1)$$

(by rearrangement of terms)

$$= \begin{vmatrix} a_1 & a_2 & a_3 \\ b_1 & b_2 & b_3 \\ c_1 & c_2 & c_3 \end{vmatrix}$$

Hence, the theorem is proved.

THEOREM 2. *If any two rows [or columns] of a determinant are interchanged, the sign of the determinant is changed.*

PROOF. Let $|A| = \begin{vmatrix} a_1 & b_1 & c_1 \\ a_2 & b_2 & c_2 \\ a_3 & b_3 & c_3 \end{vmatrix}$ be a determinant of order three.

Expanding $|A|$ along the first row, we get

$$|A| = a_1(b_2c_3 - b_3c_2) - b_1(a_2c_3 - a_3c_2) + c_1(a_2b_3 - a_3b_2)$$

$$= -a_3(b_2c_1 - b_1c_2) - b_3(a_2c_1 - a_1c_2) + c_3(a_2b_1 - a_1b_2)$$

(by rearrangement of terms)

$$= -\begin{vmatrix} a_1 & a_2 & a_3 \\ b_1 & b_2 & b_3 \\ c_1 & c_2 & c_3 \end{vmatrix} = (-1)|A|$$

THEOREM 3. *If two rows or two columns of the determinant are identical, then the value of the determinant vanishes, i.e.,*

$$|A| = \begin{vmatrix} a_1 & b_1 & c_1 \\ a_2 & b_2 & c_2 \\ a_3 & b_3 & c_3 \end{vmatrix} = 0.$$

PROOF. We have $|A|$ is a determinant of order 3 whose first and third row are identical. If we interchange the two identical rows, then obviously there will be no change in the value of $|A|$. But by theorem 2, the value of A is multiplied by –1 if we interchange two rows. Therefore, we get

$$|A| = -|A|$$

$$2|A| = 0 \qquad \text{or} \qquad |A| = 0$$

THEOREM 4. *If all the elements of any row, or any column, of a determinant are multiplied by the same number then the determinant is multiplied by that number.*

PROOF. Let $|A| = \begin{vmatrix} a_{11} & a_{12} & \cdots & a_{1n} \\ a_{21} & a_{22} & \cdots & a_{2n} \\ \cdots & \cdots & \cdots & \cdots \\ a_{n1} & a_{n2} & \cdots & a_{nn} \end{vmatrix}$ be a determinant of order n

We have $\begin{vmatrix} ma_{11} & a_{12} & \cdots & a_{1n} \\ ma_{21} & a_{22} & \cdots & a_{2n} \\ \cdots & \cdots & \cdots & \cdots \\ ma_{n1} & a_{n2} & \cdots & a_{nn} \end{vmatrix} = ma_{i1}A_{i1} + ma_{i2}A_{i2} + \ldots ma_{in}A_{in} = m|A|$

(where $A_{i1}, A_{i2} \ldots, A_{in}$ be the cofactor of elements $a_{i1}, a_{i2}, \ldots, a_{in}$ of ith row of $|A|$)

THEOREM 5. *If in the determinant, the elements of a row (or column) are added m times the corresponding elements of the another rows (or column), the value of the determinant does not change. In particular,*

$$\begin{vmatrix} a_1 + mb_1 + nc_1 & b_1 & c_1 \\ a_2 + mb_2 + nc_2 & b_2 & c_2 \\ a_3 + mb_3 + nc_3 & b_3 & c_3 \end{vmatrix} = \begin{vmatrix} a_1 & b_1 & c_1 \\ a_2 & b_2 & c_2 \\ a_3 & b_3 & c_3 \end{vmatrix}$$

PROOF. We have

$$\begin{vmatrix} a_1 + mb_1 + nc_1 & b_1 & c_1 \\ a_2 + mb_2 + nc_2 & b_2 & c_2 \\ a_3 + mb_3 + nc_3 & b_3 & c_3 \end{vmatrix} = \begin{vmatrix} a_1 & b_1 & c_1 \\ a_2 & b_2 & c_2 \\ a_3 & b_3 & c_3 \end{vmatrix} + \begin{vmatrix} mb_1 & b_1 & c_1 \\ mb_2 & b_2 & c_2 \\ mb_3 & b_3 & c_3 \end{vmatrix} + \begin{vmatrix} nc_1 & b_1 & c_1 \\ nc_2 & b_2 & c_2 \\ nc_3 & b_3 & c_3 \end{vmatrix}$$

$$= \begin{vmatrix} a_1 & b_1 & c_1 \\ a_2 & b_2 & c_2 \\ a_3 & b_3 & c_3 \end{vmatrix} + m\begin{vmatrix} b_1 & b_1 & c_1 \\ b_2 & b_2 & c_2 \\ b_3 & b_3 & c_3 \end{vmatrix} + n\begin{vmatrix} c_1 & b_1 & c_1 \\ c_2 & b_2 & c_2 \\ c_3 & b_3 & c_3 \end{vmatrix}$$

(By theorem 4)

$$= \begin{vmatrix} a_1 & b_1 & c_1 \\ a_2 & b_2 & c_2 \\ a_3 & b_3 & c_3 \end{vmatrix} + m(0) + n(0)$$

(By theorem 3)

$$= \begin{vmatrix} a_1 & b_1 & c_1 \\ a_2 & b_2 & c_2 \\ a_3 & b_3 & c_3 \end{vmatrix}$$

RECAPITULATIONS

- The value of a determinant does not change when rows and columns are interchanged.
- If any two rows [or columns] of a determinant are interchanged, the sign of the determinant is changed.
- If two rows or two columns of the determinant are identical, then the value of the determinant vanishes, *i.e.*, $|A| = \begin{vmatrix} a_1 & b_1 & c_1 \\ a_2 & b_2 & c_2 \\ a_3 & b_3 & c_3 \end{vmatrix} = 0.$
- If all the elements of any row, or any column, of a determinant are multiplied by the same number then the determinant is multiplied by that number.
- If in the determinant, the elements of row (or column) are added in and m times the corresponding elements of the another rows (or column), the value of the determinant does not change.

Solved Examples

1. *Evaluate the following determinant :*

$$\begin{vmatrix} 3 & -2 \\ 4 & 5 \end{vmatrix}.$$

SOLUTION. We have $|A| = \begin{vmatrix} 3 & -2 \\ 4 & 5 \end{vmatrix}$

$= 3 \times 5 - 4 \times (-2)$
$= 15 + 8 = 23.$

2. *Find the value of the determinant of the matrix*

$$A = \begin{bmatrix} 1 & 2 & 3 \\ 2 & 3 & 1 \\ 3 & 1 & 2 \end{bmatrix}$$

SOLUTION. We have $|A| = \begin{vmatrix} 1 & 2 & 3 \\ 2 & 3 & 1 \\ 3 & 1 & 2 \end{vmatrix}$

On expanding the determinant along the first row, we get

$$= 1\begin{vmatrix} 3 & 1 \\ 1 & 2 \end{vmatrix} - 2\begin{vmatrix} 2 & 1 \\ 3 & 2 \end{vmatrix} + 3\begin{vmatrix} 2 & 3 \\ 3 & 1 \end{vmatrix}$$

$= 1\cdot(6 - 1) - 2\cdot(4 - 3) + 3\cdot(2 - 9)$
$= -18.$

3. *Show that:*

$$\begin{vmatrix} 1 & x & y \\ 0 & \cos x & \sin y \\ 0 & \sin x & \cos y \end{vmatrix} = \cos(x + y).$$

SOLUTION. We have $\begin{vmatrix} 1 & x & y \\ 0 & \cos x & \sin y \\ 0 & \sin x & \cos y \end{vmatrix}$

On expanding the determinant along first column, we get

$$= 1\begin{vmatrix} \cos x & \sin y \\ \sin x & \cos y \end{vmatrix} - 0\begin{vmatrix} x & y \\ \sin x & \sin y \end{vmatrix} + 0\begin{vmatrix} x & y \\ \cos x & \cos y \end{vmatrix}$$

$= \cos x \cos y - \sin x \sin y = \cos(x + y)$

4. *Show that* $\begin{vmatrix} 1 & 1 & 1 \\ 1 & 1+x & 1 \\ 1 & 1 & 1+y \end{vmatrix} = xy$

SOLUTION. We have L.H.S. $= \begin{vmatrix} 1 & 1 & 1 \\ 1 & 1+x & 1 \\ 1 & 1 & 1+y \end{vmatrix}$

Applying $C_2 - C_1$ and $C_3 - C_1$ in the given determinant, we get

$$\text{L.H.S.} = \begin{vmatrix} 1 & 0 & 0 \\ 1 & x & 0 \\ 1 & 0 & y \end{vmatrix}$$

On expanding the determinant along the first row, we get

$$= 1\begin{vmatrix} x & 0 \\ 0 & y \end{vmatrix} - 0\begin{vmatrix} 1 & 0 \\ 1 & y \end{vmatrix} - 0\begin{vmatrix} 1 & x \\ 1 & 0 \end{vmatrix}$$

$= xy =$ R.H.S.

5. *Without expanding, show that*

$$\begin{vmatrix} b-c & c-a & a-b \\ c-a & a-b & b-c \\ a-b & b-c & c-a \end{vmatrix} = 0.$$

SOLUTION. We have

$$\begin{vmatrix} b-c & c-a & a-b \\ c-a & a-b & b-c \\ a-b & b-c & c-a \end{vmatrix} = \begin{vmatrix} 0 & c-a & a-b \\ 0 & a-b & b-c \\ 0 & b-c & c-a \end{vmatrix}$$

(Operating $C_1 \to C_1 + C_2 + C_3$, we get) $= 0$.

6. *Without expanding, show that*

$$\begin{vmatrix} b^2c^2 & bc & b+c \\ c^2a^2 & ca & c+a \\ a^2b^2 & ab & a+c \end{vmatrix} = 0.$$

SOLUTION. Consider

$$\begin{vmatrix} b^2c^2 & bc & b+c \\ c^2a^2 & ca & c+a \\ a^2b^2 & ab & a+c \end{vmatrix}$$

$$= \frac{abc}{abc}\begin{vmatrix} b^2c^2 & bc & b+c \\ c^2a^2 & ca & c+a \\ a^2b^2 & ab & a+b \end{vmatrix}$$

(Multiplying R_1 by a, R_2 by b and R_3 by c)

$$= \frac{1}{abc}\begin{vmatrix} ab^2c^2 & abc & ab+ca \\ bc^2a^2 & abc & bc+ab \\ ca^2b^2 & abc & ca+bc \end{vmatrix}$$

(Take abc out from C_1 and C_2)

$$= \frac{abc.abc}{abc}\begin{vmatrix} bc & 1 & ab+ca \\ ca & 1 & bc+ab \\ ca & 1 & ca+bc \end{vmatrix}$$

$$= abc\begin{vmatrix} bc & 1 & ab+bc+ca \\ ca & 1 & ca+bc+ab \\ cb & 1 & ab+ca+bc \end{vmatrix}$$

(Operate $C_3 \to C_3 + C_1$)

$$= abc(ab+bc+ca)\begin{vmatrix} bc & 1 & 1 \\ ca & 1 & 1 \\ cb & 1 & 1 \end{vmatrix}$$

$= abc(ab + bc + ca) \times 0 = 0$

7. *If a, b, c are in A.P., prove that*

$$\begin{vmatrix} x+1 & x+2 & x+a \\ x+2 & x+3 & x+b \\ x+3 & x+4 & x+c \end{vmatrix} = 0.$$

SOLUTION. Given a, b, c are in A.P. therefore

$$a + c = 2b$$

$\Rightarrow \quad a + c - 2b = 0$

Operating $R_1 \to R_1 + R_3 - 2R_2$, we get

$$\begin{vmatrix} x+1 & x+2 & x+a \\ x+2 & x+3 & x+b \\ x+3 & x+4 & x+c \end{vmatrix} = \begin{vmatrix} 0 & 0 & a+c-2b \\ x+2 & x+3 & x+b \\ x+3 & x+4 & x+c \end{vmatrix}$$

$$= \begin{vmatrix} 0 & 0 & 0 \\ x+2 & x+3 & x+b \\ x+3 & x+4 & x+c \end{vmatrix} = 0$$

8. *Prove that*
$$\begin{vmatrix} a & b & c \\ a^2 & b^2 & c^2 \\ a^3 & b^3 & c^3 \end{vmatrix} = abc\begin{vmatrix} 1 & 1 & 1 \\ a & b & c \\ a^2 & b^2 & c^2 \end{vmatrix}$$
$= abc(a-b)(b-c)(c-a)$.

SOLUTION. We have
$$|A| = \begin{vmatrix} a & b & c \\ a^2 & b^2 & c^2 \\ a^3 & b^3 & c^3 \end{vmatrix} = abc\begin{vmatrix} 1 & 1 & 1 \\ a & b & c \\ a^2 & b^2 & c^2 \end{vmatrix}$$
Now again
$$|A| = abc\begin{vmatrix} 1 & 1 & 1 \\ a & b & c \\ a^2 & b^2 & c^2 \end{vmatrix}$$
Applying $C_2 - C_1$ and $C_3 - C_1$, we get
$$= abc\begin{vmatrix} 1 & 0 & 0 \\ a & b-a & c-a \\ a^2 & b^2-a^2 & c^2-a^2 \end{vmatrix}$$
On expanding along the first row, we get
$$= abc\begin{vmatrix} b-a & c-a \\ b^2-a^2 & c^2-a^2 \end{vmatrix}$$
$$= abc[(b-a)(c^2-a^2)-(b^2-a^2)(c-a)]$$
$$= abc[(b-a)(c-a)\{(c+a)-(b+a)\}]$$
$$= abc(b-a)(c-a)(c+a-b-a) =$$
$$abc(a-b)(b-c)(c-a)$$

9. *Prove that*
$$\begin{vmatrix} a+b+2c & a & b \\ c & b+c+2a & b \\ c & a & c+a+2b \end{vmatrix}.$$
$$= 2(a+b+c)^3$$

SOLUTION. Let
$$|A| = \begin{vmatrix} a+b+2c & a & b \\ c & b+c+2a & b \\ c & a & c+a+2b \end{vmatrix}$$
Adding C_2 and C_3 in C_1, we get
$$\begin{vmatrix} 2(a+b+c) & a & b \\ 2(a+b+c) & b+c+2a & b \\ 2(a+b+c) & a & c+a+2b \end{vmatrix} =$$
$$= 2(a+b+c)\begin{vmatrix} 1 & a & b \\ 1 & b+c+2a & b \\ 1 & a & c+a+2b \end{vmatrix}$$
Applying $(R_2 - R_1)$ and $(R_3 - R_1)$, we get
$$= 2(a+b+c)\begin{vmatrix} 1 & a & b \\ 0 & b+c+a & 0 \\ 0 & 0 & c+a+b \end{vmatrix}$$
On expanding the determinant along the first column, we get
$$= 2(a+b+c)\begin{vmatrix} b+c+a & 0 \\ 0 & a+b+c \end{vmatrix}$$
$$= 2(a+b+c)(a+b+c)^2$$
$$= 2(a+b+c)^3$$

10. *Prove that*
$$\begin{vmatrix} 1+a & 1 & 1 \\ 1 & 1+b & 1 \\ 1 & 1 & 1+c \end{vmatrix} = abc\left(1+\frac{1}{a}+\frac{1}{b}+\frac{1}{c}\right)$$
[UPTU(B.PHARMA)–2000, 06]

SOLUTION. Operating $C_1 \to C_1 - C_3$ and $C_2 \to C_2 - C_3$, we get
$$\begin{vmatrix} 1+a & 1 & 1 \\ 1 & 1+b & 1 \\ 1 & 1 & 1+c \end{vmatrix} = \begin{vmatrix} a & 0 & 1 \\ 0 & b & 1 \\ -c & -c & 1+c \end{vmatrix}$$
$$= a[b\cdot(1+c)-(-c)\cdot 1]+1[0\cdot(-c)-(-c)b]$$
$$= a(b+bc+c)+bc$$
$$= abc+bc+ca+ab$$
$$= abc\left(1+\frac{1}{a}+\frac{1}{b}+\frac{1}{c}\right).$$

11. *Prove that*
$$\begin{vmatrix} a-b-c & 2a & 2a \\ 2b & b-c-a & 2b \\ 2c & 2c & c-a-b \end{vmatrix} = (a+b+c)^3.$$
[DELHI(BCA)–2010]

SOLUTION. Operating $R_1 \to R_1 + R_2 + R_3$, we get
$$= \begin{vmatrix} a+b+c & a+b+c & a+b+c \\ 2b & b-c-a & 2b \\ 2c & 2c & c-a-b \end{vmatrix}$$
$$= (a+b+c)\begin{vmatrix} 1 & 1 & 1 \\ 2b & b-c-a & 2b \\ 2c & 2c & c-a-b \end{vmatrix}$$
(Operate $C_2 \to C_2 - C_1$ and $C_3 \to C_3 - C_1$)
$$= (a+b+c)\begin{vmatrix} 1 & 0 & 0 \\ 2b & -b-c-a & 0 \\ 2c & 0 & a-b-c \end{vmatrix}$$
(expand by R_1)
$$= (a+b+c)1(-a-b-c)(-a-b-c)$$
$$= (a+b+c)^3.$$

12. *Without expanding the determinant, show that*

$$\begin{vmatrix} 0 & b & -c \\ -b & 0 & a \\ c & -a & 0 \end{vmatrix} = 0$$

[UPTU(B.PHARMA)–2001]

SOLUTION. Let $\Delta = \begin{vmatrix} 0 & b & -c \\ -b & 0 & a \\ c & -a & 0 \end{vmatrix}$

By changing columns into rows :

$$\Delta = \begin{vmatrix} 0 & -b & c \\ b & 0 & -a \\ -c & a & 0 \end{vmatrix} = (-1)^3 \begin{vmatrix} 0 & b & -c \\ -b & 0 & a \\ c & -a & 0 \end{vmatrix}$$

(taking (–1) Common from each column)

$$= (-1)^3\Delta = -\Delta.$$

$$2\Delta = 0$$

or $\Delta = 0.$

13. *Without expanding the determinant, show that* $\begin{vmatrix} 1 & a & bc \\ 1 & b & ca \\ 1 & c & ab \end{vmatrix} = \begin{vmatrix} 1 & a & a^2 \\ 1 & b & b^2 \\ 1 & c & c^2 \end{vmatrix}$ *and evaluate it.* [UPTU(B.PHARMA)–2001, 08]

SOLUTION. Let $\Delta = \begin{vmatrix} 1 & a & bc \\ 1 & b & ca \\ 1 & c & ab \end{vmatrix}$

Multiplying the 1st, 2nd and 3rd rows by a, b, c respectively. we get

$$\Delta = \frac{1}{abc}\begin{vmatrix} a & a^2 & abc \\ b & b^2 & bca \\ c & c^2 & cab \end{vmatrix}$$

$$= \frac{abc}{abc}\begin{vmatrix} a & a^2 & 1 \\ b & b^2 & 1 \\ c & c^2 & 1 \end{vmatrix}$$

Taking abc common from 3rd column

$$= \begin{vmatrix} a & 1 & a^2 \\ b & 1 & b^2 \\ c & 1 & c^2 \end{vmatrix} \quad \text{applying } C_2 \leftrightarrow C_3$$

$$= \begin{vmatrix} 1 & a & a^2 \\ 1 & b & b^2 \\ 1 & c & c^2 \end{vmatrix} \quad \text{applying } C_1 \leftrightarrow C_2$$

Applying $R_2 \to R_2 - R_1$ and $R_3 \to R_3 - R_1$, we get

$$\Delta = \begin{vmatrix} 1 & a & a^2 \\ 0 & b-a & b^2-a^2 \\ 0 & c-a & c^2-a^2 \end{vmatrix}$$

$$= \begin{vmatrix} b-a & b^2-a^2 \\ c-a & c^2-a^2 \end{vmatrix}$$

On expanding the determinant along C_1

$$= (b-a)(c-a)\begin{vmatrix} 1 & b+a \\ 1 & c+a \end{vmatrix}$$

taking $(b - a)$ common from R_1 and $(c - a)$ common from R_2

$$= (b-a)(c-a)[c + a - (b + a)]$$
$$= (b-a)(c-a)(c-b)$$
$$= (a-b)(b-c)(c-a)$$

14. *Without expanding the determinant show that* $(a + b + c)$ *is a factor of following determinant.*

$$\Delta = \begin{vmatrix} a & b & c \\ b & c & a \\ c & a & b \end{vmatrix}$$ [UPTU(B.PHARMA)–2003]

SOLUTION. Applying $C_1 \to C_1 + C_2 + C_3$, we get

$$\Delta = \begin{vmatrix} a+b+c & b & c \\ a+b+c & c & a \\ a+b+c & a & b \end{vmatrix}$$

$$= (a+b+c)\begin{vmatrix} 1 & b & c \\ 1 & c & a \\ 1 & a & b \end{vmatrix}$$

$$= (a+b+c)\begin{vmatrix} 1 & b & c \\ 0 & c-b & a-c \\ 0 & a-b & b-c \end{vmatrix}$$

Applying $R_2 \to R_2 - R_1$, $R_3 \to R_3 - R_1$

$$= (a+b+c)\begin{vmatrix} c-b & a-c \\ a-b & b-c \end{vmatrix}$$

$$= (a+b+c)\{-(b-c)^2-(a-b)(a-c)\}$$
$$= (a+b+c)(-a^2-b^2-c^2+ab+bc+ca)$$

Thus $(a + b + c)$ is a factor of Δ.

15. *Show that*

$$\begin{vmatrix} a & b & c \\ a-b & b-c & c-a \\ b+c & c+a & a+b \end{vmatrix} = a^3+b^3+c^3-3abc$$

SOLUTION. Operating $R_2 \to R_2 - R_1$ and $R_3 \to R_3 + R_1$, we get

$$= \begin{vmatrix} a & b & c \\ -b & -c & -a \\ a+b+c & a+b+c & a+b+c \end{vmatrix}$$

[Take $(a + b + c)$ out from R_3 and (-1) from R_2]

$$= -(a+b+c).\begin{vmatrix} a & b & c \\ b & c & a \\ 1 & 1 & 1 \end{vmatrix}$$

(Expand by R_3)

$$= -(a + b + c)\cdot[1\cdot(ab - c^2) - 1(a^2 - bc) + 1\cdot(ca - b^2)]$$

$$= -(a + b + c)\cdot(ab + bc + ca - a^2 - b^2 - c^2)$$

$$= (a + b + c)\cdot(a^2 + b^2 + c^2 - ab - bc - ca)$$

$$= a^3 + b^3 + c^3 - 3abc.$$

16. *Find the value of x if*

$$\begin{vmatrix} 3+x & 5 & 2 \\ 1 & 7+x & 6 \\ 2 & 5 & 3+x \end{vmatrix} = 0.$$

(NAGPUR–2014)

SOLUTION. We have $\begin{vmatrix} 3+x & 5 & 2 \\ 1 & 7+x & 6 \\ 2 & 5 & 3+x \end{vmatrix} = 0$

Applying $(R_1 - R_3)$, we get

$$\begin{vmatrix} 1+x & 0 & -1-x \\ 1 & 7+x & 6 \\ 2 & 5 & 3+x \end{vmatrix} = 0$$

Applying $C_3 \to C_3 + C_1$, we get

$$\begin{vmatrix} 1+x & 0 & 0 \\ 1 & 7+x & 7 \\ 2 & 5 & 5+x \end{vmatrix} = 0$$

On expanding the determinant along the first row, we get

$$(1+x)\begin{vmatrix} 7+x & 7 \\ 5 & 5+x \end{vmatrix} = 0$$

$$(1 + x)[(7 + x)(5 + x) - 35] = 0$$

or $$(1 + x)(x^2 + 12x) = 0$$

$$x(1 + x)(x + 12) = 0$$

$$x = 0, -1, -12.$$

17. *Evaluate:* $|A| = \begin{vmatrix} 3 & 2 & 1 & 4 \\ 15 & 29 & 2 & 14 \\ 16 & 19 & 3 & 17 \\ 23 & 39 & 8 & 38 \end{vmatrix}$

SOLUTION. Applying $C_1 \to C_1 - 3C_2$, $C_2 \to C_2 - 3C_3$, $C_4 \to C_4 - 4C_3$, we get

$$|A| = \begin{vmatrix} 0 & 0 & 1 & 0 \\ 9 & 25 & 2 & 6 \\ 7 & 13 & 3 & 5 \\ 9 & 23 & 8 & 6 \end{vmatrix}$$

On expanding the determinant along first row, we get

$$= 1\begin{vmatrix} 9 & 25 & 6 \\ 7 & 13 & 5 \\ 9 & 23 & 6 \end{vmatrix}$$

Applying $R_1 \to R_1 - R_3$, we get

$$= 1\begin{vmatrix} 0 & 2 & 0 \\ 7 & 13 & 5 \\ 9 & 23 & 6 \end{vmatrix}$$

On expanding the determinant along the first row, we get

$$= -2\begin{vmatrix} 7 & 5 \\ 9 & 6 \end{vmatrix} = -2(42 - 45) = 6$$

18. *Using properties of determinants, solve the following determinant for x.*

$$\begin{vmatrix} a+x & a-x & a-x \\ a-x & a+x & a-x \\ a-x & a-x & a+x \end{vmatrix}$$

SOLUTION. Given $\begin{vmatrix} a+x & a-x & a-x \\ a-x & a+x & a-x \\ a-x & a-x & a+x \end{vmatrix} = 0$

(Operate $C_1 \to C_1 + C_2 + C_3$)

$$\Rightarrow \begin{vmatrix} 3a-x & a-x & a-x \\ 3a-x & a+x & a-x \\ 3a-x & a-x & a+x \end{vmatrix} = 0$$

$$\Rightarrow (3a-x)\begin{vmatrix} 1 & a-x & a-x \\ 1 & a+x & a-x \\ 1 & a-x & a+x \end{vmatrix} = 0$$

(Operate $R_2 \to R_2 - R_1$, $R_3 \to R_3 - R_1$)

$$\Rightarrow (3a-x)\begin{vmatrix} 1 & a-x & a-x \\ 0 & 2x & 0 \\ 0 & 0 & 2x \end{vmatrix} = 0$$

(Expand by C_1)

$$\Rightarrow (3a-x)1.\begin{vmatrix} 2x & 0 \\ 0 & 2x \end{vmatrix} = 0$$

$$\Rightarrow (3a - x)\cdot(4x^2 - 0) = 0$$

$$\Rightarrow 4x^2(3a - x) = 0$$

$$\Rightarrow x^2 = 0 \text{ or } 3a - x = 0$$

$$\Rightarrow x = 0, 0, 3a$$

Hence, the values of x are 0, 0, $3a$.

19. *Using properties of determinant, prove that*

$$\begin{vmatrix} 1 & 1 & 1 \\ \alpha & \beta & \gamma \\ \beta\gamma & \gamma\alpha & \alpha\beta \end{vmatrix} = (\alpha-\beta)(\beta-\gamma)(\gamma-\alpha)$$

SOLUTION. Operate $C_2 \to C_2 - C_1$ and $C_3 \to C_3 - C_1$, we get

$$\begin{vmatrix} 1 & 1 & 1 \\ \alpha & \beta & \gamma \\ \beta\gamma & \gamma\alpha & \alpha\beta \end{vmatrix} = \begin{vmatrix} 1 & 0 & 0 \\ \alpha & \beta-\alpha & \gamma-\alpha \\ \beta\gamma & \gamma(\alpha-\beta) & \beta(\alpha-\gamma) \end{vmatrix}$$

[Take $(\alpha - \beta)$ out from C_2 and $(\gamma - \alpha)$ out from C_3]

$$= (\alpha-\beta)(\gamma-\alpha)\begin{vmatrix} 1 & 0 & 0 \\ \alpha & -1 & 1 \\ \beta\gamma & \gamma & -\beta \end{vmatrix}$$

(Expand by C_1)

$$= (\alpha-\beta)(\gamma-\alpha)\cdot 1\cdot\begin{vmatrix} -1 & 1 \\ \gamma & -\beta \end{vmatrix}$$

$$= (\alpha-\beta)(\gamma-\alpha)(\beta-\gamma)$$

$$= (\alpha-\beta)(\beta-\gamma)(\gamma-\alpha)$$

20. *Prove that*

$$\begin{vmatrix} a^2+1 & ab & ac \\ ab & b^2+1 & bc \\ ac & bc & c^2+1 \end{vmatrix} = 1+a^2+b^2+c^2$$

SOLUTION. We have

$$|A| = \begin{vmatrix} a^2+1 & ab & ac \\ ab & b^2+1 & bc \\ ac & bc & c^2+1 \end{vmatrix}$$

Now multiply the column 1st, 2nd and 3rd by a, b and c respectively, we get

$$|A| = \frac{1}{abc}\begin{vmatrix} a(a^2+1) & ab^2 & ac^2 \\ a^2b & b(b^2+1) & bc^2 \\ a^2c & b^2c & c(c^2+1) \end{vmatrix}$$

To take a, b, c common from 1st, 2nd and 3rd rows respectively, we get

$$= \frac{abc}{abc}\begin{vmatrix} a^2+1 & b^2 & c^2 \\ a^2 & b^2+1 & c^2 \\ a^2 & b^2 & c^2+1 \end{vmatrix}$$

Now apply $C_1 \to C_1 + C_2 + C_3$, we get

$$= \begin{vmatrix} a^2+b^2+c^2+1 & b^2 & c^2 \\ a^2+b^2+c^2+1 & b^2+1 & c^2 \\ a^2+b^2+c^2+1 & b^2 & c^2+1 \end{vmatrix}$$

$$= (a^2+b^2+c^2+1)\begin{vmatrix} 1 & b^2 & c^2 \\ 1 & b^2+1 & c^2 \\ 1 & b^2 & c^2+1 \end{vmatrix}$$

Now applying $R_2 \to R_2 - R_1$ and $R_3 \to R_3 - R_1$, we get

$$= (a^2+b^2+c^2+1)\begin{vmatrix} 1 & 0 \\ 0 & 1 \end{vmatrix}$$

$$= a^2+b^2+c^2+1$$

21. *If x, y, z are all different and*

$$\begin{vmatrix} x & x^2 & 1+x^3 \\ y & y^2 & 1+y^3 \\ z & z^2 & 1+z^3 \end{vmatrix} = 0.$$

Show that $xyz = -1$.

SOLUTION. Given $\begin{vmatrix} x & x^2 & 1+x^3 \\ y & y^2 & 1+y^3 \\ z & z^2 & 1+z^3 \end{vmatrix} = 0.$

$$\Rightarrow \begin{vmatrix} x & x^2 & 1 \\ y & y^2 & 1 \\ z & z^2 & 1 \end{vmatrix} + \begin{vmatrix} x & x^2 & x^3 \\ y & y^2 & y^3 \\ z & z^2 & z^3 \end{vmatrix} = 0$$

[Take x, y, z out from R_1, R_2 and R_3 respectively from the second determinant]

$$\Rightarrow \begin{vmatrix} 1 & x & x^2 \\ 1 & y & y^2 \\ 1 & z & z^2 \end{vmatrix} + xyz\begin{vmatrix} 1 & x & x^2 \\ 1 & y & y^2 \\ 1 & z & z^2 \end{vmatrix} = 0$$

$$\Rightarrow \begin{vmatrix} 1 & x & x^2 \\ 1 & y & y^2 \\ 1 & z & z^2 \end{vmatrix}(1+xyz) = 0$$

$$\Rightarrow (x-y)\cdot(y-z)\cdot(z-x)\cdot(1+xyz) = 0$$

$$\Rightarrow (1+xyz) = 0$$

(Because x, y, z are distinct, so $x-y \neq 0, y-z \neq 0, z-x \neq 0$).

$$\Rightarrow xyz = -1.$$

22. *Without expanding show that the value of the determinant given below is zero*

$$\begin{vmatrix} \sin\alpha & \cos\alpha & \sin(\alpha+\delta) \\ \sin\beta & \cos\beta & \sin(\beta+\delta) \\ \sin\gamma & \cos\gamma & \sin(\gamma+\delta) \end{vmatrix}$$

SOLUTION. Let $\Delta = \begin{vmatrix} \sin\alpha & \cos\alpha & \sin(\alpha+\delta) \\ \sin\beta & \cos\beta & \sin(\beta+\delta) \\ \sin\gamma & \cos\gamma & \sin(\gamma+\delta) \end{vmatrix}$

Using $\sin(A + B) = \sin A \cos B + \cos A \sin B$, we get

$$\Delta = \begin{vmatrix} \sin\alpha & \cos\alpha & \sin\alpha\cos\delta+\cos\alpha\sin\delta \\ \sin\beta & \cos\beta & \sin\beta\cos\delta+\cos\beta\sin\delta \\ \sin\gamma & \cos\gamma & \sin\gamma\cos\delta+\cos\gamma\sin\delta \end{vmatrix}$$

$$= \begin{vmatrix} \sin\alpha & \cos\alpha & 0 \\ \sin\beta & \cos\beta & 0 \\ \sin\gamma & \cos\gamma & 0 \end{vmatrix}$$

Using $C_3 \to C_3 - (\cos\delta)C_1 - (\sin\delta)C_2$

$= 0$

23. *Show that*

$$\begin{vmatrix} (b+c)^2 & a^2 & bc \\ (c+a)^2 & b^2 & ca \\ (a+b)^2 & c^2 & ab \end{vmatrix} = (a^2+b^2+c^2)(a+b+c)(b-c)(c-a)(a-b).$$

SOLUTION. Let $\Delta = \begin{vmatrix} (b+c)^2 & a^2 & bc \\ (c+a)^2 & b^2 & ca \\ (a+b)^2 & c^2 & ab \end{vmatrix}$

Applying $C_1 \to C_1 - 2C_3$, we get

$$= \begin{vmatrix} b^2+c^2+a^2 & a^2 & bc \\ c^2+a^2+b^2 & b^2 & ca \\ a^2+b^2+c^2 & c^2 & ab \end{vmatrix}$$

Operating $C_1 \to C_1 + C_2$, we get

$$= (a^2+b^2+c^2)\begin{vmatrix} 1 & a^2 & bc \\ 1 & b^2 & ca \\ 1 & c^2 & ab \end{vmatrix}$$

Operating $R_2 \to R_2 - R_1$ and $R_3 \to R_3 - R_2$

$$= (a^2+b^2+c^2)\begin{vmatrix} 1 & a^2 & bc \\ 0 & b^2-a^2 & (ca-bc) \\ 0 & c^2-a^2 & (ab-bc) \end{vmatrix}$$

$$= (a^2+b^2+c^2)(b-c)(c-a)\begin{vmatrix} 1 & a^2 & bc \\ 0 & b+a & -c \\ 0 & c+a & -b \end{vmatrix}$$

$R_3 \to R_3 - R_2$, we get

$$= (a^2+b^2+c^2)(b-a)(c-a)\begin{vmatrix} 1 & a^2 & bc \\ 0 & b+a & -c \\ 0 & c-a & c-b \end{vmatrix}$$

$$= (a^2+b^2+c^2)(b-a)(c-a)(c-b)\begin{vmatrix} 1 & a^2 & bc \\ 0 & b+a & -c \\ 0 & 1 & 1 \end{vmatrix}$$

Expanding along first column, we get

$$\Delta = (a^2+b^2+c^2)(b-a)(c-a)(c-b)(a+b+c)$$

24. *Show that*

$$\begin{vmatrix} a+b & b+c & c+a \\ b+c & c+a & a+b \\ c+a & a+b & b+c \end{vmatrix} = 2\begin{vmatrix} a & b & c \\ b & c & a \\ c & a & b \end{vmatrix}.$$

SOLUTION. Let $\Delta = \begin{vmatrix} a+b & b+c & c+a \\ b+c & c+a & a+b \\ c+a & a+b & b+c \end{vmatrix}$

Applying $C_1 \to C_1 + C_2 + C_3$, we get

$$= \begin{vmatrix} 2(a+b+c) & b+c & c+a \\ 2(a+b+c) & c+a & a+b \\ 2(a+b+c) & a+b & b+c \end{vmatrix}$$

$$= 2\begin{vmatrix} a+b+c & -a & -b \\ a+b+c & -b & -c \\ a+b+c & -c & -a \end{vmatrix}$$

Applying $C_2 \to C_2 - C_1,\ C_3 \to C_3 - C_1$

We get

$$= 2(-1)(-1)\begin{vmatrix} a+b+c & a & b \\ a+b+c & b & c \\ a+b+c & c & a \end{vmatrix}$$

Applying $C_1 \to C_1 - C_2 - C_3$, we get

$$= 2\begin{vmatrix} c & a & b \\ a & b & c \\ b & c & a \end{vmatrix}$$

Applying $C_1 \leftrightarrow C_2$, we get

$$= 2\begin{vmatrix} a & c & b \\ b & a & c \\ c & b & a \end{vmatrix} = 2\begin{vmatrix} a & b & c \\ b & c & a \\ c & a & b \end{vmatrix}$$

(On using $C_2 \leftrightarrow C_3$)

Exercise-2.1

Evaluate the following determinants (1 *to* 7):

1. $\begin{vmatrix} \frac{1}{2} & 8 \\ 4 & 2 \end{vmatrix}$ **2.** $\begin{vmatrix} -2 & 3 \\ 4 & -9 \end{vmatrix}$

3. $\begin{vmatrix} \cos\theta & -\sin\theta \\ \sin\theta & \cos\theta \end{vmatrix}$ **4.** $\begin{vmatrix} x^2-x+1 & x-1 \\ x+1 & x-1 \end{vmatrix}$

5. $\begin{vmatrix} 1 & 0 & 6 \\ 3 & 4 & 15 \\ 5 & 6 & 21 \end{vmatrix}$ **6.** $\begin{vmatrix} 23 & 12 & 11 \\ 36 & 10 & 26 \\ 63 & 26 & 37 \end{vmatrix}$

7. $\begin{vmatrix} 3 & 1 & -4 \\ 3 & 2 & 5 \\ 1 & 1 & 3 \end{vmatrix}$

Write the minor and co-factors of each element of the following determinants and also evaluate the determinants in each case (8 *to* 11):

8. $\begin{vmatrix} 5 & -10 \\ 0 & 3 \end{vmatrix}$ **9.** $\begin{vmatrix} 1 & 3 & -2 \\ 4 & -5 & 6 \\ 3 & 5 & 2 \end{vmatrix}$

10. $\begin{vmatrix} 1 & 0 & 0 \\ 0 & 1 & 0 \\ 0 & 0 & 1 \end{vmatrix}$ **11.** $\begin{vmatrix} 1 & 0 & 4 \\ 3 & 5 & -1 \\ 0 & 1 & 2 \end{vmatrix}$

12. Evaluate $\begin{vmatrix} x+1 & x+2 & x+4 \\ x+5 & x+6 & x+8 \\ x+7 & x+10 & x+14 \end{vmatrix}$

13. Evaluate $\begin{vmatrix} 1 & a & bc \\ 1 & b & ca \\ 1 & c & ab \end{vmatrix}$

14. Evaluate $\begin{vmatrix} x+\lambda & x & x \\ x & x+\lambda & x \\ x & x & x+\lambda \end{vmatrix}$

15. Evaluate $\begin{vmatrix} b+c & a & a \\ b & c+a & b \\ c & c & a+b \end{vmatrix}$

16. Prove that $\begin{vmatrix} 1 & x & x^2 \\ 1 & y & y^2 \\ 1 & z & z^2 \end{vmatrix} = (x-y)(y-z)(z-x).$

17. Prove that $\begin{vmatrix} -a^2 & ab & ac \\ ba & -b^2 & bc \\ ac & bc & -c^2 \end{vmatrix} = 4\,a^2b^2c^2.$

18. Prove that
$$\begin{vmatrix} x & x^2 & yz \\ y & y^2 & zx \\ z & z^2 & xy \end{vmatrix} = (x-y)(y-z)(z-x)(xy+yz+zx)$$

19. Using properties of determinants, prove that
$$\begin{vmatrix} y+z & x & y \\ z+x & z & x \\ x+y & y & z \end{vmatrix} = (x+y+z)(x-z)^2.$$

20. Using properties of determinants, prove that
$$\begin{vmatrix} a-b-c & 2a & 2a \\ 2b & b-c-a & 2b \\ 2c & 2c & c-a-b \end{vmatrix} = (a+b+c)^3$$

21. Solve the following determinants
$$\begin{vmatrix} x-2 & 2x-3 & 3x-4 \\ x-4 & 2x-9 & 3x-16 \\ x-8 & 2x-27 & 3x-64 \end{vmatrix} = 0$$

[UPTU(B.PHARMA)–2007]

22. Prove that using properties of determinants
$$\begin{vmatrix} 1+a^2-b^2 & 2ab & -2b \\ 2ab & 1-a^2+b^2 & 2a \\ 2b & -2a & 1-a^2-b^2 \end{vmatrix} = (1+a^2+b^2)^3$$

23. Prove that $\begin{vmatrix} x & x^2 & 1+px^3 \\ y & y^2 & 1+py^3 \\ z & z^2 & 1+pz^3 \end{vmatrix}$
$$= (1+pxyz)(x-y)(y-z)(z-x)$$

24. Prove that using properties of determinants
$$\begin{vmatrix} 3a & -a+b & -a+c \\ -b+a & 3b & -b+c \\ -c+a & -c+b & 3c \end{vmatrix} = 3(a+b+c)(ab+bc+ca)$$

25. Prove that
$$\begin{vmatrix} \sin\alpha & \cos\alpha & \cos(\alpha+\delta) \\ \sin\beta & \cos\beta & \cos(\beta+\delta) \\ \sin\gamma & \cos\gamma & \cos(\gamma+\delta) \end{vmatrix} = 0$$

Hint to Selected Problems

1. (i) $\begin{vmatrix} 1/2 & 8 \\ 4 & 2 \end{vmatrix} = \frac{1}{2}\times 2 - 8\times 4 = 1 - 32 = -31.$

3. We have $\begin{vmatrix} \cos\theta & -\sin\theta \\ \sin\theta & \cos\theta \end{vmatrix} = \cos^2\theta + \sin^2\theta = 1$

4. On expanding, we get

$$\Rightarrow (x^2 - x + 1)(x - 1) - (x - 1)(x + 1)$$
$$= (x - 1)(x^2 - x + 1 - x - 1)$$
$$= (x - 1)(x^2 - 2x)$$
$$= x^3 - 2x^2 - x^2 + 2x$$
$$|A| = x^3 - 3x^2 + 2x$$

5. $$|A| = \begin{vmatrix} 1 & 0 & 6 \\ 3 & 4 & 15 \\ 5 & 6 & 21 \end{vmatrix} = \begin{vmatrix} 1 & 0 & 3\cdot 2 \\ 3 & 4 & 3\cdot 5 \\ 5 & 6 & 3\cdot 7 \end{vmatrix}$$

$$= 3\begin{vmatrix} 1 & 0 & 2 \\ 3 & 4 & 5 \\ 5 & 6 & 7 \end{vmatrix}$$

$$= 3\begin{vmatrix} 1 & 0 & 2 \\ 3 & 2\cdot 2 & 5 \\ 5 & 2\cdot 3 & 7 \end{vmatrix} = 6\begin{vmatrix} 1 & 0 & 2 \\ 3 & 2 & 5 \\ 5 & 3 & 7 \end{vmatrix}$$

$$= 6\,[(14 - 15) + 2(9 - 10)] = -18.$$

8. $$\begin{vmatrix} 5 & -10 \\ 0 & 3 \end{vmatrix}$$

Minor of the element a_{11} is $M_{11} = |3| = 3$.

Minor of the element a_{12} is $M_{12} = 0$.

Minor of the element a_{21} is $M_{21} = -10$.

Minor of the element a_{22} is $M_{22} = 5$.

Hence cofactors are as

$$A_{11} = (-1)^{1+1}M_{11} = 3$$
$$A_{12} = (-1)^{1+2}M_{12} = 0$$
$$A_{21} = (-1)^{2+1}M_{21} = 10$$
$$A_{22} = (-1)^{2+2}M_{22} = 5$$

$$|A| = \begin{vmatrix} 5 & -10 \\ 0 & 3 \end{vmatrix} = 15 - 0 = 15$$

9. Minor of $a_{11} = \begin{vmatrix} -5 & 6 \\ 5 & 2 \end{vmatrix} = -40$

Minor of $a_{12} = \begin{vmatrix} 4 & 6 \\ 3 & 2 \end{vmatrix} = -10$

Minor of $a_{13} = \begin{vmatrix} 4 & -5 \\ 3 & 5 \end{vmatrix} = 35$

Minor of $a_{21} = \begin{vmatrix} 3 & -2 \\ 5 & 2 \end{vmatrix} = 16$

Minor of $a_{22} = \begin{vmatrix} 1 & -2 \\ 3 & 2 \end{vmatrix} = 8$

Minor of $a_{23} = \begin{vmatrix} 1 & 3 \\ 3 & 5 \end{vmatrix} = -4$

Minor of $a_{31} = \begin{vmatrix} 3 & -2 \\ -5 & 6 \end{vmatrix} = 8$

Minor of $a_{32} = \begin{vmatrix} 1 & -2 \\ 4 & 6 \end{vmatrix} = 14$

Minor of $a_{33} = \begin{vmatrix} 1 & 3 \\ 4 & -5 \end{vmatrix} = -17$

Now Cofactors are :

$$A_{11} = (-1)^{1+1}M_{11} = -40$$
$$A_{12} = (-1)^{1+2}M_{12} = 10$$
$$A_{13} = (-1)^{1+3}M_{13} = 35$$
$$A_{21} = (-1)^{2+1}M_{21} = -16$$
$$A_{22} = (-1)^{2+2}M_{22} = 8$$
$$A_{23} = (-1)^{2+3}M_{23} = 4$$
$$A_{31} = (-1)^{3+1}M_{31} = 8$$
$$A_{32} = (-1)^{3+2}M_{32} = -14$$
$$A_{33} = (-1)^{3+3}M_{33} = -17$$

12. Applying the following operations and then expanding

$$R_3 \to R_3 - R_1,\ R_2 \to R_2 - R_1$$
and $C_3 \to C_3 - C_1$, $C_2 \to C_2 - C_1$.

13. Applying $R_2 \to R_2 - R_1$ and $R_3 \to R_3 - R_1$. And expanding along a_{11}, we get the required results.

14. Applying $R_1 \to R_1 + R_2 + R_3$.

Then $C_2 \to C_2 - C_1$ and $C_3 \to C_3 - C_1$ and expending we get the required result.

17. Taking a, b, c common from the first, second and third columns respectively, we get

$$\Delta = abc\begin{vmatrix} -a & a & a \\ b & -b & b \\ c & c & -c \end{vmatrix} = a^2b^2c^2\begin{vmatrix} -1 & 1 & 1 \\ 1 & -1 & 1 \\ 1 & 1 & -1 \end{vmatrix}$$

Taking a, b, c common from 1st, 2nd and 3rd row respectively

$$= a^2b^2c^2\begin{vmatrix} -1 & 1 & 1 \\ 0 & 0 & 2 \\ 0 & 2 & 0 \end{vmatrix}$$

applying $R_2 \to R_2 + R_1$, $R_3 \to R_3 + R_1$

$$= a^2b^2c^2(-1)(-4) = 4a^2b^2c^2.$$

18. Multiplying the first, second and third rows of the determinant on the L.H.S. by x, y and z respectively. We get,

$$= \frac{1}{xyz}\begin{vmatrix} x^2 & x^3 & xyz \\ y^2 & y^3 & xyz \\ z^2 & z^3 & xyz \end{vmatrix}$$

$$= \frac{xyz}{xyz}\begin{vmatrix} x^2 & x^3 & 1 \\ y^2 & y^3 & 1 \\ z^2 & z^2 & 1 \end{vmatrix} = \begin{vmatrix} 1 & 1 & 1 \\ x^2 & y^2 & z^2 \\ x^3 & y^3 & z^3 \end{vmatrix}$$

Applying $C_2 \to C_2 - C_1$, $C_3 \to C_3 - C_1$ to the determinant. We get

$$= \begin{vmatrix} 1 & 0 & 0 \\ x^2 & y^2 - x^2 & z^2 - x^2 \\ x^3 & y^3 - x^3 & z^3 - x^3 \end{vmatrix}$$

$$= \begin{vmatrix} (y-x)(y+x) & (z-x)(z+x) \\ (y-x)(y^2+xy+x^2) & (z-x)(z^2+zx+x^2) \end{vmatrix}$$

$$= (y-x)(z-x)\begin{vmatrix} y+x & z+x \\ y^2+xy+x^2 & z^2+zx+x^2 \end{vmatrix}$$

[Taking $(y - x)$ common from the first column and $(z - x)$ from the second column]

Now Applying $C_2 \to C_2 - C_1$, We get

$$\Rightarrow (y-x)(z-x)\begin{vmatrix} y+x & z-y \\ y^2+xy+x^2 & (z^2-y^2)+zx-xy \end{vmatrix}$$

$$= (y-x)(z-x)\begin{vmatrix} y+x & z-y \\ y^2+xy+x^2 & (z-y)(x+y+z) \end{vmatrix}$$

$$= (y-x)(z-x)(z-y)\begin{vmatrix} y+x & 1 \\ y^2+xy+x^2 & x+y+z \end{vmatrix}$$

$$= (x-y)(y-z)(z-x)(xy+yz+zx)$$

20. Applying $R_1 \to R_1 + R_2 + R_3$

$C_2 \to C_2 - C_1$

$C_3 \to C_2 - C_1$ we get the required result.

21. Applying $R_2 \to R_2 - R_1$, $R_3 \to R_3 - R_1$, the given equation becomes

$$\begin{vmatrix} x-2 & 2x-3 & 3x-4 \\ -2 & -6 & -12 \\ -6 & -24 & -60 \end{vmatrix} = 0.$$

or $$\begin{vmatrix} x-2 & 2x-3 & 3x-4 \\ 1 & 3 & 6 \\ 1 & 4 & 10 \end{vmatrix} = 0.$$

Expanding the determinant along the first row, the above equation becomes :

$$(x-2)[30-24] - (2x-3)[10-6] + (3x-4)(4-3) = 0$$

$$6x - 12 - 8x + 12 + 3x - 4 = 0,\ x = 4$$

23. $$\begin{vmatrix} x & x^2 & 1+px^3 \\ y & y^2 & 1+py^3 \\ z & z^2 & 1+pz^3 \end{vmatrix} = \begin{vmatrix} x & x^2 & 1 \\ y & y^2 & 1 \\ z & z^2 & 1 \end{vmatrix} + \begin{vmatrix} x & x^2 & px^3 \\ y & y^2 & py^3 \\ z & z^2 & pz^3 \end{vmatrix}$$

$$= \begin{vmatrix} x & x^2 & 1 \\ y & y^2 & 1 \\ z & z^2 & 1 \end{vmatrix} + xyz\begin{vmatrix} 1 & x & px^2 \\ 1 & y & py^2 \\ 1 & z & pz^2 \end{vmatrix}$$

$$= \begin{vmatrix} x & x^2 & 1 \\ y & y^2 & 1 \\ z & z^2 & 1 \end{vmatrix} + pxyz\begin{vmatrix} 1 & x & x^2 \\ 1 & y & y^2 \\ 1 & z & z^2 \end{vmatrix}$$

$$= \begin{vmatrix} 1 & x & x^2 \\ 1 & y & y^2 \\ 1 & z & z^2 \end{vmatrix} + pxyz\begin{vmatrix} 1 & x & x^2 \\ 1 & y & y^2 \\ 1 & z & z^2 \end{vmatrix}$$

$$= (1+pxyz)\begin{vmatrix} 1 & x & x^2 \\ 1 & y & y^2 \\ 1 & z & z^2 \end{vmatrix}$$

$$= (1 + pxyz)(x-y)(y-z)(z-x).$$

25. $$\begin{vmatrix} \sin\alpha & \cos\alpha & \cos(\alpha+\delta) \\ \sin\beta & \cos\beta & \cos(\beta+\delta) \\ \sin\gamma & \cos\gamma & \cos(\gamma+\delta) \end{vmatrix}$$

$$= \begin{vmatrix} \sin\alpha & \cos\alpha & \cos\alpha\cos\delta - \sin\alpha\sin\delta \\ \sin\beta & \cos\beta & \cos\beta\cos\delta - \sin\beta\sin\delta \\ \sin\gamma & \cos\gamma & \cos\gamma\cos\delta - \sin\gamma\sin\delta \end{vmatrix}$$

Applying $C_3 \to C_3 + (\sin\delta)C_1 - (\cos\delta)C_2$.

We get $$\begin{vmatrix} \sin\alpha & \cos\alpha & 0 \\ \sin\beta & \cos\beta & 0 \\ \sin\gamma & \cos\gamma & 0 \end{vmatrix} = 0$$

ANSWERS

1. –31 **2.** 6 **3.** 1 **4.** $x^3 - x^2 + 2$ **5.** – 18 **6.** 0 **7.** 49

8. $M_{11} = 3, M_{12} = 0, M_{21} = -10, M_{22} = 5, A_{11} = 3, A_{12} = 0, A_{21} = 10, A_{22} = 5$; 15

9. $M_{11} = -40, M_{12} = -10, M_{13} = 35, M_{21} = 16, M_{22} = 8, M_{23} = -4, M_{31} = 8, M_{32} = 14, M_{33} = -17$
$A_{11} = -40, A_{12} = 10, A_{13} = 35, A_{21} = -16, A_{22} = 8, A_{23} = 4, A_{31} = 8, A_{32} = -14, A_{33} = -17$; –80

10. $M_{11} = 1, M_{12} = 0, M_{13} = 0, M_{21} = 0, M_{22} = 1, M_{23} = 0, M_{31} = 0, M_{32} = 0, M_{33} = 1$
$A_{11} = 1, A_{12} = 0, A_{13} = 0, A_{21} = 0, A_{22} = 1, A_{23} = 0, A_{31} = 0, A_{32} = 0, A_{33} = 1$; 1

11. $M_{11} = 11, M_{12} = 6, M_{13} = 3, M_{21} = -4, M_{22} = 2, M_{23} = 1, M_{31} = -20, M_{32} = -13, M_{33} = 5$
$A_{11} = 11, A_{12} = -6, A_{13} = 3, A_{21} = 4, A_{22} = 2, A_{23} = -1, A_{31} = 20, A_{32} = 13, A_{33} = 5$; 23

12. –24 **13.** $(a-b)(b-c)(c-a)$ **14.** $\lambda^2(3x + \lambda)$ **15.** $4abc$ **21.** $x = 4$

2.6 CRAMER'S RULE

Consider the system of linear equations

$$a_1x + b_1y + c_1z = d_1$$
$$a_2x + b_2y + c_2z = d_2$$
$$a_3x + b_3y + c_3z = d_3 \qquad \ldots(1)$$

We define Δ = determinant coefficients $= \begin{vmatrix} a_1 & b_1 & c_1 \\ a_2 & b_2 & c_2 \\ a_3 & b_3 & c_3 \end{vmatrix}$.

Now we define Δ_x which is obtained by suppressing the column of coefficients of x and replacing it by the column of constant terms d_1, d_2, d_3 on right hand side

$$\therefore \qquad \Delta_x = \begin{vmatrix} d_1 & b_1 & c_1 \\ d_2 & b_2 & c_2 \\ d_3 & b_3 & c_3 \end{vmatrix}.$$

Similarly, we obtained

$$\Delta_y = \begin{vmatrix} a_1 & d_1 & c_1 \\ a_2 & d_2 & c_2 \\ a_3 & d_3 & c_3 \end{vmatrix} \text{ and } \Delta_z = \begin{vmatrix} a_1 & b_1 & d_1 \\ a_2 & b_2 & d_2 \\ a_3 & b_3 & d_3 \end{vmatrix}$$

Now

Case I. If $\Delta \neq 0$, then solution of system (1) is given by

$$x = \frac{\Delta_x}{\Delta}, y = \frac{\Delta_y}{\Delta}, z = \frac{\Delta_z}{\Delta}$$

and system is called consistent.

Case II. $\Delta = 0$ but at least one of $\Delta_x, \Delta_y, \Delta_z \neq 0$, then, the system does not possess any common solution and system is called inconsistent.

Case III. $\Delta = 0$, also $\Delta_x = \Delta_y = \Delta_z = 0$ and at least one cofactor of $\Delta \neq 0$, then system has infinitely many solution and the system then be solved by elimination method.

Elimination of one unknown from three equations gives any one equations in two unknowns therefore two unknowns can be found in terms of the other, we give this unknown an arbitrary value.

If $\Delta = \Delta_x = \Delta_y = \Delta_z = 0$ and all cofactor of Δ, Δx, Δy and Δz are zero then system is equivalent to only one equation in three unknowns and then we give any two unknowns arbitrary values and find the remaining unknown in terms of three constants.

Solved Examples

1. *Using the Cramer's rule, solve the following system of equations*

$$x + y - 4 = 0, 2x - 3y - 3 = 0.$$

SOLUTION. The given equation is

$$x + y - 4 = 0 \qquad \ldots(1)$$
$$2x - 3y - 3 = 0 \qquad \ldots(2)$$

Here, $\Delta = \begin{vmatrix} 1 & 1 \\ 2 & -3 \end{vmatrix} = -5 \neq 0$

$$\Delta_x = \begin{vmatrix} 4 & 1 \\ 3 & -3 \end{vmatrix} = -15$$

$$\Delta_y = \begin{vmatrix} 1 & 4 \\ 2 & 3 \end{vmatrix} = -5$$

$\therefore$ By Cramer's rule

$$x = \frac{\Delta_x}{\Delta} = 3, y = \frac{\Delta_y}{\Delta} = 1$$

2. *Solve the following by Cramer's rule*

$$x + y + z = 6, x - y + z = 2,$$
$$3x + 2y - 4z = -5.$$

SOLUTION. We have

$$\Delta = \begin{vmatrix} 1 & 1 & 1 \\ 1 & -1 & 1 \\ 3 & 2 & -4 \end{vmatrix}$$

$$= \begin{vmatrix} 1 & 0 & 0 \\ 1 & -2 & 0 \\ 3 & -1 & 7 \end{vmatrix} = 14 \neq 0$$

$$\Delta_x = \begin{vmatrix} 6 & 1 & 1 \\ 2 & -1 & 1 \\ -5 & 2 & -4 \end{vmatrix}$$

$$= \begin{vmatrix} 6 & 1 & 1 \\ -4 & -2 & 0 \\ 19 & 6 & 0 \end{vmatrix} = 14$$

$$\Delta_y = \begin{vmatrix} 1 & 6 & 1 \\ 1 & 2 & 1 \\ 3 & -5 & -4 \end{vmatrix}$$

$$= \begin{vmatrix} 1 & 6 & 1 \\ 0 & -4 & 0 \\ 0 & -23 & -7 \end{vmatrix} = 28$$

$$\Delta_z = \begin{vmatrix} 1 & 1 & 6 \\ 1 & -1 & 2 \\ 3 & 2 & 5 \end{vmatrix}$$

$$= \begin{vmatrix} 1 & 1 & 6 \\ 0 & -2 & -4 \\ 0 & -1 & -23 \end{vmatrix} = 42$$

Hence, by Cramer's rule

$$x = \frac{\Delta_x}{\Delta} = 1, y = \frac{\Delta_y}{\Delta} = 2, z = \frac{\Delta_z}{\Delta} = 3.$$

Hence, solution is given by $x = 1, y = 2, z = 3$.

3. *Solve the following system equations with the help of Cramer's rule.*

$3x - 4y + 5z = -6,\ x + y - 2z = -1,$
$2x + 3y + z = 5.$[UPTU(B.PHARMA)–2004]
[DELHI (BCA) -2010]

SOLUTION. Let

$$\Delta = \begin{vmatrix} 3 & -4 & 5 \\ 1 & 1 & -2 \\ 2 & 3 & 1 \end{vmatrix} = 3(1+6)+4(1+4)$$

$$+ 5(3-2) = 46 \neq 0.$$

Since, $\Delta \neq 0$, therefore the given system has a unique solution given by

$$\frac{x}{\Delta_x} = \frac{y}{\Delta_y} = \frac{z}{\Delta_z} = \frac{1}{\Delta}$$

Now, $\Delta_x = \begin{vmatrix} -6 & -4 & 5 \\ -1 & 1 & -2 \\ 5 & 3 & 1 \end{vmatrix}$

by $R_1 \to R_1 + 4R_2, R_3 \to R_3 - 3R_2$.

$$= \begin{vmatrix} -10 & 0 & -3 \\ -1 & 1 & -2 \\ 8 & 0 & 7 \end{vmatrix} = \begin{vmatrix} -10 & -3 \\ 8 & 7 \end{vmatrix}$$

$= -70 + 24 = -46.$

$$\Delta_y = \begin{vmatrix} 3 & -6 & 5 \\ 1 & -1 & -2 \\ 2 & 5 & 1 \end{vmatrix} \text{ by } R_1 \to R_1 - 3R_2,\ R_3 \to R_3 - 2R_2$$

$$= \begin{vmatrix} 0 & -3 & 11 \\ 1 & -1 & -2 \\ 0 & 7 & 5 \end{vmatrix} = -\begin{vmatrix} -3 & 11 \\ 7 & 5 \end{vmatrix} = 92$$

$$\Delta_z = \begin{vmatrix} 3 & -4 & -6 \\ 1 & 1 & -1 \\ 2 & 3 & 5 \end{vmatrix} \text{ by } R_1 \to R_1 - 3R_2,\ R_3 \to R_3 - 2R_2$$

$$= \begin{vmatrix} 0 & -7 & -3 \\ 1 & 1 & -1 \\ 0 & 1 & 7 \end{vmatrix} = -\begin{vmatrix} -7 & -3 \\ 1 & 7 \end{vmatrix} = 46$$

The solution of the given system is

$$x = \frac{\Delta_x}{\Delta} = \frac{-46}{46} = -1,$$

$$y = \frac{\Delta_y}{\Delta} = \frac{92}{46} = 2$$

$$\text{and } z = \frac{\Delta_z}{\Delta} = \frac{46}{46} = 1$$

Hence, the required solution is $x = -1, y = 2, z = 1$.

4. *Solve using Cramer's rule*

$x + y = 5,\ y + z = 3,\ z + x = 4.$
[UPTU(B.PHARMA)–2001, 07]

SOLUTION. Let $\Delta = \begin{vmatrix} 1 & 1 & 0 \\ 0 & 1 & 1 \\ 1 & 0 & 1 \end{vmatrix}$

$= 1(1-0) - 1(0-1)$
$= 1 + 1 = 2$

Since $\Delta \neq 0$, therefore the given systems has a unique solution given by

$$\frac{x}{\Delta_x} = \frac{y}{\Delta_y} = \frac{z}{\Delta_z} = \frac{1}{\Delta}$$

Now $\Delta_x = \begin{vmatrix} 5 & 1 & 0 \\ 3 & 1 & 1 \\ 4 & 0 & 1 \end{vmatrix} = 6$

$$\Delta_y = \begin{vmatrix} 1 & 5 & 0 \\ 0 & 3 & 1 \\ 1 & 4 & 1 \end{vmatrix} = 4$$

$$\Delta_z = \begin{vmatrix} 1 & 1 & 5 \\ 0 & 1 & 3 \\ 1 & 0 & 4 \end{vmatrix} = 2.$$

The solution of the given system is

$$x = \frac{\Delta_x}{\Delta} = \frac{6}{2} = 3,\ y = \frac{\Delta_y}{\Delta} = \frac{4}{2} = 2,$$

$$z = \frac{\Delta_z}{\Delta} = \frac{2}{2} = 1.$$

5. *Solve the following by using Cramer's rule.*

$x - 2y + 3z = 2,\ 2x - 3z = 3,$

$x + y + z = 6.$ [UPTU(B.PHARMA)–2002]

SOLUTION. Let

$$\Delta = \begin{vmatrix} 1 & -2 & 3 \\ 2 & 0 & -3 \\ 1 & 1 & 1 \end{vmatrix} = \begin{vmatrix} 1 & 0 & 0 \\ 2 & 4 & -9 \\ 1 & 3 & -2 \end{vmatrix}$$

by $R_2 + 2R_1, R_3 - 3R_1$

$$= \begin{vmatrix} 4 & -9 \\ 3 & -2 \end{vmatrix} = -8 + 27 = 19 \neq 0$$

since $\Delta \neq 0$, therefore the given system has a unique solution given by

$$\frac{x}{\Delta_x} = \frac{y}{\Delta_y} = \frac{z}{\Delta_z} = \frac{1}{\Delta_x}.$$

Now $\Delta_x = \begin{vmatrix} 2 & -2 & 3 \\ 3 & 0 & -3 \\ 6 & 1 & 1 \end{vmatrix} = \begin{vmatrix} 2 & 0 & 5 \\ 3 & 3 & 0 \\ 6 & 7 & 7 \end{vmatrix}$

by $R_2 + R_1, R_3 + R_1$

$$= 2\begin{vmatrix} 3 & 0 \\ 7 & 7 \end{vmatrix} + 0 + 5$$

$$\begin{vmatrix} 3 & 3 \\ 6 & 7 \end{vmatrix} = 57.$$

$$\Delta_y = \begin{vmatrix} 1 & 2 & 3 \\ 2 & 3 & -3 \\ 1 & 6 & 1 \end{vmatrix} = \begin{vmatrix} 1 & 0 & 0 \\ 2 & -1 & -9 \\ 1 & 4 & -2 \end{vmatrix}$$

by $R_2 - 2R_1, R_3 - 3R_1$

$$= 1\begin{vmatrix} -1 & -9 \\ 4 & -2 \end{vmatrix} = 38.$$

$$\Delta_z = \begin{vmatrix} 1 & -2 & 2 \\ 2 & 0 & 3 \\ 1 & 1 & 6 \end{vmatrix} = \begin{vmatrix} 1 & 0 & 0 \\ 2 & 4 & -1 \\ 1 & 3 & 4 \end{vmatrix}$$

by $R_2 + 2R_1, R_3 - 2R_1$

$$= 1\begin{vmatrix} 4 & -1 \\ 3 & 4 \end{vmatrix} = 16 + 3 = 19.$$

The solution of the given system is

$$x = \frac{\Delta_x}{\Delta} = \frac{57}{19} = 3,\ y = \frac{\Delta_y}{\Delta} = \frac{38}{19} = 1$$

and $\quad z = \dfrac{\Delta_z}{\Delta} = \dfrac{19}{19} = 1$

Hence, the required solution is $x = 3$, $y = 2, z = 1$.

6. *Find the value of λ for which the system of equations $x + y - 2z = 0$, $2x - 3y + z = 0$, $x - 5y + 4z = \lambda$ is consistent and find the solutions for all such value of λ.*

SOLUTION. The given system of equations is

$$x - 5y + 4z = \lambda \qquad \ldots(1)$$

$$x + y - 2z = 0 \qquad \ldots(2)$$

$$2x - 3y + z = 0 \qquad \ldots(3)$$

$$\Delta = \begin{vmatrix} 1 & -5 & 4 \\ 1 & 1 & -2 \\ 2 & -3 & 1 \end{vmatrix} = \begin{vmatrix} 1 & -5 & 4 \\ 0 & 6 & -6 \\ 0 & 7 & -7 \end{vmatrix} = 0.$$

Hence, system is consistent only when $\Delta_x = \Delta_y = \Delta_z = 0$

Now $\Delta_x = \begin{vmatrix} \lambda & -5 & 4 \\ 0 & 1 & -2 \\ 0 & -3 & 1 \end{vmatrix} = -5\lambda = 0$

$\Rightarrow \quad \lambda = 0$

For $\lambda = 0$, clearly $\Delta_y = \Delta_z = 0$.

$\therefore$ System is consistent if $\lambda = 0$, then on eliminating x from (1), (2) and (3), we have

$$6y - 6z = 0,\ y - z = 0$$

and $\quad 7y - 7z = 0$ or $y = z$.

Let $y = z = k \in R$, then from (1), we have $x = 5k - 4k = k$.

Hence, solution is given by $x = y = z = k \in \boldsymbol{R}$.

7. *Solve the equations by Cramer's rule*

$$\frac{4}{x+5} + \frac{3}{y+7} = -1$$

$$\frac{6}{x+5} - \frac{6}{y+7} = -5$$

SOLUTION. The given system of equation is

$$\frac{4}{x+5} + \frac{3}{y+7} = -1$$

$$\frac{6}{x+5} - \frac{6}{y+7} = -5$$

Now putting $\dfrac{1}{x+5} = a, \dfrac{1}{y+7} = b,$

the equations becomes

$$4a + 3b = -1$$
$$6a - 6b = -5$$

$$\Delta = \begin{vmatrix} 4 & 3 \\ 6 & -6 \end{vmatrix} = -42 \neq 0$$

$$\Delta_a = \begin{vmatrix} -1 & 3 \\ -5 & -6 \end{vmatrix} = 21, \Delta_b = \begin{vmatrix} 4 & -1 \\ 6 & -5 \end{vmatrix} = -14.$$

So by Cramer's rule

$$a = \frac{\Delta_a}{\Delta} = \frac{21}{-42} = \frac{1}{2},$$

$$b = \frac{\Delta_b}{\Delta} = \frac{-14}{-42} = \frac{1}{3}$$

$\therefore$ $x + 5 = -2, y + 7 = 3$

or $x = -7, y = -4.$

Hence, the solution is

$$x = -7, y = -4.$$

8. *Using Cramer's rule solve the following equation :*

$$x + 2y + 3z = 6$$
$$2x + 4y + z = 17$$
$$3x + 2y + 9z = 2$$

SOLUTION. We have

$$\Delta = \begin{vmatrix} 1 & 2 & 3 \\ 2 & 4 & 1 \\ 3 & 2 & 9 \end{vmatrix} = -20$$

$$\Delta_x = \begin{vmatrix} 6 & 2 & 3 \\ 17 & 4 & 1 \\ 2 & 2 & 9 \end{vmatrix} = -20$$

$$\Delta_y = \begin{vmatrix} 1 & 6 & 3 \\ 2 & 17 & 1 \\ 3 & 2 & 9 \end{vmatrix} = -80$$

$$\Delta_z = \begin{vmatrix} 1 & 2 & 6 \\ 2 & 4 & 17 \\ 3 & 2 & 2 \end{vmatrix} = -20$$

Then by Cramer's rule, we have

$$x = \frac{\Delta_x}{\Delta} = \frac{-20}{-20} = 1$$

$$y = \frac{\Delta_y}{\Delta} = \frac{-80}{-20} = 4$$

$$z = \frac{\Delta_z}{\Delta} = \frac{20}{-20} = -1$$

Exercise-2.2

1. (a) Using Cramer's rule, solve the following equations

$$x + y + z = 6$$
$$2x + y - z = 1$$
$$x + y - 2z = -3$$

(b)
$$x + y + z = 6$$
$$x - y + z = 2$$
$$3x + 2y - 9z = -5$$

2. Find the value of k if the following equations are consistent :

$$x + y - 3 = 0$$
$$(1 + k)x + (2 + k)y - 8 = 0$$
$$x - (1 + k)y + (2 + k) = 0.$$

3. Find the value of k if the system of equations

$$(k + 1)^3x + (k + 2)^3y = (k + 3)^3$$
$$(k + 1)x + (k + 2)y = (k + 3)$$
$$x + y = 1 : \text{is consistent.}$$

4. If the system of equations $x + 2y = 5, 2x - y = 5, x + 3y = 6$ is consistent, solve it.

5. Solve the following by Cramer's rule

$$x + y + z = 11$$
$$2x - 6y - z = 0$$
$$3x + 4y + 2z = 0.$$

6. Show that the system of equations

$$3x - y + 4z = 3$$
$$x + 2y - 3z = -2$$
$$6x + 5y + \lambda z = -3$$

has at least one solution for any real number λ. Find the set of solution if $\lambda = -5$.

7. Using Cramer's rule to solve the following system of linear equations.

$$2x - 3y + z = 7$$
$$2x + y + z = 1$$
$$4y + 3z = -11$$

ANSWERS

1. (a) $x = 1, y = 2, z = 3$ (b) $x = \frac{9}{4}, y = 2, z = \frac{21}{12}$

2. $k = 1$ or $-5/3$ **3.** $k = -2$ **5.** $x = -8, y = -7, z = 26.$

❑❑❑❑❑❑

Chapter

3

Matrices

3.1 INTRODUCTION

Matrix is an ordered rectangular array of numbers (real or complex) in horizontal and vertical lines called rows and columns respectively. Matrix plays an important role in various branches of mathematics, electrical engineering, genetic and sociology etc. The word 'matrix' was first used by British mathematician J.J. Silvestor in 1850. Another British mathematician Arthur Cayley formulated the general theory of matrix in 1857. Matrix is useful in every branch of science and engineering.

3.2 MATRIX

Definition. *A set of mn numbers* $a_{11}, a_{12}, \ldots, a_{mn}$ *arranged in a rectangular array of m rows and n columns is called a matrix of order* $m \times n$. *Generally it is denoted by* [ ] *or* ( ) *or* || ||

A matrix of order $m \times n$ can be illustrated as follows :

$$A_{m\times n} = \begin{bmatrix} a_{11} & a_{12} & \cdots & a_{1j} & \cdots & a_{1n} \\ a_{21} & a_{22} & \cdots & a_{2j} & \cdots & a_{2n} \\ \vdots & & & & & \\ a_{i1} & a_{i2} & \cdots & a_{ij} & \cdots & a_{in} \\ \vdots & & & & & \\ a_{m1} & a_{m2} & \cdots & a_{mj} & \cdots & a_{mn} \end{bmatrix}$$

The quantities a_{ij} $(i = 1, 2, \ldots, m, j = 1, 2, \ldots, n)$ are called the elements of the matrix A. An element occurring in the ith row (horizontal lines) and j^{th} column (vertical lines) of a matrix A is called $(i, j)^{th}$ element of A and is denoted by a_{ij}.

For example: Let $A = \begin{bmatrix} 2 & 3 & -5 \\ 4 & 3 & 8 \end{bmatrix}$

Then $a_{11} = 2,\quad a_{12} = 3,\quad a_{13} = -5$

$a_{21} = 4,\quad a_{22} = 3,\quad a_{23} = 8$

3.3 KINDS OF MATRICES

(1) Horizontal Matrix : A matrix of order $m \times n$ is called a horizontal matrix if $m < n$, *i.e.*, if number of rows is less than the number of columns.

For example: The matrix $\begin{bmatrix} a & b & c \\ d & e & f \end{bmatrix}$ is a horizontal matrix because it has two rows and three columns.

(2) Vertical Matrix: A matrix of order $m \times n$ is called a vertical matrix if $m > n$, *i.e.*, if number of rows is greater than the number of columns.

For example: $\begin{bmatrix} a & b \\ c & d \\ e & f \end{bmatrix}$ is a vertical matrix because it has three rows and two columns.

(3) Square Matrix : A matrix in which number of rows is equal to number of columns is called square matrix. In such type of matrix $m = n$. [MEERUT(BCA)–2008, 09, 16, 17, 18; KANPUR–2010; RAIPUR–2008]

For example: $\begin{bmatrix} a & b \\ c & d \end{bmatrix}$ and $\begin{bmatrix} a_{11} & a_{12} & a_{13} \\ a_{21} & a_{22} & a_{23} \\ a_{31} & a_{32} & a_{33} \end{bmatrix}$ are square matrix of order 2×2 and 3×3 respectively.

- Because the matrix of order $m \times m$ is a square matrix. Therefore, we say it is of order m instead of order $m \times m$.

(4) Row Matrix or Row Vector : A matrix having only one row is called a row matrix or row vector.

For example: $\begin{bmatrix} 1 & 2 & 3 & 4 \end{bmatrix}$ and $\begin{bmatrix} a & b & c \end{bmatrix}$ are the row matrices of order 1×4 and 1×3 respectively.

(5) Column Matrix or Column Vector : A matrix having only one column is called a column matrix or column vector.

For example: $\begin{bmatrix} a \\ b \end{bmatrix}$ and $\begin{bmatrix} 1 \\ 3 \\ 5 \end{bmatrix}$ are the column matrices of order 2×1 and 3×1 respectively.

(6) Zero or Null Matrix : A matrix in which every element is zero is called the null or zero matrix. It is denoted by O.

For example: $\begin{bmatrix} 0 & 0 & 0 \end{bmatrix}$ and $\begin{bmatrix} 0 & 0 & 0 \\ 0 & 0 & 0 \\ 0 & 0 & 0 \\ 0 & 0 & 0 \end{bmatrix}$ are the null matrices of order 1×3 and 4×3 respectively.

(7) Unit or Identity Matrix : A square matrix in which all the elements along the principal diagonal are one (1) and all elements not occurring along the principal diagonal are zero. It is denoted by I. [MEERUT(BCA)-2008, 09, 12, 16, 17; DELHI-2010, RAJASTHAN-2014, PUNJAB-2006]

For example: $\begin{bmatrix} 1 & 0 \\ 0 & 1 \end{bmatrix}$, $\begin{bmatrix} 1 & 0 & 0 \\ 0 & 1 & 0 \\ 0 & 0 & 1 \end{bmatrix}$ and $\begin{bmatrix} 1 & 0 & 0 & 0 \\ 0 & 1 & 0 & 0 \\ 0 & 0 & 1 & 0 \\ 0 & 0 & 0 & 1 \end{bmatrix}$ are the unit matrices of order 2×2, 3×3 and 4×4 respectively.

In other words A square matrix $A = [a_{ij}]$ is a unit matrix if

$$a_{ij} = \begin{cases} 1 & \text{if} \quad i = j \\ 0 & \text{if} \quad i \neq j \end{cases}$$

Principal Diagonal: Every square matrix has two diagonals in which the diagonal starting from the first element down to last element is said to be main diagonal.

For example : $\begin{bmatrix} a & b & c \\ d & e & f \\ g & h & i \end{bmatrix}$ → main diagonal

- Only square matrix has diagonals. The elements lying on main diagonal are called diagonal elements.

(8) Diagonal Matrix : A square matrix which has all its elements are zero except the diagonal elements, is said to be diagonal matrix. [MEERUT BCA-2008, 09, 14, 16]

For example: $\begin{bmatrix} 3 & 0 \\ 0 & 2 \end{bmatrix}$ and $\begin{bmatrix} 1 & 0 & 0 \\ 0 & 5 & 0 \\ 0 & 0 & 7 \end{bmatrix}$ are diagonal matrices.

(9) Scalar Matrix: A square matrix is said to be scalar if all elements along the principal diagonal are equal and non-diagonal elements are zero.

For example: $\begin{bmatrix} 2 & 0 & 0 \\ 0 & 2 & 0 \\ 0 & 0 & 2 \end{bmatrix}$ and $\begin{bmatrix} a & 0 & 0 \\ 0 & a & 0 \\ 0 & 0 & a \end{bmatrix}$ are scalar matrices.

(10) Sub-matrix : The matrix obtained by leave some row and column of the given matrix is called sub matrix.

For example: $\begin{bmatrix} 1 & 2 \\ 3 & 9 \end{bmatrix}$ is the sub matrix of the matrix $\begin{bmatrix} 5 & 4 & 8 \\ 6 & 1 & 2 \\ 7 & 3 & 9 \end{bmatrix}$.

(11) Triangular Matrices

(i) Upper-Triangular Matrix : A square matrix $A = [a_{ij}]_{m \times n}$ is called an upper triangular matrix if $a_{ij} = 0 \ \forall \ i > j$. Therefore, a square matrix is said to be upper triangular if all the elements below the main diagonal are equal to zero.

For example: $\begin{bmatrix} 5 & 4 & 0 \\ 0 & 3 & 2 \\ 0 & 0 & 1 \end{bmatrix}$ and $\begin{bmatrix} 1 & 2 & 4 & 8 \\ 0 & 4 & 3 & 2 \\ 0 & 0 & 7 & 8 \\ 0 & 0 & 0 & 9 \end{bmatrix}$ are upper triangular matrices.

(ii) Lower-Triangular Matrix : A square matrix $A = [a_{ij}]$, is called a lower triangular matrix if $a_{ij} = 0$ for all $i < j$. Therefore, a square matrix is said to be lower triangular matrix if all the elements above the main diagonal are equal to zero.

For example: $\begin{bmatrix} a & 0 \\ b & c \end{bmatrix}$ and $\begin{bmatrix} 5 & 0 & 0 & 0 \\ 8 & 1 & 0 & 0 \\ 4 & 2 & 9 & 0 \\ 3 & 5 & 1 & 7 \end{bmatrix}$ are lower triangular matrices.

(12) Comparable Matrices : Two matrices A and B are said to be comparable if they are of same order.

For example: $A = \begin{bmatrix} 1 & 4 & 7 \\ 6 & 0 & 8 \end{bmatrix}$ and $B = \begin{bmatrix} 5 & 2 & 7 \\ 4 & 8 & 9 \end{bmatrix}$ are two matrices of same order 2×3.

Hence, they are comparable.

3.3.1 EQUALITY OF MATRICES

Two matrices A and B are said to be equal (*i.e.*, $A = B$) if

(i) they are of same order.

and (ii) their corresponding elements are equal.

Symbolically : Two matrices $A = [a_{ij}]_{m \times n}$ and $B = [b_{ij}]_{r \times s}$ are said to be equal if

(i) No. of rows in A = no. of rows in B.

(ii) No. of column in A = no. of column in B.

(iii) $(i, j)^{th}$ element of A = $(i, j)^{th}$ element of B, *i.e.*, $a_{ij} = b_{ij}\ \forall\ i, j$

For example: $A = \begin{bmatrix} 2 & 4 \\ 6 & 8 \end{bmatrix}$ and $B = \begin{bmatrix} 2 & 4 \\ 6 & 8 \end{bmatrix}$. Then $A = B$.

3.4 OPERATIONS ON MATRICES

(i) Addition of Matrices: Let A and B two matrices of same order say $m \times n$. Then addition of A and B denoted by $A + B$ is obtained by adding each element of A to the corresponding element of B.

If $\quad A = [a_{ij}], B = [b_{ij}], \quad i = 1, 2, ..., m;\ j = 1, 2, ..., n$

Then $\quad A + B = [a_{ij} + b_{ij}], \quad i = 1, 2, ..., m;\ j = 1, 2, ..., n$

In other words $[a_{ij}]_{m \times n} + [b_{ij}]_{m \times n} = [a_{ij} + b_{ij}]_{m \times n}$

For example:

Let $$A = \begin{bmatrix} 2 & 3 & 4 \\ 0 & 2 & -1 \end{bmatrix}, B = \begin{bmatrix} -3 & 4 & 5 \\ 6 & 2 & 9 \end{bmatrix}$$

Then $$A + B = \begin{bmatrix} 2-3 & 3+4 & 4+5 \\ 0+6 & 2+2 & -1+9 \end{bmatrix} = \begin{bmatrix} -1 & 7 & 9 \\ 6 & 4 & 8 \end{bmatrix}$$

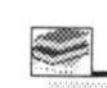

- Operation of adding is a binary operation in set of matrices of same order.

(ii) Negative of a Matrix: Let $A = [a_{ij}]_{m \times n}$ be a matrix. Negative of A is represented by $-A$ and is given by $(-a_{ij})$.

For example:

Let $A = \begin{bmatrix} 1 & 3 & 5 \\ -8 & 9 & 7 \\ 6 & -4 & 0 \end{bmatrix}$ and $-A = \begin{bmatrix} -1 & -3 & -5 \\ 8 & -9 & -7 \\ -6 & 4 & 0 \end{bmatrix}$

- If order of A is of $m \times n$ then order of $-A$ also be of $m \times n$.

(iii) Difference of Two Matrices: Let A and B be two matrices of order $m \times n$, then difference between A and B represented by $A - B$ and it is defined as $A - B = A + (-B)$. Order of $A - B$ will be same as the order of A and B. Subtract each elements of B from corresponding elements of A to get $A - B$.

For example: Let $A = \begin{bmatrix} 6 & 7 & 8 \\ -4 & 3 & 7 \\ 6 & 5 & -2 \end{bmatrix}$ and $B = \begin{bmatrix} 4 & 2 & 5 \\ 4 & 6 & 4 \\ 9 & 8 & 3 \end{bmatrix}$

Then $$A - B = \begin{bmatrix} 6-4 & 7-2 & 8-5 \\ -4-4 & 3-6 & 7-4 \\ 6-9 & 5-8 & -2-3 \end{bmatrix} = \begin{bmatrix} 2 & 5 & 3 \\ -8 & -3 & 3 \\ -3 & -3 & -5 \end{bmatrix}$$

3.5 PROPERTIES OF MATRICES ADDITION

Property 1. (Commutative law of Addition)

If A and B are two matrices of order m × n, then A + B = B + A.

Proof. Let $A = [a_{ij}]_{m \times n}$ and $B = [b_{ij}]_{m \times n}$, then

$$A + B = [a_{ij}]_{m \times n} + [b_{ij}]_{m \times n}$$

$$= [a_{ij} + b_{ij}]_{m \times n} \quad \text{(Addition rule for matrix)}$$
$$= [b_{ij} + a_{ij}]_{m \times n} \quad \text{(Commutative law of numbers)}$$
$$= [b_{ij}]_{m \times n} + [a_{ij}]_{m \times n}$$

Hence, $A + B = B + A$

Property 2. (Associative law of Addition)

If A, B and C are three matrices of order $m \times n$, then

$$A + (B + C) = (A + B) + C$$

Proof. Let $A = [a_{ij}]_{m \times n}$, $B = [b_{ij}]_{m \times n}$ and $C = [c_{ij}]_{m \times n}$, then

$$(A + B) + C = \{[a_{ij}]_{m \times n} + [b_{ij}]_{m \times n}\} + [c_{ij}]_{m \times n}$$
$$= [a_{ij} + b_{ij}]_{m \times n} + [c_{ij}]_{m \times n}$$
$$= [(a_{ij} + b_{ij}) + c_{ij}]_{m \times n}$$
$$= [a_{ij} + (b_{ij} + c_{ij})]_{m \times n}$$

(Associative rule of addition of numbers)

$$= [a_{ij}]_{m \times n} + \{[b_{ij}]_{m \times n} + [c_{ij}]_{m \times n}\}$$
$$= A + (B + C)$$

Hence, $(A + B) + C = A + (B + C)$

Property 3. (Existence of Additive Identity)

Let A be a matrix of order $m \times n$ and there exists a null matrix O such that $A + O = O + A = A$.

Proof. Let $A = [a_{ij}]_{m \times n}$ and $O = [b_{ij}]_{m \times n}$

where $b_{ij} = 0$, $i = 1, 2, ..., m$ and $j = 1, 2, ..., n$

then $A + O = [a_{ij}]_{m \times n} + [b_{ij}]_{m \times n}$

$$= [a_{ij} + b_{ij}]_{m \times n} = [a_{ij} + 0]_{m \times n} \quad [\because b_{ij} = 0]$$
$$= [a_{ij}]_{m \times n} = A$$

$\therefore$ $A + O = A$

Similarly $O + A = A$

Therefore, $A + O = O + A = A$

- Null matrix of $m \times n$ order is called additive identity for all $m \times n$ order matrices.

Property 4. (Existence of Additive Inverse) *For a matrix A*

$$A + (-A) = (-A) + A = O, \text{ where } O \text{ is null matrix.}$$

Proof. Let $A = [a_{ij}]_{m \times n}$. Then $(-A) = [-a_{ij}]_{m \times n}$

$$A + (-A) = [a_{ij}]_{m \times n} + [-a_{ij}]_{m \times n} = [a_{ij} + (-a_{ij})]_{m \times n}$$
$$= O, \text{ where } O \text{ is null matrix.}$$

So $A + (-A) = O$

Similarly, $(-A) + A = O$

Hence, $A + (-A) = (-A) + A = O$

- Matrix $(-A)$ is called additive inverse of A.

Property 5. (Cancellation law for matrix addition)

If A, B and C are three matrices of order $m \times n$. Then

(i) $A + B = A + C \Rightarrow B = C$ (Left cancellation law)

(ii) $B + A = C + A \Rightarrow B = C$ (Right cancellation law)

Proof: We have $A + B = A + C$

$\Rightarrow$ $(-A) + A + B = (-A) + A + C$

$\Rightarrow$ $(-A + A) + B = (-A + A) + C$ (Associativity)

$\Rightarrow$ $O + B = O + C$ $(-A + A = O)$

$\Rightarrow \quad B = C$

So, $A + B = A + C \Rightarrow B = C$

Similarly, we can show that

$$B + A = C + A \Rightarrow B = C$$

3.6 MULTIPLICATION OF A MATRIX BY A SCALAR

Scalar multiplication of a matrix A is obtained by multiplying of each element of matrix by the given scalar.

i.e., $kA = [ka_{ij}]$

For example: If $A = \begin{bmatrix} 1 & -3 \\ 0 & 3 \end{bmatrix}$

Then $3A = 3\begin{bmatrix} 1 & -3 \\ 0 & 3 \end{bmatrix} = \begin{bmatrix} 3 & -9 \\ 0 & 9 \end{bmatrix}$

Similarly, $-6A = -6\begin{bmatrix} 1 & -3 \\ 0 & 3 \end{bmatrix} = \begin{bmatrix} -6 & +18 \\ 0 & -18 \end{bmatrix}$

3.6.1 Properties of Scalar Multiplication

THEOREM. *In matrix addition, the scalar multiplication is distributive over addition, i.e., If A and B, are two matrices of same order and k is a scalar, then k(A + B) = kA + kB.*

PROOF. Let $A = [a_{ij}]_{m \times n}$ and $B = [b_{ij}]_{m \times n}$

$$A + B = [a_{ij} + b_{ij}]_{m \times n}$$

$$\Rightarrow \quad k(A + B) = [ka_{ij} + kb_{ij}]_{m \times n}$$

$$= [ka_{ij}]_{m \times n} + [kb_{ij}]_{m \times n}$$

$$= k[a_{ij}]_{m \times n} + k[b_{ij}]_{m \times n} = kA + kB$$

Hence, $k(A + B) = kA + kB$

For example: If $A = \begin{bmatrix} a & b \\ c & d \end{bmatrix}$ and $B = \begin{bmatrix} x & y \\ z & u \end{bmatrix}$

Then $k(A+B) = k\begin{bmatrix} a+x & b+y \\ c+z & d+u \end{bmatrix} = \begin{bmatrix} ka+kx & kb+ky \\ kc+kz & kd+ku \end{bmatrix}$

$$= \begin{bmatrix} ka & kb \\ kc & kd \end{bmatrix} + \begin{bmatrix} kx & ky \\ kz & ku \end{bmatrix} = k\begin{bmatrix} a & b \\ c & d \end{bmatrix} + k\begin{bmatrix} x & y \\ z & u \end{bmatrix} = kA + kB$$

$\Rightarrow \quad k(A + B) = kA + kB$

Solved Examples

1. *Write $A = [a_{ij}]_{2 \times 3}$ where $a_{ij} = 2i - 3j$.*

SOLUTION. Given $a_{ij} = 2i - 3j$

$$a_{11} = 2 \times 1 - 3 \times 1 = -1$$
$$a_{12} = 2 \times 1 - 3 \times 2 = -4$$
$$a_{13} = 2 \times 1 - 3 \times 3 = -7$$
$$a_{21} = 2 \times 2 - 3 \times 1 = 1$$
$$a_{22} = 2 \times 2 - 3 \times 2 = -2$$
$$a_{23} = 2 \times 2 - 3 \times 3 = -5$$

So $A = \begin{bmatrix} -1 & -4 & -7 \\ 1 & -2 & -5 \end{bmatrix}$

2. *If $\begin{bmatrix} 3x-2 & 4y-8 \\ z-2 & a+11 \end{bmatrix} = \begin{bmatrix} 10 & 8 \\ 11 & 9 \end{bmatrix}$ find x, y, z and a.*

SOLUTION. Comparing the corresponding elements

$$3x - 2 = 10 \Rightarrow x = 4$$
$$4y - 8 = 8 \Rightarrow y = 4$$
$$z - 2 = 11 \Rightarrow z = 13$$
$$a + 11 = 9 \Rightarrow a = -2$$

3. *If $A = \begin{bmatrix} 2 & 3 & -1 \\ 0 & -1 & 5 \end{bmatrix}$ and $B = \begin{bmatrix} 1 & 2 & -6 \\ 0 & -1 & +3 \end{bmatrix}$ then find*

(i) 5A + 2B (ii) 3A – 4B

SOLUTION. (i) $5A = 5\begin{bmatrix} 2 & 3 & -1 \\ 0 & -1 & 5 \end{bmatrix} = \begin{bmatrix} 10 & 15 & -5 \\ 0 & -5 & 25 \end{bmatrix}$

and $2B = 2\begin{bmatrix} 1 & 2 & -6 \\ 0 & -1 & 3 \end{bmatrix} = \begin{bmatrix} 2 & 4 & -12 \\ 0 & -2 & 6 \end{bmatrix}$

$$5A + 2B = \begin{bmatrix} 10 & 15 & -5 \\ 0 & -5 & 25 \end{bmatrix} + \begin{bmatrix} 2 & 4 & -12 \\ 0 & -2 & 6 \end{bmatrix} = \begin{bmatrix} 12 & 19 & -17 \\ 0 & -7 & 31 \end{bmatrix}$$

(ii) $3A = 3\begin{bmatrix} 2 & 3 & -1 \\ 0 & -1 & 5 \end{bmatrix} = \begin{bmatrix} 6 & 9 & -3 \\ 0 & -3 & 15 \end{bmatrix}$

and $4B = 4\begin{bmatrix} 1 & 2 & -6 \\ 0 & -1 & 3 \end{bmatrix} = \begin{bmatrix} 4 & 8 & -24 \\ 0 & -4 & 12 \end{bmatrix}$

$$3A - 4B = \begin{bmatrix} 6 & 9 & -3 \\ 0 & -3 & 15 \end{bmatrix} - \begin{bmatrix} 4 & 8 & -24 \\ 0 & -4 & 12 \end{bmatrix} = \begin{bmatrix} 2 & 1 & 21 \\ 0 & 1 & 3 \end{bmatrix}$$

4. *Find the value of x, y, z and a, for which*

$$\begin{bmatrix} x+3 & 2y+x \\ z-1 & 4a-6 \end{bmatrix} = \begin{bmatrix} 0 & -7 \\ 3 & 2a \end{bmatrix}$$

SOLUTION. $\begin{bmatrix} x+3 & 2y+x \\ z-1 & 4a-6 \end{bmatrix} = \begin{bmatrix} 0 & -7 \\ 3 & 2a \end{bmatrix}$

$x + 3 = 0 \Rightarrow x = -3$

$2y + x = -7 \Rightarrow y = -2$

$z - 1 = 3 \Rightarrow z = 4$

$4a - 6 = 2a \Rightarrow a = 3$

5. *If* $A = \begin{bmatrix} 1 & 0 & 2 \\ 0 & 2 & 3 \\ 1 & 2 & 3 \end{bmatrix}$ *and* $B = \begin{bmatrix} 3 & 1 & 1 \\ 1 & 2 & 3 \\ 0 & 1 & 2 \end{bmatrix}$

find 3A + 6B.

SOLUTION. We have

$$3A = 3\begin{bmatrix} 1 & 0 & 2 \\ 0 & 2 & 3 \\ 1 & 2 & 3 \end{bmatrix} = \begin{bmatrix} 3 & 0 & 6 \\ 0 & 6 & 9 \\ 3 & 6 & 9 \end{bmatrix}$$

and

$$6B = 6\begin{bmatrix} 3 & 1 & 1 \\ 1 & 2 & 3 \\ 0 & 1 & 2 \end{bmatrix} = \begin{bmatrix} 18 & 6 & 6 \\ 6 & 12 & 18 \\ 0 & 6 & 12 \end{bmatrix}$$

Therefore,

$$3A + 6B = \begin{bmatrix} 3 & 0 & 6 \\ 0 & 6 & 9 \\ 3 & 6 & 9 \end{bmatrix} + \begin{bmatrix} 18 & 6 & 6 \\ 6 & 12 & 18 \\ 0 & 6 & 12 \end{bmatrix} = \begin{bmatrix} 21 & 6 & 12 \\ 6 & 18 & 27 \\ 3 & 12 & 21 \end{bmatrix}$$

6. *If* $A = \begin{bmatrix} 1 & 4 & 3 & 6 \\ -3 & 7 & 0 & 2 \end{bmatrix}$ *and* $B = \begin{bmatrix} 2 & -3 & 4 & -1 \\ 0 & 6 & 5 & -7 \end{bmatrix}$ *find matrix C, if A – C = 3B.*

SOLUTION. Given, $A - C = 3B \Rightarrow C = A - 3B$

$$3B = 3\begin{bmatrix} 2 & -3 & 4 & -1 \\ 0 & 6 & 5 & -7 \end{bmatrix} = \begin{bmatrix} 6 & -9 & 12 & -3 \\ 0 & 18 & 15 & -21 \end{bmatrix}$$

$$C = \begin{bmatrix} 1 & 4 & 3 & 6 \\ -3 & 7 & 0 & 2 \end{bmatrix} - \begin{bmatrix} 6 & -9 & 12 & -3 \\ 0 & 18 & 15 & -21 \end{bmatrix} = \begin{bmatrix} -5 & 13 & -9 & 9 \\ -3 & -11 & -15 & 23 \end{bmatrix}$$

7. *Two farmers Radheyshyam and Hari Prasad cultivates three varieties of rice namely, Basmati, Permal and Naura. The sale (in Rs) of these varieties of rice by both the farmers in the month of September and October are given by the following matrices A and B.*

September sales

$$A = \begin{bmatrix} \text{Basmati} & \text{Permal} & \text{Naura} \\ 10{,}000 & 20{,}000 & 30{,}000 \\ 50{,}000 & 30{,}000 & 10{,}000 \end{bmatrix} \begin{matrix} \\ \text{Radheyshyam} \\ \text{Hari Prasad} \end{matrix}$$

October sales

$$B = \begin{bmatrix} \text{Basmati} & \text{Permal} & \text{Naura} \\ 5{,}000 & 10{,}000 & 6{,}000 \\ 20{,}000 & 10{,}000 & 10{,}000 \end{bmatrix} \begin{matrix} \\ \text{Radheyshyam} \\ \text{Hari Prasad} \end{matrix}$$

Find :

(i) What are combined sales in September and October for each farmer in each variety?

(ii) *What was the change in sales from September to October?*

(iii) *If the farmer receive 2% profit on gross rupees sales, compute the profit for each farmer and for each variety sold in October.*

SOLUTION. (i) The combined sales is given by

$$A+B=\begin{bmatrix} \text{Basmati} & \text{Permal} & \text{Naura} \\ 15{,}000 & 30{,}000 & 36{,}000 \\ 70{,}000 & 40{,}000 & 20{,}000 \end{bmatrix}\begin{matrix} \\ \text{Radheyshyam} \\ \text{Hari Prasad} \end{matrix}$$

(ii) Change in the sales from September to October is given by Now

$$A-B=\begin{bmatrix} \text{Basmati} & \text{Permal} & \text{Naura} \\ 5{,}000 & 10{,}000 & 24{,}000 \\ 30{,}000 & 20{,}000 & 0 \end{bmatrix}\begin{matrix} \\ \text{Radheyshyam} \\ \text{Hari Prasad} \end{matrix}$$

(iii) Since both the farmers receive 2% profit. Hence, profit for each farmer for each variety sold in October will be the entries of the matrix $\frac{2}{100}B$.

Now 2% of $B=\frac{2}{100}\times B = 0.02B$

$$= 0.02\begin{bmatrix} \text{Basmati} & \text{Permal} & \text{Naura} \\ 5{,}000 & 10{,}000 & 6{,}000 \\ 20{,}000 & 10{,}000 & 10{,}000 \end{bmatrix}\begin{matrix} \\ \text{Radheyshyam} \\ \text{Hari Prasad} \end{matrix}$$

$$= \begin{bmatrix} \text{Basmati} & \text{Permal} & \text{Naura} \\ 100 & 200 & 120 \\ 400 & 200 & 200 \end{bmatrix}\begin{matrix} \\ \text{Radheyshyam} \\ \text{Hari Prasad} \end{matrix}$$

Hence, in October, Radheyshyam receives Rs. 100, Rs. 200, and Rs. 120 as profit in the sales of each variety of rice respectively and Hariprasad receives profit of Rs. 400, 200 and 200 in each variety of rice respectively.

Exercise-3.1

1. (a) If a matrix has five rows and each rows contains 3 elements. Find the order of matrix.
   (b) If a matrix has 12 elements, find all possible order of matrix.
   (c) If a matrix has 5 elements, find all possible order of matrix.
2. Construct a matrix $[a_{ij}]_{2\times 2}$ where $a_{ij} = i + 2j$.
3. If $\begin{bmatrix} x & 3x-y \\ 2x+z & 3y-\omega \end{bmatrix} = \begin{bmatrix} 3 & 2 \\ 4 & 7 \end{bmatrix}$ then find x, y, z, ω.
4. Find $(A + B)$,
   if $A=\begin{bmatrix} 1 & 4 & 3 \\ 2 & 1 & 8 \\ 1 & 1 & 2 \end{bmatrix}$ and $B=\begin{bmatrix} 2 & 1 & 2 \\ 0 & 4 & 8 \\ 6 & 1 & 4 \end{bmatrix}$.
5. If $A=\begin{bmatrix} 2 & 3 & 4 \\ -3 & 0 & 2 \end{bmatrix}, B=\begin{bmatrix} 3 & -4 & -5 \\ 1 & 2 & 1 \end{bmatrix}$,
   $C=\begin{bmatrix} 5 & -1 & 0 \\ 7 & 0 & 3 \end{bmatrix}$, then find $A + B + C$.
6. Find $3A - 2B$,
   $A=\begin{bmatrix} 1 & 6 & 2 \\ 4 & 3 & -5 \end{bmatrix}, B=\begin{bmatrix} 2 & 9 & -6 \\ 4 & -5 & 3 \end{bmatrix}$.
7. Find the matrix x and y of order 2×2 where
   $2x-3y=\begin{bmatrix} 2 & 5 \\ 3 & 1 \end{bmatrix}, 3x+2y=\begin{bmatrix} 7 & 1 \\ 4 & 5 \end{bmatrix}$.
8. If $A=\begin{bmatrix} \cos^2\alpha & \sin^2\alpha \\ \cos\alpha & \sin\alpha \end{bmatrix}$ and $B=\begin{bmatrix} \sin^2\alpha & \cos^2\alpha \\ \sin\alpha & \cos\alpha \end{bmatrix}$. Find $(A + B)$.
9. If $A=\begin{bmatrix} 2 & 1 & 1 \\ 3 & -1 & 0 \\ 0 & 2 & 4 \end{bmatrix}, B=\begin{bmatrix} 9 & 7 & -1 \\ 3 & 5 & 4 \\ 2 & 1 & 6 \end{bmatrix}$
   and $C=\begin{bmatrix} 2 & -4 & 3 \\ 1 & -1 & 0 \\ 9 & 4 & 5 \end{bmatrix}$. Verify associative law for matrix addition.
10. If $A=\begin{bmatrix} -1 & 0 & 2 \\ 3 & 1 & 4 \end{bmatrix}, B=\begin{bmatrix} 0 & -2 & 5 \\ 1 & -3 & 1 \end{bmatrix}$
    and $C=\begin{bmatrix} 1 & -5 & 2 \\ 6 & 0 & -4 \end{bmatrix}$,
    then find $(2A - 3B + 4C)$.
11. Simplify :
    $\cos\theta\begin{bmatrix} \cos\theta & \sin\theta \\ -\sin\theta & \cos\theta \end{bmatrix} + \sin\theta\begin{bmatrix} \sin\theta & -\cos\theta \\ \cos\theta & \sin\theta \end{bmatrix}$
12. Find the value of x, y and z if :
    (i) $\begin{bmatrix} 3 & x \\ 4 & y \end{bmatrix} = 2\begin{bmatrix} 1.5 & 1 \\ z & 1 \end{bmatrix}$ (ii) $\begin{bmatrix} 4 & 3 \\ x & 5 \end{bmatrix} = \begin{bmatrix} y & z \\ 1 & 5 \end{bmatrix}$
13. If $A=\begin{bmatrix} 2+i & -i \\ 3 & 4i \end{bmatrix}$ and $B=\begin{bmatrix} 1-i & 2i \\ 2i & 3 \end{bmatrix}$, prove that $A+B=\begin{bmatrix} 3 & i \\ 3+2i & 4i+3 \end{bmatrix}$.

14. If $A=\begin{bmatrix}2 & 3\\ 4 & -5\end{bmatrix}, B=\begin{bmatrix}8 & 9\\ 6 & 7\end{bmatrix}$, find

(i) $4A$ (ii) $5B$

(iii) $2A + 3B$ (iv) $5A - 3B$.

15. If $x+y=\begin{bmatrix}2 & 1\\ 1 & 2\end{bmatrix}$ and $2x-y=\begin{bmatrix}1 & 2\\ 2 & 1\end{bmatrix}$, prove that $x=\begin{bmatrix}1 & 1\\ 1 & 1\end{bmatrix}$.

ANSWERS

1. (a) 5×3 (b) $1 \times 12, 2 \times 6, 3 \times 4, 4 \times 3, 6 \times 2, 12 \times 1$ (c) $1 \times 5, 5 \times 1$

2. $\begin{bmatrix}3 & 5\\ 4 & 6\end{bmatrix}$ **3.** $x = 3, y = 7, z = -2, \omega = 14$ **4.** $\begin{bmatrix}3 & 5 & 5\\ 2 & 5 & 16\\ 7 & 2 & 6\end{bmatrix}$ **5.** $\begin{bmatrix}10 & -2 & -1\\ 5 & 2 & 6\end{bmatrix}$

6. $\begin{bmatrix}-1 & 0 & 18\\ 4 & 19 & -21\end{bmatrix}$ **7.** $x=\frac{1}{13}\begin{bmatrix}25 & 13\\ 18 & 17\end{bmatrix}, y=\frac{1}{13}\begin{bmatrix}8 & -13\\ -1 & 7\end{bmatrix}$ **8.** $\begin{bmatrix}\frac{1}{\cos\alpha+\sin\alpha} & \frac{1}{\cos\alpha+\sin\alpha}\end{bmatrix}$

10. $\begin{bmatrix}2 & -14 & -3\\ 27 & 11 & -11\end{bmatrix}$ **11.** $\begin{bmatrix}1 & 0\\ 0 & 1\end{bmatrix}$ **12.** (i) 2, 2, 2 (ii) 1, 4, 3

14. (i) $\begin{bmatrix}8 & 12\\ 16 & -20\end{bmatrix}$ (ii) $\begin{bmatrix}40 & 45\\ 30 & 35\end{bmatrix}$ (iii) $\begin{bmatrix}28 & 33\\ 26 & 11\end{bmatrix}$ (iv) $\begin{bmatrix}-14 & -12\\ 2 & -46\end{bmatrix}$

3.7 MULTIPLICATION OF MATRICES

Definition. *Two matrices A and B can be multiplied only when*

No. of columns in A = No. of rows in B

In this way matrices A and B are said to be conformal to AB.

So, If $A = [a_{ik}]_{m \times p}$ and $B = [b_{kj}]_{p \times n}$ are two matrices, then order of AB is of $m \times n$ in which $(i, j)^{th}$ element is the sum of product of element in i^{th} row of A with corresponding element of jth column of B.

i.e., $AB = [a_{ik}]_{m \times p}[b_{kj}]_{p \times n}$

$$= \begin{bmatrix}a_{11} & a_{12} & \cdots & a_{1j} & \cdots & a_{1p}\\ a_{21} & a_{22} & \cdots & a_{2j} & \cdots & a_{2p}\\ \cdots & \cdots & \cdots & \cdots & \cdots & \cdots\\ a_{i1} & a_{i2} & \cdots & a_{ij} & \cdots & a_{ip}\\ \cdots & \cdots & \cdots & \cdots & \cdots & \cdots\\ a_{m1} & a_{m2} & \cdots & a_{mj} & \cdots & a_{mp}\end{bmatrix} \times \begin{bmatrix}b_{11} & b_{12} & \cdots & b_{1j} & \cdots & b_{1n}\\ b_{21} & b_{22} & \cdots & b_{2j} & \cdots & b_{2n}\\ \cdots & \cdots & \cdots & \cdots & \cdots & \cdots\\ b_{i1} & b_{i2} & \cdots & b_{ij} & \cdots & b_{ip}\\ \cdots & \cdots & \cdots & \cdots & \cdots & \cdots\\ b_{p1} & b_{p2} & \cdots & b_{pj} & \cdots & b_{pn}\end{bmatrix}$$

$$= [c_{ij}]_{m \times n}$$

where $c_{ij} = (i, j)^{th}$ element of product AB

$$= a_{i1}b_{1j} + a_{i2}b_{2j} + a_{i3}b_{3j} + \ldots + a_{ip}b_{pj} = \sum_{k=1}^{p} a_{ik}b_{kj}$$

= Row matrix of ith row of A × Column matrix of jth column of B

$$= \begin{bmatrix}a_{i1} & a_{i2} & a_{i3} & \cdots & a_{ip}\end{bmatrix}\begin{bmatrix}b_{1j}\\ b_{2j}\\ b_{3j}\\ \vdots\\ b_{pj}\end{bmatrix}$$

WORKING PROCEDURE

If matrix A and B are conformal to AB, then AB is obtained as follows :

STEP 1. The first element of AB is obtained by sum of product of element in first row of A with corresponding element of first column of B.

STEP 2. Again the second element of first row of AB is obtained by sum of product of elements in first row of A with corresponding elements of second column of B.

STEP 3. The third element of first row of AB is obtained by sum of product of elements of first row of A with corresponding elements of third column of B.

STEP 4. Continue the same procedure to find remaining elements of AB in first row.

STEP 5. As above repeat the procedure to get the elements in second, third, ... rows of AB.

For example: If $A = \begin{bmatrix} 1 & 0 & 5 \\ -1 & 2 & 4 \\ 3 & -2 & 6 \end{bmatrix}_{3\times3}, B = \begin{bmatrix} 4 & -1 \\ 2 & -2 \\ 5 & 3 \end{bmatrix}_{3\times2}$

Now
$$AB = \begin{bmatrix} 1\times4+0\times2+5\times5 & 1(-1)+0(-2)+5\times3 \\ (-1)\times4+2\times2+4\times5 & (-1)(-1)+2(-2)+4\times3 \\ 3\times4+(-2)\times2+6\times5 & 3(-1)+(-2)(-2)+6\times3 \end{bmatrix}_{3\times2}$$
$$= \begin{bmatrix} 29 & 14 \\ 20 & 9 \\ 38 & 19 \end{bmatrix}_{3\times2}$$

3.8 PROPERTIES OF MATRIX MULTIPLICATION

(1) Commutative Law

In general matrix multiplication does not obey commutative law, *i.e.*, it is not always possible that $AB = BA$.

This is clearified by following facts :

(a) If AB is well defined, then it is not necessary that BA is also defined for product *e.g.*, AB is possible for A of order 4×4 and B of order 4×3. But BA is not possible for this.

(b) If AB and BA both are possible and are of same order then it is not always possible that $AB = BA$.

- If A and B are two matrices such that AB and BA both exist. Then order of AB and BA are not necessarily equal.

(2) Associative Law

Multiplication of matrix follow associative law provided they are conformal. i.e., $A(BC) = (AB)C$ are possible only when A, B and C are of order $m \times n$, $n \times p$ and $p \times q$ respectively.

Proof. Let $A = [a_{ij}]_{m \times n}$, $B = [b_{jk}]_{n \times p}$ and $C = [c_{ki}]_{p \times q}$ be of order $m \times n$, $n \times p$ and $p \times q$ respectively.

Then first find BC which is a matrix of order $n \times q$.

$$BC = \left[\sum_{k=1}^{p} b_{jk} c_{ki} \right]$$

Similarly, by definition $A(BC)$ will be a matrix of the order $m \times q$, such that

$$A(BC) = \left[\sum_{j=1}^{n} a_{ij} \left(\sum_{k=1}^{p} b_{jk} c_{ki} \right) \right]$$

Here addition of elements follow the associative law, *i.e.*,

$$A(BC) = \left[\sum_{k=1}^{p} \left(\sum_{j=1}^{n} a_{ij} b_{jk} \right) c_{ki} \right] = (AB)C$$

So $$A(BC) = (AB)C$$

(3) Distributive Law

Multiplication of matrix is distributive over addition. i.e., $A(B + C) = AB + AC$
If A, B, C are of the order $m \times n, n \times p, n \times p$ respectively.

Proof. Let $A = [a_{ij}]_{m \times n}$, $B = [b_{jk}]_{n \times p}$ and $C = [c_{jk}]_{n \times p}$.

$$A(B+C) = \left[\sum_{j=1}^{n} a_{ij}(b_{jk} + c_{jk})\right] = \left[\sum_{j=1}^{n} a_{ij}b_{jk} + \sum_{j=1}^{n} a_{ij}c_{jk}\right]$$

$$= \left[\sum_{j=1}^{n} a_{ij}b_{jk}\right]_{m\times p} + \left[\sum_{j=1}^{n} a_{ij}c_{jk}\right]_{m\times p} = AB + AC$$

So $$A(B + C) = AB + AC$$

(4) *If product of two matrices is a null matrix then it is not necessary that one of the two matrix is null.*

If $$A = \begin{bmatrix} 0 & 1 \\ 0 & 0 \end{bmatrix}, B = \begin{bmatrix} 1 & 0 \\ 0 & 0 \end{bmatrix}$$

Then $$AB = \begin{bmatrix} 0 & 1 \\ 0 & 0 \end{bmatrix}\begin{bmatrix} 1 & 0 \\ 0 & 0 \end{bmatrix} = \begin{bmatrix} 0 & 0 \\ 0 & 0 \end{bmatrix}$$

So AB is null matrix even when both A and B are not null.

(5) Cancellation law

Cancellation law does not hold for matrix multiplication.

Proof. Let $A = \begin{bmatrix} 0 & 1 \\ 0 & 0 \end{bmatrix}, B = \begin{bmatrix} 2 & 0 \\ 0 & 0 \end{bmatrix}$ and $C = \begin{bmatrix} 1 & 0 \\ 0 & 0 \end{bmatrix}$

$$AB = \begin{bmatrix} 0 & 1 \\ 0 & 0 \end{bmatrix}\begin{bmatrix} 2 & 0 \\ 0 & 0 \end{bmatrix} = \begin{bmatrix} 0 & 0 \\ 0 & 0 \end{bmatrix}$$

$$AC = \begin{bmatrix} 0 & 1 \\ 0 & 0 \end{bmatrix}\begin{bmatrix} 1 & 0 \\ 0 & 0 \end{bmatrix} = \begin{bmatrix} 0 & 0 \\ 0 & 0 \end{bmatrix}$$

So $AB = AC$. But $B \neq C$

So cancellation law does not hold.

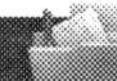

Solved Examples

1. *If $A = \begin{bmatrix} 2 & 5 \\ 1 & 3 \end{bmatrix}, B = \begin{bmatrix} 1 & -1 \\ -3 & 2 \end{bmatrix}$. Find AB and BA. Is $AB = BA$?*

SOLUTION. We have

$$AB = \begin{bmatrix} 2 & 5 \\ 1 & 3 \end{bmatrix}\begin{bmatrix} 1 & -1 \\ -3 & 2 \end{bmatrix}$$

$$= \begin{bmatrix} 2\times1+5\times(-3) & 2\times(-1)+5\times2 \\ 1\times1+3\times(-3) & 1\times(-1)+3\times2 \end{bmatrix}$$

$$\Rightarrow AB = \begin{bmatrix} -13 & 8 \\ -8 & 5 \end{bmatrix} \quad \ldots(1)$$

and

$$BA = \begin{bmatrix} 1 & -1 \\ -3 & 2 \end{bmatrix}\begin{bmatrix} 2 & 5 \\ 1 & 3 \end{bmatrix}$$

$$= \begin{bmatrix} 1\times2+(-1)\times1 & 1\times5+(-1)\times3 \\ (-3)\times2+2\times1 & (-3)\times5+2\times3 \end{bmatrix}$$

$$\Rightarrow BA = \begin{bmatrix} 1 & 2 \\ -4 & -9 \end{bmatrix} \quad \ldots(2)$$

By eqn. (1) and (2), $AB \neq BA$.

2. *If $A = \begin{bmatrix} ab & b^2 \\ -a^2 & -ab \end{bmatrix}$, show that $A^2 = 0$.*

SOLUTION. We have

$$A^2 = A \cdot A = \begin{bmatrix} ab & b^2 \\ -a^2 & -ab \end{bmatrix}\begin{bmatrix} ab & b^2 \\ -a^2 & -ab \end{bmatrix}$$

$$= \begin{bmatrix} a^2b^2 - a^2b^2 & ab^3 - ab^3 \\ -a^3b + a^3b & -a^2b^2 + a^2b^2 \end{bmatrix}$$

$$= \begin{bmatrix} 0 & 0 \\ 0 & 0 \end{bmatrix}$$

3. *Solve for the value of x and y.*

$$\begin{bmatrix} 3 & -4 \\ 1 & 2 \end{bmatrix}\begin{bmatrix} x \\ y \end{bmatrix} = \begin{bmatrix} 3 \\ 11 \end{bmatrix}$$

SOLUTION. Given $\begin{bmatrix} 3 & -4 \\ 1 & 2 \end{bmatrix}\begin{bmatrix} x \\ y \end{bmatrix} = \begin{bmatrix} 3 \\ 11 \end{bmatrix}$

$$\Rightarrow \quad \begin{bmatrix} 3x-4y \\ x+2y \end{bmatrix} = \begin{bmatrix} 3 \\ 11 \end{bmatrix}$$

$$\Rightarrow \quad 3x - 4y = 3$$

$$x + 2y = 11$$

On solving, we get

$$x = 5, y = 3.$$

4. *If* $A = \begin{bmatrix} 1 & 2 & 3 \\ 3 & 4 & 5 \end{bmatrix}$ *and* $B = \begin{bmatrix} 2 & 3 & 1 \\ 5 & 4 & 3 \\ 2 & 1 & 1 \end{bmatrix}$, *find AB. Is AB = BA?*

SOLUTION. We have

$$AB = \begin{bmatrix} 1 & 2 & 3 \\ 3 & 4 & 5 \end{bmatrix}_{2\times 3}\begin{bmatrix} 2 & 3 & 1 \\ 5 & 4 & 3 \\ 2 & 1 & 1 \end{bmatrix}_{3\times 3}$$

$$= \begin{bmatrix} 18 & 14 & 10 \\ 36 & 30 & 20 \end{bmatrix}$$

$$BA = \begin{bmatrix} 2 & 3 & 1 \\ 5 & 4 & 3 \\ 2 & 1 & 1 \end{bmatrix}_{3\times 3}\begin{bmatrix} 1 & 2 & 3 \\ 3 & 4 & 5 \end{bmatrix}_{2\times 3}$$

is not defined. So, $AB \neq BA$.

5. *If*

$$A = \begin{bmatrix} 1 & 1 & -1 \\ 2 & -3 & 4 \\ 3 & -2 & 3 \end{bmatrix}, B = \begin{bmatrix} -1 & -2 & -1 \\ 6 & 12 & 6 \\ 5 & 10 & 5 \end{bmatrix},$$

$$C = \begin{bmatrix} -1 & -1 & 1 \\ 2 & 2 & -2 \\ -3 & -3 & 3 \end{bmatrix}.$$

Prove that AB and CA are null matrices.

SOLUTION. We have

$$AB = \begin{bmatrix} 1 & 1 & -1 \\ 2 & -3 & 4 \\ 3 & -2 & 3 \end{bmatrix}\begin{bmatrix} -1 & -2 & -1 \\ 6 & 12 & 6 \\ 5 & 10 & 5 \end{bmatrix}$$

$$= \begin{bmatrix} -1+6-5 & -2+12-10 & -1+6-5 \\ -2-18+20 & -4-36+40 & -2-18+20 \\ -3-12+15 & -6-24+30 & -3-12+15 \end{bmatrix}$$

$$= \begin{bmatrix} 0 & 0 & 0 \\ 0 & 0 & 0 \\ 0 & 0 & 0 \end{bmatrix}$$

and $CA = \begin{bmatrix} -1 & -1 & 1 \\ 2 & 2 & -2 \\ -3 & -3 & 3 \end{bmatrix}\begin{bmatrix} 1 & 1 & -1 \\ 2 & -3 & 4 \\ 3 & -2 & 3 \end{bmatrix}$

$$= \begin{bmatrix} -1-2+3 & -1+3-2 & 1-4+3 \\ 2+4-6 & 2-6+4 & -2+8-6 \\ -3-6+9 & -3+9-6 & 3-12+9 \end{bmatrix}$$

$$= \begin{bmatrix} 0 & 0 & 0 \\ 0 & 0 & 0 \\ 0 & 0 & 0 \end{bmatrix}$$

6. *If* $A = \begin{bmatrix} 0 & -\tan\frac{\alpha}{2} \\ \tan\frac{\alpha}{2} & 0 \end{bmatrix}$, *and I be identity matrix of order 2 then show that*

$$(I + A) = (I - A)\begin{bmatrix} \cos\alpha & -\sin\alpha \\ \sin\alpha & \cos\alpha \end{bmatrix}$$

SOLUTION. We have

$$\cos\alpha = \frac{1-\tan^2(\alpha/2)}{1+\tan^2(\alpha/2)} = \frac{1-t^2}{1+t^2},$$

$$\sin\alpha = \frac{2\tan(\alpha/2)}{1+\tan^2(\alpha/2)} = \frac{2t}{1+t^2}$$

where $\tan\frac{\alpha}{2} = t$

Again

$$(I + A) = \begin{bmatrix} 1 & 0 \\ 0 & 1 \end{bmatrix} + \begin{bmatrix} 0 & -t \\ t & 0 \end{bmatrix} = \begin{bmatrix} 1 & -t \\ t & 1 \end{bmatrix}$$

$$(I - A) = \begin{bmatrix} 1 & 0 \\ 0 & 1 \end{bmatrix} - \begin{bmatrix} 0 & -t \\ t & 0 \end{bmatrix} = \begin{bmatrix} 1 & t \\ -t & 1 \end{bmatrix}$$

Now $(I - A)\begin{bmatrix} \cos\alpha & -\sin\alpha \\ \sin\alpha & \cos\alpha \end{bmatrix}$

$$= \begin{bmatrix} 1 & t \\ -t & 1 \end{bmatrix}\begin{bmatrix} \frac{1-t^2}{1+t^2} & \frac{-2t}{1+t^2} \\ \frac{2t}{1+t^2} & \frac{1-t^2}{1+t^2} \end{bmatrix}$$

$$= \begin{bmatrix} \frac{1-t^2}{1+t^2} + \frac{2t^2}{1+t^2} & \frac{-2t}{1+t^2} + \frac{t(1-t^2)}{1+t^2} \\ \frac{-t(1-t^2)}{1+t^2} + \frac{2t}{1+t^2} & \frac{2t^2}{1+t^2} + \frac{1-t^2}{1+t^2} \end{bmatrix}$$

$$= \begin{bmatrix} 1 & -t \\ t & 1 \end{bmatrix} = (I + A)$$

Hence,

$$(I + A) = (I - A)\begin{bmatrix} \cos\alpha & -\sin\alpha \\ \sin\alpha & \cos\alpha \end{bmatrix}$$

7. *If* $\begin{bmatrix}4\\1\\3\end{bmatrix}X = \begin{bmatrix}-4 & 8 & 4\\-1 & 2 & 1\\-3 & 6 & 3\end{bmatrix}$. *Find X.*

SOLUTION. Let $A = \begin{bmatrix}4\\1\\3\end{bmatrix}$ and $B = \begin{bmatrix}-4 & 8 & 4\\-1 & 2 & 1\\-3 & 6 & 3\end{bmatrix}$

Given $AX = B$ ...(1)

We have to find X.

Since A is a matrix of order 3×1 and B is a matrix of order 3×3 so order of X is 1×3.

Let $X = \begin{bmatrix}a & b & c\end{bmatrix}$

Now $AX = B$

$$\begin{bmatrix}4\\1\\3\end{bmatrix}\begin{bmatrix}a & b & c\end{bmatrix} = \begin{bmatrix}-4 & 8 & 4\\-1 & 2 & 1\\-3 & 6 & 3\end{bmatrix}$$

$$\begin{bmatrix}4a & 4b & 4c\\a & b & c\\3a & 3b & 3c\end{bmatrix} = \begin{bmatrix}-4 & 8 & 4\\-1 & 2 & 1\\-3 & 6 & 3\end{bmatrix}$$

Since both matrices are equal so corresponding elements must be equal.

Therefore $a = -1, b = 2, c = 1$

So, $X = \begin{bmatrix}-1 & 2 & 1\end{bmatrix}$

8. *If* $A = \begin{bmatrix}1 & 0\\1 & 1\end{bmatrix}, B = \begin{bmatrix}2 & 0\\1 & 1\end{bmatrix}$ *and* $C = \begin{bmatrix}-1 & 2\\3 & 1\end{bmatrix}$. *Then prove that* $A(B + C) = AB + AC$.

SOLUTION. Here

$$B + C = \begin{bmatrix}2 & 0\\1 & 1\end{bmatrix} + \begin{bmatrix}-1 & 2\\3 & 1\end{bmatrix} = \begin{bmatrix}1 & 2\\4 & 2\end{bmatrix}$$

$$A \cdot (B + C) = \begin{bmatrix}1 & 0\\1 & 1\end{bmatrix}\begin{bmatrix}1 & 2\\4 & 2\end{bmatrix}$$

$$= \begin{bmatrix}1 & 2\\5 & 4\end{bmatrix}_{2\times2} \quad ...(1)$$

and $AB = \begin{bmatrix}1 & 0\\1 & 1\end{bmatrix}_{2\times2} \times \begin{bmatrix}2 & 0\\1 & 1\end{bmatrix}_{2\times2}$

$$= \begin{bmatrix}2 & 0\\3 & 1\end{bmatrix}_{2\times2}$$

Now $AC = \begin{bmatrix}1 & 0\\1 & 1\end{bmatrix}_{2\times2} \times \begin{bmatrix}-1 & 2\\3 & 1\end{bmatrix}_{2\times2}$

$$= \begin{bmatrix}-1 & 2\\2 & 3\end{bmatrix}_{2\times2}$$

$$AB + AC = \begin{bmatrix}2 & 0\\3 & 1\end{bmatrix} + \begin{bmatrix}-1 & 2\\2 & 3\end{bmatrix}$$

$$= \begin{bmatrix}1 & 2\\5 & 4\end{bmatrix}_{2\times2} \quad ...(2)$$

It is clear from eq^n. (1) and (2) that

$A \cdot (B + C) = AB + AC$

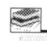

- Similarly we can prove that $(AB)C = A(BC)$

9. *If* $A = \begin{bmatrix}1 & 2 & 2\\2 & 1 & 2\\2 & 2 & 1\end{bmatrix}$ *verify that* $A^2 - 4A - 5I = 0$.

SOLUTION. We have $A = \begin{bmatrix}1 & 2 & 2\\2 & 1 & 2\\2 & 2 & 1\end{bmatrix}$

$$A^2 = A \cdot A = \begin{bmatrix}1 & 2 & 2\\2 & 1 & 2\\2 & 2 & 1\end{bmatrix}\begin{bmatrix}1 & 2 & 2\\2 & 1 & 2\\2 & 2 & 1\end{bmatrix}$$

and $= \begin{bmatrix}9 & 8 & 8\\8 & 9 & 8\\8 & 8 & 9\end{bmatrix}$

Also $4A = 4\begin{bmatrix}1 & 2 & 2\\2 & 1 & 2\\2 & 2 & 1\end{bmatrix}$

$$= \begin{bmatrix}4 & 8 & 8\\8 & 4 & 8\\8 & 8 & 4\end{bmatrix}$$

$$5I = 5\begin{bmatrix}1 & 0 & 0\\0 & 1 & 0\\0 & 0 & 1\end{bmatrix} = \begin{bmatrix}5 & 0 & 0\\0 & 5 & 0\\0 & 0 & 5\end{bmatrix}$$

$$A^2 - 4A - 5I = \begin{bmatrix}9 & 8 & 8\\8 & 9 & 8\\8 & 8 & 9\end{bmatrix} - \begin{bmatrix}4 & 8 & 8\\8 & 4 & 8\\8 & 8 & 4\end{bmatrix} - \begin{bmatrix}5 & 0 & 0\\0 & 5 & 0\\0 & 0 & 5\end{bmatrix}$$

$$= \begin{bmatrix}0 & 0 & 0\\0 & 0 & 0\\0 & 0 & 0\end{bmatrix} = 0 \quad \text{(Null matrix)}$$

10. *If* $A = \begin{bmatrix} -4 & 1 \\ 3 & 2 \end{bmatrix}$, *find f(A), if*

$f(x) = x^2 - 2x + 3.$

SOLUTION. Since, $f(x) = x^2 - 2x + 3$

Therefore, $f(A) = A^2 - 2A + 3I$

$$= \begin{bmatrix} -4 & 1 \\ 3 & 2 \end{bmatrix}\begin{bmatrix} -4 & 1 \\ 3 & 2 \end{bmatrix} - 2\begin{bmatrix} -4 & 1 \\ 3 & 2 \end{bmatrix} + 3\begin{bmatrix} 1 & 0 \\ 0 & 1 \end{bmatrix}$$

$$= \begin{bmatrix} 19 & -2 \\ -6 & 7 \end{bmatrix} - \begin{bmatrix} -8 & 2 \\ 6 & 4 \end{bmatrix} + \begin{bmatrix} 3 & 0 \\ 0 & 3 \end{bmatrix} = \begin{bmatrix} 30 & -4 \\ -12 & 6 \end{bmatrix}$$

11. *If* $A = \begin{bmatrix} \cos\theta & -\sin\theta \\ \sin\theta & \cos\theta \end{bmatrix}$ *then show that* $A^n = \begin{bmatrix} \cos n\theta & -\sin n\theta \\ \sin n\theta & \cos n\theta \end{bmatrix}$ *where n is positive integer.*

SOLUTION. For this we shall apply mathematical induction

Let $P(n): A^n = \begin{bmatrix} \cos n\theta & -\sin n\theta \\ \sin n\theta & \cos n\theta \end{bmatrix}$

For $n = 1$,

$$\text{L.H.S.} = A = \begin{bmatrix} \cos\theta & -\sin\theta \\ \sin\theta & \cos\theta \end{bmatrix}$$

$$\text{Now R.H.S.} = \begin{bmatrix} \cos\theta & -\sin\theta \\ \sin\theta & \cos\theta \end{bmatrix}$$

So, $P(1)$ is true. ...(1)

Let $P(m)$ be true

$$A^m = \begin{bmatrix} \cos m\theta & -\sin m\theta \\ \sin m\theta & \cos m\theta \end{bmatrix} \quad ...(2)$$

We have to prove that $P(m + 1)$ is true, *i.e.*,

$$A^{m+1} = \begin{bmatrix} \cos(m+1)\theta & -\sin(m+1)\theta \\ \sin(m+1)\theta & \cos(m+1)\theta \end{bmatrix} \quad ...(3)$$

Multiply both side of eq^n. (2) by matrix A

$$A^{m+1} = A\begin{bmatrix} \cos m\theta & -\sin m\theta \\ \sin m\theta & \cos m\theta \end{bmatrix}$$

$$= \begin{bmatrix} \cos\theta & -\sin\theta \\ \sin\theta & \cos\theta \end{bmatrix}\begin{bmatrix} \cos m\theta & -\sin m\theta \\ \sin m\theta & \cos m\theta \end{bmatrix}$$

$$= \begin{bmatrix} \cos\theta\cos m\theta - \sin\theta\sin m\theta & -\cos\theta\sin m\theta - \sin\theta\cos m\theta \\ \sin\theta\cos m\theta + \cos\theta\sin m\theta & -\sin\theta\sin m\theta + \cos\theta\cos m\theta \end{bmatrix}$$

$$= \begin{bmatrix} \cos(m+1)\theta & -\sin(m+1)\theta \\ \sin(m+1)\theta & \cos(m+1)\theta \end{bmatrix}$$

Therefore, $P(m + 1)$ is true. ...(4)

From eqn. (1) and (4), it is clear that $P(n)$ is true for all natural no. n.

- In the above question, if $n = 2$, then, we get $A^2 = \begin{bmatrix} \cos 2\alpha & -\sin 2\alpha \\ \sin 2\alpha & \cos 2\alpha \end{bmatrix}$

12. *In a co-operative stock there are 10 dozen Physics books, 8 dozen Chemistry books and 5 dozen Mathematics books. Selling price of each book is Rs. 8.30, 3.45 and 4.50 respectively. Using matrix, find the total sale of all books.*

SOLUTION. Let column matrix X represents the no. of books $X = 12\begin{bmatrix} 10 \\ 8 \\ 5 \end{bmatrix}\begin{matrix} \text{Physics} \\ \text{Chemistry} \\ \text{Mathematics} \end{matrix}$

$$\Rightarrow \quad X = \begin{bmatrix} 120 \\ 96 \\ 60 \end{bmatrix}$$

Now let row matrix Y represent selling price of books.

$$Y = \begin{bmatrix} \text{Physics} & \text{Chemistry} & \text{Mathematics} \\ 8.30 & 3.45 & 4.50 \end{bmatrix}$$

Therefore, total sale

$$= YX = \begin{bmatrix} 8.30 & 3.45 & 4.50 \end{bmatrix}\begin{bmatrix} 120 \\ 96 \\ 60 \end{bmatrix}$$

$= 8.30 \times 120 + 3.45 \times 96 + 4.50 \times 60$

$= 996 + 331.20 + 270 = \text{Rs. } 1597.20$

Exercise-3.2

1. Test whether the following matrices is conformal for multiplication or not:

(i) $A = \begin{bmatrix} -1 & 2 \\ 3 & 4 \end{bmatrix}, B = \begin{bmatrix} 5 \\ 6 \end{bmatrix}$

(ii) $A = \begin{bmatrix} -5 & -7 \\ 6 & -8 \end{bmatrix}, B = \begin{bmatrix} 3 & 4 \end{bmatrix}$

(iii) $A = \begin{bmatrix} 1 & 2 & 3 \\ 4 & 0 & 5 \\ 6 & 7 & 0 \end{bmatrix}, B = \begin{bmatrix} 1 & 0 & 2 & 4 \\ 3 & 7 & 0 & 0 \end{bmatrix}$

2. Find matrix B if $A = \begin{bmatrix} 1 & 4 \\ 3 & 2 \end{bmatrix}$ and $A + 2B = A2$.

3. If $A = \begin{bmatrix} 2 & 3 & 1 \\ -1 & 2 & 3 \\ 2 & 0 & 10 \end{bmatrix}$, find A^2.

4. If $A = \begin{bmatrix} 0 & 1 \\ 1 & 0 \end{bmatrix}$ and $B = \begin{bmatrix} 1 & 0 \\ 0 & -1 \end{bmatrix}$ prove that :

(i) $A^2 = B^2 = I$ (ii) $AB = -BA$

5. If $A = \begin{bmatrix} 0 & 0 & 1 \\ 2 & -3 & 0 \\ 1 & 1 & -1 \end{bmatrix}$, find $A^3 + 4A^2 - A$.

6. If $A = \begin{bmatrix} 2 & 0 & -1 \\ 2 & 3 & -2 \\ 0 & -2 & 5 \end{bmatrix}$, find $A^2 + 2A - 7I$.

7. Multiply $\begin{bmatrix} 1 & -2 & 3 \\ -4 & 2 & 5 \end{bmatrix} \times \begin{bmatrix} 2 & 3 \\ 4 & 5 \\ 2 & 1 \end{bmatrix}$.

8. If $\theta - \phi = \pi/2$, prove that

$$\begin{bmatrix} \cos^2\theta & \cos\theta\sin\theta \\ \cos\theta\sin\theta & \sin^2\theta \end{bmatrix}\begin{bmatrix} \cos^2\phi & \cos\phi\sin\phi \\ \cos\phi\sin\phi & \sin^2\phi \end{bmatrix} = 0$$

9. If $A = \begin{bmatrix} 1 & 3 & -1 \\ 2 & 2 & -1 \\ 3 & 0 & -1 \end{bmatrix}$ and $B = \begin{bmatrix} -2 & 3 & -1 \\ -1 & 2 & -1 \\ -6 & 9 & -4 \end{bmatrix}$, show that $AB = BA$.

10. If $A = \begin{bmatrix} 1 & 0 \\ 1 & 1 \end{bmatrix}, B = \begin{bmatrix} 2 & 0 \\ 1 & 1 \end{bmatrix}$ and $C = \begin{bmatrix} -1 & 2 \\ 3 & 1 \end{bmatrix}$, show that

(i) $(AB)C = A(BC)$

(ii) $A(B + C) = AB + AC$

(iii) $(B + C)A = BA + CA$

11. If $F(x) = \begin{bmatrix} \cos x & -\sin x & 0 \\ \sin x & \cos x & 0 \\ 0 & 0 & 1 \end{bmatrix}$. Show that

$$F(x)\cdot F(y) = F(x + y)$$

12. If $\begin{bmatrix} x & 0 \\ 2 & x+y \end{bmatrix}\begin{bmatrix} 1 & 0 \\ 0 & 1 \end{bmatrix} = \begin{bmatrix} 2 & 1 \\ 1 & 3 \end{bmatrix} - 2\begin{bmatrix} 0 & \frac{1}{2} \\ -\frac{1}{2} & \frac{3}{2} \end{bmatrix}$ find the value of x and y.

13. If ω is the cube root of unity, prove that

$$\left\{\begin{bmatrix} 1 & \omega & \omega^2 \\ \omega & \omega^2 & 1 \\ \omega^2 & 1 & \omega \end{bmatrix} + \begin{bmatrix} \omega & \omega^2 & 1 \\ \omega^2 & 1 & \omega \\ \omega & \omega^2 & 1 \end{bmatrix}\right\}\begin{bmatrix} 1 \\ \omega \\ \omega^2 \end{bmatrix} = \begin{bmatrix} 0 \\ 0 \\ 0 \end{bmatrix}$$

14. A manufacturer makes three items A, B, C which are sold in Delhi and Mumbai. Annual sale of these items are given as follow. If selling price of A, B and C are Rs. 2, 3 and 4 respectively then using matrix find total sale at each place.

	Items		
	A	***B***	***C***
Delhi	5,000	75,000	15,000
Mumbai	9,000	12,000	87,000

15. If $A = \begin{bmatrix} 1 & -1 \\ -1 & 1 \end{bmatrix}$ and $B = \begin{bmatrix} 1 & 1 \\ 1 & 1 \end{bmatrix}$. Prove that AB is null matrix.

16. If $A_\alpha = \begin{bmatrix} \cos\alpha & \sin\alpha \\ -\sin\alpha & \cos\alpha \end{bmatrix}$. Prove that

(i) $A_\alpha \cdot A_\beta = A_{\alpha+\beta}$ (ii) $A_\alpha \cdot A_{(-\alpha)} = I$

17. If $A = \begin{bmatrix} 1 & -1 \\ -1 & 1 \end{bmatrix}$. Prove that $A^3 = 4A$.

18. If $A = \begin{bmatrix} 3 & 3 & 5 \\ 2 & 3 & 4 \\ 5 & 2 & 3 \end{bmatrix}$. Prove that $AI_3 = I_3A$.

19. If $A = \begin{bmatrix} 2 & 0 & 0 \\ 0 & 2 & 0 \\ 0 & 0 & 2 \end{bmatrix}$ and $B = \begin{bmatrix} x_1 & y_1 & z_1 \\ x_2 & y_2 & z_2 \\ x_3 & y_3 & z_3 \end{bmatrix}$.

Prove that $AB = 2B$.

ANSWERS

1. (i) Yes (ii) No (iii) No **2.** $B = \begin{bmatrix} 6 & 4 \\ 3 & 7 \end{bmatrix}$ **3.** $\begin{bmatrix} 3 & 12 & 21 \\ 2 & 1 & 35 \\ 24 & 6 & 102 \end{bmatrix}$

5. $\begin{bmatrix} 5 & 0 & -3 \\ -6 & 14 & 0 \\ -3 & -3 & 8 \end{bmatrix}$ **6.** $\begin{bmatrix} 1 & 2 & -9 \\ 14 & 12 & -22 \\ -4 & -20 & 32 \end{bmatrix}$ **7.** $\begin{bmatrix} 0 & -4 \\ 10 & 3 \end{bmatrix}$

12. $x = 2, y = -2$ **14.** Delhi ₹ 2,95,000, Mumbai ₹ 402000

3.9 TRANSPOSE OF A MATRIX

Let A be the given matrix then the transpose of A denoted by A^T or A' is a matrix obtained by interchanging row and columns of A.

For example. Let $A = \begin{bmatrix} 1 & 2 & 3 \\ 4 & 5 & -1 \end{bmatrix}$, then $A' = \begin{bmatrix} 1 & 4 \\ 2 & 5 \\ 3 & -1 \end{bmatrix}$.

- The $(i, j)^{th}$ element of $A = (j, i)^{th}$ elements of A' and vice-versa.
- If the order of A is $m \times n$ then order of its transpose A' is $n \times m$.
- The transpose of the column matrix is a row matrix and transpose of the row matrix is a column matrix.

3.10 PROPERTIES OF THE TRANSPOSE OF MATRICES

(I) $(A + B)' = A' + B'$

(II) $(A')' = A$

(III) If $A = [a_{ij}]_{m \times n}$ and $B = [b_{jk}]_{n \times p}$, then $(AB)' = B'A'$.

Proof. Let $A = [a_{ij}]_{m \times n}$ and $B = [b_{jk}]_{n \times p}$, then

$$A' = [c_{ji}]_{n \times m} \text{ where } c_{ji} = a_{ij}$$

and

$$B' = [d_{kj}]_{p \times n} \text{ where } d_{kj} = b_{jk}$$

Clearly, AB is a matrix of order $m \times p$, therefore $(AB)'$ is a matrix of order $p \times m$ and since the order of B' is $p \times n$ and order of A' is $n \times m$, therefore the order of $B'A'$ is $p \times m$.

$\therefore$ $(AB)'$ and $B'A'$ are of the same order.

$$\therefore \quad (k, i)^{th} \text{ element of } (AB)' = (i, k)^{th} \text{ element of } AB = \sum_{j=1}^{n} a_{ij}b_{jk}$$

$$= \sum_{j=1}^{n} c_{ji}d_{kj} = \sum_{j=1}^{n} d_{kj}c_{ji} = (k, i)^{th} \text{ element of } B'A'.$$

$\because$ $(AB)'$ and $B'A'$ are of the same order and their $(k, i)^{th}$ element are equal.

Hence $(AB)' = B'A'$.

3.11 SYMMETRIC, SKEW-SYMMETRIC AND ORTHOGONAL MATRICES

1. **Symmetric Matrix:** A square matrix $A = [a_{ij}]$ is said to be a symmetric matrix if $a_{ij} = a_{ji}$, for all possible values of i and j.

   For example: The matrices $A = \begin{bmatrix} 1 & 3 & 5 \\ 3 & 2 & 0 \\ 5 & 0 & -1 \end{bmatrix}, B = \begin{bmatrix} 1 & 3 \\ 3 & 0 \end{bmatrix}$ are symmetric.

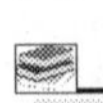

- A square matrix A is symmetric If $A' = A$.

2. **Skew-Symmetric Matrix:** A square matrix $A = [a_{ij}]$ is said to be skew-symmetric if $a_{ij} = -a_{ji}$ for all possible values of i and j.

   For example: $A = \begin{bmatrix} 0 & 2 \\ -2 & 0 \end{bmatrix}, B = \begin{bmatrix} 0 & 2 & -1 \\ -2 & 0 & -3 \\ 1 & 3 & 0 \end{bmatrix}$

- A square matrix is skew symmetric if and only if $A' = -A$.
- In skew symmetric matrix the elements of main diagonal are zero.

3. **Orthogonal Matrix:** A matrix A is said to be orthogonal if $A'A = I$ where A' is the transpose of A.

Solved Examples

1. *Write the transpose of matrix A.*

$$A = \begin{bmatrix} 5 & 1 & 2 \\ 6 & 4 & 5 \end{bmatrix}_{2\times3}$$

SOLUTION. Given $A = \begin{bmatrix} 5 & 1 & 2 \\ 6 & 4 & 5 \end{bmatrix}_{2\times3}$

$\therefore$ Transpose $A' = \begin{bmatrix} 5 & 6 \\ 1 & 4 \\ 2 & 5 \end{bmatrix}_{3\times2}$

2. *If* $A = \begin{bmatrix} 0 & 1 \\ 2 & 3 \end{bmatrix}$ *and* $B = \begin{bmatrix} 1 & 2 \\ 3 & 4 \end{bmatrix}$, *then verify* $(A + B)' = A' + B'$ *and find* $(AB)'$.

SOLUTION. We have

$$A' = \begin{bmatrix} 0 & 2 \\ 1 & 3 \end{bmatrix}, B' = \begin{bmatrix} 1 & 3 \\ 2 & 4 \end{bmatrix} \qquad \ldots(1)$$

and

$$A + B = \begin{bmatrix} 0 & 1 \\ 2 & 3 \end{bmatrix} + \begin{bmatrix} 1 & 2 \\ 3 & 4 \end{bmatrix} = \begin{bmatrix} 1 & 3 \\ 5 & 7 \end{bmatrix}$$

$$\Rightarrow \qquad (A + B)' = \begin{bmatrix} 1 & 5 \\ 3 & 7 \end{bmatrix} \qquad \ldots(2)$$

From eqn. (1),

$$A' + B' = \begin{bmatrix} 0 & 2 \\ 1 & 3 \end{bmatrix} + \begin{bmatrix} 1 & 3 \\ 2 & 4 \end{bmatrix} = \begin{bmatrix} 1 & 5 \\ 3 & 7 \end{bmatrix} \qquad \ldots(3)$$

From eqn. (2) and (3),

$(A + B)' = A' + B'$

$$(AB)' = B'A' = \begin{bmatrix} 1 & 3 \\ 2 & 4 \end{bmatrix}\begin{bmatrix} 0 & 2 \\ 1 & 3 \end{bmatrix}$$

$$= \begin{bmatrix} 0+3 & 2+9 \\ 0+4 & 4+12 \end{bmatrix} = \begin{bmatrix} 3 & 11 \\ 4 & 16 \end{bmatrix} \qquad \ldots(4)$$

3. *If* $A = \begin{bmatrix} 2 & 4 & 1 \\ -1 & 0 & 2 \end{bmatrix}, B = \begin{bmatrix} 3 & 4 \\ -1 & 2 \\ 2 & 1 \end{bmatrix}$.

Show that $(AB)' = B'A'$.

SOLUTION. We have

$$AB = \begin{bmatrix} 2 & 4 & 1 \\ -1 & 0 & 2 \end{bmatrix}_{2\times3} \begin{bmatrix} 3 & 4 \\ -1 & 2 \\ 2 & 1 \end{bmatrix}_{3\times2}$$

$$= \begin{bmatrix} 0 & 15 \\ 1 & -2 \end{bmatrix}_{2\times2}$$

$$(AB)' = \begin{bmatrix} 0 & 1 \\ 15 & -2 \end{bmatrix}_{2\times2} \qquad \ldots(1)$$

Again

$$B' = \begin{bmatrix} 3 & -1 & 2 \\ 4 & 2 & 1 \end{bmatrix}_{2\times3}, A' = \begin{bmatrix} 2 & -1 \\ 4 & 0 \\ -1 & 2 \end{bmatrix}_{3\times2}$$

$$B'A' = \begin{bmatrix} 3 & -1 & 2 \\ 4 & 2 & 1 \end{bmatrix}\begin{bmatrix} 2 & -1 \\ 4 & 0 \\ -1 & 2 \end{bmatrix}$$

$$= \begin{bmatrix} 0 & 1 \\ 15 & -2 \end{bmatrix}_{2\times2} \qquad \ldots(2)$$

From eqn. (1) and (2),

$(AB)' = B'A'$

4. *If*

$$A = \begin{bmatrix} 1 & 2 & 3 \\ -1 & 2 & 4 \\ 0 & 0 & 1 \end{bmatrix} \text{ and } B = \begin{bmatrix} -1 & -2 & 0 \\ 0 & 1 & 3 \\ -1 & 2 & 0 \end{bmatrix}.$$

Prove that $(AB)' = B'A'$.

SOLUTION. By multiplication of matrices, we have

$$AB = \begin{bmatrix} -4 & 6 & 6 \\ -3 & 12 & 6 \\ -1 & 2 & 0 \end{bmatrix}_{3\times3}$$

$$\Rightarrow \quad (AB)' = \begin{bmatrix} -4 & -3 & -1 \\ 6 & 12 & 2 \\ 6 & 6 & 0 \end{bmatrix}_{3\times3} \qquad \ldots(1)$$

Again $A' = \begin{bmatrix} 1 & -1 & 0 \\ 2 & 2 & 0 \\ 3 & 4 & 1 \end{bmatrix}$ and

$$B' = \begin{bmatrix} -1 & 0 & -1 \\ -2 & 1 & 2 \\ 0 & 3 & 0 \end{bmatrix}$$

Again by multiplication of matrices, we have

$$B'A' = \begin{bmatrix} -4 & -3 & -1 \\ 6 & 12 & 2 \\ 6 & 6 & 0 \end{bmatrix} \qquad \ldots(2)$$

From eqn. (1) and (2), it is clear

$(AB)' = B'A'$

5. *Express the following matrix as a sum of symmetric and skew-symmetric matrices.*

$$\begin{bmatrix} 1 & 3 & 5 \\ -6 & 8 & 3 \\ -4 & 6 & 5 \end{bmatrix}$$

SOLUTION. For any square matrix, we can always write

$$A = \frac{1}{2}(A + A') + \frac{1}{2}(A - A')$$

where $\frac{1}{2}(A + A')$ is symmetric matrix

and $\frac{1}{2}(A - A')$ is skew-symmetric matrix.

Given that $A = \begin{bmatrix} 1 & 3 & 5 \\ -6 & 8 & 3 \\ -4 & 6 & 5 \end{bmatrix}$

$$\therefore \quad A' = \begin{bmatrix} 1 & -6 & -4 \\ 3 & 8 & 6 \\ 5 & 3 & 5 \end{bmatrix}$$

$$\Rightarrow \frac{1}{2}(A + A') = \frac{1}{2}\begin{bmatrix} 1+1 & 3-6 & 5-4 \\ -6+3 & 8+8 & 3+6 \\ -4+5 & 6+3 & 5+5 \end{bmatrix}$$

$$= \frac{1}{2}\begin{bmatrix} 2 & -3 & 1 \\ -3 & 16 & 9 \\ 1 & 9 & 10 \end{bmatrix} = \begin{bmatrix} 1 & \frac{-3}{2} & \frac{1}{2} \\ \frac{-3}{2} & 8 & \frac{9}{2} \\ \frac{1}{2} & \frac{9}{2} & 5 \end{bmatrix}$$

which is a symmetric matrix.
Again

$$\frac{1}{2}(A - A') = \frac{1}{2}\begin{bmatrix} 1-1 & 3+6 & 5+4 \\ -6-3 & 8-8 & 3-6 \\ -4-5 & 6-3 & 5-5 \end{bmatrix}$$

$$= \frac{1}{2}\begin{bmatrix} 0 & 9 & 9 \\ -9 & 0 & -3 \\ -9 & 3 & 0 \end{bmatrix} = \begin{bmatrix} 0 & \frac{9}{2} & \frac{9}{2} \\ \frac{-9}{2} & 0 & \frac{-3}{2} \\ \frac{-9}{2} & \frac{3}{2} & 0 \end{bmatrix}$$

which is a skew symmetric matrix.

Exercise-3.3

1. If $A = \begin{bmatrix} 1 & 0 & 5 \\ 2 & -1 & 3 \\ 4 & 1 & 0 \end{bmatrix}$ and $B = \begin{bmatrix} 3 & 2 & 1 \\ 0 & 2 & 1 \\ 3 & 2 & 5 \end{bmatrix}$. Show that
(a) $(A + B)' = A' + B'$
(b) $(2A)' = 2A'$

2. If $A = \begin{bmatrix} 1 & 0 \\ 3 & 2 \end{bmatrix}$ and $B = \begin{bmatrix} 4 & 0 \\ 6 & 5 \end{bmatrix}$. Show that $(AB)' = B'A'$.

3. (i) If $A = \begin{bmatrix} 2 & 5 \\ 3 & 1 \end{bmatrix}$ and $B = \begin{bmatrix} 5 & 7 \\ 2 & 0 \end{bmatrix}$. Show that $(AB)' = B'A'$.

(ii) If $A = \begin{bmatrix} 2 & 3 \\ 0 & 1 \end{bmatrix}$ and $B = \begin{bmatrix} 3 & 4 \\ 2 & 1 \end{bmatrix}$. Prove that $(AB)' = B'A'$.

(iii) If $A = \begin{bmatrix} 2 & 4 \\ 3 & 1 \end{bmatrix}$ and $B = \begin{bmatrix} 5 & 6 \\ 2 & 0 \end{bmatrix}$. Prove that $(AB)' = B'A'$.

4. If $A = \begin{bmatrix} 3 \\ 5 \\ 4 \\ 2 \end{bmatrix}$. Then find $A'A$ and AA'.

5. If $A = \begin{bmatrix} 4 & 1 \\ 2 & 3 \end{bmatrix}$ and $B = \begin{bmatrix} 3 & 2 \\ 5 & 1 \\ 3 & 5 \end{bmatrix}$. Find AB' and BA.

6. For the following matrices, show that
(i) $(A + B)' = B' + A' = A' + B'$
(ii) $(AB)' = B'A'$

$$A = \begin{bmatrix} 1 & 0 & 5 \\ 6 & 2 & 1 \\ 7 & 1 & 5 \end{bmatrix}, B = \begin{bmatrix} 5 & 14 & 10 \\ 4 & 2 & 3 \\ 0 & 9 & 5 \end{bmatrix}.$$

7. If $A = \begin{bmatrix} 1 & -1 & 0 \\ 2 & 1 & 3 \\ 4 & 1 & 8 \end{bmatrix}$ and $B = \begin{bmatrix} 4 & 1 & 0 \\ 2 & -3 & 1 \\ 1 & 1 & -1 \end{bmatrix}$.
Show that $(AB)' = B'A'$.

8. Given that $A = \begin{bmatrix} 1 & 0 & 3 \\ 2 & -1 & 1 \end{bmatrix}, B = \begin{bmatrix} 3 & 4 & 1 \\ 0 & -1 & 5 \\ 1 & 2 & -2 \end{bmatrix}$

and $C = \begin{bmatrix} 2 \\ -1 \\ 4 \end{bmatrix}$, find

(a) $(AB)'$ (b) $B'A'$
(c) $(BC)'$ (d) $C'A'$

ANSWERS

4. $A'A = [3^2 + 5^2 + 4^2 + 2^2] = 54, AA' = \begin{bmatrix} 9 & 15 & 12 & 6 \\ 15 & 25 & 20 & 10 \\ 12 & 20 & 16 & 8 \\ 6 & 10 & 8 & 4 \end{bmatrix}$ **5.** $AB' = \begin{bmatrix} 14 & 21 & 17 \\ 12 & 13 & 21 \end{bmatrix}, BA = \begin{bmatrix} 16 & 9 \\ 22 & 8 \\ 22 & 18 \end{bmatrix}$

8. (a) $\begin{bmatrix} 6 & 7 \\ 10 & 11 \\ -5 & -5 \end{bmatrix}$ (b) $\begin{bmatrix} 6 & 7 \\ 10 & 11 \\ -5 & -5 \end{bmatrix}$ (c) $[6 \quad 21 \quad -8]$ (d) $[14 \quad 9]$

3.12 ELEMENTARY OPERATIONS (OR TRANSFORMATION) ON MATRICES

The elementary transformation on matrices are as follows:

(i) The interchange of any two rows or columns: The process to interchange i^{th} and j^{th} rows is written as R_{ij} or $R_i \leftrightarrow R_j$.

i.e., $R_{ij} \equiv$ Interchange i^{th} & j^{th} row $\equiv R_i \leftrightarrow R_j$.

Similarly $C_{ij} \equiv$ Interchange i^{th} & j^{th} column $\equiv C_i \leftrightarrow C_j$.

(ii) The multiplication of the elements of any row (or column) by a non-zero number: In symbol, if we multiply i^{th} row by a scalar k, then we write $R_i(k)$, $k \neq 0$.

i.e., $R_i(k) \equiv$ multiply i^{th} row by a scalar $k \equiv R_i \to kR_i$

Similarly, $C_i(k) \equiv$ multiply i^{th} column by a scalar $k \equiv C_i \to kC_i$

(iii) The addition to the elements of any row or column, the corresponding elements of any other row or column multiplied by a non-zero number.

i.e., $R_{ij}(k) \equiv k$ times the jth row plus i^{th} row $\equiv R_i \to R_i + kR_j$

$R_{ij}(-k) \equiv i^{th}$ row minus k times j^{th} column $\equiv R_i \to R_i - kR_j$

$R_{ij}(1) \equiv$ addition of ith and j^{th} row $\equiv R_i \to R_i + R_j$

$R_{ij}(-1) \equiv$ Subtract j^{th} row from i^{th} row $\equiv R_i \to R_i - R_j$

Similarly, $C_{ij}(k) \equiv$ Add k items the jth column to i^{th} column $\equiv C_i \to C_i + kC_j$

$C_{ij}(-k) \equiv$ Subtract k times the jth column from i^{th} column $\equiv C_i \to C_i - kC_j$

- Elementary transformations are applied either on columns or row but not on both.

3.13 EQUIVALENT MATRICES AND ELEMENTARY MATRIX

3.13.1 EQUIVALENT MATRICES

Two matrices A and B are said to be equivalent if one is obtained from other by applying finite no. of elementary operations. It is written as $A \sim B$.

For example: Let $A = \begin{bmatrix} 1 & 2 & 3 \\ 2 & 3 & 4 \\ 2 & 0 & 5 \end{bmatrix}$ and $B = \begin{bmatrix} 2 & 3 & 8 \\ 1 & 2 & 6 \\ 2 & 0 & 10 \end{bmatrix}$

Now $A = \begin{bmatrix} 1 & 2 & 3 \\ 2 & 3 & 4 \\ 2 & 0 & 5 \end{bmatrix} \sim \begin{bmatrix} 2 & 3 & 4 \\ 1 & 2 & 3 \\ 2 & 0 & 5 \end{bmatrix}$ $(R_1 \leftrightarrow R_2)$

$\sim \begin{bmatrix} 2 & 3 & 8 \\ 1 & 2 & 6 \\ 2 & 0 & 10 \end{bmatrix} = B$ $(C_3 \to 2C_3)$

Hence $A \sim B$, since B is obtained by applying two elementary operations on A.

3.13.2 ELEMENTARY MATRIX

Elementary matrix is obtained on applying only one elementary operation on identity matrix.

For example: $I = \begin{bmatrix} 1 & 0 \\ 0 & 1 \end{bmatrix}$

Then $A = \begin{bmatrix} 2 & 0 \\ 0 & 1 \end{bmatrix}$ $R_1 \to 2R_1$

Clearly, A is elementary matrix.

3.13.3 SINGULAR SQUARE MATRIX

A square matrix is said to be singular if value of its determinant is zero.
i.e., if $|A| = 0$, then A is singular.

3.13.4 NON-SINGULAR SQUARE OF A MATRIX

A square matrix is said to be non-singular if value of its determinant is non-zero.
i.e., if $|A| \neq 0$, then A is non-singular.

3.14 INVERSE MATRIX OR INVERSE OF A MATRIX

Inverse of a square matrix A (non-singular) is a square matrix which gives identity matrix on multiplying with A. In other words if for two square matrices $AB = I$, then B is said to be the inverse of A. Inverse of A is written as A^{-1}.

Similarly if $AB = I$. Then $B = A^{-1}$

$$AA^{-1} = I.$$

3.14.1 IMPORTANT PROPERTIES OF INVERSE MATRIX

(i) If A^{-1} is inverse of A, then $AA^{-1} = A^{-1}A = I$.
(ii) Inverse of a matrix is always unique.
(iii) If A and B are two invertible matrices with same order, then AB is also invertible and $(AB)^{-1} = B^{-1}A^{-1}$.
(iv) For three matrices A, B, C $(ABC)^{-1} = C^{-1}B^{-1}A^{-1}$.
(v) $(A')^{-1} = (A^{-1})'$

3.15 INVERSE OF A MATRIX BY ELEMENTARY OPERATIONS

3.15.1 ELEMENTARY OPERATION ON MATRIX

Let A, B and X be three matrices such that

$$X = AB \qquad \text{...(1)}$$

Matrix equation is valid when a row operation is applied on X (Left hand side) and pre matrix A of (Right hand side) on same row. Similarly column operation is valid on matrix equation when it is applied on X and post matrix B of right hand side on same column. Row and column operations are applied on alternate order.

By using above method we can find the inverse of a matrix A if A is invertible.

3.15.2 TO FIND A^{-1}

Let A be a n order square matrix.

Then $$A = I_n A = IA \qquad \text{...(1)}$$

Now apply only elementary row operation on $A = IA$ until left hand side A became I. A in right hand side remains same. Same row operation are applied on I on right hand side. After elementary operations it became a new matrix B.

i.e., $$I = BA$$

By definition : $$B = A^{-1}$$

Solved Examples

1. *Using elementary operation find* A^{-1}

where $A = \begin{bmatrix} 6 & -3 \\ -2 & 1 \end{bmatrix}$

SOLUTION. To find A^{-1} we use elementary row operations.
Take the matrix equation

$$A = IA$$

Then $$\begin{bmatrix} 6 & -3 \\ -2 & 1 \end{bmatrix} = \begin{bmatrix} 1 & 0 \\ 0 & 1 \end{bmatrix} A$$

$$\Rightarrow \begin{bmatrix} 1 & -1/2 \\ -2 & 1 \end{bmatrix} = \begin{bmatrix} 1/6 & 0 \\ 0 & 1 \end{bmatrix} A$$

$$\left[R_1 \to \frac{1}{6}R_1\right]$$

$$\begin{bmatrix} 1 & -1/2 \\ 0 & 0 \end{bmatrix} = \begin{bmatrix} 1/6 & 0 \\ 1/3 & 1 \end{bmatrix} A$$

$$[R_2 \to R_2 + 2R_1]$$

A^{-1} is not possible because all elements of second row of matrix in left are zero.

2. *Find the inverse of A by elementary transformation, where* $A = \begin{bmatrix} 1 & 2 & 3 \\ 1 & 3 & 5 \\ 1 & 5 & 12 \end{bmatrix}$.

SOLUTION. Considering the identity

$$A = IA$$

$$\begin{bmatrix} 1 & 2 & 3 \\ 1 & 3 & 5 \\ 1 & 5 & 12 \end{bmatrix} = \begin{bmatrix} 1 & 0 & 0 \\ 0 & 1 & 0 \\ 0 & 0 & 1 \end{bmatrix} A$$

By elementary row transformation, we get

$$\begin{bmatrix} 1 & 2 & 3 \\ 0 & 1 & 2 \\ 0 & 3 & 9 \end{bmatrix} = \begin{bmatrix} 1 & 0 & 0 \\ -1 & 1 & 0 \\ -1 & 0 & 1 \end{bmatrix} A$$

$$(R_2 \to R_2 - R_1, R_3 \to R_3 - R_1)$$

$$\begin{bmatrix} 1 & 0 & -1 \\ 0 & 1 & 2 \\ 0 & 0 & 3 \end{bmatrix} = \begin{bmatrix} 3 & -2 & 0 \\ -1 & 1 & 0 \\ 2 & -3 & 1 \end{bmatrix} A$$

$$(R_1 \to R_1 - 2R_2)$$
$$(R_3 \to R_3 - 3R_2)$$

$$\Rightarrow \begin{bmatrix} 1 & 0 & -1 \\ 0 & 1 & 2 \\ 0 & 0 & 1 \end{bmatrix} = \begin{bmatrix} 3 & -2 & 0 \\ -1 & 1 & 0 \\ 2/3 & -1 & 1/3 \end{bmatrix} A$$

$$(R_3 \to 1/3\, R_3)$$

$$\Rightarrow \begin{bmatrix} 1 & 0 & 0 \\ 0 & 1 & 0 \\ 0 & 0 & 1 \end{bmatrix} = \begin{bmatrix} 11/3 & -3 & 1/3 \\ -7/3 & 3 & -2/3 \\ 2/3 & -1 & 1/3 \end{bmatrix} A$$

$$(R_1 \to R_1 + R_3)$$
$$(R_2 \to R_2 - 2R_3)$$

$$A^{-1} = \begin{bmatrix} 11/3 & -3 & 1/3 \\ -7/3 & 3 & -2/3 \\ 2/3 & -1 & 1/3 \end{bmatrix}$$

or $$\frac{1}{3}\begin{bmatrix} 11 & -9 & 1 \\ -7 & 9 & -2 \\ 2 & -3 & 1 \end{bmatrix}$$

3. *Using elementary transformation find the inverse of the following matrix.*

$$\begin{bmatrix} 1 & 3 & -2 \\ -3 & 0 & -5 \\ 2 & 5 & 0 \end{bmatrix}$$

SOLUTION. Let $A = \begin{bmatrix} 1 & 3 & -2 \\ -3 & 0 & -5 \\ 2 & 5 & 0 \end{bmatrix}$

Now $A = I_3A$

$$\begin{bmatrix} 1 & 3 & -2 \\ -3 & 0 & -5 \\ 2 & 5 & 0 \end{bmatrix} = \begin{bmatrix} 1 & 0 & 0 \\ 0 & 1 & 0 \\ 0 & 0 & 1 \end{bmatrix} A$$

$$\begin{bmatrix} 1 & 3 & -2 \\ 0 & 9 & -11 \\ 0 & -1 & 4 \end{bmatrix} = \begin{bmatrix} 1 & 0 & 0 \\ 3 & 1 & 0 \\ -2 & 0 & 1 \end{bmatrix} A$$

$$(R_2 \to R_2 + 3R_1)$$
$$(R_3 \to R_3 - 2R_1)$$

$$\begin{bmatrix} 1 & 3 & -2 \\ 0 & 1 & 21 \\ 0 & -1 & 4 \end{bmatrix} = \begin{bmatrix} 1 & 0 & 0 \\ -13 & 1 & 8 \\ -2 & 0 & 1 \end{bmatrix} A$$

$$(R_2 \to R_2 + 8R_3)$$

$$\begin{bmatrix} 1 & 0 & -65 \\ 0 & 1 & 21 \\ 0 & 0 & 25 \end{bmatrix} = \begin{bmatrix} 40 & -3 & -24 \\ -13 & 1 & 8 \\ -15 & 1 & 9 \end{bmatrix} A$$

$$(R_1 \to R_1 - 3R_2)$$
$$(R_3 \to R_3 + R_2)$$

$$\begin{bmatrix} 1 & 0 & -65 \\ 0 & 1 & 21 \\ 0 & 0 & 1 \end{bmatrix} = \begin{bmatrix} 40 & -3 & -24 \\ -13 & 1 & 8 \\ \frac{-3}{5} & \frac{1}{25} & \frac{9}{25} \end{bmatrix} A$$

$$R_3 \to \frac{1}{25}R_3$$

$$\begin{bmatrix} 1 & 0 & 0 \\ 0 & 1 & 0 \\ 0 & 0 & 1 \end{bmatrix} = \begin{bmatrix} 1 & \frac{-2}{5} & \frac{-3}{5} \\ \frac{-2}{5} & \frac{4}{25} & \frac{11}{25} \\ \frac{-3}{5} & \frac{1}{25} & \frac{9}{25} \end{bmatrix} A$$

$$(R_1 \to R_1 + 65R_3)$$
$$(R_2 \to R_2 - 21R_3)$$

$I_3 = BA$ where

$$B = \begin{bmatrix} +1 & \frac{-2}{5} & \frac{-3}{5} \\ \frac{-2}{5} & \frac{4}{25} & \frac{11}{25} \\ \frac{-3}{5} & \frac{1}{25} & \frac{9}{25} \end{bmatrix} = A^{-1}$$

4. *Find the inverse of matrix*

$$A = \begin{bmatrix} 1 & 1 & 1 \\ 1 & -1 & 1 \\ 2 & 1 & -1 \end{bmatrix}$$

SOLUTION. Consider, $A = IA$

$$\Rightarrow \begin{bmatrix} 1 & 1 & 1 \\ 1 & -1 & 1 \\ 2 & 1 & -1 \end{bmatrix} = \begin{bmatrix} 1 & 0 & 0 \\ 0 & 1 & 0 \\ 0 & 0 & 1 \end{bmatrix} A$$

$$\Rightarrow \begin{bmatrix} 1 & 0 & -2 \\ 1 & -1 & 1 \\ 2 & 1 & -1 \end{bmatrix} = \begin{bmatrix} -1 & 0 & 1 \\ 0 & 1 & 0 \\ 0 & 0 & 1 \end{bmatrix} A$$

$R_1 \to R_3 - R_1$

$$\Rightarrow \begin{bmatrix} 1 & 0 & -2 \\ 0 & -1 & 3 \\ 0 & 1 & 3 \end{bmatrix} = \begin{bmatrix} -1 & 0 & 1 \\ 1 & 1 & -1 \\ 2 & 0 & -1 \end{bmatrix} A,$$

$R_2 \to R_2 - R_1$ and $R_3 \to R_3 - 2R_1$

$$\Rightarrow \begin{bmatrix} 1 & 0 & -2 \\ 0 & -1 & 3 \\ 0 & 0 & 6 \end{bmatrix} = \begin{bmatrix} -1 & 0 & 1 \\ 1 & 1 & -1 \\ 3 & 1 & -2 \end{bmatrix} A$$

$R_3 \to R_2 + R_3$

$$\Rightarrow \begin{bmatrix} 1 & 0 & -2 \\ 0 & -1 & 3 \\ 0 & 0 & 1 \end{bmatrix} = \begin{bmatrix} -1 & 0 & 1 \\ 1 & 1 & -1 \\ 1/2 & 1/6 & -1/3 \end{bmatrix} A$$

$R_3 \to \frac{1}{6} R_3$

$$\Rightarrow \begin{bmatrix} 1 & 0 & 0 \\ 0 & -1 & 0 \\ 0 & 0 & 1 \end{bmatrix} = \begin{bmatrix} 0 & 1/3 & 1/3 \\ -1/2 & 1/2 & 0 \\ 1/2 & 1/6 & -1/3 \end{bmatrix} A$$

$(R_1 \to R_1 + 2R_3)$
$(R_2 \to R_2 - 3R_3)$

$$\Rightarrow \begin{bmatrix} 1 & 0 & 0 \\ 0 & 1 & 0 \\ 0 & 0 & 1 \end{bmatrix} = \begin{bmatrix} 0 & 1/3 & 1/3 \\ 1/2 & -1/2 & 0 \\ 1/2 & 1/6 & -1/3 \end{bmatrix} A$$

$(R_2 \to -R_2)$

$$A^{-1} = \begin{bmatrix} 0 & 1/3 & 1/3 \\ 1/2 & -1/2 & 0 \\ 1/2 & 1/6 & -1/3 \end{bmatrix}$$

Exercise-3.4

Using elementary transformation, find the inverse of matrix A. (Qus. 1-11)

1. $A = \begin{bmatrix} 2 & 1 \\ 7 & 4 \end{bmatrix}$ **2.** $A = \begin{bmatrix} 2 & 1 \\ 1 & 1 \end{bmatrix}$

3. $A = \begin{bmatrix} 2 & 3 \\ 1 & 4 \end{bmatrix}$ **4.** $A = \begin{bmatrix} 3 & -1 \\ -4 & 2 \end{bmatrix}$

5. $A = \begin{bmatrix} 2 & 1 \\ 4 & 2 \end{bmatrix}$ **6.** $A = \begin{bmatrix} 10 & -2 \\ -5 & 1 \end{bmatrix}$

7. $A = \begin{bmatrix} -1 & 1 & 2 \\ 2 & 4 & 3 \\ 1 & 3 & 2 \end{bmatrix}$ **8.** $A = \begin{bmatrix} -1 & 2 & 1 \\ -1 & 0 & 2 \\ 2 & 1 & -3 \end{bmatrix}$

9. $A = \begin{bmatrix} 2 & -3 & 3 \\ 2 & 2 & 3 \\ 3 & -2 & 2 \end{bmatrix}$ **10.** $A = \begin{bmatrix} 2 & -1 & 3 \\ -5 & 3 & 1 \\ -3 & 2 & 3 \end{bmatrix}$

11. $A = \begin{bmatrix} 1 & 3 & 3 \\ 1 & 4 & 3 \\ 1 & 3 & 4 \end{bmatrix}$ [MEERUT(BCA)–2008, 12]

12. If $A = \begin{bmatrix} \cos\alpha & -\sin\alpha \\ \sin\alpha & \cos\alpha \end{bmatrix}$, prove that

$$A^{-1} = \begin{bmatrix} \cos\alpha & \sin\alpha \\ -\sin\alpha & \cos\alpha \end{bmatrix}.$$

13. If $A = \begin{bmatrix} 3 & -3 & 4 \\ 2 & -3 & 4 \\ 0 & -1 & 1 \end{bmatrix}$, prove that $A^3 = A^{-1}$. [MEERUT(BCA)–2009, 11]

14. If $A = \begin{bmatrix} 1 & 1 & 1 \\ 1 & 2 & 1 \\ 1 & 1 & 2 \end{bmatrix}$, then find A^{-1}.

ANSWERS

1. $A^{-1} = \begin{bmatrix} 4 & -1 \\ -7 & 2 \end{bmatrix}$ **2.** $A^{-1} = \begin{bmatrix} 1 & -1 \\ -1 & 2 \end{bmatrix}$ **3.** $A^{-1} = \begin{bmatrix} 4/5 & -3/5 \\ -1/5 & 2/5 \end{bmatrix}$ **4.** $A^{-1} = \begin{bmatrix} 1 & \frac{1}{2} \\ 2 & \frac{3}{2} \end{bmatrix}$

5. Inverse does not exist **6.** Inverse does not exist **7.** $A^{-1} = \frac{1}{4}\begin{bmatrix} -1 & 4 & -5 \\ -1 & -4 & 7 \\ 2 & 4 & -6 \end{bmatrix}$ **8.** $A^{-1} = \frac{1}{3}\begin{bmatrix} -2 & 7 & 4 \\ 1 & 1 & 1 \\ -1 & 5 & 2 \end{bmatrix}$

9. $A^{-1} = \begin{bmatrix} -\frac{2}{5} & 0 & \frac{3}{5} \\ -\frac{1}{5} & \frac{1}{5} & 0 \\ \frac{2}{5} & \frac{1}{5} & -\frac{2}{5} \end{bmatrix}$ **10.** $A^{-1} = \begin{bmatrix} -7 & -9 & 10 \\ -12 & -15 & 17 \\ 1 & 1 & -1 \end{bmatrix}$ **11.** $A^{-1} = \begin{bmatrix} 7 & -3 & -3 \\ -1 & 1 & 0 \\ -1 & 0 & 1 \end{bmatrix}$ **14.** $A^{-1} = \begin{bmatrix} 3 & -1 & -1 \\ -1 & 1 & 0 \\ -1 & 0 & 1 \end{bmatrix}$

3.16 ECHELON FROM OF A MATRIX

A matrix A is said to be in Echelon form if :

(*i*) every row of A has all its entries 0 (zero) which occurs below every row having a non-zero entry and

(*ii*) the number of zeros before the first non-zero entry in a row is less than the number of such zeros in the next row.

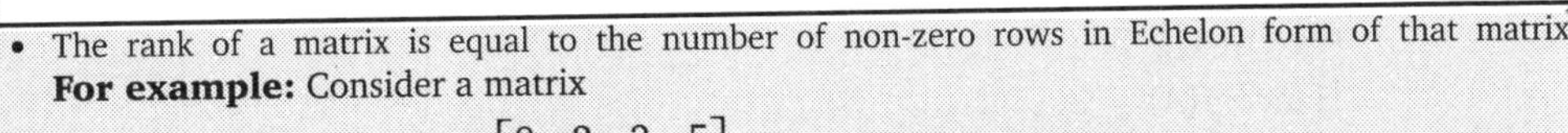

- The rank of a matrix is equal to the number of non-zero rows in Echelon form of that matrix.
  For example: Consider a matrix

$$A = \begin{bmatrix} 0 & 2 & 3 & 5 \\ 0 & 0 & 3 & 2 \\ 0 & 0 & 0 & 0 \end{bmatrix}$$

Clearly, A is in Echelon form which has 2 non-zero rows, hence the rank of A is 2.

THEOREM 1. *The rank of the transpose of a matrix is equal to the rank of that matrix.*

PROOF. Let A be a marix, then A' is its transpose and let $\rho(A) = r$, then there exists an r-rowed minor of A which is not equal to zero and all s-rowed minors of A are zero, where $s > r$. Let $|B|$ be a r-rowed minor of A such that $|B| \neq 0$. Since A' is the transpose of A, then $|B'|$ is the r-rowed minor of A' but $|B'| = |B| \neq 0$, therefore $\rho(A') \geq r$. Suppose there is an s-minor $|C|$ of A' such that $|C| \neq 0$, where $s > r$, then $|C'|$ will be an s-minor of A such that $|C'| = |C| \neq 0$, therefore $\rho(A) > r$ which is a contradiction, hence $\rho(A') = r$.

Solved Examples

1. *Find the rank of the following matrices :*

(i) $\begin{bmatrix} 3 & 0 & 0 \end{bmatrix}$ (ii) $\begin{bmatrix} 1 & 2 & 3 \\ 2 & 4 & 5 \end{bmatrix}$

(iii) $\begin{bmatrix} 1 & 2 & 3 \\ 3 & 4 & 5 \\ 4 & 5 & 6 \end{bmatrix}$ (iv) $\begin{bmatrix} 1 & 5 & 2 & 4 \\ 0 & 1 & 3 & 1 \\ 0 & 0 & 1 & 3 \end{bmatrix}$

SOLUTION. (i) Let $A = \begin{bmatrix} 3 & 0 & 0 \end{bmatrix}$, then A is the non-zero rowed matrix, therefore $\rho(A) \geq 1$. Also A is a matrix of order of 1×3, then $\rho(A) \leq 1$, hence

$$\rho(A) = 1.$$

(ii) Let $A = \begin{bmatrix} 1 & 2 & 3 \\ 2 & 4 & 5 \end{bmatrix}$

The order of A is 2×3, then

$$\rho(A) \leq 2.$$

Also there is a 2-minor $\begin{vmatrix} 2 & 3 \\ 4 & 5 \end{vmatrix}$ of A which is not equal to zero, then $\rho(A) \geq 2$, hence $\rho(A) = 2$.

(iii) Let $A = \begin{bmatrix} 1 & 2 & 3 \\ 3 & 4 & 5 \\ 4 & 5 & 6 \end{bmatrix}$. The order of A is 3×3, then $\rho(A) \leq 3$.

Now,

$$|A| = \begin{vmatrix} 1 & 2 & 3 \\ 3 & 4 & 5 \\ 4 & 5 & 6 \end{vmatrix}$$

$$= 1(24-25) - 2(18-20) + 3(15-16) = 0$$

$\therefore$ The only 3-minor $|A|$ of A is zero, thus $\rho(A) < 3$. Further, there is a 2-minor $\begin{vmatrix} 1 & 2 \\ 3 & 4 \end{vmatrix}$ of A which is not equal to zero, hence $\rho(A) = 2$.

(iv) Let $A = \begin{bmatrix} 1 & 5 & 2 & 4 \\ 0 & 1 & 3 & 1 \\ 0 & 0 & 1 & 3 \end{bmatrix}$

The order of A is 3×4, then

$\rho(A) \le 3$.

Now there is a 3-minor $\begin{vmatrix} 1 & 5 & 2 \\ 0 & 1 & 3 \\ 0 & 0 & 1 \end{vmatrix}$

of A which is not equal to zero, then $\rho(A)\ge 3$.

Hence $\rho(A) = 3$.

2. *Let A and B be two square matrices of order n. If $\rho(A)=\rho(B)= n$, then prove that $\rho(AB) = n$ and conversely.*

SOLUTION. Suppose $\rho(A) = \rho(B) = n$, then both A and B are non-singular.

$\therefore \quad |A|\ne 0$ and $|B|\ne 0$

$\Rightarrow \quad |AB|=|A|\,|B| \ne 0$

Since the order of AB is n and $|AB| \ne 0$, therefore $\rho(AB)= n$.

Conversely, suppose that

$$\rho(AB)= n$$

$\therefore \quad |AB| \ne 0$

$\Rightarrow \quad |A|\,|B| \ne 0$

$\Rightarrow \quad |A| \ne 0$ and $|B| \ne 0$

$\Rightarrow \quad \rho(A)= n,\ \rho(B)= n.$

3. *Prove that every skew-symmetric matrix of odd order has rank less than its order.*

SOLUTION. Let A be a skew-symmetric matrix of order n, where n is an odd natural number, then

$$A' = -A.$$

which implies

$$|A'| = |-A|$$

$\Rightarrow \quad |A| = |(-1)A|\ [\because |A'| = |A|]$

$\Rightarrow \quad |A| = (-1)^n|A|$

$\Rightarrow \quad |A| = -|A| \qquad [\because n \text{ is odd}]$

$\Rightarrow \quad 2|A| = 0$

$\Rightarrow \quad |A| = 0$

$\Rightarrow \quad \rho(A) \ne n$

But $\rho(A) \le n$, hence

$$\rho(A) < n.$$

4. *If A be a non-zero column and B is a non-zero row matrix, then show that $\rho(AB)=1$.*

SOLUTION. Let

$$A = \begin{bmatrix} a_{11} \\ a_{21} \\ \vdots \\ a_{m1} \end{bmatrix} \text{ and } B = \begin{bmatrix} b_{11} & b_{12} & \cdots & b_{1n} \end{bmatrix}$$

be two non-zero column and row matrices respectively.

Then we have

$$AB = \begin{bmatrix} a_{11} \\ a_{21} \\ \vdots \\ a_{m1} \end{bmatrix} \begin{bmatrix} b_{11} & b_{12} & \cdots & b_{1n} \end{bmatrix}$$

$$= \begin{bmatrix} a_{11}b_{11} & a_{11}b_{12} & \cdots & a_{11}b_{1n} \\ a_{21}b_{11} & a_{21}b_{12} & \cdots & a_{21}b_{1n} \\ \vdots & \vdots & \vdots & \vdots \\ a_{m1}b_{11} & a_{m1}b_{12} & \cdots & a_{m1}b_{1n} \end{bmatrix}$$

Clearly, AB is a matrix of order $m\times n$ and AB is a non-zero matrix since A and B are non-zero matrices,

then $\qquad \rho(AB) \ge 1 \qquad$ ..(1)

also every 2-minor of AB vanishes, then

$$\rho(AB) \le 1 \qquad ...(2)$$

From (1) and (2) we have

$$\rho(AB) = 1.$$

5. *If A is n-rowed square matrix of rank $n-1$, then show that adj A is non-zero matrix.*

SOLUTION. Since the rank of A is $n-1$, *i.e.*, $\rho(A)= n-1$, then there exists a non-zero $(n-1)$ minor of A, therefore there exists at least one element of *adj A* which is non-zero, hence *adj. A* is a non-zero matrix.

6. *Let A be a square matrix of order n. Show that $\rho(adj.\ A)$ is n or 0 in accordance with $\rho(A)$ is n or less than $n-1$.*

SOLUTION. Suppose $\rho(A) = n$, then $|A| \ne 0$

But we know that

$$|adj.\ A| = |A|^{n-1}$$

$\Rightarrow \quad |adj.\ A| \ne 0 \qquad [\because |A|\ne 0]$

$\therefore \quad \rho(adj.\ A) = n,$

since the order of *adj.* $A = n$.

Next, when $\rho(A)< n-1$, then $|A| = 0$ and every r-minor of A is zero, where $r \ge n-1$, therefore every element of *adj.* A is zero so that *adj.* A is a null matrix, hence $\rho(adj.\ A) = 0$.

7. *Find the value of x so that $\rho(A) \leq 2$, where A is the matrix given by*

$$\begin{bmatrix} 3x-8 & 3 & 3 \\ 3 & 3x-8 & 3 \\ 3 & 3 & 3x-8 \end{bmatrix}$$

SOLUTION. Since $\rho(A) \leq 2$, then $|A| = 0$ because A is a square matrix of order 3×3.

Now $\quad |A| = 0$

$$\Rightarrow \begin{vmatrix} 3x-8 & 3 & 3 \\ 3 & 3x-8 & 3 \\ 3 & 3 & 3x-8 \end{vmatrix} = 0$$

$$\Rightarrow (3x-8)\{(3x-8)(3x-8)-9\} - 3\{3(3x-8)-9\} + 3\{9-3(3x-8)\} = 0$$

$$\Rightarrow (3x-8)^3 - 9(3x-8) - 9(3x-8) + 27 + 27 - 9(3x-8) = 0$$

$$\Rightarrow (3x-8)^3 - 27(3x-8) + 54 = 0$$

$$\Rightarrow (3x-5)^2(3x-2) = 0$$

$$\Rightarrow 3x-2 = 0 \text{ or } 3x-5 = 0$$

$$\Rightarrow x = \frac{2}{3} \text{ or } x = \frac{5}{3}$$

When $x = \frac{2}{3}$, then $A = \begin{bmatrix} -6 & 3 & 3 \\ 3 & -6 & 3 \\ 3 & 3 & -6 \end{bmatrix}$,

clearly there is a 2-minor $\begin{vmatrix} -6 & 3 \\ 3 & -6 \end{vmatrix}$ of A, which is non-zero, hence $\rho(A) = 2$.

Again, when $x = \frac{5}{3}$, then

$$A = \begin{bmatrix} -3 & 3 & 3 \\ 3 & -3 & 3 \\ 3 & 3 & -3 \end{bmatrix}$$

Clearly, there is a 2-minor $\begin{vmatrix} -3 & 3 \\ 3 & -3 \end{vmatrix}$ of A, which is non-zero, hence $\rho(A) = 2$.

8. *Determine the rank of the following matrices :*

(i) $\begin{bmatrix} 2 & -1 & 3 & 4 \\ 0 & 3 & 4 & 1 \\ 2 & 3 & 7 & 5 \\ 2 & 5 & 11 & 6 \end{bmatrix}$

(ii) $\begin{bmatrix} -2 & -1 & -3 & -1 \\ 1 & 2 & 3 & -1 \\ 1 & 0 & 1 & 1 \\ 0 & 1 & 1 & -1 \end{bmatrix}$

SOLUTION. (i) Let

$$A = \begin{bmatrix} 2 & -1 & 3 & 4 \\ 0 & 3 & 4 & 1 \\ 2 & 3 & 7 & 5 \\ 2 & 5 & 11 & 6 \end{bmatrix}$$

Applying $R_3 \to R_3 - R_1$, $R_4 \to R_4 - R_1$

$$A \sim \begin{bmatrix} 2 & -1 & 3 & 4 \\ 0 & 3 & 4 & 1 \\ 0 & 4 & 4 & 1 \\ 0 & 6 & 8 & 2 \end{bmatrix}$$

Again applying

$R_3 \to R_3 - \frac{4}{3}R_2$, $R_4 \to R_4 - 2R_2$

$$A \sim \begin{bmatrix} 2 & -1 & 3 & 4 \\ 0 & 3 & 4 & 1 \\ 0 & 0 & -4/3 & -1/3 \\ 0 & 0 & 0 & 0 \end{bmatrix}$$

Again applying $R_3 \to 3R_3$

$$A \sim \begin{bmatrix} 2 & -1 & 3 & 4 \\ 0 & 3 & 4 & 1 \\ 0 & 0 & -4 & -1 \\ 0 & 0 & 0 & 0 \end{bmatrix}$$

The last equivalent matrix is in Echelon form which has 3 non-zero rows, hence $\rho(A) = 3$.

(ii) Let $A = \begin{bmatrix} -2 & -1 & -3 & -1 \\ 1 & 2 & 3 & -1 \\ 1 & 0 & 1 & 1 \\ 0 & 1 & 1 & -1 \end{bmatrix}$

Applying $R_1 \leftrightarrow R_2$

$$A \sim \begin{bmatrix} 1 & 2 & 3 & -1 \\ -2 & -1 & -3 & -1 \\ 1 & 0 & 1 & 1 \\ 0 & 1 & 1 & -1 \end{bmatrix}$$

Again applying $R_2 \to R_2 + 2R_1$, $R_3 \to R_3 - R_1$

$$A \sim \begin{bmatrix} 1 & 2 & 3 & -1 \\ 0 & 3 & 3 & -3 \\ 0 & -2 & -2 & 2 \\ 0 & 1 & 1 & -1 \end{bmatrix}$$

Again applying $R_2 \to R_2 + R_3$

$$A \sim \begin{bmatrix} 1 & 2 & 3 & -1 \\ 0 & 1 & 1 & -1 \\ 0 & -2 & -2 & 2 \\ 0 & 1 & 1 & -1 \end{bmatrix}$$

Again applying $R_3 \to R_3 + 2R_2$,
$R_4 \to R_4 - R_2$

$$A \sim \begin{bmatrix} 1 & 2 & 3 & -1 \\ 0 & 1 & 1 & -1 \\ 0 & 0 & 0 & 0 \\ 0 & 0 & 0 & 0 \end{bmatrix}$$

The last equivalent matrix is in Echelon form which has 2 non-zero rows, hence $\rho(A) = 2$.

9. *Reduce the matrix* $A = \begin{bmatrix} 1 & -1 & 2 & -3 \\ 4 & 1 & 0 & 2 \\ 0 & 3 & 0 & 4 \\ 0 & 1 & 0 & 2 \end{bmatrix}$ *to the normal form* $\begin{bmatrix} I_r & O \\ O & O \end{bmatrix}$ *and hence determine its rank.*

SOLUTION. We have $A = \begin{bmatrix} 1 & -1 & 2 & -3 \\ 4 & 1 & 0 & 2 \\ 0 & 3 & 0 & 4 \\ 0 & 1 & 0 & 2 \end{bmatrix}$

Applying $R_2 \to R_2 - 4R_1$

$$A \sim \begin{bmatrix} 1 & -1 & 2 & -3 \\ 0 & 5 & -8 & 14 \\ 0 & 3 & 0 & 4 \\ 0 & 1 & 0 & 2 \end{bmatrix}$$

Applying $C_2 \to C_2 + C_1$, $C_3 \to C_3 - 2C_1$, $C_4 \to C_4 + 3C_1$

$$A \sim \begin{bmatrix} 1 & 0 & 0 & 0 \\ 0 & 5 & -8 & 14 \\ 0 & 3 & 0 & 4 \\ 0 & 1 & 0 & 2 \end{bmatrix}$$

Applying $R_2 \leftrightarrow R_4$

$$A \sim \begin{bmatrix} 1 & 0 & 0 & 0 \\ 0 & 1 & 0 & 2 \\ 0 & 3 & 0 & 4 \\ 0 & 5 & -8 & 14 \end{bmatrix}$$

Applying $R_3 \to R_3 - 3R_2, R_4 \to R_4 - 5R_2$

$$A \sim \begin{bmatrix} 1 & 0 & 0 & 0 \\ 0 & 1 & 0 & 2 \\ 0 & 0 & 0 & -2 \\ 0 & 0 & -8 & 4 \end{bmatrix}$$

Applying $C_4 \to C_4 - 2C_2$

$$A \sim \begin{bmatrix} 1 & 0 & 0 & 0 \\ 0 & 1 & 0 & 0 \\ 0 & 0 & 0 & -2 \\ 0 & 0 & -8 & 4 \end{bmatrix}$$

Applying $C_3 \leftrightarrow C_4$

$$A \sim \begin{bmatrix} 1 & 0 & 0 & 0 \\ 0 & 1 & 0 & 0 \\ 0 & 0 & -2 & 0 \\ 0 & 0 & 4 & -8 \end{bmatrix}$$

Applying $R_4 \to R_4 + 2R_3$

$$A \sim \begin{bmatrix} 1 & 0 & 0 & 0 \\ 0 & 1 & 0 & 0 \\ 0 & 0 & -2 & 0 \\ 0 & 0 & 0 & -8 \end{bmatrix}$$

Applying $R_3 \to \frac{1}{2}R_3, R_4 \to -\frac{1}{8}R_4$

$$A \sim \begin{bmatrix} 1 & 0 & 0 & 0 \\ 0 & 1 & 0 & 0 \\ 0 & 0 & 1 & 0 \\ 0 & 0 & 0 & 1 \end{bmatrix}$$

$\therefore \quad A \sim I_4$

Hence $\rho(A) = 4$

10. *Find the rank of the matrix*

$$A = \begin{bmatrix} 2 & -2 & 0 & 6 \\ 4 & 2 & 0 & 2 \\ 1 & -1 & 0 & 3 \\ 1 & -2 & 1 & 2 \end{bmatrix}$$

by reducing it to normal form.

SOLUTION. We have $A = \begin{bmatrix} 2 & -2 & 0 & 6 \\ 4 & 2 & 0 & 2 \\ 1 & -1 & 0 & 3 \\ 1 & -2 & 1 & 2 \end{bmatrix}$

Applying $R_1 \to \frac{1}{2}R_1$

$$A \sim \begin{bmatrix} 1 & -1 & 0 & 3 \\ 4 & 2 & 0 & 2 \\ 1 & -1 & 0 & 3 \\ 1 & -2 & 1 & 2 \end{bmatrix}$$

Applying $R_2 \to R_2 - 4R_1$, $R_3 \to R_3 - R_1$, $R_4 \to R_4 - R_1$

$$A \sim \begin{bmatrix} 1 & -1 & 0 & 3 \\ 0 & 6 & 0 & -10 \\ 0 & 0 & 0 & 0 \\ 0 & -1 & 1 & -1 \end{bmatrix}$$

Applying $C_2 \to C_2 + C_1,\ C_4 \to C_4 - 3C_1$

$$A \sim \begin{bmatrix} 1 & -1 & 0 & 0 \\ 0 & 6 & 0 & -10 \\ 0 & 0 & 0 & 0 \\ 0 & -1 & 1 & 1 \end{bmatrix}$$

Applying $R_2 \leftrightarrow R_4$

$$A \sim \begin{bmatrix} 1 & 0 & 0 & 0 \\ 0 & -1 & 1 & 1 \\ 0 & 0 & 0 & 0 \\ 0 & 6 & 0 & -10 \end{bmatrix}$$

Applying $R_4 \to R_4 + 6R_2$

$$A \sim \begin{bmatrix} 1 & 0 & 0 & 0 \\ 0 & -1 & 1 & 1 \\ 0 & 0 & 0 & 0 \\ 0 & 0 & 6 & -4 \end{bmatrix}$$

Applying $C_3 \to C_3 + C_2,\ C_4 \to C_4 + C_2$

$$A \sim \begin{bmatrix} 1 & 0 & 0 & 0 \\ 0 & -1 & 0 & 0 \\ 0 & 0 & 0 & 0 \\ 0 & 0 & 6 & -4 \end{bmatrix}$$

Applying

$C_3 \to \frac{1}{6}C_3,\ C_4 \to \frac{-1}{4}C_4,\ C_2 \to (-1)C_2$

$$A \sim \begin{bmatrix} 1 & 0 & 0 & 0 \\ 0 & 1 & 0 & 0 \\ 0 & 0 & 0 & 0 \\ 0 & 0 & 1 & 1 \end{bmatrix}$$

Applying $R_3 \leftrightarrow R_4$

$$A \sim \begin{bmatrix} 1 & 0 & 0 & 0 \\ 0 & 1 & 0 & 0 \\ 0 & 0 & 1 & 1 \\ 0 & 0 & 0 & 0 \end{bmatrix}$$

Applying $C_4 \to C_4 - C_3$

$$A \sim \begin{bmatrix} 1 & 0 & 0 & 0 \\ 0 & 1 & 0 & 0 \\ 0 & 0 & 1 & 0 \\ 0 & 0 & 0 & 0 \end{bmatrix}$$

$$A \sim \begin{bmatrix} I_3 & O \\ O & O \end{bmatrix}$$

Hence $\rho(A) = 3$.

11. *Find two non-singular matrices P and Q such that PAQ is in the normal form where*

$$A = \begin{bmatrix} 1 & 1 & 1 \\ 1 & -1 & -1 \\ 3 & 1 & 1 \end{bmatrix}.$$ *Also find the rank of the matrix A.* [KURUKSHETRA–2005]

SOLUTION. We write $A = I_3 A I_3$ or

$$\begin{bmatrix} 1 & 1 & 1 \\ 1 & -1 & -1 \\ 3 & 1 & 1 \end{bmatrix} = \begin{bmatrix} 1 & 0 & 0 \\ 0 & 1 & 0 \\ 0 & 0 & 1 \end{bmatrix} A \begin{bmatrix} 1 & 0 & 0 \\ 0 & 1 & 0 \\ 0 & 0 & 1 \end{bmatrix} \quad \text{...(1)}$$

In order to find P and Q such that $PAQ = \begin{bmatrix} I_r & O \\ O & O \end{bmatrix}$ we shall reduce the matrix on LHS of (1) by using elementary transformations, while in doing so we shall apply elementary row transformation to pre-factor of A and elementary-column transformation to post-factor of A on RHS of (1).

Now applying $R_2 \to R_2 - R_1,\ R_3 \to R_3 - 3R_1$

$$\begin{bmatrix} 1 & 1 & 1 \\ 1 & -2 & -2 \\ 0 & -2 & -2 \end{bmatrix} = \begin{bmatrix} 1 & 0 & 0 \\ -1 & 1 & 0 \\ -3 & 0 & 1 \end{bmatrix} A \begin{bmatrix} 1 & 0 & 0 \\ 0 & 1 & 0 \\ 0 & 0 & 1 \end{bmatrix}$$

Applying $C_2 \to C_2 - C_1,\ C_3 \to C_3 - C_1$

$$\begin{bmatrix} 1 & 0 & 0 \\ 0 & -2 & -2 \\ 0 & -2 & -2 \end{bmatrix} = \begin{bmatrix} 1 & 0 & 0 \\ -1 & 1 & 0 \\ -3 & 0 & 1 \end{bmatrix} A \begin{bmatrix} 1 & -1 & -1 \\ 0 & 1 & 0 \\ 0 & 0 & 1 \end{bmatrix}$$

Applying $R_2 \to \left(-\frac{1}{2}\right)R_2$

$$\begin{bmatrix} 1 & 0 & 0 \\ 0 & 1 & 1 \\ 0 & -2 & -2 \end{bmatrix} = \begin{bmatrix} 1 & 0 & 0 \\ \frac{1}{2} & -\frac{1}{2} & 0 \\ -3 & 0 & 1 \end{bmatrix} A \begin{bmatrix} 1 & -1 & -1 \\ 0 & 1 & 0 \\ 0 & 0 & 1 \end{bmatrix}$$

Applying $R_3 \to R_3 + 2R_2$

$$\begin{bmatrix} 1 & 0 & 0 \\ 0 & 1 & 1 \\ 0 & 0 & 0 \end{bmatrix} = \begin{bmatrix} 1 & 0 & 0 \\ \frac{1}{2} & -\frac{1}{2} & 0 \\ -2 & -1 & 1 \end{bmatrix} A \begin{bmatrix} 1 & -1 & -1 \\ 0 & 1 & 0 \\ 0 & 0 & 1 \end{bmatrix}$$

Applying $C_2 \to C_3 - C_2$

$$\begin{bmatrix} 1 & 0 & 0 \\ 0 & 1 & 0 \\ 0 & 0 & 0 \end{bmatrix} = \begin{bmatrix} 1 & 0 & 0 \\ \frac{1}{2} & -\frac{1}{2} & 0 \\ -2 & -1 & 1 \end{bmatrix} A \begin{bmatrix} 1 & -1 & 0 \\ 0 & 1 & -1 \\ 0 & 0 & 1 \end{bmatrix}$$

or $\begin{bmatrix} I_2 & O \\ O & O \end{bmatrix} = PAQ$

where

$$\begin{bmatrix}1&0&0\\0&1&0\\0&0&0\end{bmatrix}=\begin{bmatrix}1&0&0\\\frac{1}{2}&-\frac{1}{2}&0\\-2&-1&1\end{bmatrix}A\begin{bmatrix}1&-1&0\\0&1&-1\\0&0&1\end{bmatrix}$$

$$A\sim\begin{bmatrix}I_2&O\\O&O\end{bmatrix}$$

Hence $\rho(A) = 2$.

Exercise-3.5

1. Find the rank of the following matrices :

(i) $\begin{bmatrix}0&0\\0&0\end{bmatrix}$ (ii) $\begin{bmatrix}5&10\\3&6\end{bmatrix}$

(iii) $\begin{bmatrix}1&-3&4&7\\9&1&2&0\end{bmatrix}$ (iv) $\begin{bmatrix}1&2&3\\2&1&0\\0&1&2\end{bmatrix}$

(v) $\begin{bmatrix}1&2&-7&5\\0&5&0&8\\0&0&0&-3\end{bmatrix}$ (vi) $\begin{bmatrix}0&1&2&1\\1&2&3&2\\3&1&1&3\end{bmatrix}$

(vii) $\begin{bmatrix}1&2&3&4\\2&4&6&8\\3&6&9&12\end{bmatrix}$ (viii) $\begin{bmatrix}1&5&4&6\\2&7&5&9\\3&9&6&12\end{bmatrix}$

(ix) $\begin{bmatrix}1&x&x^2\\1&y&y^2\\1&z&z^2\end{bmatrix}$ (x) $\begin{bmatrix}1&1&1&1\\1&1&1&1\\1&1&1&1\\1&1&1&1\end{bmatrix}$

2. If $A=\begin{bmatrix}0&1&0&0\\0&0&1&0\\0&0&0&1\\0&0&0&0\end{bmatrix}$, find $\rho(A)$, $\rho(A^2)$, $\rho(A^3)$ and $\rho(A^4)$.

3. Show that the rank of a matrix does not alter on affixing any number of additional rows or columns of zeros.

4. Show that the rank of a matrix is greater than or equal to the rank of its every submatrix.

5. Find the rank of A, B, $A+B$ and AB, where

$$A=\begin{bmatrix}1&1&-1\\2&-3&4\\3&-2&3\end{bmatrix} \text{ and } B=\begin{bmatrix}-1&-2&-1\\6&12&6\\5&10&5\end{bmatrix}$$

ANSWERS

1. (i) 0 (ii) 1 (iii) 2 (iv) 2 (v) 3 (vi) 3 (vii) 1 (viii) 2

(ix) Rank =3if $x \neq y \neq z$; Rank =2 if only two of x, y, z are different; Rank = 1 if $x = y = z$. (x) 1

2. $\rho(A) = 3$, $\rho(A^2) = 2$, $\rho(A^3) = 1$, $\rho(A^4) = 0$

5. $\rho(A) = 2$, $\rho(B) = 1$, $\rho(A+B) = 2$, $\rho(AB) = 0$

3.17 SYSTEM OF LINEAR EQUATIONS

In this section we shall study the nature of solutions of a system of linear equations with the help of the theory of matrices discussed in previous chapters. Before going into details of solutions of linear equations we shall try to understand the concepts of linearly dependent and independent set of vectors.

3.18 VECTORS AND THEIR DEPENDENCE AND INDEPENDENCE

An ordered set of n numbers $(x_1, x_2, x_3, ,..., x_n)$ *is known as a vector of order n.*

The n numbers $x_1, x_2, x_3, ,..., x_n$ are called the components of the vector. We denote this vector by a single letter X. Conveniently, we may write the components of a vector X in the form of a row or in the form of a column.

Therefore, we may write $X = [x_1, x_2, x_3, ,..., x_n]$

which is known as a n-dimensional row vector or it may be written as $X = \begin{bmatrix} x_1 \\ x_2 \\ x_3 \\ \vdots \\ x_n \end{bmatrix}$ which is known as an n-dimensional column vector.

If we consider an $m \times n$ matrix, then it contains m-row vectors and n-column vectors, each row vector consists of the components of an n-vector and each column vector consists of the components of an m-vector.

For example: Consider a matrix of order 3×4 given by

$$A = \begin{bmatrix} 1 & -1 & 4 & 5 \\ 2 & 3 & 0 & -7 \\ 3 & 2 & 2 & 6 \end{bmatrix}$$

Then, $R_1 = [1 \quad -1 \quad 4 \quad 5]$, $R_2 = [2 \quad 3 \quad 0 \quad -7]$, $R_3 = [3 \quad 2 \quad 2 \quad 6]$

$$C_1 = \begin{bmatrix} 1 \\ 2 \\ 3 \end{bmatrix}, C_2 = \begin{bmatrix} -1 \\ 3 \\ 2 \end{bmatrix}, C_3 = \begin{bmatrix} 4 \\ 0 \\ 2 \end{bmatrix}, C_4 = \begin{bmatrix} 5 \\ -7 \\ 6 \end{bmatrix}$$

Thus A can be written as $A = \begin{bmatrix} R_1 \\ R_2 \\ R_3 \end{bmatrix}$ or $A = \begin{bmatrix} C_1 & C_2 & C_3 & C_4 \end{bmatrix}$

Definition : *If all the components of a vector are zero, then it is called a null vector or a zero vector. It is usually denoted by capital letter O.*

For example : The vectors $\begin{bmatrix} 0 & 0 & 0 & 0 \end{bmatrix}$ and $\begin{bmatrix} 0 \\ 0 \\ 0 \\ 0 \end{bmatrix}$ are both null vectors.

3.18.1 Linear Dependence and Independence of Vectors

Let $x_1, x_2, x_3, \ldots, x_m$ be m vectors. Then they are said to be linearly independent if

$$\lambda_1 x_1 + \lambda_2 x_2 + \ldots + \lambda_m x_m = 0 \quad \Rightarrow \quad \lambda_1 = \lambda_2 = \lambda_3 = \ldots = \lambda_m = 0$$

If at least one of $\lambda_1, \lambda_2, \ldots, \lambda_m$ is non-zero, then the vectors $x_1, x_2, \ldots, x_m$ are called linearly dependent.

3.18.2 Linear Combination of Vectors

A vector X is said to be a linear combination of the vectors $x_1, x_2, \ldots, x_m$ if there exists scalars $\lambda_1, \lambda_2, \ldots, \lambda_m$ such that

$$X = \lambda_1 x_1 + \lambda_2 x_2 + \ldots + \lambda_m x_m$$

Suppose that the vectors $x_1, x_2, \ldots, x_m$ are linearly dependent, then in the equation.

$$\lambda_1 x_1 + \lambda_2 x_2 + \ldots + \lambda_m x_m = O \qquad \ldots (1)$$

there is at least one of $\lambda_1, \lambda_2, \ldots \lambda_m$ is non-zero, let it be λ_r, then equation (1) can be written as

$$\lambda_r X_r = -\lambda_1 x_1 - \lambda_2 x_2 - \ldots \lambda_{r-1} x_{r-1} - \lambda_{r+1} x_{r+1} - \ldots - \lambda_m x_m$$

$$\Rightarrow \quad X_r = \left(-\frac{\lambda_1}{\lambda_r}\right) x_1 + \left(-\frac{\lambda_2}{\lambda_r}\right) x_2 + \ldots + \left(-\frac{\lambda_{r-1}}{\lambda_r}\right) x_{r-1} + \left(-\frac{\lambda_{r+1}}{\lambda_r}\right) x_{r+1} + \ldots + \left(-\frac{\lambda_m}{\lambda_r}\right) x_m$$

$\Rightarrow \qquad X_r = k_1x_1 + k_2x_2 + ... + k_{r-1}x_{r-1} + k_{r+1}x_{r+1} + ... + k_mx_m$

It follows that X_r is a linear combination of vectors $x_1, x_2, .., x_{r-1}, x_{r+1}, ..., x_m$.

Hence if a set of vectors is linearly dependent, then at least one member of the set can be expressed as a linear combination of the remaining vectors.

3.18.3 Linear Dependence and Independence of any Matrix

Consider a matrix of order $m \times n$, given by

$$A = \begin{bmatrix} a_{11} & a_{12} & \cdots & a_{1n} \\ a_{21} & a_{22} & \cdots & a_{2n} \\ \vdots & \vdots & & \vdots \\ a_{m1} & a_{m2} & \cdots & a_{mn} \end{bmatrix}$$

Let the rank of A be r, then there exists at least one r-minor of A which is non-zero. If A_r be a square submatrix of order $r \times r$ such that $|A_r| \neq 0$, then r rows and columns of A_r are linearly independent, it follows that the matrix A has r rows and columns which are linearly independent. As the rank of A is r so that no set of $(r+1)$ rows and columns of A can be linearly independent. Hence the rank of a matrix A is defined to be the maximum number of linearly independent rows and columns of A.

Since on interchanging rows, the rank of A does not change so without loss of generality we may suppose that the first r rows of A are linearly independent. Let $x_1, x_2, x_3, ... , x_r$ denote the r independent vectors and let x_t be one of the remaining $(m - r)$ vectors, then the vectors $x_1, x_2, x_3, ... , x_r, x_t$ are linearly dependent, therefore there exists scalars $\lambda_1, \lambda_2, \lambda_3, ... \lambda_r, \lambda_t$, not all zero such that

$$\lambda_1 x_1 + \lambda_2 x_2 + ... + \lambda_r x_r + \lambda_t x_t = O$$

Since $x_1, x_2, ..., x_r$ are linearly dependent, so we take $\lambda_t \neq 0$, thus

$$x_t = \left(-\frac{\lambda_1}{\lambda_t}\right)x_1 + \left(-\frac{\lambda_2}{\lambda_t}\right)x_2 + ... + \left(-\frac{\lambda_r}{\lambda_t}\right)x_r$$

It follows that x_t is a linear combination of $x_1, x_2, ..., x_r$.

Hence if the rank of a matrix of order $m \times n$ is r, then it has a set of r linearly independent rows (or columns) and $(m - r)$ linearly dependent rows (or columns).

3.19 HOMOGENEOUS LINEAR EQUATIONS

Let us consider a system of linear homogeneous equations as follows

$$\left.\begin{array}{r} a_{11}x_1 + a_{12}x_2 + ... + a_{1n}x_n = 0 \\ a_{21}x_1 + a_{22}x_2 + ... + a_{2n}x_n = 0 \\ \cdots\cdots\cdots\cdots\cdots\cdots\cdots\cdots \\ a_{m1}x_1 + a_{m2}x_2 + ... + a_{mn}x_n = 0 \end{array}\right\} \quad ...(1)$$

These equations are m equations in n unknowns. Any set of numbers $x_1, x_2, ..., x_n$ that satisfies all the equations (1) is called a solution of (1).

3.19.1 Trivial Solution

The solution $x_1 = 0, x_2 = 0, ... x_n = 0$ of the equations (1) is called *trivial* solution.

3.19.2 Non-Trivial Solution

Any other solutions, if exists, is called a *non-trivial* solution of equation (1).

Let the coefficient matrix be
$$A = \begin{bmatrix} a_{11} & a_{12} & \cdots & a_{1n} \\ a_{21} & a_{22} & \cdots & a_{2n} \\ \vdots & \vdots & & \vdots \\ a_{m1} & a_{m2} & \cdots & a_{mn} \end{bmatrix}_{m\times n}$$

and
$$X = \begin{bmatrix} x_1 \\ x_2 \\ x_3 \\ \vdots \\ x_n \end{bmatrix}_{n\times 1}, O = \begin{bmatrix} 0 \\ 0 \\ 0 \\ \vdots \\ 0 \end{bmatrix}_{m\times 1}$$

Then the system of equation (1) can also be written as

$$AX = O \qquad \text{... (2)}$$

This equation (2) is called a *matrix equation.*

PROPERTIES

(1) If X_1 and X_2 are two non-trivial solutions of $AX = O$, then $k_1X_1 + k_2X_2$ is also a solution of $AX = O$, where k_1 and k_2 are any arbitrary numbers.

(2) If the rank of A is r, then the number of linearly independent solutions of the equation $AX = O$ which is a system of m homogeneous linear equations in n unknowns is $(n - r)$.

3.20 NATURE OF THE SOLUTION OF THE EQUATION AX = 0

Since $AX = O$ is a matrix equation of a system of m homogeneous linear equations in n unknowns and A is a coefficient matrix of order $m \times n$. Let the rank of A be r. Then obviously r cannot be greater than n. So that either r is n or r is less than n. Therefore these are some cases.

Case 1. If $r = n$, then the equation $AX = O$, will have no linearly independent solution. So in this case only trivial solution will exist.

Case 2. If $r < n$, then there will be $(n - r)$ linearly independent solution of $AX = O$ and thus in this case we shall have infinite solutions.

Case 3. Suppose the number of equations is less than number of unknowns, *i.e.*, $m < n$ and since $r \le m$, then obviously $r < n$. Thus in this case a non-zero solution will exist. Therefore, the equation $AX = O$ will have infinite solutions.

WORKING PROCEDURE

In order to determine the solutions of the equation $AX = O$, we proceed to the following steps :

STEP 1. Reduce the matrix A to Echelon form by applying E-row transformations only. The Echelon form gives the rank of A.

STEP 2. Let A be matrix of order $m \times n$ and let $\rho(A) = r$. If $r = n$, then $AX = O$ will have zero solution only. If $r < n$, then we will assign $n - r$ arbitrarily chosen values to $n - r$ unknowns.

STEP 3. Let B be the Echelon form of A, then the equation $AX = O$ is equivalent to the equation $BX = O$. Reduce $BX = O$ to a system of equations and choose $n - r$ unknowns in this system of equations for assigning arbitrary values like $c_1, c_2 ..., c_{n-r}$.

STEP 4. By back substitution of $(n - r)$ unknowns to the system of equations reduced from $BX = O$, we finally obtain the solutions. In case of $r < n$, we get infinite solutions.

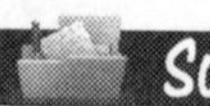

Solved Examples

1. *Find the non-trivial solutions of the equations:*

$$x + y - 6z = 0$$
$$-3x + y + 2z = 0$$
$$x - y + 2z = 0$$

SOLUTION. The given system of equations can be written as $AX = O$ ... (1)

where $A = \begin{bmatrix} 1 & 1 & -6 \\ -3 & 1 & 2 \\ 1 & -1 & 2 \end{bmatrix}$,

$$X = \begin{bmatrix} x \\ y \\ z \end{bmatrix} \text{ and } O = \begin{bmatrix} 0 \\ 0 \\ 0 \end{bmatrix}$$

Reducing the matrix A into Echelon form, we have

Applying $R_2 \to R_2+3R_1$, $R_3 \to R_3-R_1$, we get

$$A \sim \begin{bmatrix} 1 & 1 & -6 \\ 0 & 4 & -16 \\ 0 & -2 & 8 \end{bmatrix}$$

Again applying $R_2 \to \frac{1}{4}R_2$, we get

$$A \sim \begin{bmatrix} 1 & 1 & -6 \\ 0 & 1 & -4 \\ 0 & -2 & 8 \end{bmatrix}$$

Again applying $R_3 \to R_3 + 2R_2$ we get

$$A \sim \begin{bmatrix} 1 & 1 & -6 \\ 0 & 1 & -4 \\ 0 & 0 & 0 \end{bmatrix}$$

The last equivalent matrix in Echelon form with two non-zero rows, therefore $\rho(A) = 2$

Thus the given system of equations is equivalent to

$$\begin{bmatrix} 1 & 1 & -6 \\ 0 & 1 & -4 \\ 0 & 0 & 0 \end{bmatrix} \begin{bmatrix} x \\ y \\ z \end{bmatrix} = \begin{bmatrix} 0 \\ 0 \\ 0 \end{bmatrix}$$

$\Rightarrow$ $x+y-6z = 0$ ... (2)

$y - 4z = 0$ ... (3)

Let us put $z = c$ in (3), we get

$$y = 4c$$

Now putting $y = 4c$ and $z = c$ in (2), we get

$$x = 2c$$

Hence, the non-trival solutions of the given system of equatons are $x = 2c$, $y = 4c$, $z = c$, where c is a non-zero arbitrary number.

2. *Show that the only real value of λ for which the following equations have non-zero solutions is 6:*

$x + 2y + 3z = \lambda x$, $3x+y+2z = \lambda y$, $2x + 3y+z = \lambda z$

SOLUTION. The given system of equations can be rewritten as

$(1 - \lambda)x+2y+3z = 0$ ...(1)

$3x+(1 - \lambda)y+2z = 0$ ...(2)

$2x+3y+(1 - \lambda)z = 0$ ...(3)

This system of equations can be written as

$AX = O$ ... (4)

where $A = \begin{bmatrix} 1-\lambda & 2 & 3 \\ 3 & 1-\lambda & 2 \\ 2 & 3 & 1-\lambda \end{bmatrix}$,

$$X = \begin{bmatrix} x \\ y \\ z \end{bmatrix} \text{ and } O = \begin{bmatrix} 0 \\ 0 \\ 0 \end{bmatrix}$$

For non-zero solutions, we must have $|A| = 0$

i.e.,
$$\begin{vmatrix} 1-\lambda & 2 & 3 \\ 3 & 1-\lambda & 2 \\ 2 & 3 & 1-\lambda \end{vmatrix} = 0$$

$$(1-\lambda)(1-\lambda)(1-\lambda)+8+27-6(1-\lambda) -6(1-\lambda)-6(1-\lambda)=0$$

$$\Rightarrow 1-\lambda^3-3\lambda+3\lambda^2+35-18(1-\lambda)=0$$

$$\Rightarrow -\lambda^3+3\lambda^2+15\lambda+18=0$$

$$\Rightarrow \lambda^3-3\lambda^2-15\lambda-18=0$$

$$\Rightarrow (\lambda-6)(\lambda^2+3\lambda+3)=0$$

Since $\lambda^2 + 3\lambda + 3 = 0$ given imaginary roots, therefore the only real value of λ for which the system of equations is to have a non-zero solution is 6.

3. *Does the following system of equations possess a common non-zero solution?*

$$x+y+z=0$$
$$2x-y-3z=0$$
$$3x-5y+4z=0$$
$$x+17y+4z=0$$

SOLUTION. The coefficient matrix is

$$A=\begin{bmatrix}1 & 1 & 1\\ 2 & -1 & -3\\ 3 & -5 & 4\\ 1 & 17 & 4\end{bmatrix}$$

First reduce A into Echelon form.

Performing $R_2 \to R_2-2R_1$,
$R_3 \to R_3-3R_1$,
$R_4 \to R_4-R_1$

$$\sim\begin{bmatrix}1 & 1 & 1\\ 0 & -3 & -5\\ 0 & -8 & 1\\ 0 & 16 & 3\end{bmatrix}$$

Performing $R_2 \to -\frac{1}{3}R_2$

$$\sim\begin{bmatrix}1 & 1 & 1\\ 0 & 1 & \frac{5}{3}\\ 0 & -8 & 1\\ 0 & 16 & 3\end{bmatrix}$$

Performing

$R_3 \to R_3+8R_2, R_4 \to R_4-16R_4$

$$\sim\begin{bmatrix}1 & 1 & 1\\ 0 & 1 & \frac{5}{3}\\ 0 & 0 & \frac{43}{3}\\ 0 & 0 & \frac{71}{3}\end{bmatrix}$$

Performing $R_3 \to \frac{3}{43}R_3$

$$\sim\begin{bmatrix}1 & 1 & 1\\ 0 & 1 & \frac{5}{3}\\ 0 & 0 & 1\\ 0 & 0 & -\frac{71}{3}\end{bmatrix}$$

Performing $R_4 \to R_4+\frac{71}{3}R_3$

$$\sim\begin{bmatrix}1 & 1 & 1\\ 0 & 1 & \frac{5}{3}\\ 0 & 0 & 1\\ 0 & 0 & 0\end{bmatrix}$$

This is an Echleon form and having three non-zero rows so A has the rank 3. Since there are 3 number of unknown, hence a trival solution exists here, *i.e.*, $x=0, y=0, z=0$.

4. *Find all the solutions of the following system of linear homogeneous equations.*

$$x-2y+z-w=0$$
$$x+y-2z+3w=0$$
$$4x+y-5z+8w=0$$
$$5x-7y+2z-w=0$$

SOLUTION. The coefficient matrix is given by

$$A=\begin{bmatrix}1 & -2 & 1 & -1\\ 1 & 1 & -2 & 3\\ 4 & 1 & -5 & 8\\ 5 & -7 & 2 & -1\end{bmatrix}$$

Change this matrix into Echelon form as follows:

Performing

$R_2 \to R_2-R_1, R_3 \to R_3-4R_1$

and $R_4 \to R_4-5R_1$

$$\sim\begin{bmatrix}1 & -2 & 1 & -1\\ 0 & 3 & -3 & 4\\ 0 & 9 & -9 & 12\\ 0 & 3 & -3 & 4\end{bmatrix}$$

Performing $R_2 \to \frac{1}{3}R_2$

$$\sim\begin{bmatrix}1 & -2 & 1 & -1\\ 0 & 1 & -1 & \frac{4}{3}\\ 0 & 9 & -9 & 12\\ 0 & 3 & -3 & 4\end{bmatrix}$$

Performing

$R_3 \to R_3-9R_2, R_4 \to R_4-3R_2$

$$\sim\begin{bmatrix}1 & -2 & 1 & -1\\ 0 & 1 & -1 & \frac{4}{3}\\ 0 & 0 & 0 & 0\\ 0 & 0 & 0 & 0\end{bmatrix}$$

This is an Echelon form having two non-zero rows. Hence rank of $A=2$. Therefore the given system of equation is equivalent to

$$\begin{bmatrix} 1 & -2 & 1 & -1 \\ 0 & 1 & -1 & \frac{4}{3} \\ 0 & 0 & 0 & 0 \\ 0 & 0 & 0 & 0 \end{bmatrix} \begin{bmatrix} x \\ y \\ z \\ w \end{bmatrix} = 0$$

or $x - 2y + z - w = 0$ ... (1)

$y - z + \frac{4}{3}w = 0$ ... (2)

Let $z = c_1, w = c_2$

From (2) $y = c_1 - \frac{4}{3}c_2$

and from (1) $x = c_1 - \frac{5}{3}c_2$

Hence, solution is

$x = c_1 - \frac{5}{3}c_2, y - c_1 - \frac{4}{3}c_2,$

$z = c_1, w = c_2$

where c_1 and c_2 are arbitrary numbers.

Exercise-3.6

Find the solution of the following system of linear homogeneous equations:

1. $x + 2y + 3z = 0$
$3x + 4y + 4z = 0$
$7x + 10y + 12z = 0$

2. $x + y - 3z + 2w = 0$
$2x - y + 2z - 3w = 0$
$3x - 2y + z - 4w = 0$
$-4x + y - 3z + w = 0$

3. $x + y + z = 0$
$2x + 5y + 7z = 0$
$2x - 5y + 3z = 0$

4. $3x + 4y - z - 6w = 0$
$2x + 3y + 2z - 3w = 0$
$2x + y + 4z - 9w = 0$
$x + 3y + 13z + 3w = 0$

5. $2x - 3y + z = 0$
$x + 2y - 3z = 0$
$4x - y - 2z = 0$

6. $x + 2y + 3z = 0$
$2x + 3y + 4z = 0$
$7x + 13y + 19z = 0$

7. $x + 3y - 2z = 0$
$2x - y + 4z = 0$
$x - 11y + 14z = 0$

8. $2x - 2y + 5z + 3w = 0$
$4x - y + z + w = 0$
$3x - 2y + 3z + 4w = 0$
$x - 3y + 7z + 6w = 0$

ANSWERS

1. $x = 0 = y = z$ **2.** $x = 0 = y = z = w$ **3.** $x = 0 = y = z$

4. $x = 11c_1 + 6c_2, y = -8c_1 - 3c_2, z = c_1, w = c_2$ **5.** $x = 0 = y = z$ **6.** $x = c, y = -2c, z = c$

7. $x = -\frac{10}{7}c, y = \frac{8}{7}c, z = c$ **8.** $x = \frac{5}{9}c, y = 4c, z = \frac{7}{9}c, w = c$

3.21 NON-HOMOGENEOUS EQUATIONS

Let us consider a system of equations which are non-homogeneous as follows:

$$\left.\begin{aligned} a_{11}x_1 + a_{12}x_2 + \ldots + a_{1n}x_n &= b_1 \\ a_{21}x_1 + a_{22}x_2 + \ldots + a_{2n}x_n &= b_2 \\ \ldots\ldots\ldots\ldots\ldots\ldots\ldots\ldots\ldots\ldots \\ a_{m1}x_1 + a_{m2}x_2 + \ldots + a_{mn}x_n &= b_m \end{aligned}\right\} \quad \ldots (1)$$

These are m equations in n unknowns. Let

$$A = \begin{bmatrix} a_{11} & a_{12} & \cdots & a_{1n} \\ a_{21} & a_{22} & \cdots & a_{2n} \\ \vdots & \vdots & \vdots & \vdots \\ a_{m1} & a_{m2} & \cdots & a_{mn} \end{bmatrix}_{m \times n}$$

$$X = \begin{bmatrix} x_1 \\ x_2 \\ \vdots \\ x_n \end{bmatrix}_{n\times 1}, B = \begin{bmatrix} b_1 \\ b_1 \\ \vdots \\ b_m \end{bmatrix}_{m\times 1}$$

Then the system of equations (1) can also be written as

$$AX = B \quad \text{... (2)}$$

This equation is called a matrix equation. If $x_1, x_2, ... x_n$ simultaneously satisfy the equation (2), then $(x_1, x_2, ... x_n)$ is called the solution of (2).

3.21.1 CONSISTENCY AND INCONSISTENCY

When there exists one or more than one solution of the equation $AX = B$, then the equations are said to be consistent otherwise they are said to be inconsistent.

3.21.2 AUGMENTED MATRIX

The matrix of the type

$$[A \mid B] = \begin{bmatrix} a_{11} & a_{12} & \cdots & a_{1n} & b_1 \\ a_{21} & a_{22} & \cdots & a_{2n} & b_2 \\ \vdots & \vdots & \cdots & \cdots & \cdots \\ a_{m1} & a_{m2} & \cdots & a_{mn} & b_m \end{bmatrix}$$

is called the augmented matrix of the equations.

3.22 CONDITION FOR CONSISTENCY

THEOREM **(Rouche's Theorem).** *The equation $AX = B$ is consistent if and only if the rank of A and the rank of the augmented matrix $[A|B]$ are same.*

PROOF. Since the equation is $AX = B$

The matrix A can be written as $A = [c_1, c_2, ... c_n]$ ... (1)

where $c_1, c_2, ... c_n$ are column vectors. Then the equation (1) can be written as

$$[c_1, c_2, ..., c_n] \cdot \begin{bmatrix} x_1 \\ x_2 \\ \vdots \\ x_n \end{bmatrix} = B$$

or

$$x_1c_1 + x_2c_2 + ... + x_nc_n = B \quad \text{... (2)}$$

Suppose the rank of A is r, then A has r linearly independent columns. Let these columns be $c_1, c_2, ... c_r$ and these $c_1, c_2, ... c_r$ are linearly independent and remaining $(n - r)$ columns are linear combination of $c_1, c_2, ... c_r$.

Necessary condition. Suppose the equations are consistent, there must exist $k_1, k_2, ..., k_n$ such that

$$k_1c_1 + k_2c_2 + ... + k_nc_n = B \quad \text{... (3)}$$

But $c_{r+1}, c_{r+2}, ... c_n$ is a linear combination of $c_1, c_2, ... c_r$ then from (2) it is obvious that B is also a linear combination of $c_1, c_2, ... c_r$ and thus $[A|B]$ has the rank r. Hence, the rank of A is same as the rank of $[A|B]$.

Sufficient condition. Suppose rank A = rank $[A|B] = r$. This implies that $[A|B]$ has r linearly independent columns. But $c_1, c_2, ... c_r$ of $[A|B]$ are already linearly independent.

Thus B can be expressed as

$$B = k_1c_1+k_2c_2+...+ k_r\, c_r \text{ ; where } k_1, k_2, ... k_r \text{ are scalars.} \quad ...(4)$$

Now, equation (4) becomes

$$B = k_1c_1+k_2c_2+...+ k_rc_r+0.c_{r+1} +... +0.\, c_n \quad ...(5)$$

Comparing (2) and (5), we get $x_1 = k_1, x_2 = k_2, ... x_r = k_r, x_{r+1} = 0, ... = x_n = 0$ and these values of $x_1, x_2, ... x_n$ are the solution of $AX = B$. Hence, the equations are consistent.

- The n equations in n unknowns have a unique solution.
- If rank of $A <$ rank of $[A|B]$, then there is no solution.
- If $r = n$, then there will be a unique solution.
- If $r < n$, then $(n - r)$ variables can be assigned arbitrary values. Thus there will be infinite solutions and $(n - r+1)$ solutions will be linearly independent.
- If $m<n$ and $r \leq m \leq n$, then equations will have infinite solutions.

WORKING PROCEDURE

In order to determine the solutions of the equation $AX = B$, we proceed the following steps:

STEP 1. Reduce the augmented matrix $[A|B]$ to Echelon form by applying E-row transformations only. The Echelon form gives the rank of A and augmented matrix $[A|B]$.

STEP 2. (i) If the rank of A is not equal to the rank of $[A|B]$, then the system of equations has no solution, *i.e.*, equations are inconsistent.

(ii) If the rank of A is equal to the rank of $[A|B]$, then the equations are consistent and they will have unique solution if

rank of A = rank of $[A|B]$ = number of unknowns

and then will have infinite solutions if

rank of A = rank of $[A|B]$ = number of unknowns

STEP 3. Let $[A'|B']$ be the reduced Echelon form of $[A|B]$. Now reduce the equation $A'X = B'$ to a system of equations, after solving these equations we get the required solution.

Solved Examples

1. *Show that the equations*

$x + 2y - z = 3, 3x - y + 2z = 1,$

$2x - 2y + 3z = 2, x - y + z = -1$

are consistent and then solve them.

(BHILAI-2005; MADRAS-2002)

SOLUTION. The given equations can be written as:

$$\begin{bmatrix} 1 & 2 & -1 \\ 3 & -1 & 2 \\ 2 & -2 & 3 \\ 1 & -1 & 1 \end{bmatrix} \begin{bmatrix} x \\ y \\ z \end{bmatrix} = \begin{bmatrix} 3 \\ 1 \\ 2 \\ -1 \end{bmatrix}, i.e., AX = B$$

Therefore, augmented matrix is

$$[A \mid B] = \begin{bmatrix} 1 & 2 & -1 & \vdots & 3 \\ 3 & -1 & 2 & \vdots & 1 \\ 2 & -2 & 3 & \vdots & 2 \\ 1 & -1 & 1 & \vdots & -1 \end{bmatrix}$$

Performing $R_2 \to R_2 - 3R_1$, $R_3 \to R_3 - 2R_1$, $R_4 \to R_4 - R_1$

we get

$$[A \mid B] = \begin{bmatrix} 1 & 2 & -1 & \vdots & 3 \\ 0 & -7 & 5 & \vdots & -8 \\ 0 & -6 & 5 & \vdots & -4 \\ 0 & -3 & 2 & \vdots & -4 \end{bmatrix}$$

Performing $R_2 \to R_2 - R_3$

$$\sim \begin{bmatrix} 1 & 2 & -1 & \vdots & 3 \\ 0 & -1 & 0 & \vdots & -4 \\ 0 & -6 & 5 & \vdots & -4 \\ 0 & -3 & 2 & \vdots & -4 \end{bmatrix}$$

Performing $R_3 \to R_3 - 6R_2, R_4 \to R_4 - 3R_2$

$$\sim \begin{bmatrix} 1 & 2 & -1 & \vdots & 3 \\ 0 & -1 & 0 & \vdots & -4 \\ 0 & 0 & 5 & \vdots & 20 \\ 0 & 0 & 2 & \vdots & 8 \end{bmatrix}$$

Performing $R_3 \to \frac{1}{5}R_3, R_4 \to \frac{1}{2}R_4$

$$\sim\begin{bmatrix}1 & 2 & -1 & \vdots & 3\\0 & -1 & 0 & \vdots & -4\\0 & 0 & 1 & \vdots & 4\\0 & 0 & 1 & \vdots & 4\end{bmatrix}$$

Performing $R_4 \to R_4 - R_3$

$$\sim\begin{bmatrix}1 & 2 & -1 & \vdots & 3\\0 & -1 & 0 & \vdots & -4\\0 & 0 & 1 & \vdots & 4\\0 & 0 & 0 & \vdots & 0\end{bmatrix}$$

This is an Echelon form and having three non-zero rows. Thus rank A = rank of $[A|B]$ = 3. Therefore the equations are consistent

and $\begin{bmatrix}1 & 2 & -1\\0 & -1 & 0\\0 & 0 & 1\\0 & 0 & 0\end{bmatrix}\begin{bmatrix}x\\y\\z\end{bmatrix}=\begin{bmatrix}3\\-4\\4\\0\end{bmatrix}$

$x+2y-z=3, -y=-4, z=4$

Hence, the solution is $x=-1,\ y=4, z=4$.

2. *Solve the following equations by matrix method:*

$$x-2y+3z=6$$
$$3x+y-4z=-7$$
$$5x-3y+2z=5$$

SOLUTION. The given equations can be written as

$$\begin{bmatrix}1 & -2 & 3\\3 & 1 & -4\\5 & -3 & 2\end{bmatrix}\begin{bmatrix}x\\y\\z\end{bmatrix}=\begin{bmatrix}6\\-7\\5\end{bmatrix}$$

i.e., $AX = B$

∴ Argumented matrix is

$$[A\,|\,B]=\begin{bmatrix}1 & -2 & 3 & \vdots & 6\\3 & 1 & -4 & \vdots & -7\\5 & -3 & 2 & \vdots & 5\end{bmatrix}$$

Performing

$R_2 \to R_2 - 3R_1, R_3 \to R_3 - 5R_1$, we get

$$[A\,|\,B]=\begin{bmatrix}1 & -2 & 3 & \vdots & 6\\0 & 0 & -13 & \vdots & -25\\0 & 7 & -13 & \vdots & -25\end{bmatrix}$$

Performing $R_3 \to R_3 - R_2$

$$\sim\begin{bmatrix}1 & -2 & 3 & \vdots & 6\\0 & 7 & -13 & \vdots & -25\\0 & 0 & 0 & \vdots & 0\end{bmatrix}$$

This is an Echelon form and having two non-zero rows and rank A = rank $[A|B]$ =2. Thus the equations are consistent.

$$\begin{bmatrix}1 & -2 & 3\\0 & 7 & -13\\0 & 0 & 0\end{bmatrix}\begin{bmatrix}x\\y\\z\end{bmatrix}=\begin{bmatrix}6\\-25\\5\end{bmatrix}$$

i.e., $x - 2y + 3z = 6$

$7y - 13z = -25$

Let $z = c$, then $y=-\frac{25}{7}+\frac{13}{7}c$

$$x=-\frac{8}{7}+\frac{5}{7}c$$

Hence the solution is

$$x=-\frac{8}{7}+\frac{5}{7}c, y=-\frac{25}{7}+\frac{13}{7}c, z=c$$

where c is an arbitrary constant.

3. *Investigate for what values of λ, μ the simultaneous equations*

$$x+y+z=6, x+2y+3z=10,$$
$$x+2y+\lambda z=\mu$$

have (i) no solution (ii) a unique solution (iii) infinite solution.

(UKTU-2011, UPTU-2006, 14, MUMBAI-2007, ROHTAK-2004)

SOLUTION. The given equations can be written as

$$\begin{bmatrix}1 & 1 & 1\\1 & 2 & 3\\1 & 2 & \lambda\end{bmatrix}\begin{bmatrix}x\\y\\z\end{bmatrix}=\begin{bmatrix}6\\10\\\mu\end{bmatrix}$$

i.e., $AX = B$

Therefore, augmented matrix is

$$[A\,|\,B]=\begin{bmatrix}1 & 1 & 1 & \vdots & 6\\1 & 2 & 3 & \vdots & 10\\1 & 2 & \lambda & \vdots & \mu\end{bmatrix}$$

Performing

$R_2 \to R_2 - R_1, R_3 \to R_3 - R_1$, we get

$$\sim\begin{bmatrix}1 & 1 & 1 & \vdots & 6\\0 & 1 & 2 & \vdots & 4\\0 & 1 & \lambda-1 & \vdots & \mu-6\end{bmatrix}$$

Performing $R_3 \to R_3 - R_2$

$$\sim\begin{bmatrix}1 & 1 & 1 & \vdots & 6\\0 & 1 & 2 & \vdots & 4\\0 & 0 & \lambda-3 & \vdots & \mu-10\end{bmatrix}$$

If $\lambda \neq 3$, then rank A = rank $[A|B]$ = 3. Thus in this case a unique solution exists. If $\lambda = 3$ and $\mu_0 \neq 10$, then rank A=2, rank $[A|B]$ is 3. Thus rank $A \neq$ rank $[A|B]$. Hence, in this case equations are inconsistent.

If $\lambda = 3$ and $\mu = 10$, then rank A = rank $[A|B]$= 2. Thus in this case infinite solutions exist.

4. *For what values of η the equations $x+y+z=1$, $x+2y+4z = \eta$, $x+4y+10z = \eta^2$ have a solution? Solve them completely in each case.* (GBTU-2011, BHOPAL-2000, MUMBAI-2008, VTU-2006)

SOLUTION. The given system of equations can be written as $AX = B$ ... (1)

where

$$A = \begin{bmatrix} 1 & 1 & 1 \\ 1 & 2 & 4 \\ 1 & 4 & 10 \end{bmatrix}, X = \begin{bmatrix} x \\ y \\ z \end{bmatrix}, B = \begin{bmatrix} 1 \\ \eta \\ \eta^2 \end{bmatrix}$$

Augmented matrix $[A|B]$ is given by

$$\begin{bmatrix} 1 & 1 & 1 & \vdots & 1 \\ 1 & 2 & 4 & \vdots & \eta \\ 1 & 4 & 10 & \vdots & \eta^2 \end{bmatrix}$$

Applying

$R_2 \to R_2 - R_1, R_3 \to R_3 - R_1$, we get

$$\sim \begin{bmatrix} 1 & 1 & 1 & \vdots & 1 \\ 0 & 1 & 3 & \vdots & \eta - 1 \\ 0 & 3 & 9 & \vdots & \eta^2 - 1 \end{bmatrix}$$

Applying $R_3 \to R_3 - 3R_2$, we get

$$\sim \begin{bmatrix} 1 & 1 & 1 & \vdots & 1 \\ 0 & 1 & 3 & \vdots & \eta - 1 \\ 0 & 0 & 0 & \vdots & \eta^2 - 3\eta + 2 \end{bmatrix}$$

This last equivalent matrix is in Echelon form. The given system of equations will have the solutions if

rank of A = rank of $[A|B]$

For Echelon form, the rank of A is 2 and the augmented matrix $[A|B]$ will have rank 2.

if $\quad \eta^2 - 3\eta + 2 = 0$

i.e., if $\quad (\eta - 2)(\eta - 1) = 0$

i.e., if $\quad \eta = 1, 2$

The last equivalent matrix gives the system of equations as follows:

$$\begin{bmatrix} 1 & 1 & 1 \\ 0 & 1 & 3 \\ 0 & 0 & 0 \end{bmatrix} \begin{bmatrix} x \\ y \\ z \end{bmatrix} = \begin{bmatrix} 1 \\ \eta - 1 \\ \eta^2 - 3\eta + 2 \end{bmatrix}$$

$$\Rightarrow \left.\begin{aligned} x + y + z &= 1 \\ y + 3z &= \eta - 1 \end{aligned}\right\} \quad \text{... (2)}$$

Since rank of A = rank of $[A|B]$ if $\eta = 1$ and $\eta = 2$

Now we have two cases:

Case I: When $\eta = 1$

From (2), we have

$$\left.\begin{aligned} x + y + z &= 1 \\ y + 3z &= 0 \end{aligned}\right\} \quad \text{... (3)}$$

Since rank of A = rank of $[A|B]$=2 and number of unknowns is 3, therefore we will have 3 – 2 =1 unknown to be assigned.

Let us assign z to be c_1, therefore put $z = c_1$ in $y+3z=0$, we get $y= -3c_1$.

Again putting $y = -3c_1$ and $z= c_1$ in $x+y+z=1$, we get $x=1+2c_1$

Thus, in this case the solutions are

$$x = 1 + 2c_1, y = -3c_1, z = c_1$$

where c_1 is an arbitrary number.

Case II : When $\eta = 2$

From (2), we have

$$\left.\begin{aligned} x + y + z &= 1 \\ y + 3z &= 1 \end{aligned}\right\} \quad \text{...(4)}$$

Let us assign z to be c_2, therefore, putting $z= c_2$ in $y + 3z = 1$, we get $y = 1 - 3c_2$.

Again, putting $z = c_2$, $y = 1-3c_2$ in $x+y+z = 1$, we get $x = 2c_2$.

Thus, in this case the solutions are $x = 2c_2$, $y = 1-3c_2$, $z= c_2$

where c_2 is an arbitrary number.

Exercise-3.7

1. Use matrix method to solve the equations $2x - y + 3z = 9, x + y + z = 6, x - y + z = 2$.
2. Show that the equations $x - 3y - 8z + 10 = 0$, $3x + y - 4z = 0$, $2x + 5y + 6z - 13 = 0$ are consistent and solve them.
3. Examine if the system of equations $x + y + 4z = 6, 3x + 2y - 2z = 9$, $5x + y + 2z = 13$ is consistent. Find also the solution if it exists.

4. For what values of λ will the following equations fail to have a unique solution
$3x - y + \lambda z = 1, 2x + y + z = 2, x + 2y - \lambda z = -1$
Will the equations have any solution for these values of λ?

5. Solve $2x + 3y + z = 9, x + 2y + 3z = 6, 3x + y + 2z = 8$.

Solve the following equations by matrix method: (Q 6-9)

6. $5x + 3y + 7z = 4, 3x + 26y - 2z = 9, 7x + 2y + 10z = 5$. (JNTU-2005, PTU-2005, BHOPAL-2008)

7. $5x - 6y + 4z = 15, 7x + 4y - 3z = 19, 2x + y + 6z = 46$.

8. $x - y + 2z = 4, 3x + y + 4z = 6, x + y + z = 1$.

9. $x + y + z = 6, x + 2y + 3z = 4, 3x + y - 4z = 0$. (UPTU-2007)

10. $2x - y + 3z = 8, -x + 2y + z = 4, 3x + y - 4z = 0$.

11. Show that the following equations are inconsistent
$2x - y + z = 4, 3x - y + z = 6, 4x - y + 2z = 7, -x + y - z = 9$.

12. Show that the equations are inconsistent
$x - 4y + 7z = 14, 3x + 8y - 2z = 13, 7x - 8y + 26z = 5$.

13. Prove that the following system of equations have a unique solution
$5x + 3y + 14z = 4, y + 2z = 1, x - y + 2z = 0$.

14. Solve the following equations by matrix mehod: $x + y + z = 9, 2x + 5y + 7z = 52, 2x + y - z = 0$.

15. Using matrix method, show that the equations are consistant and hence find the solutions.
$3x + 3y + 2z = 1, x + 2y = 4, 10y + 3z = -2, 2x - 3y - z = 5$ are consistant and hence find the solutions. (UKTU-2010, GBTU-2010, NAGARJUNA-2008)

16. Show that the equations $2x + 6y + 11 = 0$, $6x + 20y - 6z + 3 = 0$ and $6y - 18z + 1 = 0$ are not consistent. (UKTU-2011, RAJASTHAN-2005, 13)

17. Show that the system of equations $2x - 3y + 7z = 5$; $3x + y - 3z = 13$ and $2x + 19y - 47z = 32$ is not consistent. (GBTU-2010)

18. For what value of λ, the system of equations $2x - 2y + z = \lambda x$, $2x - 3y + 2z = \lambda y$, $-x + 2y + 0z = \lambda z$ posses a non-trivial solution. Obtain its general solution. (MTU-2011)

19. Find the value of k so that the equation $x + y + 3z = 0$, $4x + 3y + kz = 0$ and $2x + y + 2z = 0$ have a non-trivial solution. (UPTU-2008)

20. Show that the system of equations $3x + 4y + 5z = a, 4x + 5y + 6z = b, 5x + 6y + 7z = c$ does not have a solution unless $a + c = 2b$. (UPTU-2008, MTU-2009, RAIPUR-2004, 14, NAGPUR-2001)

ANSWERS

1. $x = 1, y = 2, z = 3$ **2.** $x = 2c - 1, y = 3 - 2c, z = c$ **3.** Consistent; $x = 2, y = 2, z = \frac{1}{2}$

4. $\lambda \neq -\frac{7}{2}$ solution is unique; $\lambda = -\frac{7}{2}$, no solution. **5.** $x = \frac{35}{18}, y = \frac{29}{18}, z = \frac{5}{18}$ **6.** $x = \frac{7}{11}, y = \frac{3}{11}, z = 0$

7. $x = 3, y = 4, z = 6$ **8.** $x = \frac{5}{2} - \frac{3}{2}c, y = -\frac{3}{2} + \frac{1}{2}c, z = c$ **9.** $x = c - 2, y = 8 - 2c, z = c$

10. $x = 2, y = 2, z = 2$ **14.** $x = 1, y = 3, z = 4$ **15.** 2, 1, – 4

18. $\lambda = 1, x = 2k_1 - k_2, y = k_1, z = k_2, \lambda = -3, x = -k, y' = -2k, z = k$ **19.** 8

3.23 GAUSS ELIMINATION METHOD

In this method, the variables from the system of linear equations are eliminated successively and the system of equations is therefore reduced to an upper triangular system from which the variable are determined by back substitution. This method is described as follows: Let us consider a system of linear equation

$$AX = B \qquad ...(1)$$

Assuming $\det A \neq 0$. Equation (1) has the following form:

$$\left.\begin{array}{l} a_{11}x_1 + a_{12}x_2 + \ldots + a_{1n}x_n = b_1 \\ a_{21}x_1 + a_{22}x_2 + \ldots + a_{2n}x_n = b_2 \\ \ldots \quad \ldots \quad \ldots \quad \ldots \quad \ldots \quad \ldots \\ \ldots \quad \ldots \quad \ldots \quad \ldots \quad \ldots \quad \ldots \\ a_{n1}x_1 + a_{n2}x_2 + \ldots + a_{nn}x_n = b_n \end{array}\right\} \quad \ldots(2)$$

Assuming $a_{11} \neq 0$ and divide the first equation by a_{11} and then we subtract this equation multiplied by a_{21}, a_{31}, ..., a_{n1} from second, third ... nth equation of (2), we get

$$\left.\begin{array}{r} x_1 + a'_{12}x_2 + \ldots + a'_{1n}x_n = b'_1 \\ a'_{22}x_2 + \ldots + a'_{2n}x_n = b'_2 \\ \ldots \quad \ldots \quad \ldots \quad \ldots \quad \ldots \\ \ldots \quad \ldots \quad \ldots \quad \ldots \quad \ldots \\ a'_{n2}x_2 + \ldots + a'_{n2}x_n = b'_n \end{array}\right\} \quad \ldots(3)$$

Next, we divide second equation of (3) by a'_{22} (assuming $a'_{22} \neq 0$) and subtract this equation multiplied by $a'_{32}, a'_{42}, \ldots, a'_{n2}$ from third, fourth ... nth equation of (3), we get

$$\left.\begin{array}{r} x_1 + a'_{12}x_2 + \ldots + a'_{1n}x_n = b'_1 \\ x_2 + a''_{23}x_3 + \ldots + a''_{2n}x_n = b''_2 \\ a''_{33}x_3 + \ldots + a''_{3n}x_n = b''_3 \\ \ldots \quad \ldots \quad \ldots \quad \ldots \quad \ldots \\ a''_{3n}x_3 + \ldots + a''_{nn}x_n = b''_n \end{array}\right\} \quad \ldots(4)$$

Continuing in this way, we get a system of equation as follows:

$$\left.\begin{array}{r} x_1 + c_{12}x_2 + c_{13}x_3 + \ldots + c_{1n}x_n = d_1 \\ x_2 + c_{23}x_3 + \ldots + c_{2n}x_n = d_2 \\ \vdots \\ \vdots \\ c_{nn}x_n = d_n \end{array}\right\} \quad \ldots(5)$$

This is a form of upper triangular system. From back substitution we can find the solution of the system of given equations.

- The coefficient a_{11}, a'_{22} and a''_{33} are called pivots.
- This method will fail if any one of the pivots a_{11}, a'_{22} and a''_{33} becomes zero. In such cases, we rewrite the equations in a different order so that the pivots are non-zero.
- From each of the procedure, the largest coefficient of x is chosen as pivot element.

WORKING PROCEDURE

Let us consider these equations

$$\left.\begin{array}{l} a_{11}x_1 + a_{12}x_2 + a_{13}x_3 = b_1 \\ a_{21}x_1 + a_{22}x_2 + a_{23}x_3 = b_2 \\ a_{31}x_1 + a_{32}x_2 + a_{33}x_3 = b_3 \end{array}\right\} \quad \ldots(6)$$

STEP 1. First, eliminate x_1 from second and third equations. Assuming $a_{11} \neq 0$, now dividing first equation by a_{11} and then subtract from second and third after multiplied by a_{21} and respectively, we get

$$\left.\begin{aligned} x_1 + a'_{12}x_2 + a'_{13}x_3 &= b'_1 \\ a'_{22}x_2 + a'_{23}x_3 &= b'_2 \\ a'_{32}x_2 + a'_{33}x_3 &= b'_3 \end{aligned}\right\} \quad ...(7)$$

where $a'_{12} = \dfrac{a_{12}}{a_{11}}$, $a'_{13} = \dfrac{a_{13}}{a_{11}}$, $a'_{22} = a_{22} - a_{21}a'_{12}, a'_{23} = a_{23} - a_{21}a'_{13}$

$a'_{32} = a_{32} - a_{31}a'_{12}, a'_{33} = a_{33} - a_{31}a'_{13}$, $b'_1 = \dfrac{b_1}{a_{11}}, b'_2 = b_2 - a_{21}b'_1, b'_3 = b_3 - a_{31}b'_1$

STEP 2. Now eliminating x_2 from third equation in (7).
Again assuming $a'_{22} \neq 0$. Dividing second equation in (7) by a'_{22} and then subtract from third equation after multiplied by a'_{32} we get

$$\left.\begin{aligned} x_1 + a'_{12}x_2 + a'_{13}x_3 &= b'_1 \\ x_2 + a''_{23}x_3 &= b'_2 \\ a''_{33}x_3 &= b'_3 \end{aligned}\right\} \quad ...(8)$$

where $a''_{23} = \dfrac{a'_{23}}{a'_{22}}, a'_{33} = a'_{33} - a'_{32}a''_{23}$, $b''_2 = \dfrac{b'_2}{a'_{22}}, b''_3 = b_3' - a'_{32}b''_2$.

STEP 3. Evaluating x_1, x_2 and x_3 from (8) by back substitution.

Solved Examples

1. *Solve the following equations by Gauss's elimination method*

$$6x + 3y + 2z = 6$$
$$6x + 4y + 3z = 0$$
$$20x + 15y + 12z = 0.$$

SOLUTION. Here pivot element is 6. Now Divide first equation by 6, we get

$$x + \frac{1}{2}y + \frac{1}{3}z = 1 \quad ...(1)$$

Now eliminating x from second and third equation with the help of (1). Subtract (1) multiplied by 6 and 20 from second and third equation, respectively we get

$$y + z = -6 \quad ...(2)$$

$$5y + \frac{16}{3}z = -20 \quad ...(3)$$

Now eliminating y from (3) with the help of (2), we get

$$\left(\frac{16}{3} - 5\right)z = -20 + 30$$

$$\frac{1}{3}z = 10 \Rightarrow z = 30$$

Substitute the value of z into (2), we get

$$y = -6 - 30 = -36$$

and again substitute the values of y and z into (1), we get

$$x + \frac{1}{2}(-36) + \frac{1}{3}(30) = 1$$

$$x - 18 + 10 = 1 \Rightarrow x = 9$$

Hence, the solution of the equations are

$$x = 9, y = -36, z = 30.$$

2. *By Gauss's elimination method, solve the following equations*

$$5x - y - 2z = 142$$
$$x - 3y - z = -30$$
$$2x - y - 3z = -50$$

SOLUTION. The largest coefficient in first equation is 5, which is pivot element. So divide first equation by 5, we get

$$x - \frac{1}{5}y - \frac{2}{5}z = \frac{142}{5} \quad ...(1)$$

Now eliminating x from second and third equation with help of (1), we get

$$-\frac{14}{5}y - \frac{3}{5}z = -\frac{292}{5} \quad ...(2)$$

$$-\frac{3}{5}y - \frac{11}{5}z = -\frac{309}{5} \quad ...(3)$$

Eliminating y from (2) and (3), we get

or $$-\frac{145}{5}z = -\frac{3450}{5}$$

$$z = \frac{3450}{145} = 23.79$$

Substitute the value of z into (3) we get

$$-\frac{3}{5}y - \frac{11}{5}(23.79) = -\frac{309}{5}$$

$$-\frac{3}{5}y = -\frac{309}{5} + \frac{11(23.79)}{5}$$

$$-3y = -309 + 11(23.79)$$

$$-3y = -47.31$$

or $y = 15.77$

Substitute the values of y and z into (1), we get

$$x - \frac{1}{5}(15.77) - \frac{2}{5}(23.79) = \frac{142}{5}$$

or $x = 41.07$

Hence, the solution are given by

$$x = 41.07, y = 15.77, z = 23.79.$$

3. *Solve by the Gauss's elimination method.*

$$2x + y + 4z = 12$$
$$8x - 3y + 2z = 23$$
$$4x + 11y - z = 33$$

SOLUTION. Dividing first equation by 2, we get

$$x + \frac{1}{2}y + 2z = 6 \qquad ...(1)$$

Now subtract (1) after multiplied by 8 and 4 respectively from second and third equation, we get

$$-7y - 14x = -45 \qquad ...(2)$$
$$9y - 9z = 9 \qquad ...(3)$$

Now multiplying (4) by 9 and subtract from (3), we get

$$-27z = 9 - \frac{405}{7}$$

or $$-27z = -\frac{342}{7} \qquad ...(5)$$

Hence, the system of equations reduces to upper triangular form as follows:

$$\left.\begin{aligned} x + \frac{1}{2}y + 2z &= 6 \\ y + 2z &= \frac{45}{7} \\ -27z &= -\frac{342}{7} \end{aligned}\right\} \qquad ...(6)$$

By back substitution , we get

$$z = \frac{342}{189} = 1.81$$

and $$y + 2(1.81) = \frac{45}{7}$$

$$\Rightarrow \quad y = \frac{45}{7} - 2(1.81) = 6.43 - 3.62$$
$$= 2.81$$

and $$x + \frac{1}{2}(2.81) + 2(1.81) = 6$$

$$\therefore \quad x = 6 - \frac{1}{2}(2.81) - 2(1.81)$$
$$= 0.975$$

Hence, the solution is

$$x = 0.975, y = 2.81, z = 1.81.$$

Exercise-3.8

1. Solve the following equations by Gauss's elimination method :

(i) $x_1 + x_2 + 2x_3 = 4$
$3x_1 + x_2 - 3x_3 = -4$
$2x_1 - 3x_2 - 5x_3 = -5$

(ii) $2x_1 + x_2 + 4x_3 = 12$
$8x_1 - 3x_2 + 2x_3 = 20$
$4x_1 + 11x_2 - x_3 = 33$

(iii) $x_1 + x_2 + x_3 = 10$
$2x_1 + x_2 + 2x_3 = 17$
$3x_1 + 2x_2 + x_3 = 17$

(iv) $2x + 3y - z = 5$
$4x + 4y - 3z = 3$
$2x - 3y + 2z = 2$

(v) $2x + y + z = 10$
$x + 2y + 3z = 18$
$x + 4y + 9z = 16$

(vi) $2x_1 + 4x_2 + x_3 = 2$
$3x_1 + 2x_2 - 2x_3 = -2$
$x_1 - x_2 + x_3 = 6$

2. Apply Gauss's elimination method to solve the equations

$$x + 4y - z = -5$$
$$x + y - 6z = -12$$
$$3x - y - z = 4$$

3. Solve the following system by Gauss's elimination method :

$$2x + y + z = 10$$
$$3x + 2y + 3z = 18$$
$$x + 4y + 9z = 4$$

4. By Gauss's elimination method, solve

$$4x + 11y - z = 33$$
$$x + y + 4z = 12$$
$$8x - 3y + 2z = 20$$

5. Solve by Gauss's elimination method

$$x + 2y + z = 3$$
$$2x + 3y + 3z = 10$$
$$3x - y + 2z = 13$$

ANSWERS

1. (i) $x_1 = 1, x_2 = -1, x_3 = 2$ (ii) $x_1 = 3, x_2 = 2, x_3 = 1$ (iii) $x_1 = 2, x_2 = 3, x_3 = 5$
(iv) $x = 1, y = 2, z = 3$ (v) $x = 7, y = -9, z = 5$ (vi) $x_1 = 2, x_2 = -1, x_3 = 3$

2. $x = \frac{117}{71}, y = -\frac{81}{71}, z = \frac{148}{71}$

3. $x = 7, y = -9, z = 5$

4. $x = 2.856, y = 2.121, z = 1.756$

5. $x = -5, y = \frac{4}{3}, z = \frac{16}{3}$

3.24 EIGENVALUE AND EIGENVECTORS OF A MATRIX

A polynomial in indeterminate λ of the form

$$f(\lambda) = A_0 + A_1\lambda + A_2\lambda^2 + \ldots + A_n\lambda^n$$

where $A_0, A_1, A_2, \ldots, A_n$ are all square matrices of the same order, is called a matrix polynomial of degree n if $A_n \neq O$ (null matrix).

From above definition it is clear that every square matrix can be expressed as a matrix polynomial of zero degree. If A is a square matrix, then we can write

$$A = \lambda^\circ A$$

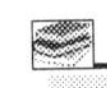

- Two matrix polynomials are said to be equal if and only if the coefficients of like powers of λ are the same.

3.25 THE CHARACTERISTIC EQUATION OF A MATRIX

Let A be a square matrix of order $n \times n$ and let

$$A = \begin{bmatrix} a_{11} & a_{12} & \cdots & a_{1n} \\ a_{21} & a_{22} & \cdots & a_{2n} \\ \vdots & \vdots & & \vdots \\ a_{n1} & a_{n2} & \cdots & a_{nn} \end{bmatrix},$$

If λ is indeterminate, then the matrix $A - \lambda I$ is called the characteristic matrix of A, where I is the unit matrix of order $n \times n$.

The determinant $|A - \lambda I| = \begin{bmatrix} a_{11} - \lambda & a_{12} & \cdots & a_{1n} \\ a_{21} & a_{22} - \lambda & \cdots & a_{2n} \\ \vdots & \vdots & & \vdots \\ a_{n1} & a_{n2} & \cdots & a_{nn} - \lambda \end{bmatrix}$ is an ordinary polynomial in λ

which is called the characteristic polynomial of A and the equation

$$|A - \lambda I| = 0$$

i.e.,

$$\begin{vmatrix} a_{11} - \lambda & a_{12} & \cdots & a_{1n} \\ a_{21} & a_{22} - \lambda & \cdots & a_{2n} \\ \vdots & \vdots & & \vdots \\ a_{n1} & a_{n2} & \cdots & a_{nn} - \lambda \end{vmatrix} = 0$$

is known as the characteristic equation of A. The roots of the equation $|A - \lambda I| = 0$ are called characteristic roots or latent roots or eigenvalues of A. The set of all eigenvalues of a matrix A is called spectrum of A.

3.26 CHARACTERISTIC VECTORS OR EIGENVECTORS OF A MATRIX

Let $A = [a_{ij}]$ be a matrix of order $n \times n$ and let $X = \begin{bmatrix} x_1 \\ x_2 \\ \vdots \\ x_n \end{bmatrix}$

be a column vector. Consider a vector equation

$$AX = \lambda X \text{ ; where } \lambda \text{ is a scalar.} \qquad ...(1)$$

It is evident that $X = O$ satisfies the equation (1) for every value of λ, thus $X = O$ is a solution of (1). A value of λ for which a non-zero vector, *i.e.*, $X \neq O$ satisfies (1) is called an eigenvalue of the matrix A and the non-zero vector X is called an eigenvector of A corresponding to that eigenvalue λ.

Now equation (1) can be written as $\qquad AX = \lambda IX$

or $\qquad (A - \lambda I)X = O \qquad ...(2)$

where I is the unit matrix of order $n \times n$. Equation (2) represents a matrix equation of a system of n homogeneous equations. The necessary and sufficient condition for the equation (2) to possess a non-zero solution, *i.e.*, $X \neq O$ is that $|A - \lambda I| = 0$, which is a characteristic equation of matrix A.

- The eigenvector is also known as proper vector.
- If X is an eigenvector of a matrix corresponding eigenvalue λ, then for any non-zero scalar kX is also an eigenvector of A corresponding to the same eigenvalue λ.
- Corresponding to an eigenvalue of a matrix A, there will be different eigenvectors of A.
- For a given eigenvector of a matrix A there corresponds one and only one eigenvalue of A.

3.27 RELATION BETWEEN EIGENVALUES AND EIGENVECTORS

THEOREM 1. *λ is an eigenvalue of a matrix A if and only if there exists a non-zero vector X such that*

$$AX = \lambda X.$$

PROOF. Suppose that λ is an eigenvalue of A, then

$$|A - \lambda I| = 0$$

$\Rightarrow \quad A - \lambda I$ is a singular matrix.

$\therefore \quad$ The matrix equation $(A - \lambda I)X = O$ has a non-zero solution, thus there exists a non-zero vector X such that

$$(A - \lambda I)X = O \text{ or } AX = \lambda X$$

Conversely, Suppose that there is a non-zero vector X such that $AX = \lambda X$

$$\Rightarrow \qquad (A - \lambda I)X = O$$

Since the matrix equation $(A - \lambda I)X = O$ has a non-zero solution, then the coefficient matrix $A - \lambda I$ is singular, therefore $\qquad |A - \lambda I| = 0$

Hence A is an eigenvalue of A.

THEOREM 2. *If X is an eigenvector of a matrix A corresponding to an eigenvalue of A, then kX is also an eigenvector of A corresponding to the same eigenvalue A, where k is any non-zero number.*

PROOF. Since X is an eigenvector of a matrix A corresponding to an eigenvalue of A, then we have

$$AX = \lambda X \qquad ...(1)$$

Since $k \neq 0$, then multipling both sides of (1) by k, we get $k(AX) = k(\lambda X)$

$$\Rightarrow \qquad A(kX) = \lambda(kX) \qquad ...(2)$$

From equation (2), it follows that kX is also an eigenvector of A corresponding to the same eigenvalue λ.

THEOREM 3. *If X is a non-zero eigenvector of a matrix A, then X cannot correspond to more than one eigenvalue of A.*

PROOF. If possible, let X be an eigenvector corresponding to eigenvalues λ_1 and λ_2, then

$$AX = \lambda_1 X \quad \text{...(1)}$$

and

$$AX = \lambda_2 X \quad \text{...(2)}$$

From (1) and (2) we have $\lambda_1 X = \lambda_2 X$

$\Rightarrow$ $(\lambda_1 - \lambda_2) X = O$

$\Rightarrow$ $\lambda_1 - \lambda_2 = 0$ $\quad \because X \neq O$

$\Rightarrow$ $\lambda_1 = \lambda_2$

IMPORTANT PROPERTIES

(1) If X_1 and X_2 be non-zero eigenvectors of a matrix A corresponding to an eigenvalue λ of A, then $k_1X_1 + k_2X_2$ is also an eigenvector of A corresponding to eigenvalue λ, where k_1 and k_2 are non-zero numbers.

(2) Let A be an $n \times n$ matrix. Then the distinct eigenvectors corresponding to distinct eigenvalues of A are linearly independent.

3.28 EIGENVALUE OF SPECIAL TYPE OF MATRICES

THEOREM 1. *The eigenvalues of a Hermitian matrix are real.* (UKTU - 2011)

PROOF. Let A be a Hermitian matrix. Let λ be an eigenvalue of A and let X be its corresponding eigenvector.

Then we have $AX = \lambda X$ ...(1)

Pre-multiplying both sides of (1) by X^θ, we have

$$X^\theta AX = X^\theta \lambda X = \lambda X^\theta X \quad \text{...(2)}$$

Taking conjugate transpose of both sides of (2), we have

$$(X^\theta AX)^\theta = (\lambda X^\theta X)^\theta$$

$\Rightarrow$ $X^\theta A^\theta (X^\theta)^\theta = \bar{\lambda} X^\theta (X^\theta)^\theta$

$\Rightarrow$ $X^\theta A^\theta X = \bar{\lambda} X^\theta X$ $\quad \because (X^\theta)^\theta = X$

$\Rightarrow$ $X^\theta AX = \bar{\lambda} X^\theta X$ $\quad [\because A \text{ is Hermitian} \Rightarrow A^\theta = A]$

$\Rightarrow$ $X^\theta \lambda X = \bar{\lambda} X^\theta X$ $\quad$ [Using (1)]

or $\lambda X^\theta X = \bar{\lambda} X^\theta X$

or $(\lambda - \bar{\lambda}) X^\theta X = O$

or $(\lambda - \bar{\lambda}) = 0$ $\quad [\because X \text{ is non-zero} \Rightarrow X^\theta X \neq O]$

or $\lambda = \bar{\lambda}$

Hence, λ is real.

THEOREM 2. *The eigenvalues of a real symmetric matrix are all real.*

PROOF. Let A be a real symmetric matrix, then

$$A' = A \quad \text{...(1)}$$

Let λ be any eigenvalue of A and let X be its corresponding eigenvector, then we have

$$AX = \lambda X \quad \text{...(2)}$$

Pre-multiplying both sides of (2) by X' we get

$$X'AX = X'\lambda X = \lambda X'X \quad \text{...(3)}$$

Taking transpose of both sides of (3), we get

$$(X'AX)' = (\lambda X'X)' \Rightarrow X'A'(X')' = \bar{\lambda} X'(X')'$$

$\Rightarrow$ $X'A'X = \bar{\lambda} X'X$ $\quad [\because (X')' = X]$

$$\Rightarrow \quad X'AX = \bar{\lambda}X'X \quad [\because A' = A]$$

$$\Rightarrow \quad X'\lambda X = \bar{\lambda}X'X \quad [\because AX = \lambda X]$$

$$\Rightarrow \quad \lambda X'X = \bar{\lambda}X'X$$

$$\Rightarrow \quad (\lambda - \bar{\lambda})X'X = O \quad \Rightarrow \quad (\lambda - \bar{\lambda}) = 0 \; [\because X \neq O \Rightarrow X'X \neq O]$$

$$\Rightarrow \quad \lambda = \bar{\lambda} \quad \Rightarrow \lambda \text{ is real.}$$

THEOREM 3. *The eigenvalues of a skew-Hermitian matrix are either purely imaginary or zero.*

PROOF. Let A be a skew-Hermitian matrix, then

$$A^{\theta} = -A$$

Now $(iA)^{\theta} = -iA^{\theta} \Rightarrow \quad (iA)^{\theta} = iA$

$\Rightarrow$ iA is a Hermitian matrix

Let λ be an eigenvalue of A and X be its corresponding eigenvector, then

$$AX = \lambda X \quad \Rightarrow \quad iAX = i\lambda X$$

$\therefore$ $i\lambda$ is an eigenvalue of a Hermitian matrix. By theorem 1, we can say that $i\lambda$ is real. It follows that either λ is purely imaginary or zero.

COROLLARY. *The eigenvalues of a real skew-symmetric matrix are either purely imaginary or zero.*

PROOF. If the elements of a skew-Hermitian matrix are all real, then it is a real skew-symmetric. Therefore, a real skew-symmetric matrix is skew-Hermitian matrix, hence the result follows from theorem 3.

THEOREM 4. *The eigenvalues of a unitary matrix are of unit modulus.* (UKTU-2010, 12)

PROOF. Let A be a unitary matrix, then

$$A^{\theta}A = I \quad \ldots(1)$$

Let λ be an eigenvalue of A and let X be its corresponding eigenvector, then

$$AX = \lambda X \quad \ldots(2)$$

Taking conjugate transpose of both sides of (2), we have

$$(AX)^{\theta} = (\lambda X)^{\theta}$$

or

$$X^{\theta}A^{\theta} = \bar{\lambda}X^{\theta} \quad \ldots(3)$$

Now $(X^{\theta}A^{\theta})(AX) = (\bar{\lambda}X^{\theta})(\lambda X)$ [Using (2) and (3)]

$$\Rightarrow \quad X^{\theta}(A^{\theta}A)X = \bar{\lambda}\lambda X^{\theta}X$$

$$\Rightarrow \quad X^{\theta}IX = \bar{\lambda}\lambda X^{\theta}X \quad \text{[Using (1)]}$$

$$\Rightarrow \quad X^{\theta}X = \bar{\lambda}\lambda X^{\theta}X$$

$$\Rightarrow \quad (1 - \bar{\lambda}\lambda)X^{\theta}X = O$$

$$\Rightarrow \quad \bar{\lambda}\lambda = 1 \quad [\because X \neq O \Rightarrow X^{\theta}X \neq O]$$

$$\Rightarrow \quad |\lambda|^2 = 1 \quad \Rightarrow \quad |\lambda| = 1$$

COROLLARY *The eigenvalues of an orthogonal matrix are of unit modulus.*

PROOF. We know that if the elements of a unitary matrix are all real, then it is an orthogonal matrix, therefore an orthogonal matrix is a unitary matrix hence, the result follows from theorem 4.

WORKING PROCEDURE

To find the eigenvalue and eigenvectors

Let A be an $n \times n$ matrix, then it will have n eigenvalues. In order to find the eigenvalues and eigenvectors of A, we use the following steps :

STEP 1. Find the roots of the characteristic equation $|A - \lambda I| = 0$, the roots of λ give the eigenvalues of A.

STEP 2. Let $X = \begin{bmatrix} x_1 \\ x_2 \\ \vdots \\ x_n \end{bmatrix} \neq O$ be an eigenvector of A corresponding to an eigenvalue λ_1 (say).

Then X can be determined from the equation $(A - \lambda_1 I) X = O$

which is a system of n homogeneous equations in $x_1, x_2, ..., x_n$. If the rank of $(A - \lambda_1 I)$ is r, then the number of linearly independent solutions is $n - r$.

Solved Examples

1. *If λ is a non-zero eigenvalue of a matrix A, then show that $\frac{1}{\lambda}$ is an eigenvalue of A^{-1}.*

SOLUTION. Let $X \neq O$ be an eigenvector corresponding to the eigenvalue λ of A, then

$$AX = \lambda X$$

$$\Rightarrow \quad A^{-1}(AX) = A^{-1}(\lambda X) \quad [\because A^{-1} \text{ exists.}]$$

$$\Rightarrow \quad (A^{-1}A)X = \lambda(A^{-1}X)$$

$$\Rightarrow \quad IX = \lambda(A^{-1}X) \quad [\because A^{-1}A = I]$$

$$\Rightarrow \quad X = \lambda(A^{-1}X) \quad [\because IX = X]$$

$$\Rightarrow \quad A^{-1}X = \left(\frac{1}{\lambda}\right)X$$

Hence, $\frac{1}{\lambda}$ is an eigenvalue of A^{-1}.

2. *Let A be an $n \times n$ matrix. Then show that zero is an eigenvalue of A iff A is singular.*

SOLUTION. Let $X \neq O$ be an eigenvector corresponding to the eigenvalue 0 of A, then

$$AX = 0X = O \quad ...(1)$$

Since (1) represents a system of homogeneous equations, it will have non-zero solution if and only if $\rho(A) < n$

i.e., iff $|A| = 0$

i.e., iff A is singular.

3. *If $\lambda_1, \lambda_2, ..., \lambda_n$ are the eigenvalues of A, then show that $k\lambda_1, k\lambda_2, ..., k\lambda_n$ are eigenvalues of kA, where k is any number.*

SOLUTION. If $k = 0$, then $kA = 0A = O$. Since each eigenvalue of a zero matrix is zero, therefore $0\lambda_1, 0\lambda_2, ..., 0\lambda_n$ are the eigenvalues of kA if $\lambda_1, \lambda_2, ..., \lambda_n$ are eigenvalues of A.

Next, suppose that $k \neq 0$, then we have

$$|kA - k\lambda I| = k^n|A - \lambda I|$$

Now $|kA - k\lambda I| = 0$ iff $|A - \lambda I| = 0$

It follows that $k\lambda$ is an eigenvalue of kA.

Hence, if $\lambda_1, \lambda_2, ..., \lambda_n$ are the eigenvalues of A then $k\lambda_1, k\lambda_2, ..., k\lambda_n$ are the eigenvalues of kA.

4. *If X be a non-zero eigenvector of an $n \times n$ matrix A, then prove that for each positive integer n, X is an eigenvector of A^n corresponding to the eigenvalue λ^n.*

SOLUTION. Since $X \neq O$ is an eigenvector corresponding eigenvalue λ of A, then we have

$$AX = \lambda X \quad ...(1)$$

Now we have to show that $A^nX = \lambda^nX$.

We shall prove this by induction on n.

If $n = 1$, then the result is true by virtue of (1).

Suppose that the result is true for $n = k$, then we have

$$A^kX = \lambda^kX \quad ...(2)$$

$$\begin{aligned} \text{Now} \quad A^{k+1}X &= (A^kA)X \\ &= A^k(AX) \\ &= A^k(\lambda X) \quad [\text{Using (1)}] \\ &= \lambda(A^kX) \\ &= \lambda(\lambda^kX) \quad [\text{Using (2)}] \\ &= \lambda^{k+1}X \end{aligned}$$

$$A^{k+1}X = \lambda^{k+1}X$$

Thus, the result is true for $n = k+1$.

Hence by induction the result is true for all positive integers n.

5. *Show that similar matrices have the same eigenvalues.*

SOLUTION. Two matrices A and B of the same order are said to be similar if there exists a non-singular matrix P such that

$$B = P^{-1}AP$$

Let λ be an eigenvalue of A, then X is a root of $|A - \lambda I| = 0$.

Now
$$B - \lambda I = P^{-1}AP - \lambda I$$
$$= P^{-1}AP - P^{-1}(\lambda I)P$$
$$[\because P^{-1}(\lambda I)P = \lambda P^{-1}P = \lambda I]$$
$$= P^{-1}(A - \lambda I)P$$
$$\Rightarrow \quad |B - \lambda I| = |P^{-1}|\,|A - \lambda I|\,|P|$$
$$\Rightarrow \quad |B - \lambda I| = |A - \lambda I|\,|P^{-1}|\,|P|$$
$$\Rightarrow \quad |B - \lambda I| = |A - \lambda I|\,|P^{-1}P|$$
$$\Rightarrow \quad |B - \lambda I| = |A - \lambda I|$$
$$[\because |P^{-1}P| = |I| = 1]$$

Since λ is a root of $|A - \lambda I| = 0$, therefore λ is also a root of $|B - \lambda I| = 0$, it follows that λ is an eigenvalue of B.

Hence, similar matrices have the same eigenvalues.

6. *Let A and B be two matrices of order n × n. Let $X \neq O$ be an eigenvector of A and B corresponding to the eigenvalues λ_1 and λ_2 respectively, then show that X is an eigenvector of AB corresponding to the eigenvalue $\lambda_1\lambda_2$ of AB.*

SOLUTION. Since $X \neq O$ is an eigenvector of A and B corresponding to the eigenvalues λ_1 and λ_2 respectively, then we have

$$AX = \lambda_1 X \quad \ldots(1)$$
and
$$BX = \lambda_2 X \quad \ldots(2)$$
Now
$$(AB)X = A(BX)$$
$$= A(\lambda_2 X) \quad [\text{Using (2)}]$$
$$= \lambda_2(AX)$$
$$= \lambda_2(\lambda_1 X) \quad [\text{Using (1)}]$$
$$= (\lambda_2\lambda_1)X$$
$$(AB)X = (\lambda_1\lambda_2)X \text{ with } X \neq O$$

It follows that X is an eigenvector of AB corresponding to the eigenvalue $\lambda_1\lambda_2$.

7. *Determine the eigenvalues of the matrix :*

$$A = \begin{bmatrix} 1 & 2 & 3 \\ 0 & -4 & 2 \\ 0 & 0 & 7 \end{bmatrix}$$

SOLUTION. The characteristic equation of A is given by
$$|A - \lambda I| = 0$$
i.e.,
$$\begin{vmatrix} 1-\lambda & 2 & 3 \\ 0 & -4-\lambda & 2 \\ 0 & 0 & 7-\lambda \end{vmatrix} = 0$$
i.e.,
$$(1-\lambda)(-4-\lambda)(7-\lambda) = 0$$

The roots of this characteristic equation are given by $\lambda = 1, -4, 7$.

These are the required eigenvalues of A.

- It is clear that the given matrix A is an upper triangular matrix so that the principal diagonal elements 1, – 4, 7 will be the eigenvalues of A.

8. *Determine the eigenvalues of the matrix :*

$$A = \begin{bmatrix} 0 & 1 & 2 \\ 1 & 0 & -1 \\ 2 & -1 & 0 \end{bmatrix}.$$

SOLUTION. The characteristic equation of A is given

$$|A - \lambda I| = 0$$
$$\begin{vmatrix} 0-\lambda & 1 & 2 \\ 1 & 0-\lambda & -1 \\ 2 & -1 & 0-\lambda \end{vmatrix} = 0$$
or
$$-\lambda(\lambda^2 - 1) - 1(-\lambda + 2) + 2(-1 + 2\lambda) = 0$$
or
$$-\lambda^3 + 6\lambda - 4 = 0$$

Solving this equation, we get

$$(\lambda - 2)(\lambda^2 + 2\lambda - 2) = 0$$
$$\Rightarrow \quad \lambda = 2 \text{ and } \lambda = -1 \pm \sqrt{3}$$

Hence, the eigenvalues of A are 2, $-1 \pm \sqrt{3}$.

9. *Determine the eigenvalues and eigenvectors of the matrix*

$$A = \begin{bmatrix} 5 & 4 \\ 1 & 2 \end{bmatrix}.$$ (BHOPAL -2008)

SOLUTION. The characteristic equation of A is given by

$$|A - \lambda I| = 0$$
or
$$\begin{vmatrix} 5-\lambda & 4 \\ 1 & 2-\lambda \end{vmatrix} = 0$$
or
$$(5-\lambda)(2-\lambda) - 4 = 0$$
or
$$\lambda^2 - 7\lambda + 10 - 4 = 0$$
or
$$\lambda^2 - 7\lambda + 6 = 0$$

The roots of this equation are $\lambda = 6, 1$.
Thus, the eigenvalues of A are 6, 1.

Eigenvector corresponding to $\lambda_1 = 6$:

Let $X_1 = \begin{bmatrix} x_1 \\ x_2 \end{bmatrix} \neq O$ be an eigenvector of A corresponding to $\lambda_1 = 6$, then we have

$$AX_1 = 6X_1$$

or $$(A - 6I)X_1 = O$$

or $$\begin{bmatrix} 5-6 & 4 \\ 1 & 2-6 \end{bmatrix}\begin{bmatrix} x_1 \\ x_2 \end{bmatrix} = \begin{bmatrix} 0 \\ 0 \end{bmatrix}$$

or $$\begin{bmatrix} -1 & 4 \\ 1 & -4 \end{bmatrix}\begin{bmatrix} x_1 \\ x_2 \end{bmatrix} = \begin{bmatrix} 0 \\ 0 \end{bmatrix} \quad \ldots(1)$$

The non-zero solution of (1) will give X_1.
Applying $R_2 \to R_2 + R_1$, we have

$$\begin{bmatrix} -1 & 4 \\ 1 & -4 \end{bmatrix}\begin{bmatrix} x_1 \\ x_2 \end{bmatrix} = \begin{bmatrix} 0 \\ 0 \end{bmatrix} \quad \ldots(2)$$

The coefficient matrix of equation (1) is of rank 1, *i.e.*, $\rho(A - 6I) = 1$, therefore the system of equations (1) will have 2 – 1 = 1 linearly independent solution.
From (2), we have

$$-x_1 + 4x_2 = 0$$

Clearly, $x_1 = 4$ and $x_2 = 1$ satisfy the above equation.
Hence, the eigenvector corresponding to eigenvalue $\lambda_1 = 6$ is

$$X_1 = \begin{bmatrix} 4 \\ 1 \end{bmatrix}$$

Eigenvector corresponding to $\lambda_2 = 1$:

Let $X_2 = \begin{bmatrix} x_1 \\ x_2 \end{bmatrix} \neq O$ be an eigenvector of A corresponding to eigenvalue $\lambda_2 = 1$, then we have

$$AX_2 = \lambda_2 X_2$$

or $$AX_2 = IX_2$$

or $$(A - I)X_2 = O$$

or $$\begin{bmatrix} 5-1 & 4 \\ 1 & 2-1 \end{bmatrix}\begin{bmatrix} x_1 \\ x_2 \end{bmatrix} = \begin{bmatrix} 0 \\ 0 \end{bmatrix}$$

or $$\begin{bmatrix} 4 & 4 \\ 1 & 1 \end{bmatrix}\begin{bmatrix} x_1 \\ x_2 \end{bmatrix} = \begin{bmatrix} 0 \\ 0 \end{bmatrix} \quad \ldots(3)$$

The non-zero solution of (3) will give X_2.

Applying $R_2 \to R_2 - \frac{1}{4}R_1$, we get

$$\begin{bmatrix} 4 & 4 \\ 0 & 0 \end{bmatrix}\begin{bmatrix} x_1 \\ x_2 \end{bmatrix} = \begin{bmatrix} 0 \\ 0 \end{bmatrix} \quad \ldots(4)$$

Clearly, $\rho(A - I) = 1$, therefore the system of equations (3) will have 2 – 1 = 1 linearly independent solution.
From (4), we get

$$4x_1 + 4x_2 = 0$$

Clearly, $x_1 = 1$ and $x_2 = -1$, satisfy above equation.
Hence, the eigenvector corresponding to eigen- value $\lambda_2 = 1$ is

$$X_2 = \begin{bmatrix} 1 \\ -1 \end{bmatrix}.$$

10. *Determine the eigenvalues and eigenvectors of the matrix*

$$A = \begin{bmatrix} 8 & -6 & 2 \\ -6 & 7 & -4 \\ 2 & -4 & 3 \end{bmatrix}. \qquad \text{(GBTU-2011)}$$

SOLUTION. The characteristic equation of A is given by

$$|A - \lambda I| = 0$$

or $$\begin{vmatrix} 8-\lambda & -6 & 2 \\ -6 & 7-\lambda & -4 \\ 2 & -4 & 3-\lambda \end{vmatrix} = 0$$

or $$(8-\lambda)((7-\lambda)(3-\lambda)-16) + 6(-18+6\lambda+8) + 2(24-14+2\lambda) = 0$$

or $$\lambda^3 - 18\lambda^2 + 45\lambda = 0$$

or $$\lambda(\lambda-3)(\lambda-15) = 0$$

The roots of this equation are $\lambda = 0, 3, 15$.
Thus, the eigenvalues of A are

$$\lambda_1 = 0, \lambda_2 = 3, \lambda_3 = 15.$$

Eigenvector corresponding to $\lambda_1 = 0$:

Let $X_1 = \begin{bmatrix} x_1 \\ x_2 \\ x_3 \end{bmatrix} \neq O$ be an eigenvector corresponding to the eigenvalue $\lambda_1 = 0$, then we have

$$AX_1 = \lambda_1 X_1$$

or $$AX_1 = 0X_1$$

or $$(A - 0I)\,X_1 = O$$

or $$\begin{bmatrix} 8 & -6 & 2 \\ -6 & 7 & -4 \\ 2 & -4 & 3 \end{bmatrix}\begin{bmatrix} x_1 \\ x_2 \\ x_3 \end{bmatrix} = \begin{bmatrix} 0 \\ 0 \\ 0 \end{bmatrix} \quad ...(1)$$

The non-zero solution of (1) will give X_1. Reducing the coefficient matrix of (1) in Echeleon form by applying elementary row transformations.

Applying $R_1 \leftrightarrow R_3$, we get

$$\begin{bmatrix} 2 & -4 & 3 \\ -6 & 7 & -4 \\ 8 & -6 & 2 \end{bmatrix}\begin{bmatrix} x_1 \\ x_2 \\ x_3 \end{bmatrix} = \begin{bmatrix} 0 \\ 0 \\ 0 \end{bmatrix}$$

Applying $R_2 \to R_2 + 3R_1$, $R_3 \to R_3 - 4R_1$, we get

$$\begin{bmatrix} 2 & -4 & 3 \\ 0 & -5 & 5 \\ 0 & 10 & -10 \end{bmatrix}\begin{bmatrix} x_1 \\ x_2 \\ x_3 \end{bmatrix} = \begin{bmatrix} 0 \\ 0 \\ 0 \end{bmatrix}$$

Applying $R_3 \to R_3 + 2R_2$, we get

$$\begin{bmatrix} 2 & -4 & 3 \\ 0 & -5 & 5 \\ 0 & 0 & 0 \end{bmatrix}\begin{bmatrix} x_1 \\ x_2 \\ x_3 \end{bmatrix} = \begin{bmatrix} 0 \\ 0 \\ 0 \end{bmatrix} \quad ...(2)$$

Clearly $\rho(A - 0.I) = 2$, therefore the system of equations (2) will have $3 - 2 = 1$ (unknowns – rank) linearly independent solution.

From (2), we have

$$2x_1 - 4x_2 + 3x_3 = 0$$
$$-5x_2 + 5x_3 = 0$$

Clearly, $x_1 = \frac{1}{2}$, $x_2 = 1$ and $x_3 = 1$ satisfy the above equations.

Hence, the eigenvector corresponding to eigenvalue $\lambda_1 = 0$ is

$$X_1 = \begin{bmatrix} 1/2 \\ 1 \\ 1 \end{bmatrix}$$

Eigenvector corresponding to $\lambda_2 = 3$:

Let $X_2 = \begin{bmatrix} x_1 \\ x_2 \\ x_3 \end{bmatrix} \neq O$ be an eigenvector of A corresponding to $\lambda_2 = 3$, then we have

$$AX_2 = \lambda_2 X_2$$

or $$(A - \lambda_2 I)X_2 = O$$

or $$(A - 3I)X_2 = O$$

or $$\begin{bmatrix} 8-3 & -6 & 2 \\ -6 & 7-3 & -4 \\ 2 & -4 & 3-3 \end{bmatrix}\begin{bmatrix} x_1 \\ x_2 \\ x_3 \end{bmatrix} = O$$

or $$\begin{bmatrix} 5 & -6 & 2 \\ -6 & 4 & -4 \\ 2 & -4 & 0 \end{bmatrix}\begin{bmatrix} x_1 \\ x_2 \\ x_3 \end{bmatrix} = O \quad ...(3)$$

The non-zero solution of (3) will give X_2.

Applying $R_1 \to R_1 + R_2$, we get

$$\begin{bmatrix} -1 & -2 & -2 \\ -6 & 4 & -4 \\ 2 & -4 & 0 \end{bmatrix}\begin{bmatrix} x_1 \\ x_2 \\ x_3 \end{bmatrix} = \begin{bmatrix} 0 \\ 0 \\ 0 \end{bmatrix}$$

Applying $R_2 \to R_2 - 6R_1$, $R_3 \to R_3 + 2R_1$, we get

$$\begin{bmatrix} -1 & -2 & -2 \\ 0 & 16 & 8 \\ 0 & -8 & -4 \end{bmatrix}\begin{bmatrix} x_1 \\ x_2 \\ x_3 \end{bmatrix} = \begin{bmatrix} 0 \\ 0 \\ 0 \end{bmatrix}$$

Applying $R_2 \to \frac{1}{8}R_2$, we get

$$\begin{bmatrix} -1 & -2 & -2 \\ 0 & 2 & 1 \\ 0 & -8 & -4 \end{bmatrix}\begin{bmatrix} x_1 \\ x_2 \\ x_3 \end{bmatrix} = \begin{bmatrix} 0 \\ 0 \\ 0 \end{bmatrix}$$

Again applying $R_3 \to R_3 + 4R_2$, we get

$$\begin{bmatrix} -1 & -2 & -2 \\ 0 & 2 & 1 \\ 0 & 0 & 0 \end{bmatrix}\begin{bmatrix} x_1 \\ x_2 \\ x_3 \end{bmatrix} = \begin{bmatrix} 0 \\ 0 \\ 0 \end{bmatrix} \quad ...(4)$$

Clearly $\rho(A - 3I) = 2$, therefore the system of equations (3) will have $3 - 2 = 1$ linearly independent solution.

From (4), we have

$$-x_1 - 2x_2 - 2x_3 = 0$$
$$2x_2 + x_3 = 0$$

Clearly, $x_1 = -2$, $x_2 = -1$ and $x_3 = 2$ satisfy the above equations.

Hence, the eigenvector corresponding to eigenvalue $\lambda_2 = 3$ is

$$X_2 = \begin{bmatrix} -2 \\ -1 \\ 2 \end{bmatrix}$$

Eigenvector corresponding to $\lambda_3 = 15$:

Let $X_3 = \begin{bmatrix} x_1 \\ x_2 \\ x_3 \end{bmatrix} \neq O$ be an eigenvector of A corresponding to $\lambda_3 = 15$, then we have

$$AX_3 = \lambda_3 X_3$$

or $(A - \lambda_3 I)X_3 = O$

or $(A - 15I)X_3 = O$

or $$\begin{bmatrix} 8-15 & -6 & 2 \\ -6 & 7-15 & -4 \\ 2 & -4 & 3-15 \end{bmatrix}\begin{bmatrix} x_1 \\ x_2 \\ x_3 \end{bmatrix} = O$$

or $$\begin{bmatrix} -7 & -6 & 2 \\ -6 & -8 & -4 \\ 2 & -4 & -12 \end{bmatrix}\begin{bmatrix} x_1 \\ x_2 \\ x_3 \end{bmatrix} = O \quad \ldots(5)$$

The non-zero solution of (5) will give X_3.

Applying $R_1 \leftrightarrow R_3$, we get

$$\begin{bmatrix} 2 & -4 & -12 \\ -6 & -8 & -4 \\ -7 & -6 & 2 \end{bmatrix}\begin{bmatrix} x_1 \\ x_2 \\ x_3 \end{bmatrix} = \begin{bmatrix} 0 \\ 0 \\ 0 \end{bmatrix}$$

Applying $R_1 \to \frac{1}{2}R_1$, we get

$$\begin{bmatrix} 1 & -2 & -6 \\ -6 & -8 & -4 \\ -7 & -6 & 2 \end{bmatrix}\begin{bmatrix} x_1 \\ x_2 \\ x_3 \end{bmatrix} = \begin{bmatrix} 0 \\ 0 \\ 0 \end{bmatrix}$$

Applying $R_2 \to R_2 + 6R_1, R_3 \to R_3 + 7R_1$, we get

$$\begin{bmatrix} 1 & -2 & -6 \\ 0 & -20 & -40 \\ 0 & -20 & -40 \end{bmatrix}\begin{bmatrix} x_1 \\ x_2 \\ x_3 \end{bmatrix} = \begin{bmatrix} 0 \\ 0 \\ 0 \end{bmatrix}$$

Applying $R_3 \to R_3 - R_2$, we get

$$\begin{bmatrix} 1 & -2 & -6 \\ 0 & -20 & -40 \\ 0 & 0 & 0 \end{bmatrix}\begin{bmatrix} x_1 \\ x_2 \\ x_3 \end{bmatrix} = \begin{bmatrix} 0 \\ 0 \\ 0 \end{bmatrix} \quad \ldots(6)$$

Clearly $\rho(A - 15I) = 2$, therefore the system of equations (5) will have $3 - 2 = 1$ linearly independent solution.

From (6), we have

$$x_1 - 2x_2 - 6x_3 = 0$$

$$-20x_2 - 40x_3 = 0$$

Clearly, $x_1 = 2$, $x_2 = -2$ and $x_3 = 1$ satisfy the above equations.

Hence, the eigenvector corresponding to eigenvalue $\lambda_3 = 15$ is

$$X_3 = \begin{bmatrix} 2 \\ -2 \\ 1 \end{bmatrix}.$$

11. *Find the eigenvalues and eigenvectors of the matrix*

$$A = \begin{bmatrix} 5 & 4 & 2 \\ 4 & 5 & 2 \\ 2 & 2 & 2 \end{bmatrix}.$$

SOLUTION. The characteristic equation of A is given by

$$|A - \lambda I| = 0$$

or $$\begin{vmatrix} 5-\lambda & 4 & 2 \\ 4 & 5-\lambda & 2 \\ 2 & 2 & 2-\lambda \end{vmatrix} = 0$$

or $$(5-\lambda)\{(5-\lambda)(2-\lambda)-4\} - 4\{4(2-\lambda)-4\} + 2\{8-2(8-\lambda)\} = 0$$

or $$-\lambda^3 + 12\lambda - 21\lambda + 10 = 0$$

or $$-(\lambda-1)^2(\lambda-10) = 0$$

The roots of this equation are 1, 1, 10.

Thus the eigenvalues of A are

$$\lambda_1 = 1, \lambda_2 = 1, \lambda_3 = 10.$$

Eigenvector corresponding to the eigenvalue $\lambda_1 = \lambda_2 = 1$

Let $X = \begin{bmatrix} x_1 \\ x_2 \\ x_3 \end{bmatrix} \neq 0$ be an eigenvector corresponding to the eigenvalue $\lambda_1 = \lambda_2 = 1$, then we have

$$AX = IX$$

or $(A - I)X = O$

or $$\begin{bmatrix} 5-1 & 4 & 2 \\ 4 & 5-1 & 2 \\ 2 & 2 & 2-1 \end{bmatrix}\begin{bmatrix} x_1 \\ x_2 \\ x_3 \end{bmatrix} = \begin{bmatrix} 0 \\ 0 \\ 0 \end{bmatrix}$$

or $$\begin{bmatrix} 4 & 4 & 2 \\ 4 & 4 & 2 \\ 2 & 2 & 1 \end{bmatrix}\begin{bmatrix} x_1 \\ x_2 \\ x_3 \end{bmatrix} = \begin{bmatrix} 0 \\ 0 \\ 0 \end{bmatrix} \quad ...(1)$$

Applying $R_1 \leftrightarrow R_3$, we get

$$\begin{bmatrix} 2 & 2 & 1 \\ 4 & 4 & 2 \\ 4 & 4 & 2 \end{bmatrix}\begin{bmatrix} x_1 \\ x_2 \\ x_3 \end{bmatrix} = \begin{bmatrix} 0 \\ 0 \\ 0 \end{bmatrix}$$

Applying $R_2 \to R_2 - 2R_1$, $R_3 \to R_3 -2R_1$, we get

$$\begin{bmatrix} 2 & 2 & 1 \\ 0 & 0 & 0 \\ 0 & 0 & 0 \end{bmatrix}\begin{bmatrix} x_1 \\ x_2 \\ x_3 \end{bmatrix} = \begin{bmatrix} 0 \\ 0 \\ 0 \end{bmatrix} \quad ...(2)$$

From (2), it is clear that $\rho(A - I) = 1$, therefore the equations (1) will have 3–1 =2 linearly independent solutions.

From (2), we have

$$2x_1 + 2x_2 + x_3 = 0$$

Since this equation has two linearly independent solutions so we take $x_2 = c_1$ and $x_3 = c_2$, where c_1 and c_2 are non-zero scalars, then $x_1 = -c - \frac{c_2}{2}$.

Therefore,

$$\begin{bmatrix} x_1 \\ x_2 \\ x_3 \end{bmatrix} = \begin{bmatrix} -c_1 - \frac{c_2}{2} \\ c_1 \\ c_2 \end{bmatrix}$$

$$= c_1\begin{bmatrix} -1 \\ 1 \\ 0 \end{bmatrix} + c_2\begin{bmatrix} -1/2 \\ 0 \\ 1 \end{bmatrix}$$

Hence, the eigenvectors corresponding to the eigenvalue $\lambda_1 = \lambda_2 = 1$ are

$$X_1 = \begin{bmatrix} -1 \\ 0 \\ 1 \end{bmatrix} \text{ and } X_2 = \begin{bmatrix} -1/2 \\ 0 \\ 1 \end{bmatrix}$$

Eigenvector corresponding to the eigenvalue $\lambda_3 = 10$:

Let $X_3 = \begin{bmatrix} x_1 \\ x_2 \\ x_3 \end{bmatrix} \neq O$ be an eigenvector corresponding to $\lambda_3 = 10$, then we have

$$AX_3 = 10X_3$$

or $\quad (A - 10I)X_3 = O$

or

$$\begin{bmatrix} 5-10 & 4 & 2 \\ 4 & 5-10 & 2 \\ 2 & 2 & 2-10 \end{bmatrix}\begin{bmatrix} x_1 \\ x_2 \\ x_3 \end{bmatrix} = \begin{bmatrix} 0 \\ 0 \\ 0 \end{bmatrix}$$

or $$\begin{bmatrix} -5 & 4 & 2 \\ 4 & -5 & 2 \\ 2 & 2 & -8 \end{bmatrix}\begin{bmatrix} x_1 \\ x_2 \\ x_3 \end{bmatrix} = \begin{bmatrix} 0 \\ 0 \\ 0 \end{bmatrix} \quad ...(3)$$

Applying $R_1 \to R_1 + R_2$, we get

$$\begin{bmatrix} -1 & -1 & 4 \\ 4 & -5 & 2 \\ 2 & 2 & -8 \end{bmatrix}\begin{bmatrix} x_1 \\ x_2 \\ x_3 \end{bmatrix} = \begin{bmatrix} 0 \\ 0 \\ 0 \end{bmatrix}$$

Applying $R_2 \to R_2 + 4R_1$, $R_3 \to R_3 + 2R_1$, we get

$$\begin{bmatrix} -1 & -1 & 4 \\ 0 & -9 & 18 \\ 0 & 0 & 0 \end{bmatrix}\begin{bmatrix} x_1 \\ x_2 \\ x_3 \end{bmatrix} = \begin{bmatrix} 0 \\ 0 \\ 0 \end{bmatrix} \quad ...(4)$$

From (4), it is clear that $\rho(A - 10I) = 2$, therefore the system of equations (3) will have 3 – 1= 2 linearly independent solutions.

From (4), we have

$$-x_1 - x_2 + 4x_3 = 0$$
$$-9x_2 + 18x_3 = 0$$

Let us take $x_3 = c$, then $x_2 = 2c$ and $x_1 = 2c$.

Therefore,

$$\begin{bmatrix} x_1 \\ x_2 \\ x_3 \end{bmatrix} = \begin{bmatrix} 2c \\ 2c \\ c \end{bmatrix} = c\begin{bmatrix} 2 \\ 2 \\ 1 \end{bmatrix}$$

Hence, the eigenvector corresponding to eigenvalue $\lambda_3 = 10$ is

$$X_3 = \begin{bmatrix} 2 \\ 2 \\ 1 \end{bmatrix}.$$

- Let A be an $n \times n$ matrix with real entries. If λ is a complex eigenvalue of A with associated eigenvector X, then $\bar{\lambda}$ is also an eigenvalue of A with associated eigenvector $\bar{X}$.

Exercise-3.9

1. Prove that a square matrix A and its transpose A' have the same set of eigenvalues.

2. Let A be an $n \times n$ matrix and let $g(x)$ be any polynomial. If λ is an eigenvalue of A, then prove that $g(\lambda)$ is an eigenvalue of $g(A)$.

3. Show that the eigenvalues of a triangular matrix are just the diagonal elements of the matrix.

4. Let A = dig. $(\lambda_1, \lambda_2, ..., \lambda_n)$ be a diagonal matrix. Prove that each λ_i $(i = 1, 2, 3, ..., n)$ is an eigenvalue of A.

5. Let A be an 3×3 matrix. If $\lambda_1, \lambda_2, \lambda_3$ are the eigenvalues of A, then find the eigenvalues of the matrix $(I + aA)^{-1}(1 + bA)$, where a, b are scalars such that $a\lambda_i \neq -1$ for $i = 1, 2, 3$.

6. Let A and B be two $n \times n$ matrices. Let X be an eigenvector of A and B both. Show that X is also an eigenvcctor of $aA + bB$, where a, b are scalars.

7. Prove that the eigenvectors of a real symmetric matrix corresponding to two distinct eigenvalues are orthogonal.

8. Prove that the eigenvectors of a Hermitian matrix corresponding to two distinct eigenvalues are orthogonal.

9. (i) If λ is an eigenvalue of a matrix A, then show that $k + \lambda$ is an eigenvalue of $A + kI$.

(ii) If the matrix A has characteristic roots $\lambda_1, \lambda_2, ..., \lambda_n$ show that the matrix A^2 has such roots as $\lambda_1^2, \lambda_2^2, ..., \lambda_n^2$.

10. (i) Find the eigenvalues of a matrix $\begin{bmatrix} 1 & 4 \\ 2 & 3 \end{bmatrix}$.

(ii) Find the eigenvalues of the matrix

$$A = \begin{bmatrix} a & h & g \\ 0 & b & f \\ 0 & 0 & c \end{bmatrix}.$$

11. Find the eigenvalues and eigenvectors of the following matrices :

(i) $\begin{bmatrix} 2 & -4 \\ -1 & -1 \end{bmatrix}$ (ii) $\begin{bmatrix} -1 & 0 \\ 0 & 1 \end{bmatrix}$

(iii) $\begin{bmatrix} 1 & 1 \\ -2 & 4 \end{bmatrix}$ (iv) $\begin{bmatrix} 10 & -18 \\ 6 & -11 \end{bmatrix}$

12. Find the eigenvalues and eigenvectors of the following matrices :

(i) $\begin{bmatrix} 0 & 1 & 0 \\ 0 & 0 & 1 \\ 1 & -3 & 3 \end{bmatrix}$ (ii) $\begin{bmatrix} 5 & 8 & 16 \\ 4 & 1 & 8 \\ -4 & -4 & -11 \end{bmatrix}$

(iii) $\begin{bmatrix} 1 & -1 & -1 \\ -1 & 1 & -1 \\ -1 & -1 & 1 \end{bmatrix}$ (iv) $\begin{bmatrix} 1 & 2 & 2 \\ 1 & 2 & -1 \\ -1 & 1 & 4 \end{bmatrix}$

(v) $\begin{bmatrix} 6 & -2 & 2 \\ -2 & 3 & -1 \\ 2 & -1 & 3 \end{bmatrix}$ (vi) $\begin{bmatrix} -2 & 2 & -3 \\ 2 & 1 & -6 \\ -1 & -2 & 0 \end{bmatrix}$

(UKTU-2011, GBTU-2010)

(vii) $\begin{bmatrix} 1 & 2 & 3 \\ 0 & 2 & 3 \\ 0 & 0 & 2 \end{bmatrix}$ (viii) $\begin{bmatrix} 1 & 1 & 0 \\ 0 & 2 & 2 \\ 0 & 0 & 3 \end{bmatrix}$

(ix) $\begin{bmatrix} 3 & 1 & 1 \\ 2 & 4 & 2 \\ 1 & 1 & 3 \end{bmatrix}$ (x) $\begin{bmatrix} 2 & 1 & 0 \\ 0 & 2 & 1 \\ 0 & 0 & 2 \end{bmatrix}$

13. Find the eigenvalues and eigenvectors of the matrix

$$A = \begin{bmatrix} 1 & 1 & 0 & 0 \\ 0 & 2 & 0 & 0 \\ 0 & 0 & 1 & 1 \\ 0 & 0 & -2 & 4 \end{bmatrix}$$

14. Find all the characteristic roots and the corresponding characteristic vectors of the matrix

$$A = \begin{bmatrix} 2 & 1 & -1 \\ 0 & 3 & -2 \\ 2 & 4 & -3 \end{bmatrix}$$

ANSWERS

5. $\frac{1+b\lambda_1}{1+a\lambda_1}, \frac{1+b\lambda_2}{1+a\lambda_2}, \frac{1+b\lambda_3}{1+a\lambda_3}$ **10.** (i) –1, 5 (ii) a, b, c **11.** (i) $\lambda_1 = -2, X_1 = \begin{bmatrix} 1 \\ 1 \end{bmatrix}; \lambda_2 = 3, X_2 = \begin{bmatrix} -4 \\ 1 \end{bmatrix}$

(ii) $\lambda_1 = 1, X_1 = \begin{bmatrix} 0 \\ 1 \end{bmatrix}; \lambda_2 = -1, X_2 = \begin{bmatrix} 1 \\ 0 \end{bmatrix}$ (iii) $\lambda_1 = 2, X_1 = \begin{bmatrix} 1 \\ 1 \end{bmatrix}; \lambda_2 = 3, X_2 = \begin{bmatrix} 1 \\ 2 \end{bmatrix}$

(iv) $\lambda_1 = -2, X_1 = \begin{bmatrix} 3 \\ 2 \end{bmatrix}; \lambda_2 = 1, X_2 = \begin{bmatrix} 2 \\ 1 \end{bmatrix}$ **12.** (i) $\lambda_1 = \lambda_2 = \lambda_3 = 1, X = \begin{bmatrix} 1 \\ 1 \\ 1 \end{bmatrix}$

(ii) $\lambda_1 = 1, X_1 = \begin{bmatrix} -2 \\ -1 \\ 1 \end{bmatrix}; \lambda_2 = -3, X_2 = \begin{bmatrix} -1 \\ 1 \\ 0 \end{bmatrix}; \lambda_3 = -3, X_3 = \begin{bmatrix} -2 \\ 0 \\ 1 \end{bmatrix}$

(iii) $\lambda_1 = -1, X_1 = \begin{bmatrix} 1 \\ 1 \\ 1 \end{bmatrix}; \lambda_2 = 2, X_2 = \begin{bmatrix} -1 \\ 1 \\ 0 \end{bmatrix}; \lambda_3 = 2, X_3 = \begin{bmatrix} -1 \\ 0 \\ 1 \end{bmatrix}$

(iv) $\lambda_1 = 1, X_1 = \begin{bmatrix} 2 \\ -1 \\ 1 \end{bmatrix}; \lambda_2 = 3, X_2 = \begin{bmatrix} 1 \\ 1 \\ 0 \end{bmatrix}; \lambda_3 = 3, X_3 = \begin{bmatrix} 1 \\ 0 \\ 1 \end{bmatrix}$

(v) $\lambda_1 = 2, X_1 = \begin{bmatrix} -1 \\ 0 \\ 2 \end{bmatrix}; \lambda_2 = 2, X_2 = \begin{bmatrix} 1 \\ 2 \\ 0 \end{bmatrix}; \lambda_3 = 8, X_3 = \begin{bmatrix} 2 \\ -1 \\ 1 \end{bmatrix}$

(vi) $\lambda_1 = -3, X_1 = \begin{bmatrix} -2 \\ 1 \\ 0 \end{bmatrix}; \lambda_2 = -3, X_2 = \begin{bmatrix} 3 \\ 0 \\ 1 \end{bmatrix}; \lambda_3 = 5, X_3 = \begin{bmatrix} 1 \\ 2 \\ 1 \end{bmatrix}$

(vii) $\lambda_1 = \lambda_2 = 1, X = \begin{bmatrix} 1 \\ 0 \\ 0 \end{bmatrix}; \lambda_3 = 2, X_1 = \begin{bmatrix} 2 \\ 1 \\ 0 \end{bmatrix}$

(viii) $\lambda_1 = 1, X_1 = \begin{bmatrix} 1 \\ 0 \\ 0 \end{bmatrix}; \lambda_2 = 2, X_2 = \begin{bmatrix} 2 \\ 1 \\ 0 \end{bmatrix}; \lambda_3 = 3, X_3 = \begin{bmatrix} 1 \\ 2 \\ 1 \end{bmatrix}$

(ix) $\lambda_1 = 2, X_1 = \begin{bmatrix} -1 \\ 1 \\ 0 \end{bmatrix}; \lambda_2 = 2, X_2 = \begin{bmatrix} -1 \\ 0 \\ 1 \end{bmatrix}; \lambda_3 = 6, X_3 = \begin{bmatrix} 1 \\ 2 \\ 1 \end{bmatrix}$ (x) $\lambda_1 = \lambda_2 = \lambda_3 = 2, X = \begin{bmatrix} 1 \\ 0 \\ 0 \end{bmatrix}$

13. $\lambda_1 = 1, X_1 = \begin{bmatrix} 1 \\ 0 \\ 0 \\ 0 \end{bmatrix}; \lambda_2 = 2, X_2 = \begin{bmatrix} 1 \\ 1 \\ 0 \\ 0 \end{bmatrix}; \lambda_3 = 2, X_3 = \begin{bmatrix} 0 \\ 0 \\ 1 \\ 1 \end{bmatrix}; \lambda_4 = 3, X_4 = \begin{bmatrix} 0 \\ 0 \\ 0 \\ 1 \end{bmatrix}$

3.29 THE CAYLEY-HAMILTON THEOREM

STATEMENT. *Every square matrix satisfies its characteristic equation.*

or let A be a square matrix of order n and the characteristic equation of A is

$$|A - \lambda I| = (-1^n)\ [\lambda^n + a_1\lambda^{n-1} + a_2\lambda^{n-2} + \ldots + a_{n-1}\lambda + a_n] = 0$$

then its matrix equation $X^n + a_1X^{n-1} + a_2X^{n-2} + \ldots + a_{n-1}X + a_nI = O$ *is satisfied by the matrix* $X = A$

i.e. $$A^n + a_1A^{n-1} + a_2A^{n-2} + \ldots + a_{n-1}A + a_nI = O$$

where I is a unit matrix of order n and O is null matrix of order n.

PROOF. Since A and I are two square matrices of order n and λ is any characteristic root of A, then the matrix $(A - \lambda I)$ is also a square matrix of order n whose elements are at most of degree one in λ. Therefore Adj. $(A - \lambda I)$ will have its elements a polynomials in λ of degree $n-1$ or less and thus Adj. $(A - \lambda I)$ can be expressed as a matrix polynomial in λ as follows :

$$\text{Adj. } (A - \lambda I) = B_0\lambda^{n-1} + B_1\lambda^{n-2} + \ldots + B_{n-2}\lambda + B_{n-1} \qquad \ldots(1)$$

where $B_0, B_1, \ldots, B_{n-1}$ are the square matrices of order n.

Since we know that $A(\text{Adj. } A) = |A| I_n$

$$\therefore \qquad (A - \lambda I) \text{ Adj. } (A - \lambda I) = |A - \lambda I| I$$

or $$(A - \lambda I) \text{ Adj. } (A - \lambda I) = (-1^n)\ (\lambda^n + a_1\lambda^{n-1} + a_2\lambda^{n-2} + \ldots + a_{n-1}\lambda + a_n)I \ \ldots(2)$$

Multiplying both sides of (1) by $(A - \lambda I)$, we get

$$(A - \lambda I) \text{ Adj.}(A - \lambda I) = (A - \lambda I)(B_0\lambda^{n-1} + B_1\lambda^{n-2} + \ldots + B_{n-2}\lambda + B_{n-1}) \ \ldots(3)$$

From (2) and (3), we get

$$(A - \lambda I)(B_0\lambda^{n-1} + B_1\lambda^{n-2} + \ldots + B_{n-2}\lambda + B_{n-1}) = (-1^n)\ (\lambda^n + a_1\lambda^{n-1} + a_2\lambda^{n-2} + \ldots + a_{n-1}\lambda + a_n)I$$

Now comparing the coefficients of like powers of λ, we get

$$\left.\begin{aligned} -IB_0 &= (-1)^n I \\ AB_0 - IB_1 &= (-1)^n a_1 I \\ AB_1 - IB_2 &= (-1)^n a_2 I \\ &\cdots\cdots\cdots\cdots \\ AB_{n-2} - IB_{n-3} &= (-1)^n a_{n-1} I \\ AB_{n-1} &= (-1)^n a_n I \end{aligned}\right\} \qquad \ldots(4)$$

Premultiplying first, second, third, etc. equations of (4) by A^n, A^{n-1}, A^{n-2}, etc. respectively and then adding, we get

$$-A^nB_0 + A^nB_0 - A^{n-1}B_1 + A^{n-1}B_1 + \ldots = (-1)^n (A^n + a_1A^{n-1} + \ldots + a_nI)$$

or $$0 = (-1)^n (A^n + a_1A^{n-1} + \ldots + a_nI)$$

Hence $$A^n + a_1A^{n-1} + \ldots + a_nI = O$$

SOME IMPORTANT PROPERTIES

(1) If A be a non-singular matrix of order $n \times n$ and its characteristic polynomial is

$$|A - \lambda I| = (-1)^n (\lambda^n + a_1\lambda^{n-1} + \ldots + a_{n-1}\lambda + a_n)$$

then $$\det(A) = (-1)^n a_n.$$

(2) If $\lambda_1, \lambda_2, ..., \lambda_n$ are eigenvalues of a square matrix of order $n \times n$, then $\det(A) = \lambda_1\lambda_2\lambda_3 ...\lambda_n$.

(3) Let A be an $n \times n$ matrix with characteristic polynomial

$$f(t) = (-1)^n(t^n + a_1t^{n-1} + ... + a_{n-1}t + a_n)$$

Then A is invertible iff $a_n \neq 0$ and its inverse is

$$A^{-1} = \left(\frac{-1}{a_n}\right)(A^{n-1} + a_1A^{n-2} + ... + a_{n-2}A + a_{n-1}I)$$

(4) If $\lambda_1, \lambda_2, ..., \lambda_n$ are the eigenvalue of a matrix A of order $n \times n$, then

$$Tr(A) = \text{Trace of } A = \sum_{i=1}^{n} \lambda_i$$

(5) *If the* characteristic equation of a matrix A of order $n \times n$ is

$$|A - \lambda I| = (-1)^n(\lambda^n + a_1\lambda^{n-1} + a_2\lambda^{n-2} + ... + a_{n-1}\lambda + a_n) = 0$$

then $\quad Tr(A) = -a_1$

(6) Let A be a matrix of order $n \times n$. If m be a positive integer such that $m \geq n$, then A_m is linearly expressible in terms of those of lower order of A.

Solved Examples

1. *Find the characteristic equation of the matrix*

$$A = \begin{bmatrix} 1 & 0 & 2 \\ 0 & 2 & 1 \\ 2 & 0 & 3 \end{bmatrix}$$

and verify that it is satisfied by A and hence find its inverse.

SOLUTION. The characteristic equation of A is given by

$$|A - \lambda I| = 0$$

or
$$\begin{vmatrix} 1-\lambda & 0 & 2 \\ 0 & 2-\lambda & 1 \\ 2 & 0 & 3-\lambda \end{vmatrix} = 0$$

or
$$(1-\lambda)\{(2-\lambda)(3-\lambda) - 0\} + 2\{0 - 2(2-\lambda)\} = 0$$

or
$$-\lambda^3 + 6\lambda^2 - 7\lambda - 2 = 0$$

or
$$\lambda^3 - 6\lambda^2 + 7\lambda + 2 = 0$$

Next we have to show that

$$A^3 - 6A^2 + 7A + 2I = O$$

Now $\quad A^2 = A.A$

$$= \begin{bmatrix} 1 & 0 & 2 \\ 0 & 2 & 1 \\ 2 & 0 & 3 \end{bmatrix}\begin{bmatrix} 1 & 0 & 2 \\ 0 & 2 & 1 \\ 2 & 0 & 3 \end{bmatrix} = \begin{bmatrix} 5 & 0 & 8 \\ 2 & 4 & 5 \\ 8 & 0 & 13 \end{bmatrix}$$

and $A^3 = A^2 . A$

$$= \begin{bmatrix} 5 & 0 & 8 \\ 2 & 4 & 5 \\ 8 & 0 & 13 \end{bmatrix}\begin{bmatrix} 1 & 0 & 2 \\ 0 & 2 & 1 \\ 2 & 0 & 3 \end{bmatrix} = \begin{bmatrix} 21 & 0 & 34 \\ 12 & 8 & 23 \\ 34 & 0 & 55 \end{bmatrix}$$

$\therefore \quad A^3 - 6A^2 + 7A + 2I$

$$= \begin{bmatrix} 21 & 0 & 34 \\ 12 & 8 & 23 \\ 34 & 0 & 55 \end{bmatrix} - 6\begin{bmatrix} 5 & 0 & 8 \\ 2 & 4 & 5 \\ 8 & 0 & 13 \end{bmatrix} + 7\begin{bmatrix} 1 & 0 & 2 \\ 0 & 2 & 1 \\ 2 & 0 & 3 \end{bmatrix} + 2\begin{bmatrix} 1 & 0 & 0 \\ 0 & 1 & 0 \\ 0 & 0 & 1 \end{bmatrix}$$

$$= \begin{bmatrix} 21-30+7+2 & 0-0+0+0 & 34-48+14+0 \\ 12-12+0+0 & 8-24+14+2 & 23-30+7+0 \\ 34-48+14+0 & 0-0+0+0 & 55-78+21+2 \end{bmatrix}$$

$$= \begin{bmatrix} 0 & 0 & 0 \\ 0 & 0 & 0 \\ 0 & 0 & 0 \end{bmatrix} = O$$

Hence,

$$A^3 - 6A^2 + 7A + 2I = O \qquad ...(1)$$

To find A^{-1} :

Since the characteristic equation of A is

$$\lambda^3 - 6\lambda^2 + 7\lambda + 2 = 0$$

$\therefore \quad |A| = (-1)^3 2 = -2 \neq 0$

$[\because |A| = (-1)^n a_n]$

$\Rightarrow \quad A^{-1}$ exist.

Premultiplying (1) by A^{-1}, we get

$$A^2 - 6A + 7I + 2A^{-1} = O$$

$$\Rightarrow A^{-1} = -\frac{1}{2}[A^2 - 6A + 7I]$$

$$\Rightarrow A^{-1} = -\frac{1}{2}\left\{\begin{bmatrix} 5 & 0 & 8 \\ 2 & 4 & 5 \\ 8 & 0 & 13 \end{bmatrix} - 6\begin{bmatrix} 1 & 0 & 2 \\ 0 & 2 & 1 \\ 2 & 0 & 3 \end{bmatrix} + 7\begin{bmatrix} 1 & 0 & 0 \\ 0 & 1 & 0 \\ 0 & 0 & 1 \end{bmatrix}\right\}$$

$$= -\frac{1}{2}\begin{bmatrix} 6 & 0 & -4 \\ 2 & -1 & -1 \\ -4 & 0 & 2 \end{bmatrix}$$

Hence,

$$A^{-1} = -\frac{1}{2}\begin{bmatrix} 6 & 0 & -4 \\ 2 & -1 & -1 \\ -4 & 0 & 2 \end{bmatrix} = \frac{1}{2}\begin{bmatrix} -6 & 0 & 4 \\ -2 & 1 & 1 \\ 4 & 0 & -2 \end{bmatrix}$$

2. *Find the characteristic equation of the matrix* $A = \begin{bmatrix} 2 & -1 & 1 \\ -1 & 2 & -1 \\ 1 & -1 & 2 \end{bmatrix}$ *and verify that it is satisfied by A and hence find* A^{-1}.

(UPTU-2006, GBTU-2012, UKTU-2011, MADRAS-2006)

SOLUTION. The characteristic equation of A is given by $|A - \lambda I| = 0$

or
$$\begin{vmatrix} 2-\lambda & -1 & 1 \\ -1 & 2-\lambda & -1 \\ 1 & -1 & 2-\lambda \end{vmatrix} = 0$$

or
$$(2-\lambda)\{(2-\lambda)(2-\lambda)-1\} + 1(-2+\lambda+2) + 1(1-2+\lambda) = 0$$

or
$$-\lambda^3 + 6\lambda^2 - 9\lambda + 4 = 0$$

or
$$\lambda^3 - 6\lambda^2 + 9\lambda - 4 = 0$$

Next we have to show that

$$A^3 - 6A^2 + 9A - 4I = O$$

Now $A^2 = A.A$

$$= \begin{bmatrix} 2 & -1 & 1 \\ -1 & 2 & -1 \\ 1 & -1 & 2 \end{bmatrix}\begin{bmatrix} 2 & -1 & 1 \\ -1 & 2 & -1 \\ 1 & -1 & 2 \end{bmatrix}$$

$$= \begin{bmatrix} 6 & -5 & 5 \\ -5 & 6 & -5 \\ 5 & -5 & 6 \end{bmatrix}$$

and $A^3 = A^2.A$

$$= \begin{bmatrix} 6 & -5 & 5 \\ -5 & 6 & -5 \\ 5 & -5 & 6 \end{bmatrix}\begin{bmatrix} 2 & -1 & 1 \\ -1 & 2 & -1 \\ 1 & -1 & 2 \end{bmatrix}$$

$$= \begin{bmatrix} 22 & -21 & 21 \\ -21 & 22 & -21 \\ 21 & -21 & 22 \end{bmatrix}$$

Now $A^3 - 6A^2 + 9A - 4I$

$$= \begin{bmatrix} 22 & -21 & 21 \\ -21 & 22 & -21 \\ 21 & -21 & 22 \end{bmatrix} - 6\begin{bmatrix} 6 & -5 & 5 \\ -5 & 6 & -5 \\ 5 & -5 & 6 \end{bmatrix} + 9\begin{bmatrix} 2 & -1 & 1 \\ -1 & 2 & -1 \\ 1 & -1 & 2 \end{bmatrix} - 4\begin{bmatrix} 1 & 0 & 0 \\ 0 & 1 & 0 \\ 0 & 0 & 1 \end{bmatrix}$$

$$= \begin{bmatrix} 22-36+18-4 & -21+30-9-0 & 21-30+9-0 \\ -21+30-9-0 & 22-36+18-4 & -21+30-9-0 \\ 21-30+9-0 & -21+30-9-0 & 22-36+18-4 \end{bmatrix}$$

$$= \begin{bmatrix} 0 & 0 & 0 \\ 0 & 0 & 0 \\ 0 & 0 & 0 \end{bmatrix} = O$$

Hence, $A^3 - 6A^2 + 9A - 4I = O$ ...(1)

Since $|A| = 2(4-1) + 1(-2+1) + 1(1-2)$

$$= 6 - 1 - 1 = 4 \neq 0$$

$\Rightarrow A^{-1}$ exist.

Premultiplying (1) by A^{-1}, we get

$$A^2 - 6A + 9I - 4A^{-1} = O$$

$$\Rightarrow A^{-1} = +\frac{1}{4}[A^2 - 6A + 9I]$$

$\Rightarrow$

$$A^{-1} = \frac{1}{4}\left\{\begin{bmatrix} 6 & -5 & 5 \\ -5 & 6 & -5 \\ 5 & -5 & 6 \end{bmatrix} - 6\begin{bmatrix} 2 & -1 & 1 \\ -1 & 2 & -1 \\ 1 & -1 & 2 \end{bmatrix} + 9\begin{bmatrix} 1 & 0 & 0 \\ 0 & 1 & 0 \\ 0 & 0 & 1 \end{bmatrix}\right\}$$

$$= \frac{1}{4}\begin{bmatrix} 6-12+9 & -5+6+0 & 5-6+0 \\ -5+6+0 & 6-12+9 & -5+6+0 \\ 5-6+0 & -5+6+0 & 6-12+9 \end{bmatrix}$$

$$\therefore \quad A^{-1} = \frac{1}{4}\begin{bmatrix} 3 & 1 & -1 \\ 1 & 3 & 1 \\ -1 & 1 & 3 \end{bmatrix}.$$

3. *Find the characteristic equation of the matrix* $A = \begin{bmatrix} 1 & 2 & 0 \\ 2 & -1 & 0 \\ 0 & 0 & -1 \end{bmatrix}$ *and hence find* A^{-1}.

SOLUTION. The characteristic equation of A is given by

$$|A - \lambda I| = 0$$

or
$$\begin{vmatrix} 1-\lambda & 2 & 0 \\ 2 & -1-\lambda & 0 \\ 0 & 0 & -1-\lambda \end{vmatrix} = 0$$

or
$$(1-\lambda)\{(-1-\lambda)(-1-\lambda)-0\} - 2\{2(-1-\lambda)-0\} = 0$$

or
$$(1-\lambda)(1+\lambda)^2 + 4(1+\lambda) = 0$$

or
$$1+\lambda^2+2\lambda-\lambda-\lambda^3-2\lambda^2+4+4\lambda = 0$$

or
$$-\lambda^3 - \lambda^2 + 5\lambda + 5 = 0$$

or
$$\lambda^3 + \lambda^2 - 5\lambda - 5 = 0$$

By Cayley-Hamilton theorem, we have

$$A^3 + A^2 - 5A - 5I = O \quad \ldots(1)$$

Since $|A - \lambda I| = -\lambda^3 - \lambda^2 + 5\lambda + 5$

$\Rightarrow$ $|A| = 5 \neq 0$ (Putting $\lambda = 0$)

$\Rightarrow$ A^{-1} exists.

Premultiplying (1) by A^{-1}, we get

$$A^2 + A - 5I - 5A^{-1} = 0$$

$$\Rightarrow \quad A^{-1} = \frac{1}{5}(A^2 + A - 5I) \quad \ldots(2)$$

Now $A^2 = A.A$

$$= \begin{bmatrix} 1 & 2 & 0 \\ 2 & -1 & 0 \\ 0 & 0 & -1 \end{bmatrix}\begin{bmatrix} 1 & 2 & 0 \\ 2 & -1 & 0 \\ 0 & 0 & -1 \end{bmatrix}$$

$$= \begin{bmatrix} 5 & 0 & 0 \\ 0 & 5 & 0 \\ 0 & 0 & 5 \end{bmatrix}$$

So

$$A^{-1} = \frac{1}{5}\left\{\begin{bmatrix} 5 & 0 & 0 \\ 0 & 5 & 0 \\ 0 & 0 & 1 \end{bmatrix} + \begin{bmatrix} 1 & 2 & 0 \\ 2 & -1 & 0 \\ 0 & 0 & -1 \end{bmatrix} - 5\begin{bmatrix} 1 & 0 & 0 \\ 0 & 1 & 0 \\ 0 & 0 & 1 \end{bmatrix}\right\}$$

$$= \frac{1}{5}\begin{bmatrix} 1 & 2 & 0 \\ 2 & -1 & 0 \\ 0 & 0 & -5 \end{bmatrix}$$

4. *Use Cayley-Hamilton theorem to express* $2A^5 - 3A^4 + A^2 - 4I$ *as a linear polynomial in A, where :*

$$A = \begin{bmatrix} 3 & 1 \\ -1 & 2 \end{bmatrix}.$$

SOLUTION. The characteristic equation of A is given by

$$|A - \lambda I| = 0$$

or
$$\begin{vmatrix} 3-\lambda & 1 \\ -1 & 2-\lambda \end{vmatrix} = 0$$

or
$$(3-\lambda)(2-\lambda) + 1 = 0$$

or
$$\lambda^2 - 5\lambda + 7 = 0$$

By Cayley-Hamilton theorem, we have

$$A^2 - 5A + 7I = O \quad \ldots(1)$$

$$\Rightarrow \quad A^2 = 5A - 7I \quad \ldots(2)$$

Now $A^3 = A^2.A$

$$= (5A - 7I)A = 5A^2 - 7A$$

$$\therefore \quad A^3 = 5A^2 - 7A \quad \ldots(3)$$

Again, $A^4 = A^3.A = (5A^2 - 7A)A$

$$= 5A^3 - 7A^2$$

$$\Rightarrow \quad A^4 = 5(5A^2 - 7A) - 7(5A - 7I)$$

[Using (2) and (3)]

$$\Rightarrow \quad A^4 = 25A^2 - 35A - 35A + 49I$$

$\Rightarrow \quad A^4 = 25(5A - 7I) - 70A + 49I$ [Using (2)]

$\Rightarrow \quad A^4 = 125A - 175I - 70A + 49I$

$\Rightarrow \quad A^4 = 55A - 126I \quad \ldots(4)$

Also $A^5 = A^4 . A = (55A - 126I)A$

$A^5 = 55A^2 - 126A$

$\Rightarrow \quad A^5 = 55(5A - 7I) - 126A$ [Using (2)]

$\therefore \quad A^5 = 149A - 385I \quad \ldots(5)$

Now $2A^5 - 3A^4 + A^2 - 4I$

$= 2(149A - 385I) - 3(55A - 126I) + 5A - 7I - 4I$

[Using (2), (4) and (5)]

$= 298A - 770I - 165A + 378I + 5A - 11I$

$= 138A - 403I$

$\therefore \quad 2A^5 - 3A^4 + A^2 - 4I = 138A - 403I$

which is a linear polynomial in A.

Exercise-3.10

1. Verify Cayley-Hamilton theorem for the matrix $A = \begin{bmatrix} 1 & 1 \\ 8 & 1 \end{bmatrix}$ and use it to find A^{-1}.

2. Use Cayley-Hamilton theorem to find the inverse of the matrix $A = \begin{bmatrix} 2 & 1 \\ 5 & 3 \end{bmatrix}$.

3. Verify Cayley-Hamilton theorem for the matrix $A = \begin{bmatrix} 0 & 0 & 0 \\ 3 & 1 & 0 \\ -2 & 1 & 4 \end{bmatrix}$ and hence find A^{-1}.

4. Verify Cayley-Hamilton theorem for the following matrix:

$$A = \begin{bmatrix} 2 & 0 \\ 0 & 1 \end{bmatrix}.$$

5. Show that the matrix $A = \begin{bmatrix} 1 & 2 \\ 1 & 1 \end{bmatrix}$ satisfies Cayley-Hamilton theorem.

6. State the Cayley-Hamilton theorem and verify it for the matrix

$$A = \begin{bmatrix} 1 & 0 & -2 \\ 0 & 0 & 0 \\ -2 & 0 & 4 \end{bmatrix}$$

7. Verify Cayley-Hamilton theorem for the matrix $A = \begin{bmatrix} 1 & 4 \\ 2 & 3 \end{bmatrix}$ and hence obtain A^{-1}.

8. Verify Cayley-Hamilton theorem for the matrix

$$A = \begin{bmatrix} 1 & 2 & 1 \\ 0 & 1 & -1 \\ 3 & -1 & 1 \end{bmatrix}$$

and hence find A^{-1}.

9. Verify that the matrix $A = \begin{bmatrix} 1 & 2 & 1 \\ -1 & 0 & 3 \\ 2 & -1 & 1 \end{bmatrix}$ satisfies its characteristic equation.

10. Show that the matrix $A = \begin{bmatrix} 2 & 2 & 1 \\ 1 & 3 & 1 \\ 1 & 2 & 2 \end{bmatrix}$ satisfies Cayley-Hamilton theorem.

11. Verify Cayley-Hamilton theorem for the matrix

$$A = \begin{bmatrix} 1 & \sqrt{2} & 0 \\ \sqrt{2} & -1 & 0 \\ 0 & 0 & 1 \end{bmatrix}$$

and hence find A^{-1}.

12. If $A = \begin{bmatrix} 1 & 2 \\ -1 & 3 \end{bmatrix}$ express $A^6 - 4A^5 + 8A^4 - 12A^3 + 14A^2$ as a linear polynomial in A.

13. Find the characteristic equation of the matrix $A = \begin{bmatrix} 2 & 1 & 1 \\ 0 & 1 & 0 \\ 1 & 1 & 2 \end{bmatrix}$ and hence compute A^{-1}. Also find the value of

$A^8 - 5A^7 + 7A^6 - 3A^5 + A^4 - 5A^3 + 8A^2 - 2A + I$

(UKTU 2010)

14. If $A = \begin{bmatrix} 1 & 0 & 0 \\ 1 & 0 & 1 \\ 0 & 1 & 0 \end{bmatrix}$, show that for every integer $n \geq 3$

$A^n = A^{n-2} + A^2 - I$ (UPTU-2009, MUMBAI-2006)

15. Verify Cayley-Hamilton theorem for the following matrices

(i) $\begin{bmatrix} 2 & 2 & 1 \\ 0 & 1 & -1 \\ 3 & -1 & 1 \end{bmatrix}$ (UPTU-2007)

(ii) $\begin{bmatrix} 1 & 0 & -4 \\ 0 & 5 & 4 \\ -4 & 4 & 3 \end{bmatrix}$ (GBTU-2010)

(iii) $\begin{bmatrix} 3 & 0 & 1 \\ 0 & 2 & 0 \\ 0 & 0 & 1 \end{bmatrix}$ (UPTU-2008)

(iv) $\begin{bmatrix} 7 & 2 & -2 \\ -6 & -1 & 2 \\ 6 & 2 & -1 \end{bmatrix}$ (UKTU-2012)

(v) $\begin{bmatrix} 2 & -1 & 1 \\ -1 & 2 & -1 \\ 1 & -1 & 2 \end{bmatrix}$ (SVTU-2008, ANNA-2009, MADRAS-2006)

(vi) $\begin{bmatrix} 3 & 2 & 4 \\ 4 & 3 & 2 \\ 2 & 4 & 3 \end{bmatrix}$ (PTU-2006)

(vii) $\begin{bmatrix} 1 & 3 & 7 \\ 4 & 2 & 3 \\ 1 & 2 & 1 \end{bmatrix}$ (ANNA-2005, BHOPAL-2008,KERALA 2005)

(viii) $\begin{bmatrix} 1 & 2 & 3 \\ 2 & 4 & 5 \\ 3 & 5 & 6 \end{bmatrix}$ (UPTU-2007)

ANSWERS

1. $A^{-1} = -\frac{1}{7}\begin{bmatrix} 1 & -1 \\ -8 & 1 \end{bmatrix}$ **2.** $A^{-1} = \begin{bmatrix} 3 & -1 \\ -5 & 2 \end{bmatrix}$ **3.** $A^{-1} = \frac{1}{5}\begin{bmatrix} 4 & 1 & -1 \\ -12 & 2 & 3 \\ 5 & 0 & 0 \end{bmatrix}$

7. $A^{-1} = -\frac{1}{3}\begin{bmatrix} 3 & -4 \\ -2 & 1 \end{bmatrix}$ **8.** $A^{-1} = \frac{1}{9}\begin{bmatrix} 0 & 3 & 3 \\ 3 & 2 & -1 \\ 3 & -7 & -1 \end{bmatrix}$ **11.** $A^{-1} = -\frac{1}{3}\begin{bmatrix} -1 & -\sqrt{2} & 0 \\ -\sqrt{2} & 1 & 0 \\ 0 & 0 & -3 \end{bmatrix}$

12. $-4A + 5I$ **13.** $A^3 - 5A^2 + 7A - 3I = 0;\ A^{-1} = \frac{1}{3}\begin{bmatrix} 2 & -1 & -1 \\ 0 & 3 & 0 \\ -1 & -1 & 2 \end{bmatrix}, \begin{bmatrix} 8 & 5 & 5 \\ 0 & 3 & 0 \\ 5 & 5 & 8 \end{bmatrix}$

□□□□□□

Chapter

4

Group, Ring and Fields

4.1 INTRODUCTION

The theory of groups, an important part in present mathematics, started early nineteenth century in connection with the solution of algebraic equations. Originally, a group was the set of all permutations of the roots of an algebraic eqation, which has the property that combinations of any two of these permutations again belong to the set. Later, the idea was generalised to the concept of an abstract group. An abstract group is essentially the study of a set with an operation defined and Group Theory has many useful applications both within and outside mathematics.

4.2 GROUPS

Let G be a non-empty set and $*$ be a binary operation defined on it, then the structure $(G,*)$ is said to be a **group** if the following axioms are satisfied:

(i) Closure Property, $a * b \in G; \forall\ a, b \in G$.

(ii) Associativity. *The opration* $*$ *is associative on G.i.e.,*

$$a* (b* c) = (a*b) * c; \forall\ a, b, c \in G$$

(iii) Existence of identity. *There exists an element* $e \in G$ *such that*

$$a*e = e*a = a; \forall a \in G$$

e is called identity of $*$ *in G.*

(iv) Existence of inverse For each element $a \in G$, there exist an element $b \in G$ such that

$$a * b = b * a = e$$

The element b is called the inverse of element a with respect to $*$ and we write $b = a^{-1}$

- When we say * is a binary operation defined on a non-empty set G, it implies that G is closed for the binary operation *, *i.e.,*

$$a* b \in G\ \forall\ a, b \in G.$$

- A group is not simply a set, but it is an algebraic structure.
- Because of the associativity, the parenthesis can be dropped in products of more than two elements of a group and instead of writing $a^* (b^* c)$ or $(a^* b) {}^*c$ we may simply write $a * b * c$. The associative law can be extended to any finite number of elements.
- We know that '.' is a binary operation on G we must have $a.b \in G\ \forall\ a, b \in G$. Hence, in our definition of a group there is no necessity of mentioning the closure axioms. We mentioned it to emphasize the fact that while showing the group postulates in a problem, one should not forgot the closure axioms.

4.3 ABELIAN OR COMMUTATIVE GROUP

A group $(G, *)$ is said to be abelian or commutative if $a * b = b * a; \forall\ a, b \in G$. The group which are not abelian are called non-abelian or non-commutative.

- An abelian group under addition is sometimes called a 'module'.
- The commutative group is also known as Abelian group after the name of famous mathematician Abel.
- The smallest group for a given composition is the set {e}, containing identity elements .
- A group consisting the identity element only, is called a trivial group, other are called non-trivial groups.

4.4 FINITE AND INFINITE GROUPS

If a group contains a finite number of elements, it is called a finite group. If the number of elements in a group is infinite, it is called an infinite group.

4.4.1 ORDER OF A GROUP

The number of elements in a finite group is called the order of the group. It is denoted by o(G).

An infinite group is called a group of infinite order.

ILLUSTRATIONS

(i) The set Z of integers is an infinite abelian group with respect to the operation of addition but Z is not a group with respect to the multiplication.
(ii) Let $G = \{1\}$, then G is an abelian group of order 1 with resepect to multilpication.
(iii) Let $G=\{0\}$, then G is an abelian group of order 1 with respect to addition.
(iv) Let $G = \{1, -1\}$, then G is an abelian group of order 2 with respect to multiplication.

4.4.2 GENERAL PROPERTIES OF GROUPS

THEOREM 1. *Let (G,∗) be a group, then*
(i) the identity element is unique.
(ii) every element of G has unique inverse in G.

PROOF. (i) Let, if possible e_1 and e_2 be two distinct identities of the group G. Then, by definition of identity, we have

$$e_1 * e_2 = e_1 \qquad \text{(if } e_2 \text{ is identity)}$$

and $$e_1 * e_2 = e_2 \qquad \text{(if } e_1 \text{ is identity)}$$

Hence, it follows that $e_1 = e_2$

$\Rightarrow$ Identity is unique.

(ii) If possible, let any element $a \in G$ have two inverses say b and c, then, we have

$$a * b = e = b * a$$

and $$a * c = e = c * a.$$

Therefore, $$b = b*e = b*(a*c) = (b*a)*c \qquad \text{(By Associativity)}$$

$$= e * c = c$$

$\Rightarrow$ $b = c$

Hence, every element of a group has unique inverse.

- The identity element has its own inverse.

THEOREM 2. *If (G, ∗) is a group, then*
(i) $(a^{-1})^{-1} = a \ \forall \ a \in G$.
(ii) $(a * b)^{-1} = b^{-1} * a^{-1}; \forall a, b \in G$ *(Reversal Rule)*

PROOF. (i) For each element $a \in G$, there exist an element $b \in G$ such that

$$ab = ba = e$$

From the symmetry of this result, we have

$$a^{-1} = b \qquad \ldots(1)$$

and $$b^{-1} = a \qquad \ldots(2)$$

Putting the value of b in equation (2), we get

$$(a^{-1})^{-1} = a$$

(ii) For all $a, b \in G$, we have

$$(a*b) * (b^{-1} * a^{-1}) = a*(b * b^{-1}) * a^{-1} \quad \text{(by Associativity)}$$
$$= a*(e) * a^{-1} = (a * e) * a^{-1} \quad \text{(by Associativity)}$$
$$= a * a^{-1} = e$$

Similarly, We can easily show that

$$(b^{-1} * a^{-1}) * (a * b) = e$$

Thus, $(b^{-1} * a^{-1}) * (a * b) = e$

Thus, $(a * b) * (b^{-1} * a^{-1}) * = e = (b^{-1} * a^{-1}) * (a * b)$

Hence, it follows that

$$(a * b)^{-1} = b^{-1} * a^{-1}$$

- The above reversal law can be generalised as follows:
"if $a_1, a_2, \ldots a_n$, are elements of a group G, then $(a_1 * a_2 * \ldots * a_n)^{-1} = a_n^{-1} * a_{n-1}^{-1} * a_{n-2}^{-1} * \ldots * a_2^{-1} * a_1^{-1}$
- In additive composition, above result can be started as follows:
(i) $-(-a) = a; \forall a \in G$ (ii) $-(a+b) = (-b) + (-a); \forall a, b \in G$.

THEOREM 3. *If a, b, c are three elements of a group (G, ∗) then*

$$a * c = b * c \Rightarrow a = b \quad \textit{(Right cancellation law)}$$
$$c * a = c * b \Rightarrow a = b \quad \textit{(Left cancellation law)}$$

PROOF. (i) $a * c = b * c \Rightarrow (a * c) * c^{-1} = (b * c) * c^{-1}$ $(\because c^{-1} \in G)$

$\Rightarrow a * (c * c^{-1}) = b * (c * c^{-1})$ (by associativity)

$\Rightarrow a * e = b * e \Rightarrow a = b.$

$c * a = c * b \Rightarrow c^{-1} * (c * a) = c^{-1} * (c * b)$

$\Rightarrow (c^{-1} * c) * a = (c^{-1} * c) * b$

$\Rightarrow e * a = e * b \Rightarrow a = b.$

THEOREM 4. *In a group G, the equation a∗x = b and y∗a = b where a, b∈ G have solutions in G.*

PROOF.

$$a * x = b$$

$\Rightarrow a^{-1} * (a * x) = a^{-1} * b$ $(\because a^{-1} \in G)$

$\Rightarrow (a^{-1} * a) * x) = a^{-1} * b$ (by associativity)

$\Rightarrow e * x = a^{-1} * b$

$\Rightarrow x = a^{-1} * b \in G$ $(\because a^{-1}, b \in G \Rightarrow a^{-1} * b \in G)$

Therefore, the equation $a * x = b$ has a solution $x = a^{-1} * b$ in G.

Similarty it can be proved that the equation $y * a = b$ has a solution $y = b * a^{-1}$ in G.

Uniqueness. Let, if possible x_1 and x_2 be any two solutions of the equation

$$a * x = b$$

so that $a * x_1 = b$ and $a * x_2 = b$

$\Rightarrow a * x_1 = a * x_2$

$\Rightarrow x_1 = x_2$

Therefore, the solution of the equation $a * x = b$ is unique. Similarly, it can be proved that the equation $y * a = b$ has a unique solution.

Hence, the given equations have unique solutions in G.

- With the help of the above theorem, we can define the group alternatively as follows:
" A set G with a binary composition ∗ is a group iff"
(i) the composition ∗ is associative.
(ii) the equations $ax = b$ and $ya = b$ have unique solutions in G.

THEOREM 5. *The left identity is also the right identity.*

PROOF. Let e be the left identity of a group G and let $a \in G$ be any element. Then

$$ea = a \quad ...(1)$$

To prove that e is also the right identity, it is sufficient to show that

$$ae = a \quad ...(2)$$

Let a^{-1} be the inverse of a , then

$$a^{-1}\, a = e \quad ...(3)$$

Now, $a^{-1}\,(ae) = (a^{-1}a)e = e.e = e = a^{-1}a$

$\Rightarrow$ $a^{-1}\,(ae) = a^{-1}a$

$\Rightarrow$ $ae = a.$ (By left cancellation law)

Hence, we have that the left identity is also the right identity of G.

THEOREM 6. *The left inverse of an elemnt is also its right inverse.*

PROOF. Let a^{-1} be the left inverse of an element a of a group G, so that

$$a^{-1}a = e \quad ...(1)$$

where e is the identity of G.

To prove that a^{-1} is also the right inverse of a, it is sufficient to show that

$$aa^{-1} = e \quad ...(2)$$

By associativity, we have

$$a^{-1}(aa^{-1}) = (a^{-1}a)\, a^{-1} = ea^{-1} \quad \text{[Using (1)]}$$

$$= a^{-1} = a^{-1}e$$

$\Rightarrow$ $aa^{-1} = e$ (By left cancellation law)

Hence, from (2), we can say that the left inverse of an element is also the right inverse of that element.

4.4.3 DEFINITION OF A GROUP BASED UPON LEFT AXIOMS

A non-empty set G with a binary operation $*$ is a group iff the following properties are satisfied:

(i) Associative law. The binary operation $*$ must be associative i.e.,

$$a * (b * c) = (a * b) * c;\ \forall a, b, c \in G.$$

(ii) Existence of left identity. There exists an element $e \in$ G (called the left identity) such that

$$e * a = a\ ;\ \forall\ a \in G.$$

(iii) Existence of left inverse. For each element $a \in$G, there exists an element $b \in G$ such that

$$b * a = e$$

b is called the left inverse of a and is denoted by a^{-1}.

4.4.4 DEFINITION OF A GROUP BASED UPON RIGHT AXIOMS

A non-empty set G with a binary operation $*$ is said to be group iff the following properties are satisfied :

(i) Associative law. The binary operation $*$ must be associative *i.e.*,

$$a * (b * c) = (a * b) * c; \quad \forall\ a, b, c \in G.$$

(ii) Existence of right identity. There exists an element $e \in G$ (called the right identity) such that

$$a * e = a;\ \forall a \in G.$$

(iii) Existence of right inverse. For each element $a \in G$, there exists an element $b \in G$ such that $a * b = e$

b is called the right inverse of a and is denoted by a^{-1} .

Solved Examples

1. *Show that the set* **Z** *of integers (positive or negative integers including 0) with additive binary operation is an infinite abelian group.*

SOLUTION. Let us apply the group-axioms to all integers :

(i) Closure property. Closure property is satisifed because the sum of any two integers is an integer.

(ii) Associativity. The associative property is satisfied, because if a, b, c are any three integers, then

$$(a + b) + c = a + (b + c)$$

(iii) Existence of identity. The axiom on identity is satisfied, because 0 is the identity element in the set **Z** such that

$$a + 0 = a;\ \forall a \in \mathbf{Z}.$$

(iv) Existence of inverse. The axiom on inverse is satisfied, because the inverse of any integer a is the integer $-a$ such that $a+(-a)=(-a)+a=0$, the identity element.

(v) Commutativity. Since, we know that $a+b = b+a$; $\forall a, b \in \mathbf{Z}$, the commutative law is satisfied.

Also, the number of elements in **Z** is infinite.

Hence, the set **Z** is an infinite abelian group with additive binary operation.

2. *Show that the set* $\{1, -1, i, -i\}$ *is an abelian finite group of order 4 under multiplication.*

SOLUTION. **(i) Closure property.** Closure property is satisfied as

$1(-1) = -1$, $1.i = i$, $i(-i)=1$, $i(-i) = -i$ etc.

(ii) Associativity. Associative property is satisfied as

$(1 . i)\cdot(-i) = 1. \{i\cdot(-i)\} = 1$, $(1, i). (-1) = 1, \{i(-1)\} = -i$ etc.

(iii) Existence of identity. Axioms on identity is satisfied, 1 being the multiplicative identity.

(iv) Existence of inverse. Axiom on inverse is satisfied since the inverse of each element of the set exists

$1\cdot1 = e = 1$, $(-1)\cdot(-1) = e = 1$, $i\cdot(-i) = e = 1$, $(-i)\cdot(i) = e = 1$.

(v) Commutativity. The commutative law is also satisfied as. $1\cdot(-1) = (-1)\times1$, $(-1)i = i(-1)$ etc.

Finally, since, there are four elements in the given set, hence it is a group of order 4.

3. *Show that the set of all positive rational numbers forms an abelian group under the composition * defined by* $a*b = \dfrac{(ab)}{2}$.

SOLUTION. Let $\mathbf{Q}^+$ be the set of all positive rational numbers. To show $(\mathbf{Q}^+, *)$ is a group.

(i) Closure Property : For every a, $b \in \mathbf{Q}^+$, $ab/2 \in \mathbf{Q}^+$

$\Rightarrow$ $\mathbf{Q}^+$ is a closed under the composition $*$.

(ii) Associativity: Let $a, b, c \in \mathbf{Q}^+$ then

$$(a*b)*c = \left(\frac{ab}{2}\right)*c = \frac{[ab/2]\cdot c}{2}$$

$$= \frac{[abc/2]}{2} = a*\left(\frac{cb}{2}\right)$$

$$= a*(b*c)$$

(iii) Existence of Identity : An element e will be the identity element if $e \in \mathbf{Q}^+$ and if

$$e*a = a = a*e; \forall\, a \in \mathbf{Q}^+$$

Now, $e*a = \dfrac{(ea)}{2} = a$

$\Rightarrow \quad a(e-2) = 0$

$\Rightarrow \quad e = 2$

Since, $a \in \mathbf{Q}^+ \Rightarrow a \neq 0$

$a \in \mathbf{Q}^+$ and we have

$2*a = (2a)/2 = a = a*2; \forall\, a \in \mathbf{Q}^+$.

Hence, 2 is the identity element.

(iv) Existence of Inverse : Let $b \in \mathbf{Q}^+$ is the inverse of a, then we must have

$b*a = e = 2$

$$\Rightarrow \frac{(ba)}{2} = 2 \Rightarrow b = \frac{4}{a}$$

Now, $a \in \mathbf{Q}^+ \Rightarrow 4/a \in \mathbf{Q}^+$

We have $(4/a) * a = \{(4/a) \times a\}/2$

$= 2 = a * (4/a)$

$\Rightarrow 4/a$ is the inverse of a

$\Rightarrow$ inverse of each element of $\mathbf{Q}^+$ exists.

(v) Commutativity: Let $a, b \in \mathbf{Q}^+$

$\Rightarrow a * b = (ab)/2 = (ba)/2 = b * a$

Hence $(\mathbf{Q}^+, *)$ is an abelian group.

4. *Show that the set* **Z** *of all integers form a group with respect to binary operation $*$ defined by $a * b = a + b + 1; \forall\ a, b \in \mathbf{Z}$ is an abelian group.*

SOLUTION. **(i) Closure property :** Let $a, b \in \mathbf{Z}$

$\Rightarrow a + b + 1 \in \mathbf{Z} \Rightarrow a * b \in \mathbf{Z}$

$\Rightarrow \mathbf{Z}$ is closed with respect to $*$.

(ii) Associativity : If $a, b, c \in \mathbf{Z}$, then

$(a * b) * c = (a + b + 1) * c$

$= (a + b + 1) + c + 1$

$= a + b + c + 2$

Also, $a * (b * c) = a * (b + c + 1) = a + \{b + c + 1) + 1\} = a + b + c + 2$

$\Rightarrow (a * b) * c = a * (b * c);\ \forall\ a, b, c \in \mathbf{Z}.$

(iii) Existence of Identity : An element $e \in \mathbf{Z}$ will be the identity if $e * a = a;\ \forall\ a \in \mathbf{Z}.$

Now, $e * a = e + a + 1$

$e + a + 1 = a \Rightarrow e = -1$

Since, $-1 \in \mathbf{Z}$ and we have for any $a \in \mathbf{Z}$

$(-1) * a = -1 + a + 1 = a$

$\Rightarrow -1$ is the identity element.

(iv) Existence of inverse : If $a \in \mathbf{Z}$, then $b \in \mathbf{Z}$ will be the inverse of a if $b * a = -1$

($\because -1$ is the identity element)

Now, $b * a = -1$

$\Rightarrow b + a + 1 = -1 \Rightarrow b = -2 - a.$

Also $a \in \mathbf{Z} \Rightarrow -2 - a \in \mathbf{Z}$

and $(-2 - a) * a = (-2 - a) + a + 1$

$= -1$, identity element.

$\therefore (-2 - a)$ is the inverse of a.

(v) Commutativity : Since, $a * b = a + b + 1 = b + a + 1 = b * a$

$\Rightarrow$ Commutativity satisfied.

Hence, **Z** is an inifinite abelian group under the given composition.

Exercise-4.1

1. Show that follwoing are groups :
   (i) Set of all even integers (including zero) under addition.
   (ii) Set of all non-zero rational numbers with respect to binary operation of multiplication.
   (iii) The set of all real numbers with respect to addition.
   (iv) The set **C** of all non-zero complex numbers with respect to multiplication.
2. Does the set of all odd integers form a group with respect to addition.
3. Show that the set of positive rational numbers does not form a group with respect to the binary operation $*$ defined by $a * b = a/b$.
4. Show that the set $A = \{a + b\sqrt{2} : a, b \in \mathbf{Q}\}$ is a group with respect to addition.
5. Show that the set of all $n \times n$ non-singular matrices having their elements as rational (real or complex) number is an infinite non-abelian group with respect to matrices multiplication.
6. Show that the matrices $A = \begin{bmatrix} \cos\alpha & -\sin\alpha \\ \sin\alpha & \cos\alpha \end{bmatrix}$ where α is a real number, form a group with respect matrix multiplication.
7. Show that the four matrices $\begin{bmatrix} 1 & 0 \\ 0 & 1 \end{bmatrix}, \begin{bmatrix} -1 & 0 \\ 0 & 1 \end{bmatrix}, \begin{bmatrix} 1 & 0 \\ 0 & -1 \end{bmatrix}, \begin{bmatrix} -1 & 0 \\ 0 & -1 \end{bmatrix}$ forms a group with respect to matrix multiplication.
8. Show that the set of all n, n^{th} roots of unity forms a finite abelian group of order n with respect to multiplication.
9. Show that the set **Z** of all integers is an abelian group with operation $*$ defined by $a * b = a + b + 2$.
10. Show that the set **Q** of all rational numbers, other than 1 with operation $*$, defined by $a * b = a + b + 2$ forms a group under binary operation $*$.
11. Show that the set $G = (1, \omega, \omega^2)$, where ω is an imaginary cube root of unity is a group with respect to multiplication.
12. Show that the set of complex numbers **C** with the condition $|z| = 1$ forms a group with respect to the operation of multiplication of complex numbers.

13. Show that the set of four transformation f_1, f_2, f_3, f_4 on the set of complex numbers denoted by $f_1(z) = z, f_2(z) = -z, f_3(z) = 1/z, f_4(z) = -1/z$ forms a finite abelian group with respect to the composition of functions.

14. Show that the set V of all vectors (defined as directed line segment) froms an infinte abelian group with respect to vector addition.

15. Show that **Q** the set of all rational numbers without 1 by the operation defined by $a * b = a+b-ab$ is an infinte abelian group.

4.5 INTEGRAL POWERS OF AN ELEMENT

Let G be a group with respect to multiplication. If $a \in G$, then aa is denoted by a^2, aaa is denoted by a^3 and so on. We have

$$a \cdot a \cdot a \ldots n \text{ times} = a^n;\ n \in \mathbf{Z}^+$$

But closure property $a^2, a^3, \ldots, a^n \in G$.

Also, if e is the identity element in G, we define $a^{\circ} = e$.

If n is a positive integer, we define

$$a^{-n} = (a^n)^{-1} \in G \text{ since } a^n = a \cdot a \cdot a \ldots n \text{ times} \in G.$$

Further, $$(a^n)^{-1} = (a \cdot a \ldots n \text{ times})^{-1} = a^{-1}a^{-1} \ldots n \text{ times} = (a^{-1})^n$$

Thus, $$a^{-n} = (a^n)^{-1} = (a^{-1})n$$

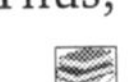

- If G is an additive group, we write na in place of a^n.
- If m is a positive integer such that $a^m = e$ then $0(a) \leq m$.
- Identity element e in a group G, is the only element whose order is one.
- The order of an element of an infinte group may be finite or infinite.

  For example: In the multiplicative group $\mathbf{Q}_0$ of non-zero rational number $1, -1 \in \mathbf{Q}_0$ such that $o(1) = 1$ and $o(-1) = 2$. The order of any other element of this group is infinite.

Solved Examples

1. *Consider the multiplicative group $G = \{1, -1, i, -i\}$ of cube roots of unity. Find the order of each element of G.*

SOLUTION. Since 1 is the identity element, therefore $o(1) = 1$.

Also, $(-1)^2 = 1 \Rightarrow o(-1) = 2$

$(i)^4 = 1 \Rightarrow o(i) = 4$

$(-i)^4 = 1 \Rightarrow o(-i) = 4$

2. *Consider the group $\mathbf{Z} = \{\ldots, -3, -2, -1, 0, 1, 2, 3, \ldots\}$ of all integers. Show that 0 is the only element of finite order.*

SOLUTION. If a be any non-zero integer, then there exists no positive integer n such that $na = (a + a + \ldots + n \text{ times}) = 0$

$\Rightarrow o(a)$ is infinite.

Hence, in **Z**, the identity 0 is the only element of finite order.

THEOREM 1. *The order of every element of a finite group is finite.*

PROOF. Let G be a finite group and $a \in G$

Consider all positive integral powers of a, i.e.,

$$a, a^2, a^3, \ldots, a^s, \ldots, a^r, \ldots$$

By closure property, these all are elements of G.

Since, G is finite, therefore all the integral powers of a cannot be distinct elements of G.

Suppose that $$a^r = a^s, \text{ where } r > s \quad \ldots(1)$$

Then, $$a^r = a^s \Rightarrow \quad a^r a^{-s} = a^s \cdot a^{-s}$$

$$\Rightarrow \quad a^{r-s} = a^0 = e$$

$$\Rightarrow \quad a^m = e, \text{ where } m = r - s > 0$$

Thus, there exists a positive integer m such that $a^m = e$. Now since every set of positive integers has a least member, it follows that the set of all positive integers m such that $a^m = e$ has a least member say n.

Thus, $$o(a) = n, \text{ which is finite.}$$

Hence, the order of every element of the finite group G is finite.

THEOREM 2. *If the element a of a group G is of order n, then $a^m = e$. iff n is a divisor of m.*

PROOF. Let $o(a) = n$ and $a^m = e$, for some positive integer m then $m \geq n$. If $m = n$ then n is a divisor of m.

If $m \geq n$, then by division algorithm, there exists two integers q and r such that $m = nq + r$, where $0 \leq r \leq n$.

Therefore, $\quad a^m = e \Rightarrow a^{nq+r} = e$

$\Rightarrow \quad a^{nq} \cdot a^r = e \Rightarrow a^r = e \qquad [\because a^{nq} = (a^n)^q = e^q = e]$

Thus, $\quad a^r = e$, where $0 < r < n$ or $r = 0$ (By division algorithm)

Now, since $o(a) = n$, n is the least positive integer such that $a^n = e$. Hence, it follows that $r = 0$.

Therefore, $\quad m = nq \Rightarrow n$ is a divisor of m.

Conversely, Let n be a divisor of m, so that

$$m = nq, \text{ for } q \in \mathbf{Z}^+$$

Hence, $\quad a^m = a^{nq} = (a^n)^q = e^q = e.$

THEOREM 3. *The order of an element of a group is the same as that of its inverse.*

PROOF. Let G be a group under multiplication and a is any element of G.

$$o(a) = m \text{ and } o(a^{-1}) = n$$

Now, $\quad o(a) = m \Rightarrow a^m = e \Rightarrow (a^m)^{-1} = e^{-1} = e$

$\Rightarrow \quad (a^{-1})^m = e$, since $(a^m)^{-1} = e^{-1} = e$

$\Rightarrow \quad o(a^{-1}) \leq m \Rightarrow n \leq m \qquad ...(1)$

Again $\quad o(a^{-1}) = n \Rightarrow (a^{-1})^n = e \Rightarrow (a^n)^{-1} = e$

$\Rightarrow \quad ((a^n)^{-1})^{-1} = e^{-1} \Rightarrow a^n = e$

$\Rightarrow \quad o(a) \leq n \Rightarrow m \leq n \qquad ...(2)$

From (1) and (2), we conclude that

$$m = n, \quad \text{i.e., } o(a) = o(a^{-1})$$

THEOREM 4. *The order of any integral power of an element a cannot exceed that order of a.*

PROOF. Let r be any integral power of a and let $o(a) = n$. Now, $o(a) = n \Rightarrow a^n = e$

$\Rightarrow \quad (a^n)^r = e^r \Rightarrow a^{nr} = e$

$\Rightarrow \quad (a^r)^n = e \Rightarrow o(a)^r \leq n$

$\Rightarrow \quad o(a^r)$ cannot exceeds the $o(a)$.

THEOREM 5. *If a and b are any two elements of a group G, then $o(a) = o(b^{-1}ab)$.*

PROOF. Let $o(a) = m$, hence m is the least positive integer, such that $a^m = e$.

Now, $\quad (b^{-1}ab)^2 = (b^{-1}ab)(b^{-1}ab) = b^{-1}a(bb^1)ab$ (By associativity)

$= b^{-1}aeab \qquad (\because bb^{-1} = e)$

$= b^{-1}a^2b \qquad (\because ae = a)$

Similarly $\quad (b^{-1}ab)^3 = b^{-1}a^3b$

⋮ ... and so on.

$(b^{-1}ab)^m = (b^{-1}ab)(b^{-1}ab)$ ... to m factors

$= b^{-1}abb^{-1}ab \ldots b^{-1}ab$ (By associativity)

$= b^{-1}a(bb^{-1})a(bb^{-1}) \ldots (bb^{-1})ab$ (By associativity)

$= b^{-1}a^mb = b^{-1}eb = b^{-1}b = e \qquad (\because a^m = e)$

Thus, we have $(b^{-1}ab)^m = b^{-1}a^mb = e$

Now, since, m is the least positive integer such that $a^m = e$, it follows that m is the least positivie integer such that

$$(b^{-1}ab)^m = e$$

Hence, $\quad o(b^{-1}ab) = m$

THEOREM 6. *For any two elements a, b of a group G, $o(ab) = o(ba)$.*

PROOF. We have

$$ba = e(ba) = (a^{-1}a)(ba) = a^{-1}(ab)(a)$$

Hence, by Theorem 5

$$o[a^{-1}(ab)a] = o(ab) \quad \Rightarrow \quad o(ba) = o(ab)$$

THEOREM 7. *The order of any integral power of an element of a group is a divisor of the order of that element.*

PROOF. Let a be any element of a group G with $o(a) = n$.

$\Rightarrow \quad a^n = e$

Let r be any integral power of a such that $o(a^r) = m$

Then $\quad (a^r)^n = a^{rn} = (a^n)^r = e^r = e$

Thus, $\quad (a^r)^n = e \quad \Rightarrow \quad o(a^r)$ divides n

Hence, $o(a^r)$ is a divisor of $o(a)$.

THEOREM 8. *If a is an element of order n and p is prime to n, then a^p is also of order n.*

PROOF. Let r be the order of a^p.

Now $\quad o(a) = n \quad \Rightarrow \quad a^n = e$

$\Rightarrow \quad (a^n)^p = e^p = e \quad \Rightarrow \quad (a^n)^p = e$

$\Rightarrow \quad o(a^n) \le n \quad \Rightarrow \quad r \le n$ ...(1)

Now, since p and n are relatively prime, there exists integers x and y such that

$$px + ny = 1$$

$\therefore \quad a = a^1 = a^{px+ny} = a^{px} \cdot a^{ny} = a^{px}(a^n)^y = a^{px}e^y$

$\quad = a^{px} \cdot e = a^{px} = (a^p)^x$

Also, $\quad a^r = [(a^n)^x]^r = (a^p)^{rx} = [(a^p)^r]^x = e^x \quad [\because o(a^p) = r \Rightarrow (a^p)^r = e]$

$\quad = e$

$\therefore \quad o(a) \le r \quad \Rightarrow \quad n \le r$ ...(2)

From (1) and (2), we conclude that

$$n = r$$

Solved Examples

1. *For any two elements a and b of a group G, show that G is abelian iff $(ab)^2 = a^2b^2$*

SOLUTION. Let us first suppose that G be abelian so that $ab = ba \ \forall \ a, b \in G$.

Consider

$(ab)^2 = (ab)(ab) = a(ba)b$ (by associativity)

$= a(ab)b$ (by commutativity)

$= (aa)(bb)$ (by associativity)

$= a^2 \cdot b^2$

Thus, $(ab)^2 = a^2b^2, \ \forall \ a, b \in G$.

Convesely, Let $(ab)^2 = a^2b^2$, $\forall \ a, b \in G$.

To show $\quad ab = ba$

Consider $(ab)^2 = a^2b^2$

$\Rightarrow \quad (ab)(ab) = (aa)(bb)$

$\Rightarrow \quad a(ba)b = a(ab)b$ (By associativity)

$\Rightarrow \quad ab = ba$

(By left and right concellation law)

Thus, we have $ab = ba, \ \forall \ a, b \in G$.

Hence, G is abelian.

2. *Show that if G is an abelian group then for all $a, b \in G$ and all integers n, $(ab)^n = a^nb^n$.*

SOLUTION. (i) Let $n = 0$

Then $(ab)^0 = e$

Also, $a^0b^0 = e \cdot e = e$

$\therefore \quad (ab)^0 = a^0b^0$

(ii) Let $n>0$

If $n = 1$, then $(ab)^1 = ab = a^1b^1$

Let us suppose that result is true for $n = r$

i.e., $\quad (ab)^r = a^rb^r$

Then $(ab)^{r+1} = (ab)^r \cdot ab = a^rb^rab$

$= a^rab^rb \quad (\because ab^r = b^ra)$

$= a^{r+1}b^{r+1}$

Then, by mathematical induction for all $n>0$, $(ab)^n = a^n \cdot b^n$

(iii) Let $n<0$

Let $n = -r$, where r is a positive integer.

Then $(ab)^n = (ab)^{-r} = [(ab)^r]^{-1}$

$= [a^rb^r]^{-1} = [b^ra^r]^{-1}$

$(\because a^mb^m = b^ma^m)$

$= [a^r]^{-1}[b^r]^{-1}$

$[\because (ab)^{-1} = b^{-1}a^{-1}]$

$= a^{-r}b^{-r} = a^n b^n$

3. *If number of elements in a group G is less than or equal to four, then group must be abelain.*

SOLUTION. (i) When $o(G) = 1$, $G = \{e\}$, where e is the identity element.

$\Rightarrow G$ is abelian, since $e \cdot e = e$

(ii) When $o(G) = 2$, Let $G = \{e, a\}$ where $a \neq e$

In this case $ae = ea = a$ (by closedness of G and hence G is abelian.

(iii) When $o(G) = 3$, Let $G = \{e, a, b\}$, then $a \neq b \neq e$

In this case we prepare the composition table as follows :

•	e	a	b
e	e	a	b
a	a	a^2	ab
b	b	ba	b^2

Since, in any row of the composition table of a group, each element appears only once.

So, $a^2 = e$ or $ab = e$ ...(1)

and $b^2 = e$ or $ba = e$ ...(2)

Now, $a^2 = e \Rightarrow ab = b$ since each element in second row occurs only once.

$\Rightarrow ab = eb \Rightarrow a = e$

This is not possible, since $a \neq e$. Thus, $a \neq e \Rightarrow ab = e$

Similarly $b^2 = e \Rightarrow b = a$, by the last row of the composition table.

$\Rightarrow ba = ea \Rightarrow b = e$

Hence, G is abelian.

(iv) Let $G = \{e, a, b, c\}$ be a group of order 4, the identity element e has its own inverse. Since G is a group of even order, there must be at least one more element in G which has its own inverse.

Let $a^{-1} = a$. If $b^{-1} = b$ and $c^{-1} = c$, then in G, every element has its own inverse.

$\Rightarrow bc = e = cb$

Also, $a^{-1} = a \Rightarrow a^2 = e$

Now, $ab = b$ or $ab = c$

($\because$ each element in the second row occurs only once.)

Since, $ab = b \Rightarrow a = e$, which is not possible so $ab = c$

Then, $ac = b$

Now, we prepare the composition table as follows :

•	e	a	b	c
e	e	a	b	c
a	a	e	c	b
b	b	c	a	e
c	c	b	e	a

From the above table we conclude that each row is identical to corresponding columns.

$\Rightarrow G$ is commutative.

Hence, G is abelian.

4. *If G is a group of even order, then show that there exists an element a, other than the identity 'e', such that $a^2 = e$*

SOLUTION. Let $o(G) = 2r$, where r is any positive integer.

Since, we know that, in a group every element possesses a unique inverse and $e^{-1} = e$. The remaining $(2r-1)$ elements should, therefore, be divided into pairs in such a way that each pair consists of two distinct elements, which are inverse of each other. But this is not possible, since $(2r-1)$ is odd.

Hence, $\exists$ an element $a \in G$, such that,

$a^{-1} = a$, where $a \neq e$

But $a = a^{-1} \Rightarrow a^2 = a^{-1}a = e$

Thus, there exists $a \in G$ such that $a \neq e$ and $a^2 = e$.

5. *In a group, if $ba = a^m b^n$, prove that the elements $a^m b^{n-2}$, $a^{m-2}b^n$, ab^{-1} have the same order.*

SOLUTION. We can write

$a^m b^{n-2} = a^m b^n b^{-2} = bab^{-2}$

$(\because ba = a^m b^m)$

$= bab^{-1}b^{-1} = (b^{-1})^{-1}(ab^{-1})b^{-1}$

In a group, we know that $o(a) = o(x^{-1}ax)$, where a, x are any two elements of the group.

$\therefore o(a^m b^{n-2}) = o[(b^{-1})^{-1}(ab^{-1})b^{-1}]$

$= o(ab^{-1})$ ...(1)

Also, $a^{m-2}b^n = a^{-2}a^m b^n = a^{-2}ba$

$$= a^{-2}ba^{2-1} = a^{-2}ba^{-1}a^2$$
$$= (a^2)^{-1}(ba^{-1})a^2$$
$$\therefore o(a^{m-2}b^n) = o[(a^2)^{-1}(ba^{-1})a^2]$$
$$= o(ba^{-1})$$
$$= o[(ba^{-1})^{-1}]$$
$$[\because o(a^{-1}) = o(a)]$$
$$= o[(a^{-1})^{-1}b^{-1}] = o(ab^{-1}) \quad ...(2)$$

Hence, from (1) and (2) we get $o(a^mb^{n-2}) = o(ab^{-1}) = o(a^{m-2}b^n)$

6. *If G is a finite abelian group with elements $a_1, a_2, ..., a_n$ show that $a_1 \cdot a_2 ... a_n$ is an element whose square is an identity.*

SOLUTION. We know that

$$(a_1a_2 ... a_n)^2 = (a_1a_2 ... a_n)(a_1a_2 ... a_n) \quad ...(1)$$

Now, each element in a group has a unique inverse. Thus each of $a_1a_2 ... a_n$ is the inverse of exactly one of them. Hence, associating each of $a_1a_2 ... a_n$ with its inverse, the relation (1) reduces to

$$(a_1 \cdot a_2 \cdots a_n)^2$$
$$= (a_1a_1^{-1})(a_2a_2^{-1})\cdots(a_na_n^{-1})$$
$$= e \cdot e \cdot e \cdot ... \text{ n times} = e$$

7. *In any group G if $a^5 = e$, $aba^{-1} = b^2$ for $a, b \in G$. Find $o(b)$.*

SOLUTION. We have

$$(aba^{-1})^2 = aba^{-1}aba^{-1} = ab(a^{-1}a)ba^{-1}$$
$$= ab(e)ba^{-1} = ab^2a^{-1} = aaba^{-1}a^{-1}$$
$$(\because aba^{-1} = b^2)$$
$$= a^2ba^{-2}$$

Therefore, $(aba^{-1})^4 = [\{aba^{-1}\}^2]^2$
$= (a^2ba^{-2})^2 = a^2ba^{-2}a^2ba^{-2}$
$= a^2b^2a^{-2} = a^2aba^{-1}a^{-2} = a^3ba^{-3}$
$\Rightarrow (aba^{-1})^8 = [(aba^{-1})^4]^2 = (a^3ba^{-3})^2$
$= a^3ba^{-3}a^3ba^{-3} = a^3b^2a^{-3}$
$= a^3aba^{-1}a^{-3} = a^4ba^{-4}$
and $(aba^{-1})^{16} = a^4aba^{-1}a^{-4} = a^5ba^{-5}$
$= ebe \qquad (\because a^5 = e \Rightarrow a^{-5} = e)$
$= b$
Hence, $\quad (aba^{-1})^{16} = b$

$\because \quad (b^2)^{16} = b$
$\Rightarrow \quad b^{32} = b$
$\Rightarrow \quad b^{31} = e$
Since, $\quad b^m = e$
$\Rightarrow \quad o(b)\,|\,m$, therefore $o(b)\,|\,31$
but 31 is prime integer, therefore $o(b) = 1$ or 31
Therefore if $b = e$, then $o(b) = 1$ and if $b \neq e$ then $o(b) = 31$.

8. *In a group G if $xy^2 = y^3x$ and $yx^2 = x^3y$, show that $x = y = e$, where e is the identiy of G.*

SOLUTION. It is given that $xy^2 = y^3x$

$\Rightarrow \quad x^2y^2 = xy^3x$
$\Rightarrow \quad x^2y = xy^3xy^{-1} = xy^2yxy^{-1}$
$= y^3xyxy^{-1} \quad ...(1)$

Further $yx^2 = x^3y$
$\Rightarrow \quad yx^2 = xx^2y$
$\Rightarrow \quad yx^2 = xy^3xyxy^{-1} \quad$ [Using (1)]
$\Rightarrow \quad x^2 = y^{-1}xy^3xyxy^{-1}$
$\Rightarrow \quad x^2y = y^{-1}xy^3xyx \quad ...(2)$

Using (1) and (2), we get
$y^3xyxy^{-1} = y^{-1}xy^3xyx$
$\Rightarrow \quad y^4xyx = xy^3xyxy = xy^2yxyxy$
$= y^3xyxyxy$
$\Rightarrow \quad yxyx = xyxyxy$
$\Rightarrow \quad (yx)^2 = (xy)^3 \quad ...(3)$

Now, since the given relation is symmetrical in x and y, so interchanging x and y in (3), we get
$$(xy)^2 = (yx)^3 \quad ...(4)$$
Hence, from (3) and (4), we have
$$(xy)^2 = (yx)^3 = (yx)^2(yx)$$
$$= (xy)^3(yx)$$
Cancelling $(xy)^2$ from both sides, we get
$$e = (xy)(yx) = xy^2x$$
$\Rightarrow \quad x^{-2} = y^2$
Now, $\quad xy^2 = y^3x \Rightarrow xx^{-2} = yx^{-2}x$
$\Rightarrow \quad x^{-1} = yx^{-1} \Rightarrow \quad y = e$
Further, $\quad yx^2 = x^3y$
$\Rightarrow \quad ex^2 = x^3e$
$\Rightarrow \quad x^2 = x^3$
$\Rightarrow \quad x = e$

Exercise-4.2

1. If a and b any elements of a group G, then show that $(bab^{-1})^n = ba^nb^{-1}$ for any $n \in \mathbf{Z}$.
2. Show that if for every element a in a group G, $a^2 = e$, then G is abelian.
3. Show that if every element of a group G has its own inverse, then G is abelian.
4. If G is group such that $(ab)^p = a^pb^p$ for three consecutive integers $p \;\forall\, a, b \in G$.

5. Show that a group G is abelian if every element of G except the identity element is of order 2.
6. Find the order of each element in the multiplicative group $G = [1, \omega, \omega^2]$ where ω is the cube root of unity.
7. If the element a, b and ab of a group are each of order 2 show that $ab = ba$.
8. Show that in a group G, we have (i) $ab = e \Rightarrow a = b^{-1}$ and $b = a^{-1}$ (ii) $ab = a$ or $ba = a \Rightarrow b = e$.
9. If a is an element of a group, prove that the integral powers of a form a multiplicative group.
10. Show that a group G is abelian iff $(ab)^{-1} = a^{-1}b^{-1} \; \forall \; a, b \in G$.
11. If in a group G, the elements a and b commutes, then prove that
    (i) a^{-1} and b^{-1} also commute
    (ii) a^{-1} and b also commute
    (iii) a and b^{-1} also commute

Hint to Selected Problems

1. Consider the three cases $n = 0, n > 0, n < 0$.
2. Prove the result for three consecutive integeral values of m *i.e.*, for $n - 1$, n, and $n+1$
3. $o(1) = 1, o(\omega)^3 = \omega^3 = 1$.
   Also $(\omega^2)^3 = \omega^6 = (\omega^3)^2 = 1 \Rightarrow o(\omega^2) = 3$.

ANSWERS

6. $o(1) = 1, (\omega) = 3, (\omega^2) = 3$

4.6 SUBGROUPS OF A GROUP

Let (G, $*$) be a group and H is any subset of G such that $H \neq \phi$. Then by properties of a group $\forall \; a, b \in H \Rightarrow a, b \in G$ for $H \subset G$.

$$\Rightarrow \quad a * b \in G \Rightarrow a * b \in H$$

If $a * b \in H$, then we say that H is stable for the composition in G and the composition in G has induced a composition in H. Now, there are two possibilities.

(i) H is itself a group with respect to the operation$*$.
(ii) H is not a group with respect to $*$.

4.6.1 COMPLEX OF A GROUP

Any non-empty subset H of G is called a complex of the group G.

4.6.2 SUBGROUP

A non-empty subset H of a group G is calld a subgroup of G if H is itself a group with respect to the operation defined in G.

- The two subgroups, G and {e} of the group G are called Improper (or trivial) subgroups of G. Any subgroup other than these two subgroups is called a proper (or non-trivial) subgroups.
- It is clear that, if H is a subgroup of G and K is a subgroup of H, then K is subgroup of G.
- Every subgroup of G is a complex of G, but every complex is not always a subgroup.

ILLUSTRATIONS

(1) ({1, –1},.) is a subgroup of ({1, –1, i, –i}, .)
(2) (**Z**, +) is a subgroup of (**Q**, +)
(3) (**Q**, +) is a sub group of (**R**, +)
(4) The set of all non-singular matrices with real elements whose determinant value are 1, is a subgroup of multiplicative group of all non-singular $n \times n$ matrices.
(5) The multiplicative group of positive rational numbers is a subgroup of the multiplicative group of all non-zero rational numbers.

- If H and K are two complexes of a group G, then
$$HK = \{x \in G : x = hk, h \in H, k \in K\}$$
Also, HK is a complex consisting of the elements of G, which obtained on multiplying each member of H to each member of K.
- Multiplication of complexes is associative.
- If H is be any complex of G, then inverse of H, *i.e.*, H^{-1} is the complex of G consisting the inverse of the elements of H. *i.e.*, H^{-1} is the complex of G consisting the inverse of the element of H, *i.e.*, $H^{-1} = \{h^{-1} : h \in H\}$

THEOREM 1. *Let H be a subgroup of G. Then*

(i) Identify of H is same as that of G.

(ii) The inverse of an element $a \in H$ is the same as the inverse of the same element a regard as an element of the group G.

(iii) The order of an element $a \in H$ is the same order of the same element regarded as an element of the Group G.

PROOF. Let H be a subgroup of G.

(i) Let e and e' be identities in H and G respectively. To show $e = e'$

Let $a \in H$

$a \in H \Rightarrow ae = a$ ($\because$ e is the identity of H) ..(1)

Also $a \in H \Rightarrow a \in G$ ($\because H \subset G$)

$ae' = a$ (e' is the identity in G) ...(2)

From (1) and (2), we have $ae = ae' \Rightarrow e = e'$.

(ii) Let e be the identity of H as well as of G. Let $a \in G$ be arbitrary. Let b be the inverse of a in H. Let c be the inverse of a in G.

To show that $b = c$

By assumption $ba = e = ca$ in G, we have $ba = ca \Rightarrow b = c$.

(iii) Let e be the identity of H as well as of G.

Let n be the order a in H and m be the order of a in G.

To show $m = n$

Since e is the identity in H $\Rightarrow a^n = e$

Since e is the identity in G $\Rightarrow a^m = e$, where n and m are positive integers.

Therefore, $a^n = a^m$

$\Rightarrow$ $a^{m-n} = e = a^0 \Rightarrow a^{m-n} = a^0$

$\Rightarrow$ $m - n = 0 \Rightarrow m = n$

THEOREM 2. *Let H and K be complexes of Group G, then $(HK)^{-1} = K^{-1}H^{-1}$.*

SOLUTION. Let x be any arbitrary element of $(HK)^{-1}$. Then

$$x = (hk)^{-1}, h \in H, k \in K$$
$$= k^{-1}h^{-1} \in K^{-1}H^{-1}$$
$$(HK)^{-1} \subseteq K^{-1}H^{-1} \quad ...(1)$$

Now, let y be any arbitrary element of $K^{-1}H^{-1}$

Then $y = k^{-1}h^{-1}, k \in K, h \in H = (hk)^{-1} \in (HK)^{-1}$

$\therefore$ $K^{-1}H^{-1} \subseteq (HK)^{-1}$ ...(2)

Now from (1) and (2), we conclude that $(HK)^{-1} = K^{-1}H^{-1}$.

THEOREM 3. *If H is any subgroup of G, then $H^{-1} = H$. Also, show that converse is not true.*

SOLUTION. Let $h^{-1} \in H$. Then $h \in H$.

Since, H is subgroup of G, therefore, $h \in H \Rightarrow h^{-1} \in H$.

Thus, $h^{-1} \in H^{-1} \Rightarrow h^{-1} \in H$

$\Rightarrow$ $h^{-1} \subseteq H$ ...(1)

Again $h \in H \Rightarrow h^{-1} \in H \Rightarrow (h^{-1})^{-1} \in H^{-1} \Rightarrow h \in H^{-1}$

$\therefore$ $h \subseteq H^{-1}$

Now, from (1) and (2), we have

$$H = H^{-1} \qquad ...(2)$$

Now, to show converse is not true.

i.e., If H is a complex of a group G and $H^{-1} = H$, then it is not necessary that H is a subgroup of G.

For example

$H = \{-1\}$ is a complex of the multiplicative group $G = \{-1, 1\}$.

Also $H^{-1} = \{-1\}$ ($\because -1$ is the inverse of -1). But H = {–1} is not a subgroup of G.

We have $(-1)(-1) = 1 \notin H$, *i.e.*, H is not closed with respect of multiplication.

4.6.3 CRITERION FOR A SUBSET TO BE SUBGROUP

It is not necessary for an arbitrary subset of H of a group G to be a subgroup. It would be interesting to find out criteria by which H can be identified as a subgroup or otherwise.

THEOREM 4. *A non-empty subset H of a group G is a subgroup of G if and only if*

(i) $a, b \in H \Rightarrow ab \in H$

(ii) $a \in H \Rightarrow a^{-1} \in H$, *where* a^{-1} *is the inverse of* $a \in G$.

PROOF. Let H be a subgroup of G, then H must be closed with respect to multiplication, *i.e.*, the composition in G.

Therefore $\qquad a \in H, b \in H \Rightarrow ab \in H.$

Conversely, suppose H is a subset of a group G such that (i) and (ii), the given conditions, holds. In order to show that H is a subgroup, all that is needed is to verify that the identify element $e \in H$ and that the associative law holds for element of H.

If $a \in H$, then by (2), $a^{-1} \in H$ and so by (1) we see that $e = aa^{-1} \in H$, again since associative law does holds in G, it holds in H, which is a subset of G, Hence, H is a subgroup of G.

THEOREM 5. *Let H be a non-empty subset of a group G. Then H is a subgroup of G iff*

$$a, b \in H \Rightarrow ab^{-1} \in H, \text{ where } b^{-1} \text{ is the inverse of } b \text{ in } G.$$

PROOF. **Necessary condition.** Let us first suppose H is a subgroup of G and $a, b \in H$. Since H is a group, each element of H must have its inverse in H. Thus if $b \in H \Rightarrow b^{-1} \in H$ and then by closure property $ab^{-1} \in H$. This proves the necessary condition.

Condition is sufficient. Let H be a subset of G for which $a, b \in H$ implies $ab^{-1} \in H$. To show that H is a subgroup of G, we must verify that H is closed, the identity element of H has an inverse in H and the associative law holds for element of H.

Let $b = a$, then we see that $a \in H \Rightarrow aa^{-1} \in H \Rightarrow e \in H$

Identify element of G also belongs to H.

Now, for the elements e and b of H, we have $eb^{-1} \in H$ and so $b^{-1} \in H$, since b is arbitrary element of H, we see that for any $b \in H$, $b^{-1} \in H$.

Now, $\qquad a, b \in H \Rightarrow a, b^{-1} \in H$

$\Rightarrow \qquad a(b^{-1})^{-1} \in H$

$\Rightarrow \qquad ab \in H$

$\Rightarrow \qquad H$ is closed.

Finally, since the associative law does hold for G, it also holds for H which is a subset of G. Hence, $(H, .)$ is a subgroup.

- In case of additive composition, the condition of the above theorem becomes

$$a, b \in H \; a - b \in H$$

- To show that a non-empty subset H of a group G is a subgroup of G, we should take any two arbitrary elements $a, b \in H$ and try to show that $ab^{-1} \in H$.

THEOREM 6. *If H, K are subgroups of a group G, then HK isa subgroup of G iff HK = KH.*

PROOF. Let H and K be two subgroups of a group G so that

$$H H^{-1} = H, K K^{-1} = K \quad \text{... (1)}$$

and

$$K^{-1} = K, H^{-1} = H \quad \text{... (2)}$$

Step I. Let HK be a subgroup of G so that

$$(HK)^{-1} = HK$$

To show $HK = KH$ ... (3)

$\because (HK)^{-1} = HK \Rightarrow K^{-1} H^{-1} = HK$ .... (4)

Using (2), we have $HK = KH$.

Step II. Let $HK = KH$

To show that HK is a subgroup of G. For this we have to prove,

$$(HK)^{-1} = HK \quad \text{... (5)}$$

Consider $(HK)\ (HK)^{-1} = (HK)(K^{-1}H^{-1}) = H(KK^{-1})\ (H^{-1})$ (By associativity)

$= HKH^{-1}$ [by (1)]

$= KHH^{-1}$ [by (4)]

$= K(HH^{-1}) = KH = HK$ [by (4)]

THEOREM 7. *If H and K are subgroups of an abeliam group G, then HK is a subgroup of G.*

PROOF. Let us suppose H and K be subgroups of an abelian group G, so that

$$H^{-1} = H, K^{-1} = L \quad \text{...(1)}$$

$$HH^{-1} = H, K K^{-1} = K \quad \text{...(2)}$$

To show that (HK) is a subgroup of G, we have to show that

$$(HK)(HK)^{-1} = HK$$

Now, since G is abelian $\Rightarrow$ $ab = ba \ \forall\ a, b \in$ G.

$\therefore \quad h \in H, \quad k \in K \Rightarrow \quad hK = kh \Rightarrow HK = KH.$

Consider $(HK)(HK)^{-1} = (HK)\ (K^{-1} H^{-1}) = H(KK^{-1})\ H^{-1}$ ...(3)

$= HKH^{-1} = (HK)H^{-1} = (KH)H^{-1} = K\ (HH^{-1})$

$= KH = HK.$

4.7 UNION AND INTERSECTION OF SUBGROUPS

THEOREM 1. *The intersection of any two subgroups of a group G is a subgroup of G.*

PROOF. Let H_1 and H_2 be two subgroups of a group G. To show that $H_1 \cap H_1$ is a subgroup of G.

Let $a, b \in H_1 \cap H_2 \Rightarrow a, b \in H_1$ and $a, b \in H_2$

Now, since H_1 and H_2 are subgroups, then

$$a, b \in H_1 \Rightarrow ab^{-1} \in H_1 \text{ and } a, b \in H_2 \Rightarrow ab^{-1} \in H_2$$

Finally, $ab^{-1} \in H_1$ and $ab^{-1} \in H_2 \Rightarrow ab^{-1} \in H_1 \cap H_2$. Hence $H_1 \cap H_2$ is a subgroup of G.

THEOREM 2. *An arbitrary intersection of subgroups of a group G is a subgroup of G.*

PROOF. Let H_r be the collection of subgroups for $r \in \mathbf{N}$.

Let $H = \bigcap_{r=1}^{\infty} H_r$

To show that H is a subgroup of G.

$$\begin{aligned} a, b \in H \quad &\Rightarrow \quad a \in \bigcap_{r=1}^{\infty} H_r \text{ and } b \in \bigcap_{r=1}^{\infty} H_r \\ &\Rightarrow \quad a \in H_r, b = H_r; \forall\ r \in N \\ &\Rightarrow \quad ab^{-1} \in \bigcap_{r=1}^{\infty} H_r = H \\ &\Rightarrow \quad ab^{-1} \in H \end{aligned}$$

Thus, we have proved that $a, b \in H \Rightarrow ab^{-1} \in H$

This declares that H is a subgroup of G.

- $H_1 \cap H_2$ is a largest subgroup of G which is contained in H_1 as well as H_2.

THEOREM 3. *The union of two subgroups of a group G is a subgroup of G iff one is contained in the other.*

PROOF. Let H_1 and H_2 be subgroups of a group G. Let us first suppose

$$H_1 \subset H_2 \text{ or } H_2 \subset H_1.$$

To show that $H_1 \cup H_2$ is a subgroup of G

$$H_1 \subset H_2 \Rightarrow H_1 \cup H_2 = H_2$$

Also, H_2 is a subgroup of $G \Rightarrow H_1 \cup H_2$ is a subgroup of G. Again

$$H_2 \subset H_1 \Rightarrow H_1 \cup H_2 = H_1$$

Also, H_1 is a subgroup of $G \Rightarrow H_1 \cup H_2$ is a subgroup of G.

Hence, $H_1 \cup H_2$ is a subgroup of G, in both cases.

Conversely, Suppose that H_1 and H_2 are subgroups of a group G such that $H_1 \cup H_2$ is a subgroup of G. To prove either $H_1 \subset H_2$ or $H_2 \subset H_1$.

Suppose the contraty. Then $H_1 \not\subset H_2$ or $H_2 \not\subset H_1$

$$H_1 \not\subset H_2 \Rightarrow \exists a \in H_1 \text{ s. t.} a \notin H_2$$

and $$H_2 \not\subset H_1 \Rightarrow \exists a \in H_2 \text{ s. t.} a \notin H_1$$

Now $a, b \in H_1 \cup H_2$ and $H_1 \cup H_2$ is a subgroup of G

$\Rightarrow$ $$ab \in H_1 \cup H_2$$

This implies $ab \in H_1$ or $ab \in H_2$

$$a \in H_1, ab \in H_1 \Rightarrow a^{-1}(ab) \in H_1 \qquad (\because H_1 \text{ is a subgroup})$$

$\Rightarrow$ $$(a^{-1}a)b \in H_1 \Rightarrow eb \in H_1 \Rightarrow b \in H_1$$

Which is a contradiction $(\because b \notin H_1)$

Also, $b \in H_2, a\,b \in H_2 \Rightarrow (ab)b^{-1} \in H_2$

$\Rightarrow$ $$a \in H_2 \qquad (\text{For } (ab)b^{-1} = a(bb^{-1}) = ae = a)$$

Again, we get a contradiction $(\because a \notin H_2)$

Hence, our initial assumption is wrong.

Consequently $$H_1 \subset H_2 \text{ or } H_2 \subset H_1$$

- The union of two subgroups is not necessarily a subgroup.

  For example: Let H_1 and H_2 be two subgroups of the group $(\mathbf{Z}, +)$ where

  $$H_1 = \{2n : n \in \mathbf{Z}\}, H_2 = \{5n : n \in \mathbf{Z}\}.$$

  Then, $$H_1 \cup H_2 = [x : x = 2n \text{ or } 5n \text{ where } n \in \mathbf{Z}]$$
  $$= [0, \pm 2, \pm 4, \pm 6, \ldots, 0, \pm 5, \pm 10, \pm 15, \ldots]$$

  $$6, 15 \in H_1 \Rightarrow 6 + 15 = 21 \neq H_1 \cup H_2$$

  $\Rightarrow$ Clossure property is not satisfied.

  Hence, $H_1 \cup H_2$ is not a subgroups of $(\mathbf{Z}, +)$.

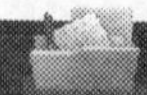

Solved Examples

1. Is **Z** a subgroup of $(\mathbf{Q}, +)$?

SOLUTION. For $\mathbf{Z} \subset \mathbf{Q}$ and the inverse of $b \in \mathbf{Q}$ is $-b$

Now, $\forall\, a, b \in \mathbf{Z}$

$\Rightarrow \quad a + (-b) = a - b \in \mathbf{Z}$

Therefore **Z** is a subgroup of **Q,** under addition.

2. Let G be the additive group of integers and $H = \{nl : n$ is a fixed integer and $l \in \mathbf{Z}\}$. Show that H is a subgroup of G.

SOLUTION. Here, we have $H \subseteq G$.

Let $a = nh$ and $b = nk$, be any two elements of H, with $h, k \in \mathbf{Z}$. Then $a+b = n\,(h+k)$ certainly belongs to H.

Thus $a, b \in H$ implies that $a + b \in H$.

Also, $-a = n(-h)$, the additive inverse of a is in H. Thus $a \in H$ implies that $-a \in H$. Hence, H is a subgroup of G.

3. If G is a group, then show that the set Z, defined by

$$Z = \{xz = zx : x \in G, z \in \mathbf{Z}\}$$

(is said to be centre of the group) is subgroup of G.

SOLUTION. Let $z_1, z_2 \in \mathbf{Z}\}$, then
$z_1 x = x z_1,\ z_2 x = x z_2,\ \forall x \in G$ ...(1)
Now, $x z_1 = z_1 x = z_1 (z_2^{-1} z_2 x), \forall x \in G$
$= z_1 z_2^{-1}(z_2 x) = z_1 z_2^{-1}(x z_2)$

$\therefore (x z_1) z_2^{-1} = z_1 z_2^{-1}(x z_2) z_2^{-1}$ [From (1)]
or $x(z_1 z_2^{-1}) = z_1 z_2^{-1} x (z_2 z_2^{-1})$
$= (z_1 z_2^{-1}) x, \forall x \in G$
Hence, $\mathbf{Z}$ is a subgroup of $\mathbf{G}$.

4.8 COSETS

Let H be a subgroup of a group $(G,.)$. Let $a \in G$ be arbitrary. We define.

$$aH = \{ah : h \in H\} \text{ and } Ha = \{ah : h \in H\}$$

Then aH is called left coset of H in G generated by a, and Ha is called right coset of H in G generated by a.

- If e the identity of G, then $e \in H$ is also identity for H.
  $$a = ae \in aH,\ a = ea \in Ha$$
  This gives that any left or right cosets of H in G is not-empty.
- Since $He = H = eH$, hence H itself is right is well as left cosets.
- If the group $(G, .)$ is abelian, then the right coset of H in G generated by a is defined as $aH = Ha$, $\forall a \in H$
- If the composition in G is additive, then the right coset of H in G generated by a is defined as $H + a = \{h + a : h \in H\}$

4.8.1 INDEX OF A SUBGROUP IN A GROUP

If H is a subgroup of a group G, then number of distinct right (or left) cosets of H in G is called index of H in G and is denoted by $[G : H]$ or by $i_G(H) = o(G)/o(H)$

4.8.2 RELATION OF CONGRUENCE MODULO A SUBGROUP IN A GROUP

Let H be a subgroup of a group G and $a, b \in G$ be arbitrary, we define

$$a \equiv b \bmod H \text{ iff } \quad ab^{-1} \in H.$$

The symbol $a \equiv b \pmod H$ is read as a is congruent to b modulo H.

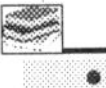

- $a \equiv b \pmod{H}$ *iff* $ab^{-1} \in H$ or $Ha = Hb$.
- $a \in Hb \Leftrightarrow ab^{-1} \in H \Leftrightarrow Ha = Hb$

THEOREM 1. *Let $a \in G$ be arbitrary and let H be a subgroup of a group G. Then $Ha = H = aH \Leftrightarrow a \in H$*

PROOF. Let H be a subgroup of G and let $a \in G$ be arbitrary.

Step I. To show that

$$Ha = H \Leftrightarrow a \in H.$$

Let us first suppose $Ha = H$. To show $a \in H$.

$$e \in H, a \in H \Rightarrow ea \in Ha \Rightarrow a \in Ha$$

$\Rightarrow$ $a \in H$. For $H = Ha$.

Now, let $a \in H$. To show $Ha = H$.

Let $xa \in H a$ $\Rightarrow x \in H$
$\Rightarrow x \in H,\ a \in H$, *for* $a \in H$
$\Rightarrow xa \in H$ ($\because$ H is a subgroup)

Thus, any $xa \in Ha$ $\Rightarrow xa \in H$.

This prove that $Ha \subset H$. ...(1)

$a \in H \Rightarrow a^{-1} \in H$. ($\because$ H is a subgroup)

For any $y \in H, a^{-1} \in H \Rightarrow ya^{-1} \in H$.
$\Rightarrow (ya^{-1})a \in Ha$.
$\Rightarrow y \in Ha$ for $ya^{-1}a = ye = y$

Thus any $y \in H$ $\Rightarrow y \in Ha$
$\Rightarrow H \subset Ha$ ...(2)

Now from (1) and (2) we get $H = Ha$.

Step II. To show $aH = H \Leftrightarrow a \in H$.

We can prove step II by making the parallel arguments as in step I.

THEOREM 2. *If a and b are arbitrary distinct elements of a group G and H is any subgroup of G, then*

$$Ha = Hb \Leftrightarrow ab^{-1} \in H$$
$$Ha = Hb \Leftrightarrow b^{-1}a \in H$$

PROOF. Let a and b be arbitrary elements of a group G such that $a \neq b$

Let e be the identity of G. Firstly, we shall show that

$$Ha = Hb \Rightarrow ab^{-1} \in H$$
$$Ha = Hb \Rightarrow (Ha)b^{-1} = (Hb)b^{-1}$$

$\Rightarrow \quad H(ab^{-1}) = H(bb^{-1}) = He = H$

$\Rightarrow \quad H(ab^{-1}) = H \Rightarrow (ab^{-1}) \in H$ (By previous theorem)

Conversely $\quad ab^{-1} \in H \Rightarrow H(ab^{-1}) = H$

$\Rightarrow \quad H(ab^{-1})(b) = Hb \Rightarrow (Ha)(b^{-1}b) = Hb$

$\Rightarrow \quad (Ha)\, e = Hb \Rightarrow Ha = Hb$

Therefore , we have

$$Ha = Hb \Leftrightarrow ab^{-1} \in H$$

THEOREM 3. *Any two left cosets of a subgroup are either disjoint or identical.*

PROOF. Let aH and bH be any two left cosets of H. To show if aH and bH have an element in common *i.e.*, If $aH \cap bH$ is not the empty set, then they are identical, *i.e.*, $aH = bH$. Let $aH \cap bH \neq \phi$ and let c be any element of $aH \cap bH$ then there exist element $h_1, h_2 \in H$ such that $c = ah_1$ and $c = bh_2$, it follows that

$$ah_1 = bh_2 \text{ so } a = bh_2(h_1)^{-1} \quad ...(1)$$

Now, let ah be any element of aH. Then

$$ah = bh_2\,(h_1)^{-1}\,h$$

Now, since H is a subgroup, $h_2(h_1)^{-1}h \in H$ and so $ah \in bH$.

This shows that every $ah \in aH$ is also is also in bH. Therefore $aH \subseteq bH$.

Similary, we can show that $bH \subseteq aH$.

Therefore, we have

$$aH = bH.$$

Hence, we have shown that any left cosets which are not disjoint are identical.

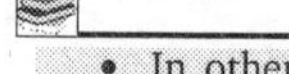

- In other words, we can state this theorem as "Any two left (right) cosets either concide or have no element in common. In symbols.

  either $\quad aH = bH$ or $aH \cap bH = \Phi$

  similarly, either $\quad Ha = Hb$ or $Ha \cap Hb = \Phi$

THEOREM 4. *There exists a one-one correspondence between a subgroup H of G and a left coset aH of H in G.*

PROOF. Consider a map $f : H \rightarrow aH$, defined by

$f(h) = ah$ for every $h \in H$.

The mapping f is clearly onto on aH, because for each $ah \in aH$ there exists $h \in H$ such that $\quad f(h) = ah$.

Now, let $h_1, h_2 \in H$ such that $f(h_1) = f(h_2)$, *i.e.*, $ah_1 = ah_2$

$\Rightarrow \quad h_1 = h_2$

$\Rightarrow \quad f$ is one-one.

Thus, f maps H such that f is one-one and onto.

Hence, there is one-to-one correspondence between H and aH.

THEOREM 5. **(Lagrange's Theorem)** *Th[illegible] order of each subgroup of a finite group is a divisor (factor) of the group.*

PROOF. Let H be a subgroup of a finite group G and let

$$o(G) = n \text{ and } o(H) = m$$

To show m is a divisor of n.

For this we have to show tha $n = mp$ for some $p \in \mathbf{N}$.

Let Ha be any right coset of H in G.

Then $\quad o(Ha) = m \quad \Rightarrow \quad \exists m$ distinct elements $h_1, h_2, ..., h_m \in H$

$\Rightarrow \quad \exists m$ distinct elements $h_1a, h_2a, ..., h_ma \in Ha$. For any map from H into Ha is one-one onto, we have

$$o(Ha) = m = o(H), a \in G.$$

$\Rightarrow$ Every right coset of H in G has m distinct elements.

Since, G finite and therefore, number of distinct right cosets of H in G will be finite say p. Also, any two right cosets of H in G will be either identical or disjoint. Hence, p disjoint right cosets of H in G will contains mp distinct elements.

$\therefore \quad G = H \cup Ha \cup Hb \cup Hc \cup ...$ where a, b, c ... p times $= mp$

$$o(G) = o(H) + o(Ha) + o(Hb) + ... = m + m + ... + p \text{ times} = mp$$

Hence, order of the subgroup of a finite group is a divisor of the group.

- The converse of the Lagrange's theorem is not true, *i.e.*, if G is a finte group of order n and m is any divisor of n then it is not necessary that G must have a subgroup of order m.

  For example: Consider the symmetric group P_4 of permutation of degree 4. Then $o(P_4) = 4! = 24$. Let A_4 be the alternating group of even permutation of degree 4. Then $o(A_4) = 24/2 = 12$. There exists no subgroup H of A_4 such that $o(H) = 6$, though 6 is a divisor of 12.
- The Lagrange's theorem has important applications in group theory. If G is a group of order 8, then there will not exist subgroups of G of order 3, 5, 6, 7. The only subgroup of G may be of order 2 and 4. Since, 2 and 4 are divisors of 8.

THEOREM 6. *The order of every element of a finite group G is a divisor of the order of the group, i.e.,* $o(a) | o(G)$.

PROOF. Let G be a finite group of order n and let $a \in G$ be arbitrary, such that $o(a) = m$.

To show m is a divisor of n.

Define $\quad H = \{a^p : p \in \mathbf{Z}\}$

$$o(a) = m$$

$\Rightarrow \quad m$ is the least positive integer such that $a^m = e$.

$$H = \{..., a^{-2}, a^{-1}, a^0, a^1, a^2, ..., a^m = e\}$$

Let $\quad x, y \in H \quad \Rightarrow \exists, p, q \in \mathbf{Z}$ such that

$\Rightarrow \quad xy^{-1} = a^{p-q} = a^r$ where $p - q = r \in \mathbf{Z}$

$\Rightarrow \quad xy^{-1} = a^r \in H$

$\Rightarrow \quad H$ is a subgroup of G.

Now, to show $\quad o(H) = m, \quad$ *i.e.*, H contains m distinct elements.

$$a, a^2, a^3, ..., a^m = e = a^0$$

Let $r, s \in \mathbf{Z}^+$ such that $s > 0$, $1 \le r \le m$, $1 \le s \le m$

Now, $\quad a^r = a^s \Rightarrow \quad a^{r-s} = e \quad \Rightarrow \quad o(a) \le r - s < m \quad \Rightarrow \quad o(a) < m$

which is a contradiction

$\therefore \quad a^r \ne a^s$ if $r \ne s$

$\Rightarrow \quad a, a^2, a^3, ..., a^m$ are distinct elements of H.

$\Rightarrow \quad o(H) = m = o(a)$

Then, by Lagrange's theorem, we have m is a divisor of n.

Hence, $o(a)$ is a divisor of $o(G)$.

THEOREM 7. *Let G be a finite group of order n and* $a \in G$ *then* $a^n = e$.

PROOF. Let G be a finite group of order n and let $a \in G$ be an element of order m so that $a^m = e$.

to show $a^n = e$. Let $H = \{a^p : p \in \mathbf{Z}\}$.
Then, by previous theorem, H is a subgroup of order m.
Using Lagrange's theorem, we have m is a divisor of n.
$\Rightarrow \quad \exists\, p \in \mathbf{N}$ such that $n/m = p \Rightarrow n = mp$
Now, $a^n = a^{mp} = (a^m)^p = (e)^p = e \Rightarrow a^n = e$

THEOREM 8. **(Fermat's Theorem).** *If a is any integer and p is prime, then* $a^p \equiv a \pmod p$

PROOF. If $a \neq 0$. Let G be a multiplicative group of residue classes modulo p, then G contains $(p-1)$ distinct elements namely

$$[1], [2], ..., [p-1]$$

$$\Rightarrow \quad o(G) = p-1 \text{ and } [e] = 1$$

Then, we have $[a^{p-1}] = [1] \Rightarrow a^{p-1} \equiv 1 \pmod p$
Now, since p is prime, hence, $a^{p-1}a \equiv 1.\, a \pmod p \Rightarrow a^p \equiv a \pmod p$.

4.8.3 EULER'S Φ FUNCTION

For any positive integer n, the Euler's Φ function is defined as follows :

$$\Phi(1) = 1$$

and for $n > 1$, $\Phi(n)$ = The number of positive integers less than n and relatively prime to n.

For example:

$\Phi(6) = 2$, since the positive integer less than 6 and relatively prime to 6 are 5 and 1 and their number is 2.

THEOREM 9. **(Euler's Theorem)** *If n is positive integer and a is any integer relatively prime to n, then* $a^{\Phi(n)} \equiv 1 \pmod n$

PROOF. Let us suppose $[X]$ denote the residue class of the set of integer mod n, for any integer n.
Now we have, the residue classes G is group of order $\Phi(n)$ with identity element, residue class $[1]$.
Now, we have

$$[a] \in G \Rightarrow [a]^{o(G)} = [1] \quad \Rightarrow [a]^{\Phi(n)} = [1]$$
$$\Rightarrow [a][a] \ldots \text{ up to } \Phi(n) \text{ times} = [1]$$
$$\Rightarrow [a \cdot a \ldots \text{ up to } \Phi(n) \text{ times}] = [1]$$
$$\Rightarrow [a^{\Phi(n)}] = [1] \quad \Rightarrow a^{\Phi(n)} \equiv 1 \pmod n$$

THEOREM 10. *Let H and K be finite subgroup of a group G, then* $o(HK) = \dfrac{o(H)\,o(K)}{o(H \cap K)}$.

PROOF. Let G be group and H and K be two subgroup of G. Then $H \cap K$ is a subset of K also. Let $D = H \cap K$, then D is a subgroup of G and $D \subseteq K$. Therefore D is a subgroup of K also. Since, K is finite therefore the number of distinct right cosets is finite. Let it be n. Then by Lagrange's theorem, we have $n = \dfrac{o(K)}{o(D)}$ ...(1)

Let $Dk_1, Dk_2, ..., Dk_n$ are some distinct right cosets of D in K, then elements in K can be written as $K = Dk_1 \cup Dk_2 \cup \ldots \cup Dk_n = \bigcup_{i=1}^{n} Dk_i$

We should see that $k_1, k_2, ..., k_n$ are some distinct elements in K.

Then, $K = Dk_1 \cup Dk_2 \cup \ldots \cup Dk_n = \bigcup_{i=1}^{n} Dk_i \qquad (\because D \subseteq H \Rightarrow HD = D)$

$$= Hk_1 \cup Hk_2 \cup \ldots \cup Hk_n$$

Now, we shall prove that the cosets $Hk_1, Hk_2, ..., Hk_n$ are pairwise distinct, we have

$$HK_i = Kk_j \Rightarrow k_i k_j^{-1} \in H \qquad (\because k_i k_j \in K \Rightarrow k_i k_j^{-1} \in K)$$

$$\Rightarrow \quad k_i k_j^{-1} \in H \cap K$$

$\Rightarrow \quad k_i k_j^{-1} \in D \quad \Rightarrow \quad Dk_i = Dk_j$

$\Rightarrow \quad k_i = k_j$ ($\because Dk_i, ..., Dk_j$ are distinct cosets)

Therefore, $Hk_1, Hk_2, ..., Hk_n$ are distinct right cosets and therefore they are pairwise distinct elements. Also, number of element in each of them in equal to o(H), *i.e.*, the number of elements in H. Now from (1).

The number of elements in $HK = n \times o(H)$

$$\Rightarrow \quad o(HK) = n \times o(H) = \frac{o(K)}{o(D)} \cdot o(H) = \frac{o(K)o(H)}{o(H \cap K)}$$

THEOREM 11. **(Cayley's Theorem)** *Every finite group G is isomorphic to a permutation group.*

PROOF. Let $a \in G$. Define a map $f_a : G \to G$ given by

$$f_a(x) = ax \; \forall \; x \in G.$$

f_a is one-one.

Let $f_a(x_1) = f_a(x_2) : x_1, x_2 \in G$

$\Rightarrow \quad ax_1 = ax_2 \quad \Rightarrow \quad x_1 = x_2.$

f_a is onto.

$f_a : G \to G$ is one-one and G is finite, therefore f is onto. Thus, f_a is one-one map of a finite set G onto itself. It means that f_a is a permutation of degree n.

Here $f_a = \begin{pmatrix} a_1 & a_2 & \cdots & a_n \\ aa_1 & aa_2 & \cdots & aa_n \end{pmatrix}$

The elements $aa_1, aa_2, ..., aa_n$ *are* all distinct elements of G.

Write $G' = \{f_a : a \in G\}$ then G' is a set of permutations of degree n.

Now, we claim that (G', .) is a group, where (.) denotes permutations multiplications.

Let $a, b, c \in G$ be arbitrary and e be the identity in G.

Let a^{-1} denote inverse of a in G so that $a^{-1}a = aa^{-1} = e$.

(i) Closure property : $f_a, f_b \in G' \Rightarrow f_a f_b \in G'$

Consider $(f_a f_b)(x) = f_a[f_b(x)] = f_a(bx)$

$= a(bx) = (ab)x,$ (By associativity in G)

$= f_{ab}(x)$

$\Rightarrow \quad f_a f_b = f_{ab}$ ...(1)

$a, b \in G \quad \Rightarrow f_{ab} \in G' \quad \Rightarrow \quad f_a f_b \in G'.$

(ii) Associativity : Let $a, b, c \in G$

$\Rightarrow \quad (ab)c = a(bc) \quad \Rightarrow f_{a(bc)}$

$\Rightarrow \quad f_{(ab)} f_c = f_a f_{bc} \Rightarrow \quad (f_a f_b) f_c = f_a (f_b f_c).$

(iii) Existence of identity : $a, e \in G \Rightarrow f_e \in G'$ and $ae = ea = a$

$\Rightarrow \quad f_{ae} = f_{ea} = f_a \quad \Rightarrow \quad f_a f_e = f_e f_a = f_a$

$\Rightarrow \quad f_e \in G'$ is identity element of G'.

(iv) Existence of inverse : $a \in G \Rightarrow a, a^{-1} \in G \Rightarrow f_a, f_a^{-1} \in G'$.

Also, $aa^{-1} = a^{-1}a = e$

$f_{aa^{-1}} = f_{a^{-1}a} = f_e$ or $f_a f_a^{-1} = f_a^{-1} f_a = f_e$

$\Rightarrow \quad f_a^{-1} \in G'$ is the inverse of $f_a \in G$.

(v) Order of G' : For $o(G) = n$, $G = \{f_a : a \in G\} \Rightarrow o(G') = n$.

Therefore, we have (G', .) is a finite group of order n.

Now we claim that $(G', .) \cong (G', .)$.

Now define a map $g : G \to G'$ such that $g(x) = f_x, \forall \; x \in G$

(i) g is one-one : For $g(x_1) = g(x_2)$; $x_1, x_2 \in G$

$\Rightarrow \quad f_{x_1} = f_{x_2}$

$\Rightarrow \quad f_{x_1}(x) = f_{x_2}(x) \; \forall \; x \in G$

$\Rightarrow \quad x_1 x = x_2 x$

$\Rightarrow \quad x_1 = x_2$

(ii) g is onto : For any $f_a \in G' \Rightarrow a \in G$ such that $g(a) = f_a$.

(iii) g preserves composition in G and G' :

For $\quad g(x_1x_2) = f_{x_1x_2}$ (where $x_1, x_2 \in G \Rightarrow x_1x_2 \in G$)

Hence, G is an isomorphism of G onto G and hence $G \cong G'$.

- Cayley's theorem can also be stated as "Any finite group is isomorphic to a transformation group" or Any finite group of order n is isomorphic to a subgroup of the symmetric group s_n.
- Cayley's theorem holds, even if G is not finite. In this case the word permutation should not exist in the statement of the theorem. In that case we state as "Every group is isomorphic to a group of one-one onto function."

4.8.4 REGULAR PERMUTATION GROUP

The permutation group to which G is isomorphic is called a regular permutation group.

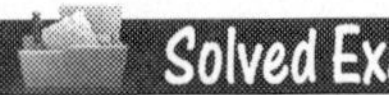

Solved Examples

1. *If G is group and $a \in G$, then show that the set $H = \{a^n : n \in \mathbf{Z}\}$ is a subgroup of G and it is the smallest subgroup of G which contains the element a.*

SOLUTION. Clearly, H is non-empty subset of G.

Let $x, y \in H$, then $x = a^p, y = a^q$, where $p, q \in \mathbf{Z}$

Thereore, xy^{-1} $(a^p)(a^q)^{-1} = a^p a^{-q}$

$= a^{p-q} \in H$

$\Rightarrow H$ is a non-empty subset of G and $x, y \in H \Rightarrow xy^{-1} \in H$. Therefore, H is a subgroup of G.

Now, if K is any subgroup of G which contain a, then by closure property in K, $a^n \in K$ for every integer n. Also every integral power of a belong to K, *i.e.*, $H \subseteq K$. Hence, H is the smallest subgroup of G which contain a.

- If G is a group $a \in G$, then the subgroup $H = \{a^n : n \in \mathbf{Z}\}$ is called the subgroup of G, generated by a.

2. *Prove that those elements of a group G which commute with the square of a given elements b of G form a subgroup of G.*

SOLUTION. Let $H = \{x \in G : xb^2 = b^2x\}$

Since, $b^2 \in G$ and $eb^2 = b^2e$, so $e \in H \Rightarrow H$ is a non-empty subset of G.

Let $x_1, x_2 \in H$ so that $x_1b^2 = b^2x_1$ and $x_2b^2 = b^2x_2$

Now, $(x_1x_2)b^2 = x_1(x_2b^2)$ (by associativity)

$= x_1(b^2x_2) \quad (\because x_2b^2 = b^2x_2)$

$= (b^2x_1)x_2 = b^2(x_1x_2) \quad (\because x_1b^2 = b^2x_1)$

$\Rightarrow x_1, x_2 \in H \Rightarrow x_1 \cdot x_2 \in H \quad ...(1)$

Also, $x_1 \in H \Rightarrow x_1b^2 = b^2x_1$

$\Rightarrow x_1^{-1}(x_1b^2)x_1^{-1} = x_1^{-1}(b^2x_1)x_1^{-1}$

$\Rightarrow (x_1^{-1}x_1)(b^2x_1^{-1}) = (x_1^{-1}b^2)(x_1x_1^{-1})$

$\Rightarrow \quad e(b^2x_1^{-1}) = (x_1^{-1}b^2)e$

$\Rightarrow \quad b^2x_1^{-1} = x_1^{-1}b^2$

Thus, $\quad x_1 \in H \Rightarrow x_1^{-1} \in H \quad ...(2)$

Hence, from (1) and (2), we conclude that H is a subgroup of G.

3. *If H is a subgroup of group G and $T = \{x \in G : xH = Hx\}$, show that T is a subgroup of G.*

SOLUTION. Since $e \in G$ and $eH = He \Rightarrow e \in T$

$\Rightarrow \quad T$ is a non-empty subset of G.

Let $x_1, x_2 \in T$ so that $x_1H = Hx_1$, $x_2H = Hx_2$

Now, $x_2 \in T \Rightarrow \quad x_2H = Hx_2$

$\Rightarrow x_2^{-1}(x_2H)x_2^{-1} = x_2^{-1}(Hx_2)x_2^{-1}$

$\Rightarrow x_2^{-1}x_2(Hx_2^{-1}) = (x_2^{-1}H)(x_2x_2^{-1})$

$\Rightarrow \quad e(Hx_2^{-1}) = (x_2^{-1}H)e$

$\Rightarrow \quad Hx_2^{-1} = x_2^{-1}H$

$\Rightarrow \quad x_2^{-1} \in T$

Thus, $\quad x_2T \Rightarrow x_2^{-1} \in T$

Also, $(x_1x_2^{-1})H = x_1(x_2^{-1}H)$

$= x_1(Hx_2^{-1}) = (x_1H)x_2^{-1} = (Hx_1)x_2^{-1}$

$= H(x_1x_2^{-1})$

$\Rightarrow \quad x_1x_2^{-1} \in T.$

Thus, T is a non-empty subset of G and $x_1, x_2 \in T \Rightarrow x_1x_2^{-1} \in T$. Hence, T is a subgroup of G.

4. *Find the regular permutation group isomorphic to the multiplicative group* $G = \{1, -1, i, -i\}$.

SOLUTION. We know by Cayley's theorem that the regular permutation group G' isomorphic to G consist the following four permutations.

$$f_1 = \begin{pmatrix} 1 & -1 & i & -i \\ 1\cdot 1 & 1\cdot(-1) & 1\cdot i & (1)\cdot(-\text{i}) \end{pmatrix}$$

$$= \begin{pmatrix} 1 & -1 & i & -i \\ 1 & -1 & i & -i \end{pmatrix} = I$$

$$f_2 = \begin{pmatrix} 1 & -1 & i & -i \\ (-1)\cdot 1 & (-1)\cdot(-1) & (-1)\cdot i & (-1)\cdot(-i) \end{pmatrix}$$

$$= \begin{pmatrix} 1 & -1 & i & -i \\ -1 & 1 & -i & i \end{pmatrix} = (1,-1),(i,-i)$$

$$f_3 = \begin{pmatrix} 1 & -1 & i & -i \\ i\cdot 1 & i\cdot(-1) & 1\cdot i & i\cdot(-i) \end{pmatrix}$$

$$= \begin{pmatrix} 1 & -1 & i & -i \\ i & -1 & i & 1 \end{pmatrix} = (1,i,-1,-i)$$

$$f_4 = \begin{pmatrix} 1 & -1 & i & -i \\ (-i)\cdot 1 & (-i)\cdot(-1) & (-i)\cdot i & (-i)\cdot(-i) \end{pmatrix}$$

$$= \begin{pmatrix} 1 & -1 & i & -i \\ -i & i & 1 & -1 \end{pmatrix} = (1,-i,-1,i)$$

Exercise-4.3

1. Let G be the additive group of integers. Then show that the set of all multiples of integers by a mixed integer m is a subgroup of G.
2. Show that the integral multiples of 5 form a subgroup of the additive group of integers.
3. Show that the 24 permutations on 4 symbols form a group with respect to permutation multiplication.
4. Use Lagrange's theorem to show that any group of prime order can have no proper subgroups.
5. Find the regular permutation group isomorphic to the group $\{1, \omega, \omega^2\}$ with respect to multiplication.
6. If a finite group G contains an element of even order, show that G must also be of even order.
7. If a finite group possesses an element of order 2, show that it possesses an odd number of such elements.
8. If $H \subseteq K$ are two subgroups of a finite group G, prove that $[G : H] = [G : K][K : H]$.
9. Show that the set of inverses of the elements of a right coset is a left coset.
10. Show that the intersection of two subgroups, each of finite index, is again of finite index.

4.9 RING

Definition. *Let R be a non-empty set. An algebraic structure (R, +, .) together with two binary operations addition and multiplication is called a ring if this structure satisfies following properties:*

(a) Addition Axioms

(i) Closed under addition: $a+b \in R, \forall a, b \in R$

(ii) Associative under addition: $a+(b+c) = (a+b)+c, \forall a,b,c \in R$

(iii) Existence of identity. If $0+a=a=a+0, \forall a \in R$ then 0 is an additive identity of R.

(iv) Existence of inverse. There exists an element $-a \in R$ such that

$$-a + a = 0 = a + (-a) \ \forall a \in R$$

then $-a$ is an additive inverse of a.

(v) Commutative under addition. $a+b = b + a \ \forall a, b \in R$

(b) Multiplication Axioms

(i) Closed under multiplication. $a.b \in R \ \forall a, b \in R$

(ii) Associative under multiplication. $a.(b.c) = (a.b).c \ \forall a, b, c \in R$

(iii) Distributive laws. (Distribution of '.' over '+')

$a.(b+c) = a.b+a.c \ \forall \ a, b, c \in R$ (Left distributive)

and $(b+c).a = b.a+c.a$ (Right distributive)

OR

An algebraic structure (R, +,.) is said to be a ring provided $a+b \in R$, $a.b \in R$ for all $a, b \in R$ and satisfies following properties:

(i) (R, +) is an abelian group.

(ii) Multiplication is associative.

(iii) Multiplication is distributive over addition.

4.9.1 Ring with Unity

A ring R is said to be a ring with unity if there exists the multiplicative identity, *i.e.*, $1 \in R$ such that $1.a = a = a.1, \ \forall a \in R$

4.9.2 Commutative Ring

A ring R is said to be a commutative ring if $a.b = b.a, \ \forall a, b \in R$

4.9.3 Special Classes of Rings

1. **Null ring (or zero ring).** A set R having a single element 0 with two binary operations, addition and multiplication defined by 0+0 =0 and 0.0 = 0 is called a null ring.
   We conclude that
   (i) The zero of a ring $(R, +, \cdot)$ can not have a multiplicative inverse unless R is the zero ring $(\{0\}, + \cdot)$
   (ii) The additive identity 0 and the multiplicative identity 1 of a ring $(R, +, \cdot)$ are not equal unless R is the zero ring.
2. **Ring of integers.** The set **Z** of all integers with respect to addition and multiplication forms a ring. This ring is called a ring of integers.
3. **Ring of real numbers.** The set **R** of all real numbers with two binary operations addition and multiplication forms a ring which is called a ring of real numbers.
4. **Ring of rational number.** The set **Q** of all rational numbers forms a commutative ring under addition and multiplication. This ring is called a ring of rational numbers.
5. **Ring of matrices.** The set M of all matrices of order $n \times n$ whose element as integers, real, complex number forms a non-commutative ring with unit element with respect to matrix addition and matrix multiplication, is called a ring of matrices.

4.10 ELEMENTARY PROPERTIES OF A RING

For all a, b, c in a ring R, we have the following property:

(1) $a0 = 0a = 0$

(2) $a(-b) = -(ab) = (-a)b$

(3) $(-a)(-b) = ab$

(4) $a(b-c) = ab - ac$

(5) $(b-c)a = ba - ca$

4.11 RING WITH AND WITHOUT ZERO DIVISORS

4.11.1 Zero Divisors

By elementary property of a ring we know that if 0 is an additive identity in R (a ring), then $a0 = 0 = 0a, \ \forall a \in R$. But in some rings it is possible that $ab = 0$ when neither $a = 0$ nor $b = 0$. Such type of elements a and b are called zero divisors.

4.11.2 Ring with Zero Divisors

A ring R is said to be ring with zero divisor if there exist non-zero elements a, b in R such that $ab = 0$, that is, if $a \neq 0$, $b \neq 0$ but $ab = 0$.

For example:

The set M of all matrices of order 2×2 having their elements as integers forms a ring with zero divisors under addition and multiplication of matrices, that is,

$$A = \begin{bmatrix} 1 & 1 \\ 1 & 1 \end{bmatrix}, B = \begin{bmatrix} -1 & -1 \\ 1 & 1 \end{bmatrix}, O = \begin{bmatrix} 0 & 0 \\ 0 & 0 \end{bmatrix}, \text{ then } AB = 0 \text{ but } A \neq 0 \text{ and } B \neq 0.$$

4.11.3 Ring without Zero Divisors

A ring R is said to be ring without zero divisor if $ab=0$, then either $a=0$ or $b=0$.

For Example

The ring of integers is a ring without zero divisors.

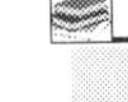

- Even though the existence of multiplicative inverses implies the absence of zero divisors, the absence of zero divisors does not guarantee the existence of multiplicative inverses, *i.e.*, in a ring, zero divisors and multiplicative inverses for all the elements (non-zero) cannot exist together.

4.12 CANCELLATION LAWS IN A RING

Let R be a ring and $a, b, c \in R$. For $a \neq 0$, if $ab = ac$ implies $b = c$, and for $a \neq 0$, if $ba = ca$ implies $b = c$. Then first is known as left cancellation law while second is known as right cancellation law.

THEOREM 1. *A ring R is without zero divisors if and only if the cancellation laws holds in R.*

PROOF. Let us first suppose that the ring R is without zero divisors, then we have to show that the cancellation laws hold in R.

Let $a \in R$ and $a \neq 0$ and we have

$$ab = ac$$

$\Rightarrow$ $ab - ac = 0$

$\Rightarrow$ $a(b - c) = 0$ (By left distributive law)

$\Rightarrow$ $b - c = 0$ ($\because$ R is of without zero divisor.)

$\Rightarrow$ $b = c$

Similarly, $ba = ca$

$\Rightarrow$ $ba - ca = 0$

$\Rightarrow$ $(b - c)\, a = 0$ (By left distributive law)

$\Rightarrow$ $b - c = 0$ ($\because$ R is of without zero divisor.)

$\Rightarrow$ $b = c$

Conversely, suppose cancellation laws hold in R, then we have to show that R is without zero divisor. Let us assume R is with zero divisor, that is

$$ab = 0, \text{ with } a \neq 0, b \neq 0$$

$\therefore$ $ab = a0$ ($\because$ $a0 = 0$)

$\Rightarrow$ $b = 0$ (By left cancellation law and $a \neq 0$)

Which is a contradiction.

Similarly, let is take $ba = 0$

$\therefore$ $ba = 0a$

$\Rightarrow$ $b = 0$ (By right cancellation law)

This gives again contradiction. Hence R is without zero divisors.

4.13 FIELD, INTEGRAL DOMAIN AND SKEW FIELD

4.13.1 Integral Domain

A commutative ring R with unit element having no zero divisors is called an integral domain.

For Example :

1. The ring of integers (**Z**, +,.) is an integral domain.
2. Let $S = \{a+b\sqrt{2} : a, b \in \mathbf{R}\}$ then (S, +, .) is an integral domain.

4.13.2 FIELD

A commutative ring R with unit element having at least two elements is called a field if every non-zero element of R possesses multiplicative inverse.

For Example

1. The ring of rational numbers (**Q**, '+', '.') is a field.
2. Let $S = (\{0, 1,2,3,4\}, +_5, \times_5)$, then S is a finite field.

- An element is a multiplicative inverse of b if $ab = 1 = ba$ for all $a \neq 0$, $b \neq 0$ in R.

4.13.3 SKEW FIELD

A ring R with unit element having at least two elements is called a skew field if every non-zero elements of R possesses their multiplicative inverse. The skew field is also known as division ring.

- We can define the field as a **commutative division ring.**
- Every field is also a divisor ring.
- Every integral domain satisfies the cancellation laws.
- Every division ring satisfies the cancellation laws.
- If R is a ring with a unity and without zero divisors, then the only solutions of $a^2 = a$, $a \in R$ are 0 and 1.
- A ring satisfies the left (right) cancellation law iff it has no left (right) divisors of zero.
- Every ring satisfies the cancellation laws with respect to addition, when we use the phrase 'the ring R satisfies the cancellation laws', we are referring to the fact that the ring R satisfies the cancellation laws with respect to multiplication.
- You must be cautious while applying the cancellation laws in a ring $ab = ac \Rightarrow b = c$ only when $a = 0$. Compare this situation with that in R, where division by a is allowed only when $a \neq 0$.

THEOREM 1. *Every field is an integral domain.*

PROOF. Let F be a field. We have to show that F is an integral domain. Since F is a field so it is commutative ring with unit element. Therefore in order to show F to be an integral domain, we only have to show that F has no zero divisors.

Let $a \in F$ and $a \neq 0$, then a^{-1} exists in F. We have $ab = 0$

$\Rightarrow \quad a^{-1}(ab) = a^{-1}0$

$\Rightarrow \quad (a^{-1}a)b = a^{-1}0$ (By associative law)

$\Rightarrow \quad 1b = a^{-1}0$ ($\because a^{-1}a = 1$)

$\Rightarrow \quad 1b = 0$ (By elementary property of ring)

$\Rightarrow \quad b = 0$ ($\because 1.a = a = a.1$)

Similarly, let $b \in F$ and $b \neq 0$

$ab = 0$

$\Rightarrow \quad (ab)b^{-1} = 0b^{-1}$

$\Rightarrow \quad a(bb^{-1}) = 0$ (By associative law and $0b^{-1} = 0 = b^{-1}0$)

$\Rightarrow \quad a1 = 0$ ($\because bb^{-1} = 1$)

$\Rightarrow \quad a = 0$ ($\because a.1 = a = 1.a$)

Thus we obained that in F, $ab = 0$, then either $a = 0$ or $b = 0$ which implies F is without zero divisors. Hence F is an integral domain.

THEOREM 2. *Disprove that every integral domain is a filed.*

PROOF. To disprove that every integral domain is a field we shall give an example. We know that the ring of integers is an integral domain but it is not field, because if $a \in \mathbf{Z}$ and $a \neq 0$, then $a^{-1} \notin \mathbf{Z}$.

THEOREM 3. *A field has no zero divisors.*

PROOF. Since field is a commutative ring with unit element in which every non-zero element possesses its multiplicative inverse. Let $a \in F$ and $a \neq 0$ (a field), then a^{-1} exists in F, is also non-zero. Let us assume

$$a^{-1} = 0$$

$\Rightarrow$ $$aa^{-1} = a0$$

$\Rightarrow$ $$1 = 0$$

This gives a contradiction. $(\because aa^{-1} = 1, a0 = 0)$

Thus $a^{-1} \neq 0$ and $aa^{-1} = 1 \neq 0$

Therefore in a field F, product of two non-zero elements is again a non-zero element. Hence F has no zero divisors.

- A skew-field has no zero divisors.

THEOREM 4. *Every finite integral domain is a field.*

PROOF. Let D be a finite integral domain. Therefore by the definition of integral domain we have that D is a commutative ring with unit element having no zero divisors. Let $D = \{a_1, a_2, ..., a_n\}$. In order to show that D is a field we only have to show that D has multiplicative inverse for every non-zero element in D. For this purpose let $a \neq 0$ be any arbitrary element of D and consider the set

$$D_1 = \{aa_1, aa_2, ..., aa_n\}$$

D_1 has n distinct products. For this let us suppose $aa_i = aa_j$ for $i \neq j$

$\Rightarrow$ $$a(a_i - a_j) = 0$$ (By left distributive law)

Since D has no zero divisors and $a \neq 0$, then

$$a_i - a_j = 0 \quad \text{for } i \neq j$$

$\Rightarrow$ $$a_i = a_j \quad \text{for } i \neq j$$

$\Rightarrow$ This is a contradiction, because D has n distinct elements $a_1, a_2, ..., a_n$.

Consequently D_1 has n distinct products. But the elements of D_1 are the elements of D placed in some order. Further D has unit element, that is ,

$$1 \in D \Rightarrow 1 \in D_1.$$

This implies that there exists an element b in D such that $ab = 1$.

But D is commutative. Therefore $ab = 1 = ba$.

Thus a^{-1} exists in D. Hence D is a field.

THEOREM 5. *A finite commutative ring without zero divisors is a field.*

PROOF. Let R be a finite commutative ring without zero divisor. We have to show that R is a field. In order to show R is a field, we only have to show that R has unit element and every non-zero element of R has its multiplicative inverse. Since R is a finite set so let us assume

$$R = \{a_1, a_2, ..., a_n\}$$

has n distinct elements. Let $a \neq 0$ be any non-zero arbitrary element of R. Then consider the set

$$R_1 = \{aa_1, aa_2, ..., aa_n\}$$

This set R_1 will have n distinct products.

Let if possible, $aa_i = aa_j$ for $i \neq j$

$\Rightarrow$ $$aa_i - aa_j = 0$$

$\Rightarrow$ $$a(a_i - a_j) = 0$$ (By left distributive law)

Since R has no zero divisors and $a \neq 0$, then

$$a_i - a_j = 0 \quad \text{for } i \neq j \qquad \text{or} \qquad a_i = a_j \quad \text{for } i \neq j.$$

This is a contradiction, because R has distinct elements. Consequently R_1 has n distinct product and these n products are the elements of R which are placed in some order. Since $a \in R$ and $a \neq 0$, so we have

$$aa_k = a \text{ for some } k$$

or $$aa_k = a.1 \qquad (\because a.1 = a)$$

$\Rightarrow$ $$a(a_k - 1) = 0$$

$\Rightarrow$ $$a_k = 1 \qquad (\because R \text{ is without zero divisor.})$$

Thus there exists an element $1 \in R$. Now we have to show that this element 1 is a multiplicative identity element of R. For this purpose let a_m be any arbitrary element of R then

$$a_m = aa_r = a_r a \text{ for some } a_r \in R$$

$$1.\ a_m = 1\ .\ (aa_r) = (1.\ a)\ a_r \qquad \text{(By associative law)}$$

$$= aa_r = a_m$$

Similarly, $a_m \cdot 1 = a_m$

Thus $a_m \cdot 1 = a_m = 1.\ a_m$. Consequently 1 is a multiplicative identity of R. Therefore there exists $b \in R$ such that $ab = 1 = ba$. Hence a^{-1} exists in R and hence R is a field.

- If the coefficient of a polynomial form an integral domain, we can solve a polynomial equation in which the polynomial can be factored into linear factors in the usual fashion by setting each factor equal to zero.

Solved Examples

1. *Show that the set R = {0,1,2,3,4,5} forms a commutative ring with respect to binary operations '$+_6$' and '$\times_6$'.*

SOLUTION. First we shall prove that (R, '$+_6$') is an abelian group. Now forming a compositioin table for '$+_6$'

$+_6$	**0**	**1**	**2**	**3**	**4**	**5**
0	0	1	2	3	4	5
1	1	2	3	4	5	0
2	2	3	4	5	0	1
3	3	4	5	0	1	2
4	4	5	0	1	2	3
5	5	0	1	2	3	4

From composition table it is clear that R is closed under '$+_6$'.

Associativity. If $a, b, c \in R$, then we have to show $a +_6 (b +_6 c) = (a +_6 b) +_6 c$

$a +_6 (b +_6 c)$ = remainder when $a + (b + c)$ is divided by 6

= remainder when $(a + b) + c$ is divided by 6

$= (a +_6 b) +_6 c$

Existence of identity. Since $0 \in R$, then $0 +_6 a = a = a +_6 0$ for $a \in R$.

Thus 0 is the identity which exists in R.

Existence of inverse. From composition table it is observed that $1 +_6 5 = 0, 2 +_6 4 = 0, 3 +_6 3 = 0$. Hence inverse of every element exists in R.

Commutativity. If $a, b \in R$, then we have to show that

$a +_6 b = b +_6 a$

$a +_6 b$ = remainder when $(a+b)$ is divided by 6

= remainder when $(b+a)$ is divided by 6

$= b +_6 a$

Thus (R, '$+_6$') is an abelian group.

Next we form a composition table for '$\times_6$' as follows :

$\times_6$	**0**	**1**	**2**	**3**	**4**	**5**
0	0	0	0	0	0	0
1	0	1	2	3	4	5
2	0	2	4	0	2	4
3	0	3	0	3	0	3
4	0	4	2	0	4	2
5	0	5	4	3	2	1

From this composition table it is observed that R is closed '$\times_6$'. Also '$\times_6$' is asociative.For this we have

$a \times_6 (b \times_6 c) = (a \times_6 b) \times_6 c$, for all $a, b, c \in R$

Now $a \times_6 (b \times_6 c)$ = remainder when $a \times (b \times c)$ is divided by 6

= remainder when $(a \times b) \times c$ is divided by 6

$= (a \times_6 b) \times_6 c$

$\therefore a \times_6 (b \times_6 c) = (a \times_6 b) \times_6 c$

Distributive laws. If $a, b, c \in R$, then $a \times_6 (b \times_6 c) = (a \times_6 b) \times_6 (a \times_6 c)$ and $(b \times_6 c) \times_6 a = (b \times_6 a) +_6 (c \times_6 a)$

Now $a \times_6 (b \times_6 c)$ = remainder when $a(b+c)$ is divided by 6.

= remainder when $ab+ac$ is divided by 6.

$= (a \times_6 b) +_6 (a \times_6 c)$

Similarly, $(b \times_6 c) \times_6 a = (b \times_6 a) +_6 (c \times_6 a)$.

Commutativity. If $a, b \in R$, then $(a \times_6 b) = (b \times_6 a)$

Now $a \times_6 b$ = remainder when $a \times b$ is divided by 6.

= remainder when $b \times a$ is divided by 6.

$= b \times_6 a$

$\therefore a \times_6 b = b \times_6 a$

Hence $(R +_6, \times_6)$ is a commutative ring.

2. *If R is a ring such that $a^2 = a$ for all $a \in R$ prove that*

(i) $a + a = 0, \forall a \in R$

(ii) $a + b = 0 \Rightarrow a = b$

(iii) *R is a commutative ring.*

SOLUTION. (i) Since $a \in R \Rightarrow a + a \in R$

Now $(a + a)^2 = (a + a)$ $\quad (\because a^2 = a)$

$\Rightarrow (a + a)(a + a) = a + a$

$\Rightarrow (a + a)a + (a + a)a = a + a$ (By left distributive law)

$\Rightarrow (a^2 + a^2) + (a^2 + a^2) = a + a$ (By right distributive law)

$\Rightarrow (a + a) + (a + a) = a + a$ $\quad (\because a^2 = a)$

$\Rightarrow (a + a) + (a + a) = (a + a) + 0$ $\quad (\because a + 0 = a)$

$\Rightarrow \quad a + a = 0$ (By left cancellation law)

(ii) $a + b = 0$ (given)

$\Rightarrow a + b = a + a \quad (\because a + a = 0)$

$\Rightarrow a = b$

(iii) If $a, b \in R \Rightarrow a + b \in R$

Now $(a + b)^2 = (a + b)$ $\quad (\because a^2 = a)$

$\Rightarrow (a + b)(a + b) = a + b$

$\Rightarrow (a + b)a + (a + b)b = a + b$ (By left distributive law)

$\Rightarrow a^2 + ba + ab + b^2 = a + b$ (By right distributive law)

$\Rightarrow a + ba + ab + b = a + b$ $\quad (\because a^2 = a)$

$\Rightarrow a + ba + ab = a$ (By right cancellation law)

$\Rightarrow ba + ab = 0$ (By left cancellation law)

$\Rightarrow ba = ab$ $\quad (\because a + b = 0 \Rightarrow a = b)$

Hence, R is a commutative ring.

- If $a^2 = a, \forall a \in R$ (Ring), then R is called a boolean ring.

Exercise-4.4

1. Show that the set **Q** of all rational numbers is a commutative ring with unity under addition and multiplication.
2. Show that the set **C** of all complex numbers is a commutative ring under the addition and multilpication of complex numbers.
3. Show that the set M of all matrices of order 2 ×2 forms a ring with zero divisors under the addition and multiplication of matrices. The elements of matrices being integers.
4. Let C be the set of ordered pairs (a, b) of real numbers. The addition and multiplication are defined as

$$(a, b) + (c, d) = (a+c, b+d)$$
$$(a, b).(c, d) = (ac - bd, bc + ad)$$

Prove that **C** is a field.

5. Define integral domain with respect to addition and multiplication.
6. Prove that the set of integers $R=\{0,1,2,3,4\}$ forms a field under addition and multiplication modulo 5.
7. Prove that the set {0,1,2,} (mod 3) is a field with respect to addition and multiplication.
8. If the two binary operations * and o on the set of integer **Z** are defined as follows :

$$a * b = a + b - 1, \; aob = a+b-ab$$

Show that $(\mathbf{Z}, *, o)$ is a field.

9. Prove that the set $R=\{0,2,4,6,8\}$ (mod 10) is a ring with unity with respect to addition and multiplication.

10. Prove that a ring R is commutative if and only if $(a+b)^2 = a^2+2ab+b^2$ $a, b \in R$.

11. If R is a ring with unity element 1, then $a = -a = a(-1)$ $\forall$ $a \in R$ and $(-1)(-1) = 1$.

12. Prove that the set $I(2)$ of numbers of the form $a + \sqrt{2}\, b$, with a as integers is an integral domain with respect to addition and multiplication. Is it a field ?

13. Give an example of a ring which is not an integral domain.

14. If R is a ring satisfying all the conditions for a ring with unity with the possible exception of $a+b = b+a$, prove that the axiom of $a+b = b+a$ must hold in R that R is thus a ring.

15. Prove that the set R = $\{a+b.\ 3^{1/3} + c\ .a^{1/3};$ $a, b, c \in \mathbf{Q}\}$ is a ring under addition and multiplication.

16. Let p be a prime number. Prove the set of integers $I_p = \{0,1,2,3, ... p-1\}$ forms a field with respect to addition and multiplication modulo p.

17. In a ring R prove that

(i) $(a+b)^2 = a^2+ab+b^2$, $\forall$ $a, b \in R$

(ii) $-(-a) = a, a \in R$.

18. Show that the set of all matrices of the form $\begin{bmatrix} 0 & a \\ 0 & b \end{bmatrix}$ where a and b are real numbers forms a ring with respect to matrix addition and matrix multiplication. Is it a commutative ring ?

Hint to the Selected Problems

1. $\mathbf{Q} = \left\{\frac{a}{b}\ ;\ b \neq 0, a, b \in R\right\}$, then prove that ($\mathbf{Q}$, '+', '.') is a commutative ring with unity.

3. We have to prove that (M, '+', '.') is a ring with zero divisors :

(i) A, B $\in$ M, A+B $\in$ M

(ii) Matrix addition is always associative.

(iii) Since $O = \begin{bmatrix} 0 & 0 \\ 0 & 0 \end{bmatrix} \in M$ such that for A $\in$ M.

$-A + A = A + O$

$\therefore$ O is the additive identity of M.

(iv) There exists a unique matrix –A corresponding to A $\in$ M such that

$-A+A = O = A + (-A)$

(v) Matrix addition is always commutative.

(vi) Since the product of two 2×2 matrix is again a 2×2 matrix so M is closed under matrix multiplication.

(vii) Matrix multiplication is always associative.

(viii) For $A, B, C \in M$, we have A. (B+C) = A . B+A . C and (B+C) . A = B . A + C . A.

Hence, $(M$, '+', '.') forms a ring.

Also let $A = \begin{bmatrix} 0 & a \\ 0 & b \end{bmatrix}$ and $B = \begin{bmatrix} c & d \\ 0 & 0 \end{bmatrix}$

which are non-zero matrices.

But AB = O, this implies that M is of with zero divisors.

6. The composition table for $+_5$ and $\times_5$ are given by

$+_5$	0	1	2	3	4
0	0	1	2	3	4
1	1	2	3	4	0
2	2	3	4	0	1
3	3	4	0	1	2
4	4	0	1	2	3

$\times_5$	0	1	2	3	4
0	0	0	0	0	0
1	0	1	2	3	4
2	0	2	4	1	3
3	0	3	1	4	2
4	0	4	3	2	1

From above tables we can easily prove the required results.

8. We have to prove that ($\mathbf{Z}$, *, .) is a commutative ring with unit elements.

(i) Since $a * b = a+ b - 1 \in \mathbf{Z}$ so $\mathbf{Z}$ is closed under '*'.

(ii) For $a, b, c \in \mathbf{Z}$, we have

$(a * b) * c = (a+b-1) * c = a+b-1 + c-1$

$= a+b+c-2$

and $a * (b * c) = a * (b+c-1)$

$= a+b + c-1-1 = a+b+c-2$

$\therefore$ $(a * b) * c = a * (b * c), \forall\ a, b, c \in \mathbf{Z}.$

Thus '*' is associative over $\mathbf{Z}$.

(iii) Identity element for '*' is $e = 1 \in \mathbf{Z}$.

(iv) Inverse element of a is $2 - a \in \mathbf{Z}$.

(v) Also, $a * b = b * a$ $\forall\ a, b \in \mathbf{Z}$.

(vi) $a \circ b = a+b-ab \in \mathbf{Z}$ so $\mathbf{Z}$ is closed under '∘'.

(vii) Also $(a \circ b) \circ c = a \circ (b \circ c), \forall\ a, b, c \in \mathbf{Z}$.

(viii) $a \circ b = b \circ a$, $\forall\ a, b \in \mathbf{Z}$

(ix) Unit element for the operation '∘' is 0 which belongs to $\mathbf{Z}$.

Hence, ($\mathbf{Z}$, '*', '∘') is a commutative ring with unity.

12. $\mathbf{I}(\sqrt{2}) = \{a+b\sqrt{2}, a, b \in \mathbf{Z}\}$, then we have to prove that this set form an integral domain. For this first we prove that $\mathbf{I}(\sqrt{2})$ forms a commutative ring with unity, which is a similar as Hint number 8.

Let $a + b\sqrt{2}$ and $c + d\sqrt{2}$ be any two elements of $\mathbf{I}(\sqrt{2})$,

and $(a+b\sqrt{2})(c+d\sqrt{2}) = 0 + 0.\sqrt{2}$

$\Rightarrow ac+2bd = 0$ and $bc+ad = 0$

These equations are possible only when either $a = 0, b = 0$ or $c = 0, d = 0$.

Thus when $(a+b\sqrt{2})$ $(c+d\sqrt{2})=0+0.\sqrt{2}$, then either $(a+b\sqrt{2}) = 0$ or $(c+d\sqrt{2}) = 0$, this shows that $\mathbf{I}(\sqrt{2})$ is of without zero divisors. Also $\mathbf{I}(\sqrt{2})$ is not a field, because for $5+3\sqrt{2} \in \mathbf{I}(\sqrt{2})$, $\frac{1}{5+3\sqrt{2}} = \frac{5}{7} + \frac{3}{7}\sqrt{3} \notin \mathbf{I}(\sqrt{2})$. That is $5 +3\sqrt{2}$ has no multiplication inverse.

ANSWERS

12. No **18.** No

4.14 SUBRINGS : RINGS WITHIN RINGS

Definition. *Let S be any non-empty subset of a ring R. Then S is said to be a subring of R if S itself is a ring for the same operations as defined on R.*

4.14.1 IMPROPER SUBRINGS

Let R be a ring. Then {0} and R itself are the subrings of R. These subrings are called improper subrings or trivial subrings.

4.14.2 PROPER SUBRINGS

Let R be a ring. Then other subrings of R except {0} and R are called proper subrings.

For Example :

(1) The ring of rational numbers is a proper subring of the ring of real numbers.

(2) The ring of even integers is a subring of the ring of integers.

4.15 PROPERTIES OF SUBRINGS

THEOREM 1. *The necessary and sufficient condition for a non-empty subset S of a ring R to be a subring is*

(i) $a \in S, b \in S \Rightarrow a - b \in S$ *(ii) $a \in S, b \in S \Rightarrow ab \in S$*

PROOF. Suppose S is a subring of a ring R, then we have to show that S is closed under addition and multiplication.

If $b \in S \Rightarrow -b \in S$ ($\because$ S is a group under multiplication.)

$\therefore$ $a \in S, -b \in S$

$\Rightarrow$ $a + (-b) \in S$ ($\because$ S is closed under addition.)

$\Rightarrow$ $a - b \in S$

Hence, $a \in S, b \in S \Rightarrow a - b \in S$ and $a \in S, b \in S \Rightarrow ab \in S$

Conversely, suppose S is any non-empty subset of a ring R and

(i) $a \in S, b \in S \Rightarrow a - b \in S$

(ii) $a \in S, b \in S \Rightarrow ab \in S$

Then we have to show that S is a subring of R.

Now, from (i) we have

$a \in S, a \in S$

$\Rightarrow$ $a - a \in S \Rightarrow 0 \in S$.

$\therefore$ Additive identity exists in S.

Again (i) we have $0 \in S, a \in S$

$\Rightarrow$ $0 - a \in S \Rightarrow -a \in S$

$\therefore$ Additive inverse exists in S.

From (i), we have $a \in S, -b \in S$

$\Rightarrow$ $a - (-b) \in S \Rightarrow a + b \in S$

$\therefore$ S is closed under addition

and from (ii) S is closed under multiplication. Further since addition and multiplication are always associative and multiplication is distributive over addition. So, S is a ring and hence S is a subring of R.

THEOREM 2. *The necessary and sufficient condition for a non-empty subset S of a ring R to be a subring of R are*

(i) $S + (-S) = S$ *(ii)* $SS \subseteq S$

PROOF. **The conditions are necessary.** Let us suppose S is a subring of R, then we shall have to show that $S + (-S) = S$ and $SS \subseteq S$.

Let $a \in S$

$\therefore$ $a = a + 0$ (By the definition of additive identity is S)

But $a + 0 \in S + (-S)$ $(\because 0 \in -S)$

$\Rightarrow$ $a \in S + (-S)$

$\Rightarrow$ $S \subseteq S + (-S)$ ...(1)

Now, let $a + (-b)$ be any arbitrary element of $S + (-S)$, then we have

$$a + (-b) \in S + (-S) \Rightarrow a \in S, -b \in (-S)$$

$\Rightarrow$ $a \in S, b \in S$

$\Rightarrow$ $a - b \in S$ ($\because$ S is a subring.)

$\therefore$ $S + (-S) \subseteq S$

Thus, from (1) and (2), we have

$$S + (-S) = S \qquad ...(2)$$

Further, since S is a subring so that it is closed under multiplication, that is,

if $a \in S, b \in S \Rightarrow ab \in S$

But $ab \subseteq SS$

$\therefore$ $SS \subseteq S$

Hence, the necessary conditions.

Sufficient conditions. Now suppose,

(i) $S + (-S) = S$ (ii) $SS \subseteq S$

Then we shall have to show that S is subring of R. To show S to be subring, we have only to prove $a - b, ab \in S$. For this we proceed as follows :

If $a \in S, b \in S \Rightarrow a \in S, -b \in (-S)$

$\Rightarrow$ $a + (-b) \in S + (-S)$

$\Rightarrow$ $a + (-b) \in S$ $(\because S + (-S) = S)$

$\Rightarrow$ $a - b \in S$

Also, $a \in S, b \in S \Rightarrow ab \in S$

Therefore, if $a - b \in S$, $ab \in S$ then S is a subring of R.

Hence, proved the theorem.

THEOREM 3. *The intersection of two subrings is again a subring.*

PROOF. Let S_1 and S_2 be two subrings of a ring R. Then we have to show that $S_1 \cap S_2$ is a subring of R. Let $a, b \in S_1 \cap S_2 \Rightarrow a, b \in S_1$ and $a, b \in S_2$ since S_1 and S_2 are subring of R, then $a - b \in S_1$, $a - b \in S_2$ and $ab \in S_1$, $ab \in S_2$.

Therefore we have

If $a - b \in S_1$ and $a - b \in S_2$, then $a - b \in S_1 \cap S_2$

And if $ab \in S_1$ and $ab \in S_2$, then $ab \in S_1 \cap S_2$

$\therefore$ $a \in S_1 \cap S_2, \ b \in S_1 \cap S_2 \Rightarrow a - b \in S_1 \cap S_2$

and $a \in S_1 \cap S_2, b \in S_1 \cap S_2 \Rightarrow ab \in S_1 \cap S_2$

Hence $S_1 \cap S_2$ is a subring of R.

Generallisation. Further, we can also prove that arbitrary intersection of subrings of a ring are again a subring.

Let $a, b \in \bigcup_{i \in \Lambda} S_i \Rightarrow a, b \in S_i, \ \forall \ i \in \Lambda.$

Since each S_i is a subring of R so we have

$$a - b \in S_i \ \ \forall \ i \in \Lambda \text{ and } ab \in S_i, \ \ \forall \ i \in \Lambda.$$

Therefore we obtain

$$a - b \in \bigcap_{i \in \Lambda} S_i \text{ and } ab \in \bigcap_{i \in \Lambda} S_i.$$

Hence $\bigcap_{i \in \Lambda} S_i$ is a subring of R.

- The union of two subrings is a subring if one is contained in the other.

THEOREM 4. *The intersection of the collection of all the subrings containing a given subset M of a ring R is the smallest subring containing M.*

PROOF. Let $\{S_\alpha : \alpha \in \Lambda\}$ be the collection of all the subring containing a given subset M of a ring R. That is, $M \subseteq S_\alpha$ for each α. Since R is itself a subring containing M so that the collection S_α is non-empty. Further, the intersection of all subrings containing M is a subring of R containing M. Also, $\cap S_\alpha$ is a smallest subring of R containing M.

4.16 SUBFIELD : FIELD WITHIN FIELD

Definition. *Let K be a non-empty subset of a field F. Then K is a subset of F if K itself is a field under the same operations as defined on F.*

For Example

(1) The field of real numbers is a subfield of the field of complex numbers.

(2) The field of real numbers is a subfield of the field of real numbers.

4.16.1 NECESSARY AND SUFFICIENT CONDITION FOR A SUBSET TO BE SUBFIELD

THEOREM 1. *The necessary and sufficient condition for a non-empty subset K of a field F to be a subfield of F are*

(i) $a \in K, b \in K \Rightarrow a - b \in K$

(ii) $a \in K, b \in K \Rightarrow ab^{-1} \in K$

PROOF. Suppose K is a subfield of F. Then

If $b \in K \Rightarrow -b \in K$

Now $a \in K, \ -b \in K$

$\Rightarrow$ $a + (-b) \in K$ ($\because$ K is closed under addition.)

$\Rightarrow$ $a - b \in K$

and if $b \in K \Rightarrow b^{-1} \in K$ ($\because$ K is a field.)

Now $a \in K, b^{-1} \in K$

$\Rightarrow$ $ab^{-1} \in K$ ($\because$ K is closed under multiplication.)

Conversely, Suppose K is a non-empty subset of F and

(i) $a \in K, b \in K \Rightarrow a - b \in K$

(ii) $a \in K, b \in K \Rightarrow ab^{-1} \in K$

Then we have to show that K is a subfield of F. For this, we have (from (i))

$$a \in K, a \in K$$

$\Rightarrow$ $a - a \in K$

$\Rightarrow$ $0 \in K$

$\therefore$ Additive identity exists in K. Also from (i), we have

$$0 \in K, a \in K$$

$\Rightarrow$ $0 - a \in K$

$\Rightarrow \quad -a \in K$

$\therefore$ Additive inverse exists in K. Also, from (ii), we have

$$a \in K, a \in K$$

$\Rightarrow \quad aa^{-1} \in K$ (By (i))

$\Rightarrow \quad 1 \in K$

$\therefore$ Multiplicative identity exists in K. Again from (ii), we have

$$1 \in K, a \in K$$

$\Rightarrow \quad 1 \,.\, a^{-1} \in K$

$\Rightarrow \quad a^{-1} \in K$

$\therefore$ Multiplicative inverse exists in K.

Further since, addition and multiplication are always associative and commutative and also multiplication is distributive over addition. Hence, K is a field and hence K is a subfield of F.

4.17 CHARACTERISTIC OF A RING

Let R be a ring with zero element '0' and suppose there exists a positive integer n such that $na = a + a + a + \ldots + a$ *(upto n terms)*$= 0, \forall\, a \in R$. *Then the smallest such positive integer n is called the characteristic of a ring.*

If there does not exist such positive integer n such that $na = 0 \;\forall\, a \in R$ and $a \neq 0$. Then the ring R is said to be of characteristic zero or infinite.

For Example :

(1) The ring of integers is of characteristic zero and the ring of rational number is also of characteristic zero.

(2) If I_6=$\{0,1,2,3,4,5,6\}$, then the ring $\{I_6, '+_6', '\times_6'\}$ is of characteristic 6, because $6a = 0$ $\forall\, a \in I_6$.

- When we say that the characteristic of R is n, we mean that n is the least positive integer for which the relation $na = 0$ is universally true in the ring.

THEOREM 1. *The characteristic of a ring with unity is zero or $n > 0$ according as the unity element 1 regarded as a member of the additive group of the ring has the order of zero or n.*

PROOF. Let R be a ring with unity element 1 and if order of 1 is zero, it is obvious that the characteristic of the ring is zero. Let us suppose that the order of 1 is finite say n, then

$$1 + 1 + 1 + \ldots + 1 \; (n \text{ times}) = 0$$

or $\quad n \,.\, 1 = 0$ ...(1)

Let a be any non-zero element of R, then we have

$$\begin{aligned} na &= a + a + a + \ldots. + a(n \text{ times}) \\ &= 1.\, a + 1.\, a + 1 \,.\, a + \ldots + 1.a \; n \text{ times} \quad (\because R \text{ is with unity.}) \\ &= [\,1 + 1 + 1 + \ldots + 1\; (n \text{ times})] \,.\, a \\ &= (n \,.\, 1)\, a = 0 \,.\, a = 0 \quad [\text{Using (1)}] \end{aligned}$$

$\Rightarrow \quad$ order of $a \leq n$.

Hence, the characteristic of R is n.

THEOREM 2. *The characteristic of an integral domain is zero or $n > 0$ according as the order of any non-zero element of the integral domain regarded as a member of additive group of the integral domain either zero or n.*

PROOF. Let D be an integral domain and let a be any non-zero element of D.

If the order of a is zero, then obviously the characteristic of D is zero.

Suppose that the order of $n > 0$, then we have

$$na = 0. \quad \ldots(1)$$

Furthermore, suppose b is any other non-zero element of D.

Mutliplying both sides of (1) by b, we have

$$(na)b = 0.\, b$$

$\Rightarrow$ $[a + a + a + ... + a(n \text{ times})]\, b = 0$ $(\because\ 0.\, b = 0)$

$\Rightarrow$ $ab + ab + ab + ... + ab(n \text{ times})] = 0$ (By right distributive law)

$\Rightarrow$ $a[b + b + b + ... + b(n \text{ times})] = 0$ (By left distributive law)

$\Rightarrow$ $a(nb) = 0$

$\Rightarrow$ $nb = 0$ $(\because\ a \neq 0)$ ...(2)

But o$(a) = n \Rightarrow n$ is the least positive integer such that $na = 0$. Also, $n\,.\,0 = 0$.

Thus (1) and (2) implies that n is the least positive integer such that $nx = 0$, $\forall\ x \in D$.

Hence, the characteristic of D is n.

THEOREM 3. *The characteristic of an integral domain is either zero or a prime number.*

PROOF. Let D be an integral domain and let a be any non-zero element of D. If the order of a is zero, then the characteristic of D is zero.

Let us suppose that the order of a is p, then the characteristic of D is p.

Now we shall show that p is prime. Let if possible p is not prime, then

$$p = p_1 p_2 \text{ with } p_1 < p,\, p_2 < p \text{ and } p_1 \neq 1,\, p_2 \neq 1$$

Since $a \neq 0$ so that $a^2 \neq 0$ and the characteristic of D is p, then

$$p(a^2) = 0$$

$\Rightarrow$ $p_1 p_2 (a^2) = 0$ $(\because\ p = p_1 p_2)$

$\Rightarrow$ $(p_1 a)(p_2 a) = 0$

$\Rightarrow$ either $p_1 a = 0$ or $p_2 a = 0$ [$\because$ D has no zero divisor.]

$\Rightarrow$ the characteristic of D is either p_1 and p_2.

But the characteristic of D is p, which is the least positive integer, therefore neither $p_1 a = 0$ nor $p_2 a = 0$, this implies that p is a prime number.

THEOREM 4. *Each non-zero element of integral domain D, regarded as a member of the additive group D is of the same order.*

PROOF. Let a be any non-zero element of D and let $o(a) = n$ (say).

Suppose b is any other non-zero element of D and $o(a) = m$ (say).

Since $o(a) = n$

$\Rightarrow$ $na = 0$

$\Rightarrow$ $nb = 0$ $(\because\ nx = 0\ \forall\ x \in D)$

$\Rightarrow$ $o(b) \leq n$

$\therefore$ $m \leq n$ ...(1)

Also, $o(b) = m$

$\Rightarrow$ $mb = 0$

$\Rightarrow$ $a(mb) = a\,.0 = 0$

$\Rightarrow$ $a[b + b + b + ... + b(m \text{ times})] = 0$

$\Rightarrow$ $ab + ab + ab + ... + ab(m \text{ times}) = 0$

$$[a + a + a + ... + (m \text{ times})]b = 0$$

$(ma)\, b = 0$ ($b \neq 0$ and D has no zero divisor.)

$$(ma) = 0$$

$$o(a) \leq m.$$

$n \leq m.$ ...(2)

From (1) and (2), we have $m = n$

$$o(b) = o(a)$$

Also, if o(a) is zero, then $o(b)$ will also be zero.

4.18 CHARACTERISTIC OF A FIELD

Since every field is an integral domain, therefore, the characteristic of a field F is zero or $n > 0$ according as any non-zero element (in particular the unit element 1) of F is order zero or n.

In order to find the characteristic of field F, we should find the order of the unit element 1 of F when regarded as a member of the additive group of F. Thus if the order of 1 is zero, then the characteristic of F is zero and if the order of 1 is finite say n, then F is a characteristic of n.

For Example:

(1) The characteristic of the field of real number is 0.

(2) If $F = \{I_7, '+_7', '\times_7'\}$ be a field, where $I_7 = \{0,1,2,3,4,5,6\}$, then the characteristic of I_7 is 7.

4.19 ORDERED INTEGRAL DOMAIN

Definition (1). *Let $(R, +, \cdot)$ be an integral domain. This integral domain is said to be ordered if* **R** *contains a subset* $\mathbf{R}^+$ *(the set of positive elements of* **R***) such that*

(i) $\mathbf{R}^+$ is closed under addition and multiplication as define on **R**.

(ii) There is one and only one $a = 0$, $a \in \mathbf{R}^+$, $-a \in \mathbf{R}^+$ for all $a \in \mathbf{R}$ holds.

For Example

The integral domain of integers is ordered.

Definition (2). *A field F is said to be ordered if it is ordered as an integral domain.*

4.20 POLYNOMIAL RINGS

Definition. *The expression of the type*

$$f(x) = a_0 + a_1x + a_2x^2 + ... + a_nx^n,\ a_n \neq 0$$

is called a polynomial of degree n and the variable x is called indeterminate.

Definition. *Let R be a ring and x be an indeterminate which does not belong to R. Then a polynomial of the form*

$$f(x) = a_0 + a_1x + a_2x^2 + ... + a_nx^n,\ a_n \neq 0$$

where a_0, a_1, a_2,..., a_n... all are in R with finite and non-zero is called a polynomial over a ring R.

4.21 SET OF ALL POLYNOMIALS OVER A RING

Let R be a ring and x be an indeterminate, then the set of all polynomial of the form $f(x) = a_0 + a_1x + a_2x^2 + ... + a_nx^n + ...$, where a_0, a_1, a_2,..., a_n... all are in R with finite number of non-zero elements is called the set of polynomials over R and it is denoted by $R[x]$.

4.21.1 ZERO POLYNOMIAL

A polynomial over a ring R of the type

$$a_0 + a_1x + a_2x^2 + ... + a_nx^n + ...$$

is called a zero polynomial if $a_n = 0\ \forall\ n$.

4.21.2 EQUALITY, SUM AND PRODUCT OF POLYNOMIALS

(i) Equality. Let R be a ring and let

$$f(x) = a_0 + a_1x + a_2x^2 + ... \text{ and } g(x) = b_0 + b_1x + b_2x^2 + ..$$

be two polynomials over R. Then they are said to be equal if $a_n = b_n$, $\forall n$.

(ii) Sum of polynomials. Let R be a ring and x be indeterminate and let

$$f(x) = a_0 + a_1x + a_2x^2 + ... \text{ and } g(x) = b_0 + b_1x + b_2x^2 + ..$$

be two polynomials over R, *i.e.*, $f(x), g(x) \in R[x]$.

Then $$f(x) + g(x) = c_0 + c_1x + c_2x^2 + ...$$

is said to be the sum of $f(x)$ and $g(x)$ if $c_n = a_n + b_n$, $\forall\ n$.

(iii) Product of polynomials. Let R be a ring and x be an indeterminate and let $f(x)$, $g(x) \in R[x]$, where,

$$f(x) = a_0 + a_1x + a_2x^2 + ... \quad \text{and} \quad g(x) = b_0 + b_1x + b_2x^2 + ..$$

Then the polynomial $f(x). g(x) = c_0 + c_1x + c_2x^2 + ..$

is said to be the product of $f(x)$ and $g(x)$ if

$$c_n = a_0b_n + a_1b_{n-1} + a_2b_{n-2} + ... + a_nb_0$$

$$= \sum_{i+j=n} a_ib_i \text{ for all } b \text{ belongs to (set of all non-negative integers).}$$

(iv) Degree of a polynomial. Let $f(x) \in R[x]$ is of the form

$$f(x) = a_0 + a_1x + a_2x^2 + ... + a_nx^n + ...$$

Then the degree of $f(x)$ is n if and only if $a_n \neq 0$ and $a_m = 0, m > n$.

4.21.3 LEADING TERM

If a polynomial $f(x)$ is of degree n, then the term a_nx^n is called the leading term, a_n is called the leading coefficient and a_0 is called the constant term.

Solved Examples

1. *Show that the set of all matrices of order 2×2 of the form* $\begin{bmatrix} a & 0 \\ b & c \end{bmatrix}$ *where a,b,c are integers is a subring of the ring M of all matrices of order 2×2 with integral elements.*

SOLUTION. Since M is a ring of all matrices of order 2×2 and let M_1 be the set of all matrices of the type $\begin{bmatrix} a & 0 \\ b & c \end{bmatrix}$, where $a, b, c, \in Z$ (set of integers). We have to show that M_1 is a subring of M. For this purpose, let A, B be any two elements of M_1, *i.e.*,

$$A = \begin{bmatrix} a_1 & 0 \\ b_1 & c_1 \end{bmatrix}, B = \begin{bmatrix} a_2 & 0 \\ b_2 & c_2 \end{bmatrix},$$

$a_1, b_1, c_1, a_2, b_2, c_2 \in \mathbf{Z}$

Then, we have

$$A - B = \begin{bmatrix} a_1 - a_2 & 0 \\ b_1 - b_2 & c_1 - c_2 \end{bmatrix}$$

since $a_1 - a_2$, $b_1 - b_2$, $c_1 - c_2$, are all in $\mathbf{Z}$. Thus $A - B \in \mathbf{M}_1$. Also, we have

$$AB = \begin{bmatrix} a_1 & 0 \\ b_1 & c_1 \end{bmatrix}\begin{bmatrix} a_2 & 0 \\ b_2 & c_2 \end{bmatrix}$$

$$= \begin{bmatrix} a_1a_2 & 0 \\ b_1a_2 + c_1b_2 & c_1c_2 \end{bmatrix}$$

It is the type of $\begin{bmatrix} a & 0 \\ b & c \end{bmatrix}$.

$\therefore$ AB $\in$ M

Hence M_1 is a subring of M.

2. *Let R be a ring of integer and let S = {mx:x∈**Z**}, m being a fixed integer. Show that S is a subring of R.*

SOLUTION. Let $a, b \in S$. Then

$a = mx$ (For some $x \in \mathbf{Z}$)

and $b = my$ (For some $y \in \mathbf{Z}$)

Now $a - b = mx - my = m(x - y)$

$\therefore$ $a - b \in S$ $(x - y \in \mathbf{Z})$

Now $ab = (mx)(my) = m(mxy)$

$\therefore$ $ab \in S$ $(\because mxy \in \mathbf{Z})$

Hence S is subring of R.

3. *Add and multiply the following polynomials over ring* $(I_5, +_5, \times_5,)$.

$f(x) = 3+4x+2x^2,$

$g(x) = 1+3x+4x^2+2x^3.$

SOLUTION. We have $f(x)+g(x)$

$= 3+4x+2x^2+ 1+3x+4x^2+2x^3$

$= 4 +7x+6x^2+2x^3$

$= 4 +2x+x^2+2x^3$

$[\because 7 \equiv 2(\text{mod } 5), 6 \equiv 1(\text{mod } 5)]$

and $f(x)g(x)$

$= (3+4x+2x^2)(1+3x+4x^2+2x^3)$

$= 3+13x+26x^2+28x^3+16x^4+4x^5$

$= 3+3x+x^2+3x^3+x^4+4x^5$

$[\because 13 \equiv 3(\text{mod } 5), 28 \equiv 3(\text{mod } 5), 16 \equiv 1(\text{mod } 5)]$

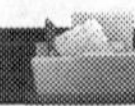

Exercise-4.5

1. Show that the set of matrices of the form $\begin{bmatrix} a & b \\ 0 & c \end{bmatrix}$ is a subring of the ring of all matrices of order 2×2 with integral elements.
2. Let M be the ring of 2×2 matrices with real elements. Show that the set of matrices of the type $\begin{bmatrix} 0 & a \\ 0 & b \end{bmatrix}$ with real elements is a subring of R.
3. Show that the set of even integers forms a subring of the ring of integers.
4. If $(R, +, .)$ is a ring, show that the set $Z(R) = \{c \in R : xy = yx, \forall y \in R\}$ is a subring of R.
5. Give an example to show that the union of two subrings is not necessarily a subring.
6. If D is an integral domain, then the polynomial ring $D[x]$ is also an integeral domain.
7. The set of integers is a subring of the ring of rational numbers.
8. Let x, y be commutative elements of a ring R of characteristic 2, show that
$$(x+y)^2 = x^2+y^2 = (x-y)^2.$$
9. Let **R** be a non-zero ring such that for all $x \in R$, $x^2 = x$. Prove that R is a commutative ring of characteristic 2.

Hints to the Selected Problems

1. Let $M = \left\{\begin{bmatrix} a & b \\ 0 & c \end{bmatrix} : a, b \in \mathbf{Z}\right\}$ then we have to prove that M is a subring of the ring of all matrices of order 2×2 with integral elements.

   Let $A = \begin{bmatrix} a_1 & b_1 \\ 0 & c_1 \end{bmatrix}, B = \begin{bmatrix} a_2 & b_2 \\ 0 & c_2 \end{bmatrix}$ be any two elements of M. Now $A - B = \begin{bmatrix} a_1 - a_2 & b_1 - b_2 \\ 0 & c_1 - c_2 \end{bmatrix}$ as $a_1 - a_2$, $b_1 - b_2$ and $c_1 - c_2$ are the integers. Similarly $AB \in$ M.

   Hence M is a subring.
3. Let $E = \{2x : x \in \mathbf{Z}\}$, then we have to prove that E form a subring of ring integers.

   For a_1, $b_1 \in E$, *i.e.*, $a_1 = 2x$, $b_1 = 2y$ for x, $y \in \mathbf{Z}$.

   $a_1 - b_1 = 2x - 2y = 2(x-y) \in E$ as $x - y \in \mathbf{Z}$.

   Also $a_1 b_1 = (2x)(2y) = 2(2xy) \in E$ as $2xy \in \mathbf{Z}$.

   Hence E forms a subring.
5. Let $(\mathbf{Z}, +, .)$ be a ring of integers and let $R_1 = 2\mathbf{Z}$, $R_2 = 3\mathbf{Z}$, then $R_1 \cup R_2$ is not a subring. But if $R_3 = 4\mathbf{Z}$, then $R_1 \cup R_3$ is a subring.
8. Since characteristic $(R) = 2$, *i.e.*, $1+1 = 0$ or $2 = 0$. Then for $x, y \in R$

   $(x+y)^2 = (x+y)(x+y) = (x+y)x + (x+y)y = x^2+yx+xy+y^2 = x^2+2xy+y^2$

   But $2 \simeq 0$. $\therefore$ $(x+y)^2 = x^2 + y^2$, similarly $(x-y)^2 = x^2 + y^2$.

❑❑❑❑❑❑

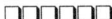

Chapter

5 Limit, Continuity and Differentiability

5.1 INTRODUCTION

Consider the following example: $\frac{1}{3} = 0.\overline{3} = 0.33333...$

We know that exact value of 0.3333... is not $\frac{1}{3}$. But as we increased the digit 3 in 0.3333... the difference between $\frac{1}{3}$ and 0.3333... will decrease. Then we say that $\frac{1}{3}$ is the limiting value of 0.3333.

Consider another example of an infinite G.P. given by

$$1+\frac{1}{2}+\frac{1}{2^2}+\frac{1}{2^3}+\frac{1}{2^4}+...\infty$$

First term of the series = 1

Sum of first two terms of this series $= 1+\frac{1}{2} = \frac{3}{2} = 1.5$

Sum of first three terms of this series $= 1+\frac{1}{2}+\frac{1}{2^2} = 1.75$

Sum of first four terms of this series $= 1+\frac{1}{2}+\frac{1}{2^2}+\frac{1}{2^3} = 1.875$

Sum of first five terms of this series $= 1+\frac{1}{2}+\frac{1}{2^2}+\frac{1}{2^3}+\frac{1}{2^4} = 1.9375$

It is very clear from above that as we increased the number of terms of this series, the sum will approaches to 2. We may decrease the difference between the sum of the series and 2 as small as we please, but the sum of the series may not be equal to 2, whatever be the number of terms we sum. Hence, we conclude that the value of a function may not be obtained but value of the function for the approximate value of the variable may be known, then such value of the function is known as limit of the function.

5.2 SOME IMPORTANT EXPLANATIONS

(i) Meaning of $x \to 0$, *i.e.*, x tends to 0

Let x be a real variable which takes the values as required. The meaning of $x \to 0$ is that x is very close to 0 but it is never equal to zero.

(ii) Meaning of $x \to \infty$, *i.e.*, x tends to ∞

The meaning of $x \to \infty$ is that

(i) x is larger than any number however large

(ii) x is not a fixed number

(iii) Meaning of $x \to a$, *i.e.*, x tends to a

By $x \to a$ we mean that x assumes successively values (either less than or greater than a) whose numerical difference from a can be made as small as we please. Here x is very close to a but not equal to a. *i.e.*, $x \to a$ implies that

(i) $x \neq a$

(ii) x assumes values nearer and nearer to a

- In the above definition x tends to a either from left or from right.

5.3 DEFINED AND UNDEFINED FUNCTIONS

(i) Defined function. Let $y = f(x)$ be a function. Putting $x = a$ in $f(x)$ to get $f(a)$. If $f(a)$ is a finite quantity, then we say that $f(x)$ is a defined function at $x = a$.

For example. Let $f(x) = 2x^3 + 5x^2 - 9x + 7$

Then value of $f(x)$ at $x = 2$, *i.e.*,

$$f(2) = 2(2)^3 + 5(2)^2 - 9 \times 2 + 7$$
$$= 16 + 20 - 18 + 7 = 25$$

$\Rightarrow f(2) = 25$, which is a finite quantity. Hence, the given function $f(x)$ is a defined function at $x = 2$.

(ii) Undefined function: A function $y = f(x)$ is said to be undefined function at a point $x = a$ if we get any one of the following indeterminate form $\frac{0}{0}, \infty \times \infty, \infty - \infty \ldots$ when we substitute $x = a$ in $f(x)$.

5.4 CONCEPT OF THE LIMIT OF A FUNCTION

Let $y = f(x)$ be a given function. Suppose that for any value of $x = a$ (say) if the value of $f(x)$, *i.e.*, $f(a)$ becomes infinite or undefined then we compute the limiting value of f(x) which is very nearer to the actual value of $f(x)$. This limiting value of the function is called limit of the function. [KANPUR(BCA)–2001, 08, 14; MEERUT(BCA)–2005, 07, 17]

5.5 LIMIT OF THE FUNCTION

Let $y = f(x)$ be a function. The value of x approaches to a quantity a after increasing from left or decreasing from right. As the value of the function will tends to a finite quantity A, then this finite quantity A is called the limit of the function.

O	$x < a$ → approaches from left	$x = a$	← $x > a$ approaches from right

Fig. 1

Symbolically it can be written as $\lim_{x \to a} f(x) = A$.

5.6 RESULTS RELATED TO LIMITS

Some results related to 'limits' are given below:

If $\lim_{x \to a} f(x) = A$ and $\lim_{x \to a} \phi(x) = B$, then

(i) $\lim_{x \to a} [f(x) \pm \phi(x)] = \lim_{x \to a} f(x) \pm \lim_{x \to a} \phi(x) = A \pm B$

(ii) $\lim_{x \to a} [kf(x)] = k \lim_{x \to a} f(x) = k \cdot A$

(iii) $\lim_{x\to a}[f(x)\cdot\phi(x)] = \lim_{x\to a} f(x)\cdot \lim_{x\to a}\phi(x) = A\cdot B$

(iv) $\lim_{x\to a}\dfrac{f(x)}{\phi(x)} = \dfrac{\lim_{x\to a} f(x)}{\lim_{x\to a}\phi(x)} = \dfrac{A}{B}$; if $B \neq 0$ (v) $\lim_{x\to a} f(x) = \lim_{h\to 0} f(a+h)$

5.7 METHOD OF FINDING THE LIMIT OF A FUNCTION

To find the limit of the function we have to calculate left hand limit (LHL) and right hand limit (RHL) of the function.

Case-I. To find the limit of rational function $f(x) = \dfrac{\phi(x)}{\psi(x)}$

(i) If at $x = a$, $\phi(a) = 0$ and $\psi(a) = 0$, then function is of the form $\dfrac{0}{0}$. In such cases use the following working steps to calculate the limit of function.

WORKING PROCEDURE

STEP 1. Factorize numerator and denominator by assuming $x \neq a$.
STEP 2. Cancel the common factors from numerator and denominator.
STEP 3. Substitute $x = a$ in the function obtained in step-2.

- If limit is of the form $\lim_{x\to a}\dfrac{f(x)}{g(x)} = \dfrac{0}{0}$, then we have, $\lim_{x\to a}\dfrac{f(x)}{g(x)} = \lim_{x\to a}\dfrac{f'(x)}{g'(x)}$ (L-Hospital Rule)

Solved Examples

1. *Find the value of* $\lim_{x\to a}\dfrac{x^3-a^3}{x-a}$

SOLUTION. We have,

$$\lim_{x\to a}\frac{x^3-a^3}{x-a}$$

$$= \lim_{x\to a}\frac{(x-a)(x^2+ax+a^2)}{(x-a)} \quad (\text{If } x \neq a)$$

$$= \lim_{x\to a}(x^2+ax+a^2)$$

$= a^2 + a\cdot a + a^2$ (Putting $x = a$)

$= 3a^2$

Aliter: We have to calculate

$$\lim_{x\to a}\frac{(x^3-a^3)}{x-a}$$

Let $x = a + h$ when $x = a$, then $h = 0$

$\therefore$ $x \to a \Rightarrow h \to 0$

Therefore,

$$\lim_{x\to a}\frac{x^3-a^3}{x-a}$$

$$= \lim_{h\to 0}\frac{(a+h)^3-a^3}{a+h-a}$$

$$= \lim_{h\to 0}\frac{a^3+3a^2h+3ah^2+h^3-a^3}{h}$$

$$= \lim_{h\to 0}\frac{h(3a^2+3ah+h^2)}{h}$$

$$= \lim_{h\to 0}(3a^2+3ah+h^2)$$

$= 3a^2 + 0 + 0$ (Putting $h = 0$)

$= 3a^2$

Case II. To find the limit of irrational functions

Let $f(x)$ be an irrational function, *i.e.*, $f(x) = \dfrac{\phi(x)}{\psi(x)}$, such that it becomes indefinite when $x = a$. To find the limit of such function, first rationalize the given function and then use the same method as in case I.

2. *Evaluate* $\lim\limits_{x \to 0} \dfrac{x}{\sqrt{(1+x)} - 1}$

SOLUTION. We have, $\lim\limits_{x \to 0} \dfrac{x}{\sqrt{(1+x)} - 1}$ (Form $\dfrac{0}{0}$)

Multiply numerator and denominator by the conjugate of denominator $\sqrt{1+x}+1$, we get

$$= \lim_{x \to 0} \frac{x[\sqrt{(1+x)}+1]}{[\sqrt{(1+x)}-1][\sqrt{(1+x)}+1]}$$

$$= \lim_{x \to 0} \frac{x[\sqrt{(1+x)}+1]}{(1+x)-1}$$

$$= \lim_{x \to 0} \frac{x[\sqrt{(1+x)}+1]}{x}$$

$$= \lim_{x \to 0} \sqrt{(1+x)}+1] = \sqrt{(1+0)}+1 = 2$$

3. *Prove* $\lim\limits_{x \to 0} \dfrac{(1+x)^{1/2} - (1-x)^{1/2}}{x} = 1$

SOLUTION. We have, $\lim\limits_{x \to 0} \dfrac{(1+x)^{1/2} - (1-x)^{1/2}}{x}$ (Form $\dfrac{0}{0}$)

Multiply numerator and denominator by the conjugate, *i.e.*, $[(1+x)^{1/2} + (1-x)^{1/2}]$

$$[(1+x)^{1/2} - (1-x)^{1/2}]$$

$$= \lim_{x \to 0} \frac{[(1+x)^{1/2} + (1-x)^{1/2}]}{x[(1+x)^{1/2} + (1-x)^{1/2}]}$$

$$= \lim_{x \to 0} \frac{(1+x)-(1-x)}{x[(1+x)^{1/2} + (1-x)^{1/2}]}$$

$$= \lim_{x \to 0} \frac{2x}{x[(1+x)^{1/2} + (1-x)^{1/2}]}$$

$$= \lim_{x \to 0} \frac{2}{(1+x)^{1/2} + (1-x)^{1/2}}$$

$$= \frac{2}{(1+0)^{1/2} + (1-0)^{1/2}}$$

(Putting $x = 0$)

$$= \frac{2}{2} = 1$$

Case III. If limit of the function $\to \infty$

To find the limit of such function, put $\dfrac{1}{z}$ for x and then use $z \to 0$

$[\because$ When $x \to \infty, \dfrac{1}{x} \to 0, i.e., z \to 0]$

5.7.1 LIMIT BASED ON THE EXPANSION OF THE FUNCTIONS

4. *Evaluate* $\lim\limits_{x \to 0} \left(\dfrac{e^x - e^{-x}}{x}\right)$

SOLUTION. We know that,

$$e^x = 1 + x + \frac{x^2}{2!} + \frac{x^3}{3!} + \frac{x^4}{4!} + \ldots\infty$$

and $e^{-x} = 1 - x + \dfrac{x^2}{2!} + \dfrac{x^3}{3!} + \dfrac{x^4}{4!} + \ldots\infty$

$$\therefore e^x - e^{-x} = 2\left(x + \frac{x^3}{3!} + \frac{x^5}{5!} + \ldots\infty\right)$$

$$= 2x\left(1 + \frac{x^2}{3!} + \frac{x^4}{5!} + \ldots\infty\right)$$

$$\therefore \frac{e^x - e^{-x}}{x} = 2\left[1 + \frac{x^2}{3!} + \frac{x^4}{5!} + \ldots\infty\right]$$

Therefore, $\lim\limits_{x \to 0} \dfrac{e^x - e^{-x}}{x}$

$$= \lim_{x \to 0} 2\left[1 + \frac{x^2}{3!} + \frac{x^4}{5!} + \ldots\infty\right]$$

$$= 2[1 + 0 + 0 + \ldots] = 2$$

5. *Evaluate* $\lim\limits_{x \to 0} \dfrac{(1+x)^{1/n} - 1}{x}$

SOLUTION. Using Binomial expansion, we have

$$(1+x)^n = 1 + nx + \frac{n(n-1)}{2!}x^2 + \ldots$$

Putting $\dfrac{1}{n}$ for n, we get

$$(1+x)^{1/n} = 1 + \frac{1}{n}x + \frac{\frac{1}{n}\left(\frac{1}{n}-1\right)}{2!}x^2 + \frac{\frac{1}{n}\left(\frac{1}{n}-1\right)\left(\frac{1}{n}-2\right)}{3!}x^3 + \ldots$$

$$\Rightarrow (1+x)^{1/n} - 1 = \frac{1}{n}x + \frac{\frac{1}{n}\left(\frac{1}{n}-1\right)}{2!}x^2 + \frac{\frac{1}{n}\left(\frac{1}{n}-1\right)\left(\frac{1}{n}-2\right)}{3!}x^3 + \ldots$$

$$\Rightarrow \frac{(1+x)^{1/n}-1}{x}$$

$$= \frac{1}{n}\left[1+\frac{\frac{1}{n}-1}{2!}x + \frac{\left(\frac{1}{n}-1\right)\left(\frac{1}{n}-2\right)}{3!}x^2+\ldots\right]$$

Therefore,

$$\lim_{x\to 0}\left[\frac{(1+x)^{1/n}-1}{x}\right]$$

$$= \lim_{x\to 0}\left[\frac{1}{n}\left\{1+\frac{\left(\frac{1}{n}-1\right)}{2!}x + \frac{\left(\frac{1}{n}-1\right)\left(\frac{1}{n}-2\right)}{3!}x^2+\ldots\right\}\right]$$

$$= \frac{1}{n}[1+0+0+\ldots]$$

$$\therefore \lim_{x\to 0}\frac{(1+x)^{1/n}-1}{x} = \frac{1}{n}$$

6. *Evaluate* $\lim_{x\to 1}\frac{\log x}{x-1}$

SOLUTION. Let $x = 1 + h$. If $x = 1$, then $h = 0$

Therefore, $x \to 1 \Rightarrow h \to 0$

$$\Rightarrow \lim_{x\to 1}\frac{\log x}{x-1} \Rightarrow \lim_{h\to 0}\frac{\log(1+h)}{1+h-1}$$

$$= \lim_{h\to 0}\frac{\log(1+h)}{h}$$

We know that, $\log(1+x)=x-\frac{1}{2}x^2+\frac{1}{3}x^3-\frac{1}{4}x^4+\ldots\infty$

Therefore, $\lim_{h\to 0}\frac{\log(1+h)}{h}$

$$= \lim_{h\to 0}\frac{h-\frac{1}{2}h^2+\frac{1}{3}h^3-\frac{1}{4}h^4+\ldots\infty}{h}$$

$$= \lim_{h\to 0}\frac{h\left[1-\frac{1}{2}h+\frac{1}{3}h^2-\frac{1}{4}h^3+\ldots\infty\right]}{h}$$

$$= \lim_{h\to 0}\left[1-\frac{1}{2}h+\frac{1}{3}h^2-\frac{1}{4}h^3+\ldots\infty\right]$$

$$= 1-0+0-0+\ldots$$

$$\therefore \lim_{x\to 1}\frac{\log x}{x-1} = 1$$

7. *Evaluate* $\lim_{x\to a}\frac{x^m-a^m}{x-a}$

SOLUTION. Consider $\lim_{x\to a}\frac{x^m-a^m}{x-a}$

Let $x = a + h$. If $x = a$, then $h = 0$

$\therefore \quad x \to a \Rightarrow h \to 0$

$$\therefore \lim_{x\to a}\frac{x^m-a^m}{x-a} = \lim_{h\to 0}\frac{(a+h)^m-a^m}{a+h-a}$$

$$= \lim_{h\to 0}\frac{a^m\left(1+\frac{h}{a}\right)^m-a^m}{h}$$

$$= \lim_{h\to 0}\frac{a^m}{h}\left[\left(1+\frac{h}{a}\right)^m-1\right]$$

(By Binomial theorem)

$$= \lim_{h\to 0}\frac{a^m}{h}\left[1+m\left(\frac{h}{a}\right)+\frac{m(m-1)}{2!}\left(\frac{h}{a}\right)^2+\ldots-1\right]$$

$$= \lim_{h\to 0}\frac{a^m}{h}\left[m\left(\frac{h}{a}\right)+\frac{m(m-1)}{2!}\left(\frac{h}{a}\right)^2+\ldots\right]$$

$$= \lim_{h\to 0}\frac{a^m}{h}m\left(\frac{h}{a}\right)\left[1+\frac{(m-1)}{2!}\left(\frac{h}{a}\right)+\ldots\right]$$

$$= \lim_{h\to 0} ma^{m-1}\left[1+\frac{(m-1)}{2!}\left(\frac{h}{a}\right)+\ldots\right]$$

$$= m\cdot a^{m-1}[1+0+0+\ldots] = ma^{m-1}$$

8. *Prove that* $\lim_{\theta\to 0}\frac{\sin\theta}{\theta} = 1$

SOLUTION.

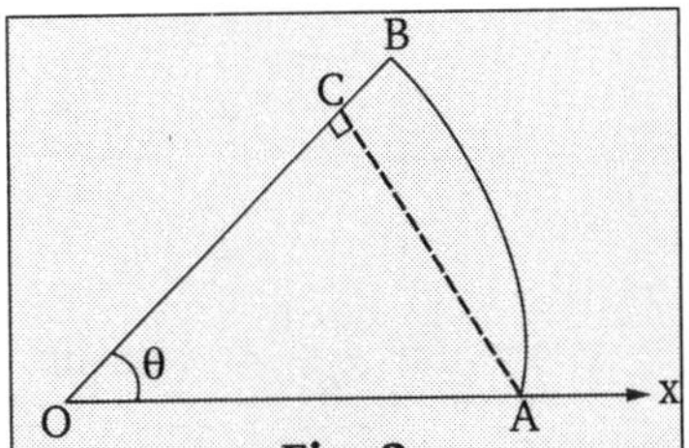

Fig. 2

Method-1 Let OA be the initial position of the imaginary axis. After rotating anticlockwise direction, it comes in the position OB when $\angle AOB = \theta$.

Draw perpendicular AC from A on OB.

$\therefore$ in ΔOAC

$$\sin\theta = \frac{AC}{OA} \text{ and } \theta = \frac{\text{Arc}}{\text{radius}} = \frac{\text{Arc } AB}{OA}$$

$$\therefore \frac{\sin\theta}{\theta} = \frac{AC}{OA} \div \frac{\text{Arc } AB}{OA}$$

$$= \frac{AC}{OA} \times \frac{OA}{\text{Arc } AB}$$

$$\therefore \frac{\sin\theta}{\theta} = \frac{AC}{\text{Arc } AB}$$

As θ decrease, the difference between AC and arc AB will decrease and at the end, they becomes equal

$$\therefore \lim_{\theta\to 0} \frac{\sin\theta}{\theta} = \lim_{\theta\to 0} \frac{AC}{AB} = \frac{AC}{AC} = 1$$

$$\therefore \lim_{\theta\to 0} \frac{\sin\theta}{\theta} = 1$$

- When imaginary line rotate in clockwise direction then θ will be negative acute angle. Let $\theta = -\alpha$ therefore,

$$\frac{\sin\theta}{\theta} = \frac{\sin(-\alpha)}{-\alpha} = \frac{-\sin\alpha}{-\alpha} = \frac{\sin\alpha}{\alpha}$$

$$\therefore \lim_{\theta\to 0} \frac{\sin\theta}{\theta} = \lim_{\alpha\to 0} \frac{\sin\alpha}{\alpha} = 1$$

Method-2 We know that (from trigonometry)

$$\sin\theta = \theta - \frac{\theta^3}{3!} + \frac{\theta^5}{5!} + \frac{\theta^7}{7!} + \ldots\infty$$

$$= \theta\left[1 - \frac{\theta^2}{3!} + \frac{\theta^4}{5!} + \frac{\theta^6}{7!} + \ldots\infty\right]$$

$$\because \frac{\sin\theta}{\theta} = 1 - \frac{\theta^2}{3!} + \frac{\theta^4}{5!} - \frac{\theta^6}{7!} + \ldots\infty$$

$$\therefore \lim_{\theta\to 0} \frac{\sin\theta}{\theta}$$

$$= \lim_{\theta\to 0}\left[1 - \frac{\theta^2}{3!} + \frac{\theta^4}{5!} - \frac{\theta^6}{7!} + \ldots\infty\right]$$

$$= 1$$

- Use the following as a formula

$$\lim_{\theta\to 0} \frac{\sin\theta}{\theta} = 1;\ \lim_{\theta\to 0} \frac{\theta}{\sin\theta} = 1;\ \lim_{\theta\to 0} \cos\theta = 1$$

9. *Evaluate* $\lim_{x\to 0} \frac{\sin ax}{\sin bx}$.

SOLUTION. We have,

$$\lim_{x\to 0} \frac{\sin ax}{\sin bx} = \lim_{x\to 0} \sin ax \lim_{x\to 0} \frac{1}{\sin bx}$$

$$= \lim_{x\to 0} \frac{\sin ax}{ax} xa. \lim_{x\to 0} \frac{bx}{bx \sin bx}$$

$$= \frac{a}{b} \lim_{x\to 0} \frac{\sin ax}{ax}. \lim_{x\to 0} \frac{bx}{\sin bx}$$

$$= \frac{a}{b}.1.1 = \frac{a}{b}$$

$$\left(\because \lim_{\theta\to 0} \frac{\sin\theta}{\theta} = 1 \text{ and } \lim_{\theta\to 0} \frac{\theta}{\sin\theta} = 1\right)$$

10. *Prove that* $\lim_{x\to 0} \frac{\tan x - \sin x}{x^3} = \frac{1}{2}$.

SOLUTION. We have, $\lim_{x\to 0} \frac{\tan x - \sin x}{x^3}$

$$= \lim_{x\to 0} \frac{\sin x - \sin x \cos x}{x^3 \cos x}$$

$$= \lim_{x\to 0} \frac{\sin x(1 - \cos x)}{x^3 \cos x}$$

$$= \lim_{x\to 0} \frac{\sin x}{x}. \lim_{x\to 0} \frac{1 - \cos x}{x^2 \cos x}$$

$$= \lim_{x\to 0} \frac{\sin x}{x} \lim_{x\to 0} \frac{1 - 1 + 2\sin^2 x/2}{x^2 \cos x}$$

$$= \lim_{x\to 0} \frac{\sin x}{x} \lim_{x\to 0} \frac{2}{4}\left(\frac{\sin x/2}{x/2}\right)^2 . \lim_{x\to 0} \frac{1}{\cos x}$$

$$= \frac{1}{2} \lim_{x\to 0} \frac{\sin x}{x} \lim_{x\to 0}\left(\frac{\sin x/2}{x/2}\right)^2 \cdot \lim_{x\to 0} \frac{1}{\cos x}$$

$$= \frac{1}{2} \times 1 \times 1 \times 1 = \frac{1}{2} \quad \left(\because \lim_{x\to 0} \frac{\sin\theta}{\theta} = 1\right)$$

11. *Evaluate* $\lim_{x\to\pi/4} \frac{\sin x - \cos x}{x - \pi/4}$.

SOLUTION. Let $x = \pi/4 + h$. If $x = \pi/4 \Rightarrow h = 0$

Therefore $x \to \frac{\pi}{4} \Rightarrow h \to 0$

$$\therefore \lim_{x\to\pi/4} \frac{\sin x - \cos x}{x - \pi/4}$$

$$= \lim_{h\to 0} \frac{\sin(\pi/4 + h) - \cos((\pi/4 + h)}{\frac{\pi}{4} + h - \frac{\pi}{4}}$$

$$= \lim_{h\to 0} \frac{(\sin\pi/4\cos h + \cos\pi/4\sin h) - (\cos\pi/4\cos h - \sin\pi/4\sin h)}{h}$$

$$= \lim_{h\to 0} \frac{1}{\sqrt{2}} \frac{(\cos h + \sin h - \cos h + \sin h)}{h}$$

$$\left(\cos\pi/4 = \sin\pi/4 = \frac{1}{\sqrt{2}}\right)$$

$$= \frac{1}{\sqrt{2}} \lim_{h\to 0} \frac{2\sin h}{h} = \sqrt{2} \lim_{h\to 0} \frac{\sin h}{h}$$

$$= \sqrt{2} \times 1 = \sqrt{2} \qquad \left(\because \lim_{h\to 0} \frac{\sin h}{h} = 1\right)$$

12. *Evaluate* $\lim_{x\to\infty} x \sin\frac{1}{x}$

SOLUTION. $\lim_{x\to\infty} x\sin\frac{1}{x} = \lim_{x\to\infty} \frac{\sin(1/x)}{1/x}$.

Let $\frac{1}{x} = \theta$. Therefore, if $x = \infty$ then $\theta = 0$

$\therefore \quad x \to \infty \Rightarrow \theta \to 0$

$$\therefore \quad \lim_{x\to\infty} \frac{\sin 1/x}{(1/x)} = \lim_{\theta\to 0} \frac{\sin\theta}{\theta} = 1$$

Exercise-5.1

Evaluate the following limits:

1. $\lim_{x\to 0} (7x^2 - 5x + 1)$
2. $\lim_{x\to 0} (6x^3 - 5x^2 - 7x + 8)$
3. $\lim_{x\to 0} \frac{\cos x}{x+1}$
4. $\lim_{x\to 1} \frac{x^2 - 1}{x - 1}$
5. $\lim_{x\to -2} \frac{x^3 + 8}{x + 2}$
6. $\lim_{x\to 0} \frac{e^x - 1}{e^x}$
7. $\lim_{x\to 0} \frac{3e^x - 3}{x}$
8. $\lim_{x\to 0} \frac{a^x - 1}{x}, a > 0$
9. $\lim_{x\to 0} \frac{\log\left(1 - \frac{x}{2}\right)}{x}$
10. $\lim_{x\to 0} \frac{1 - \cos x}{x^2}$
11. $\lim_{x\to 0} \frac{x}{\sqrt{2+x} - \sqrt{2}}$
12. $\lim_{\theta\to 0} \frac{\sin(\theta/4)}{\theta}$
13. $\lim_{x\to 0} \frac{\log(1+x)}{x}$
14. $\lim_{x\to\infty} \cos\log\left(\frac{x-1}{x}\right)$
15. $\lim_{x\to 0} \frac{\cos x}{x+2}$
16. $\lim_{x\to 0} \frac{\sin x}{x+5}$
17. $\lim_{x\to\infty} \frac{1^2 + 2^2 + 3^2 + \ldots + n^2}{n^3}$
18. $\lim_{x\to\pi/2} (\sec x - \tan x)$

Prove the following:

19. $\lim_{x\to\infty} \frac{9x^2 + 3x + 7}{5x^2 + 2x + 1} = \frac{9}{5}$
20. $\lim_{x\to 0} \frac{\log_e(1+x) - x}{x^2} = \frac{-1}{2}$
21. $\lim_{x\to 1} \frac{(2x-3)(\sqrt{x} - 1)}{(2x^2 + x - 3)} = \frac{-1}{10}$
22. $\lim_{x\to 1} \frac{x - 1}{2x^2 - 7x + 5} = -\frac{1}{3}$
23. $\lim_{x\to 0} \frac{\sqrt[3]{(1+x)} - 1}{x} = \frac{1}{3}$
24. $\lim_{x\to a} \frac{x^m - a^m}{x^n - a^n} = \frac{m}{n} a^{m-n}$ if $(m > n)$
25. $\lim_{x\to\infty} \left(1 + \frac{a}{x}\right)^x = e^a$
26. $\lim_{x\to\infty} \left[\frac{\sin x}{x}\right] = 0$
27. $\lim_{n\to\infty} \frac{1 + 2 + 3 + 4 + \ldots + n}{n^2} = \frac{1}{2}$
28. $\lim_{x\to 1} \frac{\sqrt{(4+x)} - \sqrt{5}}{x - 1} = \frac{\sqrt{5}}{10}$
29. $\lim_{x\to 0} \left[\frac{1 - \cos mx}{1 - \cos nx}\right] = \frac{m^2}{n^2}$
30. $\lim_{x\to 0} \left[\frac{a^x + a^{-x} - 2}{a^x - a^{-x}}\right] = 0$
31. $\lim_{x\to 0} \frac{a^x - b^x}{x} = \log_e\left(\frac{a}{b}\right)$

32. $\lim_{x\to 2} \frac{\sqrt{(3-x)}-1}{2-x} = \frac{1}{2}$

33. $\lim_{\theta\to 0}\left(\frac{\sin\theta}{\sin\theta/2}\right) = 2$

34. (i) $\lim_{x\to\infty}\left[\left(1+\frac{1}{x}\right)^x\right] = e$

(ii) $\lim_{x\to 0}(1+x)^{1/x} = \frac{5}{2}$

35. If $f(x) = \frac{x^2}{1+x^2}$, prove that $\lim_{x\to\infty} f(x) = 1$.

36. Prove that $\lim_{\theta\to\pi/2} \frac{2\cos\theta}{\pi - 2\theta} = 1$

37. Prove that $\lim_{x\to\infty}\left(1+\frac{2}{x}\right)^x = e^2$

38. Prove that $\lim_{x\to 0}\frac{\tan x^\circ}{x} = \frac{\pi}{180}$

39. Prove that $\lim_{n\to\infty}\left(\frac{1^2}{n^3}+\frac{2^2}{n^3}+\frac{3^2}{n^3}+\ldots+\frac{n^2}{n^3}\right) = \frac{1}{3}$

40. Prove that $\lim_{x\to 0}\frac{\sin^{-1} x}{x} = 1$.

ANSWERS

1. 1 **2.** 8 **3.** 1 **4.** 2 **5.** 12 **6.** 0 **7.** 3 **8.** $\log_e a$ **9.** $\frac{-1}{2}$

10. $\frac{1}{2}$ **11.** $2\sqrt{2}$ **12.** $\frac{1}{4}$ **13.** 1 **14.** 1 **15.** $\frac{1}{2}$ **16.** 0 **17.** $\frac{1}{3}$ **18.** 0

5.8 RIGHT AND LEFT HAND LIMIT OF A FUNCTION

Let $f(x)$ be a function defined in some interval I containing a point a but may or may not be defined at a itself. Consider the behaviour of $f(x)$ as $x \to a$. It may happen that the values of f become closer and closer to a number l as $x \to a$. Therefore, there are two methods by which x tends to a. As a result, there are two types of limits.

1. **Left hand limit:** A function $f(x)$ is said to approaches the limit l as x approaches from the left, if corresponding to an arbitrary positive number ε there exists a positive number $\delta > 0$ such that

$$|f(x) - l| < \varepsilon \text{ whenever } |x - a| < \delta$$

It is written as $\lim_{x\to a^-} f(x)$ or $f(a-0)$

Therefore $$f(a-0) = \lim_{x\to a^-} f(x)$$

WORKING PROCEDURE

- To find the limit from left, put $a - h$ for x in $f(x)$ and then take limit as $h \to 0$ *i.e.,* $\lim_{x\to a-0} f(x) = \lim_{x\to a^-} f(x) = \lim_{h\to 0} f(a-h)$

2. **Right hand limit:** A function f is said to approaches the limit l as x approaches a from the right, if corresponding to an arbitrary positive number ε there exists a positive number $\delta > 0$ such that

$$|f(x) - l| < \varepsilon \text{ whenever } |x - a| < \delta$$

We say that right hand limit of $f(x)$ as x tends to a exists and is equal to l if as x approaches a, always remaining greater than a, the value of $f(x)$ approaches a definite unique real number l.

It is written as $\lim_{x\to a^+} f(x)$ or $f(a+0)$

Therefore $$f(a+0) = \lim_{x\to a^+} f(x)$$

WORKING PROCEDURE

- To find the limit from right, put $a + h$ for x in $f(x)$ and then take limit as $h \to 0$ *i.e.*, $\lim_{x\to a+0} f(x) = \lim_{h\to 0} f(a+h) = f(a+0)$

5.9 EXISTENCE OF THE LIMIT OF A FUNCTION

Let $y = f(x)$ be a function defined in an interval I. Let $a \in I$. The limit of $f(x)$ at $x = a$ exists if

right hand limit of $f(x)$ = left hand limit of $f(x)$

i.e., $$\lim_{x\to a^-} f(x) = \lim_{x\to a^+} f(x)$$

or $$f(a - 0) = f(a + 0)$$

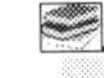

- It is clear from above that limit of a function is unique.

Solved Examples

1. *Find right hand and left hand limits of the function* $f(x) = \dfrac{2}{5+x}$ *at* $x = 2$.

SOLUTION. **Left hand limit**

$$f(x) = \frac{2}{5+x}$$

Let $x = 2 - h$

$\therefore$ when $x = 2$, $h = 0$

$\therefore$ $x \to 2 \Rightarrow h \to 0$

$$\therefore \lim_{x\to 2^-} f(x) = \lim_{h\to 0} f(2-h)$$
$$= \lim_{h\to 0} \frac{2}{5+(2-h)} = \lim_{h\to 0} \frac{2}{7-h}$$
$$= \frac{2}{7-0} = \frac{2}{7}$$
$$\therefore \quad f(2-0) = \frac{2}{7}$$

Right hand limit

$$f(x) = \frac{2}{5+x}$$

Let $x = 2 + h$

when $x = 2$, $h = 0$

$\therefore$ $x \to 2 \Rightarrow h \to 0$

$$\therefore \lim_{x\to 2^+} f(x) = \lim_{h\to 0} f(2+h)$$
$$= \lim_{h\to 0} \frac{2}{5+(2+h)} = \lim_{h\to 0} \frac{2}{7+h}$$
$$= \frac{2}{7+0} = \frac{2}{7}$$
$$\therefore \quad f(2+0) = \frac{2}{7}$$

2. *Show that right hand and left hand limits of the function* $\dfrac{\log x}{x-1}$, *when* $x \to 1$ *are equal to* 1.

SOLUTION. **Left hand limit**

$$f(x) = \frac{\log x}{x-1}$$

Let $x = 1 - h$ therefore, if $x = 1$ then $h = 0$ so $x \to 1 \Rightarrow h \to 0$

$$\therefore \lim_{x\to 1} f(x) = \lim_{h\to 0} f(1-h)$$
$$= \lim_{h\to 0} \frac{\log(1-h)}{1-h-1}$$
$$= \lim_{h\to 0} \frac{\log(1-h)}{-h}$$
$$= \lim_{h\to 0} \frac{-[h + \frac{1}{2}h^2 + \frac{1}{3}h^3 + \ldots\infty]}{-h}$$
$$\left[\because \log(1-x) = -[x + \frac{x^2}{2} + \frac{x^3}{3} + \ldots\infty]\right]$$
$$= \lim_{h\to 0} \frac{-h\left[1 + \frac{h}{2} + \frac{h^2}{3} + \frac{h^3}{4} + \ldots\infty\right]}{-h}$$
$$= \lim_{h\to 0} \left[1 + \frac{h}{2} + \frac{h^2}{3} + \frac{h^3}{4} + \ldots\infty\right]$$
$$= [1 + 0 + 0 + \ldots] = 1$$

∴ Therefore, left hand limit of the function = 1

Right hand limit

Let $x = 1 + h$

If $x = 1$, then $h = 0$

$$\therefore \lim_{x\to 1^+} f(x) = \lim_{h\to 0} f(1+h)$$

$$= \lim_{h\to 0} \frac{\log(1+h)}{(1+h-1)}$$

$$= \lim_{h\to 0} \frac{\log(1+h)}{h}$$

$$= \lim_{h\to 0} \frac{h - \frac{h^2}{2} + \frac{h^3}{3} - \frac{h^4}{4} + \ldots}{h}$$

$$= \lim_{h\to 0} \frac{h\left[1 - \frac{h}{2} + \frac{h^2}{3} - \frac{h^3}{4} + \ldots\infty\right]}{h}$$

$$= \lim_{h\to 0}\left[1 - \frac{h}{2} + \frac{h^2}{3} - \frac{h^3}{4} + \ldots\infty\right]$$

$$= 1 - 0 + 0 - 0 + \ldots = 1$$

∴ Right hand limit of the function = 1

Hence, RHL = LHL = 1

3. *Find RHL and LHL of the function* $f(x) = x\cos\left(\frac{1}{x}\right)$ *at* $x = 0$.

SOLUTION. Given $f(x) = x\cos\left(\frac{1}{x}\right)$

Left hand limit

Let $x = 0 - h$, if $x = 0 \Rightarrow h = 0$

$$\lim_{x\to 0^-} f(x) = \lim_{h\to 0} f(0-h)$$

$$= \lim_{h\to 0} (0-h)\cos\left(\frac{1}{0-h}\right)$$

$$= \lim_{h\to 0} (-h)\cos\left(\frac{1}{-h}\right)$$

$$= \lim_{h\to 0} (-h) \lim_{h\to 0} \cos\left(-\frac{1}{h}\right)$$

$= 0 \times$ {a finite quantity lying between 1 and –1}

$= 0$

Right hand limit

Let $x = 0 + h$, if $x = 0 \Rightarrow h = 0$

Therefore, $x \to 0 \Rightarrow h \to 0$

$$\lim_{x\to 0^+} f(x) = \lim_{h\to 0} f(0+h)$$

$$= \lim_{h\to 0} (0+h)\cos\left(\frac{1}{0+h}\right)$$

$$= \lim_{h\to 0} h\cos\left(\frac{1}{h}\right)$$

$$= \lim_{h\to 0} h \times \lim_{h\to 0} \cos\left(\frac{1}{h}\right)$$

$= 0 \times$ {a finite quantity lying between 1 and –1}

$= 0$

Hence, RHL = LHL = 0

4. *Prove that RHL and LHL of the function* $\frac{1+\cos x}{\tan^2 x}$ *when* $x \to \pi$ *are equal. Hence, evaluate* $\lim_{x\to\pi} \frac{1+\cos x}{\tan^2 x}$.

SOLUTION. Given that, $f(x) = \frac{1+\cos x}{\tan^2 x}$

Right hand limit

Clearly x tends to π from right

Let $x = \pi + h$, when $x = \pi$ then $h = 0$

$$\therefore \lim_{x\to \pi^+} f(x) = \lim_{h\to 0} f(\pi+h)$$

$$= \lim_{h\to 0} \frac{1+\cos(\pi+h)}{\tan^2(\pi+h)}$$

$$= \lim_{h\to 0} \frac{1-\cos h}{\tan^2 h}$$

[∵ $\cos(\pi + h) = -\cos h$ and $\tan^2(\pi + h) = (\tan h)^2 = \tan^2 h$]

$$= \lim_{h\to 0} \frac{1 - \left\{1 - \frac{h^2}{2!} + \frac{h^4}{4!} - \frac{h^6}{6!} + \ldots\infty\right\}}{\left(h + \frac{1}{3}h^3 + \frac{2}{15}h^5 + \ldots\infty\right)^2}$$

$$\left(\because \cos\theta = 1 - \frac{\theta^2}{2!} + \frac{\theta^4}{4!} - \frac{\theta^6}{6!} + \ldots\infty \text{ and } \tan\theta = \theta + \frac{\theta^3}{3} + \frac{2}{15}\theta^5 + \ldots\infty\right)$$

$$= \lim_{h\to 0} \frac{h^2\left[\frac{1}{2!} - \frac{h^2}{4!} + \ldots\infty\right]}{h^2\left[1 + \frac{h^2}{3} + \frac{2}{15}h^4 + \ldots\infty\right]^2}$$

$$= \lim_{h\to 0} \frac{\frac{1}{2!} - \frac{h^2}{4!} + \ldots\infty}{\left(1 + \frac{h^2}{3} + \frac{2}{15}h^4 + \ldots\infty\right)^2}$$

$$= \frac{\frac{1}{2!} - 0 + 0 - 0 + \ldots}{(1+0+0+\ldots)^2} = \frac{1}{2!} = \frac{1}{2}$$

Left hand limit

In this case, x tends to π from left

Let $x = \pi - h$, when $x = \pi$ then $h = 0$

$$\therefore \lim_{x\to\pi^-} f(x) = \lim_{h\to 0} f(\pi - h)$$

$$= \lim_{h\to 0} \frac{1+\cos(\pi - h)}{\tan^2(\pi - h)}$$

$$= \lim_{h\to 0} \frac{1-\cos h}{\tan^2 h}$$

$$= \lim_{h\to 0} \frac{1 - \left\{1 - \frac{h^2}{2!} + \frac{h^4}{4!} - \frac{h^6}{6!} + \ldots\infty\right\}}{\left(h + \frac{h^3}{3} + \frac{2}{15}h^5 + \ldots\infty\right)^2}$$

$$= \lim_{h\to 0} \frac{h^2\left[\frac{1}{2!} - \frac{h^2}{4!} + \ldots\infty\right]}{h^2\left(1 + \frac{h^2}{3} + \frac{2}{15}h^4 + \ldots\infty\right)^2}$$

$$= \lim_{h\to 0} \frac{\frac{1}{2!} - \frac{h^2}{4!} + \ldots\infty}{\left(1 + \frac{h^2}{3} + \frac{2}{15}h^4 + \ldots\infty\right)}$$

$$= \frac{\frac{1}{2!} - 0 + \ldots}{(1+0+\ldots)^2} = \frac{1}{2!} = \frac{1}{2}$$

Therefore when $x \to \pi$.

RHL of $f(x)$ = LHL of $f(x)$

Hence, $\lim_{x\to\pi} \frac{1+\cos x}{\tan^2 x} = \frac{1}{2}$

Miscellaneous Examples

1. *Evaluate the following limits :*

(*i*) $\lim_{x\to 1}\left(\frac{1}{x^2-1} - \frac{2}{x^4-1}\right)$

(*ii*) $\lim_{x\to a} \frac{\sqrt{a+2x}-\sqrt{3x}}{\sqrt{3a+x}-2\sqrt{x}}, a \neq 0$

SOLUTION. (i) We have,

$$\lim_{x\to 1}\left(\frac{1}{x^2-1} - \frac{2}{x^4-1}\right)$$

$$= \lim_{x\to 1}\left(\frac{1}{(x^2-1)} - \frac{2}{(x^2-1)(x^2+1)}\right)$$

$$= \lim_{x\to 1}\left[\frac{x^2+1-2}{(x^2-1)(x^2+1)}\right]$$

$$= \lim_{x\to 1} \frac{(x^2-1)}{(x^2-1)(x^2+1)} = \lim_{x\to 1} \frac{1}{x^2+1}$$

$$= \frac{1}{1^2+1} = \frac{1}{2}$$

(ii) We have,

$$\lim_{x\to a} \frac{\sqrt{a+2x}-\sqrt{3x}}{\sqrt{3a+x}-2\sqrt{x}}, a \neq 0$$

$$= \lim_{x\to a} \frac{(\sqrt{a+2x}-\sqrt{3x})\frac{(\sqrt{a+2x}+\sqrt{3x})}{(\sqrt{a+2x}+\sqrt{3x})}}{(\sqrt{3a+x}-2\sqrt{x})\frac{(\sqrt{3a+x}+2\sqrt{x})}{(\sqrt{3a+x}+2\sqrt{x})}}$$

$$= \lim_{x\to a} \left\{\frac{\frac{a+2x-3x}{\sqrt{a+2x}+\sqrt{3x}}}{\frac{3a+x-4x}{\sqrt{3a+x}+2\sqrt{x}}}\right\}$$

$$= \lim_{x\to a} \left\{\frac{(a-x)}{\sqrt{a+2x}+\sqrt{3x}} \cdot \frac{\sqrt{3a+x}+2\sqrt{x}}{3(a-x)}\right\}$$

$$= \lim_{x\to a} \frac{\sqrt{3a+x}+2\sqrt{x}}{3(\sqrt{a+2x}+\sqrt{3x})} = \frac{\sqrt{4a}+2\sqrt{a}}{3(\sqrt{3a}+\sqrt{3a})}$$

$$= \frac{4\sqrt{a}}{3\cdot 2\sqrt{3a}} = \frac{2}{3\sqrt{3}}$$

2. *Evaluate the following limits:*

(i) $\lim_{x\to 0} \frac{\sin ax}{\tan bx}$

(ii) $\lim_{x\to 0} \frac{\operatorname{cosec} x - \cot x}{x}$

SOLUTION. (i) We have,

$$\lim_{x\to 0} \frac{\sin ax}{\tan bx} = \lim_{x\to 0} \left\{ \frac{\left(\frac{\sin ax}{ax}\right).ax}{\left(\frac{\tan bx}{bx}\right)bx} \right\}$$

$$= \lim_{x\to 0} \frac{\left(\frac{\sin ax}{ax}\right)}{\left(\frac{\tan bx}{bx}\right)}.\frac{a}{b}$$

$$= \frac{1\cdot a}{1\cdot b} = \frac{a}{b}$$

$$\left(\because \lim_{x\to 0}\frac{\sin ax}{ax} = 1, \lim_{x\to 0}\frac{\tan bx}{bx} = 1\right)$$

(ii) We have,

$$\lim_{x\to 0} \frac{\operatorname{cosec} x - \cot x}{x}$$

$$= \lim_{x\to 0} \left\{ \frac{\frac{1}{\sin x} - \frac{\cos x}{\sin x}}{x} \right\}$$

$$= \lim_{x\to 0} \frac{1-\cos x}{x\sin x}$$

$$= \lim_{x\to 0} \frac{2\sin^2\frac{x}{2}}{x\cdot 2\sin\frac{x}{2}.\cos\frac{x}{2}}$$

$$= \lim_{x\to 0} \frac{\sin\frac{x}{2}}{x\sin\frac{x}{2}}.\frac{\sin\frac{x}{2}}{\cos\frac{x}{2}}$$

$$= \lim_{x\to 0} \frac{\tan\frac{x}{2}}{x} = \lim_{x\to 0} \frac{\tan\frac{x}{2}}{2\cdot\frac{x}{2}}$$

$$= \lim_{x\to 0} \frac{1}{2}\cdot\left(\frac{\tan\frac{x}{2}}{\frac{x}{2}}\right) = \frac{1}{2}$$

3. *Evaluate* $\lim_{x\to 0}\left(\frac{\tan 2x - x}{3x - \sin x}\right)$.

SOLUTION. We have,

$$\lim_{x\to 0}\left(\frac{\tan 2x - x}{3x - \sin x}\right)$$

$$= \lim_{x\to 0} \frac{\left(\frac{\tan 2x}{2x}\right)2x - x}{3x - \left(\frac{\sin x}{x}\right).x}$$

$$= \lim_{x\to 0} \frac{\left(\frac{\tan 2x}{2x}\right)2 - 1}{3 - \frac{\sin x}{x}} = \frac{2\cdot 1 - 1}{3-1} = \frac{1}{2}$$

4. *Evaluate*

$$\lim_{x\to 0} \frac{\sin(a+b)x + \sin(a-b)x + \sin 2ax}{\cos 2bx - \cos 2ax}.x$$

SOLUTION. We have,

$$\lim_{x\to 0} \frac{\sin(a+b)x + \sin(a-b)x + \sin 2ax}{\cos 2bx - \cos 2ax}.x$$

$$= \lim_{x\to 0} \left\{ \frac{\frac{\sin(a+b)x}{(a+b)x}.(a+b)x + \frac{\sin(a-b)x}{(a-b)x}.(a-b)x + \frac{\sin 2ax}{2ax}.2ax}{\frac{2\sin(a+b)x}{(a+b)x}.(a+b)x.\ \sin\frac{(a-b)x}{(a-b)x}(a-b)x} \right\}.x$$

$$= \lim_{x\to 0} \left\{ \frac{\frac{\sin(a+b)x}{(a+b)x}.(a+b) + \frac{\sin(a-b)x}{(a-b)x}.(a-b) + \frac{\sin 2ax}{2ax}.2a}{\frac{2\sin(a+b)x}{(a+b)x}.(a+b).\frac{\sin(a-b)x}{(a-b)x}(a-b)} \right\}$$

$$= \frac{1\cdot(a+b) + 1(a-b) + 1.2a}{2\cdot 1\cdot(a+b)\cdot 1\cdot(a-b)}$$

$$= \frac{4a}{2(a^2-b^2)} = \frac{2a}{(a^2-b^2)}$$

5. *Evaluate* $\lim_{x\to 0}\frac{1-\cos x\sqrt{\cos 2x}}{x^2}$.

SOLUTION. We have, $\lim_{x\to 0}\left(\frac{1-\cos x\sqrt{\cos 2x}}{x^2}\right)$

$$= \lim_{x\to 0}\left\{\frac{1-\cos x\sqrt{\cos 2x)}\,(1+\cos x\sqrt{\cos 2x)}}{x^2(1+\cos x\sqrt{\cos 2x}}\right\}$$

$$= \lim_{x\to 0}\left(\frac{1-\cos^2 x\times\cos 2x}{x^2(1+\cos x\sqrt{\cos 2x}}\right)$$

$$= \lim_{x\to 0}\left(\frac{1-(1-\sin^2 x)(1-2\sin^2 x)}{x^2(1+\cos x\sqrt{\cos 2x})}\right)$$

$$= \lim_{x\to 0}\left(\frac{1-(1-3\sin^2 x+2\sin^4 x}{x^2(1+\cos x\sqrt{\cos 2x})}\right)$$

$$= \lim_{x\to 0}\left(\frac{\sin^2 x(3-2\sin^2 x)}{x^2(1+\cos x\sqrt{\cos 2x})}\right)$$

$$= \lim_{x\to 0}\left(\frac{\sin x}{x}\right)^2\left(\frac{3-2\sin^2 x}{1+\cos x\sqrt{\cos 2x}}\right)$$

$$= 1^2\left(\frac{3}{1+1}\right) = \frac{3}{2}$$

6. *Evaluate* $\lim_{\theta\to\frac{\pi}{2}}(\sec\theta-\tan\theta)$

SOLUTION. We have,

$$\lim_{\theta\to\frac{\pi}{2}}(\sec\theta-\tan\theta)$$

$$= \lim_{\theta\to\frac{\pi}{2}}\left(\frac{1}{\cos\theta}-\frac{\sin\theta}{\cos\theta}\right) = \lim_{\theta\to\frac{\pi}{2}}\left(\frac{1-\sin\theta}{\cos\theta}\right)$$

$$= \lim_{\theta\to\frac{\pi}{2}}\left(\frac{(1-\sin\theta)\cos\theta}{\cos^2\theta}\right)$$

$$= \lim_{\theta\to\frac{\pi}{2}}\frac{(1-\sin\theta)\cos\theta}{(1-\sin^2\theta)}$$

$$= \lim_{\theta\to\frac{\pi}{2}}\frac{\cos\theta}{1+\sin\theta} = \frac{0}{1+1} = 0$$

7. *Evaluate* $\lim_{x\to 0}\left(\frac{1-\cos x\cos 2x\cos 3x}{\sin^2 2x}\right)$.

SOLUTION. We have,

$\cos x\cos 2x\cos 3x$

$$= \frac{1}{2}(2\cos x\cos 3x\cos 2x)$$

$$= \frac{1}{2}[(\cos 2x+\cos 4x)\cos 2x]$$

$$= \frac{1}{4}[(2\cos^2 2x+2\cos 4x\cos 2x)]$$

$$= \frac{1}{4}[1+\cos 4x+\cos 2x+\cos 6x]$$

Therefore,

$$\lim_{x\to 0}\left[\frac{1-\cos x\cos 2x\cos 3x}{\sin^2 2x}\right]$$

$$= \lim_{x\to 0}\left[\frac{1-\frac{1}{4}(1+\cos 4x+\cos 2x+\cos 6x}{\sin^2 2x}\right]$$

$$= \lim_{x\to 0}\left[\frac{1-\cos 2x+1-\cos 4x+1-\cos 6x}{4\sin^2 2x}\right]$$

$$= \lim_{x\to 0}\frac{2\sin^2 x+2\sin^2 2x+2\sin^2 3x}{4\sin^2 2x}$$

$$= \lim_{x\to 0}\left\{\frac{2\left(\frac{\sin x}{x}\right)^2.x^2+2\left(\frac{\sin 2x}{2x}\right)^2.4x^2+2\left(\frac{\sin 3x}{3x}\right)^2.9x^2}{4\left(\frac{\sin 2x}{2x}\right)^2.4x^2}\right\}$$

$$= \frac{28}{16} = \frac{7}{4}$$

8. *Evaluate* $\lim_{x\to y}\frac{\tan x-\tan y}{x-y}$.

SOLUTION. We have,

$$\lim_{x\to y}\frac{\tan x-\tan y}{x-y}$$

$$=\lim_{h\to 0}\frac{\tan(y+h)-\tan y}{y+h-y}$$

$$=\lim_{h\to 0}\frac{1}{h}\left[\frac{\sin(y+h)}{\cos(y+h)}-\frac{\sin y}{\cos y}\right]$$

$$=\lim_{h\to 0}\frac{\{\sin(y+h)\cos y-\cos(y+h)\sin y\}}{h\cos(y+h)\cos y}$$

$$=\lim_{h\to 0}\frac{\sin(y+h-y)}{h\cos(y+h)\cos y}$$

$$=\lim_{h\to 0}\frac{\sin h}{h}\cdot\frac{1}{\cos(y+h)\cos y}$$

$$=1\cdot\frac{1}{\cos^2 y}=\sec^2 y$$

9. *Evaluate* $\lim_{\theta\to\frac{\pi}{6}}\left(\dfrac{\sin\left(\theta-\frac{\pi}{6}\right)}{\frac{\sqrt{3}}{2}-\cos\theta}\right)$.

SOLUTION. Let $\theta=h+\dfrac{\pi}{6}$

$$\therefore\quad \lim_{\theta\to\frac{\pi}{6}}\frac{\sin\left(\theta-\frac{\pi}{6}\right)}{\frac{\sqrt{3}}{2}-\cos\theta}$$

$$=\lim_{h\to 0}\frac{\sin h}{\frac{\sqrt{3}}{2}-\cos\left(\frac{\pi}{6}+h\right)}$$

$$=\lim_{h\to 0}\frac{\sin h}{\cos\frac{\pi}{6}-\cos\left(\frac{\pi}{6}+h\right)}$$

$$=\lim_{h\to 0}\frac{\sin h}{2\sin\left(\frac{\pi}{6}+\frac{h}{2}\right)\sin\frac{h}{2}}$$

$$=\lim_{h\to 0}\left\{\frac{\left(\frac{\sin h}{h}\cdot h\right)}{2\sin\left(\frac{\pi}{6}+\frac{h}{2}\right)\left(\frac{\sin(h/2)}{h/2}\right)h/2}\right\}$$

$$=\frac{1}{\sin\frac{\pi}{6}}=2$$

10. *If α, β are the roots of the equation $ax^2+bx+c=0$, find the value of*

$$\lim_{x\to\frac{1}{\alpha}}\sqrt{\frac{1-\cos(cx^2+bx+a)}{2(1-\alpha x)^2}}.$$

SOLUTION. Since α, β are the roots of the equation $ax^2+bx+c=0$ then roots of the equation $cx^2+bx+a=0$ will be $\dfrac{1}{\alpha}$ and $\dfrac{1}{\beta}$.

$$\Rightarrow\quad cx^2+bx+a=c\left(x-\frac{1}{\alpha}\right)\left(x-\frac{1}{\beta}\right)$$

$$\therefore\quad \lim_{x\to\frac{1}{\alpha}}\sqrt{\frac{1-\cos(cx^2+bx+a)}{2(1-\alpha x)^2}}$$

$$=\lim_{x\to\frac{1}{\alpha}}\sqrt{\frac{1-\cos\left\{c\left(x-\frac{1}{\alpha}\right)\left(x-\frac{1}{\beta}\right)\right\}}{2(1-\alpha x)^2}}$$

$$=\lim_{x\to\frac{1}{\alpha}}\left|\frac{\sin\left\{\frac{c}{2}\left(x-\frac{1}{\alpha}\right)\left(x-\frac{1}{\beta}\right)\right\}}{1-\alpha x}\right|$$

$$=\lim_{x\to\frac{1}{\alpha}}\left|\frac{\sin\left\{\frac{c}{2}\left(x-\frac{1}{\alpha}\right)\left(x-\frac{1}{\beta}\right)\right\}}{\frac{c}{2}\left(x-\frac{1}{\alpha}\right)\left(x-\frac{1}{\beta}\right)}\cdot\frac{c(\alpha x-1)(\beta x-1)}{2\alpha\beta(1-\alpha x)}\right|$$

$$=\left|\frac{c}{2\alpha\beta}\left(\frac{\beta}{\alpha}-1\right)\right|=\left|\frac{c}{2\alpha}\left(\frac{1}{\alpha}-\frac{1}{\beta}\right)\right|$$

11. *Evaluate* $\lim_{x\to\theta}\dfrac{x\sin\theta-\theta\sin x}{x-\theta}$.

SOLUTION. Let $x=\theta+h\Rightarrow x\to\theta\Rightarrow h\to 0$

Now

$$\lim_{x\to\theta}\frac{x\sin\theta-\theta\sin x}{x-\theta}$$

$$=\lim_{h\to 0}\frac{(\theta+h)\sin\theta-\theta\sin(\theta+h)}{\theta+h-\theta}$$

$$=\lim_{h\to 0}\frac{\theta\sin\theta+h\sin\theta-\theta\sin(\theta+h)}{h}$$

$$= \lim_{h\to 0} \frac{\theta[\sin\theta - \sin(\theta+h)] + h\sin\theta}{h}$$

$$= \lim_{h\to 0}\left[\frac{\theta\cdot 2\cdot\cos\frac{2\theta+h}{2}\cdot\sin\left(-\frac{h}{2}\right)}{h} + \frac{h\sin\theta}{h}\right]$$

$$= \lim_{h\to 0}\left[\frac{\theta\cdot 2\cos\frac{2\theta+h}{2}\cdot\frac{\sin\left(-\frac{h}{2}\right)}{\left(-\frac{h}{2}\right)}\left(-\frac{h}{2}\right)}{h} + \sin\theta\right]$$

$$= -\theta\cos\theta + \sin\theta = \sin\theta - \theta\cos\theta$$

12. *If* $f(x) = \frac{ax^2+b}{x^2+1}$, $\lim_{x\to 0} f(x) = 1$ *and* $\lim_{x\to\infty} f(x) = 1$. *Prove that* $f(-2) = f(2) = 1$.

SOLUTION. We have, $f(x) = \frac{ax^2+b}{x^2+1}$ ...(1)

and

$$\lim_{x\to 0} f(x) = 1 \Rightarrow \lim_{x\to 0}\frac{ax^2+b}{x^2+1} = 1 \Rightarrow b = 1$$

Also $\lim_{x\to\infty} f(x) = 1 \Rightarrow \lim_{x\to\infty}\frac{ax^2+b}{x^2+1} = 1$

$$\Rightarrow \lim_{x\to\infty}\frac{a+\frac{b}{x^2}}{1+\frac{1}{x^2}} = 1 \Rightarrow a = 1$$

Now, putting the values of a and b in eqn. (1) we get

$$f(x) = \frac{x^2+1}{x^2+1} = 1$$

$\Rightarrow$ $f(2) = f(-2) = 1$

13. *Evaluate* $\lim_{n\to\infty}\left(\frac{1^2}{n^3}+\frac{2^2}{n^3}+\frac{3^2}{n^3}+\ldots+\frac{n^2}{n^3}\right)$.

SOLUTION. We have,

$$\lim_{n\to\infty}\left[\frac{1^2}{n^3}+\frac{2^2}{n^3}+\frac{3^2}{n^3}+\ldots+\frac{n^2}{n^3}\right]$$

$$= \lim_{n\to\infty}\frac{1^2+2^2+3^2+\ldots+n^2}{n^3}$$

$$= \lim_{n\to\infty}\frac{n(n+1)(2n+1)}{6n^3}$$

$$= \lim_{n\to\infty}\frac{(n+1)(2n+1)}{6n^2}$$

$$= \lim_{n\to\infty}\left(\frac{2n^2+3n+1}{6n^2}\right)$$

$$= \lim_{n\to\infty}\left(\frac{2+\frac{3}{n}+\frac{1}{n^2}}{6}\right) = \frac{2}{6} = \frac{1}{3}$$

14. *Evaluate* $\lim_{x\to\infty}(\sqrt{x^2+x+1}-x)$.

SOLUTION. We have, $\lim_{x\to\infty}(\sqrt{x^2+x+1}-x)$

$$= \lim_{x\to\infty}\frac{(\sqrt{x^2+x+1}-x)(\sqrt{x^2+1+x}+x)}{(\sqrt{x^2+x+1}+x)}$$

$$= \lim_{x\to\infty}\frac{x^2+x+1-x^2}{\sqrt{x^2+x+1}+x}$$

$$= \lim_{x\to\infty}\frac{x+1}{\sqrt{x^2+x+1}+x}$$

$$= \lim_{x\to\infty}\frac{x+1}{x\sqrt{1+\frac{1}{x}+\frac{1}{x^2}}+x}$$

$$= \lim_{x\to\infty}\frac{x\left(1+\frac{1}{x}\right)}{x\left(\sqrt{1+\frac{1}{x}+\frac{1}{x^2}}+1\right)}$$

$$= \lim_{x\to\infty}\frac{1+\frac{1}{x}}{\sqrt{1+\frac{1}{x}+\frac{1}{x^2}}+1} = \frac{1}{2}$$

15. *Evaluate* $\lim_{x\to 0}\left(\frac{1}{|x|}\right)$.

SOLUTION. By definition, when

$$x\to 0^-, |x|\to 0^+ \Rightarrow \lim_{x\to 0^-}\left(\frac{1}{|x|}\right) = \infty \qquad \ldots(1)$$

and when

$$x \to 0^+, |x| \to 0^+ \Rightarrow \lim_{x \to 0^+}\left(\frac{1}{|x|}\right) = \infty \quad \ldots(2)$$

From eqn. (1) and (2), we can say that

$$\lim_{x \to 0}\left(\frac{1}{|x|}\right) = \infty$$

16. *If* $f(x) = \begin{cases} \dfrac{e^{1/x}}{1+e^{1/x}} & , \; x \neq 0; \\ 0 & , \; x = 0 \end{cases}$ *Then find* $\lim_{x \to 0} f(x)$. [MEERUT(BCA)–2006, 10, 16]

SOLUTION. If $x < 0$, LHL $= \lim_{x \to 0-0}\left(\frac{1}{x}\right) = \infty$

$$\Rightarrow \lim_{x \to 0-0} f(x) = \lim_{x \to 0} \frac{e^{1/x}}{1+e^{1/x}}$$

$$= \frac{0}{1+0} = 0$$

$$[\because e^{-\infty} = 0] \quad \ldots(1)$$

Similarly RHL ($x > 0$)

$$\Rightarrow \lim_{x \to 0+0}\left(\frac{1}{x}\right) = \infty$$

$$\Rightarrow \lim_{x \to 0+0} f(x) = \lim_{x \to 0} \frac{e^{1/x}}{1+e^{1/x}}$$

$$= \lim_{x \to 0} \frac{1}{\frac{1}{e^{1/x}}+1} = \frac{1}{0+1} = 1$$

$$[\because \lim_{x \to 0} e^{-1/x} = 0] \quad \ldots(2)$$

From eqn. (1) and (2), we have

$$\lim_{x \to 0-0} f(x) \neq \lim_{x \to 0+0} f(x)$$

Hence, $\lim_{x \to 0} f(x)$ does not exist.

17. *If* $f(x) = \begin{cases} mx^2 + n & ; \quad x < 0 \\ nx + m & ; \quad 0 \le x \le 1 \\ nx^3 + m & ; \quad x > 1 \end{cases}$

Then for what integral values of m and n $\lim_{x \to 0} f(x)$ *and* $\lim_{x \to 1} f(x)$ *exist?* (NCERT)

SOLUTION. We have

$$f(x) = \begin{cases} mx^2 + n & ; \quad x < 0 \\ nx + m & ; \quad 0 \le x \le 1 \\ nx^3 + m & ; \quad x > 1 \end{cases}$$

Therefore

$$\lim_{x \to 0^-} f(x) = \lim_{x \to 0^-} (mx^2 + n) = n$$

and $\lim_{x \to 0^+} f(x) = \lim_{x \to 0^+} (nx + m) = m$

Clearly, for the existence of $\lim_{x \to 0} f(x)$

We must have $\lim_{x \to 0^-} f(x) = \lim_{x \to 0^+} f(x)$

i.e., m must be equal to n.

Similarly,

$$\lim_{x \to 1^-} f(x) = \lim_{x \to 1^-} (nx + m) = n + m$$

$$\lim_{x \to 1^+} f(x) = \lim_{x \to 1^+} (nx^3 + m) = n + m$$

For the existence of $\lim_{x \to 1} f(x)$, we have

$$\lim_{x \to 1^-} f(x) = \lim_{x \to 1^+} f(x)$$

Hence, for the existence of both $\lim_{x \to 0} f(x)$ and $\lim_{x \to 1} f(x)$ we must have

$$n + m = m + n \Rightarrow m = n.$$

18. *If the function f(x) satisfies* $\lim_{x \to 1} \frac{f(x)-2}{x^2-1} = \pi$, *find the value of* $\lim_{x \to 1} f(x)$. (NCERT)

SOLUTION. We have, $\lim_{x \to 1} \frac{f(x)-2}{x^2-1} = \pi \quad \ldots(1)$

Clearly, $\lim_{x \to 1}(x^2 - 1) = 0$

Therefore, if $\lim_{x \to 1} f(x) - 2 \neq 0$, then $\lim_{x \to 1} \frac{f(x)-2}{x^2-1} = \infty$ or $-\infty$ which is not possible by eqn. (1).

Therefore $\lim_{x \to 1}\{f(x) - 2\} = 0$

$$\Rightarrow \lim_{x \to 1} f(x) = 2$$

19. *If* $f(x) = \begin{cases} a + bx & ; \quad x < 1 \\ 4 & ; \quad x = 1 \\ b - ax & ; \quad x > 1 \end{cases}$ *and*

$\lim_{x\to1} f(x) = f(1)$, *find the value of a and b.* (NCERT)

SOLUTION. We have, $f(x) = \begin{cases} a+bx & ; & x<1 \\ 4 & ; & x=1 \\ b-ax & ; & x>1 \end{cases}$

$\Rightarrow \quad f(1) = 4 \quad \ldots(1)$

$\lim_{x\to1^-} f(x) = \lim_{x\to1^-} (a+bx) = a+b \quad \ldots(2)$

and $\lim_{x\to1^+} f(x) = \lim_{x\to1^+} (b-ax) = b-a \quad \ldots(3)$

It is given that $\lim_{x\to1} f(x)$ exists.

Therefore, $\lim_{x\to1^-} f(x) = \lim_{x\to1^+} f(x)$

$\Rightarrow \quad a+b = b-a$

$\Rightarrow \quad 2a = 0$

$\Rightarrow \quad a = 0$

Similarly, $\lim_{x\to1} f(x) = f(1)$

$\Rightarrow \quad a+b = 4$

$\Rightarrow \quad b = 4 \quad (\because a = 0)$

Hence, $a = 0$ and $b = 4$.

Exercise-5.2

1. Evaluate the following limits:

(i) $\lim_{x\to1} \frac{x^2+3x+2}{x^2+1}$ (ii) $\lim_{x\to64} \frac{x^{1/6}-2}{x^{1/3}-4}$

(iii) $\lim_{x\to0} \frac{\sqrt{1+x^2}-\sqrt{1+x}}{x}$

(iv) $\lim_{x\to1} \frac{x^2-\sqrt{x}}{\sqrt{x}-1}$

(v) $\lim_{x\to1} \frac{x^4-3x^2+2}{x^3-5x^2+3x+1}$

(vi) $\lim_{x\to-1} \frac{x^3-4x+1}{x-1}$

2. Evaluate the following limits:

(i) $\lim_{x\to-1} (1+x+x^2+\ldots+x^{10})$

(ii) $\lim_{x\to\pi} \left(x-\frac{22}{7}\right)$ (iii) $\lim_{x\to2} \frac{x^4-16}{x-2}$

(iv) $\lim_{x\to-3} \frac{x^3+27}{x^5+243}$ (v) $\lim_{x\to1} \frac{x^{1/3}-1}{x^{1/6}-1}$

(vi) $\lim_{x\to a} \frac{x-a}{x^{3/2}-a^{3/2}}$ (vii) $\lim_{x\to\infty} \left(1+\frac{p}{x}\right)^x$

(viii) $\lim_{x\to1} \left(\frac{1-x^{1/3}}{1-x^{-2/3}}\right)$ (ix) $\lim_{x\to3} \frac{x^n-3^n}{x-3}$

(x) $\lim_{x\to0} \left(\frac{\sqrt{a+x}-\sqrt{a}}{x\sqrt{a(a+x)}}\right)$

(xi) $\lim_{x\to2} \frac{x^3-2x^2}{x^2-5x+6}$

(xii) $\lim_{x\to1} \frac{\sqrt{x^2+8}-\sqrt{10-x^2}}{\sqrt{x^2+3}-\sqrt{5-x^2}}$

(xiii) $\lim_{x\to2} \left[\frac{1}{x-2} - \frac{2(2x-3)}{x^3-3x^2+2x}\right]$

(xiv) $\lim_{x\to1} \left[\frac{x-2}{x^2-x} - \frac{1}{x^3-3x^2+2x}\right]$

3. Evaluate the following limits:

(i) $\lim_{x\to0} \frac{\sin 2x+3x}{2x+\sin 3x}$

(ii) $\lim_{x\to0} \frac{x(\cos x+\cos 2x)}{\sin x}$

(iii) $\lim_{x\to0} \frac{\sin x-2\sin 3x+\sin 5x}{x}$

(iv) $\lim_{x\to0} \frac{\tan x-\sin x}{x^3}$ (v) $\lim_{x\to0} \frac{1-\sqrt{\cos x}}{x^2}$

(vi) $\lim_{y\to0} \frac{(x+y)\sec(x+y)-x\sec x}{y}$

(vii) $\lim_{x\to\frac{\pi}{2}} \frac{\cot x}{\frac{\pi}{2}-x}$ (viii) $\lim_{x\to\frac{\pi}{4}} \frac{\sec^2 x-2}{\tan x-1}$

(ix) $\lim_{x\to\frac{\pi}{6}} \frac{\sqrt{3}\sin x-\cos x}{x-\frac{\pi}{6}}$

(x) $\lim_{x\to0} \frac{3\sin x-\sin 3x}{x^3}$

(xi) $\lim_{x\to0} x(3\operatorname{cosec} 2x-2\cot 3x)$

(xii) $\lim_{x\to0} \frac{\cos 7x-\cos 9x}{\cos 3x-\cos 5x}$

(xiii) $\lim_{x\to0} \frac{\tan x-\sin x}{x^3}$

(xiv) $\lim_{x\to0} \frac{\cos ax-\cos bx}{\cos x-1}$

(xv) $\lim_{\theta\to 0}\frac{\sin\theta^n}{(\sin\theta)^m}, n>m>0$

(xvi) $\lim_{x\to\pi}\frac{\sin(\pi-x)}{\pi(\pi-x)}$

(xvii) $\lim_{x\to 1}(1-x)\tan\frac{\pi x}{2}$

(xviii) $\lim_{\theta\to\frac{\pi}{2}}\frac{\sec\theta-\tan\theta}{\pi-2\theta}$

4. Evaluate the following limits:

(i) $\lim_{x\to y}\frac{\sin x-\sin y}{x-y}$

(ii) $\lim_{x\to\pi}\frac{1-\sin\frac{x}{2}}{\cos\frac{x}{2}\left(\cos\frac{x}{4}-\sin\frac{x}{4}\right)}$

(iii) $\lim_{\theta\to\pi/4}\left(\frac{\sin\theta-\cos\theta}{\theta-\frac{\pi}{4}}\right)$

(iv) $\lim_{x\to a}\frac{\sin x-\sin a}{\sqrt{x}-\sqrt{a}}$

(v) $\lim_{y\to x}\frac{y\cos x-x\cos y}{y-x}$

(vi) $\lim_{\theta\to\frac{\pi}{4}}\frac{1-\tan\theta}{1-\sqrt{\tan\theta}}$

5. Evaluate the following limits:

(i) $\lim_{x\to\infty}\frac{x^3+x^2-6x+8}{4x^3+5x-8}$

(ii) $\lim_{x\to-\infty}(\sqrt{x^2+4x}-\sqrt{x^2-4x})$

(iii) $\lim_{x\to\infty}\left(\frac{1}{n^2}+\frac{2}{n^2}+\ldots+\frac{n}{n^2}\right)$

(iv) $\lim_{n\to\infty}\left(\frac{1^3}{n^4}+\frac{2^3}{n^4}+\frac{3^3}{n^4}+\ldots+\frac{n^3}{n^4}\right)$

(v) $\lim_{n\to\infty}\left[\frac{1\cdot 2+2\cdot 3+\ldots+n\cdot(n+1)}{n^3}\right]$

(vi) $\lim_{x\to-\infty}(\sqrt{x^2+ax}-\sqrt{x^2-ax})$

(vii) $\lim_{n\to\infty}\frac{2^n-1}{2^n+1}$

(viii) $\lim_{n\to\infty}\frac{(n+2)!+(n+1)!}{(n+3)!}$

(ix) $\lim_{n\to\infty}\frac{\sqrt{n^2+1}+n)^2}{(n^6+1)^{1/3}}$

(x) $\lim_{x\to\infty}\frac{(x+1)^{10}+(x+2)^{10}+(x+3)^{10}}{x^{10}+(x+3)^{10}}$

6. Evaluate the following limits: where [ ] denotes greatest integer function

(i) $\lim_{x\to\frac{\pi^-}{2}}(\tan x)$ (ii) $\lim_{x\to a^+}[x]$

(iii) $\lim_{x\to 2-0}[x]$ (iv) $\lim_{x\to a^-}\frac{|x^3|}{|x|}$

(v) $\lim_{x\to\frac{5^-}{2}}[x]$ (vi) $\lim_{x\to\frac{7}{3}}[-x]$

(vii) $\lim_{x\to 0^-}(2-\cot x)$ (viii) $\lim_{x\to 0^-}(1+\operatorname{cosec} x)$

(ix) $\lim_{x\to-3^+}\frac{[x-7]}{[x+4]}$ (x) $\lim_{x\to-2^-}\frac{x-3}{x^2-4}$

7. Let $f(x)$ be a function such that $f(-x) = -f(x)$ and $\lim_{x\to 0}f(x)$ exists, prove that

$$\lim_{x\to 0}f(x)=0$$

8. Prove that $\lim_{x\to 3^+}\left(\frac{x}{[x]}\right)\neq\lim_{x\to 3^-}\frac{x}{[x]}$.

9. Prove that $\lim_{x\to 1^+}\left(\frac{1}{x-1}\right)\neq\lim_{x\to 1^-}\left(\frac{1}{x-1}\right)$

10. If $f(x)=\begin{cases}3-x^2 & ; \quad x\le -2\\ ax+b & ; \quad -2<x<2\\ \frac{x^2}{2} & ; \quad x\ge 2\end{cases}$

then for the existence of the $\lim_{x\to 2}f(x)$ and $\lim_{x\to -2}f(x)$, prove that $a=\frac{3}{4}, b=\frac{1}{2}$.

11. A function $f(x)$ is defined as follows

$$\begin{aligned} f(x) &= x^2 && \text{when } x<1\\ &= \frac{5}{2} && \text{when } x=1\\ &= x^2+2 && \text{when } x>1 \end{aligned}$$

Does $\lim_{x\to 1}f(x)$ exists.

ANSWERS

1. (i) 3 (ii) $\frac{1}{4}$ (iii) $-\frac{1}{2}$ (iv) 3 (v) $\frac{1}{2}$ (vi) -2 **2.** (i) 1 (ii) $\left(\pi-\frac{22}{7}\right)$ (iii) 32 (iv) $\frac{1}{15}$ (v) 2 (vi) $\frac{2}{3\sqrt{a}}$ (vii) e^p (viii) $-\frac{1}{2}$ (ix) $n.3^{n-1}$ (x) $\frac{1}{2}a^{-3/2}$ (xi) -4 (xii) $\frac{2}{3}$ (xiii) $-\frac{1}{2}$ (xiv) 2 **3.** (i) 1 (ii) 2 (iii) 0 (iv) $\frac{1}{2}$ (v) $\frac{1}{4}$ (vi) $\sec x(1+x\tan x)$ (vii) 1 (viii) 2 (ix) 2 (x) 4 (xi) $\frac{5}{6}$ (xii) 2 (xiii) $\frac{1}{2}$ (xiv) a^2-b^2 (xv) 0 (xvi) $\frac{1}{\pi}$ (xvii) $\frac{2}{\pi}$ (xviii) $\frac{1}{4}$

4. (i) $\cos y$ (ii) $\frac{1}{\sqrt{2}}$ (iii) $\sqrt{2}$ (iv) $2\sqrt{a}\cos a$ (v) $\cos x + x\sin x$ (vi) 2

5. (i) $\frac{1}{4}$ (ii) 4 (iii) $\frac{1}{2}$ (iv) $\frac{1}{4}$ (v) $\frac{1}{3}$ (vi) a (vii) 1 (viii) 0 (ix) 4 (x) $\frac{3}{2}$

6. (i) ∞ (ii) $[a]$ (iii) 1 (iv) a^2 (v) 2 (vi) -3 (vii) ∞ (viii) $-\infty$ (ix) -10 (x) ∞

11. limit does not exist

5.10 CONTINUITY

Geometrically, a continuous process is one that goes on smoothly without any sudden change. Continuity of a function can also be interpreted in a similar way when we say that a function $f(x)$ is continuous at $x = a$ we mean that there is no interruption (cut) in the graph of $f(x)$ at $x = a$, *i.e.*, the graph of $f(x)$ is unbroken at $x = a$ and there is no hole, gap or jump in the graph. On the other hand, if there is a sudden jump in the value of the function at $x = a$ and the value of the function changes gradually for change in the value of the independent variable. Consider the following graph.

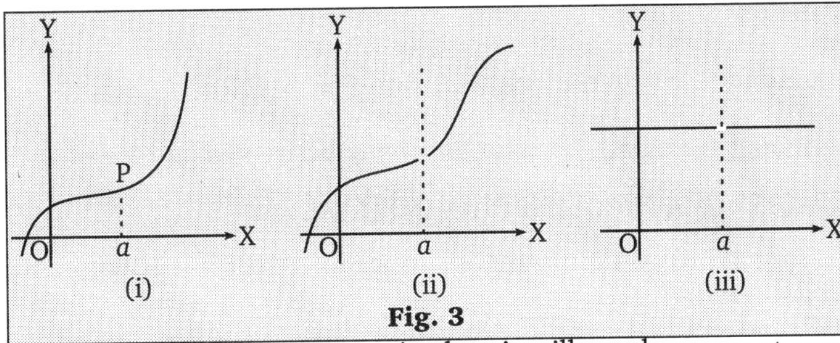

Fig. 3

If we draw a perpendicular from a on x-axis, then it will cut the curve at any point say P, *i.e.*, at $x = a$, there is no cut in the graph, but if graph of the function has a sudden cut at $x = a$, then we say that graph is broken.

The graph of the function in figure (i) proceed smoothly while in figure (ii) graph has a cut at the point $x = a$. Hence, we say that the function of fig. (i) is continuous while function of fig. (ii) is discontinuous at $x = a$.

5.11 CONTINUITY OF A FUNCTION AT A POINT

A function $f(x)$ is said to be continuous at $x = a$ if $f(x)$ is defined at $x = a$, $\lim_{x\to a} f(x)$ exists and $\lim_{x\to a} f(x) = f(a)$, *i.e.*, $f(x)$ is said to be continuous at $x = a$ if

$$\lim_{x\to a^+} f(x) = \lim_{x\to a^-} f(x) = f(a)$$

$\Rightarrow$ Right hand limit of $f(x)$ at $x = a$ = Left hand limit of $f(x)$ at $x = a$ = Value of the function at $x = a$

i.e., $f(a+0) = f(a-0) = f(a)$

WORKING PROCEDURE

To check the continuity of the function $f(x)$ at $x = a$, use the following steps :

STEP 1. Find the value of $f(x)$ at $x = a$, *i.e.*, $f(a)$

STEP 2. Evaluate LHL $= \lim_{x \to a^-} f(x) = f(a-0)$

STEP 3. Evaluate RHL $= \lim_{x \to a^+} f(x) = f(a+0)$

STEP 4. If $f(a) = f(a+0) = f(a-0)$, then $f(x)$ is said to be continuous at $x = a$.

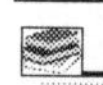

- If any of the value $f(a + 0)$, $f(a - 0)$ or $f(a)$ is different, the function is not continuous at $x = a$. Hence, to check the continuity of a function $f(x)$ at a point $x = a$ we have to calculate all three values, *i.e.*, $f(a + 0)$, $f(a - 0)$ and $f(a)$.

5.12 CONTINUITY OF THE FUNCTION FROM THE LEFT AND FROM THE RIGHT

Let $f(x)$ be a function. Then $f(x)$ is said to be continuous at $x = a$ from left if

$$\lim_{x \to a^-} f(x) = f(a)$$

Again, $f(x)$ is said to be continuous at $x = a$ from right if

$$\lim_{x \to a^+} f(x) = f(a)$$

5.13 CONTINUITY OF A FUNCTION IN ANY INTERVAL

A function $f(x)$ is said to be continuous in an interval $[a, b]$ if

(i) $f(x)$ is continuous at $x = a$ from right, *i.e.*, $\lim_{x \to a^+} f(x) = f(a)$

(ii) $f(x)$ is continuous at $x = b$ from left, *i.e.*, $\lim_{x \to b^-} f(x) = f(b)$

(iii) $f(x)$ is continuous from both sides for all x lying between a and b.

5.14 DISCONTINUITY OF A FUNCTION IN AN INTERVAL

A function $f(x)$ is said to be discontinuous in an interval I if it is not continuous at one or more points of the interval I.

5.15 PROPERTIES OF CONTINUOUS FUNCTIONS

We shall present here some theorems related to continuous functions (without proof).

(i) If $f(x)$ and $g(x)$ be two continuous functions at $x = a$, then sum and difference of $f(x)$ and $g(x)$ are also continuous at $x = a$.
i.e., $[f(x) \pm g(x)]$ is continuous at $x = a$.

(ii) If $f(x)$ and $g(x)$ be two continuous functions at $x = a$, then their product and quotient are also continuous at $x = a$, *i.e.*, $[f(x) \cdot g(x)]$ and $\left[\dfrac{f(x)}{g(x)}\right], g(a) \neq 0$, are also continuous.

(iii) If $f(x)$ is continuous at $x = a$, then $kf(x)$ is also continuous at $x = a$, $k \in \mathbf{R}$.

(iv) If $f(x)$ is continuous at $x = a$, then $\dfrac{1}{f(x)}$ is also continuous at $x = a$ provided $f(a) \neq 0$.

(v) If $f(x)$ is continuous at $x = a$ then $|f(x)|$ is also continuous at $x = a$.

(vi) Every polynomial function is continuous.

(vii) Every constant function is continuous.

(viii) If fog is defined for two continuous functions f and g then fog is also continuous.

Solved Examples

1. *Prove that $f(x)=\dfrac{1}{x-a}$ is not continuous at $x = a$.*

SOLUTION. **Left Hand Limit (LHL)**

Let $x = a - h$

If $x = a$ then $h = 0$

$\therefore x \to a \Rightarrow h \to 0$

$$\therefore \lim_{x\to a^-} f(x) = \lim_{h\to 0} f(a-h)$$

$$= \lim_{h\to 0}\frac{1}{a-h-a} = \lim_{h\to 0}\frac{1}{-h} = -\infty$$

Right Hand Limit (RHL)

Let $x = a + h$ If $x = a$ then $h = 0$

$$\therefore \lim_{x\to a} \Rightarrow \lim_{h\to 0}$$

$$\therefore \lim_{x\to a^+} f(x) = \lim_{h\to 0} f(a+h)$$

$$= \lim_{h\to 0}\frac{1}{a+h-a} = \lim_{h\to 0}\frac{1}{h}$$

$$= \infty$$

$\because$ LHL $\neq$ RHL

Hence $f(x)$ is not continuous at $x = a$.

2. *Prove that*

$$f(x)=\begin{cases} x\sin\dfrac{1}{x} & , \quad x\neq 0 \\ 0 & , \quad x=0 \end{cases}$$

is continuous at $x = 0$.

SOLUTION: Given, $f(0) = 0$ ...(1)

LHL

Let $x = 0 - h$ if $x = 0 \Rightarrow h = 0$

$$f(0-0) = \lim_{x\to 0^-} f(x) = \lim_{x\to 0} f(0-h)$$

$$= \lim_{h\to 0}(0-h)\sin\left(\frac{1}{0-h}\right)$$

$$= \lim_{h\to 0}(-h)\sin\left(\frac{1}{-h}\right) = \lim_{h\to 0} h\sin\left(\frac{1}{h}\right)$$

$$= \lim_{h\to 0} h \lim_{h\to 0}\sin\left(\frac{1}{h}\right)$$

$= 0 \times$ (a finite quantity lying between -1 and 1)

$= 0$ ...(2)

RHL

Let $x = 0 + h$ If $x = 0 \Rightarrow h = 0$

$$f(0+0) = \lim_{x\to 0^+} f(x) = \lim_{h\to 0} f(0+h)$$

$$= \lim_{h\to 0}(0+h)\sin\left(\frac{1}{0+h}\right)$$

$$= \lim_{h\to 0} h\sin\left(\frac{1}{h}\right) = \lim_{h\to 0} h\cdot \lim_{h\to 0}\sin\left(\frac{1}{h}\right)$$

$= 0 \times$ [a finite quantity lying between -1 and 1]

$= 0$ ...(3)

$\therefore f(0 + 0) = 0$

It is clear from (1), (2) and (3) that

$$f(0) = f(0-0) = f(0+0)$$

$\Rightarrow f(x)$ is continuous at $x = 0$.

3. *For what value of k, the function*

$$f(x)=\begin{cases} \dfrac{x^2-9}{x-3} & , \quad x\neq 3 \\ k & , \quad x=3 \end{cases}$$

is continuous at $x = 3$?

[MEERUT(BCA)–2008, 12; RAJ–2013; HIMACHAL–2011]

SOLUTION. Given, $f(3) = k$

LHL at $x = 3$

Let $x = 3 - h$. If $x = 3 \Rightarrow h = 0$

$$\therefore \lim_{x\to 3^-} f(x) = \lim_{h\to 0} f(3-h)$$

$$= \lim_{h\to 0}\frac{(3-h)^2-9}{3-h-3}$$

$$= \lim_{h\to 0}\frac{(3-h+3)(3-h-3)}{-h}$$

$$= \lim_{h\to 0}\frac{(6-h)(-h)}{(-h)}$$

$$= \lim_{h\to 0}(6-h) = 6 \quad (\because h = 0)$$

RHL at $x = 3$

Let $x = 3 + h$, if $x = 3 \Rightarrow h = 0$

$$\therefore \lim_{x\to 3^+} f(x) = \lim_{h\to 0}(3+h)$$

$$= \lim_{h\to 0}\frac{(3+h)^2-9}{3+h-3}$$

$$= \lim_{h\to 0} \frac{(3+h+3)(3+h-3)}{h}$$

$$= \lim_{h\to 0} \frac{(6+h)h}{h} = \lim_{h\to 0}(6+h)$$

$= 6 + 0 = 6$ $\qquad (\because h = 0)$

$\because$ $f(x)$ is continuous at $x = 3$.

$\therefore$ $f(3) = f(3-h) = f(3+h)$

$\Rightarrow$ $k = 6 = 6$

$\therefore$ $k = 6$

4. *A function f(x) is defined as follows :*

$$f(x) = \begin{cases} x, & \text{if } 0 \le x < \frac{1}{2} \\ 0, & \text{if } x = \frac{1}{2} \\ 1-x, & \text{if } \frac{1}{2} < x \le 1 \end{cases}$$

Find the value of $\lim_{x\to 1/2} f(x)$.

SOLUTION. **LHL**

Let $x = \frac{1}{2} - h$ if $x = \frac{1}{2} \Rightarrow h = 0$

$\therefore$ $\lim_{x\to\frac{1}{2}} \Rightarrow \lim_{h\to 0}$

$$\therefore \lim_{x\to\left(\frac{1}{2}\right)^-} f(x) = \lim_{h\to 0} f\left(\frac{1}{2}-h\right)$$

$$= \lim_{h\to 0}\left[\frac{1}{2}-h\right] = \left(\frac{1}{2}-0\right) = \frac{1}{2}$$

$(\because h = 0)$

RHL

Let $x = \frac{1}{2} + h$ if $x = \frac{1}{2} \Rightarrow h = 0$

$$\therefore \lim_{x\to\left(\frac{1}{2}\right)^+} f(x) = \lim_{h\to 0} f\left(\frac{1}{2}+h\right)$$

$$= \lim_{h\to 0}\left[1-\left(\frac{1}{2}+h\right)\right] = \lim_{h\to 0}\left[\frac{1}{2}-h\right]$$

$$= \left(\frac{1}{2}-0\right) = \frac{1}{2} \qquad (\because h = 0)$$

Clearly $\quad$ LHL = RHL $= \frac{1}{2}$

$$\therefore \quad \lim_{x\to\frac{1}{2}} f(x) = \frac{1}{2}$$

5. *Check the continuity of the function*

$$f(x) = \begin{cases} \frac{|x|}{x} & ,\text{if } x \ne 0 \\ 1 & ,\text{if } x = 0 \end{cases} \quad at\ x = 0.$$

SOLUTION. **LHL**

Let $x = 0 - h$, if $x = 0 \Rightarrow h = 0$

$$\therefore \lim_{x\to 0^-} f(x) = \lim_{h\to 0} f(0-h)$$

$$= \lim_{h\to 0}\frac{|0-h|}{(0-h)} = \lim_{h\to 0}\frac{|-h|}{-h} = \lim_{h\to 0}\frac{h}{-h}$$

$= -1$

RHL

Let $x = 0 + h$, if $x = 0 \Rightarrow h = 0$

$$\therefore \lim_{x\to 0^+} f(x) = \lim_{h\to 0} f(0+h)$$

$$= \lim_{h\to 0}\frac{|0+h|}{(0+h)} = \lim_{h\to 0}\frac{|h|}{h} = \lim_{h\to 0}\frac{h}{h} = 1$$

Also, the value of $f(x)$ at $x = 0$, $f(0) = 1$

$\Rightarrow$ LHL $\ne$ RHL $= f(0)$

Hence, $f(x)$ is not continuous at $x = 0$.

6. *Check the continuity of the function*

$$f(x) = \begin{cases} -x^2 & ,\text{if } x \le 0 \\ 5x-4 & ,\text{if } 0 < x \le 1 \\ 4x^2-3x & ,\text{if } 1 < x < 2 \\ 3x+4 & ,\text{if } x \ge 2 \end{cases}$$

at $x = 0, 1, 2$. [MEERUT(BCA)–2005, 12]

SOLUTION. We have to check the continuity of $f(x)$ at $x = 0$

(i) Continuity at $x = 0$

LHL

Let $x = 0 - h$ if $x = 0 \Rightarrow h = 0$

$$\therefore \lim_{x\to 0^-} f(x) = \lim_{h\to 0} f(0-h)$$

$$= \lim_{h\to 0}[-(0-h)^2]$$

$[\because$ Here $f(x) = -x^2]$

$$= \lim_{h\to 0}[-h^2] = 0 \qquad \ldots(1)$$

RHL

Let $x = 0 + h$ if $x = 0 \Rightarrow h = 0$

$$\therefore \lim_{x\to 0^+} f(x) = \lim_{h\to 0} f(0+h)$$

$$= \lim_{h\to 0}[5(0+h)-4]$$

$[\because$ Here $f(x) = 5x - 4]$

$= \lim_{h\to 0}[5h-4] = 5\times 0-4 = -4$ ...(2)

From eqn. (1) and (2) it is clear that RHL ≠ LHL

⇒ The function $f(x)$ is not continuous at $x = 0$.

(ii) Continuity at $x = 1$

LHL

Let $x = 1-h$. If $x = 1 \Rightarrow h = 0$

$\therefore \lim_{x\to 1^-} f(x) = \lim_{h\to 0} f(1-h)$

$= \lim_{h\to 0}[5(1-h)-4]$ [∵ Here $f(x) = 5x - 4$]

$= \lim_{h\to 0}(5-5h-4)$

$= \lim_{h\to 0}(1-5h) = 1-5\times 0$

$= 1-0 = 1$

RHL

Let $x = 1+h$ If $x = 1$, then $h = 0$

$\therefore \lim_{x\to 1^+} f(x) = \lim_{h\to 0} f(1+h)$

$= \lim_{h\to 0}[4(1+h)^2 - 3(1+h)]$ [∵ Here $f(x) = (4x^2 - 3x)$]

$= \lim_{h\to 0}(4h^2+8h+4-3-3h)$

$= \lim_{h\to 0}[4h^2+5h+1]$

$= 0+0+1 = 1$

At $x = 1; f(x) = 5x-4$

$\therefore f(1) = 5-4 = 1$

∴ LHL = RHL = $f(1)$

⇒ $f(x)$ is continuous at $x = 1$.

(iii) Continuity of $f(x)$ at $x = 2$

LHL

Let $x = 2-h$ If $x = 2 \Rightarrow h = 0$

$\therefore \lim_{x\to 2^-} f(x) = \lim_{h\to 0} f(2-h)$

$= \lim_{h\to 0}[4(2-h)^2 - 3(2-h)]$ [∵ Here $f(x) = (4x^2-3x)$]

$= \lim_{h\to 0}(4h^2-16h+16-6+3h)$

$= \lim_{h\to 0}[4h^2-13h+10]$

$= 0-0+10 = 10$

RHL

Let $x = 2+h$ If $x = 2 \Rightarrow h = 0$

$\therefore \lim_{x\to 2^+} f(x) = \lim_{h\to 0} f(2+h)$

$= \lim_{h\to 0}[3(2+h)+4]$ [∵ Here $f(x) = 3x + 4$]

$= \lim_{h\to 0}[10+3h] = 10+0$

$= 10$

∵ At $x = 2; f(x) = 3x+4$

$\therefore f(2) = 3\times 2+4 = 10$

∴ At $x = 2$

LHL = RHL = $f(2)$

⇒ $f(x)$ is continuous at $x = 2$.

7. *Show that* $f(x) = \begin{cases} \dfrac{|x-3|}{x-3}, & x \neq 3 \\ 0, & x = 3 \end{cases}$ *is continuous at all points except at $x = 3$.*

SOLUTION. **Continuity at $x = 3$**

LHL

Let $x = 3-h$, if $x = 3 \Rightarrow h = 0$

$\therefore \lim_{x\to 3^-} f(x) = \lim_{h\to 0} f(3-h)$

$= \lim_{h\to 0}\dfrac{|(3-h)-3|}{3-h-3}$ $\left[\text{Here } f(x) = \dfrac{|x-3|}{x-3} \because x \neq 3\right]$

$= \lim_{h\to 0}\dfrac{|-h|}{-h} = \lim_{h\to 0}\dfrac{h}{-h} = -1$

RHL

Let $x = 3+h$, if $x = 3 \Rightarrow h = 0$

$\therefore \lim_{x\to 3^+} = \lim_{h\to 0} f(3+h)$

$= \lim_{h\to 0}\dfrac{|(3+h)-3|}{3+h-3}$ $\left[\because x \neq 3 \therefore f(x) = \dfrac{|x-3|}{x-3}\right]$

$= \lim_{h\to 0}\dfrac{|h|}{h} = \lim_{x\to 0}\dfrac{h}{h} = 1$

At $x = 3, f(x) = 0$ *i.e.*, $f(3) = 0$

$\Rightarrow$ At $x = 3$, LHL $\neq$ RHL $\neq f(3)$

$\Rightarrow f(x)$ is not continuous at $x = 3$.

Now we check the continuity of $f(x)$ at $x = a$ when $a \neq 3$.

$\because \quad a \neq 3, \; f(x) = \dfrac{|x-3|}{x-3}$

$\therefore \lim_{x\to a} f(x) = \lim_{x\to a} \dfrac{|x-3|}{x-3} = \dfrac{|a-3|}{a-3}$

Again for $a \neq 3$; $f(x) = \dfrac{|x-3|}{x-3}$

$\therefore \quad f(a) = \dfrac{|a-3|}{a-3}$

$\therefore \lim_{x\to a} f(x) = f(a)$

i.e., $f(x)$ is continuous at $x = a$ while $a \neq 3$, and at $x = 3$ the function $f(x)$ is not continuous.

- If function $f(x) = \dfrac{|x-a|}{x-a}$ is continuous for all x except at $x = a$. Therefore, we have to check the continuity at $x = a$ only.

8. *Show that $f(x) = \sin x$ is continuous for all values of x.*

SOLUTION. Let a be an arbitrary value of x.

Therefore $f(a) = \sin a$

$\therefore |f(x) - f(a)| = |\sin x - \sin a|$

$= \left|2\cos\left(\dfrac{x+a}{2}\right)\sin\left(\dfrac{x-a}{2}\right)\right|$

$= \left|2\cos\left(\dfrac{x+a}{2}\right)\right|\left|\sin\left(\dfrac{x-a}{2}\right)\right|$

$< 2\left|\sin\left(\dfrac{x-a}{2}\right)\right| \quad \left[\because \left|\cos\left(\dfrac{x+a}{2}\right)\right| < 1\right]$

$< 2\left(\dfrac{x-a}{2}\right) \quad \left[\because \sin\theta < \theta \text{ and } 0 < \theta < \dfrac{\pi}{2}\right]$

$< (x-a)$

Therefore, $|f(x) - f(a)| < (x-a)$

$\therefore \quad |f(x) - f(a)| < \in$ if $|x-a| < \in$

$\therefore$ If for given $\in > 0 \, \exists \, \lambda (= \in)$ such that

$|f(x) - f(a)| < \in$ when $0 < |x-a| < \lambda$

$\Rightarrow f(x)$ is continuous at $x = a$. Now, since, a is arbitrary. Hence $f(x)$ is continuous for all x.

Exercise-5.3

1. A function $f(x)$ is defined as follows :

$$f(x) = \begin{cases} 1 & \text{if } x > 0 \\ -1 & \text{if } x < 0 \\ 0 & \text{if } x = 0 \end{cases}$$

Prove that $\lim_{x\to 0} f(x)$ does not exist.

2. Show that $\lim_{x\to 2} \dfrac{|x-2|}{(x-2)}$ does not exist.

3. A function $f(x)$ is defined as follows :

$$f(x) = \begin{cases} x^2, & \text{if } x \neq 1 \\ 1, & \text{if } x = 1 \end{cases}$$

Prove that $\lim_{x\to 1} f(x) = 1$.

4. If $f(x) = |x|$, prove that $\lim_{x\to 0} f(x) = 0$.

5. If $f(x) = \dfrac{|x-1|}{x-1}$, prove that $\lim_{x\to 1} f(x)$ does not exist.

6. If $f(x) = \dfrac{1}{|x|}$, prove that $\lim_{x\to 0} f(x)$ does not exist.

7. Prove that RHL and LHL of the function $f(x) = \dfrac{1+\cos x}{\tan^2 x}$ at $x \to \pi$ are equal. Also find the $\lim_{x\to\pi} f(x)$.

8. Find RHL and LHL of the function $f(x) = \dfrac{x^2-1}{|x-1|}$ at $x \to 1$.

9. Find RHL and LHL of the function $f(x) = \dfrac{|\sin x|}{x}$ at $x \to 0$.

10. Check the continuity of the function

$$f(x) = \begin{cases} 1+x^2, & \text{if } 0 \leq x \leq 1 \\ 1-x, & \text{if } x > 1 \end{cases} \text{ at } x = 1.$$

11. Check the continuity of the function
$$f(x) = \begin{cases} x, & \text{if } x \geq 2 \\ x^2, & \text{if } x < 2 \end{cases}.$$

12. Prove that $f(x) = \sin x$ is continuous at $x = \dfrac{\pi}{2}$.

13. If $f(x) = \begin{cases} x-4, & \text{if } x \geq 5 \\ 5x-24, & \text{if } x < 5 \end{cases}$,

prove that $f(x)$ is continuous at $x = 5$.

14. For what value of k, the function
$$f(x) = \begin{cases} kx^2, & \text{if } x \leq 2 \\ 3, & \text{if } x > 2 \end{cases}$$
is continuous?

15. For what value of k, the function
$$f(x) = \begin{cases} \dfrac{x^2-16}{x-4}, & \text{if } x \neq 4 \\ k, & \text{if } x = 4 \end{cases}$$
is continuous at $x = 4$?

16. Check the continuity of $f(x)$ at $x = 0$ if
$$f(x) = \begin{cases} x^2-1, & \text{if } x \leq 0 \\ 0, & \text{if } x > 0 \end{cases}$$

17. Check the continuity of $f(x)$ at $x = 1$ if
$$f(x) = \begin{cases} 2|x|, & \text{if } |x| \leq 1 \\ 0, & \text{if } |x| > 1 \end{cases}$$

18. Check the continuity of $f(x)$ at $x = 1$ and $x = 2$ if $f(x) = \begin{cases} 0, & \text{if } 0 < x < 1 \\ x, & \text{if } 1 \leq x < 2 \\ x^3/4, & \text{if } 2 \leq x < 3 \end{cases}$.

19. Check the continuity of $f(x)$ at $x = a$ if
$$f(x) = \begin{cases} \dfrac{x^2-a^2}{x-a}, & \text{if } x \neq a \\ 2a, & \text{if } x = a \end{cases}$$

20. Prove that the function $f(x) = x^2 - 7x + 3$ is continuous at $x = 1, x = 2, x = 3$.

21. Check the continuity of the function $f(x)$ at $x = 0$ if $f(x) = \begin{cases} x^5, & \text{if } x \neq 0 \\ 1, & \text{if } x = 0 \end{cases}$.

22. A function $f(x)$ is defined as follows
$$f(x) = \begin{cases} 1+x, & \text{if } x > 0 \\ 0, & \text{if } x = 0 \\ x^2+1, & \text{if } x < 0 \end{cases}$$
Is $f(x)$ continuous at $x = 0$? If not, what minimum correction should be made to make $f(x)$ continuous at $x = 0$?

ANSWERS

7. $\dfrac{1}{2}$ **8.** 2, –2 **9.** 1, –1 **10.** discontinuous
11. discontinuous at $x = 2$ and continuous for all other points **14.** $k = \dfrac{3}{4}$ **15.** $k = 8$
16. discontinuous **17.** discontinuous **18.** discontinuous at $x = 1$, continuous at $x = 2$
19. Continuous at $x = a$ **21.** discontinuous **22.** Take $f(0) = 1$

Miscellaneous Examples

1. *Find the point of discontinuity of the following function :*
$$f(x) = \begin{cases} x+2, & \text{if } x < 1 \\ 0, & \text{if } x = 1 \\ x-2, & \text{if } x > 1 \end{cases}$$

SOLUTION. Evidently we can say that $f(x)$ is continuous for all values of x except $x = 1$.

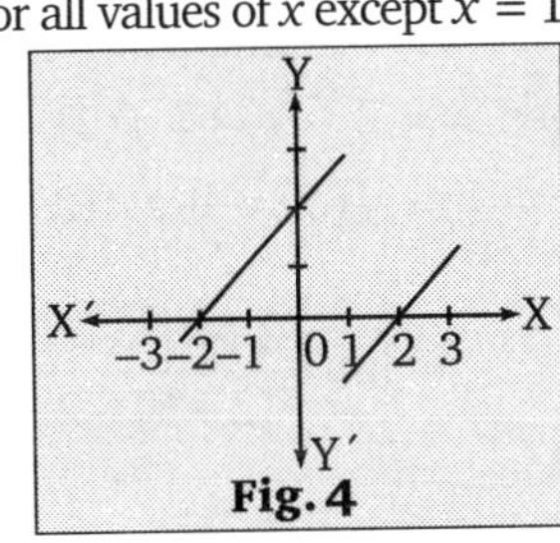

Fig. 4

Continuity at $x = 1$

$$\text{LHL} = f(1-0) = \lim_{x \to 1^-} (x+2) = 1+2 = 3$$

$$\text{RHL} = f(1+0) = \lim_{x \to 1^+} (x-2) = 1-2 = -1$$

$\Rightarrow$ $f(1+0) \neq f(1-0)$

$\Rightarrow$ $f(x)$ is not continuous at $x = 1$.

$\Rightarrow$ The only point of discontinuity of $f(x)$ is $x = 1$.

2. *Check the continuity of the function*

$$f(x)=\begin{cases}2x-1, \text{ if } x<0\\ 2x+1, \text{ if } x\geq 0\end{cases}$$

Solution. **Case-I:** When $x<0$, then $f(x)=2x-1$, which is a polynomial function and hence continuous at all point $x<0$.

Case-II: When $x>0$ then $f(x)=2x+1$, which is again a polynomial function and hence continuous for all point $x>0$.

Case-III: When $x=0$, then $f(0)=2\times 0+1=1$

and RHL $= f(0+0) = \lim\limits_{x\to 0^+} f(x)$

$$= \lim_{h\to 0} f(0+h) = \lim_{h\to 0} f(h)$$
$$= \lim_{h\to 0}(2h+1)=1$$

Similarly, LHL

$= f(0-0)$

$= \lim\limits_{x\to 0^-} f(x) = \lim\limits_{h\to 0} f(0-h) = \lim\limits_{h\to 0} f(-h)$

$= \lim\limits_{h\to 0}[(2(-h)-1)] = -1$

Clearly $f(0+0)\neq f(0-0)$

$\Rightarrow f(x)$ is not continuous at $x=0$.

3. *Check the continuity of the function* $f(x)=|x|+|x-1|$ *in the interval* $[-1,2]$.

Solution. The given function can be defined as follows:

$$f(x)=\begin{cases}1-2x; & \text{if } -1\leq x\leq 0\\ 1; & \text{if } 0<x\leq 1\\ 2x-1 & \text{if } 1<x\leq 2\end{cases}$$

We know that a polynominal function and constant function are always continuous. So $f(x)$ is continuous at $-1\leq x\leq 0, 0<x\leq 1$ and $1<x\leq 2$. So, we have to check the continuity at $x=-1,0,1$ and 2.

Case-I: At $x = -1$

RHL $= f(-1+0)$

$= \lim\limits_{x\to -1^+} f(x) = \lim\limits_{x\to -1^+}(1-2x) = 1+2 = 3$

and $f(x)=1-2x$, when $x=-1$

$\therefore f(-1)=1-2(-1)=1+2=3$

$\Rightarrow \lim\limits_{x\to -1^+} f(x) = f(-1)$

$\Rightarrow f(x)$ is continuous at $x=-1$.

Case-II: At $x = 0$

$\lim\limits_{x\to 0^-} f(x) = \lim\limits_{x\to 0^-}(1-2x) = 1-2\times 0 = 1$

and $\lim\limits_{x\to 0^+} f(x) = \lim\limits_{x\to 0^+}(1) = 1$

Also $f(0)=1$

Clearly,

$\lim\limits_{x\to 0^-} f(x) = \lim\limits_{x\to 0^+} f(x) = f(0) = 1$

$\Rightarrow f(x)$ is continuous at $x=0$.

Case-III: At $x = 1$

We have, $\lim\limits_{x\to 1^-} f(x) = \lim\limits_{x\to 1^-}(1) = 1$

and $\lim\limits_{x\to 1^+} f(x) = \lim\limits_{x\to 1^+}(2x-1) = 1$

Also, $f(1)=1$

Clearly,

$\lim\limits_{x\to 1^-} f(x) = \lim\limits_{x\to 1^+} f(x) = f(1) = 1$

Hence, $f(x)$ is continuous at $x=1$.

Case-IV: At $x = 2$

$\lim\limits_{x\to 2^-} f(x) = \lim\limits_{x\to 2^-}(2x-1) = 4-1 = 3$

and $f(2)=2\times 2-1=3$

$\Rightarrow f(x)$ is continuous at $x=2$.

$\Rightarrow f(x)$ is continuous at each point of the interval $[-1,2]$.

4. *Check the point of discontinuity of the function*

$$f(x)=\begin{cases}\dfrac{x^4-16}{x-2}, & \text{if } x\neq 2\\ 16, & \text{if } x=2\end{cases}$$

Solution. At $x\neq 2$, , $f(x)=\dfrac{x^4-16}{x-2}$ is a rational function.

$\Rightarrow f(x)$ is continuous $\forall x\in \mathbf{R}(x\neq 2)$

When $x=2$, $f(x)=f(2)=16$

Now $\lim\limits_{x\to 2^+} f(x) = \lim\limits_{h\to 0} f(2+h)$

$$= \lim_{h\to 0}\frac{(2+h)^4-16}{(2+h)-2}$$

$$= \lim_{h\to 0} \frac{2^4 + 4\times 2^3 h + 6\times 2^2 h^2 + 8h^3 + h^4 - 16}{h}$$

$$= \lim_{h\to 0} \frac{32h + 24h^2 + 8h^3 + h^4}{h}$$

$$= \lim_{h\to 0}(32 + 24h + 8h^2 + h^3) = 32$$

$\Rightarrow f(2) \neq \lim_{x\to 2^+} f(x)$

$\Rightarrow f(x)$ is not continuous at $x = 2$.

$\Rightarrow$ Point $x = 2$ is the point of discontinuity of the function $f(x)$.

5. *For what value of k, the following function is continuous at x = 2?*

$$f(x) = \begin{cases} 2x+1, & \text{if } x < 2 \\ k, & \text{if } x = 2 \\ 3x-1, & \text{if } x > 2 \end{cases}$$

SOLUTION. $\text{LHL} = \lim_{x\to 2^-} f(x) = \lim_{h\to 0} f(2-h)$

$= \lim_{h\to 0} 2(2-h)+1 = 4+1 = 5$

and

$\text{RHL} = \lim_{x\to 2^+} f(x) = \lim_{h\to 0} f(2+h)$

$= \lim_{h\to 0} 3(2+h) - 1 = 6 - 1 = 5$

Given, $f(2) = k$.

For the continuity of $f(x)$ at $x = 2$.

$\text{LHL} = \text{RHL} = f(2) = k$

$\Rightarrow \quad f(2) = 5 = k \quad \Rightarrow \quad k = 5$

6. *Prove that $\cos x$ is continuous.*

SOLUTION. Let $f(x) = \cos x$ and $a \in \mathbf{R}$

Then $f(a) = \cos a$

LHL

$f(a-0) = \lim_{x\to a^-} f(x) = \lim_{h\to 0} f(a-h)$

$= \lim_{h\to 0} \cos(a-h) = \cos a$

Similarly, RHL

$f(a+0) = \lim_{x\to a^+} f(x) = \lim_{h\to 0} f(a+h)$

$= \lim_{h\to 0} \cos(a+h) = \cos a$

Clearly $f(a) = f(a+0) = f(a-0)$

$\Rightarrow f(x)$ is continuous at $x = a$ for every value of a.

$\Rightarrow f(x)$ is continuous.

7. *Prove that $f(x) = x - [x]$ is discontinuous for all integral value of x, here $[\cdot]$ denotes the greatest integer function.*

SOLUTION. Given, $f(x) = x - [x]$

Let r be an integer, then

$$f(r) = r - [r]$$

LHL : $x < r \Rightarrow [x] = r - 1$

$\therefore$ LHL $= \lim_{x\to r^-} f(x) = \lim_{x\to r^-}(x - [x])$

$= r - (r-1) = 1$

RHL : $x > r \Rightarrow [x] = r$

$\therefore \lim_{x\to r^+} f(x) = \lim_{x\to r^+}(x - [x]) = r - r = 0$

Clearly LHL $\neq$ RHL

$\Rightarrow f(x)$ is not continuous at $x = r$ for each value of r.

8. *Prove that $|\sin x|$ is continuous.*

SOLUTION. Let $h(x) = |\sin x|$

and $f(x) = \sin x$ and $g(x) = |x|$

$\therefore (gof)(x) = g[f(x)]$

$= g(\sin x) = |\sin x|$

$\Rightarrow (gof)(x) = h(x)$

Now, since $f(x) = \sin x$ and $g(x) = |x|$ are continuous therefore *gof* is also continuous.

$\therefore \quad h(x) = |\sin x|$ is a continuous function.

9. *Find the point of discontinuity of the greatest integer function $f(x) = [x]$.*

SOLUTION. Let $f(x) = [x]$, then we have

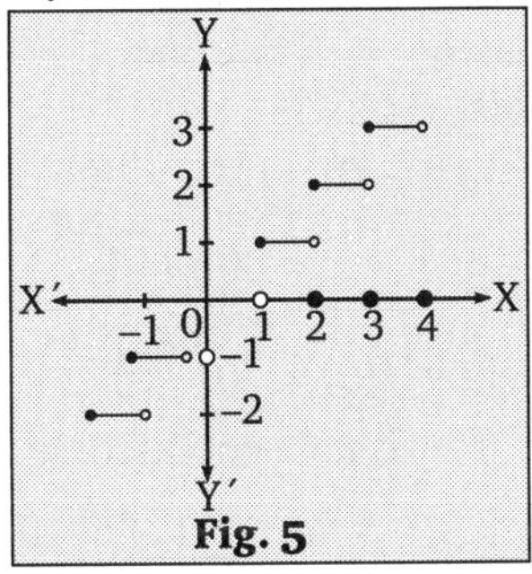

Fig. 5

$$f(x) = \begin{cases} -2 & ; & -2 \le x < -1 \\ -1 & ; & -1 \le x < 0 \\ 0 & ; & 0 \le x < 1 \\ 1 & ; & 1 \le x < 2 \\ 2 & ; & 2 \le x < 3 \\ \vdots & & \vdots \end{cases}$$

Let $x = r$ be arbitrary, then
$f(r) = [r] = r$

LHL : Here

$x < r \Rightarrow f[x] = r - 1$

$\therefore \lim_{x \to r^-} f(x) = \lim_{x \to r^-} [x] = r - 1$

RHL : Here $x > r \Rightarrow [x] = r$

Then $\lim_{x \to r^+} f(x) = \lim_{x \to r^+} [x] = r$

$\Rightarrow \lim_{x \to r^-} f(x) \ne \lim_{x \to r^+} f(x)$

$\Rightarrow f(x)$ is discontinuous at $x = r$ for all integral value of r.

$\Rightarrow$ All integers are the point of discontinuity of $f(x)$.

10. *Find the point of discontinuity of the function*

$$f(x) = \begin{cases} \dfrac{x}{|x|}, & \text{if } x < 0 \\ -1, & \text{if } x > 0 \end{cases}$$

SOLUTION. We know that,

$$|x| = \begin{cases} -x, & \text{when } x < 0 \\ x, & \text{when } x > 0 \end{cases}$$

Therefore,

$$f(x) = \begin{cases} \dfrac{-x}{x} = -1, & \text{if } x < 0 \\ \dfrac{x}{x} = 1, & \text{if } x > 0 \\ 0, & \text{if } x = 0 \end{cases}$$

$\Rightarrow$ We have to check the continuity at $x = 0$.

Now, $f(0) = 0$

$$f(0-0) = \text{LHL} = \lim_{x \to 0^-} f(x)$$
$$= \lim_{x \to 0^-} (-1) = -1$$

Clearly $f(0) \ne f(0-0)$

$\Rightarrow f(x)$ is not continuous at $x = 0$.

$\Rightarrow x = 0$ is the point of discontinuity of $f(x)$.

11. *Find the point of discontinuity of the function f defined by*

$$f(x) = \begin{cases} |x| + 3, & \text{if } x \le -3 \\ -2x, & \text{if } -3 < x < 3 \\ 6x + 2, & \text{if } x \ge 3 \end{cases}$$

SOLUTION. If $x \le -3$, then $|x| = -x$

$(\because |x| = -x;$ if $x < 0)$

$\therefore$ We can defined $f(x)$ as follows :

$$f(x) = \begin{cases} -x + 3, & \text{if } x \le -3 \\ -2x, & \text{if } -3 < x < 3 \\ 6x + 2, & \text{if } x \ge 3 \end{cases}$$

$\Rightarrow$ We have to check the continuity at $x = -3$ and $x = 3$.

(i) Continuity at $x = -3$

$f(x) = -x + 3$ if $x \le -3$

$\Rightarrow f(-3) = -(-3) + 3 = 6$

LHL: If $x < -3$ then $f(x) = -x + 3$

$$\therefore \lim_{x \to -3^-} f(x) = \lim_{x \to -3^-} (-x + 3)$$
$$= -(-3) + 3 = 6$$

RHL: When $x > -3$ then $f(x) = -2x$

$$\therefore \lim_{x \to -3^+} f(x) = \lim_{x \to -3^+} (-2x)$$
$$= -2(-3) = 6$$

It is clear that

$$\lim_{x \to -3^-} f(x) = \lim_{x \to -3^+} f(x) = f(-3)$$

$\Rightarrow f(x)$ is continuous at $x = -3$.

(ii) Continuity at $x = 3$

Given $f(x) = 6x + 2$ if $x \ge 3$

$\Rightarrow f(3) = 6 \times 3 + 2 = 20$

Now $\lim_{x \to 3^-} f(x) = \lim_{x \to 3^-} (-2x) = -6$

and $\lim_{x \to 3^+} f(x) = \lim_{x \to 3^+} (6x + 2) = 20$

$\Rightarrow \lim_{x \to 3^-} f(x) \ne f(3)$

$\Rightarrow f(x)$ is not continuous at $x = 3$.

$\Rightarrow x = 3$ is the point of discontinuity of $f(x)$.

12. *Let* $f(x) = \begin{cases} \dfrac{\sin x}{x}, & \text{if } x < 0 \\ (x+1), & \text{if } x \ge 0 \end{cases}$

Check the continuity of $f(x)$.

SOLUTION. We know that sin x and one-one function x are always continuous.

$\Rightarrow \dfrac{\sin x}{x}, x < 0$ is continuous.

Similarly, $x+1$ is continuous being the polynomial function.

Continuity at $x = 0$

$$f(0) = 0 + 1 = 1$$

$$\text{RHL} = f(0+0) = \lim_{h\to 0} f(0+h) = \lim_{h\to 0}(h+1) = 1$$

$$\text{LHL} = f(0-0) = \lim_{h\to 0} f(0-h) = \lim_{h\to 0} f(-h) = \lim_{h\to 0}\left(\frac{\sin(-h)}{-h}\right) = \lim_{h\to 0}\frac{\sin h}{h} = 1$$

$\Rightarrow f(0+0) = f(0-0) = f(0) = 1$

$\Rightarrow f(x)$ is continuous at $x = 0$.

$\Rightarrow f(x)$ is continuous at each point.

13. *Let*

$$f(x) = \begin{cases} x^2 + ax + b, & \text{if } 0 \le x < 2 \\ 3x + 2, & \text{if } 2 \le x \le 4 \\ 2ax + 5b, & \text{if } 4 < x \le 8 \end{cases}$$

Find the value of a and b if $f(x)$ is continuous in the interval $[0, 8]$.

SOLUTION. Since the given function $f(x)$ is continuous in the interval $[0,8]$, so it is also continuous in the interval $]0,2[,]2,4[$ and $]4,8[$.

$\Rightarrow f(x)$ is continuous at $x = 0$.

$$\Rightarrow \lim_{x\to 0^+} f(x) = f(0)$$

$$\Rightarrow \lim_{x\to 0^+}(x^2 + ax + b) = 0^2 + a\times 0 + b = b$$

$\because f(x)$ is continuous at $x = 2$. Therefore

$$= \lim_{x\to 2^-} f(x) = \lim_{x\to 2^+} f(x) = f(2)$$

$$\Rightarrow \lim_{x\to 2^-}(x^2 + ax + b) = \lim_{x\to 2^+}(3x+2) = 3\times 2 + 2$$

$$\Rightarrow 4 + 2a + b = 3 \times 2 + 2$$

$$\Rightarrow 2a + b = 4 \quad \ldots(1)$$

Similarly, $f(x)$ is continuous at $x = 4$.

$$\Rightarrow \lim_{x\to 4^+} f(x) = \lim_{x\to 4^-} f(x) = f(4)$$

$$\Rightarrow \lim_{x\to 4^+}(2ax + 5b) = \lim_{x\to 4^-}(3x+2) = 3\times 4 + 2$$

$$\Rightarrow 8a + 5b = 12 + 2$$

$$\Rightarrow 8a + 5b = 14 \quad \ldots(2)$$

On solving eqn. (1) and (2) we get

$$a = 3, b = -2$$

14. *Let $f(x) = |x-1| + |x+2|, x \in \mathbf{R}$. Show that the function f(x) is continuous at x = 1 and x = –2.*

SOLUTION. **(i) Right hand limit at $x = 1$**

Given $f(x) = |x-1| + |x+2|$

$\Rightarrow f(x+h) = |x+h-1| + |x+h+2|$

$\Rightarrow f(1+h) = |1+h-1| + |1+h+2|$

$$\Rightarrow \lim_{h\to 0} f(1+h) = \lim_{h\to 0}[|h| + |3+h|] = |0| + |3+0| = 3$$

(ii) Left hand limit at $x = 1$

Here,

$$f(1-h) = |1-h-1| + |1-h+2| = |-h| + |3-h|$$

$$\therefore \lim_{h\to 0} f(1-h) = \lim_{h\to 0}[|h| + |3-h|] = |0| + |3-0| = 3$$

$\Rightarrow$ RHL = LHL

and $f(1) = |1-1| + |1+2| = |0| + |3| = 3$

$$\Rightarrow f(1) = \lim_{h\to 0} f(1-h) = \lim_{h\to 0} f(1+h)$$

Hence, $f(x)$ is continuous at $x = 1$.

LHL at $x = -2$

$f(-2-h)$

$= |-2-h-1| + |-2-h+2|$

$= |-3-h| + |-h|$

$\lim_{h\to 0} f(-2-h) = \lim_{h\to 0} |3+h| + |h|$

$= |3+0| + |0| = 3$

RHL at $x = -2$

$f(-2+h)$

$= |-2+h-1| + |-2+h+2|$

$= |h-3| + |h|$

$$\Rightarrow \lim_{h\to 0} f(-2+h) = |-3| + |0| = 3$$

and $f(-2) = |-2-1| + |-2+2|$
$= |-3| + |0| = 3$

$$\Rightarrow f(-2) = \lim_{h\to 0} f(-2+h) = \lim_{h\to 0} f(-2-h)$$

Hence, we conclude that $f(x)$ is continuous at $x = -2$ also.

Exercise-5.4

1. Prove that

$f(x) = \begin{cases} x, & x \geq 0 \\ 1, & x < 0 \end{cases}$, is not continuous at $x = 0$.

2. Prove that

$f(x) = \begin{cases} \dfrac{\sin x}{x}; & x \neq 0 \\ 1; & x = 0 \end{cases}$, is continuous at $x = 0$.

[KANPUR(BCA)–2001, 07, 17; AGRA(BCA)–2008]

3. Prove that

$f(x) = \begin{cases} x+2, & x \leq 3 \\ 8-x, & x > 3 \end{cases}$, is continuous at $x = 3$.

4. Prove that

$f(x) = \begin{cases} x-1, & \text{if } x \leq 2 \\ 2x-3, & \text{if } x > 2 \end{cases}$, is continuous at every point.

5. Prove that

$f(x) = \begin{cases} \dfrac{\sin^{-1} x}{x} + e^x, & x \neq 0 \\ 2, & x = 0 \end{cases}$, is continuous at $x = 0$.

6. Let the function $f(x) = \begin{cases} 1, & \text{if } x \leq 3 \\ ax+b, & \text{if } 3 < x < 5 \\ 7, & \text{if } 5 \leq x \end{cases}$

be continuous, find the value of a and b.

7. Prove that $f(x) = 2x - |x|$ is continuous at $x = 0$.

8. Prove that $f(x) = \cos x^2$ is a continuous function.

9. Prove that $f(x) = |1 - x + |x||$ is a continuous function at $x = 0$.

10. Prove that $f(x) = x^n$, is continuous at $x = 0$.

11. If $f(x) = \begin{cases} x-4, & x \leq 5 \\ 5x-24, & x > 5 \end{cases}$ then show that $f(x)$ is continuous at $x = 5$.

12. Prove that

$f(x) = \begin{cases} \dfrac{x^2}{a} - a, & 0 < x < a \\ 0, & x = a \\ a - \dfrac{a^3}{x^2}, & x > a \end{cases}$ is continuous at $x = a$. [AGRA(BCA)–2009; MEERUT(BCA)–2000]

13. Check the continuity of the following functions:

(i) $f(x) = \begin{cases} \dfrac{1}{1-e^{1/x}}, & x \neq 0 \\ 0, & x = 0 \end{cases}$

(ii) $f(x) = \begin{cases} e^{1/x}, & x \neq 0 \\ 0, & x = 0 \end{cases}$

(iii) $f(x) = \begin{cases} \dfrac{1}{1+e^{1/x}}, & x \neq 0 \\ 0, & x = 0 \end{cases}$

14. Check the continuity of the following functions:

(i) $f(x) = \begin{cases} x \cos \dfrac{1}{x}, & x \neq 0 \\ 0, & x = 0 \end{cases}$

(ii) $f(x) = \begin{cases} \cos \dfrac{1}{x}, & x \neq 0 \\ 1, & x = 0 \end{cases}$

(iii) $f(x) = \begin{cases} \sin \dfrac{1}{x}, & x \neq 0 \\ 0, & x = 0 \end{cases}$

(iv) $f(x) = \begin{cases} \dfrac{\cos x}{\dfrac{\pi}{2} - x}, & x \neq \pi/2 \\ 1, & x = \pi/2 \end{cases}$

15. Prove that

$f(x) = \begin{cases} \dfrac{\sin^2 ax}{1}, & x \neq 0 \\ 1, & x = 0 \end{cases}$ is not continuous at $x = 0$.

16. If $f(x) = x^2 + 1$, when $x \neq 1$ and $f(x) = 3$ when $x = 1$. Prove that $f(x)$ is not continuous at $x = 1$.

17. If $f(x) = \begin{cases} 4x+a, & x < 1 \\ 6, & x = 1 \\ 3x-b, & x > 1 \end{cases}$ is continuous at $x = 1$.

Find the value of a and b.

18. Show that the function $f(x)=\frac{xe^{1/x}}{1+e^{1/x}}$, $x \neq 0, f(0) = 1$ is not continuous at $x = 0$.
[MEERUT(BCA)–2003, 09; KANPUR(BCA)–1993, 2014]

19. Show that the function $f(x)=\frac{1}{x-a}\text{cosec}\left(\frac{1}{x-a}\right)$, $x \neq 0$, $f(a) = 0$ is not continuous at $x = a$.
[MEERUT(BCA)–2011]

ANSWERS

6. $a = 3, b = -8$ **17.** $a = 2, b = -3$

5.16 DERIVATIVE OF A FUNCTION

If a function $f(x)$ is defined on nbd of a point a and

$$\lim_{h\to 0}\frac{f(a+h)-f(a)}{h}$$

exist (finitely), then the function $f(x)$ is said to be differentiable at a and this limit is called derivative of the function $f(x)$ at a.

In symbols, this derivative, is denoted by $f'(a)$ and read as the derivative of $f(x)$ at $x=a$ with respect to the variable x. The process of evaluating $f'(a)$ is called differentiation.

Graphically, $f'(a)$ means the gradient of the curve $y = f(x)$ at the point $(a, f(a))$.

Quantitatively $f'(a)$ means the rate of change of the function $f(x)$ at a, with respect to the variable x.

5.16.1 LEFT HAND DERIVATIVE

The left hand derivative (regressive derivative) of f at $x = a$ is given by

$$Lf'(a)=\lim_{h\to 0}\frac{f(a-h)-f(a)}{-h}$$

and, is denoted by $Lf'(a)$.

5.16.2 RIGHT HAND DERIVATIVE

The right hand derivative (progressive derivative) of f at $x = a$ is given by

$$Rf'(a)=\lim_{h\to 0}\frac{f(a+h)-f(a)}{h}$$

The derivative $f'(a)$ exists when $Lf'(a) = Rf'(a)$.

5.16.3 DIFFERENTIABILITY IN AN INTERVAL

(i) A function $f :]a, b[\to \mathbf{R}$ is said to be differentiable in $]a, b[$ iff it is differentiable at every point of $]a, b[$.

(ii) A function $f : [a, b]\to \mathbf{R}$ is said to be differentiable in $[a, b]$ iff $Rf'(a)$ and $Lf'(b)$ exists and f is differentiable at every point of $]a, b[$.

(iii) Let f be a function whose domain is an interval I. If I_1 be the set of all those points x of I at which f is differentiable *i.e.*, $f(x)$ exists and if $I_1 \neq \phi$, we get another function f' with domain I_1. It is called the first derivative of f. Similarly 2nd, 3rd, ...n^{th} derivative of f are defined and are denoted by $f'', f''', \ldots, f^n$ respectively of course, in order that $f^n(x)$ may be defined, it is necessary (though not sufficient) that $f^{n-1}(x)$ may be defined for all x in some open interval containing a.

- $\lim_{x \to a} \frac{f(x) - f(a)}{x - a}$ means the same thing as $\lim_{h \to 0} \frac{f(a + h) - f(a)}{h}$
- The derivative of a function at a point and the derivative of a function are two different but related concepts. The derivative of f at a point a is a number while the derivative of f is a function. However, very often the term derivative of f is used to denote both number and function and it is left to the context to distinguish what is intended.
- If $f(x)$ is derivable on interval I then $f'(x)$ at end points of I (if exists) would mean a left or right hand derivative of $f(x)$ according as it is a right or a left hand end point of I. Similar meaning holds for higher order derivatives.

5.17 CONTINUITY AND DIFFERENTIABILITY

THEOREM 1. **(A necessary condition for the existence of a finite derivative).** *Continuity is a necessary but not a sufficient condition for the existence of a finite derivative*

PROOF. Let f be differentiable at a. Then $\lim_{x \to a} \frac{f(x) - f(a)}{(x - a)}$ exists and equal to $f'(a)$.

Now we may write

$$f(x) - f(a) = \frac{f(x) - f(a)}{(x - a)}(x - a) \qquad \text{(If } x \neq a\text{)}$$

Taking limit as $x \to a$, we get

$$\lim_{x \to a} [f(x) - f(a)] = \lim_{x \to a} \left\{ \frac{f(x) - f(a)}{(x - a)}(x - a) \right\}$$

$$= \lim_{x \to a} \left\{ \frac{f(x) - f(a)}{x - a} \right\} . \lim_{x \to a} (x - a)$$

($\because$ limit of the product of two functions is equal to product of their limits)

$$= f'(a).0 = 0$$

so that $\lim_{x \to a} f(x) = f(a) \Rightarrow f(x)$ is continuous at $x = a$.

Hence, f is continuous at $x = a$. Thus continuity is a necessary condition for differentiability.

- While continuity is a necessary condition for the differentiability, it is not a sufficient condition as it is clear from the following examples :

  (i) Consider the function $f(x)$ defined on R by setting

  $$f(x) = 0 \quad \text{if} \quad x = 0$$
  $$f(x) = x \quad \text{if} \quad x \neq 0$$

  f is obviously continuous as also derivative at every point except possibly at $x=0$. At $x=0$, f is continuous but not derivable.

  (ii) Consider the function $f(x)$ such that

  $$\begin{cases} x \sin \frac{1}{x}, & x \neq 0 \\ 0, & x = 0 \end{cases}$$

  this function is continuous at $x=0$ but not differentiable at $x=0$.

  (iii) The function $f(x) = |x|$ is a continuous function, but not differentiable at $x = 0$. ($\because Lf'(0) = -1$ and $Rf'(0) = 1$)
- Continuity of a function even at every point of R has nothing to do with the differentiability of the function at any point.
- Weierstrass is considered as the first mathematician who gave in 1872 examples of functions continuous on R but no where differentiable. The examples given by Weierstrass are:

  (a) $f(x) = \sum_{n=1}^{\infty} a^n \cos b^n \pi x$, where b is an odd integer $1 > a > 0$ and $ab > 1 + \frac{3}{2}\pi$.

  (b) $f(x) = \sum_{n=1}^{\infty} \frac{1}{2^n} \cos(3^n x) \forall x \in R$.

5.18 ALGEBRA OF DERIVATIVES

(1) Let functions f and g be defined on an interval I. If f and g are differentiable at $x = a \in I$, then $f \pm g$ is also differentiable and

$$(f \pm g)'(a) = f'(a) \pm g'(a)$$

(2) Let a function $f(x)$ be differentiable at a point a and $c \in \mathbf{R}$, then the function cf is also differentiable at a and $(cf)'(a) = cf'(a)$.

(3) Let the functions f and g be defined on an interval I. If f and g are differentiable at $a \in I$, then $f.g$ is also differentiable and

$$(fg)'(a) = f'(a)g(a) + f(a)g'(a)$$

(4) If a function f is differentiable at $x=a$ and $f(a) \neq 0$, then the function $\frac{1}{f}$ is differentiable at a and $\left(\frac{1}{f}\right)'(a) = -\frac{f'(a)}{[f(a)]^2}$.

(5) Let f and g be defined on an interval I. If f and g are differentiable at $a \in I$, and if $g(a) \neq 0$, then the function f/g is also differentiable at a.

(6) Let f and g be functions such that the range of f is contained in the domain of g. If f is differentiable at a and g is differentiable at $f(a)$, then gof is differentiable at a and $(gof)' = g'(f(a)).f'(a)$ (Chain rule).

(7) **(Derivative of the inverse function).** If f is differentiable at $x = a$ and is one-one function defined on interval I with $f'(a) \neq 0$, then the inverse of the f is differentiable at $f(a)$ and its derivative at a is $\frac{1}{f'(a)}$.

THEOREM 1. **(Darboux's Theorem or Intermediate Value Theorem).** *If f is finitely differentiable in a closed interval $[a, b]$ and $f'(a)$, $f'(b)$ are of opposite sign, then there exist at least one* point $c \in\,]a, b[$ such that $f'(c) = 0$.

PROOF. Let us suppose that $f'(a) > 0$ and $f'(b) < 0$, then there exist intervals $]a, a + h[$ and $]b - h, b[$, $h > 0$ such that

$$f(x) > f(a) \ \forall x \in]a, a+h[\qquad \text{... (1)}$$

$$f(x) > f(b) \ \forall x \in]b-h, b[\qquad \text{... (2)}$$

Now, since f is finitely differentiable, then it is continuous in $[a, b]$ and hence it is bounded on $[a, b]$ and attains its supremum and infimum at least once in $[a, b]$.

[$\because$ *A* continuous function attains its supremum and infimum at least once in $[a, b]$].

Thus if M is the supremum of f in $[a, b]$, then there exist $c \in [a, b]$ such that $f(c)=M$. It is clear from (1) and (2) that the upper bound is not attained at the end points a and b so that $c \in\,]a, b[$.

Now we shall prove $f'(c) = 0$

If $f'(c) > 0$, then there exist an interval $]c, c + h[$, $h > 0$, such that $f(x) > f(c) = M$ $\forall x \in]c, c + h[$, which is not possible, since M is the supremum of the function $f(x)$ in $[a, b]$.

If $f'(c) < 0$ then there exist an interval $[c - h, c[$, $h > 0$ such that $f(x) > f(c) = M \ \forall x \in [c - h, c[$, which is not possible.

Hence, we conclude that $f'(c) = 0$

- Darboux's theorem shows that derivative do share an important property of continuous functions. Since the image of an interval under a continuous function is an interval. Darboux's theorem essentially says that the result hold even if a function is not ,continuous, provided of course, it is a derivative. That is, if a function g defined on an interval I is the derivative of some function f, then $g(I)$is an interval.

THEOREM 2. *Let f be defined and differentiable on [a, b], and if c be any number between $f'(a)$ and $f'(b)$, then there exist a real number k between a and b such that $f'(k) = c$.*

PROOF. Let g be the function defined on $[a, b]$ by setting

$$g(x) = f(x) - cx \text{ for all } x \in [a, b]$$

Now, g is differentiable on $[a, b]$ and $g'(a) = f'(a) - c$, and $g'(b) = f'(b) - c$ since c lies between $f'(a)$ and $f'(b)$. Therefore, it follows that $g'(a)$ and $g'(b)$ are of opposite signs.

Since g is differentiable on $[a, b]$, and since $g'(a)\, g'(b) < 0$, therefore there exist a number k between a and b such that $g'(k) = 0$ *i.e.*, $f'(k) = c$.

THEOREM 3. *If f is defined and differentiable on an interval, the range of f' is an interval.*

PROOF. Let the domain of f (and therefore, that of f') be an interval X and let the range of f' be Y. Also let p and q be two distinct points of Y. Then there exist two distinct points a and b in X such that $f'(a) = p$ and $f'(b) = q$.

Assume that $a < b$.

Since X is an interval and $a \in X$, $b \in X$, therefore $[a, b] \subset X$.

Now f is defined and derivable on $[a, b]$. If r be any real number between p and q, then by theorem 2, there exists a real number k between a and b such that $f'(k) = r$, that is $r \in Y$. Thus we find that if p and q are in Y, then every number between p and q is in Y, and this means that Y is an interval.

- If Y does not contain at least two distinct elements, then it is a singleton.
- If f is defined and differentiable on $[a, b]$ and $f'(x) \neq 0$ for any $x \in]a, b[$ then $f'(x)$, retains the same sign, positive or negative in $]a, b[$ *i.e.*, $f(x)$ is either positive or negative for all values of $x \in]a, b[$.

Solved Examples

1. *Prove that the function $f(x) = |x| + |x-1|$ is not differentiable at $x = 0$ and $x = 1$.*

SOLUTION. Here, we observe that

(i) $|x| = -x$ and $|x-1| = 1-x$ when $x < 0$.

(ii) $|x| = x$ and $|x-1| = 1-x$ when $0 \le x \le 1$.

(iii) $|x| = x$ and $|x-1| = x-1$ when $x > 1$.

Hence, the given function can be rewritten as

$$f(x) = \begin{cases} -x+1-x = 1-2x, & x < 0 \\ x+1-x = 1, & 0 \le x \le 1 \\ x+x-1 = 2x-1, & x > 1 \end{cases}$$

Now, firstly we check the differentiability of $f(x)$ at $x = 0$.

We have $Rf'(0) = \lim_{h \to 0} \frac{f(0+h) - f(0)}{h}$

$$= \lim_{h \to 0} \frac{f(h) - f(0)}{h}$$

$$= \lim_{h \to 0} \frac{1-1}{h} = 0$$

and $Lf'(0) = \lim_{h \to 0} \frac{f(0-h) - f(0)}{-h}$

$$= \lim_{h \to 0} \frac{f(-h) - f(0)}{-h}$$

$$= \lim_{h \to 0} \frac{1 - 2(-h) - 1}{-h}$$

$$= \lim_{h \to 0} \frac{2h}{-h} = -2$$

Thus $Rf'(0) \neq Lf'(0)$ Therefore, the given function is not differentiable at $x = 0$.

Now, we check the differentiability of $f(x)$ at $x=1$.

We have

$$Rf'(1) = \lim_{h\to 0}\frac{f(1+h)-f(1)}{h}$$

$$= \lim_{h\to 0}\frac{[2(1+h)-1]-1}{h}$$

$$= \lim_{h\to 0}\frac{2+2h-2}{h} = 2$$

and $Lf'(1) = \lim_{h\to 0}\frac{f(1-h)-f(1)}{-h}$

$$= \lim_{h\to 0}\frac{1-1}{h} = 0$$

Thus $Rf'(1) \neq Lf'(1)$. Therefore, the given function is not differentiable at $x=1$.

2. *Prove that the function $f(x) = |x|$ is continuous at $x = 0$, but not differentiable at $x = 0$, where $|x|$ is the absolute value of x.*

SOLUTION. Firstly, we check the continuity of the function $f(x)$ at $x = 0$.

We have

$$f(0) = |0| = 0$$

$$f(0+0) = \lim_{h\to 0} f(0+h) = \lim_{h\to 0} f(h)$$

$$= \lim_{h\to 0} |h| = \lim_{h\to 0} h = 0$$

and

$$f(0-0) = \lim_{h\to 0} f(0-h) = \lim_{h\to 0} f(-h)$$

$$= \lim_{h\to 0} |-h| = \lim_{h\to 0} h = 0$$

$$f(0+0) = f(0) = f(0-0)$$

Hence, $f(x)$ is continuous at $x = 0$.

Now, we check the differentiability of the function $f(x)$ at $x = 0$.

We have, $Rf'(0) = \lim_{h\to 0}\frac{f(0+h)-f(0)}{h}$

$$= \lim_{h\to 0}\frac{f(h)-f(0)}{h}$$

$$= \lim_{h\to 0}\frac{|h|-0}{h} = 1$$

and $Lf'(0) = \lim_{h\to 0}\frac{f(0-h)-f(0)}{-h}$

$$= \lim_{h\to 0}\frac{f(-h)-f(0)}{-h}$$

$$= \lim_{h\to 0}\frac{|-h|-0}{-h} = \lim_{h\to 0}\frac{h}{-h} = -1$$

$\Rightarrow Rf'(0) \neq Lf'(0)$

Hence, the function $f(x)$ is not differentiable at $x = 0$.

3. *Let the function f(x) satisfy the condition*

(i) $f(x+y) = f(x)\,f(y)\ \forall x,y$

(ii) $f(x)=1+x.g(x)$ where $\lim_{x\to 0} g(x)=1$

Show that the derivative $f'(x)$ exist and equal to $f(x)$ for all x.

SOLUTION. From condition (i), we have

$$f(x+\delta x) = f(x).f(\delta x)$$

Then

$$f(x+\delta x) - f(x) = f(x)f(\delta x) - f(x)$$

$$\Rightarrow \frac{f(x+\delta x)-f(x)}{\delta x} = \frac{f(x)[f(\delta x)-1]}{\delta x}$$

$$= \frac{f(x)\delta x\, g(\delta x)}{\delta x}$$

[By (ii)]

$$= f(x)g(\delta x)$$

$$\therefore \lim_{\delta x\to 0}\frac{f(x+\delta x)-f(x)}{\delta x} = \lim_{\delta x\to 0} f(x)g(\delta x) = f(x).1$$

$$\therefore f'(x) = f(x)$$

4. *If $f(x)$ be an even function and $f'(0)$ exists, then find the value of $f'(0)$.*

SOLUTION. Since $f(x)$ is an even function so $f(-x) = f(x)\ \forall x$

$f'(0)$ exist $\Rightarrow Rf'(0) = Lf'(0) = f'(0)$

Now $f'(0) = Rf'(0)$

$$= \lim_{h\to 0}\frac{f(h)-f(0)}{h}, h>0$$

$$= \lim_{h\to 0}\frac{f(-h)-f(0)}{h}$$

$[\because f(-x) = f(x)]$

$$= -\lim_{h\to 0}\frac{f(-h)-f(0)}{-h}$$

$$= -Lf'(0)$$

$$= -f'(0)$$

$$\Rightarrow 2f'(0) = 0 \Rightarrow f'(0) = 0$$

5. *Show that the function*

$$f(x) = \begin{cases} x\tan^{-1}\left(\frac{1}{x}\right) & , \text{ for } x \neq 0 \\ 0 & , \text{ for } x = 0 \end{cases}$$

is not differentiable at $x = 0$.

SOLUTION. Here

$$Rf'(0) = \lim_{h\to 0} \frac{f(0+h)-f(0)}{h}$$

$$= \lim_{h\to 0} \frac{f(h)-f(0)}{0}$$

$$= \lim_{h\to 0} \frac{h.\tan^{-1}\frac{1}{h} - 0}{h}$$

$$= \lim_{h\to 0} \tan^{-1}\frac{1}{h} = \tan^{-1}\infty = \frac{\pi}{2}$$

and $$Lf'(0) = \lim_{h\to 0} \frac{f(0-h)-f(0)}{-h}$$

$$= \lim_{h\to 0} \frac{f(-h)-f(0)}{-h}$$

$$= \lim_{h\to 0} \frac{-h\tan^{-1}\left(-\frac{1}{h}\right)}{-h}$$

$$= \lim_{h\to 0} \tan^{-1}\left(-\frac{1}{h}\right)$$

$$= -\tan^{-1}\infty = -\frac{\pi}{2}$$

$\Rightarrow Rf'(0) \neq Lf'(0)$

Hence, $f(x)$ is not differentiable at $x = 0$.

6. *Test the continuity and differentiability of the following function in* $-\infty < x < \infty$

$$f(x) = \begin{cases} 1 & \text{if } -\infty < x < 0 \\ 1 + \sin x & \text{if } 0 \le x < \frac{\pi}{2} \\ 2 + \left(x - \frac{\pi}{2}\right)^2 & \text{if } \frac{\pi}{2} \le x < \infty \end{cases}$$

SOLUTION. Firstly, we check the continuity and differentiability at $x = 0$.

(i) *Continuity of* $f(x)$ *at* $x = 0$.

$$f(0) = 1 + \sin 0 = 1$$

$$f(0+0) = \lim_{h\to 0} f(0+h)$$

$$= \lim_{h\to 0} f(h)$$

$$= \lim_{h\to 0} (1+\sin h) = 1$$

$$f(0-0) = \lim_{h\to 0} f(0-h)$$

$$= \lim_{h\to 0} f(-h) = \lim_{h\to 0} 1 = 1$$

$$\Rightarrow f(0+0) = f(0) = f(0-0)$$

Hence, $f(x)$ is continuous at $x = 0$.

(ii) *Differentiability of* $f(x)$ *at* $x = 0$.

$$Rf'(0) = \lim_{h\to 0} \frac{f(0+h)-f(0)}{h}$$

$$= \lim_{h\to 0} \frac{f(h)-f(0)}{h}$$

$$= \lim_{h\to 0} \frac{(1+\sin h)-(1+\sin 0)}{h}$$

$$= \lim_{h\to 0} \frac{\sin h}{h} = 1$$

and $$Lf'(0) = \lim_{h\to 0} \frac{f(0-h)-f(0)}{-h}$$

$$= \lim_{h\to 0} \frac{f(-h)-f(0)}{-h}$$

$$= \lim_{h\to 0} \frac{1-(1+\sin 0)}{-h}$$

$$= \lim_{h\to 0} \frac{0}{-h} = \lim_{h\to 0} 0 = 0$$

$\Rightarrow Rf'(0) \neq Lf'(0)$

Hence, $f(x)$ is not differentiable at $x = 0$.

Now, we shall check the continuity and differentiability at $x = \frac{\pi}{2}$.

(iii) *Continuity of* $f(x)$ *at* $x = \frac{\pi}{2}$

We have

$$f\left(\frac{\pi}{2}\right) = 2 + \left(\frac{\pi}{2} - \frac{\pi}{2}\right)^2 = 2$$

$$f\left(\frac{\pi}{2}+0\right) = \lim_{h\to 0} f\left(\frac{\pi}{2}+h\right)$$

$$= \lim_{h\to 0} \left[2\left\{\left(\frac{1}{2}\pi + h\right) - \frac{1}{2}\pi\right\}^2\right]$$

$$= \lim_{h\to 0} (2+h^2) = 2$$

and $f\left(\frac{\pi}{2}-0\right) = \lim_{h\to 0} f\left(\frac{\pi}{2}-h\right)$

$= \lim_{h\to 0}\left[1+\sin\left(\frac{\pi}{2}-h\right)\right]$

$= \lim_{h\to 0}[1+\cos h] = 1+1 = 2$

$\Rightarrow f\left(\frac{\pi}{2}+0\right) = f\left(\frac{\pi}{2}\right) = f\left(\frac{\pi}{2}-0\right)$

Hence, $f(x)$ is continuous at $x = \frac{\pi}{2}$.

(iv) *Differentiability of f(x) at* $x = \frac{\pi}{2}$

$$Rf'\left(\frac{\pi}{2}\right) = \lim_{h\to 0}\frac{f\left(\frac{\pi}{2}+h\right)-f\left(\frac{\pi}{2}\right)}{h}$$

$$= \lim_{h\to 0}\frac{\left\{\left[2+\left\{\frac{\pi}{2}+h-\frac{\pi}{2}\right\}^2\right] - \left[2+\left(\frac{\pi}{2}-\frac{\pi}{2}\right)^2\right]\right\}}{h}$$

$$= \lim_{h\to 0}\frac{2+h^2-2}{h} = \lim_{h\to 0} h = 0$$

$$Lf'\left(\frac{\pi}{2}\right) = \lim_{h\to 0}\frac{f\left(\frac{\pi}{2}-h\right)-f\left(\frac{\pi}{2}\right)}{-h}$$

$$= \lim_{h\to 0}\frac{1+\sin\left(\frac{\pi}{2}-h\right)-2}{-h}$$

$$= \lim_{h\to 0}\frac{-1+\cos h}{-h}$$

$$= \lim_{h\to 0}\frac{1-\cos h}{h}$$

$$= \lim_{h\to 0}\frac{2\sin^2(h/2)}{h}$$

$$= \lim_{h\to 0}\left[\frac{\sin h/2}{h/2}.\sin h/2\right]$$

$$= \lim_{h\to 0}\left[\frac{\sin h/2}{h/2}\right].\lim_{h\to 0}[\sin h/2]$$

$= 1\times 0 = 0$

Therefore, $Rf'\left(\frac{\pi}{2}\right) = Lf'\left(\frac{\pi}{2}\right)$

$\Rightarrow f(x)$ is differentiable at $x = \frac{\pi}{2}$.

7. *If* $f(x) = \begin{cases} x^2\sin\frac{1}{x} & , \text{ if } x \neq 0 \\ 0 & , \text{ if } x = 0 \end{cases}$

then, show that f(x) is continuous and differentiable everywhere.

SOLUTION. We have

$f(0+0) = \lim_{h\to 0} f(0+h)$

$= \lim_{h\to 0}(0+h)^2\sin\frac{1}{0+h}$

$= \lim_{h\to 0} h^2\sin\frac{1}{h} = 0$

$f(0-0) = \lim_{h\to 0} f(0-h)$

$= \lim_{h\to 0}(0-h)^2\sin\frac{1}{0-h}$

$= -\lim_{h\to 0} h^2\sin\frac{1}{h} = 0$

and $f(0) = 0$

$\Rightarrow f(0+0) = f(0) = (0-0)$

Hence, the function is continuous at $x = 0$.

Now $Rf'(0) = \lim_{h\to 0}\frac{f(0+h)-f(0)}{h}$

$= \lim_{h\to 0}\frac{f(h)-f(0)}{h}$

$= \lim_{h\to 0}\frac{h^2\sin\frac{1}{h}-0}{h}$

$= \lim_{h\to 0} h\sin\frac{1}{h} = 0$

and $Lf'(0) = \lim_{h\to 0}\frac{f(0-h)-f(0)}{-h}$

$= \lim_{h\to 0}\frac{f(-h)-f(0)}{-h}$

$= \lim_{h\to 0}\frac{(-h)^2\sin\left(-\frac{1}{h}\right)-0}{-h}$

$= \lim_{h\to 0} h\sin\frac{1}{h} = 0$

$\Rightarrow Rf'(0) = Lf'(0)$

Hence, $f(x)$ is differentiable at $x = 0$.

8. *Draw the graph of the function $y=|x-1|+|x-2|$ in the interval [0, 3] and discuss the continuity and differentiability of the function in this interval.*

SOLUTION. Here, we observe that

$y = 1-x+2-x = 3-2x$ when $x \le 1$

$= x-1+2-x = 1$ when $1 \le x \le 2$

$= x-1+x-2 = 2x-3$ when $x \ge 2$

Hence, the graph consists of the segments of the three straight lines $y = 3-2x$, $y = 1$ and $y = 2x-3$ corresponding to the intervals [0, 1], [1, 2], [2, 3] respectively.

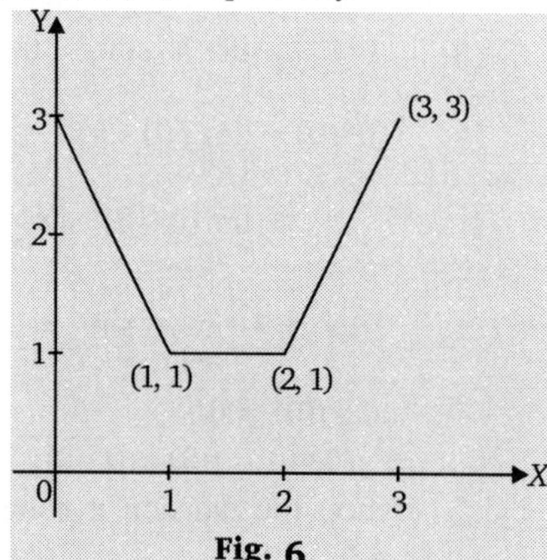

Fig. 6

The graph shows that the function is continuous throughout the interval and differentiable at all points of the interval [0, 3] except possibly at $x = 1$ and at $x = 2$.

(i) *Differentiability of f(x) at x = 1.*

Here, $$Rf'(1) = \lim_{h\to 0}\frac{f(1+h)-f(1)}{h} = \lim_{h\to 0}\frac{1-1}{h} = 0$$

and $$Lf'(1) = \lim_{h\to 0}\frac{f(1-h)-f(1)}{-h} = \lim_{h\to 0}\frac{3-2(1-h)-1}{-h} = -2$$

$\Rightarrow Rf'(1) \ne Lf'(1)$

$\Rightarrow f(x)$ is not differentiable at $x = 2$

(ii) *Differentiability of f(x) at x = 2*

$$Rf'(2) = \lim_{h\to 0}\frac{f(2+h)-f(2)}{h} = \lim_{h\to 0}\frac{2(2+h)-3-1}{h} = 2$$

$$Lf'(2) = \lim_{h\to 0}\frac{f(2-h)-f(2)}{h} = \lim_{h\to 0}\frac{1-1}{h} = 0$$

$\Rightarrow Rf'(2) \ne Lf'(2)$.

Hence, $f(x)$ is not differentiable at $x = 2$.

9. *Show that the function*

$$f(x) = \begin{cases} x\left[\dfrac{e^{1/x}-e^{-1/x}}{e^{1/x}+e^{-1/x}}\right], & if\ x \ne 0 \\ 0, & if\ x = 0 \end{cases}$$

is continuous but not differentiable at x = 0.

SOLUTION. (i) *Continuity of f(x) at x = 0.*

We have

$$\text{RHL} = f(0+0) = \lim_{h\to 0} f(0+h) = \lim_{h\to 0} f(h) = \lim_{h\to 0} h\left[\frac{e^{1/h}-e^{-1/h}}{e^{1/h}+e^{-1/h}}\right] = \lim_{h\to 0} h\left[\frac{1-e^{-2/h}}{1+e^{-2/h}}\right] = 0\times\frac{1-0}{1+0} = 0\times 1 = 0$$

and

$$\text{LHL} = f(0-0) = \lim_{h\to 0} f(0-h) = \lim_{h\to 0} f(-h) = \lim_{h\to 0} -h\left[\frac{e^{1/-h}-e^{-1/-h}}{e^{1/-h}+e^{-1/-h}}\right] = \lim_{h\to 0} -h\left[\frac{e^{-2/h}-1}{e^{-2/h}+1}\right] = 0\times\frac{0-1}{0+1} = 0$$

$\Rightarrow f(0+0) = f(0-0) = f(0)$.

Hence, f is continuous at $x = 0$.

(ii) *Differentiability of f(x) at x = 0.*

Here, we have

$$Rf'(0) = \lim_{h\to 0}\frac{f(0+h)-f(0)}{h} = \lim_{h\to 0}\frac{f(h)-f(0)}{h}$$

$$= \lim_{h\to 0} \frac{\left[h\dfrac{e^{1/h}-e^{-1/h}}{e^{1/h}+e^{-1/h}} - 0\right]}{h}$$

$$= \lim_{h\to 0} \frac{1-e^{-2/h}}{1+e^{-2/h}} = \frac{1-0}{1+0} = 1$$

and $Lf'(0) = \lim_{h\to 0} \dfrac{f(0-h)-f(0)}{-h}$

$$= \lim_{h\to 0} \frac{f(-h)-f(0)}{-h}$$

$$= \lim_{h\to 0} \frac{\left[(-h)\dfrac{e^{-1/h}-e^{1/h}}{e^{-1/h}+e^{1/h}} - 0\right]}{-h}$$

$$= \lim_{h\to 0} \frac{e^{-2/h}-1}{e^{2/h}+1} = \frac{0-1}{0+1} = -1$$

$Rf'(0) \neq Lf'(0)$

Hence, the function $f(x)$ is not differentiable at $x=0$.

10. *Let* $f(x) = \begin{cases} e^{-1/x^2} \sin\dfrac{1}{x} & , \text{ when } x \neq 0 \\ 0 & , \text{ when } x = 0 \end{cases}$

Show that at every point, $f(x)$ is differentiable and f' is continuous at $x = 0$.

SOLUTION. (i) *Differentiability at $x = 0$.*

Here, we have

$$Rf'(0) = \lim_{h\to 0} \frac{e^{-1/h^2}\sin\dfrac{1}{h} - 0}{h}$$

$$= \lim_{h\to 0} \frac{\sin\dfrac{1}{h}}{he^{1/h^2}}$$

$$= \lim_{h\to 0} \frac{\sin 1/h}{h\left[1+\dfrac{1}{h^2}+\dfrac{1}{2!}\dfrac{1}{h^4}+\right]}$$

$$= \lim_{h\to 0} \frac{\sin\dfrac{1}{h}}{h+\dfrac{1}{h}+\dfrac{1}{2!}\dfrac{1}{h^3}+\ldots}$$

$$= \frac{\text{a finite quantity lying between } -1 \text{ and } 1}{\infty} = 0$$

Similarly, $Lf'(0)=0$

Hence, the function $f(x)$ is differentiable at $x = 0$ and $f'(0) = 0$.

(ii) *Continuity of f'*

$$f'(x) = \left(\frac{2}{x^3}\right)e^{-1/x^2}\sin\frac{1}{x} - \left(\frac{1}{x^2}\right)e^{-1/x^2}\cos(1/x)$$

$$= \left\{\left(\frac{2}{x}\right)\sin\frac{1}{x} - \cos\left(\frac{1}{x}\right)\right\}\left(\frac{1}{x^2}\right)\left(\frac{1}{e^{1/x^2}}\right) \quad \ldots(1)$$

Now $f'(0+0) = \lim_{h\to 0} f'(0+h)$

$$= \lim_{h\to 0}\left(\frac{2}{h}\sin\frac{1}{h} - \cos\frac{1}{h}\right).\frac{1}{h^2 e^{1/h^2}}$$

$$= \lim_{h\to 0}\left[\frac{2\sin(1/h)}{h^3 e^{1/h^2}} - \frac{\cos(1/h)}{h^2 e^{1/h^2}}\right]$$

$$= \lim_{h\to 0}\left[\frac{2\sin(1/h)}{h^3\left[1+\dfrac{1}{h^2}+\dfrac{1}{2!\,h^4}+\ldots\right]} - \frac{\cos(1/h)}{h^2\left[1+\dfrac{1}{h^2}+\dfrac{1}{2!\,h^4}+\ldots\right]}\right]$$

$$= \frac{\text{A finite quantity}}{\infty} - \frac{\text{A finite quantity}}{\infty}$$

$= 0$

Similarly, $f'(0-0) = 0$

Hence f' is continuous at $x = 0$.

11. *Let* $f(x) = \begin{cases} -x-1 & , \quad -2 \le x \le 0 \\ x-1 & , \quad 0 < x \le 2 \end{cases}$

and $g(x) = f(|x|) + |f(x)|$.

Test the differentiability of $g(x)$ in the inteval]–2, 2[.

SOLUTION. Here, we have

$|x| = -x$, when $-2 \le x \le 0$

$|x| = x$, when $0 < x \le 2$

Therefore,

$$f(|x|) = \begin{cases} x-1 & , \quad -2 \le x \le 0 \\ -x-1 & , \quad 0 < x \le 2 \end{cases}$$

and $|f(x)| = \begin{cases} 1 & , \quad -2 \le x \le 0 \\ -x+1 & , \quad 0 < x \le 1 \\ x-1 & , \quad 1 < x \le 2 \end{cases}$

so $g(x) = f(|x|) + |f(x)|$

$$= \begin{cases} -x & , \quad -2 \le x \le 0 \\ 0 & , \quad 0 < x \le 1 \\ 2x-2 & , \quad 1 < x \le 2 \end{cases}$$

It is obvious that $g(x)$ is differentiable $\forall\, x \in\,]-2, 2[$ except possibly at $x = 0$ and 1.

At $x = 0$.

$$Rg'(0) = \lim_{h\to 0} \frac{g(0+h)-g(0)}{h}$$

$$= \lim_{h\to 0} \frac{g(h)-g(0)}{h} = \lim_{h\to 0} \frac{0-0}{h} = 0$$

and

$$Lg'(0) = \lim_{h\to 0} \frac{g(0-h)-g(0)}{-h}$$

$$= \lim_{h\to 0} \frac{g(-h)-g(0)}{-h}$$

$$= \lim_{h\to 0} \frac{h-0}{-h} = -1$$

Thus $Rg'(0) \ne Lg'(0)$

Hence, $g(x)$ is not differentiable at $x = 0$.

At $x = 1$.

$$Rg'(1) = \lim_{h\to 0} \frac{g(1+h)-g(1)}{h}$$

$$= \lim_{h\to 0} \frac{2(1+h)-2-0}{h} = 2$$

$$Lg'(1) = \lim_{h\to 0} \frac{g(1-h)-g(1)}{-h}$$

$$= \lim_{h\to 0} \frac{0-0}{-h} = 0$$

Thus, $Rg'(1) \ne Lg'(1)$. Therefore $g(x)$ is not differentiable at $x = 1$.

12. *Let* $f(x) = \begin{cases} \dfrac{x}{1+e^{1/x}} & , \text{ if } \quad x \ne 0 \\ 0 & , \text{ if } \quad x = 0 \end{cases}$

Show that f is continuous at x= 0, but f′(0) does not exist.

SOLUTION. We have

$$\text{LHL} = f(0-0) = \lim_{h\to 0} f(0-h)$$

$$= \lim_{h\to 0} f(-h), h > 0$$

$$= \lim_{h\to 0} \frac{-h}{1+e^{-1/h}} = \frac{0}{1+0} = 0$$

$$\text{RHL} = f(0+0) = \lim_{h\to 0} f(0+h)$$

$$= \lim_{h\to 0} f(h), h > 0$$

$$= \lim_{h\to 0} \frac{h}{1+e^{1/h}} = 0.\frac{0}{1+\infty} = 0.0 = 0$$

and $f(0) = 0$ (given)

Therefore $f(0+0) = f(0) = f(0-0)$

Hence, $f(x)$ is continuous at $x = 0$.

Now $Rf'(0) = \lim_{h\to 0} \dfrac{f(0+h)-f(0)}{h}$

$$= \lim_{h\to 0} \frac{f(h)-f(0)}{h}, h > 0$$

$$= \lim_{h\to 0} \frac{\frac{h}{1+e^{1/h}} - 0}{h}$$

$$= \lim_{h\to 0} \frac{1}{1+e^{1/h}} = \frac{1}{1+\infty} = 0$$

and $Lf'(0) = \lim_{h\to 0} \dfrac{f(0-h)-f(0)}{-h}$

$$= \lim_{h\to 0} \frac{f(-h)-f(0)}{-h}$$

$$= \lim_{h\to 0} \frac{\frac{-h}{1+e^{1/h}} - 0}{-h} = \lim_{h\to 0} \frac{1}{1+e^{-1/h}}$$

$$= \frac{1}{1+e^{-\infty}} = \frac{1}{1+0} = 1$$

$\Rightarrow \quad Rf'(0) \ne Lf'(0)$

Hence, $f'(0)$ does not exist.

13. *Show that the function* $f(x) = x|x|$ *is differentiable at the origin.*

PROOF. Here, we have

$$Rf'(0) = \lim_{h\to 0} \frac{f(0+h)-f(0)}{h}$$

$$= \lim_{h\to 0} \frac{f(h)-f(0)}{h}, \; h > 0$$

$$= \lim_{h\to 0} \frac{h|h|-0}{h} = \lim_{h\to 0} h = 0$$

and $Lf'(0) = \lim_{h\to 0} \dfrac{f(0-h)-f(0)}{-h}$

$$= \lim_{h\to 0} \frac{f(-h)-f(0)}{-h}$$

$$= \lim_{h\to 0} \frac{-h|h|-0}{-h} = \lim_{h\to 0} h = 0$$

$\Rightarrow Rf'(0) = Lf'(0)$

Hence, $f(x)$ is differentiable at $x = 0$.

14. *Let* $f\left(\frac{x+y}{2}\right) = \frac{f(x)+f(y)}{2} \forall x$ *and* y.

If $f'(0)$ *exists and equal* -1 *and* $f(0) = 1$, *find* $f(3)$.

SOLUTION. We have

$$f\left(\frac{x+y}{2}\right) = \frac{f(x)+f(y)}{2}$$

$$\Rightarrow f\left(\frac{x+0}{2}\right) = \frac{f(x)+f(0)}{2}$$

$$\Rightarrow \quad f\left(\frac{x}{2}\right) = \frac{1}{2}[f(x)+f(0)]$$

$$= \frac{1}{2}[f(x)+1]$$

$$\Rightarrow \quad f(x) = 2f\left(\frac{x}{2}\right) - 1 \qquad ...(1)$$

Now $f'(x) = \lim_{h\to 0} \frac{f(x+h)-f(x)}{h}$

$$= \lim_{h\to 0} \frac{f\left(\frac{2x+2h}{2}\right) - f(x)}{h}$$

$$= \lim_{h\to 0} \frac{\frac{1}{2}[f(2x)+f(2h)] - f(x)}{h}$$

$$= \lim_{h\to 0} \frac{f(h)-1}{h} \qquad \text{[Using (1)]}$$

$$= \lim_{h\to 0} \frac{f(0+h)-f(0)}{h}$$

$$= f'(0) = -1 \qquad \text{[Given]}$$

$$\Rightarrow f(x) = -x + c \qquad ...(2)$$

Putting $x = 0$ in (2), we have $c = f(0) = 1$

Therefore, $f(3) = -3 + 1 = -2$

15. *If f is differentiable at a point c then show that* $|f|$ *is also differentiable at c provided* $f(c) \neq 0$.

SOLUTION. Since f is differentiable at $c \Rightarrow f$ is continuous at c.

If $f(c) \neq 0$ then either $f(c) > 0$ or $f(c) < 0$.

If $f(c) > 0$ then there exists $\delta_1 > 0$ such that $f(x) > 0 \ \forall x \in]c - \delta_1, c + \delta_1[$

If $f(c) < 0$ then there exists $\delta_2 > 0$ such that $f(x) < 0 \ \forall x \in]c - \delta_2, c + \delta_2[$.

Therefore, we have

$$f(x) > 0 \ \forall x \in]c - \delta_1, c + \delta_1[$$

$$f(x) < 0 \ \forall x \in]c - \delta_2, c + \delta_2[$$

$$\Rightarrow |f(x)| = \begin{cases} f(x); \text{if } x \in]c-\delta_1, c+\delta_1[\\ -f(x); \text{if } x \in]c-\delta_2, c+\delta_2[\end{cases}$$

Now since f is given to be differentiable at $x = c$.

Hence, from above $|f|$ is also differentiable at $x = c$.

- The above result does not hold if $f(c) = 0$.

Exercise-5.5

1. Let $f(x) = \begin{cases} -1 & , \ -2 \le x \le 0 \\ x-1 & , \ 0 < x \le 2 \end{cases}$

Test the differentiability of $f(x)$.

2. Find $f'(1)$ if $f(x) = \begin{cases} \dfrac{x-1}{2x^2-7x+5}, \text{when } x \neq 1 \\ -1/3, \text{when } x = 1 \end{cases}$

3. Investigate the following function from the point of view of its differentiability. Does the differential coefficient of the function exist at $x = 0$ and $x = 1$?

$$f(x) = \begin{cases} -x & , \text{ if } x < 0 \\ x^2 & , \text{ if } 0 \le x \le 1 \\ x^3 - x + 1 & , \text{ if } x > 1 \end{cases}$$

4. Determine the set of all points where the function $f(x) = \dfrac{x}{1+|x|}$ is differentiable.

5. Show that $f(x) = |x - 1|$, $0 \le x \le 2$ is not differentiable at $x = 1$.

6. Show that $f(x) = \begin{cases} -x & , \text{ when } x < 0 \\ x & , \text{ when } x \ge 0 \end{cases}$ is not differentiable at $x = 0$.

7. Show that the function

$$f(x) = \begin{cases} 2+x, & \text{if } x \ge 0 \\ 2-x, & \text{if } x < 0 \end{cases}$$

is not differentiable at $x = 0$.

8. Show that the function $f(x) = |x-1| + 2|x-2| + 3|x-3|$ is not differentiable at the point 1, 2 and 3.

9. Show that the function

$$f(x)=\begin{cases} x & , \ 0\le x<1 \\ 2-x & , \ x\ge 1\end{cases}$$

is not differentiable at $x = 1$.

10. The following limits are derivatives of certain functions at a certain point. Determine these functions and points.

(i) $\lim\limits_{x\to 2}\dfrac{\log x-\log 2}{x-2}$ (ii) $\lim\limits_{h\to 0}\dfrac{\sqrt{(a+h)}-\sqrt{a}}{h}$

11. Let $f(x)=x^2\sin(x^{-4/3})$ except when $x=0$ and $f(0)=0$. Prove that $f(x)$ has zero as a derivative at $x=0$.

12. Discuss the differentiability of the functions

$$f(x)=\begin{cases} x^2 & \text{for} \quad x<-2 \\ 4 & \text{for} \quad -2\le x\le 2 \\ x^2 & \text{for} \quad x>2\end{cases}$$

13. Discuss the existence of $f'(x)$ at $x = 0, 1, 2,$ where $f(x)$ is defined as follows:

$$f(x)=\begin{cases} 1+x & \text{for} \quad x\le 0 \\ x & \text{for} \quad 0<x<1 \\ 2-x & \text{for} \quad 1\le x\le 2 \\ 3x-x^2 & \text{for} \quad x>2\end{cases}$$

14. Show that

$$f(x)=\begin{cases} x\left[1+\frac{1}{8}\sin(\log x^2)\right] & \text{, for} \quad x\ne 0 \\ 0 & \text{, for} \quad x=0\end{cases}$$

is not differentiable at $x = 0$.

15. Show that the function

$$f(x)=\begin{cases} x\sin\dfrac{1}{x} & , \quad x\ne 0 \\ 0 & , \quad x=0\end{cases}$$

is not differential at $x = 0$.

16. What do you understand by the derivative of a real valued function at the point $a\in R$? Apply your definition, discuss the differentiability of $f(x) = |x|$, $x\in R$ at $x=0$.

ANSWERS

1. Not differentiable

2. –2/9

3. Not differentiable at $x = 0$, differentiable at $x = 1$

4. Differentiable in $]-\infty, \infty[$

10. (i) $f(x) = \log x$, point is $x=2$ (ii) $f(x)=\sqrt{x}$, point is $a = 2$

12. Not differentiable at $x = -2$ and 2

13. Not differentiable at $x=0, 1, 2$

15. Not differentiable

❑❑❑❑❑❑

Chapter

6

Differentiation

6.1 INTRODUCTION

Let $y = f(x)$ be a function where x is an independent variable and y is dependent variable. Let δx be any increment in the value of independent variable x and δy be the corresponding increment in the value of dependent variable y, then $\frac{\delta y}{\delta x}$ is known as the rate of change of y with respect to x.

Definition. *Derivative of a function f(x) is the limiting value of* $\frac{\delta y}{\delta x}$ *as* $\delta x \to 0$ *provided the limit exist finitely. It is denoted by* $\frac{dy}{dx}$.

Thus, $\frac{dy}{dx} = \lim_{\delta x \to 0} \frac{\delta y}{\delta x} = \lim_{\delta x \to 0} \frac{f(x+\delta x) - f(x)}{\delta x}$, provided the limit exist.

Here, the increments δx and δy can be positive or negative.

- The differential coefficient and instantaneous rate of change are also used for derivative.
- $\frac{dy}{dx}, \frac{d}{dx}(y), y', y_1, \frac{d}{dx}(f(x)), f'(x)$ or $Df(x)$ have the same meaning.
- The derivative of a function $f(x)$ at a point $x = a$ is denoted by $f'(a)$ or $\left[\frac{d}{dx} f(x)\right]_{x=a}$.

6.2 METHOD FOR FINDING THE DERIVATIVE USING FIRST PRINCIPLES

Working Procedure

To find the derivative of a function from the first principles, we use the following steps.

Step 1. First we take the function in the form of $y = f(x)$.

Step 2. Take the small increment δx in x and let corresponding increment in y is δy such that $y + \delta y = f(x + \delta x)$.

Step 3. Find out the increment $\delta y = f(x+\delta x) - f(x)$.

Step 4. Now dividing both sides of $\delta y = f(x+\delta x) - f(x)$ by δx and takes the limit $\delta x \to 0$, we get

$$\frac{dy}{dx} = \lim_{\delta x \to 0} \frac{\delta y}{\delta x} = \lim_{\delta x \to 0} \frac{f(x+\delta x) - f(x)}{\delta x}$$

6.2.1 Differential Coefficient or Derivative of $y = x^n$

Let $y = f(x) = x^n$ so $f(x+\delta x) = (x+\delta x)^n$

$\therefore$ $\frac{dy}{dx} = \lim_{\delta x \to 0} \frac{f(x+\delta x) - f(x)}{\delta x} = \lim_{\delta x \to 0} \frac{(x+\delta x)^n - x^n}{\delta x}$

$$= \lim_{\delta x \to 0} x^n \left[\frac{\left(1+\frac{\delta x}{x}\right)^n - 1}{\delta x} \right] = \lim_{\delta x \to 0} x^n \frac{\left[1+n\frac{\delta x}{x}+\frac{n(n-1)}{2!}\left(\frac{\delta x}{x}\right)^2+\ldots-1\right]}{\delta x}$$

$$= \lim_{\delta x \to 0} x^n \left[\frac{n}{x}+\frac{n(n-1)\delta x}{x^2}+\ldots\right] = x^n \frac{n}{x} = nx^{n-1}$$

So, $\mathbf{\frac{d}{dx}(x^n) = nx^{n-1}}$

6.2.2 Differential Coefficient or Derivative of a Constant Function

Let $y = f(x) = c$, where c is a constant.

So, $f(x+\delta x) = c$

$$\therefore \quad \frac{dy}{dx} = \lim_{\delta x \to 0} \frac{f(x+\delta x)-f(x)}{\delta x} = \lim_{\delta x \to 0} \frac{c-c}{\delta x} = 0.$$

So, $\mathbf{\frac{d(c)}{dx} = 0.}$

Hence, derivative of a constant function is always zero.

6.2.3 Derivative of the Product of a Constant with a Function

The derivate of the product of a constant with a function is equal to the product of constant and the derivative of the function.

Let $y = Cf(x)$, where C is a constant.

So, $$\frac{dy}{dx} = \lim_{\delta x \to 0}\left(\frac{Cf(x+\delta x)-Cf(x)}{\delta x}\right) = C \lim_{\delta x \to 0} \frac{f(x+\delta x)-f(x)}{\delta x} = C\frac{d[f(x)]}{dx}$$

Hence, $\mathbf{\frac{d}{dx}[Cfx] = C\frac{d}{dx}[f(x)].}$

6.2.4 Derivative of sin x

Let $y = f(x) = \sin x$, then $f(x + \delta x) = \sin(x + \delta x)$

So, $$\frac{dy}{dx} = \lim_{\delta x \to 0} \frac{f(x+\delta x)-f(x)}{\delta x} = \lim_{\delta x \to 0} \frac{\sin(x+\delta x)-\sin x}{\delta x}$$

$$= \lim_{\delta x \to 0} \frac{2\cos\left(x+\frac{\delta x}{2}\right)\sin\frac{\delta x}{2}}{\delta x} \quad \left[\because \sin C - \sin D = 2\cos\left(\frac{C+D}{2}\right)\sin\left(\frac{C-D}{2}\right)\right]$$

$$= \lim_{\delta x \to 0} \frac{\cos\left(x+\frac{\delta x}{2}\right)\sin\frac{\delta x}{2}}{\frac{\delta x}{2}} = \lim_{\delta x \to 0} \cos\left(x+\frac{\delta x}{2}\right) \lim_{\delta x \to 0} \frac{\sin\frac{\delta x}{2}}{\frac{\delta x}{2}}$$

$$= \cos x \cdot 1 = \cos x \qquad \left[\text{Since} \lim_{x \to 0} \frac{\sin x}{x} = 1\right]$$

$\therefore \quad \mathbf{\frac{d}{dx}(\sin x) = \cos x}$

6.2.5 Derivative of cos x

Let $y = f(x) = \cos x$, then $f(x+\delta x) = \cos(x+\delta x)$

So $$\frac{dy}{dx} = \lim_{\delta x \to 0} \frac{f(x+\delta x)-f(x)}{\delta x} = \lim_{\delta x \to 0} \frac{\cos(x+\delta x)-\cos x}{\delta x}$$

$$= \lim_{\delta x \to 0} \frac{2\sin\left(x + \frac{\delta x}{2}\right)\sin\left(-\frac{\delta x}{2}\right)}{\delta x}$$

$$\left[\text{Since } \cos C - \cos D = \sin\left(\frac{C+D}{2}\right)\sin\left(\frac{D-C}{2}\right)\right]$$

$$= \lim_{\delta x \to 0}\left[\frac{-\sin\left(x + \frac{\delta x}{2}\right)\sin\left(\frac{\delta x}{2}\right)}{\frac{\delta x}{2}}\right]$$

$$= \lim_{\delta x \to 0}\left[-\sin\left(x + \frac{\delta x}{2}\right)\right] \lim_{\delta x \to 0} \frac{\sin\frac{\delta x}{2}}{\frac{\delta x}{2}} = -\sin x \cdot 1 = -\sin x$$

Hence, $\boldsymbol{\frac{d}{dx}(\cos x) = -\sin x}$

6.2.6 DERIVATIVE OF tan x

Let $y = f(x) = \tan x$, then $f(x + \delta x) = \tan(x + \delta x)$

So, $$\frac{dy}{dx} = \lim_{\delta x \to 0} \frac{f(x + \delta x) - f(x)}{\delta x}$$

$$= \lim_{\delta x \to 0} \frac{\tan(x + \delta x) - \tan x}{\delta x} = \lim_{\delta x \to 0}\left[\frac{\frac{\sin(x + \delta x)}{\cos(x + \delta x)} - \frac{\sin x}{\cos x}}{\delta x}\right]$$

$$= \lim_{\delta x \to 0}\left[\frac{\sin(x + \delta x)\cos x - \cos(x + \delta x)\sin x}{\delta x \cos(x + \delta x)\cos x}\right]$$

$$= \lim_{\delta x \to 0} \frac{\sin(x + \delta x - x)}{\cos(x + \delta x)\cos x . \delta x} \quad [\text{Since} \sin A \cos B - \cos A \sin B = \sin(A - B)]$$

$$= \lim_{\delta x \to 0}\left(\frac{\sin \delta x}{\delta x}\right)\frac{1}{\cos(x + \delta x)\cos x}$$

$$= \lim_{\delta x \to 0}\left(\frac{\sin \delta x}{\delta x}\right)\lim_{\delta x \to 0} \frac{1}{\cos(x + \delta x)\cos x} = 1\frac{1}{\cos^2 x} = \sec^2 x$$

Hence, $\boldsymbol{\frac{d}{dx}(\tan x) = \sec^2 x}$.

6.2.7 DERIVATIVE OF COT x

Let $y = f(x) = \cot x$, then $f(x + \delta x) = \cot(x + \delta x)$

So, $\frac{dy}{dx} = \lim_{\delta x \to 0} \frac{f(x + \delta x) - f(x)}{\delta x} = \lim_{\delta x \to 0}\left(\frac{\cot(x + \delta x) - \cot x}{\delta x}\right)$.

Proceeding in the same way, we may get

$$\boldsymbol{\frac{d}{dx}(\cot x) = -\operatorname{cosec}^2 x}.$$

6.2.8 DERIVATIVE OF SEC X

Let $y = f(x) = \sec x$ then $f(x + \delta x) = \sec(x + \delta x)$

So, $\frac{dy}{dx} = \lim_{\delta x \to 0} \frac{f(x + \delta x) - f(x)}{\delta x}$

$$= \lim_{\delta x \to 0} \frac{\sec(x+\delta x) - \sec x}{\delta x} = \lim_{\delta x \to 0} \frac{\left(\frac{1}{\cos(x+\delta x)} - \frac{1}{\cos x}\right)}{\delta x}$$

$$= \lim_{\delta x \to 0} \frac{\cos x - \cos(x+\delta x)}{\delta x \cos x \cos(x+\delta x)} = \lim_{\delta x \to 0} \frac{2\sin\left(x+\frac{\delta x}{2}\right)\sin\frac{\delta x}{2}}{\delta x \cos x \cos(x+\delta x)}$$

$$= \lim_{\delta x \to 0} \frac{\sin\left(x+\frac{\delta x}{2}\right)}{\cos x \cos(x+\delta x)} \lim_{\delta x \to 0} \frac{\sin\frac{\delta x}{2}}{\frac{\delta x}{2}} = \frac{\sin x}{\cos^2 x} = \sec x \tan x$$

Hence, $\mathbf{\frac{d}{dx}(\sec x) = \sec x \tan x}$.

6.2.9 DERIVATIVE OF e^x

Let $y = f(x) = e^x$ then $f(x + \delta x) = e^{x + \delta x}$

So, $$\frac{dy}{dx} = \lim_{\delta x \to 0} \frac{f(x+\delta x) - f(x)}{\delta x} = \lim_{\delta x \to 0} \frac{e^{x+\delta x} - e^x}{\delta x}$$

$$= \lim_{\delta x \to 0} \frac{e^x e^{\delta x} - e^x}{\delta x} = \lim_{\delta x \to 0} \frac{e^x[e^{\delta x} - 1]}{\delta x} = \lim_{\delta x \to 0} e^x \left[1 + \frac{(\delta x)}{2!} + \frac{(\delta x)^2}{3!} + \ldots\right]$$

$$= e^x$$

Hence, $\mathbf{\frac{d}{dx}(e^x) = e^x}$.

6.2.10 DERIVATIVE OF $\log_e x$

Let $y = f(x) = \log_e x$, then $f(x+\delta x) = \log_e(x+\delta x)$

So, $$\frac{dy}{dx} = \lim_{\delta x \to 0} \frac{f(x+\delta x) - f(x)}{\delta x} = \lim_{\delta x \to 0} \frac{\log_e(x+\delta x) - \log x}{\delta x}$$

$$= \lim_{\delta x \to 0} \frac{\log_e\left(\frac{x+\delta x}{x}\right)x - \log_e x}{\delta x} = \lim_{\delta x \to 0} \frac{\log_e x\left(1+\frac{\delta x}{x}\right) - \log_e x}{\delta x}$$

$$= \lim_{\delta x \to 0} \frac{\log_e x + \log\left(1+\frac{\delta x}{x}\right) - \log_e x}{\delta x} = \lim_{\delta x \to 0} \frac{\log_e\left(1+\frac{\delta x}{x}\right)}{\delta x}$$

$$= \lim_{\delta x \to 0}\left[\frac{1}{x} - \frac{1}{2}\frac{\delta x}{x^2} + \ldots\right] \qquad \left[\text{Since, } \log(1+x) = x - \frac{x^2}{2} + \frac{x^3}{3} - \ldots\right]$$

$$= \frac{1}{x}$$

Hence, $\mathbf{\frac{d}{dx}(\log_e x) = \frac{1}{x}}$.

6.2.11 DERIVATIVE OF $\log_a x$

Let $y = f(x) = \log_a x$

We know $\log_a x = \log_e x . \log_a e$

So, $\frac{d}{dx}(\log_a x) = \frac{d}{dx}[\log_e x . \log_a e] = \log_a e \frac{d}{dx}[\log_e x] = \log_a e \frac{1}{x}$

Hence, $\mathbf{\frac{d}{dx}(\log_a x) = \frac{1}{x}\log_a e}$.

6.2.12 DERIVATIVE OF a^x

Let $y = f(x) = a^x$ or $f(x) = e^{x\log a}$

then $f(x+\delta x) = e^{(x+\delta x)\log a}$

So, $$\frac{dy}{dx} = \lim_{\delta x\to 0} \frac{e^{(x+\delta x)\log a} - e^{x\log a}}{\delta x}$$

$$= \lim_{\delta x\to 0} \frac{e^{x\log a}\cdot e^{\delta x\log a} - e^{x\log a}}{\delta x} = \lim_{\delta x\to 0} \frac{e^{x\log a}[e^{\delta x\log a} - 1]}{\delta x}$$

$$= \lim_{\delta x\to 0} \frac{e^{x\log a}\left[\dfrac{\delta x\log a}{1!} + \dfrac{(\delta x)^2(\log a)^2}{2!} + \dots\right]}{\delta x} = \lim_{\delta x\to 0} e^{x\log a}\left[\log a + \frac{\delta x(\log a)^2}{2!} + \dots\right]$$

$$= e^{x\log a}\cdot\log a = a^x \log a$$

Hence, $$\boldsymbol{\frac{d}{dx}(a^x) = a^x \cdot \log_e a}.$$

6.3 DERIVATIVE OF THE SUM OF TWO FUNCTIONS

"The derivative of the sum of two functions is equal to the sum of their derivatives."

Let $$y = f(x) = \phi_1(x) + \phi_2(x), \text{ then}$$

$$f(x+\delta x) = \phi_1(x+\delta x) + \phi_2(x+\delta x)$$

So, $$\frac{dy}{dx} = \frac{df(x)}{dx} = \lim_{\delta x\to 0} \frac{f(x+\delta x) - f(x)}{\delta x}$$

$$= \lim_{\delta x\to 0} \frac{\{\phi_1(x+\delta x) + \phi_2(x+\delta x)\} - \{\phi_1(x) + \phi_2(x)\}}{\delta x}$$

$$= \lim_{\delta x\to 0} \frac{\{\phi_1(x+\delta x) - \phi_1(x)\} + \{\phi_2(x+\delta x) - \phi_2(x)\}}{\delta x}$$

$$= \lim_{\delta x\to 0} \frac{\phi_1(x+\delta x) - \phi_1(x)}{\delta x} + \lim_{\delta x\to 0} \frac{\phi_2(x+\delta x) - \phi_2(x)}{\delta x}$$

$$= \frac{d}{dx}\phi_1(x) + \frac{d}{dx}\phi_2(x).$$

Hence, $$\boldsymbol{\frac{d}{dx}\{\phi_1(x) + \phi_2(x)\} = \frac{d}{dx}\phi_1(x) + \frac{d}{dx}\phi_2(x)}.$$

- The above result can be generalized as follows:
$$\frac{d}{dx}[\phi_1(x) + \phi_2(x) + \dots + \phi_n(x)] = \frac{d}{dx}\phi_1(x) + \frac{d}{dx}\phi_2(x) + \dots + \frac{d}{dx}\phi_n(x)$$

6.4 DERIVATIVE OF THE DIFFERENCE OF TWO FUNCTIONS

"The derivative of the difference of two functions is the difference of their derivatives."

Let $$f(x) = \phi_1(x) - \phi_2(x), \text{ then}$$

$$f(x+\delta x) = \phi_1(x+\delta x) - \phi_2(x+\delta x)$$

So, $$\frac{df(x)}{dx} = \lim_{\delta x\to 0} \frac{f(x+\delta x) - f(x)}{\delta x}$$

$$\lim_{\delta x\to 0} \frac{\{\phi_1(x+\delta x) - \phi_2(x+\delta x)\} - \{\phi_1(x) - \phi_2(x)\}}{\delta x}$$

$$= \lim_{\delta x\to 0} \frac{\{\phi_1(x+\delta x) - \phi_1(x)\} - \{(\phi_2(x+\delta x) - \phi_2(x)\}}{\delta x}$$

$$= \lim_{\delta x \to 0} \frac{\phi_1(x+\delta x) - \phi_1(x)}{\delta x} - \lim_{\delta x \to 0} \frac{\phi_2(x+\delta x) - \phi_2(x)}{\delta x}$$

$$= \frac{d}{dx}\phi_1(x) - \frac{d}{dx}\phi_2(x)$$

Hence, $\mathbf{\frac{d}{dx}\{\phi_1(x) - \phi_2(x)\} = \frac{d}{dx}\phi_1(x) - \frac{d}{dx}\phi_2(x)}$.

- The above result can be generalized as follows
  $\frac{d}{dx}\{f_1(x) - f_2(x) - ... - f_n(x)\} = \frac{d}{dx}f_1(x) - \frac{d}{dx}f_2(x) - ... - \frac{d}{dx}f_n(x)$.
- From the above discussion, we have, if $y = f(x) \pm g(x) \pm h(x)...$ then
  $\frac{dy}{dx} = \frac{d[f(x)]}{dx} \pm \frac{d[g(x)]}{dx} \pm \frac{d[h(x)]}{dx} \pm ...$

SUMMARY OF STANDARD DERIVATIVES

	Function	Derivative		Function	Derivative
1.	x^n	nx^{n-1}	**14.**	$\log\lvert\operatorname{cosec} x - \cot x\rvert$	$\operatorname{cosec} x$
2.	e^x	e^x	**15.**	$\sin^{-1} x$	$\frac{1}{\sqrt{1-x^2}}$
3.	$\log\lvert x\rvert$	$1/x$	**16.**	$\cos^{-1} x$	$-1/\sqrt{1-x^2}$
4.	a^x	$a^x \log_e a,\ a > 0,\ a \neq 1$	**17.**	$\tan^{-1} x$	$1/(1+x^2)$
5.	$\cos x$	$-\sin x$	**18.**	$\cot^{-1} x$	$-1/(1+x^2)$
6.	$\sin x$	$\cos x$	**19.**	$\sec^{-1} x$	$1/(x\sqrt{x^2-1})$
7.	$\tan x$	$\sec^2 x$	**20.**	$\operatorname{cosec}^{-1} x$	$-1/(x\sqrt{x^2-1})$
8.	$\cot x$	$-\operatorname{cosec}^2 x$	**21.**	$\sin^{-1}(x/a)$	$1/\sqrt{a^2-x^2}$
9.	$\sec x$	$\sec x \tan x$	**22.**	$\cos^{-1}(x/a)$	$-1/\sqrt{a^2-x^2}$
10.	$\operatorname{cosec} x$	$-\operatorname{cosec} x \cot x$	**23.**	$(1/a)\tan^{-1}(x/a)$	$1/(a^2+x^2)$
11.	$\log\lvert\sin x\rvert$	$\cot x$	**24.**	$(1/a)\cot^{-1}(x/a)$	$-1/(a^2+x^2)$
12.	$-\log\lvert\cos x\rvert$	$\tan x$	**25.**	$(1/a)\sec^{-1}(x/a)$	$1/(x\sqrt{x^2-a^2})$
13.	$\log\lvert\sec x + \tan x\rvert$	$\sec x$	**26.**	$(1/a)\operatorname{cosec}^{-1}(x/a)$	$-1/(x\sqrt{x^2-a^2})$

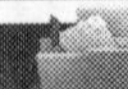

Solved Examples

1. *Find the differential coefficient of $\frac{1}{3x+4}$ from the first principles.*

SOLUTION. Let $y = f(x) = \frac{1}{3x+4}$

$$\Rightarrow y + \delta y = \frac{1}{3(x+\delta x)+4}$$

$$\therefore \quad \delta y = (y+\delta y) - y$$

$$= \frac{1}{3(x+\delta x)+4} - \frac{1}{3x+4}$$

$$= \frac{3x+4-3x-3\delta x-4}{[3(x+\delta x)+4](3x+4)}$$

$$= \frac{-3\delta x}{[3(x+\delta x)+4](3x+4)}$$

$$\therefore \quad \frac{\delta y}{\delta x} = \frac{-3}{[3(x+\delta x)+4](3x+4)}$$

Now,

$$\lim_{\delta x \to 0} \frac{\delta y}{\delta x} = \lim_{\delta x \to 0} \frac{-3}{[3(x+\delta x)+4](3x+4)}$$

$$= \frac{-3}{[3(x+0)+4](3x+4)}$$

$$\therefore \quad \frac{dy}{dx} = \frac{-3}{(3x+4)^2}$$

2. *From the first principles, find the differential coefficient of* $\frac{1}{\sqrt{x}}$.

SOLUTION. Let $\quad y = \frac{1}{\sqrt{x}}$

$$\therefore \quad y + \delta y = \frac{1}{\sqrt{x+\delta x}}$$

$$\therefore \quad \delta y = \frac{1}{\sqrt{x+\delta x}} - \frac{1}{\sqrt{x}}$$

$$= \frac{\sqrt{x} - \sqrt{x+\delta x}}{\sqrt{x}\sqrt{x+\delta x}} \times \frac{\sqrt{x} + \sqrt{x+\delta x}}{\sqrt{x} + \sqrt{x+\delta x}}$$

(Rationalising the numerator)

or $\frac{\delta y}{\delta x}$

$$= \frac{x-(x+\delta x)}{\delta x(\sqrt{x}\sqrt{x+\delta x})(\sqrt{x}+\sqrt{x+\delta x})}$$

$$= \frac{-\delta x}{\delta x(\sqrt{x}\sqrt{x+\delta x})(\sqrt{x}+\sqrt{x+\delta x})}$$

Taking the limit as $\delta x \to 0$. We get

$$\lim_{\delta x \to 0} \frac{\delta y}{\delta x}$$

$$= \lim_{\delta x \to 0} \frac{-1}{(\sqrt{x}\sqrt{x+\delta x})(\sqrt{x}+\sqrt{x+\delta x})}$$

$$\therefore \frac{dy}{dx} = \frac{-1}{(\sqrt{x}\sqrt{x+0})(\sqrt{x}+\sqrt{x+0})}$$

$$= \frac{-1}{x \times 2\sqrt{x}} = \frac{-1}{2x^{3/2}}$$

3. *Differentiate* $\tan^{-1} x^2$ *from first principles.*

SOLUTION. Let $\quad y = \tan^{-1} x^2 \Rightarrow x^2 = \tan y$

Let $\quad t = \tan y$

$$\Rightarrow t + \delta t = \tan(y + \delta y)$$

$$\Rightarrow \quad \delta t = \tan(y+\delta y) - \tan y$$

$$\Rightarrow \frac{\delta t}{\delta y} = \frac{\sin(y+\delta y)\cos y - \sin y \cos(y+\delta y)}{\delta y \cos y . \cos(y+\delta y)}$$

$$= \frac{\sin(y+\delta y - y)}{\delta y \cos y \cos(y+\delta y)}$$

$$\Rightarrow \frac{\delta y}{\delta t} = \frac{\delta y \cos y \cdot \cos(y+\delta y)}{\sin \delta y}$$

Taking limit as $\delta t \to 0$, we get

$$\frac{dy}{dt} = \lim_{\delta t \to 0} \frac{\delta y}{\delta t}$$

$$= \lim_{\delta t \to 0} \left[\frac{\delta y}{\sin \delta y} \cdot \cos(y+\delta y) \cdot \cos y\right]$$

$$= \left[\lim_{\delta x \to 0} \frac{\delta y}{\sin \delta y}\right] \left[\lim_{\delta y \to 0} \cos(y+\delta y)\right] \cos y$$

$$\frac{dy}{dt} = 1 \cdot \cos y \cdot \cos y = \cos^2 y$$

$$\Rightarrow \frac{dy}{dx} = 2x \cos^2 y$$

$$[\because x^2 = t \Rightarrow 2x dx = dt]$$

$$= \frac{2x}{\sec^2 y} = \frac{2x}{1+\tan^2 y} = \frac{2x}{1+(x^2)^2}$$

Hence $\quad \frac{d}{dx}(\tan^{-1} x^2) = \frac{2x}{1+x^4}$.

6.5 DERIVATIVE OF THE PRODUCT TO TWO FUNCTIONS

Let $\quad y = f(x) = \phi_1(x)\phi_2(x)$, then

$$f(x+\delta x) = \phi_1(x+\delta x)\phi_2(x+\delta x).$$

So, $$\frac{dy}{dx} = \frac{df(x)}{dx} = \lim_{\delta x \to 0} \frac{f(x+\delta x) - f(x)}{\delta x}$$

$$= \lim_{\delta x \to 0} \frac{\phi_1(x+\delta x)\phi_2(x+\delta x) - \phi_1(x)\phi_2(x) + \phi_1(x+\delta x)\phi_2(x) - \phi_1(x+\delta x)\phi_2(x)}{\delta x}$$

[Adding and subtracting $\phi_1(x+\delta x)\phi_2(x)$]

$$= \lim_{\delta x \to 0} \frac{\{\phi_1(x+\delta x)\phi_2(x) - \phi_1(x)\phi_2(x)\} + \{\phi_1(x+\delta x)\phi_2(x+\delta x) - \phi_1(x+\delta x)\phi_2(x)\}}{\delta x}$$

$$= \lim_{\delta x \to 0} \frac{\{\phi_1(x+\delta x) - \phi_1(x)\}\phi_2(x) + \phi_1(x+\delta x)\{\phi_2(x+\delta x) - \phi_2(x)\}}{\delta x}$$

$$= \lim_{\delta x \to 0} \frac{\phi_1(x+\delta x) - \phi_1(x)}{\delta x}\phi_2(x) + \lim_{\delta x \to 0} \phi_1(x+\delta x)\left\{\frac{\phi_2(x+\delta x) - \phi_2(x)}{\delta x}\right\}$$

$$= \frac{d\phi_1(x)}{dx}\phi_2(x) + \phi_1(x)\frac{d}{dx}\phi_2(x) = \phi_1(x)\frac{d\phi_2(x)}{dx} + \frac{d\phi_1 x}{dx}\phi_2(x).$$

Thus $\dfrac{d}{dx}\{\phi_1(x)\cdot\phi_2(x)\} = \phi_1(x)\dfrac{d[\phi_2(x)]}{dx} + \dfrac{d}{dx}\phi_1(x)\cdot\phi_2(x).$

Hence, The derivative of the product of two functions

= First function × derivative of the second function

+ derivative of the first function × second function.

6.6 DERIVATIVE OF THE QUOTIENT OF TWO FUNCTIONS

Let $y = f(x) = \dfrac{\phi_1(x)}{\phi_2(x)}$ then $y = f(x+\delta x) = \dfrac{\phi_1(x+\delta x)}{\phi_2(x+\delta x)}$

So, $$\frac{dy}{dx} = \frac{df(x)}{dx} = \lim_{\delta x \to 0} \frac{f(x+\delta x) - f(x)}{\delta x} = \lim_{\delta x \to 0} \frac{\dfrac{\phi_1(x+\delta x)}{\phi_2(x+\delta x)} - \dfrac{\phi_1(x)}{\phi_2(x)}}{\delta x}$$

$$= \lim_{\delta x \to 0} \frac{\dfrac{\phi_1(x+\delta x)}{\phi_2(x+\delta x)} - \dfrac{\phi_1(x)}{\phi_2(x+\delta x)} + \dfrac{\phi_1(x)}{\phi_2(x+\delta x)} - \dfrac{\phi_1(x)}{\phi_2(x)}}{\delta x}$$

$$\left[\text{Adding and subtracting } \frac{\phi_1(x)}{\phi_2(x+\delta x)}\right]$$

$$= \lim_{\delta x \to 0} \frac{\dfrac{1}{\phi_2(x+\delta x)}\{\phi_1(x+\delta x) - \phi_1(x)\} - \dfrac{\phi_1(x)}{\phi_2(x+\delta x)\phi_2(x)}\{\phi_2(x+\delta x) - \phi_2(x)\}}{\delta x}$$

$$= \lim_{\delta x \to 0} \frac{1}{\phi_2(x+\delta x)}\left\{\frac{\phi_1(x+\delta x) - \phi_1(x)}{\delta x}\right\} - \lim_{\delta x \to 0} \frac{\phi_1(x)}{\phi_2(x+\delta x)\phi_2(x)}\left\{\frac{\phi_2(x+\delta x) - \phi_2(x)}{\delta x}\right\}$$

$$= \frac{1}{\phi_2(x)}\frac{d}{dx}\phi_1(x) - \frac{\phi_1(x)}{\phi_2(x)\phi_2(x)}\frac{d}{dx}\phi_2(x)$$

$$= \frac{\phi_2(x)\dfrac{d}{dx}\phi_1(x) - \phi_1(x)\dfrac{d}{dx}\phi_2(x)}{[\phi_2(x)]^2}$$

Thus, $$\frac{d}{dx}\left[\frac{\phi_1(x)}{\phi_2(x)}\right] = \frac{\phi_2(x)\dfrac{d}{dx}\phi_1(x) - \phi_1(x)\dfrac{d}{dx}\phi_2(x)}{[\phi_2(x)]^2}.$$

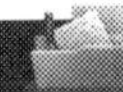

Solved Examples

1. *Find the derivative of the following functions.*

(i) $y = x^6$ (ii) $y = x^3 + 2x$

(iii) $y = -2x^2 + 4x + 6$

SOLUTION. (i) Here, we have $y = x^6$

So, $\frac{dy}{dx} = \frac{d}{dx}(x^6) = 6x^5$

$$\left[\because \frac{d}{dx}(x^n) = nx^{n-1}\right]$$

(ii) Here, we have $y = x^3 + 2x$

$$\frac{dy}{dx} = \frac{d}{dx}(x)^3 + 2\frac{d}{dx}x$$

$$= 3x^2 + 2 \quad \left[\because \frac{d}{dx}(x) = 1\right]$$

(iii) Here, $y = -2x^2 + 4x + 6$

$$\frac{dy}{dx} = -2\frac{d}{dx}(x^2) + 4\frac{d}{dx}(x) + \frac{d}{dx}(6)$$

$$= -4x + 4 \quad \left[\because \frac{d}{dx}(6) = 0\right]$$

2. *Find the differential coefficients or derivatives of the following functions :*

(i) ax^7 (ii) $8e^x$

(iii) $4\log x$ (iv) $5\log_{10} x$

(v) 10^x

SOLUTION. (i) Here, $y = ax^7$.

So, $\frac{dy}{dx} = a\frac{d}{dx}(x^7) = 7ax^6$

(ii) Here, $y = 8e^x$

So, $\frac{dy}{dx} = 8\frac{d}{dx}e^x = 8e^x$.

(iii) Here, $y = 4\log x$.

So, $\frac{dy}{dx} = 4\frac{d}{dx}(\log x) = \frac{4}{x}$

(iv) Here, $y = 5\log_{10} x$

So, $\frac{dy}{dx} = 5\frac{d}{dx}\log_{10} x$

$$= 5\frac{1}{x}\log_{10}(e)$$

(v) Here, $y = 10^x$

So, $\frac{dy}{dx} = \frac{d}{dx}(10^x) = 10^x \log_e 10$

3. *Find the differential coefficient of the following functions.*

(i) $a^x + \log x + a^2 e^x$

(ii) $x^3 \sin x$ (iii) $x^3 \log x$

(iv) $x^{-5} \cot x$ (v) $e^x \cos x$

SOLUTION. (i) $\frac{d}{dx}(a^x + \log x + a^2 e^x)$

$$= \frac{d}{dx}a^x + \frac{d}{dx}\log x + a^2 \frac{d}{dx}e^x$$

$$= a^x \log_e a + \frac{1}{x} + a^2 e^x$$

(ii) $\frac{d}{dx}(x^3 \sin x)$

$$= x^3 \frac{d}{dx}\sin x + \sin x \frac{d}{dx}(x^3)$$

$$= x^3 \cos x + 3x^2 \sin x.$$

(iii) $\frac{d}{dx}(x^3 \log x)$

$$= x^3 \frac{d}{dx}(\log x) + \log x \frac{d}{dx}(x^3)$$

$$= x^3 \frac{1}{x} + 3x^2 \log x$$

$$= x^2 + 3x^2 \log x = x^2.(1 + 3\log x)$$

(iv) $\frac{dy}{dx}(x^{-5} \cot x)$

$$= x^{-5} \frac{d}{dx}\cot x + \frac{d}{dx}(x^{-5})\cot x$$

$$= x^{-5}(-\text{cosec}^2 x) - 5x^{-6} \cot x$$

$$= x^{-5} \text{cosec}^2 x - 5x^{-6} \cot x$$

$$= -x^6(x\,\text{cosec}^2 x + 5\cot x).$$

(v) $\frac{d}{dx}(e^x \cos x)$

$$= e^x \frac{d}{dx}\cos x + \cos x \frac{d}{dx}(e^x)$$

$$= e^x(-\sin x) + e^x \cos x$$

$$= e^x(\cos x - \sin x)$$

4. *Find the differential coefficient or derivative of the following functions.*

(i) $\dfrac{\log x}{x}$ (ii) $\dfrac{\sin x}{x^2}$

(iii) $\tan x$ (iv) $\dfrac{x}{(x+1)^2}$.

SOLUTION. (i) $\dfrac{d}{dx}\left(\dfrac{\log x}{x}\right)$

$$= \frac{x\dfrac{d}{dx}(\log x) - \log x \dfrac{d}{dx}(x)}{x^2}$$

$$= \frac{x\dfrac{1}{x} - \log x \cdot 1}{x^2} = \frac{1 - \log x}{x^2}.$$

(ii) $\dfrac{d}{dx}\left(\dfrac{\sin x}{x^2}\right)$

$$= \frac{x^2 \dfrac{d}{dx}\sin x - \sin x \dfrac{d}{dx}x^2}{x^4}$$

$$= \frac{x^2 \cos x - \sin x 2x}{x^4}$$

$$= \frac{x(x\cos x - 2\sin x)}{x^4}$$

$$= \frac{x\cos x - 2\sin x}{x^3}$$

(iii) $\dfrac{d}{dx}(\tan x)$

$$= \frac{d}{dx}\left(\frac{\sin x}{\cos x}\right)$$

$$= \frac{\cos x \dfrac{d}{dx}\sin x - \sin x \dfrac{d}{dx}\cos x}{\cos^2 x}$$

$$= \frac{\cos^2 x + \sin^2 x}{\cos^2 x} = \frac{1}{\cos^2 x}$$

$$= \sec^2 x$$

$(\because \sin^2 x + \cos^2 x = 1)$

(iv) $\dfrac{d}{dx}\left(\dfrac{x}{(x+1)^2}\right)$

$$= \frac{(x+1)^2 \dfrac{d}{dx}(x) - x\dfrac{d}{dx}(x+1)^2}{(x+1)^4}$$

$$= \frac{(x+1)^2 1 - x.2(x+1)}{(x+1)^4}$$

$$= \frac{(x+1) - 2x}{(x+1)^3} = \frac{1-x}{(x+1)^3}.$$

6.7 DERIVATIVE OF FUNCTIONS OF A FUNCTION (CHAIN RULE)

If y is a function of u, say $y = f(u)$, where u is a function of x, say $u = g(x)$, then y is called a function of a function or a composite function of x.

WORKING PROCEDURE

To find the derivative of a composite function of x, say $y = f[g(x)]$, we use the following steps

STEP 1. Put inner function $g(x) = u$, *i.e.*, $y = f(u)$.

STEP 2. Differentiate with respect to u, find $\dfrac{dy}{du}$.

STEP 3. Differentiate u with respect to x and find $\dfrac{du}{dx}$.

STEP 4. Multiply $\dfrac{dy}{du}$ and $\dfrac{du}{dx}$ and find $\dfrac{dy}{dx} = \dfrac{dy}{du} \cdot \dfrac{du}{dx}$.

STEP 5. Put the value of $u = g(x)$, we get the required derivative.

THEOREM 1. *If y is a function of u and u is a function of x, then*

$$\frac{dy}{dx} = \frac{dy}{du} \cdot \frac{du}{dx}.$$

PROOF. Here, y is a function of u and u is a function of x.

i.e., $y = f(u)$ where $u = g(x)$.

To find the derivative of $y = f[g(x)]$. Let δx be the increment in the value of x

and δy be the corresponding increment in the value of y. Now, since $y = f(u)$ then $y + \delta y = f(u + \delta u)$

$$\Rightarrow \qquad \delta y = f(u + \delta u) - f(u)$$

So,
$$\frac{\delta y}{\delta x} = \frac{f(u+\delta u) - f(u)}{\delta u} \cdot \frac{\delta u}{\delta x}.$$

Taking $\delta u \neq 0$ when $\delta x \neq 0$ if $\delta x \to 0$ then δu is also tends to 0.

Then, we have

$$\lim_{\delta x \to 0} \frac{\delta y}{\delta x} = \lim_{\delta x \to 0} \frac{f(u+\delta u) - f(u)}{\delta u} \lim_{\delta x \to 0} \frac{\delta u}{\delta x}$$

$$\Rightarrow \qquad \frac{dy}{dx} = \frac{d}{du}[f(u)]\frac{du}{dx} = \frac{dy}{du} \cdot \frac{du}{dx}$$

Hence,
$$\frac{dy}{dx} = \frac{dy}{du} \cdot \frac{du}{dx}.$$

- The above result can be generalised as follows:

If y is a function of u, u is a function of v, v is a function of w and so on, then we have

$$\frac{dy}{dx} = \frac{dy}{du} \cdot \frac{du}{dv} \cdot \frac{dv}{dw} \cdots \frac{d}{dx}.$$

6.7.1 PARAMETRIC EQUATIONS

If both x and y are the function of the third variable u, such that $x = f(u)$ and $y = g(u)$ where u is a parameter then the above two relations is known as parametric equations.

In parametric equations the value of $\frac{dy}{dx}$ is $\frac{dy/du}{dx/du}$

i.e.,
$$\frac{dy}{dx} = \frac{dy/du}{dx/du},$$

where u is a parameter.

THEOREM 2. *If x is a function of t, i.e., $x = f(t)$ and y is also a function of t, i.e., $y = g(t)$ then*

$$\frac{dy}{dx} = \frac{dy/dt}{dx/dt}, \text{ where } t \text{ is a parameter.}$$

PROOF. Let δt be the increment in the value of t and let δx and δy be the corresponding increment in x and y. Now, if $\delta t \to 0$ then $\delta x \to 0$ and $\delta y \to 0$. Now, we have

$$\frac{\delta y}{\delta x} = \frac{\delta y}{\delta t} \cdot \frac{\delta t}{\delta x}.$$

Take the limit as $\delta t \to 0$ then $\delta x \to 0$ and $\delta y \to 0$, we have

$$\lim_{\delta x \to 0} \frac{\delta y}{\delta x} = \lim_{\delta t \to 0} \frac{\delta y/\delta t}{\delta x/\delta t} = \frac{\lim_{\delta t \to \infty} \delta y/\delta t}{\lim_{\delta t \to 0} \delta x/\delta t}$$

So,
$$\frac{dy}{dx} = \frac{dy/dt}{dx/dt}.$$

Solved Examples

1. *Find the derivative of the following functions.*

(i) $\log \sin x$ (ii) $\cos x^3$

(iii) $\sin 5x$.

SOLUTION. (i) Here, $y = \log \sin x$.

Let $\sin x = t$

then $y = \log t$.

Now, $\frac{dy}{dt} = \frac{1}{t}$ and $\frac{dt}{dx} = \cos x$

So, $\frac{dy}{dx} = \frac{dy}{dt}\frac{dt}{dx} = \frac{\cos x}{t}$

$= \frac{\cos x}{\sin x} = \cot x$

(ii) Here, $y = \cos x^3$.

Put $x^3 = t$ then $y = \cos t$

Now, $\frac{dy}{dt} = -\sin t$ and $\frac{dt}{dx} = 3x^2$

So, $\frac{dy}{dx} = \frac{dy}{dt}\cdot\frac{dt}{dx} = -\sin t 3x^2$

$= -3x^2 \sin t = -3x^2 \sin x^3$

(iii) Here, $y = \sin 5x$

Put $5x = t$ then $y = \sin t$

Now, $\frac{dy}{dt} = \cos t$ and $\frac{dt}{dx} = 5$

So, $\frac{dy}{dx} = \frac{dy}{dt}\frac{dt}{dx} = \cos t \cdot 5$

$= 5\cos 5x.$

2. *Find the differential coefficient (or derivative) of the following with respect to x:*

(i) $\tan^3 x$

(ii) $(3x^3 - 5x + 8)^3$.

SOLUTION. (i) Here, $y = \tan^3 x$

Put $\tan x = t$ then; $y = t^3$

Now, $\frac{dy}{dt} = 3t^2$ and $\frac{dt}{dx} = \sec^2 x$

Therefore,

$\frac{dy}{dx} = \frac{dy}{dt}\frac{dt}{dx} = 3t^2 \sec^2 x$

$= 3\tan^2 x \sec^2 x$

(ii) Here, $y = (3x^3 - 5x^2 + 8)^3$

Put $t = 3x^3 - 5x^2 + 8$;

then $y = t^3$.

Now, $\frac{dy}{dt} = 3t^2$

and $\frac{dt}{dx} = 9x^2 - 10x$.

So, $\frac{dy}{dx} = \frac{dy}{dt}\frac{dt}{dx}$

$= 3t^2(9x^2 - 10x)$

Hence,

$\frac{dy}{dx} = 3(3x^3 - 5x^2 + 8)^2(9x^2 - 10x)$

3. *Find $\frac{dy}{dx}$ of the following functions:*

(i) $x = at^2, y = 2at$

(ii) $x = a\cos t, y = a\sin t$

(iii) $x = a(\cos t + \log\tan\frac{t}{2}), y = a\sin t$

[MEERUT(BCA)–2002, 06, 07, 11, 14, 15; DELHI–2009]

(iv) $x = a\cos^2 t, y = a\sin^2 t$.

SOLUTION. (i) Here $x = at^2$ and $y = 2at$

then, $\frac{dx}{dt} = 2at$ and $\frac{dy}{dt} = 2a$.

Therefore,

$\frac{dy}{dx} = \frac{dy/dt}{dx/dt} = \frac{2a}{2at} = \frac{1}{t}$.

(ii) Here, $x = a\cos t$ and $y = a\sin t$.

Now, $\frac{dx}{dt} = -a\sin t$

and $\frac{dy}{dt} = a\cos t$.

So, $\frac{dy}{dx} = \frac{dy/dt}{dx/dt} = \frac{a\cos t}{-a\sin t} = -\cot t$

(iii) Here,

$x = a(\cos t + \log\tan\frac{t}{2}), y = a\sin t$.

Now,

$$\frac{dx}{dt} = a\left(-\sin t + \frac{1}{\tan\frac{t}{2}}\frac{d}{dx}(\tan\frac{t}{2})\right)$$

and $\frac{dy}{dt} = a\cos t$

$$= a\left(-\sin t + \frac{1}{\tan t/2}\sec^2 t/2\cdot\frac{1}{2}\right)$$

$$= a\left(-\sin t + \frac{1}{2\tan t/2\cos^2 t/2}\right)$$

$$= a\left(-\sin t + \frac{1}{2\sin t/2\cos t/2}\right)$$

$$= a\left(-\sin t + \frac{1}{\sin t}\right)$$

$$= a\left(\frac{1-\sin^2 t}{\sin t}\right) = \frac{a\cos^2 t}{\sin t}$$

So, $\frac{dy}{dx}=\frac{dy/dt}{dx/dt}=\frac{a\cos t}{\frac{a\cos^2 t}{\sin t}}$

$=\frac{\sin t}{\cos t}=\tan t.$

(iv) Here, $x=a\cos^2 t, y=a\sin^2 t$

Now $\frac{dx}{dt}=2a\cos t\frac{d}{dt}\cos t$

$=2a\cos t(-\sin t)$

$=-a2\sin t\cos t=-a\sin 2t$

and $\frac{dy}{dt}=2a\sin t\left(\frac{d}{dt}\sin t\right)$

$=2a\sin t\cos t=a\sin 2t$

So, $\frac{dy}{dx}=\frac{dy/dt}{dx/dt}=\frac{a\sin 2t}{-a\sin 2t}=-1$

So, $\frac{dy}{dx}=-1$

6.8 DIFFERENTIATION OF IMPLICIT FUNCTIONS

A function which can be expressed in terms of independent variable x is known as explicit function. On the other hand, a function which is not explicit, is known as implicit function, or we can say a function which cannot be expressed directly in terms of independent variable x is implicit function. For example, $x^y+y^x=a$ is an implicit function, because this function cannot be expressed in terms of x. To find the $\frac{dy}{dx}$ of implicit function, we differentiate each term with respect to x treating y as a function of x and then separating $\frac{dy}{dx}$. A method by which we find the $\frac{dy}{dx}$ of implicit function is known as implicit differentiation.

Solved Examples

1. *Find $\frac{dy}{dx}$ of the implicit function*

$ax^2+2hxy+by^2+2gx+2fy+c=0.$

SOLUTION. Differentiating the given equation with respect to x, we get

$$2ax+2h\left(x\frac{dy}{dx}+y\right)+2by\frac{dy}{dx}+2g+2f\frac{dy}{dx}=0$$

$\Rightarrow \frac{dy}{dx}(hx+by+f)=-(ax+hy+g)$

$\Rightarrow \frac{dy}{dx}=-\frac{ax+hy+g}{hx+by+f}.$

2. *Find $\frac{dy}{dx}$ of the function* $x\sqrt{1+y}+y\sqrt{1+x}=0$.

SOLUTION. Here, $x\sqrt{1+y}+y\sqrt{1+x}=0$

$\Rightarrow x\sqrt{1+y}=-y\sqrt{1+x}.$

On squaring, we get

$x^2(1+y)=y^2(1+x)$

or $(x^2-y^2)+(x^2y-xy^2)=0$

$\Rightarrow (x^2-y^2)+xy(x-y)=0$

$\Rightarrow (x+y)(x-y)+xy(x-y)=0$

$\Rightarrow x+y+xy=0$

or $y(1+x)+x=0$

$\Rightarrow y=-\frac{x}{1+x}.$

Now, differentiating both sides, with respect to x, we get

$$\frac{dy}{dx}=\frac{(1+x)\frac{d}{dx}(-x)-(-x)\frac{d}{dx}(1+x)}{(1+x)^2}$$

$$=\frac{-(1+x)+x}{(1+x)^2}=-\frac{1}{(1+x)^2}.$$

3. *Find $\frac{dy}{dx}$ of the function $y=x^{x^{x\ldots\infty}}$*

[MEERUT(BCA)–2004, 14; HIMACHAL–2011]

SOLUTION. Here, $y=x^{x^{x\ldots\infty}}$

$\Rightarrow y=x^y \Rightarrow \log y=y\log x$

Now, differentiating with respect to x, we get

$$\frac{1}{y}\frac{dy}{dx}=y\frac{d}{dx}(\log x)+\frac{dy}{dx}\log x$$

or $\frac{1}{y}\frac{dy}{dx}=y\frac{1}{x}+\frac{dy}{dx}\log x$

$$\Rightarrow \left(\frac{1}{y}-\log x\right)\frac{dy}{dx}=\frac{y}{x}$$

$$\Rightarrow \frac{dy}{dx}=\frac{y^2}{(1-y\log x)x}.$$

4. *Find* $\frac{dy}{dx}$ *of the function* $\log xy = x^2+y^2$.

SOLUTION. Here, $\log(xy) = x^2+y^2$

or $\log x+\log y = x^2+y^2$.

Now, differentiating both sides with respect to x, we get

$$\frac{1}{x}+\frac{1}{y}\frac{dy}{dx}=2x+2y\frac{dy}{dx}$$

or $\left(\frac{1}{y}-2y\right)\frac{dy}{dx}=2x-\frac{1}{x}$

or $\frac{(1-2y^2)}{y}\frac{dy}{dx}=\frac{(2x^2-1)}{x}$.

Therefore, $\frac{dy}{dx}=\frac{(2x^2-1)y}{(1-2y^2)x}$.

5. *If* $x^3+y^3=3axy$; *find* $\frac{dy}{dx}$.

SOLUTION. We have $x^3+y^3=3axy$

Differentiating both sides with respect to x, we get

$$\frac{d}{dx}x^3+\frac{d}{dx}y^3=\frac{d}{dx}(3axy)$$

$$3x^2+3y^2\frac{dy}{dx}=3a\left\{x\frac{dy}{dx}+y\cdot 1\right\}$$

$$\Rightarrow (3y^2-3ax)\frac{dy}{dx}=3ay-3x^2$$

$$\Rightarrow 3(y^2-ax)\frac{dy}{dx}=3(ay-x^2)$$

Hence, $\frac{dy}{dx}=\frac{ay-x^2}{y^2-ax}$

6. *Find* $\frac{dy}{dx}$ *when x and y are connected by the following relations :*

(*i*) $\tan(x+y)+\tan(x-y)=1$

(*ii*) $xy\log(x+y)=1$

SOLUTION. (i) We have

$$\tan(x+y)+\tan(x-y)=1$$

Differentiating both sides with respect to x, we get

$$\sec^2(x+y)\left[1+\frac{dy}{dx}\right]+\sec^2(x-y)\left[1-\frac{dy}{dx}\right]=0$$

$$\Rightarrow \frac{dy}{dx}[\sec^2(x+y)-\sec^2(x-y)=-[\sec^2(x+y)+\sec^2(x-y)]$$

$$\Rightarrow \frac{dy}{dx}=-\frac{[\sec^2(x+y)+\sec^2(x-y)]}{\sec^2(x+y)-\sec^2(x-y)}$$

(ii) $xy\log(x+y)=1$

Differentiating both sides w.r.t x, we get

$$xy\cdot\frac{1}{x+y}\left[1+\frac{dy}{dx}\right]+x\log(x+y)\frac{dy}{dx}+y\cdot\log(x+y)=0$$

$$\Rightarrow \frac{dy}{dx}\left[\frac{xy}{x+y}+x\log(x+y)\right]=\frac{-xy}{x+y}-y\log(x+y)$$

$$\Rightarrow \frac{dy}{dx}[xy+x(x+y)\log(x+y)]=-[xy+y(x+y)\log(x+y)]$$

$$\Rightarrow \frac{dy}{dx}=\frac{-[xy+y(x+y)\log(x+y)]}{[xy+(x+y)x\log(x+y)]}$$

7. *If* $\sqrt{1-x^2}+\sqrt{1-y^2}=a(x-y)$, *then prove that* $\frac{dy}{dx}=\frac{\sqrt{1-y^2}}{\sqrt{1-x^2}}$.

[MEERUT(BCA)–2003, 10, 11; KANPUR–2010; RAJASTHAN–2008; GARHWAL–2009]

SOLUTION. We have $\sqrt{1-x^2}+\sqrt{1-y^2}=a(x-y)$

Putting $x=\sin\theta$ and $y=\sin\phi$, we get

$$\sqrt{1-\sin^2\theta}+\sqrt{1-\sin^2\phi}=a(\sin\theta-\sin\phi)$$

$$\Rightarrow \cos\theta+\cos\phi=a(\sin\theta-\sin\phi)$$

$$\Rightarrow 2\cos\left(\frac{\theta+\phi}{2}\right)\cos\left(\frac{\theta-\phi}{2}\right)=a\left\{2\cos\left(\frac{\theta+\phi}{2}\right)\sin\left(\frac{\theta-\phi}{2}\right)\right\}$$

$$\Rightarrow \cot\left(\frac{\theta-\phi}{2}\right)=a$$

$$\Rightarrow \frac{\theta-\phi}{2}=\cot^{-1}a$$

$$\Rightarrow \sin^{-1}x-\sin^{-1}y=2\cot^{-1}a$$

Differentiating w.r.t. x, we get

$$\frac{1}{\sqrt{1-x^2}}-\frac{1}{\sqrt{1-y^2}}\frac{dy}{dx}=0$$

$$\frac{dy}{dx}=\sqrt{\frac{1-y^2}{1-x^2}}$$

8. *Find* $\frac{dy}{dx}$; *if* $x^m y^n=(x+y)^{m+n}$.

[MEERUT(BCA)–2003, 12, 14]

SOLUTION. We have $x^m y^n=(x+y)^{m+n}$

Taking log on both sides, we get

$m\log x+n\log y=(m+n)\log(x+y)$

Differentiating w.r.t. x both sides, we get

$$\frac{m}{x}+\frac{n}{y}\frac{dy}{dx}=(m+n).\frac{1}{x+y}\left(1+\frac{dy}{dx}\right)$$

$$\Rightarrow \left(\frac{n}{y}-\frac{m+n}{x+y}\right)\frac{dy}{dx}=\frac{m+n}{x+y}-\frac{m}{x}$$

$$\frac{n(x+y)-(m+n)y}{y(x+y)}\frac{dy}{dx}=\frac{(m+n)x-m(x+y)}{x(x+y)}$$

$$\Rightarrow \frac{nx-my}{y}\frac{dy}{dx}=\frac{nx-my}{x}$$

$$\frac{dy}{dx}=\frac{y}{x}$$

9. *If* $\sin y=x\sin(a+y)$, *then prove that* $\frac{dy}{dx}=\frac{\sin^2(a+y)}{\sin a}$.

SOLUTION. We have $\sin y=x\sin(a+y)$ ...(1)

Differentiating w.r.t x both sides, we get

$$\Rightarrow \cos y\frac{dy}{dx}=1\cdot\sin(a+y)+x\cos(a+y)\cdot\frac{d}{dx}(a+y)$$

$$\Rightarrow \cos y\frac{dy}{dx}=\sin(a+y)+x\cos(a+y)\frac{dy}{dx}$$

$$\Rightarrow \{\cos y-x\cos(a+y)\}\frac{dy}{dx}=\sin(a+y)$$

$$\Rightarrow \left\{\cos y-\frac{\sin y}{\sin(a+y)}\cos(a+y)\right\}\frac{dy}{dx}=\sin(a+y)$$

[From (1)]

$$\Rightarrow \left\{\frac{\cos y\sin(a+y)-\sin y\cos(a+y)}{\sin(a+y)}\right\}\frac{dy}{dx}=\sin(a+y)$$

$$\Rightarrow \frac{\sin(a+y-y)}{\sin(a+y)}\frac{dy}{dx}=\sin(a+y)$$

$$\Rightarrow \frac{dy}{dx}=\frac{\sin^2(a+y)}{\sin a}$$

10. *Find* $\frac{dy}{dx}$, *if* $y^x=x^{\sin y}$

[MEERUT(BCA)–2002, 10; ASSAM–2006]

SOLUTION. We have $y^x=x^{\sin y}$

Taking log on both sides, we get

$x\log y=\sin y\cdot\log x$ ...(1)

Differentiating w.r.t x both sides, we get

$$1\cdot\log y+\frac{x}{y}\frac{dy}{dx}=\frac{\sin y}{x}+\log x\cdot\cos y\cdot\frac{dy}{dx}$$

$$\Rightarrow \frac{dy}{dx}\left(\frac{x}{y}-\log x.\cos y\right)=\frac{\sin y}{x}-\log y$$

$$\Rightarrow \frac{dy}{dx}\left(\frac{x-y\log x.\cos y}{y}\right)=\frac{\sin y-x\log y}{x}$$

Hence, $\frac{dy}{dx}=\frac{y(\sin y-x\cdot\log y)}{x(x-y\log x\cdot\cos y)}$

11. *If* $x^2+y^2=t-\frac{1}{t}$ *and* $x^4+y^4=t^2+\frac{1}{t^2}$ *then prove that* $\frac{dy}{dx}=\frac{1}{x^3y}$.

SOLUTION. We have $x^2+y^2=t-\frac{1}{t}$

On Squaring

$$(x^2+y^2)^2=\left(t-\frac{1}{t}\right)^2=t^2+\frac{1}{t^2}-2$$

$$x^4+y^4+2x^2y^2=x^4+y^4-2$$

$$\Rightarrow 2x^2y^2=-2$$

$$\Rightarrow \qquad x^2y^2 = -1$$

$$\Rightarrow \qquad y^2 = -\frac{1}{x^2}$$

Differentiating w.r.t. x both sides, we get $2y\frac{dy}{dx} = +\frac{2}{x^3}$

$$\frac{dy}{dx} = \frac{1}{x^3 y}$$

12. *If* $\sqrt{y+x} + \sqrt{y-x} = c$ *then prove that*

$$\frac{dy}{dx} = \frac{y}{x} - \sqrt{\frac{y^2}{x^2} - 1}.$$

SOLUTION. We have $\sqrt{y+x} + \sqrt{y-x} = c$

Differentiating both sides w.r.t. x, we get $\frac{1}{2\sqrt{y+x}}\frac{d}{dx}(y+x)$

$$+\frac{1}{2\sqrt{y-x}}\frac{d}{dx}(y-x) = 0$$

$$\Rightarrow \frac{1}{2\sqrt{y+x}}\left(\frac{dy}{dx}+1\right) + \frac{1}{2\sqrt{y-x}}\left(\frac{dy}{dx}-1\right) = 0$$

$$\frac{dy}{dx}\left\{\frac{1}{\sqrt{y+x}} + \frac{1}{\sqrt{y-x}}\right\} = \frac{1}{\sqrt{y-x}} - \frac{1}{\sqrt{y+x}}$$

$$\Rightarrow \frac{dy}{dx}\left\{\frac{\sqrt{y-x}+\sqrt{y+x}}{\sqrt{y^2-x^2}}\right\} = \frac{\sqrt{y+x}-\sqrt{y-x}}{\sqrt{y^2-x^2}}$$

$$\Rightarrow \frac{dy}{dx} = \frac{\sqrt{y+x}-\sqrt{y-x}}{\sqrt{y+x}+\sqrt{y-x}} \times \frac{\sqrt{y+x}-\sqrt{y-x}}{\sqrt{y+x}-\sqrt{y-x}}$$

$$= \frac{(y+x)+(y-x)-2\sqrt{y^2-x^2}}{(y+x)-(y-x)}$$

$$= \frac{2y-2\sqrt{y^2-x^2}}{2x}$$

$$= \frac{y}{x} - \sqrt{\frac{y^2}{x^2}-1}$$

13. *If* $x^{2/3} + y^{2/3} = 2$ *find* $\frac{dy}{dx}$ *at* (1, 1).

SOLUTION. We have $x^{2/3} + y^{2/3} = 2$

Differentiating both sides w.r.t. x, we get

$$\frac{2}{3}x^{-1/3} + \frac{2}{3}y^{-1/3}\frac{dy}{dx} = 0$$

$$\Rightarrow \qquad x^{-1/3} + y^{-1/3}\frac{dy}{dx} = 0$$

$$\frac{dy}{dx} = \frac{-x^{-1/3}}{y^{-1/3}} = -\left(\frac{y}{x}\right)^{1/3}$$

$$\Rightarrow \left(\frac{dy}{dx}\right)_{(1,1)} = -\left(\frac{1}{1}\right)^{1/3} = -1$$

14. *If* $y = \cos^{-1}\left(\frac{2\cos x + 3\sin x}{\sqrt{13}}\right)$, *find* $\frac{dy}{dx}$. [MEERUT(BCA)–2002, 06, 08, 14; GARHWAL-2013; KANPUR-2007; NAGPUR-2009]

SOLUTION. Differentiating the given function w.r.t. x, we get

$$\frac{dy}{dx} = \frac{-1}{\sqrt{\left\{1 - \frac{1}{13}(2\cos x + 3\sin x)^2\right.}} \cdot \left.\frac{1}{\sqrt{13}}(-2\sin x + 3\cos x)\right\}$$

$$= -\frac{(-2\sin x + 3\cos x)}{\sqrt{13}\sqrt{\frac{13-(4\cos^2 x + 9\sin^2 x + 12\sin x\cos x)}{13}}}$$

$$= -\frac{(-2\sin x + 3\cos x)}{\sqrt{13 - 4 - 5\sin^2 x - 12\sin x\cos x}}$$

$$= -\frac{(-2\sin x + 3\cos x)}{\sqrt{9 - 5\sin^2 x - 12\sin x\cos x}}$$

$$= -\frac{(-2\sin x + 3\cos x)}{\sqrt{(9\cos^2 x + 4\sin^2 x - 12\sin x\cos x)}}$$

$$= \frac{(2\sin x - 3\cos x)}{\sqrt{(2\sin x - 3\cos x)^2}}$$

$$= \frac{2\sin x - 3\cos x}{2\sin x - 3\cos x} = 1$$

6.9 LOGARITHMIC DIFFERENTIATION

To find the derivative of a function, which is of the form of the product of functions or quotient of function or a function of the form $(f(x))^{g(x)}$. In this case, we take the logarithms on both sides and then differentiate. This process is known as Logarithmic differentiation.

Solved Examples

1. *Find $\frac{dy}{dx}$ of the function $y = x^{x^x}$.*

SOLUTION. Here, $y = x^{x^x}$.

Taking log on both sides, we get

$\log y = \log(x^{x^x})$ or $\log y = x^x \log x$.

Now, differentiating w.r. to x, we get

$$\frac{1}{y}\frac{dy}{dx} = x^x \frac{d}{dx}(\log x) + \frac{d}{dx}(x^x)\log x$$

$$\frac{1}{y}\frac{dy}{dx} = x^x \frac{1}{x} + x^x(1+\log x)\log x$$

$$\left[\because \frac{d}{dx}(x^x) = x^x(1+\log x)\right]$$

$$\frac{dy}{dx} = y[x^{x-1} + x^x \log x(1+\log x)].$$

Hence,

$$\frac{dy}{dx} = x^{x^x}[x^{x-1} + x^x \log x(1+\log x)]$$

2. *Find $\frac{dy}{dx}$ of the following functions :*

(i) $y = ax^{-3} + bx^3 + cx^{9/2}\sin x$

(ii) $y = x^x$

(iii) $y = (1+x)^x$

(iv) $y = (ax+b)^x$

(v) $y = (\cos x)^{\log x}$

SOLUTION. (i) We have,

$$y = ax^{-3} + bx^3 + cx^{9/2}\sin x$$

So,

$$\frac{dy}{dx} = \frac{d}{dx}(ax^{-3} + bx^3 + cx^{9/2}\sin x)$$

$$= a\frac{d}{dx}(x^{-3}) + b\frac{d}{dx}(x^3) + c\frac{d}{dx}(x^{9/2}\sin x)$$

$$= -3ax^{-4} + 3bx^2 + c\left(x^{9/2}\frac{d}{dx}\sin x + \frac{d}{dx}(x^{9/2})\sin x\right)$$

$$= -3ax^{-4} + 3bx^2 + c(x^{9/2}\cos x + \frac{9}{2}x^{7/2}\sin x)$$

(ii) Here, $y = x^x$.

Taking log on both sides, we get

$$\log y = x\log x.$$

Now, differentiating w.r. to x, we get

$$\frac{1}{y}\frac{dy}{dx} = x\frac{d}{dx}(\log x) + \frac{d}{dx}(x)\log x$$

or $$\frac{1}{y}\frac{dy}{dx} = x\frac{1}{x} + 1\log x$$

or $$\frac{dy}{dx} = y(1+\log x)$$

Hence, $$\frac{dy}{dx} = x^x(1+\log x)$$

(iii) Here, $y = (1+x)^x$.

Taking log on both sides, we get

$$\log y = x\log(1+x).$$

Now, differentiating both sides with respect to x, we get

$$\frac{1}{y}\frac{dy}{dx} = x\frac{d}{dx}[\log(1+x)] + \frac{d}{dx}(x)\log(1+x)$$

$$\Rightarrow \frac{1}{y}\frac{dy}{dx} = x\frac{1}{1+x} + 1.\log(1+x)$$

$$\Rightarrow \frac{dy}{dx} = y\left[\frac{x}{1+x} + \log(1+x)\right].$$

Hence,

$$\frac{dy}{dx} = (1+x)^x\left(\frac{x}{x+1} + \log(1+x)\right).$$

(iv) Here, $y = (ax+b)^x$

Taking log on both sides, we get

$$\log y = x\log(ax+b)$$

Now, differentiating both sides w.r. to x, we get

$$\frac{1}{y}\frac{dy}{dx} = x\frac{d}{dx}\log(ax+b) + \frac{d}{dx}(x)\cdot\log(ax+b)$$

or $$\frac{1}{y}\frac{dy}{dx} = x\frac{1}{(ax+b)}\frac{d}{dx}(ax+b) + 1\cdot\log(ax+b)$$

or $$\frac{1}{y}\frac{dy}{dx} = x\frac{1}{(ax+b)}a + \log(ax+b)$$

or $$\frac{dy}{dx} = y\left[\frac{ax}{ax+b} + \log(ax+b)\right].$$

Hence, $$\frac{dy}{dx} = (ax+b)^x\left[\frac{ax}{ax+b} + \log(ax+b)\right].$$

(v) Here, $y = (\cos x)^{\log x}$.

Taking log on both sides, we get

$$\log y = \log x \log(\cos x).$$

Now, differentiating both sides w.r. to x, we get

$$\frac{1}{y}\frac{dy}{dx} = \log x\frac{d}{dx}\log(\cos x) + \frac{d}{dx}\log x\cdot\log(\cos x)$$

or $$\frac{1}{y}\frac{dy}{dx} = \log x\frac{1}{\cos x}\frac{d}{dx}(\cos x) + \frac{1}{x}\log(\cos x)$$

or $$\frac{1}{y}\frac{dy}{dx} = -\log x\frac{\sin x}{\cos x} + \frac{1}{x}\log(\cos x)$$

$$\Rightarrow \frac{1}{y}\frac{dy}{dx} = \frac{1}{x}\log(\cos x) - \tan x\log x$$

or $$\frac{dy}{dx} = (\cos x)^{\log x}\left[\frac{1}{x}\log(\cos x) - \tan x\log x\right]$$

3. *Find* $\frac{dy}{dx}$ *of the following functions :*

(*i*) $xy + \tan y = \log x$

(*ii*) $y = \frac{x^2\sqrt{(4x+3)}}{3x+1}$.

SOLUTION. (i) We have,

$$xy + \tan y = \log x$$

Differentiating both sides w.r. to x, we get

$$x\frac{dy}{dx} + y + \sec^2 y\frac{dy}{dx} = \frac{1}{x}$$

or $$(x + \sec^2 y)\frac{dy}{dx} = \frac{1}{x} - y$$

or $$\frac{dy}{dx} = \frac{1-xy}{x(x+\sec^2 y)}.$$

(ii) Here, $y = \frac{x^2\sqrt{4x+3}}{3x+1}$.

Taking log on both sides, we get

$$\log y = \log x^2 + \log\{\sqrt{(4x+3)}\} - \log(3x+1)$$

or $$\log y = 2\log x + \frac{1}{2}\log(4x+3) - \log(3x+1).$$

Now, differentiating both sides with respect to x, we get

$$\frac{1}{y}\frac{dy}{dx} = 2\frac{d}{dx}\log x + \frac{1}{2}\frac{d}{dx}\log(4x+3) - \frac{d}{dx}[\log(3x+1)]$$

or $$\frac{1}{y}\frac{dy}{dx} = 2\frac{1}{x} + \frac{1}{2}\frac{1}{(4x+3)}\frac{d}{dx}(4x+3) - \frac{1}{3x+1}\frac{d}{dx}(3x+1)$$

or $$\frac{1}{y}\frac{dy}{dx} = \frac{2}{x} + \frac{2}{4x+3} - \frac{3}{3x+1}$$

or $$\frac{dy}{dx} = \frac{x^2\sqrt{(4x+3)}}{3x+1}\left[\frac{2}{x} + \frac{2}{4x+3} - \frac{3}{3x+1}\right]$$

4. *Find the derivative (or differential coefficient) of the following functions.*

(i) $(ax)^n + b$

(ii) $\frac{2}{x^2} - \frac{a}{x} + be^x + (ax)^m$

(iii) $x\log x + e^x \sin x + 2x$

SOLUTION. (i) We have, $y = (ax)^n + b.$

$$\text{So, } \frac{dy}{dx} = \frac{d}{dx}(ax)^n + \frac{d}{dx}b = n(ax)^{n-1}\frac{d}{dx}(ax) + 0 = n(ax)^{n-1}a = na^n x^{n-1}$$

(ii) We have, $y = \frac{2}{x^2} - \frac{a}{x} + be^x + (ax)^m.$

$$\text{So, } \frac{dy}{dx} = 2\frac{d}{dx}x^{-2} - a\frac{d}{dx}x^{-1} + b\frac{d}{dx}e^x + \frac{d}{dx}(ax)^m$$
$$= 2(-2x^{-3}) - a(-x^{-2}) + be^x + m(ax)^{m-1}a$$
$$= -4x^{-3} + ax^{-2} + be^x + ma^m x^{m-1}$$

(iii) We have, $y = x\log x + e^x \sin x + 2x$

$$\text{So, } \frac{dy}{dx} = \frac{d}{dx}(x\log x) + \frac{d}{dx}(e^x \sin x) + 2\frac{d}{dx}(x)$$
$$= x\frac{d}{dx}(\log x) + \frac{d}{dx}(x)\log x + e^x\frac{d}{dx}\sin x + \frac{d}{dx}(e^x)\sin x + 2$$
$$= x\frac{1}{x} + \log x + e^x \cos x + e^x \sin x + 2$$
$$= 3 + \log x + e^x(\cos x + \sin x)$$

5. *Find the derivative of the following functions.*

(i) $(x^n + a)(x^m + b)$

(ii) $\log_e x \log_a x.$

SOLUTION. (i) We have, $y = (x^n + a)\cdot(x^m + b)$

$$\text{So, } \frac{dy}{dx} = \frac{d}{dx}\{(x^n + a)(x^m + b)\}.$$
$$= (x^n + a)\frac{d}{dx}(x^m + b) + \frac{d}{dx}(x^n + a).(x^m + b)$$
$$= (x^n + a)mx^{m-1} + nx^{n-1}(x^m + b)$$

(ii) Here, $y = \log_e x \log_a x.$

$$\text{So, } \frac{dy}{dx} = \frac{d}{dx}(\log_e x \log_a x)$$
$$= \log_e x \frac{d}{dx}(\log_a x) + \frac{d}{dx}(\log_e x)\log_a x$$
$$= \log_e x \frac{1}{x}\log_a(e) + \frac{1}{x}\log_a x$$
$$= \frac{1}{x}[\log_e x \log_a e + \log_a x].$$

6. *Find the* $\frac{dy}{dx}$ *of the following functions.*

(i) $e^x \log\sin 2x$

(ii) $\frac{1+\cos x}{\sin x}$

(iii) $\sin x(x^2 + 3)$

(iv) 3^{x+8}.

SOLUTION. (i) Here, $y = e^x \log\sin 2x$

$$\frac{dy}{dx} = \frac{d}{dx}(e^x \log\sin 2x)$$
$$= e^x \frac{d}{dx}(\log\sin 2x) + \frac{d}{dx}(e^x)\log\sin 2x$$
$$= e^x \frac{1}{\sin 2x}\frac{d}{dx}\sin 2x + e^x \log\sin 2x$$
$$= e^x \frac{1}{\sin 2x}\cos 2x \frac{d}{dx}(2x) + e^x \log\sin 2x$$
$$= 2e^x \cot 2x + e^x \log\sin 2x.$$

(ii) Here, $y = \frac{1+\cos x}{\sin x}$

$$\text{So, } \frac{dy}{dx} = \frac{d}{dx}\left(\frac{1+\cos x}{\sin x}\right)$$

$$= \frac{\sin x \frac{d}{dx}(1+\cos x) - (1+\cos x)\frac{d}{dx}\sin x}{(\sin x)^2}$$

$$= \frac{\sin x(-\sin x)-(1+\cos x)(\cos x)}{(\sin x)^2}$$

$$= \frac{-\sin^2 x - \cos x - \cos^2 x}{(\sin x)^2}$$

$$= \frac{-(1+\cos x)}{1-\cos^2 x}$$

$$= \frac{-(1+\cos x)}{(1+\cos x)(1-\cos x)} = \frac{-1}{1-\cos x}$$

(iii) Here, $y = \sin x(x^2+3)$.

So, $\frac{dy}{dx} = \frac{d}{dx}[\sin x(x^2+3)]$

$$= \sin x \frac{d}{dx}(x^2+3) + (x^2+3)\frac{d}{dx}(\sin x)$$

$$= \sin x \cdot 2x + \cos x(x^2+3)$$

$$= 2x\sin x + (x^2+3)\cos x$$

(iv) Here, $y = 3^{x+8}$

So, $\frac{dy}{dx} = \frac{d}{dx}(3^{x+8}) = 3^{x+8} \cdot \log_e 3$

7. *Find $\frac{dy}{dx}$ of the following functions.*

(*i*) $y = \sin x^3 - 4\cos x^2$

(*ii*) $y = x^4 \sec x + e^x \operatorname{cosec} x$

(*iii*) $y = \log(\log x)$.

SOLUTION. (i) Here, $y = \sin x^3 - 4\cos x^2$

$$\frac{dy}{dx} = \frac{d}{dx}(\sin x^3 - 4\cos x^2)$$

$$= \frac{d}{dx}(\sin x^3) - 4\frac{d}{dx}(\cos x^2)$$

$$= \cos x^3 \frac{d}{dx} x^3 - 4(-\sin x^2)\frac{d}{dx}(x^2)$$

$$= 3x^2\cos x^3 + 4(2x)\sin x^2$$

$$= 3x^2\cos x^3 + 8x\sin x^2$$

(ii) Here, $y = x^4 \sec x + e^x \operatorname{cosec} x$

$$\frac{dy}{dx} = \frac{d}{dx}(x^4 \sec x) + \frac{d}{dx}(e^x \operatorname{cosec} x)$$

$$= x^4 \frac{d}{dx}(\sec x) + \frac{d}{dx}(x^4)\sec x + e^x \frac{d}{dx}(\operatorname{cosec} x) + \frac{d}{dx}e^x \operatorname{cosec} x$$

$$= x^4 \sec x \tan x + 4x^3 \sec x + e^x(-\operatorname{cosec} x \cot x) + e^x \operatorname{cosec} x$$

$$= x^3 \sec x(x\tan x + 4) + e^x \operatorname{cosec} x(1-\cot x)$$

(iii) Here $y = \log(\log x)$.

So, $\frac{dy}{dx} = \frac{d}{dx}[\log(\log x)]$

$$= \frac{1}{(\log x)}\frac{d}{dx}(\log x)$$

$$= \frac{1}{(\log x)}\frac{1}{x} = \frac{1}{(\log x)}.$$

8. *Find $\frac{dy}{dx}$ of the following functions:*

(*i*) $x^3 + y^3 = 3ax^2$

(*ii*) $\frac{x^m}{a^m} + \frac{y^m}{b^m} = 1$

(*iii*) $x = a(t - \sin t), y = a(1-\cos t)$

SOLUTION. (i) Here, the given equation is

$$x^3 + y^3 = 3ax^2.$$

Differentiating both sides, w.r. to x, we get

$$3x^2 + 3y^2\frac{dy}{dx} = 6ax$$

or $$3y^2\frac{dy}{dx} = 6ax - 3x^2 = 3x(2a-x)$$

or $$\frac{dy}{dx} = \frac{x(2a-x)}{y^2}.$$

(ii) Here, the given equation is

$$\frac{x^m}{a^m} + \frac{y^m}{b^m} = 1.$$

Differentiating both sides w.r. to x, we get

$$\frac{1}{a^m}\frac{d}{dx}(x^m) + \frac{1}{b^m}\frac{d}{dx}(y^m) = \frac{d}{dx}(1)$$

$$\frac{mx^{m-1}}{a^m} + \frac{1}{b^m}my^{m-1}\frac{dy}{dx} = 0.$$

or $b^m mx^{m-1} + a^m my^{m-1}\frac{dy}{dx} = 0$

or $\frac{dy}{dx} = -\frac{b^m mx^{m-1}}{a^m my^{m-1}}$

$= -\left(\frac{b}{a}\right)^m \left(\frac{x}{y}\right)^{m-1}$

or $\frac{dy}{dx} = -\left(\frac{b}{a}\right)^m \left(\frac{x}{y}\right)^{m-1}$.

(iii) Here, $x = a(t - \sin t)$
and $y = a(1 - \cos t)$

So, $\frac{dx}{dt} = a(1 - \cos t)$

and $\frac{dy}{dt} = a[-(-\sin t)]$

or $\frac{dy}{dt} = a \sin t.$

So, $\frac{dy}{dx} = \frac{dy/dt}{dx/dt} = \frac{a \sin t}{a(1-\cos t)}$

$= \frac{\sin t}{1 - \cos t}$

$= \frac{2\sin t/2 \cos t/2}{2\sin^2 t/2}$

$= \frac{\cos t/2}{\sin t/2} = \cot\frac{t}{2}.$

So, $\frac{dy}{dx} = \cot\frac{t}{2}.$

9. *If* $y = Ax^2e^x - x + 8$ *and for* $x = 1, \frac{dy}{dx} = 2$, *then obtain the value of A.*

SOLUTION. Here $y = Ax^2e^x - x + 8$ and for $x = 1, \frac{dy}{dx} = 2$

So, $\frac{dy}{dx} = A\frac{d}{dx}(x^2e^x) - \frac{d}{dx}(x) + \frac{d}{dx}(8)$

$= A\left\{x^2\frac{d}{dx}e^x + \frac{d}{dx}x^2e^x\right\} - 1$

or $\frac{dy}{dx} = A\{x^2e^x + 2xe^x\} - 1$

Now, put $x = 1, \frac{dy}{dx} = 2$

$2 = A\{e + 2e\} - 1$

$\Rightarrow A = \frac{3}{3e} = \frac{1}{e} \Rightarrow A = \frac{1}{e}.$

10. *Find* $\frac{dy}{dx}$ *of the following functions.*

(*i*) $y = \log\tan\left(\frac{\pi}{4} + \frac{x}{2}\right)$

(*ii*) $y = \tan^{-1}(\sec x + \tan x)$

(*iii*) $y = e^{\sin x}$

(*iv*) $y = \log(x^2 + x)$

SOLUTION. (i) Here, $y = \log\tan\left(\frac{\pi}{4} + \frac{x}{2}\right)$.

So,

$\frac{dy}{dx} = \frac{d}{dx}\left[\log\tan\left(\frac{\pi}{4} + \frac{x}{2}\right)\right]$

$= \frac{1}{\tan\left(\frac{\pi}{4} + \frac{x}{2}\right)} \frac{d}{dx}\left[\tan\left(\frac{\pi}{4} + \frac{x}{2}\right)\right]$

$= \frac{1}{\tan\left(\frac{\pi}{4} + \frac{x}{2}\right)} \sec^2\left(\frac{\pi}{4} + \frac{x}{2}\right)\frac{d}{dx}\left(\frac{\pi}{4} + \frac{x}{2}\right)$

$= \frac{\sec^2\left(\frac{\pi}{4} + \frac{x}{2}\right)}{\tan\left(\frac{\pi}{4} + \frac{x}{2}\right)} \frac{1}{2}$

$= \frac{1}{2\cos\left(\frac{\pi}{4} + \frac{x}{2}\right)\sin\left(\frac{\pi}{4} + \frac{x}{2}\right)}$

$= \frac{1}{\sin 2\left(\frac{\pi}{4} + \frac{x}{2}\right)} = \frac{1}{\sin\left(\frac{\pi}{2} + x\right)}.$

(ii) $y = \tan^{-1}(\sec x + \tan x)$

So, $\frac{dy}{dx} = \frac{d}{dx}[\tan^{-1}(\sec x + \tan x)]$

$= \frac{1}{1 + (\sec x + \tan x)^2} \frac{d}{dx}(\sec x + \tan x)$

$= \frac{1}{1 + (\sec x + \tan x)^2} (\sec x \tan x + \sec^2 x)$

(iii) Here, $y = e^{\sin x}$.

$$\text{So, } \frac{dy}{dx} = \frac{d}{dx}(e^{\sin x}) = e^{\sin x}\frac{d}{dx}\sin x = e^{\sin x}\cos x.$$

(iv) Here, $y = \log(x^2 + x)$.

$$\text{So, } \frac{dy}{dx} = \frac{d}{dx}[\log(x^2 + x)] = \frac{1}{(x^2+x)}\frac{d}{dx}(x^2+x) = \frac{1}{(x^2+x)}(2x+1) = \frac{2x+1}{(x^2+x)}$$

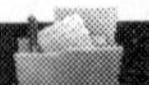

Miscellaneous Examples

1. *Find the derivative of the following functions.*

(i) $y = \dfrac{(1-x^2)}{\sqrt{(1+x^2)}}$

(ii) $y = \tan^{-1}\left(\dfrac{2x}{1-x^2}\right)$

(iii) $y = \dfrac{\sin x + \cos x}{\sin x - \cos x}$

(iv) $y = \sin^{-1}\left(\dfrac{2x}{1+x^2}\right)$

SOLUTION. (i) Here, $y = \dfrac{(1-x^2)}{\sqrt{(1+x^2)}}$

$$\text{So, } \frac{dy}{dx} = \frac{d}{dx}\left(\frac{1-x^2}{\sqrt{1+x^2}}\right)$$

$$= \frac{\sqrt{1+x^2}\dfrac{d}{dx}(1-x^2) - (1-x^2)\dfrac{d}{dx}\sqrt{1+x^2}}{(1+x^2)}$$

$$= \frac{\sqrt{1+x^2}(-2x) - (1-x^2)\dfrac{1}{2}(1+x^2)^{-1/2}}{(1+x^2)}$$

$$= \frac{-2x\sqrt{1+x^2} - \dfrac{1}{2}\dfrac{(1-x^2)}{\sqrt{1+x^2}}}{(1+x^2)}$$

$$= \frac{-2x(1+x^2) - \dfrac{1}{2}(1-x^2)}{(1+x^2)^{3/2}}$$

$$= \frac{\left(-2x - 2x^3 - \dfrac{1}{2} + \dfrac{1}{2}x^2\right)}{(1+x^2)^{3/2}}$$

(ii) Here, $y = \tan^{-1}\left(\dfrac{2x}{1-x^2}\right)$.

Differentiating with respect to x, we get

$$\frac{dy}{dx} = \frac{1}{1+\left(\dfrac{2x}{1-x^2}\right)^2}\frac{d}{dx}\frac{2x}{(1-x^2)}$$

$$= \frac{(1-x^2)^2}{\{(1-x^2)^2 + 4x^2\}} \cdot \frac{(1-x^2)\dfrac{d}{dx}(2x) - 2x\dfrac{d}{dx}(1-x^2)}{(1-x^2)^2}$$

$$= \frac{(1-x^2)^2\{2(1-x^2) + 4x^2\}}{\{(1-x^2)^2 + 4x^2\}(1-x^2)^2}$$

$$= \frac{2+2x^2}{\{(1-x^2)^2 + 4x^2\}}$$

$$= \frac{2(1+x^2)}{(1+x^4 - 2x^2 + 4x^2)}$$

$$= \frac{2(1+x^2)}{1+x^4+2x^2} = \frac{2(1+x^2)}{(1+x^2)^2}$$

$$= \frac{2}{1+x^2}.$$

(iii) Here, $y = \dfrac{\sin x + \cos x}{\sin x - \cos x}$

So, $\dfrac{dy}{dx} = \dfrac{d}{dx}\left(\dfrac{\sin x + \cos x}{\sin x - \cos x}\right)$

$$= \frac{(\sin x - \cos x)\dfrac{d}{dx}(\sin x + \cos x) - (\sin x + \cos x)\dfrac{d}{dx}(\sin x - \cos x)}{(\sin x - \cos x)^2}$$

$$= \frac{(\sin x - \cos x)(\cos x - \sin x) - (\sin x + \cos x)(\cos x + \sin x)}{(\sin x - \cos x)^2}$$

$$= \frac{-(\sin x - \cos x)^2 - (\sin x + \cos x)^2}{(\sin x - \cos x)^2}$$

$$= \frac{-(\sin^2 x + \cos^2 x - 2\sin x \cos x) - (\sin^2 x + \cos^2 x + 2\sin x \cos x)}{(\sin x - \cos x)^2}$$

$$= \frac{-1-1}{(\sin x - \cos x)^2} = \frac{-2}{(\sin x - \cos x)^2}.$$

(iv) Here, $y = \sin^{-1}\left(\dfrac{2x}{1+x^2}\right)$.

Differentiating w.r.t. x, we get

$$\frac{dy}{dx} = \frac{d}{dx}\left\{\sin^{-1}\left(\frac{2x}{1+x^2}\right)\right\}$$

$$= \frac{1}{\sqrt{1-\left(\dfrac{2x}{1+x^2}\right)^2}}\frac{d}{dx}\left(\frac{2x}{1+x^2}\right)$$

$$= \frac{(1+x^2)}{\sqrt{(1+x^2)^2 - 4x^2}} \cdot \frac{(1+x^2)\dfrac{d}{dx}(2x) - 2x\dfrac{d}{dx}(1+x^2)}{(1+x^2)^2}$$

$$= \frac{\{2(1+x^2) - 4x^2\}}{\sqrt{(1-x^2)^2}(1+x^2)}$$

$$= \frac{2-2x^2}{(1-x^2)(1+x^2)}$$

$$= \frac{2(1-x^2)}{(1-x^2)(1+x^2)} = \frac{2}{1+x^2}.$$

2. *Find* $\dfrac{dy}{dx}$ *of the following functions*

(i) $y = \dfrac{1-\tan x}{1+\tan x}$ (ii) $y = \dfrac{x\sin x}{1+\cos x}$

(iii) $y = x\log x + e^x \sin x - a^x x^3$

SOLUTION. (i) Here, $y = \dfrac{1-\tan x}{1+\tan x}$

Differentiating w.r.t. x, we get

$$\frac{dy}{dx} = \frac{(1+\tan x)\dfrac{d}{dx}(1-\tan x) - (1-\tan x)\dfrac{d}{dx}(1+\tan x)}{(1+\tan x)^2}$$

$$= \frac{-(1+\tan x)\sec^2 x - (1-\tan x)\sec^2 x}{(1+\tan x)^2}$$

$$= \frac{-2\sec^2 x}{(1+\tan x)^2}.$$

(ii) Here, $y = \dfrac{x\sin x}{1+\cos x}$.

Differentiating w.r.t. to x, we get

$$\frac{dy}{dx} = \frac{(1+\cos x)\dfrac{d}{dx}(x\sin x) - x\sin x\dfrac{d}{dx}(1+\cos x)}{(1+\cos x)^2}$$

$$= \frac{(1+\cos x)\left\{x\dfrac{d}{dx}\sin x + \dfrac{d}{dx}(x)\sin x\right\} + x\sin^2 x}{(1+\cos x)^2}$$

$$= \frac{(1+\cos x)\{x\cos x + \sin x\} + x\sin^2 x}{(1+\cos x)^2}$$

$$= \frac{x\cos x + \sin x + x\cos^2 x + \sin x\cos x + x\sin^2 x}{(1+\cos x)^2}$$

$$= \frac{x\cos x + \sin x + \sin x\cos x + x}{(1+\cos x)^2}$$

$$= \frac{\cos x(x+\sin x) + 1(x+\sin x)}{(1+\cos x)^2}$$

$$= \frac{(\cos x + 1)(x + \sin x)}{(1 + \cos x)^2}$$

$$= \frac{x + \sin x}{(1 + \cos x)}.$$

(iii) Here,

$$y = x \log x + e^x \sin x - a^x x^3.$$

Differentiating w.r.t. x, we get

$$\frac{dy}{dx} = \frac{d}{dx}(x \log x) + \frac{d}{dx}(e^x \sin x) - \frac{d}{dx}(a^x x^3)$$

$$= x\frac{d}{dx}(\log x) + \frac{d}{dx}(x)\log x + e^x \frac{d}{dx}(\sin x) + \frac{d}{dx}(e^x)\sin x - \left(a^x \frac{d}{dx}(x^3) + \frac{d}{dx}(a^x)x^3\right)$$

$$= x\frac{1}{x} + \log x + e^x \cos x + e^x \sin x - (3a^x x^2 + x^3 a^x \log_e a)$$

$$= 1 + \log x + e^x \cos x + e^x \sin x - 3a^x x^2 + x^3 \log_e a \cdot a^x$$

$$= 1 + \log x + e^x(\sin x + \cos x) - a^x(3x^2 + x^3 \log_e a)$$

3. *Find the differential coefficient at $x = 0$, if $y = a^x + \sqrt{\frac{1+x}{1-x}}$.*

SOLUTION. We have $y = a^x + \sqrt{\frac{1+x}{1-x}}$

Differentiating w.r.t. x, we get

$$\frac{dy}{dx} = a^x \log a + \frac{1}{2}\left(\frac{1+x}{1-x}\right)^{-1/2} \left\{\frac{1(1-x)-(1+x)(-1)}{(1-x)^2}\right\}$$

$$= a^x \log a + \frac{1}{2}\sqrt{\frac{1-x}{1+x}}\left\{\frac{1-x+1+x}{(1-x)^2}\right\}$$

$$= a^x \log a + \frac{1}{2}\sqrt{\frac{1-x}{1+x}}\left\{\frac{2}{(1-x)^2}\right\}$$

Putting $x = 0$

$$\left(\frac{dy}{dx}\right)_{x=0} = a^0 \log a + \frac{1}{2}\sqrt{\frac{1-0}{1+0}}\left\{\frac{2}{(1-0)^2}\right\}$$

$$= \log a + \frac{1}{2}\cdot\frac{2}{1^2} = \log a + 1$$

4. *If $\sqrt{x} + \sqrt{y} = 5$, prove that*

$$\left[\frac{dy}{dx}\right]_{(4,\,9)} = -\frac{3}{2}$$

SOLUTION. We have $\sqrt{x} + \sqrt{y} = 5$

Differentiating w.r.t. x, we get

$$\frac{1}{2\sqrt{x}} + \frac{1}{2\sqrt{y}}\frac{dy}{dx} = 0$$

$$\Rightarrow \quad \frac{dy}{dx} = -\sqrt{\frac{y}{x}}$$

Thus $$\left[\frac{dy}{dx}\right]_{(4,\,9)} = -\sqrt{\frac{9}{4}} = -\frac{3}{2}$$

5. *Differentiate* $\tan^{-1}\left(\frac{2x}{1-x^2}\right)$ *w.r.t.* $\sin^{-1}\left(\frac{2x}{1+x^2}\right)$. [MEERUT(BCA)–2001, 06, 07,08, 12, 13, 15, 17; BIKANER–2009]

SOLUTION. Let $y = \tan^{-1}\left(\frac{2x}{1-x^2}\right)$

Put $x = \tan\theta$

$$\Rightarrow \frac{2x}{1-x^2} = \frac{2\tan\theta}{1-\tan^2\theta} = \tan 2\theta$$

Also $y = \tan^{-1}(\tan 2\theta) = 2\theta = 2\tan^{-1} x$

$$\therefore \quad \frac{dy}{dx} = \frac{2}{1+x^2} \qquad \ldots(1)$$

Further let $z = \sin^{-1}\frac{2x}{1+x^2}$

Putting $x = \tan\theta$

$$\therefore \quad \frac{2x}{1+x^2} = \frac{2\tan\theta}{1+\tan^2\theta} = \sin 2\theta$$

$$\Rightarrow \sin^{-1}(\sin 2\theta) = 2\tan^{-1} x$$

Thus $$\frac{dz}{dx} = 2\cdot\frac{1}{1+x^2}$$

From (1) and (2) we conclude that

$$\frac{dy}{dz}=\frac{dy/dx}{dz/dx}=1$$

Hence, $\dfrac{dy}{dz}=1$

6. *Differentiate* $\sin^{-1}\left(\dfrac{1-x}{1+x}\right)$ *w.r.t.* $\sqrt{x}$.

[MEERUT(BCA)–2004]

SOLUTION. Let $u=\sin^{-1}\left(\dfrac{1-x}{1+x}\right), v=\sqrt{x}$

Differentiating w.r.t. x

$$\frac{du}{dx}=\frac{1}{\sqrt{1-\left(\frac{1-x}{1+x}\right)^2}}\frac{-(1+x)-(1-x)}{(1+x)^2}$$

$$=\frac{1+x}{\sqrt{(1+x)^2-(1-x)^2}}\left(\frac{-2}{(1+x)^2}\right),$$

$$=-\frac{1}{\sqrt{x}(1+x)},\frac{dv}{dx}=\frac{1}{2\sqrt{x}}$$

Therefore, $\dfrac{du}{dv}=-\dfrac{\frac{1}{\sqrt{x}(1+x)}}{\frac{1}{2\sqrt{x}}}=\dfrac{-2}{1+x}$

7. *Find the derivative of* $\tan^{-1}\dfrac{\sqrt{1+x^2}-1}{x}$ *w.r.t.* $\tan^{-1}x$.

SOLUTION. Let $u=\tan^{-1}\left(\dfrac{\sqrt{1+x^2}-1}{x}\right)$

and $v=\tan^{-1}x$

Putting $x=\tan\theta$, we have

$$u=\tan^{-1}\left[\frac{\sqrt{1+\tan^2\theta}-1}{\tan\theta}\right]$$

$$=\tan^{-1}\left[\frac{\sec\theta-1}{\tan\theta}\right]$$

$$=\tan^{-1}\left[\left(\frac{1}{\cos\theta}-1\right)\cdot\frac{\cos\theta}{\sin\theta}\right]$$

$$=\tan^{-1}\left[\frac{1-\cos\theta}{\sin\theta}\right]$$

$$=\tan^{-1}\left[\frac{1-\left(1-2\sin^2\frac{\theta}{2}\right)}{2\sin\frac{\theta}{2}\cdot\cos\frac{\theta}{2}}\right]$$

$$=\tan^{-1}\left(\tan\frac{\theta}{2}\right)=\frac{\theta}{2}$$

Also $v=\tan^{-1}(\tan\theta)=\theta$

$\Rightarrow\quad u=\dfrac{v}{2}$

Hence $\dfrac{du}{dv}=\dfrac{1}{2}$

8. *Find the derivative of* $(\log x)^{\tan x}$ *w.r.t.* $\sin(m\cos^{-1}x)$.

SOLUTION. Let $u=(\log x)^{\tan x}$

$\Rightarrow \log u=\tan x\log(\log x)$

Diff. w.r.t. x, we get

$$\frac{1}{u}\cdot\frac{du}{dx}=\tan x\cdot\frac{1}{\log x}\cdot\frac{1}{x}+[\log(\log x)]\sec^2 x$$

$$\Rightarrow \frac{du}{dx}=u\left[\frac{\tan x}{x\cdot\log x}+\sec^2 x\log(\log x)\right]$$

$$=(\log x)^{\tan x}\left[\frac{\tan x}{x\cdot\log x}+\sec^2 x\log(\log x)\right]$$

Further, let $v=\sin(m\cos^{-1}x)$

$$\Rightarrow \frac{dv}{dx}=\cos(m\cos^{-1}x)\cdot m\left(\frac{-1}{\sqrt{1-x^2}}\right)$$

$$=-\frac{m}{\sqrt{1-x^2}}\cos(m\cos^{-1}x)$$

Hence $\dfrac{du}{dv}=\dfrac{du}{dx}\cdot\dfrac{dx}{dv}$

$$=\frac{(\log x)^{\tan x}\left[\frac{\tan x}{x\cdot\log x}+\sec^2 x\cdot\log(\log x)\right]}{-\frac{m}{\sqrt{1-x^2}}\cos(m\cos^{-1}x)}$$

9. *If* $y=\sqrt{\dfrac{x}{a}}+\sqrt{\dfrac{a}{x}}$. *Then show that*

$$\frac{dy}{dx}=\frac{x-a}{2x\sqrt{ax}}$$

[MEERUT(BCA)–2007, 10, 12, 15; GARHWAL–2009]

SOLUTION. We have $y = \sqrt{\frac{x}{a}} + \sqrt{\frac{a}{x}}$

Differentiating w.r.t. x, we get

$$\frac{dy}{dx} = \frac{1}{\sqrt{a}}\frac{1}{2\sqrt{x}} + \sqrt{a}\left(-\frac{1}{2x^{3/2}}\right)$$

$$= \frac{1}{2x^{3/2}a^{1/2}}(x-a) = \frac{x-a}{2x\sqrt{ax}}.$$

10. $y = e^{x+e^{x+e^{x+\cdots\infty}}}$, *then show that*

$$\frac{dy}{dx} = \frac{y}{1-y}.$$

[MEERUT(BCA)–2007, 10, 12; DELHI(BCA)–2011]

SOLUTION. We have $y = e^{x+e^{x+e^{x+\cdots\infty}}}$

$$y = e^{x+y} \quad \ldots(1)$$

Diff. w.r.t. x, we get

$$\frac{dy}{dx} = e^{x+y}\left(1+\frac{dy}{dx}\right) = y\left(1+\frac{dy}{dx}\right)$$

[From (1)]

$$\frac{dy}{dx}(1-y) = y$$

$$\frac{dy}{dx} = \frac{y}{1-y}$$

11. (a) *Find* $\frac{dy}{dx}$ *if* $y = \tan^{-1}\sqrt{\frac{1-\cos x}{1+\cos x}}$

(b) *Find* $\frac{dy}{dx}$ *if* $y = x^{\sin x} + (\sin x)^x$

(c) *If* $y = (x+\sqrt{(x^2-1)})^m$. *Prove that* $(x^2-1)\left(\frac{dy}{dx}\right)^2 = m^2y^2$

[MEERUT(BCA)–2009, 12]

SOLUTION. (a) We have $y = \tan^{-1}\sqrt{\frac{1-\cos x}{1+\cos x}}$

$$\left(\because \cos x = 1-2\sin^2\frac{x}{2},\ \cos x = 2\cos^2\frac{x}{2}-1\right)$$

$$= \tan^{-1}\sqrt{\frac{1-\left(1-2\sin^2\frac{x}{2}\right)}{1+\left(2\cos^2\frac{x}{2}-1\right)}}$$

$$= \tan^{-1}\sqrt{\frac{\sin^2\frac{x}{2}}{\cos^2\frac{x}{2}}}$$

$$= \tan^{-1}\left(\tan\frac{x}{2}\right)$$

$$\Rightarrow y = \frac{x}{2}$$

Diff. w.r.t. x, we get

$$\frac{dy}{dx} = \frac{1}{2}$$

(b) We have

$$y = x^{\sin x} + (\sin x)^x$$

Diff. w.r.t. x, we get

$$\frac{dy}{dx} = \frac{d}{dx}(x^{\sin x}) + \frac{d}{dx}(\sin x)^x \quad \ldots(1)$$

Let $u = x^{\sin x}$

Taking logarithm of both sides, we get

$$\log u = \sin x \log x$$

Differentiating w.r.t. x, we get

$$\frac{1}{u}\cdot\frac{du}{dx} = \cos x \log x + \frac{\sin x}{x}$$

or $$\frac{du}{dx} = x^{\sin x}\left(\cos x \log x + \frac{\sin x}{x}\right) \quad \ldots(2)$$

and $v = \sin x^x$

$$\Rightarrow \log v = x \log \sin x$$

Differentiating w.r.t. x, we get

$$\frac{1}{v}\frac{dv}{dx} = \log \sin x + \frac{x}{\sin x}\cos x$$

or $$\frac{dv}{dx} = \sin x^x(\log \sin x + x\cot x) \quad \ldots(3)$$

Substituting (2) and (3) in (1), we get

$$\frac{dy}{dx} = x^{\sin x}\left(\cos x \log x + \frac{\sin x}{x}\right) + \sin x^x(\log \sin x + x\cot x)$$

(c) We have $y = \left(x+\sqrt{x^2-1}\right)^m$

Differentiating w.r. to x, we get

$$\frac{dy}{dx} = m\left(x+\sqrt{x^2-1}\right)^{m-1}\left(1+\frac{x}{(x^2-1)^{1/2}}\right)$$

$$= m\left(x+\sqrt{x^2-1}\right)^{m-1}\left(\frac{x+\sqrt{x^2-1}}{\sqrt{x^2-1}}\right)$$

$$\text{or} \left(\sqrt{x^2-1}\right)\frac{dy}{dx} = m(x+\sqrt{x^2-1})^m$$

$$\text{or} \left(\sqrt{x^2-1}\right)\frac{dy}{dx} = my$$

$$[\because y = (x+\sqrt{x^2-1})^m]$$

Squaring, we get

$$(x^2-1)\left(\frac{dy}{dx}\right)^2 = m^2y^2$$

Exercise-6.1

1. Find the derivatives (or differential coefficients) of the following functions :

(i) $y = \frac{(x+1)(x+2)}{(x+3)(x+4)}$

(ii) $y = \log \sin x^2$

(iii) $y = \frac{x^4 - 5x^2}{5x^6 + 7x}$ (iv) $y = \frac{1+\tan x}{1-\tan x}$

2. Find dy/dx of the following functions :

(i) $y = \sqrt{\left(\frac{1-x}{1+x}\right)}$ (ii) $y = \sqrt{\left(\frac{1+x}{x}\right)}$

(iii) $y = \log[\sqrt{(x+1)} - \sqrt{(x-1)}]$

(iv) $y = (2x^2 + 5x + 7)^{-2}$.

3. Find the derivatives of the following functions :

(i) $y = (x-2)(x+2)(x-3)(x+3)$

(ii) $y = (x+1)(2x^3 - 21)$

(iii) $y = \sin^{-1}(\tan x)$ (ii) $y = (\tan x)^x$.

4. Differentiate the following functions:

(i) $y = (\sin x)^{\cos x}$

(ii) $y = \sin(e^x) + \frac{1}{x} + \log(x^2 + x)$

(iii) $y = \sin x \log x$ (iv) $y = e^x \tan^4 x$

5. Find $\frac{dy}{dx}$ of the following functions :

(i) $y = \log \sin x + \cos^{-1}(e^x) + x^4 \sec x$

(ii) $y = (\log x)^x$ (iii) $\log\left(\frac{x}{y}\right) = x + y$

(iv) $y = \sec(x^2 - 2x + 1)$

6. Find the derivatives of the following functions:

(i) $e^{2x} \cos 3x$ (ii) $\log(\sin^{-1} x^4)$

(iii) $x^3 - y^3 - 3axy = 0$.

Hints to the Selected Problems

1. (i) $y = \frac{(x+1)(x+2)}{(x+3)(x+4)}$

Taking log on both sides, we get

$$\log y = \log(x+1) + \log(x+2) - \log(x+3) - \log(x+4),$$

Diff. w.r.t. x,

$$\frac{1}{y}\frac{dy}{dx} = \frac{1}{(x+1)} + \frac{1}{(x+2)} - \frac{1}{(x+3)} - \frac{1}{(x+4)}$$

$$\Rightarrow \frac{dy}{dx} = y\left\{\frac{2x+3}{(x+1)(x+2)} - \frac{2x+7}{(x+3)(x+4)}\right\}$$

(ii) $y = \log \sin x^2$

Diff.w.r.t. x we get

$$\frac{dy}{dx} = \frac{1}{\sin x^2} \cdot (\cos x^2) 2x = 2x \cot x^2$$

(iv) $y = \frac{1+\tan x}{1-\tan x}$

Diff. both sides by Quotient rule, we get

$$\frac{dy}{dx} = \frac{\sec^2(1-\tan x) + \sec^2(1+\tan x)}{(1-\tan x)^2}$$

$$= \frac{2\sec^2 x}{(1-\tan x)^2}$$

2. (i) $y = \sqrt{\left(\frac{1-x}{1+x}\right)} = \frac{(1-x)^{1/2}}{(1+x)^{1/2}}$

Diff. both sides by Quotient Rule

$$\frac{dy}{dx} = \frac{-\frac{1}{2}\frac{1}{\sqrt{1-x}}\sqrt{1+x} - \frac{1}{2}\sqrt{1-x}\frac{1}{\sqrt{1+x}}}{(1+x)}$$

$$= -\frac{1}{2}\frac{\{(1+x)+(1-x)\}}{(1+x)\sqrt{1-x^2}} = \frac{-1}{(1+x)\sqrt{1-x^2}}$$

(ii) Do as Question No.2 (i)

(iii) $y = \log[\sqrt{x+1} - \sqrt{x-1}]$, diff. w.r.t. x both sides we have

$$\frac{dy}{dx} = \frac{1}{\sqrt{x+1} - \sqrt{x-1}}\left(\frac{1}{2\sqrt{x+1}} - \frac{1}{2\sqrt{x-1}}\right)$$

$$= \frac{1}{2}\frac{-(\sqrt{x+1} - \sqrt{x-1})}{(\sqrt{x+1} - \sqrt{x-1})\sqrt{x^2-1}} = \frac{1}{2\sqrt{x^2-1}}$$

(iv) $y = (2x^2 + 5x + 7)^{-2}$, diff, both sides w.r.t. x

$$\frac{dy}{dx} = \frac{-2}{(2x^2+5x+7)^3}(4x+5)$$

$$= \frac{-2(4x+5)}{(2x^2+5x+7)^3}$$

3. (i) $y = (x-2)(x+2)(x-3)(x+3)$

$$= (x^2-4)(x^2-9)$$

Diff. w.r.t. x by product rule

$$\frac{dy}{dx} = 2x(x^2-9) + 2x(x^2-4)$$

$$= 4x^3 - 26x$$

(ii) Do as in above Question

(iii) $y = \sin^{-1}(\tan x)$, diff w.r.t. x

$$\frac{dy}{dx} = \frac{1}{\sqrt{1-\tan^2 x}}\sec^2 x$$

$$= \frac{\cos x}{\sqrt{\cos^2 x - \sin^2 x}}\sec^2 x$$

$$= \frac{\sec x}{\sqrt{\cos 2x}} = \sec x\sqrt{\sec 2x}$$

(iv) $y = (\tan x)^x$, take log on both the sides

$$\log y = x\log(\tan x),$$

Diff w.r.t. x

$$\frac{1}{y}\frac{dy}{dx} = \log(\tan x) + \frac{x}{\tan x}\sec^2 x$$

$$\frac{dy}{dx} = y\{\log\tan x + x\sec x\operatorname{cosec} x\}$$

$$= (\tan x)^x\{\log\tan x + x\sec x\operatorname{cosec} x\}$$

4. (i) $y = (\sin x)^{\cos x}$ taking log on both the sides

$$\log y = \cos x\log\sin x,$$

diff. both the sides w.r.t. x, we get

$$\frac{1}{y}\frac{dy}{dx} = -\sin x\log\sin x + \cos x\frac{\cos x}{\sin x}$$

$$\frac{dy}{dx} = y(\cos x\cot x - \sin x\log\sin x)$$

$$= (\sin x)^{\cos x}(\cos x\cot x - \sin x\log\sin x)$$

(ii) $y = \sin(e^x) + \frac{1}{x} + \log(x^2+x)$, diff w.r.t. x

$$\frac{dy}{dx} = \cos(e^x)e^x - \frac{1}{x^2} + \frac{1+2x}{x^2+x}$$

(iii) $y = \sin x(\log x)$, diff w.r.t. x by product rule

$$\frac{dy}{dx} = \frac{\sin x}{x} + \cos x(\log x)$$

(iv) $y = e^x\tan^4 x$, diff w.r.t. x by product rule

$$\frac{dy}{dx} = e^x\tan^4 x + 4\tan^3 x\sec^2 x\, e^x$$

$$= e^x\tan^x(\tan^3 x + 4\sec^2 x)$$

5. (i) $y = \log\sin x + \cos^{-1}(e^x) + x^4\sec x$,

diff. w.r.t. x

$$\frac{dy}{dx} = \frac{\cos x}{\sin x} - \frac{e^x}{\sqrt{1-e^{2x}}} + 4x^3\sec x + x^4\sec x\tan x$$

$$= \cot x - \frac{e^x}{\sqrt{1-e^{2x}}} + x^3\sec x(x\tan x + 4)$$

(ii) $y = (\log x)^x$

Taking log on both sides

$$\log y = x\log(\log x)$$

Diff. w.r.t. x, we get

$$\frac{1}{y}\frac{dy}{dx} = \frac{x}{\log x}\left(\frac{1}{x}\right) + \log(\log x)$$

$$\frac{dy}{dx} = y\left\{\frac{x}{\log x} + \log(\log x)\right\}$$

(iii) $$\log\left(\frac{x}{y}\right) = x + y$$

$$\log x - \log y = x + y,$$

Diff. both the sides w.r.t. x, we get

$$\frac{1}{x} - \frac{1}{y}\frac{dy}{dx} = 1 + \frac{dy}{dx}$$

$$\frac{dy}{dx}\left(1 + \frac{1}{y}\right) = -1 + \frac{1}{x}$$

$$\frac{dy}{dx} = \frac{y\,(1-x)}{x\,(1+y)}$$

(iv) $y = \sec(x^2 - 2x + 1)$, diff. w.r.t. x both sides

$$\frac{dy}{dx} = 2(x-1)\sec(x^2-2x+1)\tan(x^2-2x+1)$$

$$= 2(x-1)\sec(x-1)^2\tan(x-1)^2$$

6. (i) $y = e^{2x}\cos 3x$, diff. w.r.t. x

$$\frac{dy}{dx} = 2e^{2x}\cos 3x + (-3\sin 3x)e^{2x}$$

$$= e^{2x}(2\cos 3x - 3\sin 3x)$$

(ii) Let $y = \log(\sin^{-1} x^4)$ diff. both sides w.r.t. x

$$\frac{dy}{dx} = \frac{1}{\sin^{-1} x^4} \times \frac{4x^3}{\sqrt{1-x^8}}$$

$$= \frac{4x^3}{\sin^{-1} x^4 \sqrt{1-x^8}}$$

(iii) $x^3 - y^3 - 3axy = 0$, diff. w.r.t. x

$$3x^2 - 3y^2\frac{dy}{dx} - 3a\left(y + x\frac{dy}{dx}\right) = 0$$

$$-\frac{dy}{dx}(y^2 + ax) + x^2 - ay = 0$$

$$\frac{dy}{dx} = \frac{x^2 - ay}{y^2 + ax}.$$

ANSWERS

1. (i) $\frac{4x^2+20x+22}{(x^2+7x+12)^2}$ (ii) $2x\cot x^2$ (iii) $\frac{x^2(-10x^7+100x^5+21x^2-35)}{(5x^6+7x)^2}$

(iv) $\frac{2\sec^2 x}{(1-\tan x)^2}$ **2.** (i) $-\frac{1}{\sqrt{(1-x^2)}}$ (ii) $-\frac{1}{2x\sqrt{x(x+1)}}$ (iii) $\frac{-1}{2\sqrt{x^2-1}}$

2. (iv) $\frac{-2(4x+5)}{(2x^2+5x+7)^3}$ **3.** (i) $4x^3-26x$ (ii) $8x^3+6x^2-21$ (iii) $\sec x\sqrt{(\sec 2x)}$

3. (iv) $(\tan x)^x(x\sec x\,\mathrm{cosce}\,x+\log\tan x)$ **4.** (i) $(\sin x)^{\cos x}(\cos x\cot x-\sin x\log\sin x)$

4. (ii) $e^x\cos(e^x)-\frac{1}{x^2}+\frac{2x+1}{x^2+x}$ (iii) $\frac{\sin x}{x}+\cos x\log x$ (iv) $e^x\tan^3 x(4\sec^2 x+\tan x)$

5. (i) $\cot x-\frac{e^x}{\sqrt{1-e^{2x}}}+x^3\sec x(x\tan x+4)$ (ii) $(\log x)^x\left[\frac{1}{\log x}+\log(\log x)\right]$ (iii) $\frac{(1-x)y}{(1+y)x}$

5. (iv) $2(x-1)\sec(x^2-2x+1)\tan(x^2-2x+1)$ **6.** (i) $e^{2x}(2\cos 3x-3\sin 3x)$

6. (ii) $\frac{4x^3}{\sin^{-1}x^4\sqrt{(1-x^8)}}$ (iii) $\frac{x^2-ay}{ax+y^2}$.

Exercise-6.2

Find $\frac{dy}{dx}$ for the following implicit functions.

1. $xy = x + y$ **2.** $(x^2+y^2)^2 = xy$

3. $\sin(xy) + \frac{x}{y^2} = x^2 - y$

4. $ye^x + 2^x\sin x = \cos y$

5. $\sin(x+y) = \log(x+y)$

6. $e^{x-y} = \log\left(\frac{x}{y}\right)$ **7.** $x\cdot 2^y + 2^x = y$

8. $\tan^{-1}(x^2+y^2) = 9$

9. $3\sin(xy) + 4\cos(xy) = 5$

10. $y\cos x = x - y$

11. If $\sqrt{\frac{y}{x}}+\sqrt{\frac{x}{y}}=6$, show that $\frac{dy}{dx} = \frac{x-17y}{17x-y}$.

12. If $\sin y = x\cos(a+y)$, prove that

$$\frac{dy}{dx} = \frac{\cos^2(a+y)}{\cos a}$$

13. If $\sqrt{1-x^6}+\sqrt{1-y^6} = a(x^3-y^3)$ prove that

$$\frac{dy}{dx} = \frac{x^2\sqrt{1-y^6}}{y^2\sqrt{1-x^6}}$$

[KANPUR(BCA)–2005; MADRAS–2006; NAGPUR–2009]

14. If $\log\sqrt{x^2+y^2} = \tan^{-1}\frac{y}{x}$, prove that

$$\frac{dy}{dx} = \frac{x+y}{x-y}$$

15. If $e^x + e^y = e^{x+y}$, prove that $\frac{dy}{dx} = -\frac{e^x(e^y-1)}{e^y(e^x-1)}$

16. If $\cos y = x\cos(b+y)$, show that

$$\frac{dy}{dx} = \frac{\cos^2(b+y)}{\sin b}$$

[KANPUR(BCA)–2003; LUCKNOW–2010]

17. If $y = \sqrt{\sin x\sqrt{\sin x\sqrt{\sin x \ldots\infty}}}$, show that

$$\frac{dy}{dx} = \frac{\cos x}{2y-1}$$

[ROHILKHAND(BCA)–2001, 05, 14; BHOPAL–2006]

Hint to Selected Problems

1. $xy = x + y$

$\Rightarrow \; y = \dfrac{x}{x-1} = 1 + \dfrac{1}{x-1}$

Diff. w.r.t. x $\quad \dfrac{dy}{dx} = -\dfrac{1}{(x-1)^2}$

2. $(x^2 + y^2)^2 = xy$

Diff.w.r.t.x $2(x^2+y^2)\left\{2x + 2y\dfrac{dy}{dx}\right\} = x\dfrac{dy}{dx} + y$

$\Rightarrow \; \{4y(x^2+y^2) - x\}\dfrac{dy}{dx} = y - 4x(x^2+y^2)$

$$\frac{dy}{dx} = \frac{y - 4x(x^2+y^2)}{4y(x^2+y^2) - x}$$

3. $\sin(xy) + \dfrac{x}{y^2} = x^2 - y \qquad \ldots(1)$

Diff. w.r.t x

$\cos(xy)\left(y + x\dfrac{dy}{dx}\right) + \dfrac{1}{y^2} - \dfrac{2x}{y^3}\dfrac{dy}{dx} = 2x - \dfrac{dy}{dx}$

$\Rightarrow \left(x\cos(xy) - \dfrac{2x}{y^3} + 1\right)\dfrac{dy}{dx} = 2x - \dfrac{1}{y^2} - y\cos(xy)$

$\Rightarrow \left(xy^2\cos(xy) - 2\dfrac{x}{y} + y^2\right)\dfrac{dy}{dx}$

$= 2xy^2 - 1 - y^3\cos(xy)$

(Multiplying by y^2)

$\Rightarrow \; \{xy^2\cos(xy) - 2(xy^2 - y^2$

$- y\sin(xy) + y^2)\dfrac{dy}{dx}$

$= 2xy^2 - 1 - y^3\cos(xy)$

Putting the value of $\dfrac{x}{y}$ from (1)

$$\Rightarrow \frac{dy}{dx} = \frac{2xy^2 - y^3\cos(xy) - 1}{2y\sin(xy) + xy^2\cos(xy) - 2xy^2 + 3y^2}$$

4. $ye^x + 2^x\sin x = \cos y$

Diff. w.r.t. x

$ye^x + e^x\dfrac{dy}{dx} + 2^x\log 2\sin x + 2^x\cos x$

$= -\sin y\dfrac{dy}{dx}$

$$\Rightarrow \frac{dy}{dx} = \frac{-[ye^x + 2^x\cos x + 2^x\sin x\log 2}{(e^x + \sin y)}$$

5. $\sin(x+y) = \log(x+y)$

Diff w.r.t. x

$\cos(x+y)\left\{1 + \dfrac{dy}{dx}\right\} = \dfrac{1}{x+y}\left\{1 + \dfrac{dy}{dx}\right\}$

$\Rightarrow \; \left\{\cos(x+y) - \dfrac{1}{x+y}\right\}\dfrac{dy}{dx}$

$= -\left\{\cos(x+y) - \dfrac{1}{x+y}\right\}$

$\Rightarrow \; \dfrac{dy}{dx} = -1$

6. $e^{x-y} = \log\dfrac{x}{y} = \log x - \log y$

Diff w.r.t x, we have

$e^{x-y}\left(1 - \dfrac{dy}{dx}\right) = \dfrac{1}{x} - \dfrac{1}{y}\dfrac{dy}{dx}$

$\dfrac{dy}{dx}\left(\dfrac{1}{y} - e^{x-y}\right) = \dfrac{1}{x} - e^{x-y}$

$$\frac{dy}{dx} = \frac{y(1 - xe^{x-y})}{x(1 - ye^{x-y})}$$

7. $x \cdot 2^y + 2^x = y$

Diff w.r.t. x, we have

$2^y + x2^y\log 2\dfrac{dy}{dx} + 2^x\log 2 = \dfrac{dy}{dx}$

$2^y + 2^x\log 2 = \dfrac{dy}{dx}(1 - x\cdot 2^y\log 2)$

$$\frac{dy}{dx} = \left[\frac{2^y + 2^x\log 2}{1 - x2^y\log 2}\right]$$

8. $\tan^{-1}(x^2+y^2) = 9 \Rightarrow x^2 + y^2 = \tan 9$

Diff. w.r.t. x, we get

$2x + 2y\dfrac{dy}{dx} = 0 \Rightarrow \dfrac{dy}{dx} = -\dfrac{x}{y}$

9. $3\sin(xy) + 4\cos(xy) = 5$

Diff. w.r.t. x

$3\cos(xy)\left\{y + x\dfrac{dy}{dx}\right\}$

$-4\sin(xy)\left\{y + x\dfrac{dy}{dx}\right\} = 0$

$\dfrac{dy}{dx}\{3x\cos(xy) - 4x\sin(xy)$

$= -y\{3\cos(xy) - 4\sin(xy)\}$

$\dfrac{dy}{dx} = -\left(\dfrac{y}{x}\right)$

10. $y\cos x = x - y \qquad \ldots(1)$

Diff. w.r.t. x

$-y\sin x + (\cos x)\dfrac{dy}{dx} = 1 - \dfrac{dy}{dx}$

$\dfrac{dy}{dx}(1 + \cos x) = 1 + y\sin x$

$\dfrac{dy}{dx} = \dfrac{1 + y\sin x}{1 + \cos x}$

$= \left(1 + \dfrac{x\sin x}{1 + \cos + x}\right)\dfrac{1}{(1 + \cos x)}$

$= \dfrac{1 + x\sin x + \cos x}{(1 + \cos x)^2}$

11. $\sqrt{\frac{x}{y}}+\sqrt{\frac{y}{x}}=6$

$\Rightarrow y+x=6\sqrt{xy} \Rightarrow x^2+y^2-34xy=0$

Diff. w.r.t. x

$$2x+2y\frac{dy}{dx}-34\left(x\frac{dy}{dx}+y\right)=0$$

$$\frac{dy}{dx}=\frac{x-17y}{17x-y}$$

12. $\sin y = x\cos(a+y)$ ...(1)

Diff. w.r.t. x

$$\frac{dy}{dx}(\cos y)=\cos(a+y)-x\sin(a+y)\left(\frac{dy}{dx}\right)$$

$$\frac{dy}{dx}\{\cos y+x\sin(a+y)\}=\cos(a+y)$$

$$\frac{dy}{dx}\left\{\cos y+\frac{\sin y}{\cos(a+y)}\sin(a+y)\right\}=\cos(a+y)$$

From(1)

$$\frac{dy}{dx}\{\cos(a+y)\cos y+\sin y\sin(a+y)\}$$
$$=\cos^2(a+y)$$

$$\frac{dy}{dx}=\frac{\cos^2(a+y)}{\cos a}$$

14. $\frac{1}{2}\log(x^2+y^2)=\tan^{-1}\frac{y}{x}$

$$\frac{1}{2(x^2+y^2)}\left(2x+2y\frac{dy}{dx}\right)=\frac{1}{1+\frac{y^2}{x^2}}\left(\frac{x\frac{dy}{dx}-y}{x^2}\right)$$

$$x+y\frac{dy}{dx}=x\frac{dy}{dx}-y$$

$$\frac{dy}{dx}=\frac{x+y}{x-y}$$

15. $e^x+e^y=e^{x+y}$,

Diff w.r.t. x

$$e^x+e^y\frac{dy}{dx}=e^{x+y}\left\{1+\frac{dy}{dx}\right\}$$

$$e^x-e^{x+y}=\frac{dy}{dx}(-e^y+e^{x+y})$$

$$\frac{dy}{dx}=\frac{e^x(1-e^y)}{e^y(e^x-1)}$$

ANSWERS

1. $\frac{1-y}{x-1}$ or $\frac{-1}{(x-1)^2}$ **2.** $\frac{y-4x(x^2+y^2)}{4y(x^2+y^2)-(x)}$ **3.** $\frac{2xy^2-y^3\cos(xy)-1}{2y\sin xy+xy^2\cos xy-2xy^2+3y^2}$

4. $\frac{-[ye^x+2^x\cos x+2^x\sin x\log 2]}{e^x+\sin y}$ **5.** -1 **6.** $\frac{y}{x}\left[\frac{xe^{x-y}-1}{ye^{x-y}-1}\right]$

7. $\left[\frac{2^y+2^x\log 2}{1-x2^y\log 2}\right]$ **8.** $(-x/y)$ **9.** $-(y/x)$ **10.** $\frac{1+y\sin x}{1+\cos x}$

6.10 SECOND ORDER DERIVATIVES

It is known that derivative of y w.r.t. x (if exists) is denoted by $\frac{dy}{dx}$ and is called the first derivative of y,

Further, derivative of $\frac{dy}{dx}$ w.r.t. x (if it exists) is denoted by $\frac{d^2y}{dx^2}$ and is called the second derivative of y,

Thus, $$\frac{d^2y}{dx^2}=\frac{d}{dx}\left(\frac{dy}{dx}\right)=\text{ second derivative of } y \text{ w.r.t. } x.$$

Similarly, $$\frac{d^3y}{dx^3}=\frac{d}{dx}\left(\frac{d^2y}{dx^2}\right)=\text{derivative of }\frac{d^2y}{dx^2}\text{ w.r.t. } x.$$

In general $\frac{d^ny}{dx^n}$ denoted the nth derivative of y w.r.t. x.

OTHER SYMBOLS

(1) $\frac{dy}{dx}$ is also denoted by y_1 or y'. (2) $\frac{d^2y}{dx^2}$ is also denoted by y_2 or y''.

(3) $\frac{dy}{dx}$ is also denoted by Dy, where D is the operator $\frac{d}{dx}$.

$\frac{d^2y}{dx^2}$ is also denoted by D^2y, where D^2 is the operator $\frac{d^2}{dx^2}$,

(4) Let $f(x)$ be a differentiable function, then $f'(x)$ denotes the first derivative of $f(x)$ w.r.t. x.

Thus $f'(x) = \frac{d}{dx}\{f(x)\}$

Similarly $f''(x) = \frac{d}{dx}\{f'(x)\} = \frac{d^2\{f(x)\}}{dx^2}$ = second derivative of $f(x)$ w.r.t. x.

WORKING PROCEDURE

To Find the Higher Ordered Derivatives use the following steps:

STEP 1. Let the given function be y.

STEP 2. (i) Differentiate the given function w.r.t x to get $\frac{dy}{dx}$.

(ii) If both base and power in the given function are variables, then first take logarithm and then differentiate to get $\frac{dy}{dx}$.

STEP3. Now differentiate $\frac{dy}{dx}$ w.r.t. x to get $\frac{d^2y}{dx^2}$.

STEP 4. If a particular expression is to be obtained, simplify the expression involved after obtaining first derivative making use of the given relation between x and y and if required also use the expression for first derivative obtained.

After simplification find the higher derivative.

Solved Examples

1. *Find the second derivatives of the following functions*

(*i*) $y = x^3 \log x$

(*ii*) $e^{6x} \cos 3x$

SOLUTION. (i) Let $y = x^3 \log x$

Differentiating w.r.t. x we get

$$\therefore \frac{dy}{dx} = x^3 \cdot \frac{1}{x} + 3x^2 \cdot \log x$$

$$= x^2 + 3x^2 \log x$$

Again differentiating w.r.t. x, we get

$$\frac{d^2y}{dx^2} = 2x + 3x^2 \cdot \frac{1}{x} + 6x \cdot \log x$$

$$= 5x + 6x \log x$$

(ii) Let $y = e^{6x} \cos 3x$ ...(1)

Differentiating (1) w.r.t x, we get

$$\therefore \frac{dy}{dx} = e^{6x} \cdot 6\cos 3x + e^{6x}(-\sin 3x) \cdot 3$$

$$= 6e^{6x} \cos 3x - 3e^{6x} \sin 3x \qquad ...(2)$$

Again differentiating (2) w.r.t. x, we get

$$\frac{d^2y}{dx^2} = 6[e^{6x} \cdot 6\cos 3x + e^{6x}(-3\sin 3x)] - 3[e^{6x} \cdot 6\sin 3x + e^{6x} \cdot 3\cos 3x]$$

$$= e^{6x}[36\cos 3x - 18\sin 3x - 18\sin 3x - 9\cos 3x]$$

$$= e^{6x}(27\cos 3x - 36\sin 3x)$$

2. *If $y = e^{\tan x}$, prove that*

$$\cos^2 x \frac{d^2y}{dx^2} - (1 + \sin 2x)\frac{dy}{dx} = 0$$

SOLUTION. Given, $y = e^{\tan x}$

$\therefore \quad \log y = \tan x \quad \ldots(1)$

$\therefore \quad \frac{1}{y}\frac{dy}{dx} = \sec^2 x$

or $\quad \frac{dy}{dx} = y\sec^2 x \quad \ldots(2)$

or $\quad \cos^2 x\frac{dy}{dx} = y \quad \ldots(3)$

Differentiating again w.r.t. x, we get

$$\cos^2 x\frac{d^2y}{dx^2} - 2\cos x\sin x\frac{dy}{dx} = \frac{dy}{dx}$$

or $\cos^2 x\frac{d^2y}{dx^2} - (1+\sin 2x)\frac{dy}{dx} = 0.$

3. *If* $y = a\cos(\log x) + b\sin(\log x)$, *show that* $x^2\frac{d^2y}{dx^2} + x\frac{dy}{dx} + y = 0$.

SOLUTION. Given $y = a\cos(\log x) + b\sin(\log x) \quad \ldots(1)$

Differentiating (1) w.r.t x, we get

$\therefore \frac{dy}{dx} = -a\sin(\log x)\cdot\frac{1}{x} + b\cos(\log x)\cdot\frac{1}{x}$

or $x\cdot\frac{dy}{dx} = -a\sin(\log x) + b\cos(\log x)$

Again differentiating w.r.t. x, we get

$$x\frac{d^2y}{dx^2} + 1\cdot\frac{dy}{dx} = -a\cos(\log x)\cdot\frac{1}{x} - b\sin(\log x)\cdot\frac{1}{x}$$

or $x^2\frac{d^2y}{dx^2} + x\frac{dy}{dx} = -[a\cos(\log x) + b\sin(\log x)]$

$= -y \quad$ [From (1)]

or $\quad x^2\frac{d^2y}{dx^2} + x\frac{dy}{dx} + y = 0.$

4. *If* $y = (\sin^{-1} x)^2$, *prove that*

$$(1-x^2)\frac{d^2y}{dx^2} = x\frac{dy}{dx} + 2.$$

SOLUTION. Given $y = (\sin^{-1} x)^2 \quad \ldots(1)$

Differentiating (1) w.r.t. x, we get

$\therefore \frac{dy}{dx} = 2\sin^{-1} x\cdot\frac{1}{\sqrt{1-x^2}}$

or $\sqrt{1-x^2}\frac{dy}{dx} = 2\sin^{-1} x$

Squaring, we get

$$(1-x^2)\left(\frac{dy}{dx}\right)^2 = 4(\sin^{-1} x)^2 = 4y$$

[From (1)]

Again differentiating both sides w.r.t. x, we get

$$(1-x^2)2\frac{dy}{dx}\cdot\frac{d^2y}{dx^2} + (-2x)\left(\frac{dy}{dx}\right)^2 = 4\frac{dy}{dx}$$

Dividing both sides by $2\frac{dy}{dx}$, we have

$$(1-x^2)\frac{d^2y}{dx^2} = x\cdot\frac{dy}{dx} + 2.$$

5. *If* $y = e^{ax}\sin bx$, *prove that*

$$\frac{d^2y}{dx^2} - 2a\frac{dy}{dx} + (a^2+b^2)y = 0.$$

SOLUTION. Given, $y = e^{ax}\sin bx \quad \ldots(1)$

$\therefore \frac{dy}{dx} = e^{ax}\cdot b\cos bx + a\cdot e^{ax}\cdot\sin bx$

$= be^{ax}\cos bx + ay \quad$ [From (1)] $\quad \ldots(2)$

Again differentiating both sides w.r.t. x, we have

$$\frac{d^2y}{dx^2} = bae^{ax}(\cos bx) + be^{ax}\cdot b(-\sin bx) + a\frac{dy}{dx}$$

$$= a(be^{ax}\cos bx) - b^2(e^{ax}\sin bx) + a\frac{dy}{dx}$$

$$= a\left(\frac{dy}{dx} - ay\right) - b^2y + a\frac{dy}{dx}$$

[From (1) and (2)]

$$= 2a\frac{dy}{dx} - (a^2+b^2)y$$

$$\therefore \frac{d^2y}{dx^2} - 2a\frac{dy}{dx} + (a^2+b^2)y = 0.$$

6. *If* $x = a(\cos t + t\sin t), y = a(\sin t - t\cos t)$. *Find* $\frac{d^2y}{dx^2}$. [MEERUT(BCA)–2008, 12; HIMACHAL–2010]

SOLUTION. We have $x = a(\cos t + t\sin t)$

$$y = a(\sin t - t\cos t)$$

$$\frac{dx}{dt} = a(-\sin t + t\cos t + \sin t) = at\cos t$$

$$\frac{dy}{dt} = a(\cos t + t\sin t - \cos t) = at\sin t$$

$$\frac{dy}{dx} = \frac{dy/dt}{dx/dt} = \frac{at\sin t}{at\cos t} = \tan t$$

$$\frac{d^2y}{dx^2} = \frac{d}{dx}\left(\frac{dy}{dx}\right) = \frac{d}{dt}\left(\frac{dy}{dx}\right)\cdot\frac{dt}{dx}$$

$$= \frac{d}{dt}(\tan t)\cdot\frac{1}{at\cos t}$$

$$= \sec^2 t\cdot\frac{1}{at\cos t}$$

$$\frac{d^2y}{dx^2} = \frac{\sec^3 t}{at}$$

Exercise-6.3

1. Find the second order derivative of the following functions :
   (i) $\log x$ (ii) $x^2 + 3x + 2$
   (iii) $x\cos x$ (iv) $e^x \sin 5x$
   (v) $\sin(\log x)$
2. If $x = a(\theta - \sin\theta), y = a(1 - \cos\theta)$, find $\frac{dy}{dx}$.
   Also find $\frac{d^2y}{dx^2}$.
3. If $\cos x = \frac{1-t^2}{1+t^2}$ and $\sin y = \frac{2t}{1+t^2}, 0 \le t \le 1$.
   Show that $\frac{d^2y}{dx^2}$ is independent of t.
4. If $x = 3\sin t - \sin 3t, y = 3\cos t - \cos 3t$,
   find $\frac{d^2y}{dx^2}$ at $t = \frac{\pi}{3}$.
5. If $y = x^3 + \tan x$, show that
   $$\frac{d^2y}{dx^2} = 6x + 2\sec^2 x\tan x$$

ANSWERS

1. (i) $-\frac{1}{x^2}$ (ii) 2 (iii) $-x\cos x - 2\sin x$ (iv) $2e^x(5\cos 5x - 12\sin 5x)$

1. (v) $\frac{-\sin(\log x) + \cos(\log x)}{x^2}$ **2.** $\frac{dy}{dx} = \cot\frac{\theta}{2}, \frac{d^2y}{dx^2} = -\frac{1}{4a}\text{cosec}\frac{4\theta}{2}$ **4.** $-\frac{8}{9}$.

□□□□□□

Chapter

7

Successive Differentiations

7.1 INTRODUCTION

Let $y = f(x)$ be a function, then the differential coefficient of $f(x)$ denoted by $f'(x)$ is defined as follows

$$f'(x) = \lim_{\delta x \to 0} \frac{f(x+\delta x) - f(x)}{\delta x} = \frac{dy}{dx}$$

If the limit exists (*i.e.*, limit is finite and unique), then $f'(x)$ is called *first differential coefficient of $f(x)$ with respect to x*. Similarly, if $f(x)$ is differentiable twice, it is denoted by $f''(x)$, if it is differentiable thrice, it is denoted by $f'''(x)$, *i.e.*,

$$f''(x) = \frac{d}{dx}\left(\frac{dy}{dx}\right) = \frac{d^2y}{dx^2}$$

$$f'''(x) = \frac{d}{dx}\left(\frac{d^2y}{dx^2}\right) = \frac{d^3y}{dx^3}$$

If $y = f(x)$ be a function of x, then we adopt the following notations.

$$y_1 = f'(x) = \frac{dy}{dx} = Df(x) = \frac{d}{dx}(f(x))$$

$$y_2 = f''(x) = \frac{d^2y}{dx^2} = D^2f(x) = \frac{d^2}{dx^2}(f(x))$$

$$y_3 = f'''(x) = \frac{d^3y}{dx^3} = D^3f(x) = \frac{d^3}{dx^3}(f(x))$$

$$\cdots \quad \cdots \quad \cdots \quad \cdots \quad \cdots$$

$$\cdots \quad \cdots \quad \cdots \quad \cdots \quad \cdots$$

$$y_n = f^n(x) = \frac{d^ny}{dx^n} = D^nf(x) = \frac{d^n}{dx^n}(f(x))$$

Definition. *This process of finding the differential coefficients of a function is called successive differentiation.*

7.2 n^{th} DIFFERENTIATION OF SOME STANDARD FUNCTIONS

(i) $y = f(x) = x^n$.

We have

$$y = f(x) = x^n$$

$$y_1 = f'(x) = nx^{n-1}$$

$$y_2 = f''(x) = n(n-1)x^{n-2}$$

$$y_3 = f'''(x) = n(n-1)(n-2)x^{n-3}$$

....

....

$$y_n = f^n(x) = n(n-1)(n-2)\ldots 3.2.1.x^0$$

$$\Rightarrow \quad \frac{d^n}{dx^n}(x^n) = y_n = n!$$

(ii) $\mathbf{y = f(x) = x^m}$.

We have $y_1 = f'(x) = mx^{m-1}$, $y_2 = f''(x) = m(m-1)x^{m-2}$,

$$y_3 = f'''(x) = m(m-1)(m-2)x^{m-3}, \ldots,$$

$$y_n = f^n(x) = m(m-1)(m-2)\ldots(m-n+1).x^{m-n}$$

$$= \left[\frac{m(m-1)(m-2)\ldots(m-n+1)(m-n)\ldots 3.2.1}{(m-n)(m-n-1)\ldots 3.2.1}\right]x^{m-n}$$

$$\Rightarrow \quad y_n = \frac{d^n}{dx^n}(x^m) = \frac{m!}{(m-n)!}x^{m-n}$$

(iii) $\mathbf{y = f(x) = \dfrac{1}{(ax+b)}}$.

We have $y_1 = f'(x) = -\dfrac{a}{(ax+b)^2}$, $y_2 = f''(x) = \dfrac{a^2.2}{(ax+b)^3}$,

$$y_3 = f'''(x) = -\frac{a^3.2.3}{(ax+b)^4}, \ldots, y_n = f^n(x) = \frac{(-1)^n a^n.2.3.4\ldots n}{(ax+b)^{n+1}}$$

$$\Rightarrow \quad y_n = \frac{d^n}{dx^n}\left(\frac{1}{ax+b}\right) = \frac{(-1)^n.a^n.n!}{(ax+b)^{n+1}}$$

(iv) $\mathbf{y = f(x) = \dfrac{1}{(ax+b)^m}}$.

We have $y_1 = f'(x) = -\dfrac{a.m}{(ax+b)^{m+1}}$, $y_2 = f''(x) = \dfrac{a^2.m(m+1)}{(ax+b)^{m+2}}$,

$$y_3 = f'''(x) = -\frac{a^3.m(m+1)(m+2)}{(ax+b)^{m+3}}, \ldots,$$

$$y_n = f^n(x) = (-1)^n\frac{a^n.m(m+1)(m+2)\ldots(m+n-1)}{(ax+b)^{m+n}}$$

$$\Rightarrow \quad y_n = \frac{d^n}{dx^n}\left(\frac{1}{(ax+b)^m}\right) = (-1)^n\frac{a^n.(m+n-1)!}{(m-1)!(ax+b)^{m+n}}$$

(v) y = f(x) = sin (ax + b).

We have $y_1 = f'(x) = a\cos(ax+b) = a\sin\left(\frac{\pi}{2}+ax+b\right),$

$$y_2 = f''(x) = a^2\cos\left(\frac{\pi}{2}+ax+b\right) = a^2\sin\left(2.\frac{\pi}{2}+ax+b\right)$$

$$y_3 = f'''(x) = a^3\cos\left(2.\frac{\pi}{2}+ax+b\right) = a^3\sin\left(3.\frac{\pi}{2}+ax+b\right)$$

....

....

$$y_n = f^n(x) = a^n\cos\left((n-1)\frac{\pi}{2}+ax+b\right) = a^n\sin\left(n.\frac{\pi}{2}+ax+b\right)$$

$$\Rightarrow \quad y_n = \frac{d^n}{dx^n}[\sin(ax+b)] = a^n\sin\left(\frac{n\pi}{2}+ax+b\right)$$

(vi) y = f(x) = cos (ax + b).

We have $y_1 = f'(x) = -a\sin(ax+b) = a\cos\left(\frac{\pi}{2}+ax+b\right),$

$$y_2 = f''(x) = -a^2\sin(\frac{\pi}{2}+ax+b) = a^2\cos\left(\frac{2\pi}{2}+ax+b\right)$$

$$y_3 = f'''(x) = -a^3\sin(2.\frac{\pi}{2}+ax+b) = a^3\cos\left(3.\frac{\pi}{2}+ax+b\right)$$

....

....

$$y_n = f^n(x) = -a^n\sin\left((n-1)\frac{\pi}{2}+ax+b\right) = a^n\cos\left(\frac{n\pi}{2}+ax+b\right)$$

$$\Rightarrow \quad y_n = \frac{d^n}{dx^n}[\cos(ax+b)] = a^n\cos\left(\frac{n\pi}{2}+ax+b\right)$$

(vii) y = f(x) = e^{ax+b}.

We have $y_1 = f'(x) = a.e^{ax+b}$

$$y_2 = f''(x) = a^2.e^{ax+b}$$

$$y_3 = f'''(x) = a^3.e^{ax+b}$$

....

....

$$y_n = f^n(x) = a^n.e^{ax+b}$$

$$\Rightarrow \quad y_n = \frac{d^n}{dx^n}(e^{ax+b}) = a^n e^{ax+b}$$

(viii) y = f(x) = log (ax + b).

We have $y_1 = f'(x) = \frac{a}{ax+b}$

Now using result (iii), we get

$$y_n = f^n(x) = (-1)^{n-1}\frac{a^n(n-1)!}{(ax+b)^n}$$

$$\Rightarrow \qquad y_n = \frac{d^n}{dx^n}[\log(ax+b)] = (-1)^{n-1}\frac{a^n(n-1)!}{(ax+b)^n}$$

(ix) $y = f(x) = e^{ax}\sin(bx+c)$.

We have $\quad y_1 = f'(x) = ae^{ax}.\sin(bx+c) + be^{ax}\cos(bx+c)$

$$= e^{ax}[a\sin(bx+c) + b\cos(bx+c)]$$

Put $\quad a = r\cos\theta, b = r\sin\theta \;\Rightarrow\; r^2 = a^2 + b^2$ and $\tan\theta = b/a$ *i.e.*, $\theta = \tan^{-1} b/a$

Therefore, $\quad y_1 = f'(x) = r.e^{ax}\sin(bx+c+\theta)$

$$= (a^2+b^2)^{1/2}.e^{ax}\sin\left(bx+c+\tan^{-1}\frac{b}{a}\right)$$

Similarly, $\quad y_2 = f''(x) = (a^2+b^2)^{1/2}(a^2+b^2)^{1/2}.e^{ax}\sin(bx+c+\tan^{-1}b/a+\tan^{-1}b/a)$

$$= (a^2+b^2)^{2/2}.e^{ax}\sin(bx+c+2\tan^{-1}b/a)$$

$$y_3 = f'''(x) = (a^2+b^2)^{3/2}.e^{ax}\sin(bx+c+3\tan^{-1}b/a)$$

....

....

$$y_n = f^n(x) = (a^2+b^2)^{n/2}.e^{ax}\sin(bx+c+n\tan^{-1}b/a)$$

$$\Rightarrow \qquad y_n = \frac{d^n}{dx^n}[e^{ax}\sin(bx+c)] = (a^2+b^2)^{n/2}.e^{ax}\sin(bx+c+n\tan^{-1}b/a)$$

(x) $y = f(x) = e^{ax}\cos(bx+c)$.

We have $\quad y_1 = f'(x) = ae^{ax}.\cos(bx+c) - be^{ax}\sin(bx+c)$

$$= e^{ax}[a\cos(bx+c) - b\sin(bx+c)]$$

Put $\; a = r\cos\theta,\; b = r\sin\theta \Rightarrow \; \theta = \tan^{-1} b/a\;$ and $r = (a^2 + b^2)^{1/2}$

$\therefore \qquad y_1 = f'(x) = r.e^{ax}[\cos\theta\cos(bx+c) - \sin\theta\sin(bx+c)]$

$$= re^{ax}\cos(bx+c+\theta) = (a^2+b^2)^{1/2}.e^{ax}\cos(bx+c+\tan^{-1}b/a)$$

Similarly, $\quad y_2 = f''(x) = (a^2+b^2)^{2/2}.e^{ax}\cos(bx+c+2\tan^{-1}b/a)$

$$y_3 = f'''(x) = (a^2+b^2)^{3/2}.e^{ax}\cos(bx+c+3\tan^{-1}b/a)$$

....

....

$$y_n = f^n(x) = (a^2+b^2)^{n/2}.e^{ax}\cos(bx+c+n\tan^{-1}b/a)$$

$$\Rightarrow \qquad y_n = \frac{d^n}{dx^n}[e^{ax}\cos(bx+c)] = (a^2+b^2)^{n/2}.e^{ax}\cos(bx+c+n\tan^{-1}b/a)$$

RECAPITULATIONS

- $\frac{d^n}{dx^n}(x^n) = n!$
- $\frac{d^n}{dx^n}(e^{ax+b}) = a^n e^{ax+b}$
- $\frac{d^n}{dx^n}(x^m) = \frac{m!}{(m-n)!}x^{m-n}$
- $\frac{d^n}{dx^n}[\log(ax+b)] = (-1)^{n-1}\frac{a^n(n-1)!}{(ax+b)^n}$
- $\frac{d^n}{dx^n}\left(\frac{1}{(ax+b)^m}\right) = (-1)^n \frac{a^n(m+n-1)!}{(m-1)!(ax+b)^{m+n}}$
- $\frac{d^n}{dx^n}[e^{ax}\sin(bx+c)] = (a^2+b^2)^{n/2}.e^{ax}.\sin(bx+c+n\tan^{-1}b/a)$
- $\frac{d^n}{dx^n}(\sin(ax+b)) = a^n \sin\left(\frac{n\pi}{2}+ax+b\right)$
- $\frac{d^n}{dx^n}[e^{ax}\cos(bx+c)] = (a^2+b^2)^{n/2}.e^{ax}.\cos(bx+c+n\tan^{-1}b/a)$
- $\frac{d^n}{dx^n}(\cos(ax+b)) = a^n \cos\left(\frac{n\pi}{2}+ax+b\right)$

Solved Examples

1. *Find the nth differential coefficient of $\tan^{-1}\frac{x}{a}$.*

SOLUTION. We have $y = \tan^{-1}\frac{x}{a}$

$$\Rightarrow y_1 = \frac{a}{x^2+a^2} = \frac{a}{(x+ia)(x-ia)}$$

Let us suppose

$$\frac{a}{(x+ia)(x-ia)} = \frac{A}{(x+ia)} + \frac{B}{(x-ia)}$$

(Using partial fractions)

$\Rightarrow a = A(x - ia) + B(x + ia)$

To find the value of A, put $x = -ia$

We get $A = -\frac{1}{2i}$

and for B, put $x = ia$, which gives $B = \frac{1}{2i}$ therefore, we have

$$y_1 = \frac{1}{2i}\left[\frac{1}{x-ia} - \frac{1}{x+ia}\right]$$

$$= \frac{1}{2i}[(x-ia)^{-1} - (x+ia)^{-1}]$$

Differentiating $(n - 1)$ times, we get

$$y_n = \frac{1}{2i}[(-1)^{n-1}(n-1)!(x-ia)^{-n} - (-1)^{n-1}(n-1)!(x+ia)^{-n}]$$

$$= \frac{(-1)^{n-1}(n-1)!}{2i}[(x-ia)^{-n} - (x+ia)^{-n}]$$

Put $x = r\cos\theta$, $a = r\sin\theta$, we have

$$y_n = \frac{(-1)^{n-1}(n-1)!}{2i}[r^{-n}(\cos\theta - i\sin\theta)^{-n} - r^{-n}(\cos\theta + i\sin\theta)^{-n}]$$

$$= \frac{(-1)^{n-1}(n-1)!}{2i}r^{-n}[(\cos n\theta + i\sin n\theta) - (\cos n\theta - i\sin n\theta)]$$

$$= \frac{(-1)^{n-1}(n-1)!}{2i}r^{-n}.2i\sin n\theta$$

$[\because \sin(-n\theta) = -\sin n\theta]$

$$= (-1)^{n-1}(n-1)!r^{-n}.\sin n\theta$$

$$= (-1)^{n-1}(n-1)!\left(\frac{a}{\sin\theta}\right)^{-n}\sin n\theta$$

$$\left[\text{since } r = \frac{a}{\sin\theta}\right]$$

$$= (-1)^{n-1}(n-1)!a^{-n}\sin^n\theta.\sin n\theta$$

2. *Find the nth differential coefficient of $\log(ax + x^2)$.*

SOLUTION. Let $y = \log(ax + x^2) = \log[x(a + x)]$

$= \log x + \log(a + x)$

Differentiating n times, we get

$$y_n = \frac{d^n}{dx^n}(\log x) + \frac{d^n}{dx^n}\log(a+x)$$

$$= \frac{(-1)^{n-1}(n-1)!.1^n}{x^n} + \frac{(-1)^{n-1}(n-1)!.1^n}{(x+a)^n}$$

$$= (-1)^{n-1}(n-1)!\left[\frac{1}{x^n} + \frac{1}{(x+a)^n}\right].$$

3. *Find the nth differential coefficients of*

(i) $e^{ax} \sin bx \cos cx$

(ii) $e^{2x} \sin^3 x$

SOLUTION. (i) Let $y = e^{ax} \sin bx \cos cx$

$$= \frac{1}{2} e^{ax} [2 \sin bx \cos cx]$$

$$= \frac{1}{2} e^{ax} [\sin(bx+cx) + \sin(bx-cx)]$$

$$= \frac{1}{2} [e^{ax} \sin(b+c)x + e^{ax} \sin(b-c)x] \quad \ldots(1)$$

Differentiating (1) n times, we get

$$\frac{d^n}{dx^n}[y] = y_n$$

$$= \frac{1}{2} [\{a^2+(b+c)^2\}^{n/2} e^{ax} \sin\{(b+c)x + n \tan^{-1}(b+c)/a\} + \{a^2+(b-c)^2\}^{n/2} e^{ax} \sin\{(b-c)x + n \tan^{-1}(b-c)/a\}]$$

(ii) Let $y = e^{2x} \sin^3 x$.

Now using the result

$$\text{Sin}3x = 3 \sin x - 4 \sin^3 x$$

We have

$$\sin^3 x = \frac{1}{4}(3 \sin x - \sin 3x)$$

Therefore,

$$y = \frac{1}{4} e^{2x} [3 \sin x - \sin 3x]$$

$$= \frac{3}{4} e^{2x} \sin x - \frac{1}{4} e^{2x} \sin 3x.$$

Now, differentiating n times, we get

$$y_n = \frac{3}{4} [(2^2+1^2)^{1/2}]^n e^{2x} \sin[x + n \tan^{-1} 1/2] - \frac{1}{4} [(2^2+3^2)^{1/2}]^n e^{2x} \sin[3x + n \tan^{-1} 3/2].$$

4. *Find the nth differential coefficients of $\sin^5 x \cos^3 x$.*

SOLUTION. First we reduce $\sin^5 x \cos^3 x$ into a function consisting sine function of multiple of x.

Let $z = \cos x + i \sin x$.

The $z^{-1} = \cos x - i \sin x$

$\therefore z + z^{-1} = 2 \cos x$ and $z - z^{-1} = 2i \sin x$

Also, by De-Moivre's theorem, we have

$$z^m + z^{-m} = 2 \cos mx$$

and $z^m - z^{-m} = 2i \sin mx$

Now $(2i \sin x)^5 (2 \cos x)^3$

$$= (z - z^{-1})^5 + (z + z^{-1})^3$$

$\Rightarrow 2^8 i \sin^5 x \cos^3 x$

$$= (z^8 - z^{-8}) - 2(z^6 - z^{-6}) - 2(z^4 - z^{-4}) + 6(z^2 - z^{-2})$$

$$= 2i \sin 8x - 4i \sin 6x - 4i \sin 4x + 12 i \sin 2x$$

$$\Rightarrow \sin^5 x \cos^3 x = 2^{-7}[\sin 8x - 2 \sin 6x - 2 \sin 4x + 6 \sin 2x].$$

Dfferentiating both sides n times w.r.t. x, we get

$$D^n(\sin^5 x \cos^3 x)$$

$$= 2^{-7}\left[8^n \sin\left(8x + \frac{n\pi}{2}\right) - 2.6^n \sin\left(6x + \frac{n\pi}{2}\right) - 2.4^n \sin\left(4x + \frac{n\pi}{2}\right) + 6.2^n \sin\left(2x + \frac{n\pi}{2}\right)\right]$$

7.3 USE OF PARTIAL FRACTIONS

To determine the nth derivative of any rational function, we have to split it into partial fractions.

Partial fractions for

(i) $$\frac{f(x)}{(x-a)(x-b)(x-c)} = \frac{A}{(x-a)} + \frac{B}{(x-b)} + \frac{C}{(x-c)}$$

(ii) $$\frac{f(x)}{(x-a)^2(x-b)} = \frac{A}{(x-a)} + \frac{B}{(x-a)^2} + \frac{C}{(x-b)}$$

(iii) $\dfrac{f(x)}{(x-a)^3(x-b)} = \dfrac{A}{(x-a)} + \dfrac{B}{(x-a)^2} + \dfrac{C}{(x-a)^3} + \dfrac{D}{(x-b)}$

(iv) $\dfrac{f(x)}{(x-a)(x-b)(px^2+qx+r)} = \dfrac{A}{(x-a)} + \dfrac{B}{(x-b)} + \dfrac{Cx+D}{(px^2+qx+r)}$

To find *A*, *B*, *C*, *D* etc., we put each linear factor of LCM equal to zero. The remaining constants are obtained by comparing coefficients of like powers on both sides.

- Forming partial fractions is converse process of taking LCM.
- To resolve a fraction into partial fractions, the degree of the numerator must be less than the degree of denominator.

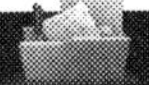

Solved Examples

1. *Find the nth differential coefficients of*

(*i*) $\dfrac{1}{1-5x+6x^2}$

(*ii*) $\dfrac{x^2}{[(x+2)(2x+3)]}$

SOLUTION. (i) Let $y = \dfrac{1}{1-5x+6x^2}$

$= \dfrac{1}{(3x-1)(2x-1)}$

$= \dfrac{2}{2x-1} - \dfrac{3}{3x-1}$

(By resolving into partial fractions)

$= 2(2x-1)^{-1} - 3(3x-1)^{-1}$

Differentaittng, *n* times, we get

$y_n = 2(-1)^n n! 2^n (2x-1)^{-n-1} - 3(-1)^n n! 3^n (3x-1)^{-n-1}$

$= (-1)^n . n! [2^{n+1}(2x-1)^{-n-1} - 3^{n+1}(3x-1)^{-n-1}]$

(ii) Let $y = \dfrac{x^2}{[(x+2)(2x+3)]}$

Since, the given fraction is not a proper one so, divide the Nr. by Dr., we observe that the quotient will be 1/2.

So let

$\dfrac{x^2}{(x+2)(2x+3)} = \dfrac{1}{2} + \dfrac{A}{x+2} + \dfrac{B}{2x+3}$

which gives $A = -4, B = 9/2$

Therefore,

$y = \dfrac{1}{2} - \dfrac{4}{x+2} + \dfrac{9}{2(2x+3)}$

$= \dfrac{1}{2} - 4(x+2)^{-1} + \dfrac{9}{2}(2x+3)^{-1}$

Differentiating *n* times, we get

$y_n = -4(-1)^n n! (x+2)^{-n-1} + \dfrac{9}{2}(-1)^n . n! 2^n (2x+3)^{-n-1}$

$= (-1)^n n! \left[\dfrac{9.2^{n-1}}{(2x+3)^{n+1}} - \dfrac{4}{(x+2)^{n+1}}\right]$

- If none of the standard formulae is applicable to find y_n in any problem, then find y_1, y_2, y_3 and then generalise.

More Solved Examples

1. *If* $y = \sqrt{x+a}$, *find* y_n.

SOLUTION. We have

$y = \sqrt{x+a} = (x+a)^{1/2}$

$y_1 = \dfrac{1}{2}(x+a)^{-1/2}$

$y_2 = \left(\dfrac{1}{2}\right)\left(-\dfrac{1}{2}\right)(x+a)^{-3/2}$

$y_3 = \left(\dfrac{1}{2}\right)\left(-\dfrac{1}{2}\right)\left(-\dfrac{3}{2}\right)(x+a)^{-5/2}$

$= (-1)^2 \dfrac{1.3}{2^3}(x+a)^{-5/2}$

....

....

$$y_n = (-1)^{n-1} \frac{1.3.5\ldots\text{upto } (n-1) \text{ times}}{2^n} (x+a)^{-\frac{(2n-1)}{2}}$$

$$y_n = (-1)^{n-1} \frac{1.3\ldots(2n-3)}{2^n} (x+a)^{-\left(\frac{2n-1}{2}\right)}$$

2. *If* $y = \tan^{-1}\left\{\frac{\sqrt{(1+x^2)}-1}{x}\right\}$, *show that*

$$y_n = \frac{1}{2}(-1)^{n-1}(n-1)!\sin^n\theta\sin n\theta,$$

where $\theta = \cot^{-1}x$.

SOLUTION. We have $y = \tan^{-1}\left\{\frac{\sqrt{(1+x^2)}-1}{x}\right\}$.

Put $x = \tan\phi$, then

$$y = \tan^{-1}\left\{\frac{\sqrt{(1+\tan^2\phi)}-1}{\tan\phi}\right\}$$

$$= \tan^{-1}\left[\frac{\sec\phi - 1}{\tan\phi}\right]$$

$$= \tan^{-1}\left(\frac{1-\cos\phi}{\sin\phi}\right)$$

$$= \tan^{-1}\left(\frac{2\sin^2(\phi/2)}{2\sin(\phi/2)\cos(\phi/2)}\right)$$

$$= \tan^{-1}\tan(\phi/2) = \phi/2 = \frac{1}{2}\tan^{-1}x$$

$$\Rightarrow y_1 = \frac{1}{2(1+x^2)} = \frac{1}{2(x-i)(x+i)}$$

$$= \frac{1}{4i}\left(\frac{1}{x-i} - \frac{1}{x+i}\right)$$

Differentiating (n–1) times, we get

$$y_n = \frac{(-1)^{n-1}(n-1)!}{4i}[(x-i)^{-n} - (x+i)^{-n}]$$

Now putting $x = r\cos\theta$, $1 = r\sin\theta$, we have

$$y_n = \frac{(-1)^{n-1}(n-1)!}{4i}\left[r^{-n}(\cos\theta - i\sin\theta)^{-n} - r^{-n}(\cos\theta + i\sin\theta)^{-n}\right]$$

$$= \frac{(-1)^{n-1}(n-1)!}{4i}r^{-n}\left[(\cos n\theta + i\sin n\theta) - (\cos n\theta - i\sin n\theta)\right]$$

$$= \frac{1}{2}(-1)^{n-1}(n-1)!r^{-n}\sin n\theta$$

$$= \frac{1}{2}(-1)^{n-1}(n-1)!\left(\frac{1}{\sin\theta}\right)^{-n}\sin n\theta$$

$$\left[\because r = \frac{1}{\sin\theta}\right]$$

$$= \frac{1}{2}(-1)^{n-1}(n-1)!\sin^n\theta\sin n\theta$$

$$\text{where } \theta = \tan^{-1}\frac{1}{x} = \cot^{-1}x.$$

3. *If* $y = \sin mx + \cos mx$, *prove that* $y_n = m^n\,[1 + (-1)^n \sin 2mx]^{1/2}$. [MTU–2012]

SOLUTION. We have

$$y_n = \frac{d^n}{dx^n}(\sin mx) + \frac{d^n}{dx^n}(\cos mx)$$

$$= m^n\sin\left(mx + n\frac{\pi}{2}\right) + m^n\cos\left(mx + n\frac{\pi}{2}\right)$$

$$= m^n\left[\left\{\sin\left(mx+n\frac{\pi}{2}\right) + \cos\left(mx+n\frac{\pi}{2}\right)\right\}^2\right]^{1/2}$$

$$= m^n\left[1 + 2\sin\left(mx+n\frac{\pi}{2}\right).\cos\left(mx+n\frac{\pi}{2}\right)\right]^{1/2}$$

$$= m^n[1+\sin(2mx+n\pi)]^{1/2}$$

$$= m^n[1 \pm \sin 2mx]^{1/2}$$

$$= m^n[1 + (-1)^n\sin 2mx]^{1/2}.$$

Similar Problems

(1) Find the nth differential coefficient of $\log[(ax+b)(cx+d)]$.

(2) Find the nth derivative of $y = \cos^4 x$.

4. *If* $y = x\log\frac{x-1}{x+1}$, *show that*

$$y_n = (-1)^{n-2}(n-2)!\left[\frac{x-n}{(x-1)^n} - \frac{x+n}{(x+1)^n}\right].$$

SOLUTION. Let $y = x\log\dfrac{x-1}{x+1}$

$\Rightarrow\ y = x\log(x-1) - x\log(x+1)$ ...(1)

Differentiating (1) w.r.t. x we get

$$y_1 = \frac{x}{x-1} + \log(x-1) - \frac{x}{x+1} - \log(x+1)$$

$$= 1 + \frac{1}{x-1} + \log(x-1) - 1 + \frac{1}{x+1} - \log(x+1)$$

$$= \frac{1}{x-1} + \frac{1}{x+1} + \log(x-1) - \log(x+1) \quad ...(2)$$

Differentiating both sides of (2) w.r.t. x, $(n-1)$ times we get

$$y_n = \frac{(-1)^{n-1}(n-1)!}{(x-1)^n} + \frac{(-1)^{n-1}(n-1)!}{(x+1)^n} + \frac{(-1)^{n-2}(n-2)!}{(x-1)^{n-1}} - \frac{(-1)^{n-2}(n-2)!}{(x+1)^{n-1}}$$

$$= (-1)^{n-2}(n-2)!\left\{-\frac{(n-1)+x-1}{(x-1)^n}\right\} + (-1)^{n-2}(n-2)!\left\{\frac{-(n-1)-(x+1)}{(x+1)^n}\right\}$$

$$\Rightarrow\ y_n = (-1)^{n-2}(n-2)!\left\{\frac{x-n}{(x-1)^n} - \frac{x+n}{(x+1)^n}\right\}$$

5. *Find the nth derivative of* $\dfrac{1}{x^2+a^2}$. [UKTU–2011]

SOLUTION. Let $y = \dfrac{1}{x^2+a^2} = \dfrac{1}{(x+ia)(x-ia)}$

$$= \frac{1}{2ia}\left[\frac{1}{x-ia} - \frac{1}{x+ia}\right] \quad ...(1)$$

Differentiating (1) n times w.r.t. x we get

$$y_n = \frac{1}{2ia}\left[\frac{(-1)^n n!}{(x-ia)^{n+1}} - \frac{(-1)^n n!}{(x+ia)^{n+1}}\right]$$

$$= \frac{(-1)^n.n!}{2ia}\left[\frac{1}{(x-ia)^{n+1}} - \frac{1}{(x+ia)^{n+1}}\right] \quad ...(2)$$

Let $x = r\cos\theta$ and $a = r\sin\theta$ *i.e.*, $\theta = \tan^{-1}\dfrac{a}{x}$ in (2), we get

$$y_n = \frac{(-1)^n.n!}{2iar^{n+1}}\left[\frac{1}{(\cos\theta - i\sin\theta)^{n+1}} - \frac{1}{(\cos\theta + i\sin\theta)^{n+1}}\right]$$

$$= \frac{(-1)^n.n!}{2iar^{n+1}}\left[\frac{1}{\cos(n+1)\theta - i\sin(n+1)\theta} - \frac{1}{\cos(n+1)\theta + i\sin(n+1)\theta}\right]$$

$$= \frac{(-1)^n.n!}{2iar^{n+1}}\left[\{\cos(n+1)\theta + i\sin(n+1)\theta\} - \{\cos(n+1)\theta - i\sin(n+1)\theta\}\right]$$

$$= \frac{(-1)^n.n!}{2iar^{n+1}}\left[2i\sin(n+1)\theta\right]$$

$$= \frac{(-1)^n.n!\sin(n+1)\theta}{a\left(\dfrac{a^{n+1}}{\sin^{n+1}\theta}\right)} \quad [\because a = r\sin\theta]$$

$$= \frac{(-1)^n.n!\sin(n+1)\theta\sin^{n+1}\theta}{a^{n+2}},$$

$\theta = \tan^{-1}\dfrac{a}{x}$.

Exercise-7.1

1. Find the nth derivatives of

(i) $\sin 3x$ (ii) $\cos x\cos 2x\cos 3x$

(iii) $e^{ax}\cos 2x\sin x$ [SVTU–2009]

(iv) $\sin 5x\cos 3x$ (v) $\sin ax\cos bx$

(vi) $\sin 2x\sin 2x$

2. Find the nth derivatives of

(i) $\dfrac{x^4}{(x-1)(x-2)}$ (ii) $\dfrac{x}{1+3x+2x^2}$

(iii) $\dfrac{1}{(x-2)(x-1)^3}$ (iv) $\dfrac{1}{x^2-a^2}$

(v) $\dfrac{x^2}{(x-a)(x-b)}$

(vi) $\dfrac{17x^2+26x-42}{6x^3-25x^2-29x+20}$

3. Find the nth derivatives of

(i) $\tan^{-1}\left(\frac{1+x}{1-x}\right)$ (ii) $\tan^{-1}\left(\frac{2x}{1-x^2}\right)$

4. Show that the value of the nth differential coefficients of $\frac{x^3}{x^2-1}$ for $x = 0$, is zero if n is even and is $-n!$, if n is odd and greater than 1.

5. If $y = x(a^2 + x^2)^{-1}$, show that

$$y_n = (-1)^n n! a^{-n-1} \sin^{n+1}\theta \cos(n+1)\theta$$

where $\theta = \tan^{-1}\left(\frac{a}{x}\right)$. [MUMBAI–2007]

6. (i) If $x = a(t - \sin t)$ and $y = a(1 + \cos t)$, prove that

$$\frac{d^2y}{dx^2} = \frac{1}{4a}\text{cosec}^4\left(\frac{t}{2}\right).$$

(MADURAI–1990, 2004)

(ii) If $x = a(\cos\theta + \theta\sin\theta)$, $y = a(\sin\theta - \theta\cos\theta)$, find $\frac{d^2y}{dx^2}$.

(iii) If $y = \sin(\sin x)$, show that

$$\left(\frac{d^2y}{dx^2}\right) + \left(\frac{dy}{dx}\right)\tan x + y\cos^2 x = 0.$$

(iv) If $y = A\sin mx + B\cos mx$, show that

$$\frac{d^2y}{dx^2} + m^2 y = 0.$$

(v) If $y = e^{ax}\sin bx$, show that

$$\frac{d^2y}{dx^2} - 2a\frac{dy}{dx} + (a^2 + b^2)y = 0.$$

7. If $p^2 = a^2\cos 2\theta + b^2\sin 2\theta$, prove that

$$p + \frac{d^2p}{d\theta^2} = \frac{a^2.b^2}{p^3}.$$

8. Prove that the value when $x = 0$ of $\frac{d^n}{dx^n}(\tan^{-1}x)$ is 0, $(n-1)!$ or $-(n-1)!$ according as n is of the form $2p$, $4p+1$ or $4p+3$ respectively.

Hint to the Selected Problems

2. (i) Resolving into partial fractions, we get

$$y = (x^2 + 3x + 7) + \frac{15x - 14}{(x-1)(x-2)}.$$

Now differentiate successively.

(ii) $y = \frac{1}{(1+x)} - \frac{1}{(1+2x)}$. Now differentiate successively.

3. (i) $y = \tan^{-1}\frac{1+x}{1-x} \Rightarrow y_1 = \frac{1}{(1+x^2)}$

$$= \frac{1}{(x-i)(x+i)} = \frac{1}{2i}\left(\frac{1}{x-i} + \frac{1}{x+i}\right)$$

Then differentiate successively.

4. The given function can be written as

$$y = x + \frac{1}{2}\left(\frac{1}{x-1} + \frac{1}{x+1}\right).$$

5. The given function can be written as

$$y = \frac{1}{2}\left(\frac{1}{x-ai} + \frac{1}{x+ai}\right).$$

6. (i) Find $\frac{dx}{dt}$ and $\frac{dy}{dt}$ such that

$$\frac{dx}{dt} = a(1-\cos t) \text{ and } \frac{dy}{dt} = -a\sin t.$$

Then $\frac{dy}{dx} = \frac{dy/dt}{dx/dt} = \frac{-a\sin t}{a(1-\cos t)}$

$= -\cot t/2.$

Now differentiate successively.

8. Let $y = \tan^{-1}x$. Then $y_1 = \frac{1}{1+x^2}$

$$= \frac{1}{(x-i)(x+i)} = \frac{1}{2i}\left[\frac{1}{x-i} - \frac{1}{x+i}\right].$$

Now differentiate successively.

ANSWERS

1.(i) $y_n = \frac{3}{4}\sin\left(x + \frac{n\pi}{2}\right) - \frac{1}{4}.3^n\sin\left(3x + \frac{n\pi}{2}\right)$

(ii) $y_n = \frac{1}{4}\left\{6^n\cos\left(6x + \frac{1}{2}n\pi\right) + 4^n\cos\left(4x + \frac{n\pi}{2}\right) + 2^n\cos\left(2x + \frac{n\pi}{2}\right)\right\}$

(iii) $y_n = \frac{1}{4}[(a^2+1)^{n/2}e^{ax}\sin\{x + n\tan^{-1}1/a\} + (a^2+9)^{n/2}e^{ax}\sin(3x + n\tan^{-1}3/a)]$

(iv) $y_n = 2^{-7}\left[8^n\sin\left(8x + \frac{1}{2}n\pi\right) - 2.6^n\sin\left(6x + \frac{1}{2}n\pi\right) - 2.4^n\sin\left(4x + \frac{1}{2}n\pi\right) + 6.2^n\sin\left(2x + \frac{1}{2}n\pi\right)\right]$

(v) $y_n = \frac{1}{2}\left[(a+b)^n \sin\left\{(a+b)x + \frac{1}{2}n\pi\right\} + (a-b)^n \sin\left\{(a-b)x + \frac{1}{2}n\pi\right\}\right]$

(vi) $y_n = 2^{n-1}\sin\left(2x + \frac{1}{2}n\pi\right) - 4^{n-1}\sin\left(4x + \frac{1}{2}n\pi\right)$

2.(i) $y_n = (-1)^n n![16(x-2)^{-n-1} - (x-1)^{-n-1}]$ (ii) $y_n = (-1)^n n!\left[\frac{1}{(x+1)^{n+1}} - \frac{2^n}{(2x+1)^{n+1}}\right]$

(iii) $y_n = (-1)^{n+1}.n!\left[\frac{(n+2)(n+1)}{2(x-1)^{n+3}} + \frac{(n+1)}{(x-1)^{n+2}} + \frac{1}{(x-1)^{n+1}} - \frac{1}{(x-2)^{n+1}}\right]$

(iv) $y_n = \frac{1}{2a}(-1)^n.n!\{(x-a)^{-n-1} - (x+a)^{-n-1}\}$

(v) $y_n = \frac{(-1)^n.n!}{(a-b)}\left[\frac{a^2}{(x-a)^{n+1}} - \frac{b^2}{(x-b)^{n+1}}\right]$

(vi) $y_n = (-1)^n.n!\left[\frac{2^n}{(2x-1)^{n+1}} - \frac{2.3^n}{(3x+4)^{n+1}} + \frac{3}{(x-5)^{n+1}}\right]$

3.(i) $y_n = (-1)^{n-1}.(n-1)!\sin^n\theta \sin n\theta$, where $\theta = \tan^{-1}\frac{1}{x}$

(ii) $y_n = 2(-1)^{n-1}(n-1)!\sin^n\theta \sin n\theta$, where $\theta = \tan^{-1}\frac{1}{x}$ **6.** (ii) $y_2 = \frac{1}{a}.\frac{\sec^3\theta}{\theta}$

7.4 LEIBNITZ'S THEOREM

This theorem help us to find the nth differential coefficient of the product of two functions in terms of the successive derivatives of the functions.

Statement. *If u, v be two functions of x, having derivative of nth order, then*

$$D^n(nv) = u_n v + {}^nC_1 u_{n-1}v_1 + {}^nC_2 u_{n-2}v_2 + \ldots + {}^nC_r u_{n-r}v_r + \ldots + {}^nC_n uv_n$$

where suffixes of u and v denote differentiations w.r.t. x.

Step 1. Let $y = uv$

$\Rightarrow$ $y_1 = u_1 v + uv_1$

and $y_2 = u_2 v + u_1 v_1 + u_1 v_1 + uv_2 = u_2 v + 2u_1 v_1 + uv_2$

$= u_2 v + {}^2C_1 u_1 v_1 + {}^2C_2 uv_2.$

Thus the theorem is true for $n = 1, 2$.

Step 2. Let us assume that the theorem is true for a particular value of n say m, then we have

$$y_m = u_m v + {}^mC_1 u_{m-1}v_1 + {}^mC_2 u_{m-2}v_2 + \ldots + {}^mC_{r-1}u_{m-r+1}v_{r-1} + {}^mC_r u_{m-r}v_r + \ldots + {}^mC_m uv_m. \quad \ldots(1)$$

Step 3. Now, differentiating (1), we have

$$y_{m+1} = u_{m+1}v + u_m v_1 + {}^mC_1 u_m v_1 + {}^mC_1 u_{m-1}v_2 + {}^mC_2 u_{m-1}v_2 + {}^mC_2 u_{m-2}v_3 + \ldots$$
$$+ {}^mC_{r-1}u_{m-r+2}v_{r-1} + {}^mC_{r-1}u_{m-r+1}v_r + {}^mC_r u_{m-r+1}v_r$$
$$+ {}^mC_r u_{m-r}v_{r+1} + \ldots + {}^mC_m u_1 v_m + {}^mC_m uv_{m+1}.$$
$$= u_{m+1}.v + ({}^mC_1 + 1)u_m v_1 + ({}^mC_2 + {}^mC_1)u_{m-1}v_2 + \ldots + ({}^mC_r + {}^mC_{r-1})u_{m-r+1}v_r$$
$$+ \ldots + {}^mC_m uv_{m+1}.$$

Now using Pascal's law, given by ${}^mC_{r-1} + {}^mC_r = {}^{m+1}C_r$

For $r = 1, 2, 3, \ldots$

We have
$$^mC_0 + {}^mC_1 = {}^{m+1}C_1 \Rightarrow 1 + {}^mC_1 = {}^{m+1}C_1$$
$$^mC_1 + {}^mC_2 = {}^{m+1}C_2$$
....

....

and
$$^mC_m = 1 = {}^{m+1}C_{m+1}$$

Therefore,

$$y_{m+1} = u_{m+1}.v + {}^{m+1}C_1 u_m v_1 + {}^{m+1}C_2 u_{m-1} v_2 + \ldots + {}^{m+1}C_r u_{m-r+1} v_r + \ldots + {}^{m+1}C_{m+1} u v_{m+1}$$

$\Rightarrow$ If the theorem is true for $n = m$, then it is also true for the next higher value $n = m + 1$.

Then, by the principle of Mathematical induction, we can say that theorem is true for any positive integer n.

Solved Examples

1. *Find the nth derivative of $x^2 \sin x$.*

SOLUTION. Let $u = \sin x$ and $v = x^2$.

Then, $u_n = \sin\left[x + \frac{n\pi}{2}\right]$

$$u_{n-1} = \sin\left(x + (n-1)\frac{\pi}{2}\right)$$

$$u_{n-2} = \sin\left[x + (n-2)\frac{\pi}{2}\right]$$

Also, $v_1 = 2x$, $v_2 = 2$, $v_3 = 0$

Now, by Leibnitz's theorem, we have

$$\frac{d^n}{dx^n}(uv) = u_n.v + {}^nC_1 u_{n-1}.v_1 + {}^nC_2 u_{n-2}.v_2$$

$$\Rightarrow \frac{d^n}{dx^n}(x^2 \sin x) = \sin\left(x + \frac{n\pi}{2}\right)x^2 + {}^nC_1 \sin\left[x + (n-1)\frac{\pi}{2}\right]2x + {}^nC_2 \sin\left[x + (n-2)\frac{\pi}{2}\right]2$$

$$= x^2 \sin\left(x + \frac{n\pi}{2}\right) + 2nx \sin\left[x + (n-1)\frac{\pi}{2}\right] + n(n-1)\sin\left[x + (n-2)\frac{\pi}{2}\right]$$

Similar Problem

(1) Find the nth derivative of $x^3 \cos x$.

2. *Find the nth derivative of $x^{n-1} \log x$.*

[UPTU–2010, 12]

SOLUTION. Let $y = x^{n-1} \log x$ ...(1)

Differentiating (1) w.r.t. x we get

$$y_1 = x^{n-1}.\frac{1}{x} + (n-1)x^{n-2}\log x$$

$$= x^{n-1}.\frac{1}{x} + (n-1)\frac{x^{n-1}}{x}\log x$$

$$\Rightarrow xy_1 = x^{n-1} + (n-1)y \quad \ldots(2)$$

Finally, differentiating (2) both the sides $(n-1)$ times w.r.t. x, we get

$$y_n x + (n-1)y_{n-1}.1 = (n-1)! + (n-1)y_{n-1}$$

Hence, $y_n = \frac{(n-1)!}{x}$.

3. *If $y = a \cos(\log x) + b \sin(\log x)$, show that $x^2y_2 + xy_1 + y = 0$ and $x^2y_{n+2} + (2n+1)xy_{n+1} + (n^2+1)y_n = 0$.*

[MADRAS–2000]

SOLUTION. We have

$$y = a\cos(\log x) + b\sin(\log x) \quad ...(1)$$

Differentiating (1) with respect to x, we have

$$y_1 = -\frac{a}{x}\sin(\log x) + \frac{b}{x}\cos(\log x)$$

$$xy_1 = -a\sin(\log x) + b\cos(\log x)$$

Again, differentiating w.r.t. x, we get

$$xy_2 + y_1 = -\frac{a}{x}\cos(\log x) - \frac{b}{x}\sin(\log x)$$

$$\Rightarrow \quad x^2y_2 + xy_1 = -a\cos(\log x) - b\sin(\log x) = -y$$

$$\Rightarrow \quad x^2y_2 + xy_1 + y = 0 \quad ...(2)$$

Now, differentiating (2) both sides n times by Leibnitz's theorem, we get

$$D^n(x^2y_2) + D^n(xy_1) + D^n(y) = 0$$

$$\Rightarrow (D^ny_2)x^2 + {}^nC_1(D^{n-1}y_2)(Dx^2) + {}^nC_2(D^{n-2}y_2)(D^2x^2) + (D^ny_1)x + {}^nC_1(D^{n-1}y_1)(Dx) + D^ny = 0$$

$$\Rightarrow x^2y_{n+2} + 2nxy_{n+1} + \frac{n(n-1)}{2}2y_n + xy_{n+1} + ny_n + y_n = 0$$

$$\Rightarrow x^2y_{n+2} + (2n+1)xy_{n+1} + (n^2+1)y_n = 0$$

4. *If* $y = e^{a\sin^{-1}x}$, *show that* $(1-x^2)y_{n+2} - (2n+1)xy_{n+1} - (n^2+a^2)y_n = 0.$

(MDU–1998, VTU–2003, KU–1999)

SOLUTION. We have

$$y = e^{a\sin^{-1}x}$$

$$\Rightarrow y_1 = e^{a\sin^{-1}x}.\frac{a}{\sqrt{1-x^2}}$$

$$y_1\sqrt{1-x^2} = ae^{a\sin^{-1}x} = ay$$

$$\Rightarrow y_1^2(1-x^2) = a^2y^2 \quad ...(1)$$

Now differentiating (1) with respect to x, we get

$$2y_1y_2(1-x^2) + y_1^2(-2x) = 2a^2yy_1$$

$$\Rightarrow 2y_1[y_2(1-x^2) - xy_1 - a^2y] = 0 \quad [\because 2y_1 \neq 0]$$

$$\Rightarrow [y_2(1-x^2) - xy_1 - a^2y] = 0 \quad ...(2)$$

Using Leibnitz's theorem, differentiating (2), n times, we get

$$D^n[y_2(1-x^2)] - D^n(y_1x) - a^2D^ny = 0$$

$$\Rightarrow \left[\begin{array}{l} y_{n+2}(1-x^2) + ny_{n+1}(-2x) \\ + \frac{n(n-1)}{2}y_n(-2) \end{array}\right] - [y_{n+1}x + ny_n] - a^2y_n = 0$$

$$\Rightarrow (1-x^2)y_{n+2} - (2n+1)xy_{n+1} - (n^2+a^2)y_n = 0$$

5. *If* $\cos^{-1}\left(\frac{y}{b}\right) = \log\left(\frac{x}{n}\right)^n$. *Prove that* $x^2y_{n+2} + (2n+1)xy_{n+1} + 2n^2y_n = 0.$

SOLUTION. We have

$$\cos^{-1}\left(\frac{y}{b}\right) = \log\left(\frac{x}{n}\right)^n = n\log\frac{x}{n} = n(\log x - \log n)$$

Now, differentiating with respect to x, we get

$$-\frac{1}{\sqrt{\left[1-\frac{y^2}{b^2}\right]}}\frac{y_1}{b} = \frac{n}{x}$$

or $$-\frac{y_1}{\sqrt{b^2-y^2}} = \frac{n}{x}$$

or $$y_1^2x^2 = n^2(b^2-y^2)$$

Again, differentiating, with respect to x, we get

$$2x^2y_1y_2 + 2xy_1^2 = -2n^2yy_1$$

or $$y_2x^2 + y_1x + n^2y = 0. \quad [\because 2y_1 \neq 0]$$

Using Leibnitz's theorem, differentiating n times, we get

$$y_{n+2}x^2 + {}^nC_1y_{n+1}(2x) + {}^nC_2y_n(2) + y_{n+1}x + {}^nC_1y_n + n^2y_n = 0$$

$$\Rightarrow x^2y_{n+2} + (2n+1)xy_{n+1} + 2n^2y_n = 0.$$

6. *If* $y = (x^2-1)^n$, *Prove that* $(x^2-1)y_{n+2} + 2xy_{n+1} - n(n+1)y_n = 0.$

[VTU–2010]

Hence if $P_n = \frac{d^n}{dx^n}(x^2-1)^n$ *show that*

$$\frac{d}{dx}\left\{(1-x^2)\frac{dP_n}{dx}\right\}+n(n+1)P_n = 0$$

SOLUTION. We have $y = (x^2-1)^n$ ...(1)

Therefore $y_1 = n(x^2-1)^{n-1}.2x$

or $(x^2-1)y_1 = n(x^2-1)^n.2x$

$\Rightarrow (x^2-1)y_1 = 2nxy.$ ...(2)

Differentiating (2), $(n+1)$ times by Leibnitz's theorem, we get

$$D^{n+1}[y_1(x^2-1)]-2nD^{n+1}(yx) = 0$$

or $y_{n+2}(x^2-1)+(n+1)y_{n+1}.2x + \frac{n(n+1)}{2}.y_n.2-2ny_{n+1}.x - 2n(n+1)y_n.1 = 0$

or $(x^2-1)y_{n+2}+2xy_{n+1}-n(n+1)y_n=0$

Hence, the first result. From (2), we get

$$(x^2-1)D^2y_n+2xDy_n-n(n+1)y_n=0. \quad ...(3)$$

Putting $y_n = \frac{d^n}{dx^n}(x^2-1)^n = P_n;$

equation (3) becomes

$$(x^2-1)D^2P_n+2xDP_n-n(n+1)P_n = 0$$

or $-(1-x^2)D^2P_n+2xD(P_n) - n(n+1)P_n = 0$

or $-\frac{d}{dx}\{(1-x^2)DP_n\}-n(n+1)P_n=0$

or $\frac{d}{dx}\left\{(1-x^2)\frac{d}{dx}P_n\right\}+n(n+1)P_n = 0$

7. *If* $y = \sin(m\sin^{-1}x)$, *Prove that*

$$(1-x^2)y_2-xy_1+m^2y = 0$$

and $(1-x^2)y_{n+2}-(2n+1)xy_{n+1} - (n^2-m^2)y_n = 0$

[GBTU–2011]

SOLUTION. Let $y = \sin(m\sin^{-1}x)$ ...(1)

Differentiating w.r.t. x we get

$$y_1 = \cos(m\sin^{-1}x).\frac{m}{\sqrt{1-x^2}}$$

$\Rightarrow y_1\sqrt{1-x^2} = m\cos(m\sin^{-1}x)$

$\Rightarrow y_1{}^2(1-x^2) = m^2\cos^2(m\sin^{-1}x)$

$= m^2[1-\sin^2(m\sin^{-1}x)]$

$= m^2(1-y^2)$ ...(2)

Again, differentiating both sides of (2) w.r.t. x we get

$$(1-x^2)2y_1y_2-2xy_1{}^2 = -2m^2yy_1$$

$\Rightarrow (1-x^2)y_2-xy_1 = -m^2y$

$\Rightarrow (1-x^2)y_2-xy_1+m^2y = 0$ ...(3)

Finally, differentiating (3) n times, by Leibnitz's theorem, we get

$$\begin{bmatrix} y_{n+2}(1-x^2)+{}^nC_1y_{n+1}(-2x) \\ +{}^nC_2y_n(-2) \end{bmatrix} - \left[y_{n+1}x+{}^nC_1y_n\right]+m^2y_n = 0$$

$\Rightarrow (1-x^2)y_{n+2}-2nxy_{n+1} - n(n+1)y_n-xy_{n+1} - ny_n+m^2y_n = 0$

or $(1-x^2)y_{n+2}-(2n+1)xy_{n+1} - (n^2-m^2)y_n = 0$

8. *If* $\cos^{-1}\left(\frac{y}{b}\right) = \log\left(\frac{x}{m}\right)^m$, *Show that*

$x^2y_{n+2}+(2n+1)xy_{n+1} + (n^2+m^2)y_n = 0.$

SOLUTION. We have $\cos^{-1}\left(\frac{y}{b}\right) = \log\left(\frac{x}{m}\right)^m$

$\Rightarrow y = b\cos\left(m\log\left(\frac{x}{m}\right)\right)$

$\therefore y_1=-b\sin\left(m\log\left(\frac{x}{m}\right)\right).m\frac{1}{(x/m)}.\frac{1}{m}$

$\Rightarrow xy_1 = -bm\sin\left(m\log\left(\frac{x}{m}\right)\right)$

Again differentiating, we get

$$xy_2+y_1 = -bm\cos\left\{m\log\left(\frac{x}{m}\right)\right\}.m.\frac{1}{(x/m)}.\frac{1}{m}$$

$\Rightarrow x^2y_2+xy_1=-m^2b\cos\left\{m\log\left(\frac{x}{m}\right)\right\} = -m^2y$

$\therefore x^2y_2+xy_1+m^2y = 0$

Differentiating both sides of the above equation, n times by Leibnitz's theorem, we get

$$[y_{n+2}.x^2 + {}^nC_1 y_{n+1}(2x) + {}^nC_2 y_n(2)]$$
$$+[y_{n+1}(x) + {}^nC_1 y_n(1)] + m^2 y_n = 0$$

$$\Rightarrow \quad x^2 y_{n+2} + (2n+1)xy_{n+1} + (n^2 + m^2)y_n = 0$$

Similar Problems

(1) If $x = \cosh\left(\frac{1}{m}\log y\right)$, prove that $(x^2-1)y_{n+2} + (2n+1)xy_{n+1} + (n^2 - m^2)y_n = 0.$

(2) If $y = \sin\log(x^2 + 2x + 1)$, prove that $(1+x^2)y_{n+2} + (2n+1)(1+x)y_{n+1} - (n^2+4)y_n = 0.$

9. *If $x = \tan(\log y)$, prove that* $(1+x^2)y_{n+1} + (2nx-1)y_n + n(n-1)y_{n-1} = 0.$

SOLUTION. Let $x = \tan(\log y)$

$$\Rightarrow \quad y = e^{\tan^{-1}x} \quad \ldots(1)$$

$$\Rightarrow \quad y_1 = e^{\tan^{-1}x}.\frac{1}{(1+x^2)}$$

$$\therefore \quad (1+x^2)y_1 = y \quad \ldots(2)$$

Differentiating (2) n times by Leibnitz's theorem, we get

$$y_{n+1}(1+x^2) + {}^nC_1 y_n(2x) + {}^nC_2 y_{n-1}(2) = y_n$$

$$\Rightarrow (1+x^2)y_{n+1} + (2nx-1)y_n + n(n-1)y_{n-1} = 0$$

10. *If $y = (1-x)^{-\alpha}e^{-\alpha x}$, prove that* $(1-x)y_{n+1} - (n + \alpha x)y_n - n\alpha y_{n-1} = 0.$ [UKTU–2011]

SOLUTION. We have $y = (1-x)^{-\alpha}e^{-\alpha x}$ ...(1)

$$\Rightarrow \quad y_1 = (1-x)^{-\alpha}(-\alpha e^{-\alpha x}) + e^{-\alpha x}(-\alpha)(1-x)^{-\alpha-1}(-1)$$

$$= e^{-\alpha x}(1-x)^{-\alpha}\left(-\alpha + \frac{\alpha}{1-x}\right)$$

$$\Rightarrow \quad y_1(1-x) = \alpha xy \quad \ldots(2)$$

Differentiating (2) n times by Leibnitz's theorem, we get

$$y_{n+1}(1-x) + {}^nC_1 y_n(-1) = \alpha[y_n(x) + {}^nC_1 y_{n-1}(1)]$$

$$\therefore \quad (1-x)y_{n+1} + (-n - \alpha x)y_n - n\alpha y_{n-1} = 0.$$

$$\Rightarrow \quad (1-x)y_{n+1} - (n + \alpha x)y_n - n\alpha y_{n-1} = 0$$

11. *If $y = \tan^{-1}\left(\frac{a+x}{a-x}\right)$, prove that* $(a^2 + x^2)y_{n+2} + 2(n+1)xy_{n+1} + n(n+1)y_n = 0.$ (GBTU–2012)

SOLUTION. We have $y = \tan^{-1}\left(\frac{a+x}{a-x}\right)$ ...(1)

Differentiating (1) w.r.t. x, we get

$$y_1 = \frac{a}{(a^2+x^2)} \Rightarrow (a^2+x^2)y_1 = a$$

Again differentiating w.r.t. x, we get

$$(a^2+x^2)y_2 + 2xy_1 = 0 \quad \ldots(2)$$

Now, differentiating (2), n times by Leibnitz's theorem, we get

$$[(x^2+a^2)y_{n+2} + {}^nC_1(2x)y_{n+1} + {}^nC_2(2)y_n] + [2xy_{n+1} + {}^nC_1.2.y_n] = 0$$

$$\Rightarrow (x^2+a^2)y_{n+2} + 2nxy_{n+1} + n(n-1)y_n + 2xy_{n+1} + 2ny_n = 0$$

$$\Rightarrow (x^2+a^2)y_{n+2} + 2x(n+1)y_{n+1} + [n(n-1) + 2n]y_n = 0$$

$$\Rightarrow \quad (x^2+a^2)y_{n+2} + 2x(n+1)y_{n+1} + n(n+1)y_n = 0$$

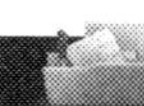

Exercise-7.2

1. Use Leibnitz's theorem, to find y_n in the following cases :

(i) x^3e^{ax} (ii) x^2e^x

(iii) $x^3\sin ax$ (iv) $x^3\log x$

(v) $x^2e^x\cos x$ (vi) $e^x\log x$

(vii) $x^n\log x$ (viii) $x^2\tan^{-1}x$

2. If $I_n = \frac{d^n}{dx^n}(x^n\log x)$, prove that $I_n = nI_{n-1} + (n-1)!$ and hence show that

$$I_n = n!\left(\log x + 1 + \frac{1}{2} + \frac{1}{3} + \ldots + \frac{1}{n}\right)$$

(MTU–2011, VTU–2001, MUMBAI–2008)

3. If $y = e^{\tan^{-1} x}$, prove that
$$(1+x^2)y_{n+2}+[2(n+1)x-1]y_{n+1}+n(n+1)y_n=0.$$

4. If $y = (\sin^{-1} x)^2$, prove that
$$(1-x^2)y_2 - xy_1 - 2 = 0$$
and $(1-x^2)y_{n+2} - x(2n+1)y_{n+1} - n^2 y_n = 0.$

5. If $y = \dfrac{\sin^{-1} x}{\sqrt{(1-x^2)}}$, prove that
$$(1-x^2)y_{n+1} - (2n+1)xy_n - n^2 y_{n-1} = 0.$$

6. If $y = [\log\{x+\sqrt{(1+x^2)}\}]^2$, prove that
$$(1+x^2)y_{n+2} + (2n+1)xy_{n+1} + n^2 y_n = 0.$$
(VTU–2007, BHILLAI–2005, GBTU(AG)–2010)

7. Differentiating n times the equation :

(i) $(1+x^2)\dfrac{d^2y}{dx^2} - x\dfrac{dy}{dx} + a^2 y = 0.$

(ii) $x^2\dfrac{d^2y}{dx^2} + x\dfrac{dy}{dx} + y = 0.$

8. If $y = [x+\sqrt{(1+x^2)}]^m$, prove that
$$(1+x^2)y_{n+2}+(2n+1)xy_{n+1}+(n^2-m^2)y_n=0.$$
(VTU–2009, MADRAS–2000, 2004)

9. If $y^{1/m} + y^{-1/m} = 2x$, prove that
$$(x^2-1)y_{n+2}+(2n+1)xy_{n+1}+(n^2-m^2)y_n=0.$$
(VTU–2008, SVTU–2007, SRM–2006, 10, MUMBAI–2007)

10. If $y = \cos(\log x)$, prove that
$$x^2 y_{n+2} + (2n+1)xy_{n+1} + (n^2+1)y_n = 0.$$

11. If $x + y = 1$, prove that
$$\frac{d^n}{dx^n}(x^n y^n) = n![y^n - ({}^nC_1)^2 y^{n-1}x + ({}^nC_2)^2 y^{n-2}x^2 ... + (-1)^n x^n].$$

12. If $y = x\cos(\log x)$, prove that
$$x^2 y_{n+2} + (2n+1)xy_{n+1} + (n^2-2n+2)y_n = 0.$$

13. If $y = \left(\dfrac{1+x}{1-x}\right)^{1/2}$, prove that
$$(1-x^2)y_n - [2(n-1)x+1]y_{n-1} - (n-1)(n-2)y_{n-2} = 0.$$

14. If $y = \dfrac{\sinh^{-1} x}{\sqrt{1+x^2}}$, prove that
$$(1+x^2)y_{n+2} + (2n+3)xy_{n+1} + (n+1)^2 y_n = 0.$$

15. If $x = \sin t$, $y = \cos pt$, prove that
$$(1-x^2)y_2 - xy_1 + p^2 y = 0.$$
Hence, show that
$$(1-x^2)y_{n+2} - (2n+1)xy_{n+1} - (n^2-p^2)y_n = 0.$$
(VTU 2005, RAIPUR– 2005)

16. If $y = \sinh[m\log(x+\sqrt{x^2+1})]$, prove that
$$(x^2+1)y_{n+2}+(2n+1)xy_{n+1}+(n^2-m^2)y_n=0.$$
(VTU– 2010)

17. If $\sin^{-1} y = 2\log(x+1)$, prove that
$$(x+1)^2 y_{n+2} + (2n+1)(x+1)y_{n+1} + (x^2+4)y_n = 0$$
(VTU –2003)

18. Prove the following
$$\frac{d^n}{dx^n}\left[\frac{\log x}{x}\right] = \frac{(-1)^n.n!}{x^{n+1}}\left(\log x - 1 - \frac{1}{2} - \frac{1}{3} - ... - \frac{1}{n}\right)$$
(VTU –2006)

Hint to Selected Problems

2. Since
$$I_n = \frac{d^n}{dx^n}(x^n \log x)$$
$$\Rightarrow I_n = \frac{d^{n-1}}{dx^{n-1}}\left[\frac{d}{dx}(x^n \log x)\right] = nI_{n-1} + (n-1)!$$
Now replace $(n-1)$, $(n-2)$ in place of n successively.

3. $y = e^{\tan^{-1} x} \Rightarrow y_1 = e^{\tan^{-1} x}.\dfrac{1}{(1+x^2)}$

$\Rightarrow y_1(1+x^2) = y.$

Differentiating, we get

$(1 + x^2)y_2 + (2x - 1)y_1 = 0.$

Now apply Leibnitz theorem.

4. $y = (\sin^{-1}x)^2 \Rightarrow y_1 = 2\sin^{-1} x.\dfrac{1}{\sqrt{1-x^2}}$

$\Rightarrow y_1^2 = \dfrac{4(\sin^{-1} x)^2}{(1-x^2)}$

$\Rightarrow (1-x^2)y_1^2 = 4(\sin^{-1} x)^2$

$\Rightarrow (1-x^2)y_1^2 = 4y$. Again differentiating, we get

$(1-x^2)2y_1.y_2 - 2xy_1^2 = 4y_1$

$\Rightarrow (1-x^2)y_2 - xy_1 - 2 = 0.$

Now apply Leibnitz's theorem.

5. $$y = \frac{\sin^{-1} x}{\sqrt{1-x^2}}$$

$$\Rightarrow y_1 = \frac{1}{(1-x^2)} + \frac{x}{(1-x^2)} \frac{\sin^{-1} x}{\sqrt{1-x^2}}$$

$$\Rightarrow \quad (1-x^2)y_1 = 1 + xy.$$

Now apply Leibnitz's theorem.

6. $$y = [\log\{x + \sqrt{1+x^2}\}]^2$$

$$\Rightarrow \sqrt{1+x^2}\, y_1 = 2[\log\{x + \sqrt{1+x^2}\}]$$

On squaring, we get

$$(1+x^2)y_1 = 4[\log\{x + (1+x^2)\}]^2$$

$$\Rightarrow (1+x^2){y_1}^2 = 4y.$$

Again differentiating, we get

$$(1+x^2)y_2 + xy_1 - 2 = 0.$$

Now applying Leibnitz's theorem.

7. Apply directly Leibnitz's theorem.

8. $$y = [x + \sqrt{1+x^2}]^m$$

$$\Rightarrow y_1 = \frac{m[x + \sqrt{1+x^2}]^m}{\sqrt{1+x^2}}$$

$$\Rightarrow \sqrt{1+x^2}\, y_1 = my.$$

On squaring, we get $(1+x^2){y_1}^2 = m^2y^2$

Again differentiating, we get

$$(1+x^2)y_2 + xy_1 - m^2y = 0.$$

Now apply Leibnitz theorem.

9. $y^{1/m} + y^{-1/m} = 2x \Rightarrow 2xy^{1/m} = y^{2/m} + 1$

Let $t = y^{1/m}$. Then $t^2 + 1 = 2xt$.

Solving for t, we get

$$t = x \pm \sqrt{x^2 - 1} \Rightarrow y = [x + \sqrt{x^2-1}]^m.$$

On differentiating, we get

$$y_1 = \frac{m[x + \sqrt{x^2-1}]^m}{\sqrt{x^2-1}}.$$

Differentiating w.r.t. x after squaring, we get

$$(x^2 - 1)y_2 + xy_1 - m^2y = 0.$$

Now apply Leibnitz theorem.

10. $y = \cos(\log x)$

$$\Rightarrow y_1 = -\sin(\log x).\frac{1}{x} \Rightarrow xy_1 = -\sin(\log x).$$

Again differentiating, we get

$$xy_2 + y_1 = -\cos(\log x).\frac{1}{x}$$

$$\Rightarrow \quad x^2y_2 + xy_1 + y = 0.$$

Now apply Leibnitz's theorem.

ANSWERS

1. (i) $e^{ax}a^{n-3}[a^3x^3 + 3na^2x^2 + 3n(n-1)ax + n(n-1)(n-2)]$ (ii) $e^x[x^2 + 2nx + n(n-1)]$

(iii) $a^{n-3}\left[a^3x^3 \sin\left(ax + \frac{n\pi}{2}\right) + 3na^2x^2 \sin\left(ax + (n-1)\frac{\pi}{2}\right) + 3n(n-1)ax \sin\left\{ax + (n-2)\frac{\pi}{2}\right\}\right.$
$\left. + n(n-1)(n-2)\sin\left(ax + (n-3)\frac{\pi}{2}\right)\right]$

(iv) $\frac{(-1)^{n-1}n!}{x^{n-3}}\left[\frac{1}{n} - \frac{3}{n-1} + \frac{3}{n-2} - \frac{1}{n-3}\right]$

(v) $e^x\left[2^{n/2}x^2\cos\left(x + \frac{n\pi}{4}\right) + 2^{(n-1)/2}2nx\cos\left(x + (n-1)\frac{\pi}{4}\right) + 2^{(n-2)/2}n(n-1)\cos\left(x + (n-2)\frac{\pi}{4}\right)\right]$

(vi) $e^x[\log x + {}^nC_1x^{-1} - {}^nC_2x^{-2} + {}^nC_3 2!x^{-3} - \ldots + {}^nC_n(-1)^{n-1}(n-1)!x^{-n}]$ (vii) $y_{n+1} = \frac{n!}{x}$

(viii) $(-1)^{n-1}(n-3)![(n-1)(n-2)x^2\sin^n\phi\sin n\phi - 2n(n-1)\sin^{n-1}\phi\sin(n-1)\phi$
$+ n(n-1)\sin^{n-2}\phi\sin(n-2)\phi]$ where $\phi = \tan^{-1}\frac{1}{x}$

7. (i) $(1-x^2)y_{n+2} - (2n+1)xy_{n+1} - (n^2 - a^2)y_n = 0$

(ii) $x^2y_{n+2} + (2n+1)xy_{n+1} + (n^2+1)y_n = 0.$

7.5 DETERMINATION OF THE VALUE OF nth DERIVATIVE OF A FUNCTION AT X = 0

WORKING PROCEDURE

STEP 1. Put the given function equal to y.

STEP 2. Find $y_1 = \frac{dy}{dx}\cdot$ Then

(i) Take L.C.M. (if required).

(ii) Square both sides, if square roots are there.

(iii) Try to get y in R.H.S. (if possible).

STEP 3. Again differentiating both sides w.r.t. x and get an equation in y_2, y_1 and y.

STEP 4. Differentiate both sides n times w.r.t. x by Leibnitz's theorem.

STEP 5. Put $x = 0$ in equations of step 1, 2, 3, 4.

STEP 6. Put $n = 1, 2, 3, 4, \ldots$ in last equation of step 5.

STEP 7. Discuss the two cases, when n is even and when n is odd.

Solved Examples

1. *If* $y = e^{a\cos^{-1}x}$, *show that*

$$(1-x^2)y_{n+2} - (2n+1)xy_{n+1} - (n^2+a^2)y_n = 0$$

and hence calculate y_n *at* $x = 0$.

[GBTU–2010, MDU–1997]

SOLUTION. We have $y = e^{a\cos^{-1}x}$ ...(1)

$$\therefore \quad y_1 = e^{a\cos^{-1}x}.\frac{-a}{\sqrt{1-x^2}}$$

$$= -\frac{ya}{\sqrt{1-x^2}} \quad \ldots(2)$$

$$\Rightarrow \quad y_1\sqrt{1-x^2} = -ya$$

Now squaring both sides we get

$$y_1^2(1-x^2) = y^2a^2$$

Differentiating w.r.t. x, we have

$$(1-x^2)2y_1y_2 - 2xy_1^2 = 2a^2yy_1$$

$$\Rightarrow \quad (1-x^2)y_2 - xy_1 = a^2y \quad \ldots(3)$$

Now, using Leibnitz's theorem, differentiating (3), n times, we get

$$(1-x^2)y_{n+2} - 2nxy_{n+1} - n(n-1)y_n - xy_{n+1} - ny_n = a^2y_n$$

$$\Rightarrow \quad (1-x^2)y_{n+2} - (2n+1)xy_{n+1} - (n^2+a^2)y_n = 0 \quad \ldots(4)$$

By putting $x = 0$ in (1), (2), (3) and (4), we get

$$y(0) = e^{a.\pi/2}$$

$$y_1(0) = -ae^{a.\pi/2}$$

$$y_2(0) = a^2y(0) = a^2.e^{a.\pi/2}$$

$$\Rightarrow \quad y_{n+2}(0) = (n^2+a^2)y_n(0) \quad \ldots(5)$$

Put $n - 2$ for n in (5), we get

$$y_n(0) = [(n-2)^2 + a^2]y_{n-2}(0) \quad \ldots(6)$$

Again put $n - 4$ for n in (5), we get

$$y_{n-2}(0) = [(n-4)^2 + a^2]y_{n-4}(0) \quad \ldots(7)$$

From (6) and (7), we get

$$y_n(0) = [(n-2)^2 + a^2][(n-4)^2 + a^2]y_{n-4}(0) \quad \ldots(8)$$

Again put $n - 6$ for n in (5), we get

$$y_{n-4}(0) = [(n-6)^2 + a^2]y_{n-6}(0) \quad \ldots(9)$$

From (8) and (9), we get

$$y_n(0) = [(n-2)^2 + a^2][(n-4)^2 + a^2][(n-6)^2 + a^2]y_{n-6}(0) \quad \ldots(10)$$

Now there are following two cases :

Case I. When n is even.

$$y_n(0) = [(n-2)^2 + a^2][(n-4)^2 + a^2][(n-6)^2 + a^2]\ldots[2^2 + a^2]a^2e^{a\pi/2}$$

Case II. When n is odd.

$$y_n(0) = [(n-2)^2 + a^2][(n-4)^2 + a^2][(n-6)^2 + a^2]\ldots[1^2 + a^2](-ae^{a\pi/2})$$

2. *If $y = \tan^{-1} x$, prove that*

$$(1+x^2)y_{n+1} + 2nxy_n + n(n-1)y_{n-1} = 0.$$

Hence, determine the values of all the derivatives of y with respect to x when $x = 0$. (MUMBAI–2008)

SOLUTION. We have $y = \tan^{-1} x$. ...(1)

$$\therefore \quad y_1 = \frac{1}{1+x^2} \quad ...(2)$$

$\Rightarrow \quad y_1(1+x^2) = 1.$

Differentiating, n times by Leibnitz's theorem, we have

$$y_{n+1}(1+x^2) + ny_n.2x + \frac{n(n-1)}{2} y_{n-1}.2 = 0$$

$$\Rightarrow \quad (1+x^2)y_{n+1} + 2nxy_n + n(n-1)y_{n-1} = 0 \ldots (3)$$

Putting $x = 0$ in (1), (2) and (3), we get

$$y(0) = 0$$
$$y_1(0) = 1$$

....

$$y_{n+1}(0) = -n(n-1)y_{n-1}(0) \quad ...(4)$$

Put $n = 1$ in (4), we get

$$y_2(0) = 0.$$

Put $n - 1$ for n in (4), we get

$$y_n(0) = -(n-1)(n-2)y_{n-2}(0) \quad ...(5)$$

Put $n - 3$ for n in (4), we get

$$y_{n-2}(0) = -(n-3)(n-4)y_{n-4}(0) \quad ...(6)$$

From (5) and (6), we get

$$y_n(0) = (n-1)(n-2)(n-3)(n-4)y_{n-4}(0) \quad ...(7)$$

There arise following two cases :

Case I. When n is even.

$$y_n(0) = (-1)^{(n-2)/2}(n-1)(n-2)(n-3)(n-4)\ldots4.2y_2(0)$$
$$= (-1)^{(n-2)/2}(n-1)(n-2)(n-3)(n-4)\ldots3.2.0$$
$$= 0 \qquad [\because y_2(0) = 0]$$

Case II. When n is odd.

$$y_n(0) = (-1)^{(n-1)/2}(n-1)(n-2)(n-3)\ldots3.2.1y_1(0)$$
$$= (-1)^{(n-1)/2}(n-1)!\,y_1(0)$$
$$= (-1)^{(n-1)/2}(n-1)! \qquad [\because y_1(0) = 1]$$

3. *If $y = [x + \sqrt{1+x^2}]^m$, find $(y_n)_0$.*

SOLUTION. We have $y = [x + \sqrt{1+x^2}]^m$. ...(1)

Differentiating both sides w.r.t. x, we get

$$y_1 = m[x + \sqrt{1+x^2}]^{m-1}\left(1 + \frac{x}{\sqrt{1+x^2}}\right)$$

or $\quad y_1 = \dfrac{m}{\sqrt{1+x^2}}[x + \sqrt{1+x^2}]^m$

or $\quad \sqrt{1+x^2} \cdot y_1 = m[x + \sqrt{1+x^2}]^m$

or $\quad \sqrt{1+x^2} \cdot y_1 = my.$

Squaring both sides, we get

$$y_1^2(1+x^2) = m^2y^2. \quad ...(2)$$

Again differentiating both sides, we get

$$2y_1(1+x^2)y_2 + 2xy_1^2 = 2m^2yy_1.$$

or $\quad (1+x^2)y_2 + xy_1 - m^2y = 0.$ ...(3)

Applying Leibnitz's theorem to differentiate n times, we get

$$D^n[(1+x^2)y_2] + D^n(xy_1) - m^2D^2y = 0$$

$$(1+x^2)y_{n+2} + {}^nC_1y_{n+1}D(1+x^2) + {}^nC_2y_nD^2(1+x^2) + xy_{n+1} + {}^nC_1y_nD(x) - m^2y_n = 0$$

or $\quad (1+x^2)y_{n+2} + ny_{n+1}2x + \dfrac{n(n-1)}{2}y_n.2 + xy_{n+1} + ny_n - m^2y_n = 0$

or $\quad (1+x^2)y_{n+2} + x(2n+1)y_{n+1} + (n^2 - m^2)y_n = 0 \ldots(4)$

Putting $x = 0$ in (1), (2), (3) and (4), we get

$$(y)_0 = 1$$

$$(y_1)_0 = m(y_0) = m$$
$$(y_2)_0 = m^2(y)_0 = m^2$$
and $$(y_{n+2})_0 = (m^2 - n^2)(y_n)_0. \quad ...(5)$$

Put $n - 2$ for n in (5), we get

$$(y_n)_0 = [m^2 - (n-2)^2](y_{n-2})_0 \quad ...(6)$$

Put $n - 4$ for n in (5), we get

$$(y_{n-2})_0 = [m^2 - (n-4)^2](y_{n-4})_0 \quad ...(7)$$

From (6) and (7), we get

$$(y_n)_0 = [m^2 - (n-2)^2][m^2 - (n-4)^2](y_{n-4})_0 .. (8)$$

There arise two cases :

Case I. When n is even.

$$(y_n)_0 = [m^2 - (n-2)^2][m^2 - (n-4)^2] ...(m^2 - 2^2)(y_2)_0$$
$$= [m^2 - (n-2)^2][m^2 - (n-4)^2] ...[m^2 - 2^2]m^2$$
$$[\because (y_2)_0 = m^2]$$

Case II. When n is odd.

$$(y_n)_0 = [m^2 - (n-2)^2][m^2 - (n-4)^2] ...(m^2 - 1^2)(y_1)_0$$
$$= [m^2 - (n-2)^2][m^2 - (n-4)^2] ...(m^2 - 1^2)m$$
$$[\because (y_1)_0 = m]$$

4. *If $y = \sin(a\sin^{-1} x)$, then, prove that $(1-x^2)y_2 - xy_1 + a^2y = 0$ and $(1-x^2)y_{n+2} - (2n+1)xy_{n+1} + (a^2 - n^2)y_n = 0.$*

Hence, find $y_n(0)$.

<u>SOLUTION.</u> We have $y = \sin(a\sin^{-1} x) \quad ...(1)$

Differentiating (1) w.r.t. x we get

$$y_1 = \cos(a\sin^{-1} x).\frac{a}{\sqrt{1-x^2}}$$
$$\Rightarrow y_1 = \frac{a}{\sqrt{1-x^2}}\cos(a\sin^{-1} x)$$
$$\Rightarrow (\sqrt{1-x^2})y_1 = a\cos(a\sin^{-1} x)$$
$$\Rightarrow (1-x^2){y_1}^2 = a^2\cos^2(a\sin^{-1} x) = a^2(1-\sin^2(a\sin^{-1} x))$$
$$\Rightarrow (1-x^2){y_1}^2 = a^2(1-y^2) \quad ...(2)$$
(Using (1))

Differentiating (2) w.r.t. x, we get

$$(1-x^2)2y_1y_2 - 2x{y_1}^2 = a^2(-2yy_1)$$
$$\Rightarrow (1-x^2)y_2 - xy_1 + a^2y = 0 \quad ...(3)$$

Now differentiating (3) n times by Leibnitz's theorem, we get

$$[(1-x^2)y_{n+2} + {}^nC_1(-2x)y_{n+1} + {}^nC_2(-2)y_n] - \left[xy_{n+1} + {}^nC_1(1)y_n\right] + a^2y_n = 0$$
$$\Rightarrow (1-x^2)y_{n+2} + n(-2x)y_{n+1} + \frac{n(n-1)}{2}(-2)y_n - xy_{n+1} - n.1.y_n + a^2y_n = 0$$
$$\Rightarrow (1-x^2)y_{n+2} - (2n+1)xy_{n+1} + (a^2 - n^2 - n + n)y_n = 0$$
$$\Rightarrow (1-x^2)y_{n+2} - (2n+1)xy_{n+1} + (a^2 - n^2)y_n = 0 \quad ...(4)$$

From (1),
$$y(0) = \sin(a\sin^{-1} 0) = 0$$
From (2),
$$y_1(0) = \frac{a}{\sqrt{1-0}}\cos(a\sin^{-1} 0) = a\cos 0 = a$$
From (3),
$$(1-0^2)y_2(0) - 0.y_1(0) + a^2y(0) = 0$$
$$\Rightarrow \quad y_2(0) = 0$$
Form (4),
$$(1-0^2)y_{n+2}(0) - (2n+1).0 + (a^2 - n^2)y_n(0) = 0$$
$$\Rightarrow \quad y_{n+2}(0) = (n^2 - a^2)y_n(0) \quad ...(5)$$

Case I. If n is even.

Put $n = 2$ in equation (5), we get

$$y_4(0) = (2^2 - a^2)y_2(0) = 0$$

Put $n = 4$ in equation (5), we get

$$y_6(0) = (4^2 - a^2)y_4(0) = 0$$

Put $n = 6$ in equation (5), we get

$$y_8(0) = (6^2 - a^2)y_6(0) = 0$$

$\Rightarrow \quad y_n(0) = 0$, if n is even

Case II. If n is odd.

Put $n = 1$ in equation (5), we get

$$y_3(0) = (1^2 - a^2)y_1(0) = (1^2 - a^2).a$$

Put $n = 3$ in equation (5), we get

$$y_5(0) = (3^2 - a^2)y_3(0) = (1^2 - a^2)(3^2 - a^2).a$$

Put $n = 5$ in equation (5), we get

$$y_7(0) = (5^2 - a^2)y_5(0) = (1^2 - a^2)(3^2 - a^2)(5^2 - a^2).a$$

$$\Rightarrow y_n(0) = (1^2 - a^2)(3^2 - a^2)(5^2 - a^2) \ldots[(n-2)^2 - a^2)]a$$

if n is odd and $n \neq 1$

Hence,

$$y_n(0) = \begin{cases} 0 & \text{if } n \text{ is even} \\ (1^2 - a^2)(3^2 - a^2)(5^2 - a^2)\ldots[(n-2)^2 - a^2]a & \text{if } n \text{ is odd and } n \neq 1 \end{cases}$$

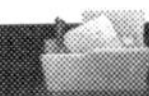

Exercise-7.3

1. If $y = \sin^{-1}x$, prove that
$$(1 - x^2)y_{n+2} - (2n+1)xy_{n+1} - n^2y_n = 0$$
and also find the value of $y_n(0)$. (SVTU–2009)

2. (i) If $y = [\log\{x + \sqrt{(1 + x^2)}\}]^2$, find all the derivatives of y w.r.t. x when $x = 0$.

   (ii) If $y = (\sinh^{-1} x)^2$, prove that
$$(1 + x^2)y_{n+2} + (2n+1)xy_{n+1} + n^2y_n = 0$$
Hence, find $y_n(0)$.

3. If $y = [x + \sqrt{1 + x^2}]^m$, find $y_n(0)$.

4. (i) If $y = \sin(m \sin^{-1}x)$, then prove that $y_{n+2}(0) = (n^2 - m^2)(y_n)_0$ and find $y_n(0)$. [MUMBAI–2008]

   (ii) If $y = \cos(m \sin^{-1}x)$, find $y_n(0)$. [COCHIN–2005]

5. If $y = e^{a \sin^{-1} x}$, show that
$$(1 - x^2)y_{n+2} - x(2n+1)y_{n+1} - (n^2 + a^2)y_n = 0$$
and hence, find the value of $y_n(0)$.

6. If $x = \sin\left(\frac{1}{a}\log y\right)$, find $(y_n)_0$.

Hint to Selected Problems

1. $y = \sin^{-1} x \Rightarrow y_1 = \frac{1}{\sqrt{1 - x^2}} \Rightarrow (1 - x^2)y_1^2 = 1$

   Differentiating, we get $(1 - x^2)y_2 - xy_1 = 0$

   Now apply Leibnitz's theorem and put $x = 0$.

2. (i) $y = [\log x + \sqrt{1 + x^2}]^2$

$$\Rightarrow \quad y_1 = \frac{2}{\sqrt{1+x^2}}\log(x + \sqrt{1 + x^2})$$

$$\Rightarrow (1 + x^2)y_1^{\,2} = 4y$$

   Again differentiating, we get

   $(1 + x^2)y2 + xy1 - 2 = 0.$

   Now apply Leibnitz's theorem to find y_n and then put $x = 0$.

3. $y = [x + \sqrt{1 + x^2}]^m \Rightarrow y_1 = \frac{m[x + \sqrt{1+x^2}]^m}{\sqrt{1+x^2}}$

   i.e., $(1 + x^2)y_1^{\,2} = m^2y^2$.

   Again differentiating, we get

$$(1 + x^2)y_2 + xy_1 - m^2y = 0$$

   Now apply Leibnitz's theorem.

4. (i) $y = \sin(m \sin^{-1}x)$

$$\Rightarrow y_1 = \frac{m\cos(m\sin^{-1} x)}{\sqrt{1-x^2}}$$

$$\Rightarrow y_1\sqrt{(1 - x^2)} = m\cos(m\sin^{-1} x)$$

Again differentianting, we get

$$(1-x^2)y_2 - xy_1 - m^2y = 0$$

Now apply Leibnitz's theorem.

5. $y = e^{a\sin^{-1}x}$

$$\Rightarrow y_1 = \frac{ay}{\sqrt{1-x^2}} \Rightarrow (1-x^2){y_1}^2 = a^2y^2$$

Differentiating w.r.t. x, we get

$$(1-x^2)y_2 - xy_1 - a^2y = 0$$

Now apply Leibnitz's theorem.

ANSWERS

1. When n is even, $y_n(0) = 0$; When n is odd $y_n(0) = 1^2.3^2.5^2...(n-2)^2$

2. (i),(ii) when n is even, $y_n(0) = (-1)^{n/2-1}.2.2^2.4^2...(n-2)^2$, when n is odd $y_n(0) = 0$

3. When n is even, $y_n(0) = [m^2-(n-2)^2][m^2-(n-4)^2]...(m^2-2^2)m^2$

When n is odd, $y_n(0) = [m^2-(n-2)^2][m^2-(n-4)^2]...(m^2-1^2)m$

4. (i) When n is even, $y_n(0) = 0$,

When n is odd, $y_n(0) = [(n-2)^2-m^2][(n-4)^2-m^2][(n-6)^2-m^2]...[(3^2-m^2)(1^2-m^2)]m$

(ii) When n is even, $y_n(0) = -[(n-2)^2-m^2][(n-4)^2-m2]...[(2^2-m^2)m^2$;

When n is odd, $y_n(0) = 0$

5. When n is even, $y_n(0) = [(n-2)^2+a^2][(n-4)^2+a^2]...(4^2+a^2)(2^2+a^2).a^2$

When n is odd, $y_n(0) = [(n-2)^2+a^2][(n-4)^2+a^2]...(3^2+a^2)(1^2+a^2).a$

❑❑❑❑❑❑

Chapter

8 Mean Value Theorems and Expansion of Functions

8.1 INTRODUCTION

In this chapter we shall discuss some important theorems namely, Rolle's, Lagrange's, Cauchy mean value and Taylor's theorem. We shall also discuss Maclaurin's series expansion of some standard functions like e^x, $\log(1+x)$, $\sin x$, $\cos x$ etc.

8.2 ROLLE'S THEOREM

If a function $f(x)$ defined on $[a,b]$ is such that it is
(i) continuous in $[a,b]$, *(ii) differentiable in $]a,b[$ and* *(iii) $f(a) = f(b)$,*

then there exists at least one vlaue of x, say $c,(a<c<b)$ such that $f'(c) = 0$.

[KANPUR(BCA)–2001, 04, 06, 08, 12, 13; DELHI–2009]

PROOF. Since, thc function $f(x)$ is continuous on $[a, b]$

$\Rightarrow$ $f(x)$ is bounded. [$\because$ Every continuous function is bounded.]

$\Rightarrow$ $f(x)$ attains its bounds [$\because$ A function, which is continuous on a closed bounded interval $[a, b]$, then it attains its bound on $[a, b]$.]

Let M and m are the supremum and infimum of $f(x)$ respectively.

Now there are two possibilities

(i) If $M=m$, then obviously $f(x)$ is a constant function, and therefore its derivative is zero, *i.e.*, $f'(x)= 0\ \forall\ x \in\ ]a, b[$.

(ii) If $M \neq m$, then at least one of the numbers M and m must be different from the equal values $f(a)$ and $f(b)$.

Let us assume $M \neq f(a)$.

Now, since, every continuous function on a closed interval attains its supremum, therefore, there exists a real number c in $[a,b]$ such that $f(c)=M$. Also since $f(a)\neq M\neq f(b)$.Therefore $c\neq a$ and $c\neq b$, this implies that $c\in]a,b[$.

Now, $f(c)$ is the supremum of f on $[a, b]$

$$\therefore \quad f(x) \le f(c)\ \forall x\in[a, b] \quad ...(1)$$

[By the definition of supremum]

In particular, $f(c-h) \le f(c) \quad h>0$

$$\Rightarrow \quad \frac{f(c-h)-f(c)}{-h} \ge 0 \quad ...(2)$$

Since $f'(x)$ exists at each point of $]a, b[$, and hence, $f'(c)$ exists.

Therefore, from (2)

$$Lf'(c) \ge 0 \quad ...(3)$$

Similarly, from (1)

$$f(c+h) \leq f(c) \quad h>0$$

Then by the same arguments

$$Rf'(c) \leq 0. \qquad \ldots(4)$$

Since $f(x)$ is differentiable in $]a, b[$ $\Rightarrow f'(c)$ exist

$$\Rightarrow \quad Lf'(c) = f'(c) = Rf'(c) \qquad \ldots(5)$$

Now from (3), (4) and (5) $\quad f'(c)=0.$

Similarly we can consider the case $M=f(a) \neq m$.

- Converse of Rolle's theorem is not true, *i.e.*, $f'(x)$ may vanish at a point $c \in]a, b[$ without $f(x)$ satisfying the three conditions of Rolle's theorem.
- There may be more than one point like c at which $f'(x)$ vanishes but Rolle's theorem ensures the existence of at least one such c.
- Rolle's theorem will not hold good if
  - (a) $f(x)$ is discontinuous at some point in the interval $[a, b]$
  - (b) $f'(x)$ does not exist at some point in the interval $]a, b[$
  - (c) $f(a) \neq f(b)$
- The hypothesis of Rolle's theorem cannot be weakened.

For example, if $f(x)=1-|x|, -1 \leq x \leq 1$, then $f(-1)=f(1)=0$ and f is continuous on $[-1,1]$. Also if $f'(x)$ exist $\forall\, x \in]-1, 1[$ except at $x=0$. Then, f satisfies all the condition of Rolle's theorem except that f is not differentiable at $x=0$. For this f, there is no c in $]-1,1[$ for which $f'(c)=0$.

8.2.1 Geometrical Interpretation of Rolle's Theorem

Geometrically, Rolle's theorem means that if the curve $y=f(x)$ is continuous from $x=a$ to $x=b$, has a definite tangent at each point of $]a,b[$ and the ordinates at the extremities are equal, then there exists at least one point between a and b at which the tangent is parallel to x-axis.

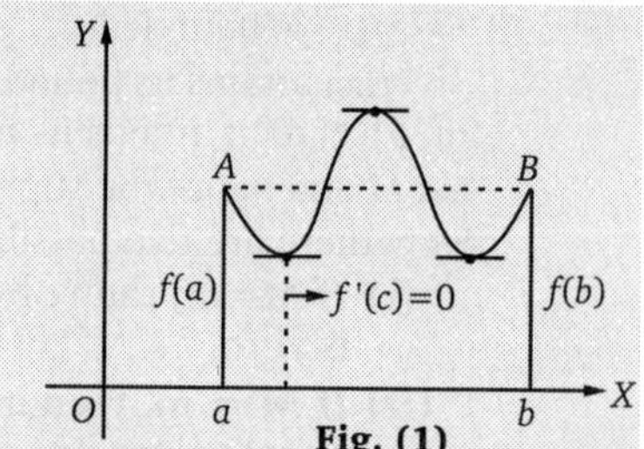

Fig. (1)

8.2.2 Algebraic Interpretation of Rolle's Theorem

Algebraically, Rolle's theorem means that if $f(x)$ is a polynomial function in x and $x=a$ and $x=b$ are two roots of the equation $f(x)=0$, then, there is at least one root of the equation $f'(x)=0$ which lies between a and b.

8.3 LAGRANGE'S MEAN VALUE THEOREM

Let f be a function defined on $[a, b]$ such that

(i) f is continuous on $[a, b]$, (ii) f is differentiable on $]a, b[$.

Then, there exists a real number $c \in]a,b[$ such that $\dfrac{f(b)-f(a)}{b-a} = f'(c)$

[MEERUT(BCA)–2011, 15; KANPUR(BCA)–2005, 08, 16; ROHILKHAND–2011]

PROOF. Let us define a function $F(x)$ such that

$$F(x) = f(x) + Ax \;\forall\, x \in [a, b] \qquad \ldots(1)$$

where A is a constant to be suitably chosen such that $F(a)=F(b)$.

Now

(i) Since, f is continuous on $[a,b]$ and Ax is continuous on $[a,b]$ therefore, F is continuous on $[a,b]$ [$\because$ Sum of two continuous functions is again continuous.]

(ii) Similarly F is differentiable on (a, b)

(iii) $F(a) - F(b) \quad \Rightarrow \qquad -A = \dfrac{f(b)-f(a)}{b-a}$ ...(2)

Hence, we find that F satisfy all the conditions of Rolle's Theorem on $[a,b]$ and consequently, there exists a real number $c \in]a,b[$ such that $F'(c)=0$, this gives

$$f'(c) + A = 0$$

$$\Rightarrow \qquad -A = f'(c). \qquad \text{...(3)}$$

Now, from (2) and (3), we have

$$\frac{f(b)-f(a)}{b-a} = f'(c)$$

- If we take $b=a+h$ and c can be written as $a+\theta h$, where θ is some real number such that $0<\theta<1$. Lagrange's theorem then read as follows :
  "Let f be defined and continuous on $[a, a+h]$ and differentiable on $]a, a+h[$, then for some real number $\theta(0<\theta<1)$
  $$\frac{f(a+h)-f(a)}{h} = f'(a+\theta h).$$
- The hypothesis of the Lagrange's mean value theorem cannot be weakened, as it is clear from the following examples :
  " Let f be the function defined on $[-1,2]$ by setting $f(x)=|x|$, $\forall x \in [-1,2]$.
  Here, f is continuous on $[-1,2]$ and differentiable at all points of $]-1, 2[$ except at $x=0$ (so that second condition is violated.)
  Now $\quad f'(x) = \begin{cases} -1 & \text{if } x \in]-1,0[\\ 1 & \text{if } x \in]0,2[\end{cases}$; $\quad$ Also $\dfrac{f(2)-f(-1)}{2-(-1)} \neq f'(x)$ for any x in $]-1, 2[$.
- Lagrange's mean value theorem is known as first mean value theorem.
- The result $f(b)-f(a)=f(b-a)f'(c)$ is also known as the formula for finite increment.
- For $f(a)=f(b)$, the Lagrange's mean value theorem yields Rolle's theorem.

8.3.1 GEOMETRICAL INTERPRETATION OF LAGRANGE'S MEAN VALUE THEOREM

If the curve $y=f(x)$ is continuous from $x=a$ and $x=b$ and has a tangent at each point on the curve between $x=a$ and $x=b$, then, geometrically, the first mean value theorem means that there is at least one point between $x=a$ and $x=b$ on the curve where the tangent to the curve parallel to the chord joining the points $(a, f(a))$ and $(b, f(b))$.

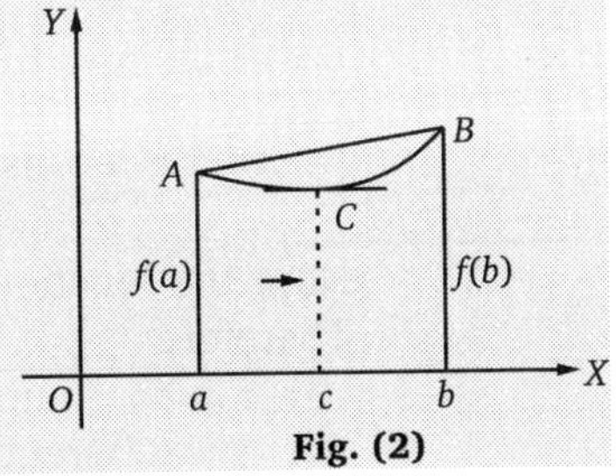

Fig. (2)

Let ACB be the graph of the function $y= f(x)$ then the co-ordinate of the points A and B are given by $(a, f(a))$ and $(b, f(b))$ respectively. If the chord AB makes an angle θ with the x-axis, then

$$\tan\theta = \frac{f(b)-f(a)}{b-a} = f'(c), \text{ where } a < c < b.$$

8.3.2 DEDUCTIONS FROM THE FIRST MEAN VALUE THEOREM

THEOREM 1. *If a function $f(x)$ satisfies the conditions of mean value theorem then*

(i) $f'(x)= 0 \ \forall \ x \in]a, b[\Rightarrow f$ is constant on $[a, b]$.

(ii) $f'(x)>0\ \forall x\in]a,b[\Rightarrow f$ *is strictly increasing on* $[a,b]$.

and *(iii)* $f'(x)<0\ \forall x\in]a,b[\Rightarrow f$ *is strictly decreasing on* $[a,b]$.

PROOF. (i) Let x_1, x_2 (where $x_1>x_2$) be any two distinict points of $[a,b]$, then by Lagrange's mean value theorem,

$$\frac{f(x_2)-f(x_1)}{x_2-x_1} = f'(c) = 0,\ x_1 < c < x_2 \qquad ...(1)$$

$\Rightarrow$ $f(x_2)=f(x_1)$.

$\Rightarrow$ function keeps the same value. Therefore $f(x)$ is constant on $[a,b]$.

(ii) From (1), we have

$$\frac{f(x_2)-f(x_1)}{x_2-x_1} = f'(c) \text{ for some } c \in]x_1,\ x_2[$$

But $f'(c) > 0$ $[\because f'(x) > 0\ \forall\ x \in [a, b]]$

$\Rightarrow$ $f(x_2)-f(x_1)>0$

$\Rightarrow$ $f(x_2)>f(x_1)$

Thus $x_2>x_1 \Rightarrow f(x_2)>f(x_1)\ \forall x_1,x_2\in[a,b]$

Hence, f is strictly increasing on $[a,b]$.

(iii) Same as (ii).

- For a strictly increasing function f, the derivative $f'(x)$ need not be strictly positive. For example, consider $f(x)=x^3$, $x \in]-1, 1[$. Here, $f(x)$ is strictly increasing but $f'(x)=3x^2$, which is zero at $x = 0 \in]-1, 1[$.

8.4 CAUCHY'S MEAN VALUE THEOREM

Let f and g be two functions defined on $[a,b]$ *such that*

(i) f and g are continuous on $[a, b]$, *(ii)* f and g are differentiabfe on $]a, b[$,

and *(iii)* $g'(x)\neq 0$ for any point of $]a, b[$. [PTU–2007, 11; VTU–2006; KANPUR(BCA)–2008]

Then, there exists a real number $c \in]a, b[$ *such that*

$$\frac{f(b)-f(a)}{g(b)-g(a)} = \frac{f'(c)}{g'(c)}$$

PROOF. Let us define a function

$$F(x) = f(x) + A.g(x) \qquad ...(1)$$

where A is a constant, to be suitably chosen such that

$$F(a) = F(b) \qquad ...(2)$$

Now, the function F is the sum of two continuous and differentiable functions. Therefore

(i) F is continuous on $[a,b]$,

(ii) F is differentiable on $]a,b[$,

and (iii) $F(a)=F(b)$.

Then, by Rolle's theorem, there must exists a real number c between a and b such that

$$F'(c) = 0$$

Here, $F'(x) = f'(x)+Ag'(x)$

$F'(c) = 0 \quad \Rightarrow \quad f'(c)+Ag'(c)=0$

$$\Rightarrow \qquad -A = \frac{f'(c)}{g'(c)} \qquad ...(3)$$

Now $F(a) = F(b) \Rightarrow f(a)+Ag(a)=f(b) + Ag(b)$

$$\Rightarrow \quad -A = \frac{f(b)-f(a)}{g(b)-g(a)} \quad ...(4)$$

From (3) and (4), we have $\frac{f(b)-f(a)}{g(b)-g(a)} = \frac{f'(c)}{g'(c)}$.

- If we put $b=a+h$, then c can be written as $a+\theta h$, where $\theta \in R$ such that $0 < \theta < 1$, then Cauchy's mean value theorem can be restated as
  "If f and g are continuous on $[a, a+h]$ and are differentiable on $]a, a+h[$ and $g'(x) \neq 0$ for any $x \in]a, a+h[$ then, $\exists$ a $\theta \in R: 0 < \theta < 1$ such that
  $$\frac{f(a+h)-f(a)}{g(a+h)-g(a)} = \frac{f'(a+\theta h)}{g'(a+\theta h)}.$$
- If we take $g(a)=g(b)$, then the function g would satisfy all the conditions of Rolle's theorem and consequently for some x in $]a,b[$, we would have $g'(x)=0$. In view of this we take $g(a) \neq g(b)$.
- In some cases, the Lagrange's mean value theorem is a particular case of Cauchy's mean value theorem (e.g., take $g(x)=k$).
- Cauchy's mean value theorem cannot be deduced by applying Lagrange's mean value theorem to two functions f and g seperately and then dividing. It can be easily seen that the desired result cannot be obtained in this manner. In this way, we get
  $$\frac{f(b)-f(a)}{g(b)-g(a)} = \frac{f'(c_1)}{g'(c_2)}$$
  where $a < c_1 < b$, and $a < c_2 < b$. But, it is not necessary that c_1 and c_2 are equal.
  Hence, Cauchy's means value theorem is not directly deduceable from the first one.
- The conditions in the theorem are sufficient one. The conclusion may still hold even when the function involved do not satisfy the condition on $[a,b]$.

8.4.1 GEOMETRICAL INTERPRETATION OF CAUCHY'S MEAN VALUE THEOREM

(1) Under suitable conditions, Cauchy's mean value theorem geometrically means that there is an ordinate $x=c$ between $x=a$ and $x=b$, such that the tangents at the points where $x=c$ cut the graphs of the function $f(x)$ and $\frac{f(b)-f(a)}{g(b)-g(a)} g(x)$ are mutually parallel.

(2) The ratio of the mean rates of increase of two functions in an interval is equal to the ratio of the actual rates of increase of the functions at some point within the interval.

Solved Examples

1. *Discuss the applicability of Rolle's theorem in the interval* $[-1,1]$ *to the function* $f(x)=|x|$.

SOLUTION. Here, we have $f(x)=|x|$

$\Rightarrow$ $f(-1)=1$ and $f(1)=1$

$\Rightarrow$ $f(1) = f(-1)$

Now, the function $f(x)$ is continuous throughout the closed interval $[-1,1]$ but $f(x)$ is not differentiable at $x = 0 \in]-1, 1[$. Hence, Rolle's theorem is not satisfied (due to the second condition).

2. *Verify Rolle's theorem the function* $f(x) = x^3 - 4x$ *on* $[-2, 2]$.

[KANPUR(BCA)-2008; MEERUT(BCA)-2007, 14]

SOLUTION. The function $f(x)=x^3-4x$ is a polynomial and so it is continuous and differentiable at all $x \in R$. In particular it is continuous in the closed interval $[-2,2]$ and differentiable in the open interval $]-2,2[$. Also $f(-2)=0=f(2)$.

Thus, $f(x)$ satisfies all the three conditions of Rolle's theorem in $[-2,2]$. Therefore, there must exist at least one real number 'x' in the open interval $]-2,2[$ for which

$$f'(x)=0.$$

Now $f'(x)=0$ gives $3x^2-4=0$

or $$x=\pm\frac{2}{\sqrt{3}}=\pm 1.55.$$

Both these values lie in the open interval $]-2, 2[$ and thus the conclusion of Rolle's theorem is verified.

3. *Discuss the applicability of Rolle's theorem to the function* $f(x) = \log\left[\frac{x^2+ab}{(a+b)x}\right]$ *in the interval* $[a, b]$.

[VTU–2005]

SOLUTION. Here, we have

$$f(a)=\log\left[\frac{a^2+ab}{(a+b)a}\right]=\log 1=0$$

and $$f(b)=\log\left[\frac{b^2+ab}{(a+b)b}\right]=\log 1=0$$

Also, it can be easily seen that $f(x)$ is continuous on $[a,b]$ and differentiable on $]a,b[$.

Thus all the three conditions of Rolle's theorem are satisfied. Hence $f'(x)=0$ for at least one value of x in $]a, b[$.

Now $$f'(x)=0 \Rightarrow \frac{2x}{x^2+ab}-\frac{1}{x}=0$$

$\Rightarrow 2x^2-(x^2+ab)=0$

$\Rightarrow$ $x^2 = ab$ or $x=\sqrt{ab}$.

Obviously $\sqrt{ab}\in]a,b[$

[Being the geometric mean of a and b]

Hence, the Rolle's theorem is verified.

4. *Verify Rolle's theorem for the function* $f(x)=2x^3+x^2-4x-2$.

SOLUTION. Since, $f(x)$ is a rational integral function of x, therefore it is continuous and differentiable for all real values of x.

Hence, the first two conditions of Rolle's theorem are satisfied in any interval.

Hence, $f(x) = 0$ gives $2x^3+x^2-4x-2=0$

i.e., $$x=\pm\sqrt{2},-\frac{1}{2}$$

$$\Rightarrow f(\sqrt{2})=f(-\sqrt{2})=f\left(-\frac{1}{2}\right)=0$$

Now take the interval $[-\sqrt{2},\sqrt{2}]$, then, all the conditions of Rolle's theorem are satisfied in this interval. Then, $\exists$ at least one value of c in $]-\sqrt{2},\sqrt{2}[$ such that $f'(c)=0$

$f'(x)=0 \Rightarrow 6x^2+2x-4=0$

$\Rightarrow x=-1, 2/3$

Since, both the points -1 and $2/3$ lies in the open interval $]-\sqrt{2},\sqrt{2}[$.

Hence, Rolle's theorem is verified.

5. *Show that there is no real number p for which the equation* $x^3-3x+p=0$ *has two distinct roots in* $]0,1[$.

SOLUTION. Let, if possible, there are two distinct roots a and b of the given equation in $]0, 1[$, such that $0 < a < b < 1$.

Now, let $f(x) = x^3-3x+p$

Obviously, $f(x)$ is continuous and differentiable for all values of x (Being a polynomial).

Also, we have

$$f(a) = f(b) = 0$$

$\Rightarrow f$ satisfies all the conditions of Rolle's theorem in $[a,b]$ hence, $\exists$ a point $c\in]a, b[$ such that $f'(c)=0$.

Now $f'(x) = 0 \Rightarrow 3x^2-3 = 0$

$\Rightarrow x = \pm 1$

which is a contradiction

($\because a < c < b$ as $0 < a < b < 1$)

$\Rightarrow$ our assumption is wrong. Hence, there cannot be two distinct roots of $f(x) = 0$ in $]0, 1[$ for any value of p.

6. *If* $a + b + c = 0$, *then show that the quadratic equation* $3ax^2+2bx+c = 0$ *has at least one root in* $]0, 1[$.

SOLUTION. Let us define a function $f(x)$ such that

$$f(x) = ax^3+bx^2+cx+d.$$

Here we have $f(0) = d$

and $f(1) = a+b+c+d = d$

($\because a+b+c = 0$)

Obviously, $f(x)$ is continuous and differentiable in $]0, 1[$ (Being a polynomial).

Thus, $f(x)$ satisfies all the three conditions of Rolle's theorem in $[0, 1]$. Hence, there is at least one value of x in the open interval $]0, 1[$ where $f'(x) = 0$

i.e., $3ax^2+2bx+c = 0$ has at least one root in $]0, 1[$.

Similar Problems

(1) Verify the Rolle's theorem for the function $f(x) = x^2$ in $[-1, 1]$.
(2) Verify the Rolle's theorem for the function $f(x) = x^3 - 3x + 2$ in $[1, 2]$.
(3) Verify the Rolle's theorem for the function $f(x) = x^{2/3}$ in $[-1, 1]$.
(4) Verify the Rolle's theorem for the function $f(x) = x^3 - 6x + 11x - 6$.
(5) Verify the Rolle's theorem for the function $f(x) = 10x - x^2$.

7. *Discuss the applicability of Rolle's theorem to the function*

$$f(x)=\begin{cases} x^2+1 \text{ , when } 0\le x<1 \\ 3-x \text{ , when } 1<x\le 2\end{cases}$$

SOLUTION. Here $f(0)=0^2+1$ and $f(2)=3-2=1$.

We shall show that $f(x)$ is continuous for all x in the range (0,2) except at $x = 1$.

Also $f(1)=1^2+1=2$

Again, $f(1+0)=\lim\limits_{x\to 1+0}(3-x)$

$$=\lim_{x\to 1+h}\left[3-(1+h)\right], \text{ when } h\to 0$$

$$=\lim_{h\to 0}(2-h)=2$$

and $f(1-0)=\lim\limits_{x\to 1-0}\left(x^2+1\right)$

$$=\lim_{x\to(1-h)}\left[(1-h)^2+1\right], \text{ when } h\to 0$$

$$=\lim_{h\to 0}\left(2-2h+h^2\right)=2$$

Hence, $f(1-0)=f(1)=f(1+0)$ and so the function $f(x)$ is continuous at $x=1$ and the continuous in the whole interval (0,2).

Again, $f'(x)=\begin{cases} 2x \text{ , when } 0\le x<1 \\ -1 \text{ , when } 1<x\le 2\end{cases}$

$\therefore$ $f(x)$ is differentiable in the interval (0,2) except at $x=1$.

Now $Rf'(1)$

$$=\lim_{h\to 0}\frac{f(1+h)-f(1)}{h}$$

$$=\lim_{h\to 0}\frac{\{3-(1+h)\}-2}{h}$$

$$=\lim_{h\to 0}\frac{2-h-2}{h}=\lim_{h\to 0}(-1)=-1$$

and $Lf'(1)$

$$=\lim_{h\to 0}\frac{f(1-h)-f(1)}{-h}$$

$$=\lim_{h\to 0}\frac{\left[(1-h)^2+1\right]-2}{-h}$$

$$=\lim_{h\to 0}\frac{2h-h^2}{h}=\lim_{h\to 0}(2-h)=2$$

$\therefore$ Thus $Rf'(1)\ne Lf'(1)$ and so $f'(1)$ does not exist.

Hence, the function $f(x)$ is not differentiable in the entire range (0, 2) and therefore Rolle's theorem is not applicable to the given function $f(x)$ in (0, 2).

8. *Find 'c' of the mean value theorem, if $f(x) = x(x-1).(x-2); a = 0, b = 1/2$.*

[GORAKHPUR–1999]

SOLUTION. Here, we have $f(a)=f(0)=0$

and $f(b)=f\left(\frac{1}{2}\right)=\frac{3}{8}$

$$\therefore \quad \frac{f(b)-f(a)}{b-a}=\frac{\frac{3}{8}-0}{\frac{1}{2}-0}=\frac{3}{4}$$

Now $f(x)=x^3-3x^2+2x$

$\therefore$ $f'(x)=3x^2-6x+2$

$\Rightarrow$ $f'(c)=3c^2-6c+2$

Putting all these values in the Lagrange's mean value theorem

$$\frac{f(b)-f(a)}{b-a}=f'(c), (a<c<b)$$

We get $\frac{3}{4}=3c^2-6c+2$ or $c=1\pm\frac{\sqrt{21}}{6}$

Hence, $c=\frac{1-\sqrt{21}}{6}$ lies in the open interval $]0, \frac{1}{2}[$ therefore, it is the required value.

9. *If $f(x)=\log x$, find all numbers strictly between e^2 and e^3 such that*

$$f'(x)=\frac{f(e^3)-f(e^2)}{e^3-e^2}$$ [BURDWAN–2003; MEERUT(BCA)–2008, 12; KANPUR(BCA)–2003; KURUKSHETRA–2009]

SOLUTION. Obviously $f(x)=\log x$ is continuous in $[e^2, e^3]$ and differentiable in $]e^2, e^3[$.

Then by Lagrange's mean value theorem. There exist $c\in]e^2, e^3]$, such that

$$f'(c)=\frac{f(e^3)-f(e^2)}{e^3-e^2}$$

$$\Rightarrow \quad \frac{1}{c}=\frac{3-2}{e^3-e^2}$$

$$\therefore \quad c=(e^3-e^2).$$

There exists only one value $c=(e^3-e^2)$ in $]e^2, e^3[$.

10. *Use the function $f(x)=x^{1/x}$, $x>0$ show that $e^{\pi}>\pi^{e}$.*

SOLUTION. Here $f(x) = x^{1/x}, x > 0$

$$\therefore \log f(x)=\frac{1}{x}\log_e x$$

Differentiating w.r.t. x, we get

$$\frac{1}{f(x)}f'(x)=\frac{1}{x}.\frac{1}{x}-\frac{1}{x^2}\log_e x$$

$$f'(x)=\frac{x^{1/x}}{x^2}[1-\log_e x]$$

For $x > e, f'(x) < 0$ $[\because \log_e x>1 \text{ for } x>e]$

$\therefore f(x)$ is a decreasing function of x for $x>e$.

Hence

$$\pi<e\Rightarrow f(\pi)<f(e)\Rightarrow \pi^{1/\pi}<e^{1/e}$$

$$\Rightarrow \left(\pi^{1/\pi}\right)^{e\pi}<\left(e^{1/e}\right)^{e\pi}$$

$$\Rightarrow \pi^e<e^\pi$$

$$\Rightarrow e^\pi>\pi^e$$

11. *Show that* $\frac{x}{1+x}<\log(1+x)<x$, *for* $x>0$.

[MUMBAI–2008; MEERUT(BCA)–2008, 11, 15; ROHILKHAND(BCA)–2005]

SOLUTION. Let, $f(x)=\log(1+x)-\frac{x}{1+x}$

Obviously, $f(0)=0$.

and $f'(x)$

$$=\frac{1}{1+x}-\frac{1.(1+x)-x.1}{(1+x)^2}$$

$$=\frac{1}{1+x}-\frac{1}{(1+x)^2}=\frac{x}{(1+x)^2}$$

Here, we observe that $f'(x)>0$, for $x>0$.

$\Rightarrow f(x)$ is monotonically increasing in the interval $[0,\infty[$. Therefore

$$f(x)>f(0), \text{ for } x>0$$

$$\Rightarrow \left[\log(1+x)-\frac{x}{1+x}\right]>0, \text{ for } x>0$$

$$\Rightarrow \quad \log(1+x)>\frac{x}{1+x}, \text{ for } x>0 \quad ...(1)$$

Now let $F(x) = x-\log(1+x)$

Obviously $F(0)=0$

Then $F'(x)=1-\frac{1}{1+x}=\frac{x}{1+x}$

Here, we observe that $F'(x)>0$, for $x>0$. Hence $F(x)$ is monotonically increasing in the interval $[0,\infty[$.

$\therefore \quad F(x)>F(0), \quad$ for $x>0$

$\Rightarrow [x-\log(1+x)]>0, \quad$ for $x>0$

$\Rightarrow \quad x>\log(1+x), \quad$ for $x>0 \quad ...(2)$

Now from (1) and (2), we get

$$\frac{x}{1+x}<\log(1+x)<x, \text{ for } x>0$$

12. *Prove that $(1+x)<e^x<1+xe^x$, $\forall x>0$.*

[MEERUT(BCA)–2005]

SOLUTION. Let us consider the function $f(x)=e^x$ in $[0, x]$.

Obviously $f(x)$ is continuous as well as differentiable in $]0, x[$.

Then, by Lagrange's theorem $\exists c\in]0, x[$, such that

$$f'(c)=\frac{f(x)-f(0)}{x-0}$$

or $$e^c=\frac{e^x-1}{x} \quad ...(1)$$

$$0<c<x \Rightarrow e^0<e^c<e^x$$

($\because e^x$ is an increasing function.) ...(2)

Now, from (1) and (2), we have

$$e^0<\frac{e^x-1}{x}<e^x, \forall x>0$$

$$\Rightarrow \quad 1<\frac{e^x-1}{x}<e^x \Rightarrow x<e^x-1<xe^x$$

$\Rightarrow (1+x)<e^x<xe^x$

13. *Let f be continuous on $[a-h, a+h]$ and differentiable $]a-h, a+h[$. Prove that there is a real number θ between 0 and 1 such that*

$f(a+h)-2f(a)+f(a-h)=h[f'(a+\theta h)-f'(a-\theta h)]$.

SOLUTION. Consider the function ϕ defined on $[0, 1]$ by $\phi = f(a+ht)+f(a-ht)\ \forall t \in [0, 1]$.

Obviously ϕ is continuous on $[0, 1]$ and differentiable on $]0, 1[$.

Then, by Lagrange's mean value theorem, there is a number θ lying between 0 and 1 such that

$$\phi(1)-\phi(0)=(1-0)\phi'(\theta)$$

i.e., $f(a+h)-2f(a)+f(a-h)$

$$=h[f'(a+\theta h)-f'(a-\theta h)].$$

which is the required result.

14. *Show that Lagrange's mean value theorem does not holds for the function $f(x)=|x|$ in the interval $[-1,1]$.*

SOLUTION. Since $f(x)=|x|$ is a continuous function on $[-1,1]$ but it is not differentiable at $x = 0 \in\ ]-1, 1[$. Hence, Lagrange's mean value theorem does not hold for the function $f(x)=|x|$ in the interval $[-1,1]$.

15. *Verify Lagrange's mean value theorem for the function $f(x)=\sin x$ in $\left[0, \frac{\pi}{2}\right]$.*

[NAGPUR–2008]

SOLUTION. The function $f(x)= \sin x$ is continuous and differentiable on R. Hence it is continuous as well as differentiable in $[0, \pi/2]$. Then, by Lagrange's mean value theorem, there must exist at least one c in $]0,\pi/2[$ such that

$$\frac{f(\pi/2)-f(0)}{\pi/2-0} = f'(c) \qquad \ldots(1)$$

Here $f(0)=0, f(\pi/2)=1$

$$f'(x)= \cos x \Rightarrow f'(c)= \cos c$$

Put all these values in (1), we have

$$\frac{1-0}{\pi/2} = \cos c \Rightarrow \cos c = \frac{2}{\pi}$$

$$\Rightarrow c = \cos^{-1}\left(\frac{2}{\pi}\right)$$

Since, $0<2/\pi<1$, therefore the value of $c = \cos^{-1}\left(\frac{2}{\pi}\right)$ lies in $\left]0, \frac{\pi}{2}\right[$, which is the required value of c. Hence, Lagrange's mean value theorem is satisfied.

16. *If $f''(x)$ exists for all points in $[a, b]$ and $\frac{f(c)-f(a)}{c-a} = \frac{f(b)-f(c)}{b-c}$ where $a < c < b$, then, there is a number l such that $a < l < b$ and $f''(l) = 0$.*

SOLUTION. Since $f''(x)$ exist for all points in $[a, b]$,

$\Rightarrow f'(x)$ is continuous in $[a, b]$

$\Rightarrow f(x)$ is continuous in $[a, b]$.

Now, applying Lagrange's mean value theorem to $f(x)$ in $[a, c]$ and $[c, b]$ respectively, we get

$$\frac{f(c)-f(a)}{c-a} = f'(l_1),\ a<l_1<c \quad \ldots(1)$$

and $$\frac{f(b)-f(c)}{b-c} = f'(l_2),\ c<l_2<b \quad \ldots(2)$$

Then, from (1) and (2), we get

$$f'(l_1)=f'(l_2)$$

$$\left[\because \frac{f(c)-f(a)}{c-a} = \frac{f(b)-f(c)}{b-c}\right]$$

Now $f'(x)$ satisfies all the conditions of Rolle's theorem in the interval $[l_1, l_2]$.

Hence, $f''(l)=0$ where $l \in\ ]l_1, l_2[$ and $l \in\ ]a, b[$.

17. *Verify Cauchy's mean value theorem for the functions $f(x)=x^2-2x+3$, $g(x) = x^3-7x^2+26x-5$ in the interval $[-1, 1]$.*

SOLUTION. Since $f(x)$ and $g(x)$ are polynomial in x, so these are continuous in the closed interval $[-1, 1]$ and also differentiable and continuous in the open interval $(-1,1)$.

Also
$$g'(x)=3x^2-14x+26$$
$$g'(-1)=3(-1)^2-14(-1)+26$$
$$=43=+\text{ve}$$
$$g'(1)=3(1)^2-14(1)+26$$
$$=15=+\text{ve}.$$

Therefore, $g'(x)\neq 0$ for any value of x in $(-1,1)$.

Hence all the conditions of Cauchy mean value theorem are satisfied.

Then, by using,

$$\frac{f(b)-f(a)}{g(b)-g(a)} = \frac{f'(c)}{g'(c)}$$

Putting $a=-1$, $b=1$ (given), we have

$$\frac{f(1)-f(-1)}{g(1)-g(-1)}=\frac{f'(c)}{g'(c)}$$

$$\frac{\left[1^2-2(1)+3\right]-\left[(-1)^2-2(-1)+3\right]}{\left[1^3-7(1)^2+26(1)-5\right]-\left[(-1)^3-7(-1)^2+26(-1)-5\right]}$$

$$=\frac{2c-2}{3c^2-14c+26} \qquad [\because f'(x)=2x-2]$$

or $\dfrac{2-6}{15-(-39)}=\dfrac{2c-2}{3c^2-14c+26}$

or $-4(3c^2-14c+26)=54\times 2(c-1)$

or $3c^2+14c+26=-27(c-1)$

or $3c^2+13c-1=0$

$\Rightarrow \quad c=\dfrac{-13\pm\sqrt{(181)}}{6}=\dfrac{-13\pm 13.454}{6}$

i.e., $c=0.076,-4.409$

Since the value 0.076 lies in $[-1,1]$. Hence, Cauchy mean value theorem is verified.

18. *Verify Cauchy's mean value theorem for the function x^2 and x^3 in the interval* $[1,2]$.

SOLUTION. Let us suppose $f(x)=x^2$ and $g(x)=x^3$. Then, obviously $f(x)$ and $g(x)$ are continuous in $[1,2]$ and differentiable in $]1,2[$.

Also $g'(x)=3x^2\neq 0$ for any point in $]1,2[$.

Then, by Cauchy's mean value theorem there exists at least one real number $c\in]1,2[$, such that

$$\frac{f(2)-f(1)}{g(2)-g(1)}=\frac{f'(c)}{g'(c)} \qquad ...(1)$$

After solving, we get $c=\dfrac{14}{9}$, which lies in the open interval $]1,2[$. Hence, Cauchy's mean value theorem is verified.

19. *If in the Cauchy's mean value theorem, we write f(x)=ex and g(x)=e–x, show that 'c' is the arithmetic mean between a and b.* (MUMBAI-2008)

SOLUTION. Since, we have

$$f(x)=e^x \text{ and } g(x)=e^{-x}$$

$$\therefore \quad \frac{f(b)-f(a)}{g(b)-g(a)}=\frac{e^b-e^a}{e^{-b}-e^{-a}}$$

$$=-e^ae^b=-e^{a+b}$$

and $\dfrac{f'(x)}{g'(x)}=\dfrac{e^x}{-e^{-x}}$

so that $\dfrac{f'(c)}{g'(c)}=\dfrac{e^c}{-e^{-c}}=-e^{2c}$

After putting all these values in Cauchy's mean value theorem, we get

$-e^{a+b}=-e^{2c} \quad \Rightarrow \quad a+b=2c$

$\Rightarrow \quad c=\dfrac{a+b}{2}$

Hence, c is the arithmetic mean between a and b.

20. *If f(x), g(x) and h(x) are functions such that*

(i) *f(x), g(x) and h(x) are continuous on $[a,b]$*

(ii) *f(x), g(x) and h(x) are differentiable on $]a,b[$, then show that*

$$\begin{vmatrix} f'(c) & g'(c) & h'(c) \\ f(b) & g(b) & h(b) \\ f(a) & g(a) & h(a) \end{vmatrix}=0 \quad \text{where } c\in]a,b[$$

SOLUTION. Consider the function $F(x)$ such that

$$F(x)=\begin{vmatrix} f(x) & g(x) & h(x) \\ f(b) & g(b) & h(b) \\ f(a) & g(a) & h(a) \end{vmatrix}=0 \qquad ...(1)$$

Obviously, $F(x)$ is of the form $A\,f(x)+B\,g(x)+C\,h(x)$, where A, B, C are some real numbers. From the condition (i) and (ii), $F(x)$ is continuous on. $[a,b]$ and differentiable on $]a,b[$.

Also $F(a)=F(b)=0$.

$\Rightarrow F(x)$ satisfies all the conditions of Rolle's theorem. Hence, there exists a $c\in]a,b[$ such that $F'(c)=0$

i.e., $\begin{vmatrix} f'(c) & g'(c) & h'(c) \\ f(b) & g(b) & h(b) \\ f(a) & g(a) & h(a) \end{vmatrix}=0.$

21. *Verify Cauchy's mean value for f(x) = sin x and g(x) = cos x in* $\left[-\frac{\pi}{2},0\right]$.

(JNTU–2006)

SOLUTION. It can be easily seen that $f(x)$ and $g(x)$ both are continuous on $\left[-\frac{\pi}{2},0\right]$ and differentiable on $\left]-\frac{\pi}{2},0\right[$.

Also, $g'(x)=-\sin x \neq 0$ for any point in the interval $\left]-\frac{\pi}{2},0\right[$.

Then, by Cauchy's mean value theorem, $\exists$ at least one $c \in \left]-\frac{\pi}{2},0\right[$ such that

$$\frac{f(0)-f\left(-\frac{\pi}{2}\right)}{g(0)-g\left(-\frac{\pi}{2}\right)}=\frac{f'(c)}{g'(c)}$$

Putting all the values and after simplification, we have

$$\cot c=-1 \Rightarrow c=-\pi/4.$$

Since $c=-\pi/4$ lies in $]-\pi/2,0[$, hence, Cauchy mean value theorem is verified.

Similar Problems

(1) Show that the function f and g defined on $\left[0,\frac{1}{2}\right]$, by $f(x) = x(x-1)(x-2)$ and $g(x) = x(x-2)(x-3)$ satisfy the condition of Cauchy's mean value theorem.

(2) Find 'c' of Cauchy's mean value theorem for the functions $f(x)=\sqrt{x}$, $\phi(x)=\frac{1}{x}$ in $[a,b]$ and show that it is the G.M. of a and b.

8.5 TAYLOR'S THEOREM

[KANPUR(BCA)–1997, 2012]

Let $f(x)$ be a single valued function defined on $[a,a+h]$ such that

(i) all the derivative of $f(x)$ upto $(n-1)^{th}$ order are continuous in $[a, a+h]$, and

(ii) $f^n(x)$ exists in $]a,a+h[$, then there exists a real number $\theta, 0<\theta<1$, such that

$$f(a+h)=f(a)+hf'(a)+\frac{h^2}{2!}f''(a)+\ldots+\frac{h^{n-1}}{(n-1)!}f^{n-1}(a)+\frac{h^n(1-\theta)^{n-p}}{p(n-1)!}f^n(a+\theta h)$$

where p is a given positive integer.

PROOF. Since, f^n exists, all the derivative $f', f'' \ldots f^{n-1}$ exist and continuous on $[a, a+h]$, consider a function f defined on $[a, a+h]$ such that

$$\phi(x)=f(x)+(a+h-x)f'(x)+\frac{(a+h-x)^2}{2!}f''(x)+\ldots+\frac{(a+h-x)^{n-1}}{(n-1)!}f^{n-1}(x)+A(a+h-x)^p \quad \ldots(1)$$

where A is a constant to be determined such that $\phi(a+h)=\phi(a)$

Now $\quad \phi(a)=f(a)+hf'(a)+\frac{h^2}{2!}f''(a)+\ldots+\frac{h^{n-1}}{(n-1)!}f^{n-1}(a)+Ah^p$

and $\quad \phi(a)=f(a+h)$

$$\Rightarrow \quad f(a+h)=f(a)+hf'(a)+\frac{h^2}{2!}f''(a)+\ldots+\frac{h^{n-1}}{(n-1)!}f^{n-1}(a)+Ah^p \quad \ldots(2)$$

Now (i) $f, f', f'', \ldots, f^{n-1}$ being all continuous on $[a, a+h]$ the function ϕ is continuous on $[a, a+h]$,

(ii) Similarly the function ϕ is differentiable on $]a, a+h[$,

and (iii) $\phi(a+h)=\phi(a)$

Thus, the function ϕ satisfies all the conditions of Rolle's theorem and hence $\exists$ a real number $\theta(0<\theta<1)$ such that $\quad \phi'(a+\theta h)=0.$

Here $\phi'(x) = f'(x)+(-f'(x)+(a+h-x)f''(x)]$

$$+\frac{1}{2!}\left[-2(a+h-x)f''(x)+(a+h-x)^2f'''(x)\right]+\ldots+\frac{1}{(n-1)!}[-(n-1)$$

$$(a+h-x)^{n-2}f^{n-1}(x)+(a+h-x)^{n-1}f^n(x)]-Ap(a+h-x)]^{p-1}$$

$$= \frac{(a+h-x)^{n-1}}{(n-1)!} f^n(x) - Ap(a+h-x)^{p-1} \text{ [Other terms canceled in pairs]}$$

$$\therefore \quad 0 = \phi'(a+\theta h) = \frac{h^{n-1}(1-\theta)^{n-1}}{(n-1)!} f^n(a+\theta h) - Aph^{p-1}(1-\theta)^{p-1}$$

$$\Rightarrow \quad A = \frac{h^{n-p}(1-\theta)^{n-p}}{p(n-1)!} f^n(a+\theta h), h \neq 0, \theta \neq 1$$

Now, putting the values of A in (2), we get

$$f(a+h) = f(a) + hf'(a) + \frac{h^2}{2!} f''(a) + \ldots + \frac{h^{n-1}}{(n-1)!} f^{n-1}(a) + \frac{h^n(1-\theta)^{n-p}}{p(n-1)!} f^n(a+\theta h)$$

8.5.1 Forms of Remainder After n Terms

(i) The term $Rn = \frac{h^n(1-\theta)^{n-1}}{p(n-1)!} f^n(a+\theta h)$ which occur after n terms, is called the Taylor's remainder after n terms. The theorem with this form of remainder is called Taylor's theorem with Schlomilch and Roche form of remainder.

(ii) For $p=1$, we get

$$R_n = \frac{h^n(1-\theta)^{n-1}}{p(n-1)!} f^n(a+\theta h)$$

Then, R_n is called Cauchy's form of remainder.

(iii) For $p=n$, we get

$$R_n = \frac{h^n}{n!} f^n(a+\theta h)$$

then, R_n is called Lagrange's form of remainder.

8.5.2 Another Form of Taylor's Theorem

Replacing h by $(x–a)$ in Taylor's theorem, we get

$$f(x) = f(a) + (x-a) f'(a) + \frac{(x-a)^2}{2!} f''(a) + \ldots + \frac{(x-a)^{n-1}}{(n-1)!} f^{n-1}(a) + \frac{(x-a)^n}{p(n-1)!} f^n(1-\theta)^{n-p}$$

The remainder, after n terms can be written as

$$R_n = \frac{(x-a)^n(1-\theta)^{n-p}}{p(n-1)!} f^n(c), a<c<x.$$

8.5.3 Deductions

Putting $a=0$ in second form of Taylor's theorem, we get (Maclaurin's theorem)

$$f(x) = f(0) + x f'(0) + \frac{x^2}{2!} f''(0) + \ldots + \frac{x^{n-1}}{(n-1)!} f^{n-1}(0) + R_n \quad \ldots(1)$$

(i) If $R_n = \frac{x^n(1-\theta)^{n-1}}{p(n-1)!} f^n(\theta x)$, then (1) is known as Maclaurin's theorem with Schlomilch and Roche's form of remainder.

(ii) For $p=1$, $R_n = \frac{x^n(1-\theta)^{n-1}}{p(n-1)!} f^n(\theta x)$ is called Cauchy's form of remainder.

(iii) For $p=n$, $R_n = \frac{x^n}{n!} f^n(\theta x)$, is called Lagrange's form of remainder.

8.5.4 TAYLOR'S SERIES

Let $f(x)$ possesess continuous derivatives of all orders in the interval $[a, a+h]$, then for every positive integral value of n, we have

$$f(a+h)= f(a)+hf'(a)+\frac{h^2}{2!}f''(a)+...+\frac{h^{n-1}}{(n-1)!}f^{n-1}(a)+R_n$$

where, $$R_n=\frac{h^n}{n!}f^n(a+\theta h),(0<\theta<1). \quad ...(1)$$

Equation (1) can also be written as

$$S_n= f(a)+hf'(a)+\frac{h^2}{2!}f''(a)+...+\frac{h^{n-1}}{(n-1)!}f^{n-1}(a)$$

Then $f(a+h)=S_n+R_n$.

Let us suppose $R_n\to 0$ as $n\to\infty$, then $\lim_{n\to\infty} S_n = f(a+h)$

i.e., the series $f(a)+hf'(a)+\frac{h^2}{2!}f''(a)+...+\frac{h^{n-1}}{(n-1)!}f^{n-1}(a)+...$ converges to $f(a+h)$.

Thus,

(i) If f possess a continuous derivative of every order in $[a, a+h]$.

(ii) The remainder after n terms $R_n\to 0$ as $n\to\infty$, then

$$f(a+h)= f(a)+hf'(a)+\frac{h^2}{2!}f''(a)+...+\frac{h^n}{n!}f^n(a)+...$$

This series is known as Taylor's series for the expansion of $f(a+h)$ as a power series in h.

8.5.5 MACLAURIN'S SERIES

If we put $a=0$ and replace h by x in Taylor's series, we get

$$f(x)= f(0)+x f'(0)+\frac{x^2}{2!}f''(0)+...+\frac{x^n}{n!}f^n(0)+...$$

This Series is known as Maclaurin's series for the expansion of $f(x)$ as a power series in x.

- Maclaurin's series is a particular case of Taylor's series.
- Maclaurin's expansions of $f(x)$ fails if any of the functions $f(x), f'(x), f''(x)$... becomes infinite or discontinuous at any point of the interval $[0, x]$ or if R_n does not tends to zero as n tends to infinity.

8.6 MACLAURIN'S THEOREM

Let f(x) be a function of x which possesses continuous derivatives of all orders in the interval [0, x] and can be expanded as an infinite series in x, then

$$f(x)= f(0)+x f'(0)+\frac{x^2}{2!}f''(0)+...+\frac{x^n}{n!}f^n(0)+...$$

PROOF. Let us define

$$f(x) = A_0+A_1x+A_2x^2+A_3x^3+... \quad ...(1)$$

Let the expression (1) be differentiable term by term any number of times. Then by successive differentiation, we have

$$f'(x)= A_1+2A_2x+3A_3x^2+4A_4x^3+...$$

$$f''(x)= 2.1.A_2+3.2.A_3x+4.3.A_4x^2+...$$

$$f'''(x)= 3.2.A_3+4.3.2.A_4x+...$$

....

Putting $x=0$, we get

$$f(0)=A_0, f'(0)=A_1, f''(0)=2!A_2, f'''(0)=3!A_3....$$

$$\Rightarrow \qquad A_0 = f(0), A_1 = f'(0), A_2 = \frac{f''(0)}{2!}, A_3 = \frac{f'''(0)}{3!} \ldots$$

Substitute all these values in (1), we get

$$f(x) = f(0) + x f'(0) + \frac{x^2}{2!} f''(0) + \ldots + \frac{x^n}{n!} f^n(0) + \ldots$$

- The Maclaurin's theorem is a particular case of Taylor's Theorem, and can be obtained by replacing $a=0$ and $h=x$ in Taylor's theorem.
- If the function $f(x)$ is denoted by y, then the expansion may be written in the form

$$y = y(0) + x y_1(0) + \frac{x^2}{2!} y_2(0) + \ldots + \frac{x^n}{n!} y_n(0) + \ldots$$

where $y(0), y_1(0), y_2(0), \ldots, y_n(0)$ etc. denotes values of $y, y_1, y_2, \ldots, y_n$ respectively for $x = 0$.

8.7 FAILURE OF TAYLOR'S AND MACLAURIN'S THEOREM

(a) *Taylor's theorem fails to expand $f(a+h)$ in an infinite power series in the following cases :*

- If any of the function $f(x), f'(x), f''(x)\ldots$ become infinite or does not exist for any value of x in the given interval.
- If R_n does not tends to zero as $n \to \infty$.

(b) *Maclaurin's theorem fails to expand $f(x)$ in an infinite power series in the following cases :*

- If any of the function $f(x), f'(x), f''(x)\ldots$ becomes infinite or does not exist in interval $[0, x]$.
- If R_n does not tends to zero as $n \to \infty$.

- Before expanding a given function as an infinite Taylor's or Maclaurin's series, it is essential to examine the behaviour of R_n as $n \to \infty$, which is not simple in many cases. We, therefore, generally obtain the expansion by assuming the possibility of expanding it in an infinite series by assuming that $R_n \to 0$ as $n \to \infty$.

8.8 POWER SERIES EXPANSION OF SOME STANDARD FUNCTIONS

WORKING PROCEDURE

To find the power series expansion we shall use the following procedure :

STEP 1. Put the given function equal to $f(x)$.

STEP 2. Differentiate $f(x)$, a number of times and obtain $f'(x), f''(x), f'''(x)\ldots$ and so on.

STEP 3. Put $x = 0$ and find $f(0), f'(0), f''(0)\ldots$ and so on.

STEP 4. Now substitute the values of $f(0), f'(0), f''(0), f'''(0), \ldots$ in

$$f(x) = f(0) + x f'(0) + \frac{x^2}{2!} f''(0) + \ldots$$

(i) Expansion of e^x. (COCHIN–2005)

Let $\qquad f(x) = e^x \ \forall x \in \mathbf{R}$

Then $\qquad f^n(x) = e^x \ \forall x \in \mathbf{R}$

Thus, for each positive n, f^n is defined in the interval $[-h, h]$.

Writing, Lagrange's form of remainder, after n terms

$$R_n(x) = \frac{x^n}{n!} f^n(\theta x), \ \theta \in \mathbf{R}, \ 0 < \theta < 1 = \frac{x^n}{n!} e^{\theta x}$$

Now, we shall show that $\lim_{n\to\infty} R_n(x) = 0$. Here, it is enough to show that $e^{\theta x}$ is bounded in $[-h, h]$ and $\lim_{n\to\infty} \frac{x^n}{n!} = 0$.

Since, $0 < \theta < 1$ and $x \in [-h, h]$, therefore $|\theta x| < h$ and consequently, $0 < e^{\theta x} < e^h$, hence $e^{\theta x}$ is bounded.

Now, let us write $\quad a_n = \frac{x^n}{n!} \; \forall n \in \mathbf{N}$

Then $\quad \frac{a_{n+1}}{a_n} = \frac{x}{n+1} \Rightarrow \lim_{n\to\infty} \frac{a_{n+1}}{a_n} = 0$

$\Rightarrow \lim_{n\to\infty} a_n$ exists and equal to zero.

Now, $$\lim_{n\to\infty} R_n(x) = e^{\theta x}\left[\lim \frac{x^n}{n!}\right] = 0$$

Hence, we find that the function $f(x)$ has a Maclaurin's series expansions for each $x \in [-h,h]$. This implies

$$f(x) = f(0) + xf'(0) + \frac{x^2}{2!}f''(0) + \ldots + \frac{x^{n-1}}{(n-1)!}f^{n-1}(0) + \ldots \; \forall x \in \mathbf{R}.$$

Substituting $f(x)=e^x, f'(x)=e^x, \ldots, f^n(x)=e^x$, we have

$$e^x = 1 + x + \frac{x^2}{2!} + \frac{x^3}{3!} + \ldots + \frac{x^{n-1}}{(n-1)!} + \ldots \quad \forall x \in \mathbf{R}$$

(ii) Expansion of sin *x*. (PTU–2005)

Let $\quad f(x) = \sin x, \; \forall x \in \mathbf{R}$

$\Rightarrow \quad f^n(x) = \sin\left(x + \frac{n\pi}{2}\right), \; \forall x \in \mathbf{R}$

Writing, Lagrange's form of remainder after n terms, we have

$$R_n(x) = \frac{x^n}{n!} f^n(\theta x), \text{ where } 0<\theta<1 = \frac{x^n}{n!}\sin\left(\theta x + \frac{n\pi}{2}\right)$$

Now, for all $x \in$ R,

$$|R_n(x)| \le \left|\frac{x^n}{n!}\right| \quad \text{and} \quad \lim_{n\to\infty} \frac{x^n}{n!} = 0 \qquad \text{[As in (i)]}$$

Thus, we find that, the function $f(x)$ has a Maclaurin's series expansions for each x in $[-h,h]$. Hence, we have

$$f(x) = f(0) + xf'(0) + \frac{x^2}{2!}f''(0) + \ldots + \frac{x^{n-1}}{(n-1)!}f^{n-1}(0) + \ldots \quad \forall x \in \mathbf{R}.$$

Now, substituting $f(x)=\sin x,\; f^n(x) = \sin\frac{n\pi}{2}$, we have

$$\sin x = x - \frac{x^3}{3!} + \frac{x^5}{5!} - \ldots \quad \forall x \in \mathbf{R}.$$

(iii) Expansion of cos *x*. (ROHILKHAND(BCA)–2003, 05)

Let $\; f(x) = \cos x, \; \forall x \in \mathbf{R}$, then $\quad f^n(x) = \cos\left(x + \frac{n\pi}{2}\right)$

Thus, for eaeh n, f^n is defined in every interval $[-h, h]$.

Writing, Lagrange's remainder after n terms, we have

$$R_n(x) = \frac{x^n}{n!} f^n(\theta x) = \frac{x^n}{n!}\cos\left(\theta x + \frac{n\pi}{2}\right), \quad \text{where } 0<\theta<1$$

Now, for all $x \in \mathbf{R}$,

$$|R_n(x)| \le \left|\frac{x^n}{n!}\right| \quad \text{and} \quad \lim_{n\to\infty} \frac{x^n}{n!} = 0 \qquad \text{[As in (i)]}$$

Thus, we find that, the function f has a Maclaurin's series expansions for each $x \in [-h, h]$, which gives

$$f(x) = f(0) + x f'(0) + \frac{x^2}{2!} f''(0) + \ldots + \frac{x^n}{n!} f^n(0) + \ldots \quad \forall x \in \mathbf{R}.$$

Now, substituting $f(x) = \cos x \ldots$, $f^n(0) = \cos\frac{n\pi}{2}$, we have $\cos x = 1 - \frac{x^2}{2!} + \frac{x^4}{4!} - \ldots \quad \forall x \in \mathbf{R}.$

(iv) Expansion of $(1+x)^m$. (ROHILKHAND(BCA)–2002, 12)

Case (i). Let m is a positive integer, then letting

$$f(x) = (1+x)^m, \ \forall x \in \mathbf{R}$$

We find that for each $n \in \mathrm{N}$, $f^n(x)$ exists for all $x \in \mathbf{R}$, and whenever $n > m$, $f^n(x) = 0 \ \forall x \in \mathrm{R}$.

$\Rightarrow$ $$R_n(x) = 0, \text{ whenever } n > m$$

Hence, $\lim_{n \to \infty} R_n(x) = 0$ and for all $x \in \mathrm{R}$, we have

$$f(x) = f(0) + x f'(0) + \ldots + \frac{x^m}{m!} f^m(0),$$

($\because$ All other terms must vanish.)

Substituting the value of $f(x), f(0), \ldots, f^m(0)$, We have

$$(1+x)^m = 1 + mx + \frac{m(m-1)}{2!} x^2 + \ldots + x^m.$$

Case (ii). Let m not be a positive integer (may be a fraction or negative integer). Here, we find that, if we write

$$f(x) = (1+x)^m, \text{ whenever } x \neq -1$$

then $$f^n(x) = m(m-1)\ldots(m-n+1)(1+x)^{m-n}, \text{ whenever } x \neq -1$$

Thus, for each positive integer n, f^n is defined in $[-h,h]$ for each h between 0 and 1. Now, writing Cauchy's form of remainder after n terms, we have

$$R_n(x) = \frac{x^n(1-\theta)^{n-1}}{(n-1)!} f^n(\theta x), \text{where } 0 < \theta < 1$$

$$= \frac{x^n(1-\theta)^{n-1}}{(n-1)!} m(m-1)\ldots(m-n+1)(1+\theta x)^{m-n}$$

$$= \frac{m(m+1)\ldots(m+n+1)}{(n-1)!} x^n \left(\frac{1-\theta}{1+\theta x}\right)^{n-1} .(1+\theta x)^{m-1}$$

Now, we observe that

(a) $\lim_{n \to \infty} \frac{m(m-1)\ldots(m-n+1)}{(n-1)!} x^n = 0$

If we write $$a_n = \frac{m(m+1)\ldots(m-n+1)}{(n-1)!} x^n$$

Then, we have $$\frac{a_{n+1}}{a_n} = \frac{(m-n)x}{n} \Rightarrow \lim_{n \to \infty} \frac{a_{n+1}}{a_n} = -x$$

If follows that if $|x| < 1$, then $\lim_{n \to \infty} a_n = 0$.

(b) $\lim_{n \to \infty} \left(\frac{1-\theta}{1+\theta x}\right)^{n-1} = 0$

In fact, since $0 < \theta < 1$ and $-1 < x < 1$, therefore, $0 < \left[\frac{1-\theta}{1+\theta x}\right] < 1$ and hence

$$\lim_{n \to \infty} \left[\frac{1-\theta}{1+\theta x}\right]^{(n-1)} = 0$$

(c) If $m > 1$, then $$(1+\theta x)^{m-1} < (1-|x|)^{m-1}$$

For (a), (b) and (c), we find that for all x in $]-1,1[$ $\lim_{n \to \infty} R_n(x) = 0$

Thus, we find that for each h between 0 and 1, the function f has Maclaurin's series expansion for all $x \in [-h,h]$.
Hence, we have

$$f(x) = f(0) + xf'(0) + \frac{x^2}{2!}f''(0) + \ldots + \frac{x^{n-1}}{(n-1)!}f^{n-1}(0) + \ldots \quad \forall x \in]-1,1[.$$

Substituting the values of $f(x), f'(0), \ldots, f^{n-1}(0)$, we have

$$(1+x)^m = 1 + mx + \frac{m(m-1)}{2!}x^2 + \frac{m(m-1)(m-2)}{3!}x^3 + \ldots$$
$$+ \frac{m(m-1)\ldots(m-n+1)}{n!}x^n + \ldots \text{whenever } -1 < x < 1$$

(v) Expansion of $\log_e(1+x)$.

Let $\qquad f(x) = \log(1+x), \; -1<x<1.$

Then $\qquad f^n(x) = \dfrac{(-1)^{n-1}(n-1)!}{(1+x)^n}$, whenever $x > -1$.

Now, we shall consider the following cases :

Case (a) Let $0 \le x \le 1$. Writing Lagrange's form of remainder after n terms, we have

$$R_n = \frac{x^n}{n!}f^n(\theta x) = \frac{x^n}{n!}(-1)^{n-1}\frac{(n-1)!}{(1+\theta x)^n} = \frac{(-1)^{n-1}}{n}\cdot\left(\frac{x}{1+\theta x}\right)^n$$

Since, $0 \le x \le 1, 0 < \theta < 1$, therefore

$$0 < \frac{x}{1+\theta x} < 1$$

$\therefore \qquad |R_n| < \dfrac{1}{n}$, and $\dfrac{1}{n} \to 0$ as $n \to \infty$

Therefore $\qquad \lim\limits_{n\to\infty} R_n = 0.$

Case (b) Let $-1<x<0$. Since in this case $\left|\dfrac{x}{1+\theta x}\right|$ need not be less than unity, therefore, we may not be able to show easily that $R_n \to 0$ as $n \to \infty$ by considering Lagrange's remainder.

Now, writing Cauchy's form of remainder, we have

$$R_n = \frac{x^n}{(n-1)!}(1-\theta)^{n-1}f^n(\theta x)$$
$$= (-1)^{n-1}x^n\left(\frac{1-\theta}{1+\theta x}\right)^{n-1}\cdot\frac{1}{1+\theta x}$$

since $|x|<1$

therefore $\left|\dfrac{1-\theta}{1+\theta x}\right| < 1$, so that $\left|\left(\dfrac{1-\theta}{1+\theta x}\right)^{n-1}\right| < 1$ and $\left|\dfrac{1}{1+\theta x}\right| < \dfrac{1}{1-|x|}$

Thus $\qquad |R_n| < \dfrac{|x|^n}{1-|x|}$

This implies that $\lim\limits_{n\to\infty} R_n = 0.$, since $|x|<1$. Thus we find that if $-1 \le x \le 1$,

RECAPITULATIONS

- $e^x = 1 + x + \dfrac{x^2}{2!} + \dfrac{x^3}{3!} + \ldots + \dfrac{x^n}{n!} + \ldots$
- $\cos x = 1 - \dfrac{x^2}{2!} + \dfrac{x^4}{4!} - \dfrac{x^6}{6!} + \ldots$
- $\sin x = x - \dfrac{x^3}{3!} + \dfrac{x^5}{5!} - \ldots$
- $(1+x)^m = 1 + mx + \dfrac{m(m-1)}{2!}x^2 + \ldots$
- $\log_e(1+x) = x - \dfrac{x^2}{2} + \dfrac{x^3}{3} - \dfrac{x^4}{4} + \ldots$
- $a^x = 1 + x\log_e a + \dfrac{x^2}{2!}(\log_e a)^2 + \ldots$

then $\lim_{n\to\infty} R_n = 0.$

$$f(x)= f(0)+xf'(0)+\frac{x^2}{2!}f''(0)+...+\frac{x^{n-1}}{(n-1)!}f^{n-1}(0)+... \text{ whenever } -1< x \le 1.$$

Substituting the values of $f(x), f(0), f'(0), ..., f^{n-1}(0), ...$, we get

$$\log(1+x) = x-\frac{x^2}{2}+\frac{x^3}{3}-..., \text{ whenever } -1<x\le 1.$$

Solved Examples

1. *Show that*

$$a^x = 1+x\log a+\frac{x^2}{2!}(\log a)^2+... +\frac{x^{n-1}}{(n-1)!}(\log a)^{n-1} +\frac{x^n}{n!}a^{\theta x}(\log a)^n, 0<\theta<1.$$

SOLUTION. Let $f(x)=a^x$ ...(1)

Then $f^n(x)=a^x(\log a)^n$ $\forall n\in N$ and $\forall x\in R$ ...(2)

Now, putting $x=0$, in (1) and (2), we get

$$f(0)=1, f^n(0)=(\log a)^n \ \forall\ n\in N$$

From (2), $f^n(\theta x)=a^{\theta x}(\log a)^n$

Now, by Maclaurin's series with Lagrange's form of remainder after n terms we have

$$f(x)= f(0)+xf'(0)+\frac{x^2}{2!}f''(0)+... +\frac{x^{n-1}}{(n-1)!}f^{n-1}(0)+\frac{x^n}{n!}a^{\theta x}(\log a)^n... \quad ...(3)$$

Now, substituting the above values in (3), we get

$$a^x= 1+x\log a+\frac{x^2}{2!}(\log a)^2+... +\frac{x^{n-1}}{(n-1)!}(\log a)^{n-1}+\frac{x^n}{n!}a^{\theta x}(\log a)^n.$$

Here, Lagrange's form of remainder after n terms

$$R_n=\frac{x^n}{n!}a^{\theta x}(\log a)^n \text{ where } 0<\theta<1.$$

2. *Expand $e^{a\sin^{-1}x}$ by Maclaurin's series and find the general term. Hence, show that* $e^{\theta}=1+\sin\theta+\frac{1}{2!}\sin^2\theta+\frac{2}{3!}\sin^3\theta+...$

SOLUTION. Here $y= e^{a\sin^{-1}x}$ ...(1)

Then $y_1= e^{a\sin^{-1}x}.\frac{a}{\sqrt{1-x^2}}=\frac{ay}{\sqrt{1-x^2}}$ ...(2)

$$\Rightarrow \left(\sqrt{1-x^2}\right)y_1 = ay$$

$$\Rightarrow \left(1-x^2\right){y_1}^2-a^2y^2=0 \quad ...(3)$$

Now, differentiating both the sides, we have

$$\Rightarrow \left(1-x^2\right)2y_1y_2-2x{y_1}^2-2a^2yy_1=0$$

$$2y_1\left[\left(1-x^2\right)y_2-xy_1-a^2y\right]=0 \quad ...(4)$$

Since $2y_1\neq 0$ hence

$$[(1-x^2)y_2-xy_1-a^2y]=0.$$

Now, differentiating n times by Leibnitz's theorem, we get

$$\left(1-x^2\right)y_{n+2}+ny_{n+1}(-2x) +\frac{n(n-1)}{2}y_n(-2)-y_{n+1}x -ny_n.1-a^2y_n=0$$

$$\Rightarrow (1-x^2)y_{n+2}-(2n+1)xy_{n+1} -(n^2+a^2)y_n=0 \quad ...(5)$$

Now, we can easily find, (from (1) to (5)) the following values

$$(y)_0=1, (y_1)_0=a, (y_2)_0=a^2$$

$$(y_{n+2})_0=(n^2+a^2)(y_n)_0 \quad ...(6)$$

Replacing n by $(n-2)$ in (6), we get

$$(y_n)_0=[(n-2)^2+a^2](y_{n-2})_0$$

$$=[(n-2)^2+a^2][(n-4)^2+a^2](y_{n-4})_0$$

If n is odd, then

$$(y_n)_0=[(n-2)^2+a^2][(n-4)^2+a^2] ...(3^2+a^2)(1^2+a^2)(y_1)_0$$

$$=[(n-2)^2+a^2][(n-4)^2+a^2] ...[(3^2+a^2)(1^2+a^2)].a$$

If n is even, then

$$(y_n)_0=[(n-2)^2+a^2][(n-4)^2+a^2]\ldots(4^2+a^2)(2^2+a^2)(y_2)_0$$
$$=[(n-2)^2+a^2][(n-4)^2+a^2]\ldots[(4^2+a^2)(2^2+a^2)].a^2$$

Hence,

$$y_n(0)=\begin{cases} a(1^2+a^2)(3^2+a^2)\ldots[(n-2)^2+a^2], \text{ if } n \text{ is odd}\\ a^2(2^2+a^2)(4^2+a^2)\ldots[(n-2)^2+a^2], \text{if } n \text{ is even}\end{cases}$$

Putting $n = 1, 2, 3, 4, \ldots$ in (6), we get

$(y_3)_0 = (3^2+a^2)(1^2+a^2)a,$

$(y_6)_0 = (4^2+a^2)(2^2+a^2)a^2$ etc.

Now putting all these values in the Maclaurin's theorem

$$y=(y)_0+x.(y_1)_0+\frac{x^2}{2!}(y_2)_0+\ldots+\frac{x^n}{n!}(y_n)_0+\ldots$$

We have

$$e^{a\sin^{-1}x}=1+ax+\frac{a^2}{2!}x^2+\frac{a(1^2+a^2)}{3!}x^3+\frac{a(2^2+a^2)}{4!}x^4+\ldots$$

The general term is $\frac{x^n}{n!}(y_n)_0$.

Now putting $x=\sin\theta$ and $a=1$, in the above equation, we get

$$e^{\theta}=1+\sin\theta+\frac{1}{2!}\sin^2\theta+\frac{2}{3!}\sin^3\theta+\ldots$$

3. *Expand log sin(x+h) in powers of h by Taylor's theorem.*

SOLUTION. Let $f(x)=\log\sin(x)$

$\Rightarrow$ $f(x+h)=\log\sin(x+h)$

Expanding $f(x+h)$ by Taylor's theorem in powers of h, we have

$$f(x+h)=f(x)+hf'(x)+\frac{h^2}{2!}f''(x)+\frac{h^3}{3!}f'''(x)+\ldots \quad \ldots(1)$$

Now $f(x)=\log\sin x$

$\Rightarrow$ $f'(x)=\cot x$

$f''(x)=-\text{cosec}^2x$

$\Rightarrow$ $f'''(x)=2\,\text{cosec}^2x\cot x$ etc.

Substituting all these values in equation (1), we get

log sin(x+h)

$$=\log\sin x+h\cot x-\frac{h^2}{2!}\text{cosec}^2x+\frac{2h^3}{3!}\text{cosec}^2x\cot x+\ldots$$

Exercise-8.1

1. Discuss the applicability of,Rolle's theorem of the following functions :

(a) $f(x)=2+(x-1)^{2/3}$ in the interval [0,2]

(b) $f(x)=x^2$ in $2\le x\le 3$

(c) $f(x)=\tan x$ in $0\le x\le\pi$

(d) $f(x)=x^4-3x^2+4$ in the interval [–4,4]

(e) $f(x)=1/(x^2+1)$ in the interval [–3,3]

(f) $f(x)=e^x\sin x$ in the interval $[0,\pi]$ (JNTU–2003)

(g) $f(x)=|x|$ in the interval [–1,1]

(h) $f(x)=(x-2)\sqrt{x}$ in the interval [0,2]

(i) $f(x)=(x-a)^m(x-b)^n, m,n\in\mathbf{Z}^+$ in the interval $[a,b]$. (VTU–2010, NAGARJUNA–2008)

2. Show that between any two roots of $e^x\cos x = 1$, there.exists at least one root of $e^x\sin x-1=0$.

3. Let $\frac{a_0}{n+1}+\frac{a_1}{n}+\frac{a_2}{n-1}+\ldots+\frac{a_{n-1}}{2}+a_n=0.$

Show that there exists at least one real x between 0 and 1 such that $a_0x^n+a_1x^{n-1}+\ldots+a_n=0$.

4. Verify the Rolle's theorem for the following functions:

(a) $f(x)=x^4-1$ on the interval [–1,1]

(b) $f(x)=e^x(\sin x-\cos x)$ in $\left(\frac{\pi}{4},\frac{5\pi}{4}\right)$

5. If $f(x)=\begin{vmatrix}\sin x & \sin\alpha & \sin\beta\\ \cos x & \cos\alpha & \cos\beta\\ \tan x & \tan\alpha & \tan\beta\end{vmatrix}$ where $0<\alpha<\beta<\frac{\pi}{2}$. Show that $f'(l)=0$, where $\alpha<l<\beta$.

6. A function $f(x)$ is continuous in the closed interval [0,1] and differentiable in the open interval]0,1[prove that

$$f'(x_1)=f(1)-f(0),\ 0<x_1<1.$$

7. Show that the set of all x for which $\log(1+x)\le x$ is equal to $[0,\infty[$.

8. Compute the value of θ in the first mean value theorem $f(x+h)=f(x)+hf'(x+\theta h)$ if $f(x)=ax^2+bx+c$.

9. Show that $x^n - a = 0$ has atmost one real positive root if n is a positive integer.

10. Show that the function f', if it exists in an interval, cannot have an ordinary or removable discontinuity in that interval.

11. Verify the Lagrange's mean value theorem for the following functions :

(a) $f(x)=x^3$ in $[-1,1]$ [MEERUT(BCA)–2005]

(b) $f(x)=\sin x$ in $[0,\pi/2]$ [NAGPUR–2008]

(c) $f(x)=x^n$ in $[-1,1]$, $n\in Z^+$

(d) $f(x)=2x^2-7x+10, x\in[2,5]$

12. Find the value of c, of mean value theorem, when

(a) $f(x)=\sqrt{x^2-4}$ in the interval $[2,4]$

(b) $f(x)=2x^2+3x+4$ in the interval $[1,2]$

(c) $f(x)=x(x-1)$ in the interval $[1,2]$

13. (a) If $f(x)=\sqrt{x}$ and $g(x)=1/\sqrt{x}$, then show by Cauchy's mean value theorem that c is the geometric mean between a and b.

(b) If $f(x)=\dfrac{1}{x^2}$ and $g(x)=\dfrac{1}{x}$, then show that c is the harmonic mean between a and b.

14. If f'' exists and continuous on $[a,b]$ and differentiable on $]a,b[$, then prove that

$$f(b)-f(a)-\frac{1}{2}(b-a)\{f'(a)-f'(b)\} = -\frac{(b-a)^3}{12}f''(d)$$

where $d\in R$ such that $d\in]a,b[$.

15. Prove that

$$\sin ax = ax-\frac{a^3x^3}{3!}+\frac{a^5x^5}{5!}-\ldots+\frac{a^{n-1}x^{n-1}}{(n-1)!}\sin\left(\frac{n-1}{2}.\pi\right)+\frac{a^nx^n}{n!}\sin\left(a\theta x+\frac{n\pi}{2}\right)$$

16. If $f(x)=f(0)+xf'(0)+\dfrac{x^2}{2!}f''(\theta x)$ find the value of θ as $x\to1$, $f(x)$ being $(1-x)^{5/2}$.

17. Show that the number θ which occurs in the Taylor's Theorem with Lagrange's form of remainder after n terms approaches the limit $\dfrac{f^{n+1}(a)}{(n+1)}$ as $h\to0$ provided that $f\ n+1(x)$ is continuous and different from zero as $x\to a$.

18. Show that the function x^3-3x^2+3x+2 is monotonically increasing in every interval.

19. Obtain by Maclaurin's theorem the expansion of $e^{\sin x}$.

20. If $f(x)=\exp\left[-\dfrac{1}{x^2}\right]$, for $x\neq0$ and $f(0)=0$, then show that :

(i) $f^n(0)=0\ \forall n=0,1,2,\ldots$ and

(ii) The Taylor's series for f about 0 agrees with $f(x)$ only at $x=0$.

21. Expand "log sec x" by Maclaurin's series expansion, upto the term containing x^6. [VTU–2009; MUMBAI–2000]

22. If $x>0$, show that

$$x-\frac{x^2}{2}+\frac{x^3}{3(1+x)}<\log(1+x)<x-\frac{x^2}{2}+\frac{x^3}{3}.$$

Hints to the Selected Problems

1. (a) Since $f'(x)$ does not exist at $x=1$, the second condition of Rolle's theorem is not satisfied.

2. Let a,b be two distinct roots of $e^x\cos x-1=0$. Then $e^a\cos a=1$ and $e^b\cos b=1$
Define a function $f(x)=e^{-x}-\cos x$.

5. $f(x)$ can be written as

$$f(x)=(\cos\alpha\tan\beta-\cos\beta\tan\alpha)\sin x -(\sin\alpha\tan\beta-\sin\beta\tan\alpha)\cos x +(\sin\alpha\cos\beta-\sin\beta\cos\alpha)\tan x$$

Since $\sin x, \cos x, \tan x$ have finite derivatives in $]0,\pi/2[$

$\Rightarrow f'(x)$ exists.

Also, $f(\alpha)=f(\beta)$. Hence, all the conditions of Rolle's theorem are satisfied.

7. Let us suppose $f(x)=\log(1+x)-x$

$\Rightarrow f(0)=0$

$$f'(x)=\frac{1}{1+x}-1=\frac{-x}{1+x}\le0$$

$\Rightarrow f(x)$ is a decreasing function.

$\Rightarrow f(x)\le f(0)\ \forall x\ge0$

$\Rightarrow \log(1+x)-x\le0$

$\Rightarrow \log(1+x)\le x$

9. $f'(x)=nx^{n-1}$. Clearly $f(x)$ is an increasing function.

Let $x_1, x_2\in]0,\infty[$ and $0<x<r<x_2$ such that $f(r)=0$.

Then $f(x_1)<f(r)<f(x_2)\Rightarrow f(x_1)<0<f(x_2)$

$\Rightarrow$ If $x\neq r$, $f(x)\neq0$ on $(0,\infty)$.

$\Rightarrow x^n-a$ has at most one real positive root.

14. Define two functions $g(x)$ and $h(x)$ such that

$$g(x) = f(x) - f(a) - \frac{1}{2}(x-a)$$
$$\{f'(a) + f'(x)\} + A(x-a)^3$$

and $h(x) = \frac{1}{2}[f'(x) - f'(a)]^{-1/2}$
$$(x-a)f''(x) + 3A(x-a)^2$$

Clearly, $g(x)$ and $h(x)$ satisfying all conditions of Rolle's theorem. Then use Rolle's theorem for both the above functions.

18. Since $f'(x) \geq 0$ in $]-\infty, 1]$. Hence, it is monotonically increasing.

22. $f'(x) = \frac{1}{1+x} - 1 + x - \frac{3x^2 + 2x^3}{3(1+x^2)}$
$$= \frac{x^3}{3(1+x)^2} > 0$$

f is increasing $\Rightarrow f(x) > f(0) = 0$ for $x > 0$
$$x - \frac{x^2}{2} + \frac{x^3}{3(1+x)} < \log(1+x) \text{ if } x > 0$$

Now, $g'(x) = 1 - x + x^2 - \frac{1}{1+x} = \frac{x^3}{1+x} > 0$

g is increasing $\Rightarrow g(x) > g(0)$
$$\log(1+x) < x - \frac{x^2}{2} + \frac{x^3}{3}$$

ANSWERS

1.(a) Not applicable (b) Not applicable (c) Not applicable (d) Verified (e)Verified (f) Verified (g) Not applicable (h) Verified (i) Verified **4.**(a)Verified (b)Verified

8. $\theta = \frac{1}{2}$ **11.** (a) Verified (b) Verified (c) Verified (d) Verified **12.** (a) $c = \sqrt{6}$ (b) $c = 3/2$

16. $\theta = \frac{9}{25}$ **19.** $y = 1 + x + \frac{x^2}{2} - \frac{x^4}{8} + \ldots$ **21.** $y = \frac{x^2}{2} + \frac{x^4}{12} + \frac{x^6}{45} + \ldots$

8.9 SOME MORE PROBLEMS BASED ON EXPANSIONS

1. *Expand $\tan^{-1} x$.*

SOLUTION. Let $f(x) = \tan^{-1} x \Rightarrow f(0) = 0$

$$f'(x) = \frac{1}{1+x^2} \Rightarrow f'(0) = 1$$
$$= (1+x^2)^{-1} = 1 - x^2 + x^4 - x^6 + \ldots$$
(By binomial expansion)
$$f''(x) = -2x + 4x^3 - 6x^5 + \ldots$$
$$\Rightarrow f''(0) = 0$$
$$f'''(x) = -2 + 12x^2 - 30x^4 + \ldots$$
$$\Rightarrow f'''(0) = -2$$
$$f^{iv}(x) = 24x - 120x^3 + \ldots \Rightarrow f^{iv}(0) = 0$$
$$f^{v}(x) = 24 - 360x^2 + \ldots \Rightarrow f^{v}(0) = 24$$
....

Put all these vaiues in Maclaurin's series, we get
$$\tan^{-1} x = x - \frac{x^3}{3} + \frac{x^5}{5} - \frac{x^7}{7} + \ldots$$

- To expand an alone inverse function, find its first derivative, expand by binomial theorem and then find other derivatives.
- The expansion of $\tan^{-1} x$ is valid only if $-1 < x < 1$.
- This expansion for $\tan^{-1} x$ known as Gregory's series, which is very useful in finding the value of π.
- In a like manner, we may get
$$\sin^{-1} x = x + \frac{1}{2}.\frac{x^3}{3} + \frac{1.3}{2.4}.\frac{x^5}{5} + \frac{1.3.5}{2.4.6}.\frac{x^7}{7} + \ldots$$

2. *Expand $\tan x$ by Macluarin's theorem as far as x^5 and hence find the value of tan 46°30′ upto four decimal places.*

(VTU–2006)

SOLUTION. Let $f(x) = \tan x$

$$\Rightarrow f(0) = 0$$
$$f'(x) = \sec^2 x = 1 + \tan^2 x$$
$$\Rightarrow f'(0) = 1$$
$$f''(x) = 2\tan x \sec^2 x$$
$$= 2\tan x(1 + \tan^2 x)$$
$$= 2\tan x + 2\tan^3 x$$

$\Rightarrow f''(0)=0$

$$f'''(x)=2\sec^2 x+6\tan^2 x\sec^2 x$$
$$=2(1+\tan^2 x)+6\tan^2 x(1+\tan^2 x)$$
$$=2+8\tan^2 x+6\tan^4 x$$

$\Rightarrow f'''(0)=2$

$$f^{iv}(x)=16\tan x\sec^2 x+24\tan^3 x\sec^2 x$$
$$=8\sec^2 x(2\tan x+3\tan^3 x)$$
$$=8(1+\tan^2 x)(2\tan x+3\tan^3 x)$$
$$=16\tan x+40\tan^3 x+24\tan^5 x$$

$\Rightarrow f^{iv}(0)=0$

and $f^{v}(x)=16\sec^2 x+120\tan^2 x\sec^2 x+120\tan^4 x\sec^2 x$

$$=8\sec^2 x(2+15\tan^2 x+15\tan^4 x)$$

$\Rightarrow \quad f^{v}(0)=16$

Now, putting all these values in Maclaurin's series'

$$f(x)=f(0)+xf'(0)+\frac{x^2}{2!}f''(0)+\frac{x^3}{3!}f'''(0)+\frac{x^4}{4!}f^{iv}(0)+\frac{x^5}{5!}f^{v}(0)+\ldots$$

we get

$$\tan x=0+x+\frac{x^3}{3!}.2+\frac{x^5}{5!}.16+\ldots$$

$$\Rightarrow \tan x=x+\frac{x^3}{3}+\frac{2}{15}x^5+\ldots$$

Deduction. Here

$x=46°30'$

$$=\left(46\frac{1}{2}\right)^\circ=\left(\frac{93}{2}\right)^\circ=\frac{93}{2}\times\frac{\pi}{180}\text{ Radians}$$

$$=\frac{31}{120}\times\frac{22}{7}=\frac{31\times 11}{60\times 7}=\frac{314}{420}=0.812$$

Now, putting $x=46°30'=0.812$ in (1), we get $\tan 46°30'$

$$=0.812+\frac{(0.812)^3}{3}+\frac{2}{15}(0.812)^5$$
$$=0.812+0.1784+0.047$$
$$=1.0374$$

3. *Expand* $\log\{x+\sqrt{(1+x^2)}\}$ *in ascending powers of x and find the general term.*

SOLUTION. Let $y=\log\{x+\sqrt{(1+x^2)}\}$ ...(1)

$$\Rightarrow \quad y_1=\frac{1}{x+\sqrt{1+x^2}}.\left[1+\frac{2x}{2\sqrt{(1+x^2)}}\right]$$

$$=\frac{1}{\sqrt{1+x^2}} \quad ...(2)$$

$\Rightarrow y_1^2(1+x^2)-1=0.$

Differentiating again w.r.t. x, we get

$$2y_1[(1+x^2)y_2+xy_1]=0$$

$$\Rightarrow \quad [(1+x^2)y_2+xy_1]=0 \quad (\because 2y_1\neq 0) \quad ...(3)$$

Using Leibnitz's theorem, differentiating (3) n times, we get

$$(1-x^2)y_{n+2}+n.y_{n+1}.2x+\frac{n(n-1)}{1.2}y_2.2+y_{n+1}.x+n.y_n=0$$

$$\Rightarrow (1+x^2)y_{n+2}+(2n+1)xy_{n+1}+n^2y_n=0 \quad ...(4)$$

Putting $x=0$ in (1), (2), (3) and (4), we have

$$y(0)=0,\ y_1(0)=1,\ y_2(0)=0$$
$$y_{n+2}(0)=-n^2y_n(0) \quad ...(5)$$

From (5), we have

$y_3(0)=-1^2y_1(0)=-1^2$

$y_5(0)=(-3^2)y_3(0)=(-3^2)(-1^2)=3^2.1^2$

$y_7(0)=(-5^2)y_5(0)=(-5^2)(-3^2)(-1^2)$

$=-5^2.3^2.1^2$ .... and so on.

Putting $n-2$ for n in (5), we get

$$y_n(0)=\{-(n-2)^2\}y_{n-2}(0) \quad ...(6)$$
$$=[-(n-2)^2][-(n-4)^2]y_{n-4}(0).$$

Here we observe that

If n is odd, then

$$y_n(0)=[-(n-2)^2][-(n-4)^2]-\ldots(-5^2)(-3^2)(-1^2).1$$
$$=[-1]^{(n-1)/2}(n-2)^2(n-4)^2\ldots5^2.3^2.1^2 \quad ...(7)$$

Also from (5), we get

$y_4(0)=-2^2.y_2(0)=0$

$y_6(0)=-4^2.y_4(0)=0$ ... and so on.

If n is even,

then, $y_n(0)=0.$

Putting all these values in Maclaurin's series

$$y=y(0)+\frac{x}{1!}y_1(0)+\frac{x^2}{2!}y_2(0)+\frac{x^3}{3!}y_3(0)+\ldots$$

we get $\log\left[x+\sqrt{(1+x^2)}\right]$

$$=x-\frac{x^3}{3!}.1^2+\frac{x^5}{5!}(3^2.1^2)-\frac{x^7}{7!}(5^2.3^2.1^2)+\ldots$$

The general term $= \frac{x^n}{n!} y_n(0)$ where

$$y_n(0) = \begin{cases} (-1)^{(n-1)/2}(n-2)^2 \\ (n-4)^2 \ldots 5^2.3^2.1^2, \text{if } n \text{ is odd} \\ 0 \quad , \text{if } n \text{ is even} \end{cases}$$

4. *Expand log sin (x+h) in power of h by Taylor's theorem.*

SOLUTION. Let $f(x+h) = \log \sin (x+h)$

$$\left.\begin{aligned} \Rightarrow \quad & f(x) = \log \sin x \\ & f'(x) = \frac{1}{\sin x}.\cos x = \cot x \\ & f''(x) = -\operatorname{cosec}^2 x \\ & f'''(x) = 2 \operatorname{cosec} x \operatorname{cosec} x \cot x \\ & \qquad = 2 \operatorname{cosec}^2 x \cot x \\ & \ldots \quad \ldots \quad \ldots \quad \ldots \quad \ldots \quad \ldots \end{aligned}\right\} \ldots(1)$$

Now by Taylor's theorem, we have

$$f(x+h) = f(x) + hf'(x) + \frac{h^2}{2!} f''(x) + \frac{h^3}{3!} f'''(x) + \ldots \quad \ldots(2)$$

Putting all the values from (1) in (2), we get

$$\log \sin(x+h) = \log \sin x + h \cot x - \frac{h^2}{2} \operatorname{cosec}^2 x + \frac{h^3}{3} \operatorname{cosec}^2 \cot x + \ldots$$

Similar Problem

(1) Expand $\sin x$ in powers of $\left(x - \frac{\pi}{2}\right)$ by using Taylor's series.

5. *Prove by Maclaurin's theorem, that*

$$e^{\sin x} = 1 + x + \frac{x^2}{1.2} - \frac{3.x^4}{1.2.3.4} + \ldots$$

(VTU–2011, BHOPAL–2009)

SOLUTION. Let $f(x) = e^{\sin x} \Rightarrow f(0) = e^0 = 1$

$f'(x) = e^{\sin x}.\cos x \Rightarrow f'(0) = e^0 \cos 0 = 1$

$f''(x) = e^{\sin x}(-\sin x) + \cos x\, e^{\sin x} \cos x$

$= e^{\sin x}[\cos^2 x - \sin x]$

$\Rightarrow f''(0) = e^0[1-0] = 1$

$f'''(x) = e^{\sin x}[2 \cos x(-\sin x) - \cos x]$

$+ e^{\sin x} \cos x.[\cos^2 x - \sin x]$

$= e^{\sin x} \cos x[-2\sin x - 1 + \cos^2 x - \sin x]$

$= -e^{\sin x} \cos x[3 \sin x + \sin^2 x]$

$\Rightarrow \quad f'''(0) = 0$

$f^{iv}(x) = -e^{\sin x} \cos x[3 \cos x + 2 \sin x \cos x]$

$+ e^{\sin x} \sin x[3 \sin x + \sin^2 x]$

$-[3 \sin x + \sin^2 x] \cos x\, e^{\sin x} \cos x$

$\Rightarrow \quad f^{iv}(0) = -3$

Putting all these values in Maclaurin's theorem, given by

$$f(x) = f(0) + xf'(0) + \frac{x^2}{2!} f''(0) + \frac{x^3}{3!} f'''(0) + \frac{x^4}{4!} f^{iv}(0) + \ldots$$

We get, $e^{\sin x} = 1 + x + \frac{x^2}{1.2} - \frac{3.x^4}{1.2.3.4} + \ldots$

6. *Expand* $e^{a \sin^{-1} x}$ *by Macluarin's theorem and find the general term. Hence, show that*

$$e^{\theta} = 1 + \sin\theta + \frac{1}{2!} \sin^2\theta + \frac{2}{3!} \sin^3\theta + \ldots$$

SOLUTION. Let $y = e^{a \sin^{-1} x} \Rightarrow y(0) = 1$

$$y_1 = e^{a \sin^{-1} x}.\frac{a}{\sqrt{1-x^2}} \Rightarrow y_1(0) = a$$

Similarly, $y_2(0) = a^2$

and $\quad y_{n+2}(0) = (n^2 + a^2) y_n(0) \quad \ldots(1)$

Putting $n = 1,2,3,\ldots$in (1), we get

$y_3(0) = (1^2 + a^2) y_1(0) = (1^2 + a^2) a$

$y_4(0) = (2^2 + a^2) y_2(0) = (2^2 + a^2) a^2$

$y_5(0) = (3^2 + a^2) y_3(0)$

$= (3^2 + a^2)(1^2 + a^2) a$

$$y_6(0)=(4^2+a^2)y_4(0)$$
$$=(4^2+a^2)(2^2+a^2)a....\text{so on}$$

In general

$$y_n(0)=\begin{cases} a^2(2^2+a^2)(4^2+a^2) \\ \quad ...[(n-2)^2+a^2], \text{if } n \text{ is even} \\ a(1^2+a^2)(3^2+a^2) \\ \quad ...[(n-2)^2+a^2], \text{ if } n \text{ is odd} \end{cases} \quad ...(2)$$

Substituting these values in Maclaurin's series

$$y = y(0)+x\,y_1(0)+\frac{x^2}{2!}y_2(0)+...$$
$$+\frac{x^n}{n!}y_n(0)+...$$

we get $e^{a\sin^{-1}x} = 1+ax+\frac{a^2}{2!}x^2$

$$+\frac{a(1^2+a^2)}{3!}x^3$$
$$+\frac{a^2(2^2+a^2)}{4!}x^4+...$$

General term : The general term= $\frac{x^n}{n!}y_n(0)$ where $y_n(0)$ is given by (2).

Now, putting $x=\sin\theta$ and $a=1$ in (3), we get

$$e^{\theta}=1+\sin\theta+\frac{1}{2!}\sin^2\theta+\frac{2}{3!}\sin^3\theta+...$$

Similar Problem

(1) If $f(x)=x^3-2x+5$, find the value of $f(2.001)$ with the help of Taylor's theorem. Find the approximate change in the value of $f(x)$ when x changes from 2 to 2.001.

7. *Expand log (1+sin x) by Maclaurin's theorem in ascending power of x upto first five terms.* [SVTU–2009; JNTU–2006; MEERUT(BCA)–2002, 04, 08,]

SOLUTION. Let $y=f(x)=\log(1+\sin x)$

By Maclaurin's expansion for $f(x)$, we have

$$y=f(x)=(y)_0+\frac{x}{1!}(y_1)_0+\frac{x^2}{2!}(y_2)_0+\frac{x^3}{3!}(y_3)_0+\frac{x^4}{4!}(y_4)_0+... \quad ...(1)$$

Now $y=\log(1+\sin x)$

$\therefore$ $(y)_0=0$

$$y_1=\frac{\cos x}{1+\sin x}\Rightarrow (y_1)_0=1$$

$$y_2=\frac{-\sin x(1+\sin x)-\cos^2 x}{(1+\sin x)^2}$$
$$=-\frac{(1+\sin x)}{(1+\sin x)^2}=-\frac{1}{1+\sin x}$$

$\Rightarrow$ $(y_2)_0=-1$

$$y_3=\frac{\cos x}{(1+\sin x)^2}=\frac{\cos x}{(1+\sin x)}\cdot\frac{1}{(1+\sin x)}$$
$$=-y_1y_2$$

$\Rightarrow (y_3)_0=-1(-1)=1$

$$y_4=-y_1y_3-y_2^{\,2}$$
$$\Rightarrow (y_4)_0=-1.1-(-1)^2=-1-1=-2$$
$$y_5=-y_1y_4-y_2y_3-2y_2y_3$$
$$=-y_1y_4-3y_2y_3$$
$$\Rightarrow (y_5)_0=-1.(-2)-3(-1).1=2+3=5$$

and so on.

Therefore, $\log(1+\sin x)$

$$=0+\frac{x}{1!}.1+\frac{x^2}{2!}.(-1)+\frac{x^3}{3!}.1+\frac{x^4}{4!}.(-2)+...$$
$$=x-\frac{x^2}{2}+\frac{x^3}{6}-\frac{x^4}{12}+\frac{x^5}{24}...$$

8. *Expand sin (π/4+θ) in powers of θ.* [MEERUT(BCA)–2003, 06, 09, 10]

SOLUTION. Let $f(\theta)=\sin(\pi/4+\theta)$

$\Rightarrow$ $f(0)=\sin\pi/4=1/\sqrt{2}$

$f'(\theta)=\cos(\pi/4+\theta)$

$\Rightarrow$ $f'(0)=\cos\pi/4=1/\sqrt{2}$

$f''(\theta)=-\sin(\pi/4+\theta)$

$\Rightarrow$ $f''(0)=-\sin\pi/4=-1/\sqrt{2}$

$f'''(\theta)=-\cos(\pi/4+\theta)$

$\Rightarrow$ $f'''(0)=-\cos\pi/4=-1/\sqrt{2}$

$f^{iv}(\theta)=\sin(\pi/4+\theta)$

$\Rightarrow f^{iv}(0) = 1/\sqrt{2}$ and so on.

The nth derivative of $f(\theta)$ is given by

$$f^n(\theta) = \sin\left(\theta + \frac{\pi}{4} + \frac{n\pi}{4}\right)$$

The Maclaurin's expansion of $f(\theta)$ with Lagrange's form of remainder is

$$f(\theta) = f(0) + \frac{\theta}{1!}f'(0) + \frac{\theta^2}{2!}f''(0) + \frac{\theta^3}{3!}f'''(0) + \ldots + \frac{\theta^{n-1}}{(n-1)!}f^{n-1}(0) + R_n \quad \ldots(1)$$

where $R_n = \frac{\theta^n}{n!}f^n(t.\theta)$

$$= \frac{\theta^n}{n!}\sin\left(t.\theta + \frac{\pi}{4} + \frac{n\pi}{2}\right), \quad 0<t<1.$$

Now

$$|R_n| = \left|\frac{\theta^n}{n!}\sin\left(t.\theta + \frac{\pi}{4} + \frac{n\pi}{2}\right)\right|$$

$$= \left|\frac{\theta^n}{n!}\right| . \left|\sin\left(t.\theta + \frac{\pi}{4} + \frac{n\pi}{2}\right)\right| \le \left|\frac{\theta^n}{n!}\right|$$

$$\therefore \lim_{n\to\infty}|R_n| \le \lim_{n\to\infty}\left|\frac{\theta^n}{n!}\right| = 0$$

$$\left[\because \lim_{n\to\infty}\frac{\theta^n}{n!} = 0\right]$$

$$\therefore \lim_{n\to\infty} R_n = 0$$

Thus all the conditions of Maclaurin's series expansion are satisfied. Hence, from (1), the expansion of $\sin(\theta+\pi/4)$ is given by

$$\sin\left(\theta+\frac{\pi}{4}\right) = \frac{1}{\sqrt{2}} + \frac{\theta}{1!}\frac{1}{\sqrt{2}} + \frac{\theta^2}{2!}\left(-\frac{1}{\sqrt{2}}\right) + \frac{\theta^3}{3!}\left(-\frac{1}{\sqrt{2}}\right) + \ldots$$

$$\sin\left(\theta+\frac{\pi}{4}\right) = \frac{1}{\sqrt{2}}\left[1 + \frac{\theta}{1!} - \frac{\theta^2}{2!} - \frac{\theta^3}{3!} + \frac{\theta^4}{4!} + \frac{\theta^5}{5!} - \frac{\theta^6}{6!} - \frac{\theta^7}{7!} + \ldots\right]$$

Exercise-8.2

1. Expand the following functions by Maclaurin's theorem :

(i) $\sec x$ (ii) $e^{x\cos x}$

(iii) $e^x \sec x$

(iv) $\log_e(1+e^x)$ (BHOPAL–2008)

(v) $\log(1+\tan x)$ [MEERUT(BCA)–2005]

2. Apply Maclaurin's theorem to prove that

$$\log \sec x = \frac{1}{2}x^2 + \frac{1}{12}x^4 + \frac{1}{45}x^6 + \ldots$$

3. If $y = \sin^{-1}x = a_0 + a_1x + a_2x^2 + \ldots$ Prove that

$$(n+1)(n+2)a_{n+2} = n^2a_n.$$

4. Show that :

(i) $e^x \cos x$

$$= 1 + x - \frac{2x^3}{3!} + \frac{2^2x^4}{4!} + \frac{2^2x^5}{5!} + \frac{2^3x^7}{7!} + \ldots + \cos\left(\frac{n\pi}{4}\right)\frac{2^{n/2}}{n!}x^n + \ldots$$

(ii) $$e^x \sin x = x + x^2 - \frac{2x^3}{3!} + \frac{2^2x^5}{5!} - \ldots + \sin\left(\frac{n\pi}{4}\right)\frac{2^{n/2}}{n!}x^n + \ldots$$

(iii) $$e^{ax}\sin bx = bx + abx^2 + \frac{3a^2b - b^3}{3!}x^3 + \ldots + \frac{\left(a^2+b^2\right)^{\frac{n}{2}}}{n!}x^n \sin\left(n\tan^{-1}\frac{b}{a}\right) + \ldots$$

(iv) $$e^{ax}\cos bx = 1 + ax + \frac{a^2-b^2}{2!}x^2 + \frac{a\left(a^2-3b^2\right)}{3!}x^3 + \ldots + \frac{\left(a^2+b^2\right)^{\frac{n}{2}}}{n!}x^n \cos\left(n\tan^{-1}\frac{b}{a}\right) + \ldots$$

5. Expand the following :

(i) $\tan^{-1}x$ in powers of $\left(x-\frac{\pi}{4}\right)$.

(ii) $2x^3+7x^2+x-1$ in powers of $x-2$. (BURDWAN–2003)

(iii) $\sin^{-1}(x+h)$ in power of x.

(iv) $\log \sin x$ in power of $(x-a)$.

6. Show that

$$\log(x+h)=\log h+\frac{x}{h}-\frac{x^2}{2h^2}+\frac{x^3}{3h^3}-\ldots$$

7. Use Taylor's theorem to prove that

$$\tan^{-1}(x+h)=\tan^{-1}x+h\sin\theta\frac{\sin\theta}{1}-(h\sin\theta)^2\frac{\sin 2\theta}{2}+(h\sin\theta)^3\frac{\sin 3\theta}{3}+\ldots+(-1)^{n-1}(h\sin\theta)^n\frac{\sin n\theta}{n}+\ldots$$

where $\theta=\cot^{-1}x$.

8. If $y=e^{\tan^{-1}x}$, show that

$$(1+x^2)y_{n+2}+[2(n+1)x-1]y_{n+1}+n(n+1)y_n=0.$$

Hence, or otherwise, find out the coefficient of x^5 if $e^{\tan^{-1}x}$ is expanded in powers of x.

9. Expand $(\sin^{-1}x)^2$ in ascending powers of x and deduce that

$$\theta^2=2.\frac{\sin^2\theta}{2!}+2^2.\frac{2\sin^4\theta}{4!}+2^2.4^2\frac{2\sin^6\theta}{6!}+\ldots$$

10. If $y=e^{m\tan^{-1}x}=a_0+a_1x+a_2x^2+\ldots+a_nx^n+\ldots$, show that $(n+1)a_{n+1}+(n-1)a_{n-1}=ma_n$.

11. If $e^{e^x}=a_0+a_1x+a_2x^2+\ldots+a_nx^n+\ldots$ show that

$$a_{n+1}=\frac{1}{n+1}\left[a_n+\frac{a_{n-1}}{1!}+\frac{a_{n-2}}{2!}+\ldots+\frac{a_{n-r}}{r!}+\ldots\frac{a_0}{n!}\right]$$

12. Show that

$$f(mx)=f(x)+(m-1)xf'(x)+\frac{(m-1)^2}{2!}x^2f''(x)+\frac{(m-1)^3}{3!}x^3f'''(x)+\ldots$$

13. By Maclaurin's theorem find the expansion of $y=\sin(e^x-1)$ upto and including the term in x. Find also the first non-vanishing terms in the expansion of x as a series ascending powers of y.

14. Prove that

$$f\left(\frac{x^2}{1+x}\right)=f(x)-\frac{x}{1+x}f'(x)+\left(\frac{x}{1+x}\right)^2\frac{1}{2!}f''(x)-\left(\frac{x}{1+x}\right)^3f'''(x)+\ldots$$

15. Calculate the approximate value of :

(i) $\sqrt{17}$ to four decimal places.

(ii) $\sqrt{26}$ to three decimal places

by Taylor's expansion.

Hint to Selected Problems

1. (i) $y=\sec x \Rightarrow y_1=\sec x\tan x=y\tan x$

$$\Rightarrow y_1^2=y^2\tan^2x=y^2(\sec^2x-1)$$
$$=y^2(y^2-1)=y^4-y^2.$$

Again differentiating, we get

$$2y_1y_2=4y^3y_1-2yy_1\Rightarrow y_2=2y^3-y$$

Similarly
$$y_3=6y^2y_1-y_1$$
$$y_4=12yy_1^3+6y^2y_2-y_2$$
$$y_5=12y_1^3-36y_1y_2-y_3$$
$$\ldots\ \ldots\ \ldots\ \ldots$$

Now putting $x=0$ in the above equation and use Maclaurin's series.

2. $y=\log\sec x \Rightarrow y_1=\tan x$

$$y_2=\sec^2x=1+\tan^2x=1+y_1^2$$
$$y_3=2y_1y_2$$
$$y_4=2y_2^2+2y_1y_3$$
$$y_5=4y_2y_3+2y_2y_3+2y_1y_4$$
$$y_6=8y_2y_4+6y_3^2+2y_1y_5$$
$$\ldots\ \ldots\ \ldots\ \ldots\ \ldots$$

Now putting $x=0$ in the above equations and use Maclaurin's series.

3. $y=\sin^{-1}x$

$$\Rightarrow y_1=\frac{1}{\sqrt{1-x^2}}\Rightarrow(1-x^2)y_1^2=1$$

Again differentiating, we get

$$(1-x^2)y_2-xy_1=0$$

Now apply Leibnitz's theorem to differentiating n times.

4. $y=e^x\cos x$

$$\Rightarrow y_1=e^x\cos x-e^x\sin x=e^x(\cos x-\sin x)$$
$$=re^x(\cos\theta\cos x-\sin\theta\sin x),$$

where $r=\sqrt{2}$, $\theta=\frac{\pi}{4}$

$\Rightarrow \quad y_1=re^x\cos(x+\theta)$

$\Rightarrow \quad y_2=r^2e^x\cos(x+2\theta)$

... ...

$$y_n=r^ne^x\cos(x+n\theta)=(2)^{n/2}e^x\cos\left(x+\frac{n\pi}{4}\right)$$

Now putting $x=0$ and use Maclaurin's series.

(ii) Here $\quad y_n=2^{n/2}e^x\sin\left(x+\frac{n\pi}{4}\right)$

(iii) $y_n=\left(a^2+b^2\right)^{n/2}e^{ax}\sin\left[bx+n\tan^{-1}\left(\frac{b}{a}\right)\right]$

5. (i) $y=f(x)=\tan^{-1}x$

$$\Rightarrow y_1=f'(x)=\frac{1}{1+x^2} \quad \Rightarrow y_2=\frac{-2.x}{\left(1+x^2\right)^2}$$

Putting $x=\pi/4$ and find $f(\pi/4)$, $f'(\pi/4)$, $f''(\pi/4)$... and so on.

Now $\quad f(x)=f\left(\frac{\pi}{4}+x-\frac{\pi}{4}\right)$

Then expand by Taylor's theorem.

6. $\quad y=f(x)=\log x$

$\Rightarrow \quad f(x+h)=\log(x+h)$

$$\Rightarrow \quad f'(x)=\frac{1}{x}, f''(x)=-\frac{1}{x^2}, f'''(x)=\frac{2}{x^3}...$$

and so on.

$\Rightarrow$Now putting $x=h$ in above derivatives and expand $f(x+h)$ by Taylor's theorem.

7. Take $\quad y=f(x)=\tan^{-1}x$

$$\Rightarrow f'(x)=\frac{1}{1+x^2}=\frac{1}{2i}\left(\frac{1}{x-i}-\frac{1}{x+i}\right)$$

$$\Rightarrow f''(x)=\frac{1}{2i}\left[(-1)(x-i)^2-(-1)(x+i)^{-2}\right]$$

... ...

$$f^n(x)=\frac{1}{2i}\left[(-1)^{n-1}(n-1)!(x-i)^{-n} -(-1)^{n-1}(n-1)!(x+i)^{-n}\right]$$

Put $\theta=\cot^{-1}x$, we get

$$f^n(x)=(-1)^{n-1}(n-1)!\,\sin^n\theta\,\sin n\theta$$

Now use Taylor's series.

8. $y=f(x)=e^{\tan^{-1}x}$

$$\Rightarrow y_1=\frac{e^{\tan^{-1}x}}{1+x^2}=\frac{y}{1+x^2}\Rightarrow\left(1+x^2\right)y_1=y$$

$$(1+x^2)y_2+(2x-1)y_1=0$$

Now to find y_n, use Leibnitz's theorem.

9. Let $\quad y=f(x)=(\sin^{-1}x)^2$

$$\Rightarrow \quad y_1=\frac{2\sin^{-1}x}{\sqrt{1-x^2}}\Rightarrow\left(1-x^2\right)y_1^2$$

$$=4\left(\sin^{-1}x\right)^2=4y$$

Now differentiating n times by Leibnitz's rule.

10. $y=f(x)=e^{m\tan^{-1}x}$

$$\Rightarrow \quad y_1=\frac{me^{\tan^{-1}x}}{1+x^2}\Rightarrow\left(1+x^2\right)y_1=my$$

Now differentiating n times by using Leibnitz's theorem.

11. Let $\quad y=f(x)=e^{e^x} \Rightarrow y_1=e^xe^{e^x}=e^x.y$

Now to find nth derivative, using Leibnitz's theorem.

12. Write $f(mx)=f[x+(m-1)x]$. Now expand by Taylor's theorem.

13. $y=f(x)=\sin(e^x-1) \quad \Rightarrow \quad y_1=e^x\cos(e^x-1)$ Now differentiating successively.

14. Write

$$f\left(\frac{x^2}{1+x}\right)=f\left(\frac{x^2}{1+x}-x+x\right)=f\left(x-\frac{x}{1+x}\right)$$

Now expand by Taylor's theorem.

15. Let $\quad y=f(17)=\sqrt{17}=\sqrt{x}$

$\quad y=f(16+1)$.

Now expand by Taylor's theorem.

ANSWERS

1. (i) $1+\frac{x^2}{2!}+\frac{5x^4}{4!}+\frac{61x^6}{6!}+...$ $\quad$ (ii) $1+x+\frac{x^2}{2}-\frac{x^3}{3}-\frac{11x^4}{24}-\frac{x^5}{5}+...$

(iii) $1+x+\frac{2x^2}{2!}+\frac{4x^3}{3!}+...$ (iv) $\log 2+\frac{x}{2}+\frac{x^2}{8}-\frac{x^4}{192}+...$

(v) $x-\frac{x^2}{2}+\frac{2}{3}x^3-\frac{7x^4}{12}+...$

5. (i) $\tan^{-1}\left(\frac{\pi}{4}\right)+\left(x-\frac{\pi}{4}\right)\Big/\left(1+\frac{\pi^2}{16}\right)-\pi\left(x-\frac{\pi}{4}\right)^2\Big/\left[4\left(1+\frac{\pi^2}{16}\right)^2\right]+...$

(ii) $45+53(x-2)+19(x-2)^2+2(x-2)^3+...$

(iii) $\sin^{-1}h+x\left(1-h^2\right)^{-1/2}+\frac{x^2}{2!}h\left(1-h^2\right)^{-3/2}+\frac{x^3}{3!}\left[\left(1-h^2\right)^{-5/2}\left(1+2h^2\right)\right]+...$

(iv) $\log\sin a+(x-a)\cot a-\frac{(x-a)^2}{2!}\operatorname{cosec}^2 a+\frac{(x-a)^3}{3!}2\operatorname{cosec}^2 a\cot a+...$

8. $\frac{1}{24}$ **9.** $2.\frac{x^2}{2!}+\frac{2.2^2}{4!}x^4+\frac{2.2^2.4^2}{6!}x^6+...+\frac{2.2^2.4^2...(2n-2)^2}{(2n)!}x^{2n}+...$

13. $x+\frac{x^2}{2!}-\frac{5x^4}{24}+...,y-\frac{y^2}{2}+...$ **15.** (i) 4.123 (ii) 5.099

❑❑❑❑❑❑

Chapter

9

Indeterminate Forms

9.1 INTRODUCTION

When a function involves the independent variable in such a manner that for a certain assigned value of that variable, its value cannot be found by simply substituting that value of the variable, the function is said to take an indeterminate form.

The most common cases occuring is that of a fraction whose numerator and denominator both vanish for the value of the variable involved.

As $f(x) \to 0$ and $g(x) \to 0$ when $x \to a$, then the quotient $\frac{f(x)}{g(x)}$ is said to have attained the indeterminate form $\frac{0}{0}$. Similarly if $\lim_{x\to a} f(x) = \infty$ and $\lim_{x\to a} g(x) = \infty$, then the fraction $\frac{f(x)}{g(x)}$ is said to have attained the indeterminate form $\frac{\infty}{\infty}$.

The other important indeterminate forms are $0 \times \infty$, $\infty - \infty$, 0°, 1^∞ and ∞^0.

- The limiting value of the indeterminate forms is also called the true value.
- The most standard form among all indeterminate forms is $\frac{0}{0}$. We reduce all other cases of limits to this form.
- It will always be assumed that $f(x)$, $g(x)$, etc. and their respective derivatives are all continuous functions.
- The true value of the indeterminate form $\frac{0}{0}$ and $\frac{\infty}{\infty}$ is determined by the application of L' Hospital Rule.

9.2 L'HOSPITAL RULE FOR INDETERMINATE FORM $\frac{0}{0}$

To find $\lim_{x\to a} \frac{f(x)}{g(x)}$ *when* $\lim_{x\to a} f(x) = 0 = \lim_{x\to a} g(x)$.

Let us assume $f(x)$ and $g(x)$ be continuous at $x = a$, then, we have

$$f(a) = \lim_{x\to a} f(x) = 0,\ g(a) = \lim_{x\to a} g(x) = 0$$

By Taylor's theorem, we have

$$f(a+h) = f(a) + hf'(a+\theta_1 h) = hf'(a+\theta_1 h),\ 0 < \theta_1 < 1$$

$$g(a+h) = g(a) + hg'(a+\theta_2 h) = hg'(a+\theta_2 h),\ 0 < \theta_2 < 1$$

Therefore

$$\lim_{x\to a} \frac{f(x)}{g(x)} = \lim_{h\to 0} \frac{f(a+h)}{g(a+h)} = \lim_{h\to 0} \frac{hf'(a+\theta_1 h)}{hg'(a+\theta_2 h)} = \lim_{h\to 0} \frac{f'(a+\theta_1 h)}{g'(a+\theta_2 h)} = \frac{f'(a)}{g'(a)} \qquad \text{(Provided } g'(a) \neq 0\text{)}$$

$$= \lim_{x \to a} \frac{f'(x)}{g'(x)}$$

$$\Rightarrow \quad \lim_{x \to a} \frac{f(x)}{g(x)} = \lim_{x \to a} \frac{f'(x)}{g'(x)}, \text{ provided } g'(a) \neq 0.$$

If $g'(a) = 0$, then this argument fails. The case when $g'(a) = 0$ but $f'(0) \neq 0$.

$$\lim_{x \to a} \frac{f'(x)}{g'(x)} \to +\infty \text{ or } -\infty$$

If $f'(a) = 0 = g'(a)$, then by Taylor's theorem, we have

$$f(a+h) = f(a) + hf'(a) + \frac{h^2}{2!} f''(a+\theta_3 h) = \frac{h^2}{2!} f''(a+\theta_3 h), \quad 0 < \theta_3 < 1$$

$$g(a+h) = g(a) + hg'(a) + \frac{h^2}{2!} g''(a+\theta_4 h) = \frac{h^2}{2!} g''(a+\theta_4 h), \quad 0 < \theta_4 < 1$$

$$\Rightarrow \quad \lim_{x \to a} \frac{f(x)}{g(x)} = \lim_{h \to a} \frac{f(a+h)}{g(a+h)} = \lim_{h \to a} \frac{f''(a+\theta_3 h)}{g''(a+\theta_4 h)} = \frac{f''(a)}{g''(a)}, \text{ provided } g''(a) \neq 0.$$

The case of failure, when $g''(a) = 0$, the limit can be determined as before.

Now, in general if

$$f(a) = f'(a) = f''(a) = \ldots = f^{n-1}(a) = 0$$

$$g(a) = g'(a) = g''(a) = \ldots = g^{n-1}(a) = 0$$

and $\quad g^n(a) \neq 0.$

Then, by Taylor's theorem, we get

$$f(a+h) = f(a) + hf'(a) + \ldots + \frac{h^{n-1}}{(n-1)!} f^{n-1}(a) + \frac{h^n}{n!} f^n(a+\theta_n h),$$

$$= \frac{h^n}{n!} f^n(a+\theta_n h). \qquad 0 < \theta_n < 1$$

and

$$g(a+h) = g(a) + hg'(a) + \ldots + \frac{h^{n-1}}{(n-1)!} g^{n-1}(a) + \frac{h^n}{n!} g^n(a+\theta_n' h),$$

$$= \frac{h^n}{n!} g^n(a+\theta_n' h). \qquad 0 < \theta_n' < 1$$

Therefore,

$$\lim_{x \to a} \frac{f(x)}{g(x)} = \lim_{h \to a} \frac{f(a+h)}{g(a+h)} = \lim_{h \to a} \frac{f^n(a+\theta_n h)}{g^n(a+\theta_n' h)} = \frac{f^n(a)}{g^n(a)}, \text{ if } g^n(a) \neq 0$$

$$\Rightarrow \quad \lim_{x \to a} \frac{f(x)}{g(x)} = \lim_{x \to a} \frac{f^n(x)}{g^n(x)}, \text{ provided } g^n(a) \neq 0.$$

9.3 L'HOSPITAL RULE FOR INDETERMINATE FORM $\frac{\infty}{\infty}$

If $\lim_{x \to a} f(x) = \infty$ *and* $\lim_{x \to a} g(x) = \infty$, *then to prove that*

$$\lim_{x \to a} \frac{f(x)}{g(x)} = \lim_{x \to a} \frac{f'(x)}{g'(x)} \textit{ provided } \lim_{x \to a} \frac{f'(x)}{g'(x)} \textit{ exists.}$$

Proof. Consider $\lim_{x \to a} \frac{f(x)}{g(x)} = \lim_{x \to a} \frac{\frac{1}{g(x)}}{\frac{1}{f(x)}} = \lim_{x \to a} \left\{ \frac{-\frac{g'(x)}{[g(x)]^2}}{-\frac{f'(x)}{[f(x)]^2}} \right\}$ $\left[\frac{0}{0} \text{form}\right]$

[By L ' Hospital rule]

$$\Rightarrow \qquad \lim_{x \to a} \frac{f(x)}{g(x)} = \lim_{x \to a} \frac{g'(x)}{f'(x)} . \lim_{x \to a} \left[\frac{f(x)}{g(x)}\right]^2 \qquad ...(1)$$

Now, let $\lim_{x \to a} \frac{f(x)}{g(x)} = l.$ ...(2)

Then there are following three cases :

Case (i) If $l \neq 0$ and $l \neq \infty$.

In this case, (1) becomes

$$l = \lim_{x \to a} \frac{g'(x)}{f'(x)} . l^2 \quad \Rightarrow \quad \frac{1}{l} = \lim_{x \to a} \frac{g'(x)}{f'(x)}$$

$$\Rightarrow \qquad \lim_{x \to a} \frac{f'(x)}{g'(x)} = l = \lim_{x \to a} \frac{f(x)}{g(x)}$$ [Using (2)]

Case (ii) If $l = 0$.

In this case, adding 1 to each side of (2), we get

$$l + 1 = \lim_{x \to a} \frac{f(x)}{g(x)} + 1 = \lim_{x \to a} \frac{f(x) + g(x)}{g(x)} = \lim_{x \to a} \frac{f'(x) + g'(x)}{g'(x)}$$ [By case (i)]

$$= \lim_{x \to a} \frac{f'(x)}{g'(x)} + 1 \quad \Rightarrow \quad l = \lim_{x \to a} \frac{f'(x)}{g'(x)}$$

Case (iii) Let $l = \infty$

In this case, by reciprocating, we have

$$\lim_{x \to a} \frac{g(x)}{f(x)} = 0$$

By case (ii) $0 = \lim_{x \to a} \frac{g(x)}{f(x)} = \lim_{x \to a} \frac{g'(x)}{f'(x)}$

Therefore, $\lim_{x \to a} \frac{f'(x)}{g'(x)} = \infty$

Hence, the result $\lim_{x \to a} \frac{f(x)}{g(x)} = \lim_{x \to a} \frac{f'(x)}{g'(x)}$ has been established in every case.

- The above result can be extended to the case when $x \to \infty$, *i.e.*, we can show that

$$\lim_{x \to \infty} \frac{f(x)}{g(x)} = \lim_{x \to \infty} \frac{f'(x)}{g'(x)}$$

Let $x = \frac{1}{y}$ then

$$\lim_{x\to\infty}\frac{f(x)}{g(x)}=\lim_{y\to 0}\frac{f\left(\frac{1}{y}\right)}{g\left(\frac{1}{y}\right)}=\lim_{y\to 0}\frac{f'\left(\frac{1}{y}\right)\left(-\frac{1}{y^2}\right)}{g'\left(\frac{1}{y}\right)\left(-\frac{1}{y^2}\right)}=\lim_{y\to 0}\frac{f'\left(\frac{1}{y}\right)}{g'\left(\frac{1}{y}\right)}=\lim_{x\to\infty}\frac{f'(x)}{g'(x)}$$

- While evaluating $\lim_{x\to\infty}\frac{f(x)}{g(x)}$ when it is of the form $\frac{\infty}{\infty}$, care must be taken to change over to the form $\frac{0}{0}$ as early as possible, otherwise process of differentiating the numerator and denominator may never terminate.
- While appplying L' Hospital rule, we are not to differentiate $\frac{f(x)}{g(x)}$ by the rule for finding the differential coefficient of the quotient of two functions, but we are to differentiate the numerator and denominator separately.
- It must be remember that $\log 1 = 0$, $\log 0 = -\infty$, and $\log \infty = \infty$.

Solved Examples

1. *Find* $\lim_{x\to 0}\frac{e^x-e^{\sin x}}{x-\sin x}$.

SOLUTION. We have $\lim_{x\to 0}\frac{e^x-e^{\sin x}}{x-\sin x}$ $\left|\frac{0}{0}\right.$ form

$$=\lim_{x\to 0}\frac{e^x-e^{\sin x}.\cos x}{1-\cos x}\quad\left|\frac{0}{0}\right.\text{ form}$$

$$=\lim_{x\to 0}\frac{e^x-[\cos x\cdot e^{\sin x}\cdot\cos x+e^{\sin x}(-\sin x)]}{\sin x}$$

$$=\lim_{x\to 0}\frac{e^x-e^{\sin x}[\cos^2 x-\sin x]}{\sin x}$$

$\left|\frac{0}{0}\right.$ form

$$=\lim_{x\to 0}\frac{\{e^x-e^{\sin x}[2\cos x(-\sin x)-\cos x]-[(\cos^2 x-\sin x)e^{x\sin x}\cos x]\}}{\cos x}$$

$$=\lim_{x\to 0}\frac{e^x-e^{\sin x}[-\sin 2x-\cos x+\cos^3 x-\sin x\cos x]}{\cos x}$$

$$=\frac{1-1(-1+1)}{1}=\frac{1}{1}=1$$

2. *Find* $\lim_{x\to 0}\frac{x\cos x-\log(1+x)}{x^2}$

[KANPUR(BCA)-2008; MEERUT(BCA)-2009, 12]

SOLUTION. We have $\lim_{x\to 0}\frac{x\cos x-\log(1+x)}{x^2}$

$$=\lim_{x\to 0}\frac{x\left(1-\frac{x^2}{2!}+\frac{x^4}{4!}-....\right)-\left(x-\frac{x^2}{2}+\frac{x^3}{3}-...\right)}{x^2}$$

$\left|\frac{0}{0}\right.$ form

$$=\lim_{x\to 0}\left(\frac{\frac{x^2}{2}-\frac{5}{6}x^3+....}{x^2}\right)$$

$$=\lim_{x\to 0}\left(\frac{1}{2}-\frac{5}{6}x+\text{terms containing } x\right)$$

$$=\frac{1}{2}.$$

3. *Find* $\lim_{x\to 0}\frac{\cosh x-\cos x}{x\sin x}$.

SOLUTION. Since we have $\lim_{x\to 0}\frac{\cosh x-\cos x}{x\sin x}$

$\left|\frac{0}{0}\right.$ form

$$=\lim_{x\to 0}\left[\left(\frac{\cosh x-\cos x}{x^2}\right)\left(\frac{x}{\sin x}\right)\right]$$

$$= \lim_{x \to 0} \frac{\cosh x - \cos x}{x^2} \qquad \left| \frac{0}{0} \text{ form} \right.$$

$$= \lim_{x \to 0} \frac{\sinh x + \sin x}{2x} \qquad \left| \frac{0}{0} \text{ form} \right.$$

$$= \lim_{x \to 0} \frac{\cosh x + \cos x}{2} = \frac{1+1}{2} = 1.$$

4. *Find* $\lim_{x \to 0} \frac{(1+x)^{1/x} - e}{x}$.

[MEERUT(BCA)–2003, 12, 13]

SOLUTION. We have $\lim_{x \to 0} \frac{(1+x)^{1/x} - e}{x} \quad \left| \frac{0}{0} \text{ form} \right.$

$$\lim_{x \to 0} \frac{(1+x)^{1/x} - e}{x}$$

$$= \lim_{x \to 0} \frac{e\left[1 - \frac{1}{2}x + \frac{11}{24}x^2 + \ldots\right] - e}{x}$$

$$= \lim_{x \to 0} \frac{e\left[-\frac{1}{2}x + \frac{11}{24}x^2 + \ldots\right]}{x} = -\frac{1}{2}e.$$

5. *Find* $\lim_{x \to 0} \frac{\log \sin 2x}{\log \sin x}$.

[MEERUT(BCA)–2011, 17]

SOLUTION. We have $\lim_{x \to 0} \frac{\log \sin 2x}{\log \sin x} \quad \left| \frac{\infty}{\infty} \text{ form} \right.$

$$= \lim_{x \to 0} \frac{\left(\frac{2}{\sin 2x}\right) \cos 2x}{\left(\frac{1}{\sin x}\right) . \cos x}$$

$$= \lim_{x \to 0} \frac{2 \cot 2x}{\cot x} \qquad \left| \frac{\infty}{\infty} \text{ form} \right.$$

$$= \lim_{x \to 0} \frac{-4 \operatorname{cosec}^2 2x}{-\operatorname{cosec}^2 x} \qquad \left| \frac{\infty}{\infty} \text{ form} \right.$$

$$= \lim_{x \to 0} \frac{4 \sin^2 x}{\sin^2 2x} \qquad \left| \frac{0}{0} \text{ form} \right.$$

$$= \lim_{x \to 0} \frac{4 \sin^2 x}{(2 \sin x \cos x)^2}$$

$$= \lim_{x \to 0} \frac{1}{\cos^2 x} = 1.$$

6. *Find* $\lim_{x \to 0} \frac{\log \log (1 - x^2)}{\log \log \cos x}$.

SOLUTION. We have $\lim_{x \to 0} \frac{\log \log (1 - x^2)}{\log \log \cos x}$

$$\left| \frac{\infty}{\infty} \text{ form} \right.$$

$$= \lim_{x \to 0} \frac{\frac{1}{\log (1 - x^2)} \cdot \frac{1}{(1 - x^2)} (-2x)}{\frac{1}{\log \cos x} \cdot \frac{1}{\cos x} \cdot (-\sin x)}$$

$$= 2 \lim_{x \to 0} \frac{x \cos x \log \cos x}{\sin x (1 - x^2) \log (1 - x^2)}$$

$$= \left(2 \lim_{x \to 0} \frac{x}{\sin x}\right)\left(\lim_{x \to 0} \frac{\cos x}{1 - x^2}\right) \cdot \left(\lim_{x \to 0} \frac{\log \cos x}{\log (1 - x^2)}\right)$$

$$= 2 \times 1 \times 1 \times \lim_{x \to 0} \frac{\log \cos x}{\log (1 - x^2)} \qquad \left| \frac{0}{0} \text{ form} \right.$$

$$= 2 \lim_{x \to 0} \frac{\frac{1}{\cos x} \cdot (-\sin x)}{\frac{1}{(1 - x^2)} \cdot (-2x)}$$

$$= 2 \times \frac{1}{2} \cdot \lim_{x \to 0} \left(\frac{\sin x}{x} \cdot \frac{1 - x^2}{\cos x}\right) = 1.$$

7. *Find* $\lim_{x \to \infty} \frac{x^n}{e^x}$, *where n is a positive integer.*

SOLUTION. We have $\lim_{x \to \infty} \frac{x^n}{e^x}$

$$= \lim_{x \to \infty} \frac{n x^{n-1}}{e^x} \qquad \left| \frac{\infty}{\infty} \text{ form} \right.$$

$$= \lim_{x \to \infty} \frac{n(n-1) x^{n-2}}{e^x} \qquad \left| \frac{\infty}{\infty} \text{ form} \right.$$

Repeating this process, we get

$$= \lim_{x \to \infty} \frac{[n(n-1)(n-2) \ldots n \text{ factors}]}{e^x}$$

$$= \lim_{x\to\infty} \frac{n!}{e^x} = \frac{n!}{e^\infty} = \frac{n!}{\infty} = 0.$$

8. *Find* $\lim_{x\to\frac{\pi}{2}} \dfrac{\log\left(x-\frac{\pi}{2}\right)}{\tan x}$.

SOLUTION. We have $\lim_{x\to\frac{\pi}{2}} \dfrac{\log\left(x-\frac{\pi}{2}\right)}{\tan x}$

$$= \lim_{x\to\frac{\pi}{2}} \left(\frac{\frac{1}{x-\pi/2}}{\sec^2 x}\right) \qquad \left|\frac{\infty}{\infty}\right. \text{ form}$$

$$= \lim_{x\to\frac{\pi}{2}} \left(\frac{\frac{1}{x-\pi/2}}{\frac{1}{\cos^2 x}}\right) = \lim_{x\to\frac{\pi}{2}} \left(\frac{\cos^2 x}{x-\pi/2}\right) \qquad \left|\frac{0}{0}\right. \text{ form}$$

$$= \lim_{x\to\frac{\pi}{2}} \left(\frac{-2\cos x \sin x}{1}\right)$$

$$= -2\cos\frac{\pi}{2}.\sin\frac{\pi}{2} = 0.$$

9. *Find the following limits :*

(*i*) $\lim_{x\to 0} \dfrac{\log x}{\cot x}$ [MEERUT(BCA)–2000, 01]

(*ii*) $\lim_{x\to 0} \dfrac{\tan x - x}{x^2 \tan x}$

[MEERUT(BCA)–2003, 07, 10]

SOLUTION. (i) We have $\lim_{x\to 0} \dfrac{\log x}{\cot x}$ $\left|\frac{\infty}{\infty}\right.$ form

$$= \lim_{x\to 0} \frac{1/x}{-\text{cosec}^2 x} = -\lim_{x\to 0} \frac{\sin^2 x}{x}$$

$$= -\lim_{x\to 0} \left(\frac{\sin x}{x}\right)\cdot \sin x$$

$$\left[\because \lim_{x\to 0}\left(\frac{\sin x}{x}\right) = 1\right]$$

$$= -1\times 0 = 0.$$

(ii) We have $\lim_{x\to 0} \dfrac{\tan x - x}{x^2 \tan x}$

$$\left[\because \tan x = x + \frac{x^3}{3} + \frac{2}{15}x^5 + \ldots\right]$$

$$= \lim_{x\to 0} \frac{\left(x + \frac{x^3}{3} + \frac{2}{15}x^5 + \ldots\right) - x}{x^2\left(x + \frac{x^3}{3} + \frac{2}{15}x^5 + \ldots\right)}$$

$$= \lim_{x\to 0} \frac{\frac{x^3}{3} + \frac{2}{15}x^5 + \ldots}{x^3 + \frac{x^5}{3} + \frac{2}{15}x^7 + \ldots}$$

$$= \lim_{x\to 0} \frac{x^3\left(\frac{1}{3} + \frac{2}{15}x^2 + \ldots\right)}{x^3\left(1 + \frac{x^2}{3} + \frac{2}{15}x^4 + \ldots\right)}$$

$$= \lim_{x\to 0} \frac{\frac{1}{3} + \frac{2}{15}x^2 + \ldots}{1 + \frac{x^2}{3} + \frac{2}{15}x^4 + \ldots} = \frac{\frac{1}{3}}{1} = \frac{1}{3}.$$

10. *Evaluate :* $\lim_{x\to 1} \dfrac{x^x - x}{x - 1 - \log x}$.

SOLUTION. $\lim_{x\to 1} \dfrac{x^x - x}{x - 1 - \log x}$ $\left|\frac{0}{0}\right.$ form

$$= \lim_{x\to 1} \frac{x^x(1+\log x) - 1}{1 - \frac{1}{x}}$$

(By L' Hospital Rule)

$\left|\frac{0}{0}\right.$ form

$$= \lim_{x\to 1} \frac{\frac{d}{dx}(x^x)(1+\log x) + x^x\left(\frac{1}{x}\right) - 0}{1/x^2}$$

$$= \lim_{x\to 1} \frac{x^x(1+\log x)^2 + x^x\left(\frac{1}{x}\right)}{x^{-2}}$$

$$= \frac{1.(1+0)^2 + 1.1}{1} = 2.$$

Exercise-9.1

1. Evaluate the following limits :

(i) $\lim_{x\to 0}\frac{x-\sin x}{x^3}$ [MEERUT(BCA)–2009, 11]

(ii) $\lim_{x\to 0}\frac{1-\cos x}{x^2}$

(iii) $\lim_{x\to 0}\frac{a^x-b^x}{x}$ [KANPUR(BCA)–2011, 14; ROHILKHAND(BCA)–2005, 12]

(iv) $\lim_{x\to 1}\frac{\log x}{x-1}$

(v) $\lim_{x\to 0}\frac{(1+x)^n-1}{x}$

(vi) $\lim_{x\to 0}\frac{xe^x-\log(1+x)}{x^2}$ [VTU–2004; OSMANIA–2000; KANPUR(BCA)–1999, AGRA(BCA)–2006]

(vii) $\lim_{x\to a}\frac{a^x-x^a}{x^x-a^a}$

(viii) $\lim_{x\to 0}\frac{5\sin x-7\sin 2x+3\sin 3x}{\tan x-x}$

(ix) $\lim_{x\to 0}\frac{\sin 2x+a\sin x}{x^2}$

(x) $\lim_{x\to 0}\frac{[\cosh x+\log(1-x)-1+x]}{x^2}$

(xi) $\lim_{x\to 1}\frac{x^5-2x^3-4x^2+9x-4}{x^4-2x^3+2x-1}$ [ROHILKHAND(BCA)–2002, 12]

2. Evaluate $\lim_{x\to 0}\frac{\sin x\sin^{-1}x-x^2}{x^6}$. [MEERUT(BCA)–2006; KANPUR(BCA)–1992, 2004]

3. Evaluate $\lim_{x\to 0}\frac{(1+x)^{1/x}-e+\frac{1}{2}ex}{x^2}$.

4. Evaluate the following limits :

(i) $\lim_{x\to\infty}\frac{a^{1/x}-b^{1/x}}{\log\left(\frac{x}{x-1}\right)}$

(ii) $\lim_{x\to\pi/2}\frac{\left(\frac{\pi}{2}-x\right)^2\sin x}{\cos^2 x}$

(iii) $\lim_{x\to 0}\frac{e^x+\log\left(\frac{1-x}{e}\right)}{\tan x-x}$

(iv) $\lim_{x\to 0+}\frac{3^x-2^x}{\sqrt{x}}$

5. (i) If $\lim_{y\to 0}\frac{re^y-q\cos y+pe^{-y}}{y\tan y}=3$, find the vlaues of p, q, and r. (MUMBAI–2009)

(ii) Find the values of a and b in order that

$$\lim_{x\to 0}\frac{x(1+a\cos x)-b\sin x}{x^3}$$

may be equatl to 1. (MUMBAI–2007)

(iii) If $\lim_{x\to 0}\frac{\sin 2x+a\sin x}{x^3}$ be finite, find the value of a and the limit. (NAGPUR–2009)

6. Evaluate the following limits :

(i) $\lim_{x\to 0}\frac{\log x^2}{\cot x^2}$

(ii) $\lim_{x\to a}\frac{\log(x-a)}{\log(e^x-e^a)}$

(iii) $\lim_{x\to 1-0}\frac{\log(1-x)}{\cot\pi x}$

(iv) $\lim_{x\to\infty}\frac{\log x}{a^x}, a>1$

(v) $\lim_{x\to\pi/2}\frac{\tan x}{\tan 3x}$

Hints to the Selected Problems

1. (i) $\lim_{x\to 0}\frac{x-\sin x}{x^3}=\lim_{x\to 0}\frac{x-\left(x-\frac{x^3}{3!}+\frac{x^5}{5!}-\ldots\right)}{x^3}$

$$=\lim_{x\to 0}\left\{\frac{\frac{x^3}{3!}-\frac{x^5}{5!}+\ldots}{x^3}\right\}$$

$$= \lim_{x\to 0}\left[\frac{1}{3!}-\frac{x^2}{5!}+\ldots\right] = \frac{1}{3!} = \frac{1}{6}.$$

(vii) $\lim_{x\to a}\frac{a^x - x^a}{x^x - a^a} = \lim_{x\to a}\frac{a^x \log a - a.x^{a-1}}{x^x(1+\log x)}$

$$= \frac{a^a \log a - a^a}{a^a(1+\log a)}$$

$$= \frac{\log a - 1}{\log a + 1}.$$

5. (i) If $r - q + p = 0$, ...(1)

we obtained $\frac{0}{0}$ form, Then we have

$$\lim_{y\to 0}\frac{re^y + q\sin y + pe^{-y}}{y\sec^2 y + \tan y}$$

Again if $r - p = 0$, ...(2)

We obtained $\frac{0}{0}$ form. Then we have

$$\lim_{y\to 0}\frac{re^y + q\cos y + pe^{-y}}{\sec^2 y + 2y\sec^2 y\tan y + \sec^2 y}$$

$\Rightarrow \quad r + q + p = 6$ ...(3)

Now solving (1), (2) and (3).

6. (iv) $\lim_{x\to\infty}\frac{\log x}{a^x}, a > 1$ $\quad\left|\text{form } \frac{\infty}{\infty}\right.$

$$= \lim_{x\to\infty}\frac{1/x}{a^x \log a} = \frac{1}{\log a}\lim_{x\to\infty}\frac{1}{xa^x}$$

$$= \frac{1}{\log a}.0 = 0.$$

ANSWERS

1. (i) $\frac{1}{6}$ (ii) $\frac{1}{2}$ (iii) $\log\frac{a}{b}$ (iv) 1 (v) n (vi) $\frac{3}{2}$ (vii) $\frac{\log a - 1}{\log a + 1}$ (viii) – 15 (ix) $\begin{cases}\infty \text{ if } a \neq -2\\ 0 \text{ if } a = -2\end{cases}$ (x) 0 (xi) 4

2. $\frac{1}{18}$ **3.** $\frac{11e}{24}$ **4.** (i) $\log\frac{a}{b}$ (ii) 1 (iii) $-\frac{1}{2}$ (iv) 0

5. (i) $p = \frac{3}{2}, q = 3, r = \frac{3}{2}$ (ii) $a = -\frac{5}{2}, b = -\frac{3}{2}$ (iii) $\begin{cases}-1 \text{ if } a = -2\\ \infty \text{ if } a \neq -2\end{cases}$ **6.** (i) 0 (ii) 1 (iii) 0 (iv) 0 (v) 3

9.4 THE INDETERMINATE FORM $0\times\infty$

To find $\lim_{x\to a}[f(x).g(x)]$, *when* $\lim_{x\to a} f(x) = 0$ *and* $\lim_{x\to a} g(x) = \infty$.

To determine this limit, the product may be transformed into the form $\frac{0}{0}$ or $\frac{\infty}{\infty}$, using any one of the following relations

$$f(x)\cdot g(x) = \frac{f(x)}{\frac{1}{g(x)}} \quad \text{or} \quad f(x)\cdot g(x) = \frac{g(x)}{\frac{1}{f(x)}}$$

and then apply previous method.

Solved Examples

1. *Evaluate* $\lim_{x\to 0^+}(x\log x)$.

SOLUTION. $\lim_{x\to 0^+}(x\log x) = \lim_{x\to 0^+}\frac{\log x}{1/x}$ $\left|\frac{\infty}{\infty}\right.$ form

$$= \lim_{x\to 0^+}\frac{1/x}{-1/x^2}$$

$$= \lim_{x\to 0^+}(-x) = 0.$$

2. *Evaluate* $\lim_{x\to 0} x\log\sin x$.

SOLUTION. $\lim_{x\to 0} x\log\sin x$ $\quad |0\times\infty$ from

$$= \lim_{x\to 0}\left(\frac{\log\sin x}{1/x}\right) \quad \left|\frac{\infty}{\infty}\right. \text{ form}$$

$$= \lim_{x \to 0} \frac{(1/\sin x)\cdot\cos x}{-1/x^2} \qquad \left|\frac{\infty}{\infty}\right. \text{form}$$

$$= \lim_{x \to 0} \frac{-x^2 \cos x}{\sin x} \qquad \left|\frac{0}{0}\right. \text{form}$$

$$= \lim_{x \to 0} \frac{x^2 \sin x - 2x\cos x}{\cos x} = 0.$$

9.5 THE INDETERMINATE FORM ∞ − ∞

To determine $\lim_{x \to a} [f(x) - g(x)]$, *when* $\lim_{x \to a} f(x) = \infty = \lim_{x \to \infty} g(x)$.

Here, this can be reduced to the form $\frac{0}{0}$ by the relation

$$f(x) - g(x) = \left\{ \frac{\left[\dfrac{1}{g(x)} - \dfrac{1}{f(x)}\right]}{\dfrac{1}{f(x)\cdot g(x)}} \right\}$$

and then evaluate by previous method

WORKING PROCEDURE

STEP 1. Change all trigonometric-ratio into $\sin x$ and $\cos x$ (if *T*-ratio are present)

STEP 2. Take L.C.M.

Now the indeterminate form is reduced into $\frac{0}{0}$ form.

Solved Examples

1. *Evaluate* $\lim_{x \to 0} \left(\frac{1}{x^2} - \frac{1}{\sin^2 x} \right)$.

[KANPUR(BCA)–1996, 2006, 09, 13; MEERUT(BCA)–2000, 06, 13]

SOLUTION. $\lim_{x \to 0} \left(\frac{1}{x^2} - \frac{1}{\sin^2 x} \right) \qquad |\infty - \infty$ form

$$= \lim_{x \to 0} \frac{\sin^2 x - x^2}{x^2 \sin^2 x} \qquad \left|\frac{0}{0}\right. \text{form}$$

$$= \lim_{x \to 0} \frac{\left(x - \dfrac{x^3}{3!} + \ldots\right)^2 - x^2}{x^2 \left(x - \dfrac{x^3}{3!} + \ldots\right)^2}$$

$$= \lim_{x \to 0} \frac{-\dfrac{2x^4}{3!} + \text{terms containing higher powers of } x}{x^4 + \text{terms containing higher power of } x}$$

$$= \lim_{x \to 0} \frac{-\dfrac{2}{3!} + \text{terms containing } x \text{ in the numerator}}{1 + \text{terms containing } x \text{ in the numerator}}$$

$$= -\frac{2}{3!} = -\frac{1}{3}$$

2. *Evaluate* $\lim_{x \to \pi/2} (\sec x - \tan x)$.

SOLUTION. We have $\lim_{x \to \pi/2} (\sec x - \tan x) \qquad |\infty - \infty$ form

$$= \lim_{x \to \pi/2} \left(\frac{1}{\cos x} - \frac{\sin x}{\cos x} \right) \qquad \left|\frac{0}{0}\right. \text{form}$$

$$= \lim_{x \to \pi/2} \left(\frac{1 - \sin x}{\cos x} \right)$$

$$= \lim_{x \to \pi/2} \frac{-\cos x}{-\sin x}$$

$$= \lim_{x \to \pi/2} \cot x = 0.$$

3. *Evaluate* $\lim_{x\to\pi/2}\left(\sec x - \frac{1}{1-\sin x}\right)$.

SOLUTION. We have $\lim_{x\to\pi/2}\left(\sec x - \frac{1}{1-\sin x}\right)$

| $\infty - \infty$ form

$$= \lim_{x\to\pi/2}\left(\frac{1}{\cos x} - \frac{1}{1-\sin x}\right)$$

| $\infty - \infty$ form

$$= \lim_{x\to\pi/2}\left(\frac{1-\sin x-\cos x}{\cos x - \cos x\sin x}\right)$$

$\left|\frac{0}{0}\right.$ form

$$= \lim_{x\to\pi/2}\frac{-\cos x+\sin x}{-\sin x+\sin^2 x-\cos^2 x}$$

$$= \frac{-0+1}{-1+1-0} = \infty.$$

9.6 THE INDETERMINATE FORM $0^\circ, 1^\infty, \infty^\circ$

To determine $\lim_{x\to a}[f(x)]^{g(x)}$ *when the limit is of the form* 0°, 1^∞, ∞°

Let $\quad y = [f(x)]^{g(x)}$

Taking logs; $\quad \log y = g(x)\log f(x)$

The RHS assumes the indeterminate forms $0 \times \infty$ in each of these above cases. The limit can, therefore, be determined by the method used in the article 9.4.

Suppose $\lim_{x\to a}[g(x)\log f(x)] = l$ (say)

$$\Rightarrow \lim_{x\to a}\log y = l \Rightarrow \lim_{x\to a}[\log y] = l$$

$$\Rightarrow \lim_{x\to a} y = e^l \Rightarrow \lim_{x\to a}[f(x)]^{g(x)} = e^l.$$

WORKING PROCEDURE

STEP 1. Let the given limit = y.

STEP 2. Take logs on both sides to get the forms $0 \times \infty$ and proceed by the method of the type $0 \times \infty$.

Solved Examples

1. *Evaluate* $\lim_{\theta\to\frac{\pi}{2}}(\cos\theta)^{\cos\theta}$.

[MEERUT(BCA)-2001, 02, 06, 14; BIKANER-2014]

SOLUTION. Let $y = (\cos\theta)^{\cos\theta}$ $\quad$ |0° form

Taking logs,

$\log y = \cos\theta \log\cos\theta$

$$\therefore \lim_{\theta\to\frac{\pi}{2}}(\log y) = \lim_{\theta\to\frac{\pi}{2}}\cos\theta\log\cos\theta$$

|$0 \times \infty$ form

$$= \lim_{\theta\to\frac{\pi}{2}}\frac{\log\cos\theta}{\sec\theta} \quad \left|\frac{\infty}{\infty}\right. \text{ form}$$

$$= \lim_{\theta\to\frac{\pi}{2}}\frac{\frac{1}{\cos\theta}\times -\sin\theta}{\sec\theta\tan\theta}$$

$$= \lim_{\theta\to\frac{\pi}{2}}(-\cos\theta) = 0$$

$$\Rightarrow \lim_{\theta\to\frac{\pi}{2}}(\log y) = 0$$

$$\Rightarrow \log\left(\lim_{\theta\to\frac{\pi}{2}} y\right) = 0 \Rightarrow \lim_{\theta\to\frac{\pi}{2}} y = e^0 = 1$$

$$\Rightarrow \lim_{\theta\to\frac{\pi}{2}}(\cos\theta)^{\cos\theta} = 1.$$

2. *Find* $\lim_{x\to 0}\left(\frac{\tan x}{x}\right)^{1/x^2}$.

[KANPUR(BCA)–1997, 2009, 13; MEERUT(BCA)–2000, 03, 07, 16]

SOLUTION. Let $y = \left(\frac{\tan x}{x}\right)^{1/x^2}$

$|1^\infty$ form for $x = 0$

$$\Rightarrow \log y = \frac{1}{x^2}\log\frac{\tan x}{x}$$

$$\Rightarrow \lim_{x\to 0}\log y = \lim_{x\to 0}\frac{1}{x^2}\log\frac{\tan x}{x}$$

$$= \lim_{x\to 0}\frac{\log\frac{\tan x}{x}}{x^2} \qquad \left|\frac{0}{0}\right. \text{ form}$$

$$= \lim_{x\to 0}\left\{\frac{1\left[\frac{x\sec^2 x - \tan x}{x^2}\right]}{\frac{\left(\frac{\tan x}{x}\right)}{2x}}\right\}$$

$$= \lim_{x\to 0}\frac{x\sec^2 x - \tan x}{2x^3}$$

$$\left|\therefore \lim_{x\to 0}\frac{\tan x}{x} = 1\right|$$

$$= \lim_{x\to 0}\frac{x.2\sec x\sec x\tan x + \sec^2 x - \sec^2 x}{6x^2}$$

$$= \lim_{x\to 0}\frac{2x\tan x\sec^2 x}{6x^2}$$

$$= \lim_{x\to 0}\frac{\tan x\sec^2 x}{3x}$$

$$= \lim_{x\to 0}\left(\frac{1}{3}\cdot\frac{\tan x}{x}\cdot\sec^2 x\right)$$

$$= \lim_{x\to 0}\frac{1}{3}\times 1\times\sec^2 x = \frac{1}{3}$$

$$\therefore \qquad \lim_{x\to 0} y = e^{1/3}$$

$$\Rightarrow \lim_{x\to 0}\left(\frac{\tan x}{x}\right)^{1/x^2} = e^{1/3}.$$

3. *Evaluate* $\lim_{x\to 0}\left(\frac{\sin x}{x}\right)^{1/x}$.

[ROHILKHAND(BCA)–2005; MEERUT(BCA)–2005, 08, 11; KURUKSHETRA–2010]

SOLUTION. Let $\quad y = \lim_{x\to 0}\left(\frac{\sin x}{x}\right)^{1/x}$

$$\therefore \log y = \lim_{x\to 0}\left(\frac{1}{x}\log\frac{\sin x}{x}\right)$$

$$= \lim_{x\to 0}\frac{1}{x}\log\left\{\frac{x - \frac{x^3}{3!} + \frac{x^5}{5!} - \ldots}{x}\right\}$$

$$= \lim_{x\to 0}\frac{1}{x}\log\left(1 - \frac{x^2}{3!} + \frac{x^4}{5!} - \ldots\right)$$

$$= \lim_{x\to 0}\frac{1}{x}\log\left[1 - \left(\frac{x^2}{6} - \frac{x^4}{120} + \ldots\right)\right]$$

$$= \lim_{x\to 0}\frac{1}{x}\log(1 - z)$$

where $z = \frac{x^2}{6} - \frac{x^4}{120} + \ldots$

$$= \lim_{x\to 0}\frac{1}{x}\left(-z - \frac{z^2}{2} - \ldots\right)$$

$$= \lim_{x\to 0}\frac{1}{x}\left[-\left(\frac{x^2}{6} - \frac{x^4}{120} + \ldots\right) - \frac{1}{2}\left(\frac{x^2}{6} - \frac{x^4}{120} + \ldots\right)^2 - \ldots\right]$$

$$= \lim_{x\to 0}\frac{1}{x}\left[-\frac{x^2}{6} + \left(\frac{x^4}{120} - \frac{x^4}{72}\right) + \ldots\right]$$

$$= \lim_{x\to 0}\frac{1}{x}\left[-\frac{x^2}{6} + \frac{x^4}{180} + \ldots\right]$$

$$= \lim_{x\to 0}\left[-\frac{x}{6} + \frac{x^3}{180} + \ldots\right] = 0$$

Hence, $\qquad y = e^0 = 1.$

4. *Evaluate* $\lim_{x\to 0}(\operatorname{cosec} x)^{1/\log x}$.

SOLUTION. We have

$$y = \lim_{x\to 0}(\operatorname{cosec} x)^{1/\log x} \qquad |\infty^\circ \text{ form}$$

$$\therefore \log y = \lim_{x\to 0}\frac{1}{\log x}(\log\operatorname{cosec} x)$$

$$\left|\frac{\infty}{\infty}\right. \text{ form}$$

$$= \lim_{x\to 0} \frac{\left(\frac{1}{\operatorname{cosec} x}\right)(-\operatorname{cosec} x \cot x)}{1/x}$$

$$= \lim_{x\to 0} \left(-\frac{x}{\tan x}\right) \qquad \left|\frac{0}{0}\right. \text{ form}$$

$$= \lim_{x\to 0} \left(-\frac{1}{\sec^2 x}\right) = -1$$

$$\Rightarrow y = e^{-1} = \frac{1}{e}.$$

5. *Evaluate the following limits :*

(*i*) $\lim_{x\to 0} (\cos x)^{\cot x}$

[KANPUR(BCA)–2001, 04, 13]

(*ii*) $\lim_{x\to 0} \frac{e^x - e^{-x} - 2\log(1+x)}{x \sin x}$

[MEERUT(BCA)–2006]

SOLUTION. (i) Let $y = \lim_{x\to 0} (\cos x)^{\cot x}$

$$\log y = \lim_{x\to 0} \log(\cos x)^{\cot x}$$

$$= \lim_{x\to 0} \cot \log \cos x$$

$$\log y = \lim_{x\to 0} \frac{\log \cos x}{\tan x}$$

$$= \lim_{x\to 0} \frac{(-\sin x)}{\cos x \cdot \sec^2 x}$$

$$= \lim_{x\to 0} \frac{-\sin x}{\sec x}$$

$$= \lim_{x\to 0} -\sin x \cos x$$

$$= \lim_{x\to 0} -\frac{\sin 2x}{2\cdot x}.x$$

$$= -\lim_{x\to 0}\left(\frac{\sin 2x}{2x}\right)\cdot \lim_{x\to 0} x$$

$$= -1\times 0.$$

$$\therefore \log y = 0 \Rightarrow y = e^0 \Rightarrow y = 1.$$

(ii) We have

$$\lim_{x\to 0} \frac{e^x - e^{-x} - 2\log(1-x)}{x \sin x}$$

$$\left|\frac{0}{0}\right. \text{ form}$$

$$= \lim_{x\to 0} \frac{e^x + e^{-x} - \frac{2}{1+x}}{x\cos x + \sin x} \qquad \left|\frac{0}{0}\right. \text{ form}$$

$$= \lim_{x\to 0} \frac{e^x - e^{-x} + \frac{2}{(1+x)^2}}{2\cos x - x \sin x}$$

$$= \frac{e^0 - e^0 + \frac{2}{(1+0)^2}}{2\cdot \cos 0 - 0}$$

$$= \frac{1 - 1 + \frac{2}{(1+0)^2}}{2\cdot\cos 0 - 0} = \frac{2}{2} = 1.$$

6. *Find* $\lim_{x\to 0}\left(\frac{\tan x}{x}\right)^{1/x^3}$.

SOLUTION. Let $y = \lim_{x\to 0}\left(\frac{\tan x}{x}\right)^{1/x^3}$

$$\log y = \lim_{x\to 0} \frac{1}{x^3} \log_e\left(\frac{\tan x}{x}\right)$$

$$= \lim_{x\to 0} \frac{\log_e \tan x - \log_e x}{x^3} \qquad \left|\frac{0}{0}\right. \text{ form}$$

$$= \lim_{x\to 0} \frac{\frac{\sec^2 x}{\tan x} - \frac{1}{x}}{3x^2} = \lim_{x\to 0} \frac{\frac{2x}{\sin 2x} - \frac{1}{x}}{3x^2}$$

$$= \lim_{x\to 0} \frac{2x - \sin 2x}{3x^2 \sin 2x} \qquad \left|\frac{0}{0}\right. \text{ form}$$

$$= \lim_{x\to 0} \frac{2 - 2\cos 2x}{6x^2 \sin 2x + 6x^3 \cos 2x}$$

$$\left|\frac{0}{0}\right. \text{ form}$$

$$= \lim_{x\to 0} \frac{2\sin 2x}{15x^2 \cos 2x + 6x \sin 2x - 6x^3 \sin 2x}$$

$$\left|\frac{0}{0}\right. \text{ form}$$

$$= \lim_{x\to 0} \frac{4\cos 2x}{-30x^2\sin 2x + 30x\cos 2x + 6\sin 2x + 12x\cos 2x - 18x^2\sin 2x - 12x^3\cos 2x}$$

$$= \frac{4}{0} = \infty$$

Hence, $y = e^{\infty} = \infty$.

Exercise-9.2

1. Evaluate the following limits :

(i) $\lim\limits_{x\to 0} x\log\tan x$ (ii) $\lim\limits_{x\to 0} \tan\left(\frac{\pi}{2} - x\right)$

(iii) $\lim\limits_{x\to\infty} 2^x \sin\frac{a}{2^x}$ (iv) $\lim\limits_{x\to\infty} (a^{1/x} - 1)\cdot x$

(v) $\lim\limits_{x\to 1} \sec\frac{\pi}{2x}\log x$

[MEERUT(BCA)–2002, 13]

(vi) $\lim\limits_{x\to 0} x^m(\log x)^n \ m; n \in \mathbf{Z}^+$.

2. Evaluate the following limits :

(i) $\lim\limits_{x\to 0}\left[\frac{1}{x} - \frac{1}{x^2}\log(1+x)\right]$

(ii) $\lim\limits_{x\to 2}\left[\frac{1}{x-2} - \frac{1}{\log(x-1)}\right]$

(iii) $\lim\limits_{x\to 0}\left[\frac{1}{x^2} - \operatorname{cosec}^2 x\right]$

(iv) $\lim\limits_{x\to 0}\left(\frac{1}{x^2} - \cot^2 x\right)$

[KANPUR(BCA)–1990; MEERUT(BCA)–2003, 09]

(v) $\lim\limits_{x\to 0}\left(\frac{1}{x^2} - \frac{1}{x\tan x}\right)$

(vi) $\lim\limits_{x\to 0}\left(\operatorname{cosec} x - \frac{1}{x}\right)$.

3. Evaluate the following limits :

(i) $\lim\limits_{x\to 0}\left(\frac{1}{x}\right)^{\tan x}$ (ii) $\lim\limits_{x\to 0} x^x$

(iii) $\lim\limits_{x\to\infty}\left(\frac{\pi}{2} - \tan^{-1} x\right)^{1/x}$

(iv) $\lim\limits_{x\to 0}\left(\frac{\tan x}{x}\right)^{1/x}$ (v) $\lim\limits_{x\to \pi/2} (\sin x)^{\tan x}$

(vi) $\lim\limits_{x\to \pi/4} (\tan x)^{\tan 2x}$ [VTU–2004]

(vii) $\lim\limits_{x\to 0}\left[\frac{2(\cosh x - 1)}{x^2}\right]^{1/x^2}$

(viii) $\lim\limits_{x\to 0} (\operatorname{cosec} x)^{1/\log x}$

(ix) $\lim\limits_{x\to \alpha}\left(2 - \frac{x}{a}\right)^{\tan\left(\frac{\pi x}{2a}\right)}$

(VTU–2010, NAGPUR–2009)

(x) $\lim\limits_{x\to\infty}\left(1 + \frac{k}{x}\right)^x$

4. Evaluate the following limits :

(i) $\lim\limits_{x\to 0}\left[\frac{a^x + b^x}{2}\right]^{1/x}$ (VTU–2007)

(ii) $\lim\limits_{x\to 0}\left[\frac{a_1^x + a_2^x + \ldots + a_n^x}{n}\right]^{1/x}$ (VTU–2011)

(iii) $\lim\limits_{x\to\infty}\left(1 + \frac{a}{x}\right)^x$. [MEERUT(BCA)–2005, 06]

Hint to Selected Problems

1. (iii) $\lim\limits_{x\to\infty} 2^x . \sin\frac{a}{2^x} = \lim\limits_{x\to\infty} \frac{\sin\left(\frac{a}{2^x}\right)}{\frac{1}{2^x}}$

$$= a\lim_{x\to\infty}\left[\frac{\sin\left(\frac{a}{2^x}\right)}{\frac{a}{2^x}}\right] = a\cdot 1 = a.$$

(v) $\lim\limits_{x\to 1} \sec\left(\frac{\pi}{2x}\right). \log x = \lim\limits_{x\to 1} \frac{\log x}{\cos\left(\frac{\pi}{2x}\right)}$

$$= \lim_{x\to 1} \frac{\frac{1}{x}}{\frac{\pi}{2x^2}\sin\left(\frac{\pi}{2}x\right)} = \lim_{x\to 1} \frac{2x}{\pi\sin\left(\frac{\pi}{2x}\right)}$$

$$= \frac{2 \times 1}{\pi \cdot \sin\left(\frac{\pi}{2}\right)} = \frac{2}{\pi}.$$

2. (v) $\lim_{x \to 0} \left(\frac{1}{x^2} - \frac{1}{x \tan x} \right) = \lim_{x \to 0} \frac{\tan x - x}{x^2 \tan x}$

$$= \lim_{x \to 0} \frac{\left(x + \frac{x^3}{3} + \frac{2}{15} x^5 + \ldots \right) - x}{x^2 \left(x + \frac{x^3}{3} + \frac{2}{15} x^5 + \ldots \right)}$$

$$= \lim_{x \to 0} \frac{x^3 \left(\frac{1}{3} + \frac{2}{15} x^2 + \ldots \right)}{x^3 \left(1 + \frac{x^2}{3} + \frac{2}{15} x^4 + \ldots \right)}$$

$$= \lim_{x \to 0} \frac{\frac{1}{3} + \frac{2}{15} x^2 + \ldots}{1 + \frac{x^2}{3} + \frac{2}{15} x^4 + \ldots} = \frac{1}{3}$$

3. (i) $\log y = \lim_{x \to 0} \left(\frac{1}{x} \right)^{\tan x}$

$$\Rightarrow \log y = \lim_{x \to 0} \tan x \log \left(\frac{1}{x} \right)$$

$$= - \lim_{x \to 0} \tan x \log x = - \lim_{x \to 0} \frac{\log x}{\cot x}$$

$$= - \lim_{x \to 0} \frac{1/x}{-\text{cosec}^2 x} = \lim_{x \to 0} \frac{\sin^2 x}{x}$$

$$= \lim_{x \to 0} \left(\frac{\sin x}{x} \right). \sin x = 1 \times 0 = 0$$

$$\Rightarrow y = e^0 = 1.$$

ANSWERS

1. (i) 0 (ii) ∞ (iii) a (iv) $\log a$ (v) $-\frac{2}{\pi}$ (vi) 0.

2. (i) $\frac{1}{2}$ (ii) $-\frac{1}{2}$ (iii) $-\frac{1}{3}$ (iv) $\frac{2}{3}$ (v) $\frac{1}{3}$ (vi) 0.

3. (i) 1 (ii) 1 (iii) 1 (iv) 1 (v) 1 (vi) $\frac{1}{e}$ (vii) $e^{1/12}$

(viii) $\frac{1}{e}$ (ix) $e^{2/\pi}$ (x) e^k. **4.** (i) $\sqrt{ab}$ (ii) $(a_1 . a_2 \ldots . a_n)^{1/n}$ (iii) e^a.

❑❑❑❑❑❑

Chapter

10

Maxima and Minima

10.1 INTRODUCTION

If $y = f(x)$ be a continuous function. At a point $x = x_1$, if the function $f(x)$ does not increase and begins to decrease then $f(x)$ has its maximum value at $x = x_1$ and if at a point $x = x_2$, $f(x)$ does not decrease and begins to increase, then $f(x)$ has its minimum value at $x = x_2$.

If $f(x)$ is maximum at a point $x = x_1$ then $f(x)$ is an increasing function for the preceding values of x_1 and is a decreasing function for those value of x just below x_1 or we can say derivative of the function $\left(i.e., \dfrac{dy}{dx}\right)$ will be positive before $x = x_1$ and will be negative after $x = x_1$. But $\dfrac{dy}{dx}$ is a continuous function and $\dfrac{dy}{dx}$ changes the sign from positive to negative. So, $\dfrac{dy}{dx}$ will be zero at any point.

Therefore, for a maximum value of $y = f(x)$ at a point, we have $\dfrac{dy}{dx} = 0$ and $\dfrac{dy}{dx}$ changes the sign from positive to negative. On the other hand, for a minimum value of $y = f(x)$ at point we have $\dfrac{dy}{dx} = 0$ and $\dfrac{dy}{dx}$ changes the sign negative to positive.

- If $\dfrac{dy}{dx}$ changes the sign positive to negative; it means that $f(x)$ is a decreasing function of x, *i.e.*, $\dfrac{d^2y}{dx^2} < 0$.
- If $\dfrac{dy}{dx}$ changes the sign from negative to positive, it means that the $f(x)$ is an increasing function of x, *i.e.*, $\dfrac{d^2y}{dx^2} > 0$.
- A function may have more than one maximum and minimum value.
- Any minimum value of the function $f(x)$ can be greater than any maximum value.
- Maximum and minimum values of the function occur alternately.
- Maximum and minimum values of the function are sometimes known as extreme value.
- From the definition of maxima and minima, it is clear that $\dfrac{dy}{dx} = 0$ is the necessary condition for maximum or minimum.
- $\dfrac{d^2y}{dx^2} < 0$ is sufficient condition for maximum and $\dfrac{d^2y}{dx^2} > 0$ is sufficient condition for minimum.

WORKING PROCEDURE

STEP 1. Find the derivative of the given function *i.e.*, $\frac{dy}{dx}$.

STEP 2. Put $\frac{dy}{dx} = 0$ and find all the real values of x. (say x_1, x_2, x_3 ...).

STEP 3. Find $\frac{d^2y}{dx^2}$.

STEP 4. Put $x = x_i$ in $\frac{d^2y}{dx^2}$ and find the result. If result is negative then the function $f(x)$ is maximum at $x = x_i$ and max. $f(x)=f(x_i)$. On the other hand, if result is positive then the function $f(x)$ is minimum at $x = x_i$ and minimum $f(x)= f(x_i)$.

- In a continuous function, maxima and minima values occur alternately, *i.e.*, between two successive maxima there is one minimum and between two successive minima, there is one maximum.
- If $\frac{d^2y}{dx^2}$ is equal to 0 at any point $x = x_i$ then find $\frac{d^3y}{dx^3}, \frac{d^4y}{dx^4}$, and find the values of these derivatives at $x = x_i$ successively and check the sign.

Solved Examples

1. *Find the value of x for which $f(x)= y = x^4+2x^3-3x^2-4x+4$ is maximum or minimum and also find those value of $f(x)$.*

SOLUTION. Here, the given function is

$$y = f(x) = x^4 + 2x^3 - 3x^2 - 4x + 4 \quad ...(1)$$

So $$\frac{dy}{dx} = 4x^3 + 6x^2 - 6x - 4$$

$$= 2(x+2)(2x+1)(x-1)$$

Now, put $\frac{dy}{dx} = 0$, we have

$$2\,(x+2)(2x+1)(x-1) = 0$$

So, $x = -2, -\frac{1}{2}, 1$

Again differentiating (2) *w.r.t.* to x, we get

$$\frac{d^2y}{dx^2} = 12x^2 + 12x - 6$$

At $x = -2$, we have

$$\frac{d^2y}{dx^2} = 12(-2)^2 + 12(-2) - 6$$

$$= 48 - 24 - 6 = 18 > 0$$

Since, $\frac{d^2y}{dx^2} > 0$ (*i.e.*, positive). So $f(x)$ is minimum at $x = -2$. The minimum value of $f(x)$ at $x=-2$ is given by

$$f(-2) = (-2)^4 + 2(-2)^3 - 3(-2)^2 - 4(-2) + 4 = 0$$

Now, at $x = -\frac{1}{2}$, we have

$$\frac{d^2y}{dx^2} = 12\left(-\frac{1}{2}\right)^2 + 12\left(-\frac{1}{2}\right) - 6$$

$$= 3 - 6 - 6 = -9 < 0$$

Since, $\frac{d^2y}{dx^2} < 0$ (*i.e.*, negative). So, $f(x)$ is maximum at $x = -\frac{1}{2}$ and maximum value of $f(x)$ at $x = -\frac{1}{2}$ is

$$f\left(-\frac{1}{2}\right) = \left(-\frac{1}{2}\right)^4 + 2\left(-\frac{1}{2}\right)^3 - 3\left(-\frac{1}{2}\right)^2 - 4\left(-\frac{1}{2}\right) + 4$$

$$= \frac{1}{16} - \frac{1}{4} - \frac{3}{4} + 2 + 4 = \frac{81}{16}$$

Similarly, at $x = 1$, we have

$$\frac{d^2y}{dx^2} = 12(1)^2 + 12(1) - 6$$
$$= 12 + 12 - 6 = 18 > 0$$

Since, $\frac{d^2y}{dx^2} > 0$ (*i.e.*, positive). So $f(x)$ is minimum at $x = 1$ and minimum value of $f(x)$ at $x = 1$ is

$$f(1) = (1)^4 + 2(1)^3 - 3(1)^2 - 4(1) + 4$$
$$= 1 + 2 - 3 - 4 + 4 = 0.$$

2. *Find the maximum and minimum value of the function*

$$y = f(x) = x^3 - 12x^2 + 36x + 21$$

SOLUTION. Here, the given function is

$$y = x^3 - 12x^2 + 36x + 21$$

Now, differentiating *w.r.t.* x, we get

$$\frac{dy}{dx} = 3x^2 - 24x + 36$$

Puting $\frac{dy}{dx} = 0$, we get

$$3x^2 - 24x + 36 = 0$$

or $x^2 - 8x + 12 = 0$

or $(x-2)(x-6) = 0$ or $x = 2, 6$

Again, differentiating *w.r.t.* x, we get

$$\frac{d^2y}{dx^2} = 6x - 24$$

At $x = 2$, we have

$$\frac{d^2y}{dx^2} = 6(2) - 24 = -12 < 0$$

Since, $\frac{d^2y}{dx^2} < 0$ so $f(x)$ is maximum at $x = 2$. The maximum value of $f(x)$ at $x = 2$ is given by

$$f(2) = (2)^3 - 12(2)^2 + 36(2) + 21$$
$$= 8 - 48 + 72 + 21 = 53.$$

Similarly, at $x = 6$, we have

$$\frac{d^2y}{dx^2} = 6 \times 6 - 24 = 36 - 24 = 12 > 0$$

Since, $\frac{d^2y}{dx^2} > 0$ so, $f(x)$ is minimum at $x = 6$ and minimum value of $f(x)$ at $x = 6$ is

$$f(6) = (6)^3 - 12(6)^2 + 36(6) + 21$$
$$= 216 - 432 + 216 + 21$$
$$= 453 - 432 = 21$$

3. *Investigate for maximum and minimum values, the function* ($\sin x + \cos 2x$).

[MEERUT(BCA)–2005, 12]

SOLUTION. Let $y = \sin x + \cos 2x$,

$$\Rightarrow \quad \frac{dy}{dx} = \cos x - 2\sin 2x$$
$$= \cos x - 4\sin x \cos x$$

For stationary point

$$\frac{dy}{dx} = 0$$

$$\Rightarrow \cos x(1 - 4\sin x) = 0$$

$$\Rightarrow \quad \cos x = 0 \text{ or } 1 - 4\sin x = 0$$

$$\Rightarrow \quad x = \frac{\pi}{2} \text{ or } \sin x = \frac{1}{4}$$

For maxima or minima

$$\frac{d^2y}{dx^2} = -\sin x - 4\cos 2x$$
$$= -\sin x - 4(1 - 2\sin^2 x)$$
$$= -\sin x - 4 + 8\sin^2 x$$

(i) At $x = \frac{\pi}{2}$,

$$\left(\frac{d^2y}{dx^2}\right) = -1 - 4 + 8 = 3$$

(which is positive.)

So, given function is minimum at $x = \frac{\pi}{2}$ and min. value of y at $x = \frac{\pi}{2}$ is given by

$$\sin\frac{\pi}{2} + \cos 2 \times \frac{\pi}{2} = 1 - 1 = 0.$$

(ii) At $\sin x = \frac{1}{4}$,

$$\left(\frac{d^2y}{dx^2}\right) = -\frac{1}{4} - 4 + 8.\frac{1}{16}$$
$$= -\frac{1}{4} - 4 + \frac{1}{2}$$
$$= \frac{-1 - 16 + 2}{4}$$
$$= \frac{-15}{4} \text{(which is negative)}.$$

Hence, given function is maximum at $x = \sin^{-1}\frac{1}{4}$ and max. value at

$\sin x = \frac{1}{4}$ is, $\frac{1}{4} + \left[1 - 2\times\left(\frac{1}{4}\right)^2\right] = \frac{7}{8}$.

4. *Find the maximum value of (x – 1) (x – 2)(x – 3).* [ROHILKHAND(BCA)–2005]

SOLUTION. Let $f(x) = (x-1)(x-2)(x-3)$

$$= x^3 - 6x^2 + 11x - 6$$

then $f'(x) = 3x^2 - 12x + 11$

For a maximum or minimum value of $f(x)$, we must have $f'(x) = 0$

$$\Rightarrow \quad 3x^2 - 12x + 11 = 0$$

i.e., $x = \dfrac{12 \pm \sqrt{144 - 4\times3\times11}}{6}$

$$= \frac{6 \pm \sqrt{(36-33)}}{3}$$

$$= 2 \pm \frac{1}{\sqrt{3}}.$$

Also $f''(x) = 6x - 12$

Now $f''[2 + (1/\sqrt{3})] = +\text{ve}$, therefore $f(x)$ has minimum value at

$x = 2 + (1/\sqrt{3})$.

Again $f''[2 - (1/\sqrt{3})] = -\text{ve}$

therefore $f(x)$ has a maximum value at $x = 2 - (1/\sqrt{3})$. The maximum value of $f(x)$ is

$= f[2 - (1/\sqrt{3})]$

$= [1 - (1/\sqrt{3})](-1/\sqrt{3})[-1 - (1/\sqrt{3})]$

$= (1 - 1/3)(1/\sqrt{3}) = 2/3\sqrt{3}$

5. *Show that $\sin x(1 + \cos x)$ is a maximum at $x = \pi/3$.* [MEERUT(BCA)–2009, 13; KANPUR(BCA)–2004, 08, 10, 15]

SOLUTION. Let $f(x) = \sin x(1 + \cos x)$

$$= \sin x + \frac{1}{2}\sin 2x$$

Then $f'(x) = \cos x + \cos 2x$

For a maximum or a minimum value of $f(x), f'(x) = 0$

i.e., $\cos x + \cos 2x = 0$

$\Rightarrow 2\cos^2 x + \cos x - 1 = 0$

$(2\cos x - 1)(\cos x + 1) = 0$

$\therefore \quad \cos x = 1/2, -1 \Rightarrow x = \pi/3, \pi$

Now $f''(x) = -\sin x - 2\sin 2x$

$\therefore \quad f''\left(\frac{\pi}{3}\right) = -\sin\left(\frac{\pi}{3}\right) - 2\sin\left(\frac{2\pi}{3}\right)$

$= -ve$

Hence $f(x)$ is maximum at $x = \pi/3$.

6. *Find the maximum value of $(1/x)^x$.* [ROHILKHAND(BCA)–2005, 06]

SOLUTION. Let $y = (1/x)^x$

$\Rightarrow \log y = x(\log 1 - \log x) = -x\log x$

$\Rightarrow \dfrac{1}{y}\dfrac{dy}{dx} = -1\log x - x(1/x)$

$$= -(1 + \log x)$$

$\Rightarrow \dfrac{dy}{dx} = -y(1 + \log x)$

$$= -(1/x)^x(1 + \log x)$$

For a maximum or a minimum of y, we must have $\dfrac{dy}{dx} = 0$

$\Rightarrow \quad -(1/x)^x(1 + \log x) = 0$

$\Rightarrow 1 + \log x = 0 \Rightarrow x = 1/e$

$\Rightarrow \dfrac{d^2y}{dx^2} = -\dfrac{dy}{dx}(1 + \log x) - y(1/x)$

$$= -\frac{dy}{dx}(1 + \log x) - (1/x)^x.(1/x)$$

Therefore, when $x = 1/e$,

$$\frac{d^2y}{dx^2} = 0 - (e)^{1/e}.e = -\text{ve}$$

$\Rightarrow y$ is maximum at $x = 1/e$.

Thus the maximum value of y is given by $e^{1/e}$.

7. *Show that the semi-vertical angle of the right circular cone of given total surface (including area of the base) and maximum value is $\sin^{-1}(1/3)$.* [KANPUR(BCA)-2006; MEERUT(BCA)-2002, 03, 11; ROHILKHAND(BCA)-2004, 09]

SOLUTION. Let x be the radius of the base, h be the height and y the slant height of the cone. Then the total surface of the cone = constant

$\Rightarrow \quad \pi x^2 + \pi xy = \text{constant} \quad ...(1)$

Now V = volume of the cone

$$= \frac{1}{3}\pi x^2 h = \frac{1}{3}\pi x^2 (y^2 - x^2)^{1/2}$$

Since, $h=\sqrt{y^2-x^2}$, therefore

$$V^2=\frac{1}{9}\pi^2x^4(y^2-x^2).$$

Now, V is maximum or minimum according as V^2 or $\frac{9V^2}{\pi^2}$ is maximum or minimum.

Let $\quad S=\frac{9V^2}{\pi^2}=x^4(y^2-x^2).$

Then S can be regarded as a function of x because y is connected with x by (1).

We have $\frac{dS}{dx}=4x^3(y^2-x^2)$

$$+x^4\left\{2y\left(\frac{dy}{dx}\right)-2x\right\} \quad ...(2)$$

Differentiating (1) w.r. to x, we get

$$\pi\left(2x+y+x\frac{dy}{dx}\right)=0$$

or $\quad \frac{dy}{dx}=-\frac{2x+y}{x}$

Substituting this value of $\frac{dy}{dx}$ in (2), we get

$$\frac{dS}{dx}=4x^3y^2-4x^5+x^4\left[-2y\frac{(2x+y)}{x}-2x\right]$$

$$=2x^3y^2-6x^5-4x^4y$$

For a maximum or a minimum of S, we must have $\frac{dS}{dx}=0$

Now $\frac{dS}{dx}=0$

$\Rightarrow\ 2x^3(y^2-2xy-3x^2)=0$

$\Rightarrow 2x^3(y-3x)(y+x)=0$

i.e., $y=3x$ since $x\neq 0$ and $y\neq -x$.

Again $\frac{d^2S}{dx^2}=6x^2y^2+4x^3y\frac{dy}{dx}$

$$-30x^4+16x^3y-4x^4\frac{dy}{dx}$$

When $y=3x, \frac{dy}{dx}=-5$,

so when $y=3x$, we have

$$\frac{d^2S}{dx^2}<0$$

Therefore S is maximum when $y=3x$.

8. *In a submarine telegraph cable the speed of signalling varies as $\log x^2\log(1/x)$, where x is the ratio of the radius of the core to that of the covering. Show that the greatest speed is attained when this ratio is $1:\sqrt{e}$.*

[MEERUT(BCA)–2002, 04, 14]

SOLUTION. Let S be the speed of signalling.

Then $S=\mu x^2\log(1/x)=-\mu x^2\log x$

where μ is a constant.

For a maximum or a minimum of S, we have $\frac{dS}{dx}=0$

i.e., $x(2\log x+1)=0$

$\Rightarrow\quad x=0$ or $\log x=-1/2$

But $x=0$ is inadmissible. Therefore

$\log x=-1/2$ or $x=e^{-1/2}=1/\sqrt{e}$

Now $\frac{d^2S}{dx^2}=-\mu(2\log x+1)-\mu x(2/x)$

$$=-\mu(2\log x+1)=-2\mu$$

When $x=1/\sqrt{e}$, we have $2\log x+1=0$, when $x=1/\sqrt{e}$, we have $\frac{d^2S}{dx^2}=-2\mu$ which is negative.

Hence, S is maximum, when $x=1/\sqrt{e}$.

9. *Show that maximum rectangle that can be inscribed in a circle is square.*

[MEERUT(BCA)–2005, 09, 16]

SOLUTION. Let $ABCD$ be the rectangle inscribed in circle with centre O and radius a. Also, let $AB=2x$ and $BC=2y$. Then

$$a^2=x^2+y^2 \quad ...(1)$$

Area of rectangle $ABCD$

$$A=(2x)(2y)=4xy$$

$$=4x\sqrt{a^2-x^2} \quad \text{[From (1)]}$$

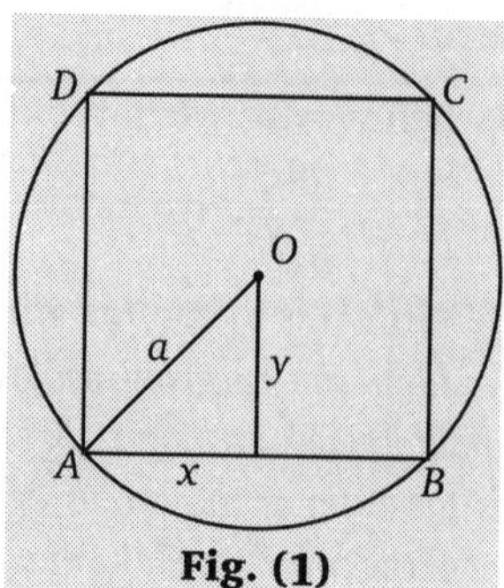

Fig. (1)

For maximum or minimum area,

$$\frac{dA}{dx} = 0$$

$$\Rightarrow \quad 4\left\{\sqrt{a^2 - x^2} - \frac{x^2}{\sqrt{a^2 - x^2}}\right\} = 0$$

$$\Rightarrow \quad 4\left\{\frac{a^2 - 2x^2}{\sqrt{a^2 - x^2}}\right\} = 0$$

$$\Rightarrow \quad a^2 - 2x^2 = 0 \Rightarrow x = \frac{a}{\sqrt{2}}$$

Now $\frac{d^2A}{dx^2} = 4\left\{(-4x)(a^2 - x^2)^{1/2} + (a^2 - 2x^2)\left(-\frac{1}{2}\right)(a^2 - x^2)^{-3/2}(-2x)\right\}$

$$= 4\left[\frac{-4x}{\sqrt{a^2 - x^2}} + \frac{x(a^2 - 2x^2)}{(a^2 - x^2)^{3/2}}\right]$$

$$\Rightarrow \quad \left(\frac{d^2A}{dx^2}\right)_{x = a/\sqrt{2}} = -16$$

(which is negative.)

Thus A is max. when $x = \frac{a}{\sqrt{2}}$.

From (1), $y = \frac{a}{\sqrt{2}}$.

Therefore $x = y = \frac{a}{\sqrt{2}}$

Hence, area is maximum when $x = y = \frac{a}{\sqrt{2}}$ *i.e.*, rectangle is square.

10. *Show that the height of the closed cylinder of given surface and greatest volume is equal to its diameter.* [MEERUT(BCA)–2005]

SOLUTION. Let r be radius of base and h the height of a closed cylinder of given surface S, then

$$S = 2\pi r^2 + 2\pi rh \Rightarrow h = \frac{S - 2\pi r^2}{2\pi r} \quad ...(1)$$

If V be volume of cylinder then

$$V = \pi r^2 h = \pi r^2\left(\frac{S - 2\pi r^2}{2\pi r}\right)$$

$$= \frac{rS - 2\pi r^3}{2}$$

$$\Rightarrow \frac{dV}{dr} = \frac{S}{2} - 3\pi r^2 \quad ...(2)$$

For max or min we have $\frac{dV}{dr} = 0$

$$\frac{S}{2} - 3\pi r^2 = 0 \Rightarrow S = 6\pi r^2$$

$$\Rightarrow 2\pi r^2 + 2\pi rh = 6\pi r^2$$

$$\Rightarrow \quad h = 2r$$

From (2) $\frac{d^2V}{dr^2} = -6\pi r$, (–ve) for any positive value of r.

Hence V is maximum when $h = 2r$, *i.e.*, when the height of cylinder is equal is diameter of base.

11. *Prove that a conical tent of a given capacity will required the least amount of canvas when the height is $\sqrt{2}$ times the radius of the base.* [MEERUT(BCA)–2006]

SOLUTION. Let us suppose h be the height, r be the radius of the base l the slant height of the conical tent. Let V be the given capacity (*i.e.* volume) and S denote the area of the curved surface of the tent.

We know that $\quad V = \frac{1}{3}\pi r^2 h \quad ...(1)$

and $\quad S = \pi lr = \pi(\sqrt{h^2 + r^2})r$

$$\Rightarrow S^2 = \pi^2 r^2(h^2 + r^2) = u\text{(say)} \quad ...(2)$$

From (1) and (2), we get

$$u = \pi^2 r^2\left[\frac{9V^2}{\pi^2 r^4} + r^2\right] = \frac{9V^2}{r^2} + \pi^2 r^4$$

$$\therefore \frac{du}{dr} = -\frac{18V^2}{r^3} + 4\pi^2 r^3$$

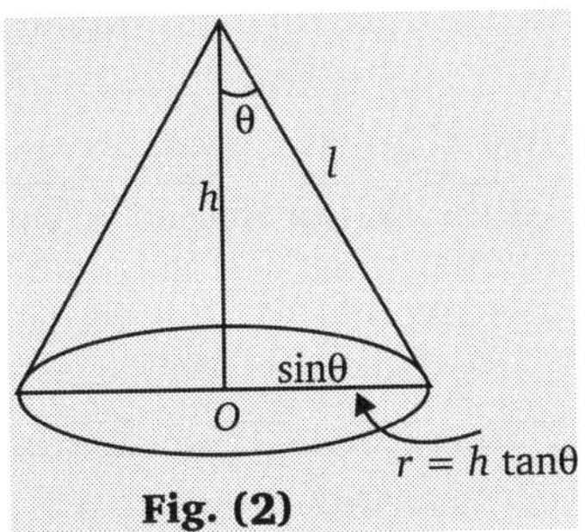

Fig. (2)

and $\dfrac{d^2u}{dr^2} = \dfrac{54V^2}{r^4} + 12\pi^2 r^2$

Now $\dfrac{du}{dr} = 0 \Rightarrow V = \left(\dfrac{2}{3\sqrt{2}}\right)\pi r^3$

for $V = \left(\dfrac{2}{3\sqrt{2}}\right)\pi r^3, \dfrac{d^2u}{dr^2} > 0$

i.e., u is minimum when $V = \dfrac{2}{3\sqrt{2}}\pi r^3$

i.e., when $\dfrac{2}{3\sqrt{2}}\pi r^3 = \dfrac{1}{3}\pi r^2 h$

i.e., $h = r\sqrt{2}$

$\Rightarrow$ u is minimum, when $h = r\sqrt{2}$.

12. *Show that the radius of the right circular cylinder of greatest curved surface which can be inscribed in a given cone is half that of the cone.*

SOLUTION. Suppose r is the radius and H is the height of the given cone

i.e., $OB = r$, $OA = H$

where O is the centre of the base circle. Suppose x is the radius and h is the height of the cylinder inscribed in the given cone.

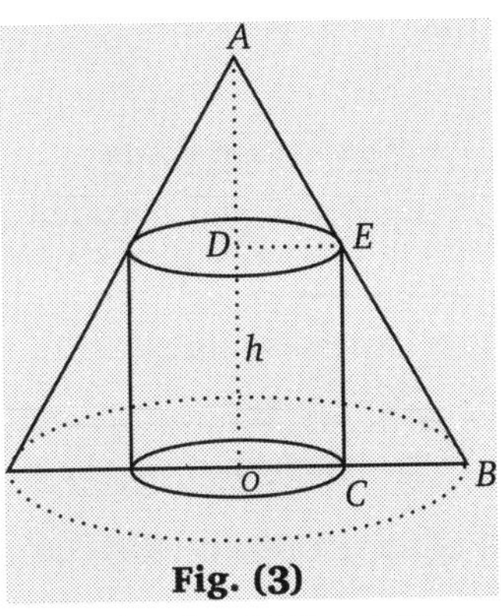

Fig. (3)

Now triangles AOB and ADE are similar, therefore

$$\frac{AD}{AO} = \frac{DE}{OB} \text{ or } \frac{H-h}{H} = \frac{x}{r}$$

$$\Rightarrow \quad 1 - \frac{h}{H} = \frac{x}{r} \Rightarrow \frac{h}{H} = 1 - \frac{x}{r}$$

$$\Rightarrow \quad h = H\left(1 - \frac{x}{r}\right)$$

Now the curved surface of the cylinder

$$\Rightarrow \quad S = 2\pi . x . h = 2\pi x H\left(1 - \frac{x}{r}\right)$$

$$\Rightarrow \quad S = \frac{2\pi H}{r}(rx - x^2)$$

$$\Rightarrow \quad \frac{dS}{dx} = \frac{2\pi H}{r}(r - 2x)$$

So $\dfrac{dS}{dx} = 0$, we get $r - 2x = 0$ or $x = \dfrac{r}{2}$

Also $\dfrac{d^2S}{dx^2} = \dfrac{2\pi H}{r}(-2) < 0$

$\Rightarrow S$ is greatest, when $x = \dfrac{r}{2}$

i.e., when radius of the cylinder is half of that can be inscribed in a sphere of radius x.

10.2 MAXIMA AND MINIMA OF A FUNCTION OF SEVERAL INDEPENDENT VARIABLES

Let $f(x, y, z, ...)$ be a function of several independent variables x, y, z.... If f is continuous and finite for all values of $x, y, z, ...$ in the neighbourhood of $x = a, y = b, z = c, ...$ respectively, then the value of $(a, b, c, ...)$ is said to be a maximum or minimum if $f(a+h, b+k, c+l, ...)$ is less than or greater than $f(a, b, c, ...)$ for all values of $h, k, l, ...$ (where $h, k, l, ...$) are sufficiently small, may be positive or negative provided they are not all zero.

In other words we can say, the value of $f(a, b, c, ...)$ is said to be a maximum or minimum if $f(a+h, b+k, c+l, ...) - f(a, b, c, ...)$ maintain an invariant sign (may be positive or negative) for all values of h, k , l, ... positive or negative provided they are taken sufficiently small and finite.

10.2.1 STATIONARY AND EXTREME POINTS

A point $(a_1, a_2, ..., a_n)$ is called a stationary point, if all the first order partial derivatives of the function $f(x_1, x_2, ..., x_n)$ vanish at the point. A stationary point, if it is maximum or minimum is known as extreme point and the value of the function at an extreme point is known as an extreme value.

- A stationary point may be a maximum or minimum or neither of these two.

10.3 NECESSARY CONDITION FOR THE EXISTENCE OF MAXIMA OR MINIMA

Let $f(x, y, z, ...)$ be a function of several independent variables $x, y, z,$... It is clear from the definition of maxima and minima that maximum or minimum of $f(x, y, z, ..)$ will occur for those values of $x, y, z, ...,$ for which the expression $f(x+h, y+k, z+l, ...) - f(x, y, z, ...)$ maintain an invariant sign for all sufficiently small and finite values of $h, k, l,$ ... positive or negative.

Now, expanding $f(x+h, y+k, z+l, ...)$ by Taylor's theorem, we have

$$f(x+h, y+k, z+l...) = f(x, y, z) + \left(h\frac{\partial f}{\partial x} + k\frac{\partial f}{\partial y} + l\frac{\partial f}{\partial z} + ...\right)$$

+ terms of second and higher order.

$$\Rightarrow \quad f(x+h, y+k, z+l...) - f(x, y, z, ...) = \left(h\frac{\partial f}{\partial x} + k\frac{\partial f}{\partial y} + l\frac{\partial f}{\partial z} + ...\right)$$

+ terms of second and higher orders. ...(1)

Now, since h, k , l, ... are sufficiently small, the first degree expression

$$\left(h\frac{\partial f}{\partial x} + k\frac{\partial f}{\partial y} + l\frac{\partial f}{\partial z} + ...\right)$$

of the equation (1) can be made to govern the sign of right hand side and hence, of the left hand side as well as. Thus, by changing the sign of the left hand side of the equation (1) will also change.

Since, left hand side is to preserve an invariable sign for maxima or minima, therefore, as a necessary condition for maximum and minimum values, we must have

$$h\frac{\partial f}{\partial x} + k\frac{\partial f}{\partial y} + l\frac{\partial f}{\partial z} + ... = 0 \qquad ...(2)$$

Now, since $h, k, l,$ ... are arbitrary and independent of each other, we must have

$$\frac{\partial f}{\partial x} = 0, \frac{\partial f}{\partial y} = 0, \frac{\partial f}{\partial z} = 0, \text{ etc.} \qquad ...(3)$$

If the number of independent variables be n, we shall get n simultaneous equations in these n variables, which will give the values $a, b, c,$ ... of the n variables $x, y, z,$ .... respectively for which $f(x, y, z, ...)$ will have a maximum or a minimum values.

- The necessary condition for a function $f(x, y, z, ...)$ of the independent variables $x, y, z,$ ... to be maximum or minimum is given by

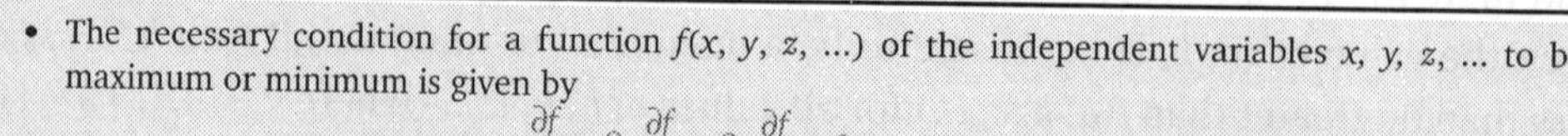

$$\frac{\partial f}{\partial x} = 0, \frac{\partial f}{\partial y} = 0, \frac{\partial f}{\partial z} = 0,$$

- The conditions given above is only a necessary condition for the maxima and minima of the function $f(x, y, z, ...)$. These conditions are not sufficient.

10.3.1 MAXIMA AND MINIMA FOR A FUNCTION OF TWO INDEPENDENT VARIABLES

(1) *To find the condition which governs the sign of a quadratic expression.*
Consider, a binary expression

$$I = ax^2 + 2hxy + by^2$$

of two variables x and y. Then I can be written as

$$I = ax^2 + 2hxy + by^2 = \frac{1}{a}[(ax+hy)^2 + (ab-h^2)y^2].$$

If $(ab - h^2)$ is positive, the sign of I will be the same as that of a.
But if $(ab - h^2)$ is negative, then, the expression within the brackets may be positive or negative and therefore we cannot say anything about the sign of expression I.

(2) *Stationary and extreme points (For the function of two independent variables)*:
Let $f(x, y)$ be a function of two independent variables x and y. A point (a, b) is called a stationary point, if both the first order partial derivatives $\left(\frac{\partial f}{\partial a} \text{ and } \frac{\partial f}{\partial b}\right)$ of the function $f(x, y)$ at (a, b) vanish.
A stationary point which is either a maximum or minimum is called an extreme point.

- A stationary point is not necessarily an extreme point, hence a stationary point may be a maximum or a minimum or neither of these two.
- The value of the function at extreme point is called extreme value.
- A point at which function is neither maximum nor minimum, is known as saddle point.

10.4 NECESSARY CONDITION FOR MAXIMA AND MINIMA

Let $f(x, y)$ be a function of two independent variables x and y.Then, we have the maximum or minimum of $f(x, y)$ at $x = a$ and $x = b$ if the expression $f(a+ h, b + k) - f(a, b)$ is of invariable sign for all sufficiently small independent variables h and k provided both of them are not equal to zero.

We observe that,

(i) If the sign of $f(a+h, b+k) - f(a, b)$ is negative, then we have a maximum of $f(x, y)$ at $x = a, y = b$.

(ii) If the sign of $f(a+h, b+k) - f(a, b)$ is positive, we have a minimum of $f(x, y)$ at $x = a, y = b$.
Expand $f(a+h, b+k)$ by Taylor's theorem, we have

$$f(a+h,b+k) = f(a,b) + \left(h\frac{\partial f}{\partial x} + k\frac{\partial f}{\partial y}\right)_{\substack{x=a\\y=b}} + \frac{1}{2!}\left(h^2\frac{\partial^2 f}{\partial x^2} + 2hk\frac{\partial^2 f}{\partial x\,\partial y} + k^2\frac{\partial^2 f}{\partial y^2}\right)_{\substack{x=a\\y=b}} + \ldots \quad \ldots(1)$$

$$\Rightarrow \quad f(a+h,b+k) - f(a,b) = h\left(\frac{\partial f}{\partial x}\right)_{\substack{x=a\\y=b}} + k\left(\frac{\partial f}{\partial y}\right)_{\substack{x=a\\y=b}} + \text{term of the second and higher}$$

orders in h and k.

Now, since h and k are sufficiently small, the expression $h\left(\frac{\partial f}{\partial x}\right)_{\substack{x=a\\y=b}} + k\left(\frac{\partial f}{\partial y}\right)_{\substack{x=a\\y=b}}$ of the equation (1) can be made to govern the sign of right hand side and hence of the left hand side as well. Thus by changing the sign of h and k, the sign of the left hand side of the equation (1) will also change.

Since L.H.S. is to preserve an invariable sign for maximum or minimum, therefore as a necessary condition for maximum and minimum values, we must have

$$h\left(\frac{\partial f}{\partial x}\right)_{\substack{x=a\\y=b}} + k\left(\frac{\partial f}{\partial y}\right)_{\substack{x=a\\y=b}} = 0. \qquad ...(2)$$

If $k = 0$, we find that if $\left(\frac{\partial f}{\partial x}\right)_{\substack{x=a\\y=b}} \neq 0$, the R.H.S. of (2) changes sign when h changes sign.

Therefore $f(x, y)$ cannot have a maximum or minimum at $x = a$, $y = b$ if $\left(\frac{\partial f}{\partial x}\right)_{\substack{x=a\\y=b}} \neq 0$.

Similarly, taking $h = 0$, we see that $f(x, y)$ cannot have a maximum or a minimum at $x = a$, $y = b$ if $\left(\frac{\partial f}{\partial y}\right)_{\substack{x=a\\y=b}} \neq 0$.

Thus, a set of necessary conditions that $f(x, y)$ should have a maximum or minimum at $x=a, y=b$ is that

$$\left(\frac{\partial f}{\partial x}\right)_{\substack{x=a\\y=b}} = 0 \text{ and } \left(\frac{\partial f}{\partial y}\right)_{\substack{x=a\\y=b}} = 0.$$

10.5 SUFFICIENT CONDITION FOR MAXIMA AND MINIMA: THE LAGRANGE'S CONDITION

Let $f(x, y)$ be a function of two variables x and y.

Let $r = \frac{\partial^2 f}{\partial x^2}, s = \frac{\partial^2 f}{\partial x \partial y}, t = \frac{\partial^2 f}{\partial y^2}$ at $x = a$ and $y = b$.

As a set of necessary conditions for a maximum or minimum at (a, b) we have

$$\frac{\partial f}{\partial x} = 0 \text{ and } \frac{\partial f}{\partial y} = 0 \text{ at } (a, b)$$

then
$$f(a + h, b + k) - f(a, b) = \frac{1}{2!}[rh^2 + 2shk + tk^2] + R \qquad ...(1)$$

Where R consists of terms of third and higher order of small quantities h and k.

Now, by taking h and k sufficiently small, the second degree terms in R.H.S. of (1) may be made to govern the sign of R.H.S. and therefore of the L.H.S. also *i.e.*, for sufficiently small values of h and k, the sign of $\frac{1}{2}(rh^2 + 2shk + tk^2) + R$ is same as that of $rh^2 + 2shk + tk^2$.

If the sign is negative, then the function is maximum at (a, b) and if the sign is positive, then the function is minimum at (a, b).

Case (i) *If* $(rt - s^2) > 0$.

Then, neither r nor t can be zero. Hence, we can write

$$rh^2 + 2shk + tk^2 = \frac{1}{2}[r^2h^2 + 2rshk + rtk^2] = \frac{1}{2}[(rh + sk)^2 + (rt - s^2)k^2]$$

since $rt - s^2 > 0$, therefore $(rh + sk)^2 + (rt - s^2)k^2 > 0$ for all values of h and k except when $rh + sk = 0$, $k = 0$ *i.e.*, at $h = 0$, $k = 0$, which is not possible.

Hence, in this case the expression $rh^2 + 2shk + tk^2$ will have the same sign for all values of h and k, and the sign is determined by the sign of r.

Thus, the function $f(x, y)$ will have a maximum or minimum at $x = a$ and $y = b$. If $rt - s^2 > 0$. The function $f(x, y)$ is maximum or minimum according as r is negative or positive.

Case (ii) *If* $(rt - s^2) < 0$.

If $rt - s^2$ is negative, we are not sure about the sign of second degree term of R.H.S. of (1) and hence there is neither a maximum nor a minimum value.

Case (iii) *If* $rt - s^2 = 0$.

If $rt = s^2$, then quadratic expression $rh^2 + 2shk + tk^2$ becomes $\frac{1}{r}(hr + ks)^2$.

So that, the quadratic expression will be of the same sign as that of r or t unless

$$\frac{h}{k} = -\frac{s}{r} = \alpha \text{ (say) } i.e., \; rh + sk = 0.$$

If this condition is safisfied, then the second degree expression in R.H.S. of (1) vanishes and hence, the sign of the R.H.S. of (1) depends upon third degree expression in h and k, which change sign with the change of sign of h and k and hence, the sign of L.H.S. of (1) will also change and hence, there will be neither maximum nor minimum.

Thus, the necessary condition for the existence of maxima and minima now is that the cubic terms must vanish collectively in R.H.S. of (1) when $\frac{h}{k} = -\frac{s}{r} = \alpha$; and then the biquadratic terms of R.H.S. of (1) must collectively be of the same sign as r and t, when

$$\frac{h}{k} = -\frac{s}{r} = \alpha \quad i.e., \; hr + ks = 0$$

Hence, the case is doubtful.

Thus, if $rt - s^2 = 0$, the case is doubtful and further, investigation is needed to determine the maxima and minima of $f(x, y)$ at (a, b).

WORKING PROCEDURE

To discuss the maxima and minima at $x = a, y = b$, we must find

$$r = \left(\frac{\partial^2 u}{\partial x^2}\right)_{\substack{x=a\\y=b}}, \; s = \left(\frac{\partial^2 u}{\partial x \partial y}\right)_{\substack{x=a\\y=b}}, \; t = \left(\frac{\partial^2 u}{\partial y^2}\right)_{\substack{x=a\\y=b}}$$

Then, calculate $rt - s^2$.

Now following cases arise :

(i) If $rt - s^2 > 0$, then

  (A) If r is negative then, $f(x, y)$ is maximum at $x = a, y = b$.

  (B) If r is positive then, $f(x, y)$ is minimum at $x = a, y = b$.

(ii) If $rt - s^2 < 0$, $f(x, y)$ is neither maximum nor minimum at $x = a, y = b$.

(iii) If $rt - s^2 = 0$, *the case is doubtful, and further investigation will be required.*

- While solving problems, we frequently used the identity, given by Lagrange.
  $\{(a^2 + b^2 + c^2)(p^2 + q^2 + r^2) - (ap + bq + cr)^2\} = \{(br - cq)^2 + (cp + ar)^2 + (aq - bp)^2\}$.

Solved Examples

1. *Find all maximum or minimum values of the function :*

$$f(x, y) = y^2 + x^2 y + x^4.$$

SOLUTION. Since, we have

$$f(x, y) = y^2 + x^2 y + x^4.$$

$$\therefore \frac{\partial f}{\partial x} = 2xy + 4x^3 \text{ and } \frac{\partial f}{\partial y} = 2y + x^2.$$

For a maximum or minimum of $f(x, y)$, we must have

$$\frac{\partial f}{\partial x} = 0 \text{ and } \frac{\partial f}{\partial y} = 0$$

$$\therefore \frac{\partial f}{\partial x} = 0 \Rightarrow 2xy + 4x^3 = 0$$

$$\Rightarrow 2x(y + 2x^2) = 0 \qquad ...(1)$$

$$\frac{\partial f}{\partial y} = 0 \Rightarrow 2y + x^2 = 0$$

Solving (1) and (2), we get $x = 0, y = 0$. Thus (0, 0) is the only point of maximum or minimum.

Now $r = \left(\frac{\partial^2 f}{\partial x^2}\right)_{(0,0)} = [2y + 12x^2]_{(0,0)} = 0$

$s = \left(\frac{\partial^2 f}{\partial x \partial y}\right)_{(0,0)} = [2x]_{(0,0)} = 0$

and $t = \left(\frac{\partial^2 f}{\partial y^2}\right)_{(0,0)} = [2]_{(0,0)} = 2$

$\therefore rt - s^2 = 0\,(2) - 0^2 = 0.$

Thus, the case is doubtful and further investigation will be required.

2. *Find the maximum or minimum values of the function $x^3 y^2(1-x-y)$.* (ANNA–2009, JNTU–2006, 08, BHOPAL–2012)

SOLUTION. Let $u = x^3 y^2 (1-x-y)$

$$\Rightarrow \frac{\partial u}{\partial x} = 3x^2y^2(1-x-y) - x^3y^2$$

and $\dfrac{\partial u}{\partial y} = 2x^3y(1-x-y) - x^3y^2.$

For a maximum or minimum of u, we must have $\dfrac{\partial u}{\partial x} = 0$ and $\dfrac{\partial u}{\partial y} = 0$

$\Rightarrow 3x^2y^2(1-x-y) - x^3y^2 = 0$ ...(1)

and $2x^3y(1-x-y) - x^3y^2 = 0.$ ...(2)

Now, subtracting (2) from (1), we have

$$x^2y(1-x-y)(3y-2x) = 0$$

which gives $y = \dfrac{2}{3}x.$

Putting the value of y in (1), we get

$$x = \frac{1}{2}$$

So $\left(\dfrac{1}{2}, \dfrac{1}{3}\right)$ be the point of maxima or minima.

Now $r = \dfrac{\partial^2 u}{\partial x^2} = 6xy^2 - 12x^2y^2 - 6xy^3$

$$= -\frac{1}{9}, \text{ at } \left(\frac{1}{2}, \frac{1}{3}\right)$$

$$t = \frac{\partial^2 u}{\partial y^2} = 2x^3 - 2x^4 - 6x^3y$$

$$= -\frac{1}{8}, \text{ at } \left(\frac{1}{2}, \frac{1}{3}\right)$$

$$s = \frac{\partial^2 u}{\partial x \partial y} = 6x^2y - 8x^3y - 9x^2y^2$$

$$= -\frac{1}{12} \text{ at } \left(\frac{1}{2}, \frac{1}{3}\right).$$

Now, $rt - s^2$ = positive.

Also, r is negative, hence the function u has a maximum at $x = \dfrac{1}{2}, y = \dfrac{1}{3}.$

The maximum value is

$$= \left(\frac{1}{2}\right)^3 \left(\frac{1}{3}\right)^2 \left(1 - \frac{1}{2} - \frac{1}{3}\right) = \frac{1}{432}.$$

3. *Discuss the maximum or minimum values of u, where*

$$u = 2a^2xy - 3ax^2y - ay^3 + x^3y + xy^3.$$

SOLUTION. We have

$$u = 2a^2xy - 3ax^2y - ay^3 + x^3y + xy^3$$

which gives

$$\frac{\partial u}{\partial x} = 2a^2y - 6axy + 3x^2y + y^3$$

and $\dfrac{\partial u}{\partial y} = 2a^2x - 3ax^2 - 3ay^2 + x^3 + 3xy^2$

For a maximum and minima of u, we have

$$\frac{\partial u}{\partial x} = 0, \frac{\partial u}{\partial y} = 0$$

which gives,

$$y(2a^2 - 6ax + 3x^2 + y^2) = 0 \quad ...(1)$$

and $2a^2x - 3ax^2 - 3ay^2 + x^3 + 3xy^2 = 0$ ...(2)

Equation (1) and (2) gives the following values of x and y :

$x = 0, y = 0; x = a, y = 0;$

$x = 2a, y = 0; x = \dfrac{3}{2}a, y = \pm\dfrac{1}{2}a;$

$x = a, y = a, x = \dfrac{1}{2}a, y = \dfrac{1}{2}a;$

$x = a, y = -a; x = \dfrac{1}{2}a, y = -\dfrac{1}{2}a.$

Then, we get the following pairs of values of x and y which make the function u stationary.

$$(0,0), (a,0), (2a,0), \left(\frac{3}{2}a, \frac{1}{2}a\right), \left(\frac{3}{2}a, -\frac{1}{2}a\right), (a,a), \left(\frac{1}{2}a, \frac{1}{2}a\right), (a,-a),, \left(\frac{1}{2}a, -\frac{1}{2}a\right).$$

Also $r = \dfrac{\partial^2 u}{\partial x^2} = -6ay + 6xy,$

$$s = \frac{\partial^2 u}{\partial x \partial y} = 2a^2 - 6ax + 3x^2 + 3y^2,$$

and $$t = \frac{\partial^2 u}{\partial y^2} = -6ay + 6xy.$$

For (0, 0).

$$r = 0, s = 2a^2, t = 0$$

$\Rightarrow$ $rt - s^2$, is negative.

Therefore, we have neither maximum nor a minimum of u at (0, 0).

Similarly, we can easily shown that u has neither a maximum nor a minimum at $(a, 0)$, $(2a, 0)$, (a, a), $(a, -a)$.

For $\left(\frac{3a}{2}, \frac{a}{2}\right)$.

$$r = \frac{3}{2}a^2, s = \frac{1}{2}a^2, t = \frac{3}{2}a^2,$$

$\Rightarrow$ $rt - s^2$ is positive.

Here, since r is positive, therefore u has minimum at $\left(\frac{3a}{2}, \frac{a}{2}\right)$.

Similarly, we can check the maxima and minima at all other points.

- The point $\left(\frac{x_1 + x_2 + x_3}{3}, \frac{y_1 + y_2 + y_3}{3}\right)$ is the centroid of the given triangle.

4. *Show that the minimum value of* $u = xy + \left(\frac{a^3}{x}\right) + \left(\frac{a^3}{y}\right)$ *is* $3a^2$.

SOLUTION. We have $u = xy + \left(\frac{a^3}{x}\right) + \left(\frac{a^3}{y}\right)$

$$\Rightarrow \frac{\partial u}{\partial x} = y - \frac{a^3}{x^2} \text{ and } \frac{\partial u}{\partial y} = x - \frac{a^3}{y^2}.$$

For a maximum or minimum of u, we have $\frac{\partial u}{\partial x} = 0$ and $\frac{\partial u}{\partial y} = 0$

Now, $\frac{\partial u}{\partial x} = 0 \Rightarrow y - \frac{a^3}{x^2} = 0$ ...(1)

and $\frac{\partial u}{\partial y} = 0 \Rightarrow x - \frac{a^3}{y^2} = 0.$ ...(2)

Solving (1) and (2), we get, $x = a, y = a$

Now $r = \frac{\partial^2 u}{\partial x^2} = \frac{2a^3}{x^3}$, $s = \frac{\partial^2 u}{\partial x \partial y} = 1$

and $t = \frac{\partial^2 u}{\partial y^2} = \frac{2a^3}{y^3}$.

At $x = y = a$, we have

$$r = 2, s = 1, t = 2$$

$\Rightarrow$ $rt - s^2 = 3 > 0.$

Thus, at (a, a), $rt - s^2 > 0$ and $r > 0$. Therefore u is minimum at $x = a$, $y = a$.

The minimum value of

$$u = a.a + \left(\frac{a^3}{a}\right) + \left(\frac{a^3}{a}\right) = 3a^2.$$

5. *Determine the points where a function* $x^3 + y^3 - 3axy$ *has maximum or minimum.*

SOLUTION. Here, we have $u = x^3 + y^3 - 3axy$

$$\Rightarrow \frac{\partial u}{\partial x} = 3x^2 - 3ay \text{ and } \frac{\partial u}{\partial y} = 3y^2 - 3ax.$$

For a maximum or minimum of u, we must have

$$\frac{\partial u}{\partial x} = 0 \text{ and } \frac{\partial u}{\partial y} = 0$$

which gives, $x^2 - ay = 0$ ...(1)

and $y^2 - ax = 0$ ...(2)

Solving (1) and (2), we get

$$x = 0, y = 0; x = a, y = a.$$

Thus (0, 0) and (a, a) are the stationary points of u.

Now $r = \frac{\partial^2 u}{\partial x^2} = 6x$, $s = \frac{\partial^2 u}{\partial x \partial y} = -3a$,

$$t = \frac{\partial^2 u}{\partial y^2} = 6y.$$

For $x = 0, y = 0$

$$r = 0, s = -3a \text{ and } t = 0$$

$\therefore rt - s^2 = -9a^2 < 0$, for all values of a.

$\Rightarrow u$ is neither maximum nor minimum at $x = 0, y = 0$.

For $x = a, y = a$

$$r = 6a, s = -3a \text{ and } t = 6a$$

$\Rightarrow rt - s^2 = 27a^2 > 0$, for all values of a.

Also $r = 6a$, which is positive if $a > 0$.

Thus (i) u is maximum at $x = a, y = a$ if $a < 0$

and (ii) u is minimum at $x = a, y = a$ if $a > 0$.

6. *Discuss the maxima and minima of the function $u = \sin x \sin y \sin (x+y)$.*

[UPTU–2009]

SOLUTION. Here, we have $u = \sin x \sin y \sin (x + y)$

$$\Rightarrow \frac{\partial u}{\partial x} = \sin y[\sin x \cos(x+y) + \cos x \sin(x+y)]$$

and $$\frac{\partial u}{\partial y} = \sin x[\sin y \cos(x+y) + \cos y \sin(x+y)].$$

For a maxima and minima of u, we must have

$$\frac{\partial u}{\partial x} = 0 \text{ and } \frac{\partial u}{\partial y} = 0.$$

$\Rightarrow \sin y\ [\sin x \cos (x + y) + \cos x \sin (x+y)] = 0$

and $\sin x\ [\sin y \cos (x + y) + \cos y \sin (x+y)] = 0$.

Equation (1) and (2) gives

$$\tan (x + y) = - \tan x \qquad ...(1)$$

$\Rightarrow \qquad \tan x = \tan y$

and $\tan (x + y) = - \tan y \qquad ...(2)$

$\Rightarrow \qquad x = y$

From (1) and (2), we have

$\tan 2x = - \tan x = \tan (\pi - x)$

$\Rightarrow 2x = \pi - x$

$\Rightarrow 3x = \pi \Rightarrow x = \frac{\pi}{3} = y.$

Moreover,

$$\frac{\partial u}{\partial x} = 0, \text{ gives } \sin y = 0 \Rightarrow y = 0$$

and $$\frac{\partial u}{\partial y} = 0, \text{ gives } \sin x = 0 \Rightarrow x = 0.$$

Thus, we get the following pair of values, which makes the function u stationary $(0,0), \left(\frac{\pi}{3}, \frac{\pi}{3}\right)$.

Now $$r = \frac{\partial^2 u}{\partial x^2} = 2\sin y \cos(2x + y),$$

$$s = \frac{\partial^2 u}{\partial x \partial y} = \sin 2(x + y),$$

and $$t = \frac{\partial^2 u}{\partial y^2} = 2\sin x \cos(2y + x).$$

For (0, 0).

$$r = 0, s = 0, t = 0$$

$\Rightarrow \qquad rt - s^2 = 0.$

$\therefore$ this case is doubtful and need further investigation.

For $\left(\frac{\pi}{3}, \frac{\pi}{3}\right)$.

$$r = 2\sin\frac{1}{3}\pi . \cos\pi = -\sqrt{3},$$

$$s = \sin\left(\frac{4\pi}{3}\right) = -\sin\frac{\pi}{3} = -\frac{\sqrt{3}}{2},$$

and $$t = 2\sin\frac{1}{3}\pi\cos\pi = -\sqrt{3}.$$

$$\therefore \quad rt - s^2 = \frac{9}{4} = \text{positive}.$$

Also $r = -\sqrt{3}$.

Hence, u has a maximum value at $\left(\frac{\pi}{3}, \frac{\pi}{3}\right)$.

7. *Find a point within a triangle such that the sum of the squares of its distances from the vertices is a minimum.*

SOLUTION. Let us suppose $[(x_r, y_r) : r = 1, 2, 3]$ be the vertices of the triangle and (x, y) be any point inside the triangle.

Now, let us define a function

$$u = \sum_{r=1}^{3} [(x - x_r)^2 + (y - y_r)^2].$$

Then, we have

$$\frac{\partial u}{\partial x} = \Sigma\, 2(x - x_r)$$
$$= 2[(x - x_1) + (x - x_2) + (x - x_3)]$$

and $$\frac{\partial u}{\partial y} = \Sigma 2(y - y_r)$$
$$= 2[(y - y_1) + (y - y_2) + (y - y_3)].$$

For a maximum or minimum of u, we must have

$$\frac{\partial u}{\partial x} = 0$$

$\Rightarrow (x - x_1) + (x - x_2) + (x - x_3) = 0$

$\Rightarrow x = \dfrac{x_1 + x_2 + x_3}{3}$

and $$\frac{\partial u}{\partial y} = 0$$

$\Rightarrow (y - y_1) + (y - y_2) + (y - y_3) = 0$

$\Rightarrow y = \dfrac{y_1 + y_2 + y_3}{3}.$

Thus, we have

$$\left(\frac{x_1 + x_2 + x_3}{3}, \frac{y_1 + y_2 + y_3}{3}\right)$$

is the only point at which u have a maximum or minimum.

Now $r=\frac{\partial^2 u}{\partial x^2}=6, s=\frac{\partial^2 u}{\partial x \partial y}=0, t=\frac{\partial^2 u}{\partial y^2}=6.$

Now, at $\left[\frac{x_1+x_2+x_3}{3}, \frac{y_1+y_2+y_3}{3}\right]$

$$r = 6, s = 0, t = 6$$

$\Rightarrow$ $rt - s^2 = 36 > 0.$

Also, since $r > 0.$

Therefore u have a minimum value at

$$\left[\frac{x_1+x_2+x_3}{3}, \frac{y_1+y_2+y_3}{3}\right].$$

Hence, the point

$$\left(\frac{x_1+x_2+x_3}{3}, \frac{y_1+y_2+y_3}{3}\right)$$

is the required point at which u is minimum.

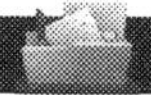

Similar Problems

(1) Discuss the maxima and minima of the function $u = x^2y^2 - 5x^2 - 8xy - 5y^2$.

(2) Find the minimum value of $x^2 + y^2 + z^2$ when $ax + by + cz = p$.

(3) Find the stationary point of $x^4 + y^4 - 2x^2 + 4xy - 2y^2$ and determine their nature. [JNTU–2009]

(4) Test the function $u = x^2y - y^2x - x + y$ for maximum and minimum.

8. *Show that distance l of any point (x, y, z) on the plane $2x+3y-z=12$ from the origin is given by*

$$l=\sqrt{[x^2+y^2+(2x+3y-12)^2]}.$$

Hence, find the point on the plane that is nearest to the origin.

SOLUTION. If l is the distance from (0, 0, 0) of any point (x, y, z) then $l=\sqrt{(x^2+y^2+z^2)}.$ If the point (x, y, z) lies on the plane $2x + 3y - z = 12$, then

$$l=\sqrt{[x^2+y^2+(2x+3y-12)^2]}$$

[$\because z = 2x + 3y - 12$, from the equation of the plane]

$$\therefore \quad l^2 = x^2+y^2+(2x+3y-12)^2$$

$$= 5x^2+10y^2+12xy - 48x+72y+144 = u\text{(say)}.$$

Now l is maximum or minimum according as l^2 *i.e.*, u is maximum or minimum.

For a maximum or minimum of u, we get

$$\frac{\partial u}{\partial x} = 10x+12y-48=0$$

and $\frac{\partial u}{\partial y} = 20y+12x-72=0$

Solving these equations, we get

$$x=\frac{12}{7} \text{ and } y=\frac{18}{7}.$$

Also

$$r=\frac{\partial^2 u}{\partial x^2}=10, \; s=\frac{\partial^2 u}{\partial x \partial y}=12$$

and $t=\frac{\partial^2 u}{\partial y^2}=20.$

Therefore $rt - s^2 = 10 \times 20 - (12)^2 =$ + ve, since $rt - s^2 > 0$ and $r > 0$, then u is minimum and hence l is minimum.

When $x=\frac{12}{7}$ and $y=\frac{18}{7}$. Putting these values of x and y in the equation of the plane, we get

$$z=2\cdot\left(\frac{12}{7}\right)+3\cdot\left(\frac{18}{7}\right)-12=-\frac{6}{7}.$$

Hence, the required point is

$$\left(\frac{12}{7}, \frac{18}{7}, -\frac{6}{7}\right).$$

9. *Find the points on $z^2 = xy + 1$ nearest to the origin.*

SOLUTION. Let l be the distance from the origin (0, 0, 0) of any point (x, y, z) on the surface $z^2 = xy + 1$ ...(1)

Then $l=\sqrt{x^2+y^2+z^2}$

$$=\sqrt{(x^2+y^2+xy+1)}$$

[Using equation (1)]

Since l is always greater than zero, therefore l is maximum or minimum according as l^2, *i.e.*, u is maximum or minimum, where $u = l^2$.

For a maximum or minimum of u, we must have

$$\frac{\partial u}{\partial x} = 2x + y = 0 \quad ...(2)$$

and $$\frac{\partial u}{\partial y} = 2y + x = 0. \quad ...(3)$$

Solving the equation (2) and (3), we get $x = 0, y = 0$

Also $r = \frac{\partial^2 u}{\partial x^2} = 2,\ s = \frac{\partial^2 u}{\partial x\,\partial y} = 1,$

$$t = \frac{\partial^2 u}{\partial y^2} = 2.$$

$\therefore\ rt - s^2 = 2.\ 2 - 1 = 3 > 0.$

Since at $x = 0, y = 0$, then $rt - s^2 > 0$ and $r > 0$.

Therefore u is minimum at $x = 0, y = 0$.

Hence l is minimum, when $x = 0, y = 0$.

Putting $x = 0,\ y = 0$ in the equation (1), we get $z^2 = 1$ *i.e.*, $z = \pm 1$.

Hence, the required points are (0, 0, 1) and (0, 0, –1).

Exercise-10.1

1. Discuss the maxima and minima of the function $f(x,y) = x^2 + y^2 + \frac{2}{x} + \frac{2}{y}$.
2. Find the values of x and y for which the expression $$(a_1x + b_1y + c_1)^2 + (a_2x + b_2y + c_2)^2 + ... + (a_nx + b_ny + c_n)^2$$ is minimum.
3. Examine for maximum and minimum values of the function $f(x, y) = x^2 - 3xy + y^2 + 2x$.
4. Examine the function $f(x, y) = x^2y - y^2x - x + y$ for maxima and minima.
5. Discuss the maxima and minima of the function $$f(x,y) = 2\sin\frac{1}{2}(x+y)\cos\frac{1}{2}(x-y) + \cos(x+y).$$
6. Find the maximum and minimum values of $u = 6xy + (47 - x - y)(4x + 3y)$.
7. Examine for extreme values
   (i) $x^2 + y^2 + 6x + 12$ [GBTU–2012]
   (ii) $x^3 + y^3 - 63(x+y) + 12xy$ [UKTU–2011]

Hints to the Selected Problems

5. $\frac{\partial f}{\partial x} = \cos x - \sin(x+y),\ \frac{\partial f}{\partial y} = \cos y - \sin(x+y)$

$\frac{\partial f}{\partial x} = 0,\ \frac{\partial f}{\partial y} = 0$, we get $\cos x = \sin(x+y)$, and $\cos y = \sin(x+y)$.

The extreme points are given by

$$\left(-\frac{\pi}{2}, \frac{\pi}{2}\right), \left(\frac{3\pi}{2}, \frac{\pi}{2}\right) \text{ and } \left(\frac{\pi}{2}, \frac{\pi}{2}\right).$$

Answers

1. $f(x, y)$ is minimum at (1, 1). 2. $f(x, y)$ is minimum for the value of x and y which are obtained by $\Sigma(a_1^2)x + (a_1b_1)y + a_1c_1 = 0$ and $\Sigma(a_1b_1)x + (b_1^2)y + b_1c_1 = 0$.
3. Stationary point is $x = \frac{4}{5}, y = \frac{6}{5}$. The function $f(x, y)$ is neither maximum nor minimum at $\left(\frac{4}{5}, \frac{6}{5}\right)$. 4. At (1, 1) and (–1, –1) function is neither maximum nor minimum.
5. $x = y = 2n\pi \pm \pi/2$; neither maximum nor minimum ; $x = y = n\pi + (-1)^n \pi/6$; f is maximum.
6. Maximum value is 3384.
7. (i) At x = –3, y = 0, minimum (ii) max at (–7, –7) min. at (3, 3) neither max nor min. at (5, –1) and (–1, 5).

10.6 MAXIMA AND MINIMA OF THE FUNCTION OF THREE INDEPENDENT VARIABLES

(1) *To find the condition, which governs the sign of the quadratic equation of three independent variables.*

Let I be the expression of three independent variables x, y and z given by

$$I = ax^2 + by^2 + cz^2 + 2fyz + 2gzx + 2hxy$$

I can be written as

$$I = \frac{1}{a}\left[a^2x^2 + aby^2 + acz^2 + 2afyz + 2agzx + 2ahxy\right](a \neq 0)$$

$$= \frac{1}{a}\left[a^2x^2 + 2ax(gz + hy) + aby^2 + acz^2 + 2afyz\right]$$

$$= \frac{1}{a}\left[(ax + hy + gz)^2 + aby^2 + acz^2 + 2afyz - (gz + hy)^2\right]$$

$$= \frac{1}{a}\left[(ax + hy + gz)^2 + \left(ab - h^2\right)y^2 + 2yz(af - gh) + \left(ac - g^2\right)z^2\right]$$

Here, we observe that I be of the same sign as provided the expression within the square brackets is positive which will of course be so if $ab-h^2$ and $\{(ab-h^2)(ac-g^2)-(af-gh)^2\}$ are positive *i.e.,* if

$$ab-h^2 \text{ and } a[abc+2fgh-af^2-bg^2-ch^2] \text{ are both positive.}$$

Hence, I will be positive if

$$a, \begin{vmatrix} a & h \\ h & b \end{vmatrix}, \begin{vmatrix} a & h & g \\ h & b & f \\ g & f & c \end{vmatrix}$$

be all positive and will be negative if these three expression are alternately negative and positive.

10.7 MAXIMA AND MINIMA FOR A FUNCTION OF THREE INDEPENDENT VARIABLES : THE LAGRANGE'S CONDITION

Let $f(x,y,z)$ be a given function of three independent variables x, y and z.

Let A, B, C, F, G, H stand for $\frac{\partial^2 f}{\partial x^2}, \frac{\partial^2 f}{\partial y^2}, \frac{\partial^2 f}{\partial z^2}, \frac{\partial^2 f}{\partial y \partial z}, \frac{\partial^2 f}{\partial z \partial x}, \frac{\partial^2 f}{\partial x \partial y}$ respectively.

Let a set of the values of x, y, z obtained by solving the equations

$$\frac{\partial f}{\partial x} = \frac{\partial f}{\partial y} = \frac{\partial f}{\partial z} = 0 \text{ be } a, b, c.$$

By Taylor's theorem, we have

$$f(a+h, b+k, c+l), -f(a,b,c) = \frac{1}{2!}\left[Ah^2 + Bk^2 + Cl^2 + 2Fkl + 2Glh + 2Hhk\right] + R \quad ...(1)$$

where, remainder term R consist of third and higher order of same quantity (*i.e.,* h, k, l).

Now, by taking h, k, l sufficiently small, the second term of R.H.S. of (1) can be made to govern the sign of R.H.S. and therefore of L.H.S. also.

If for all such values of h, k and l, these terms be of permanent sign, then we shall have a maximum or minimum of $f(x,y,z)$ according as that sign is negative or positive.

Hence, the function will be minimum if the expression

$$A, \begin{vmatrix} A & H \\ H & B \end{vmatrix}, \begin{vmatrix} A & H & G \\ H & B & F \\ G & F & C \end{vmatrix} \text{ be all positive.}$$

The function will have a maximum value, if the above three quantities are alternately negative and positive. If these conditions are not satisfied, we have neither a maximum nor a minimum.

WORKING PROCEDURE

Let $f(x, y, z)$ be a function of three independent variables x,y and z. Find the values of triads (a,b,c) of the value x,y and z by putting $\frac{\partial f}{\partial x} = 0, \frac{\partial f}{\partial y} = 0, \frac{\partial f}{\partial z} = 0$ .The values of triads (a,b,c) will give the stationary values of $f(x, y, z)$.

Now, to discuss maximum and minimum values, at (a, b, c) we find the following six partial derivatives of second order

$$A = \frac{\partial^2 f}{\partial x^2}, B = \frac{\partial^2 f}{\partial y^2}, C = \frac{\partial^2 f}{\partial z^2}, F = \frac{\partial^2 f}{\partial y \partial z}, G = \frac{\partial^2 f}{\partial z \partial x}, and\ H = \frac{\partial^2 f}{\partial x \partial y}$$

Now, we have the following cases :

Case (i) The function $f(x,y,z)$ will be minimum at (a,b,c) if the expressions

$$A, \begin{vmatrix} A & H \\ H & B \end{vmatrix}, \begin{vmatrix} A & H & G \\ H & B & F \\ G & F & C \end{vmatrix}$$ be all positive at (a, b, c).

Case (ii) The function $f(x, y, z)$ will be maximum at (a, b, c) if the expressions

$$A, \begin{vmatrix} A & H \\ H & B \end{vmatrix}, \begin{vmatrix} A & H & G \\ H & B & F \\ G & F & C \end{vmatrix}$$

be alternately negative and positive.

Case (iii) If the expression, using in case (i) and (ii) neither be all positive nor having alternately negative and positive sign at (a,b,c). Then $f(x, y, z)$ is neither maximum nor minimum at (a,b,c).

- To find the maximum and minimum of the function at stationary point, it is sufficient to find the value of a second order partial derivative of function with respect to any of the independent variables. Then, the value of the function is maximum or minimum according as the value of this second order partial derivative at the stationary point under consideration is negative or positive.

Solved Examples

1. *Find the maximum value of u, where*

$$u = \frac{xyz}{(a+x)(x+y)(y+z)(z+b)}.$$

SOLUTION. We have

$$u = \frac{xyz}{(a+x)(x+y)(y+z)(z+b)}$$

Taking, log of both the sides, we have

$$\log u = \log x + \log y + \log z - \log(a+x) - \log(x+y) - \log(y+z) - \log(z+b).$$

Differentiating w.r.t. x, we have

$$\frac{1}{u}\frac{\partial u}{\partial x} = \frac{1}{x} - \frac{1}{a+x} - \frac{1}{x+y} = \frac{ay - x^2}{x(a+x)(x+y)}$$

$$\Rightarrow \quad \frac{\partial u}{\partial x} = \frac{(ay - x^2)u}{x(a+x)(x+y)}$$

Similarly $$\frac{\partial u}{\partial y} = \frac{(xz - y^2)u}{y(x+y)(y+z)}$$

and $$\frac{\partial u}{\partial z} = \frac{(by - z^2)u}{z(y+z)(z+b)}$$

For, a maxima and minima of u, we must have

$$\frac{\partial u}{\partial x} = 0 \Rightarrow ay - x^2 = 0; \quad \frac{\partial u}{\partial y} = 0 \Rightarrow xz - y^2 = 0$$

and $$\frac{\partial u}{\partial z} = 0 \Rightarrow by - z^2 = 0$$

Here, we observe that $x^2 = ay$, $y^2 = xz$, $z^2 = by$ which implies that a, x, y, z and b are in G.P. Let r be the common ratio of this G.P.

Then $ar^4 = b$ or $r = \left(\frac{b}{a}\right)^{1/4}$

Also $x=ar, y=ar^2, z=ar^3$.

Hence, we have

$$u=\frac{ar.ar^2.ar^3}{a(1+r)ar(1+r)ar^2(1+r)ar^3(1+r)}$$

$$=\frac{1}{a(1+r)^4}=\frac{1}{a\left[1+\left(\frac{b}{a}\right)^{1/4}\right]^4}$$

$$=\frac{1}{\left(a^{1/4}+b^{1/4}\right)^4}$$

which gives a stationary value of u. Now, to decide whether this value of u is a maximum or a minimum, we proceed to find the second order partial derivative of u.

Here $$\frac{\partial^2 u}{\partial x^2}=\frac{-2ux}{x(a+x)(x+y)}+(ay-x^2)\frac{\partial}{\partial x}\left[\frac{u}{x(a+x)(x+y)}\right]$$

When $x=ar, y=ar^2, z=ar^3$, we have

$$A=\frac{\partial^2 u}{\partial x^2}=-\frac{2u}{a^2r(1+r)^2}<0$$

Hence, the above stationary value of u is maximum.

2. *Find the maxima and minima value of the function*

$$u = \sin x \sin y \sin z$$

where x,y and z are the vertex angles of a triangle.

SOLUTION. Here, we have

$$u= \sin x \sin y \sin z \text{ ; where } x+y+z= \pi \quad ...(1)$$

$$\therefore \quad u= \sin x \sin y \sin [\pi-(x+y)]$$

$$= \sin x \sin y \sin(x+y)$$

$$\therefore \quad \frac{\partial u}{\partial x}= \cos x \sin y \sin(x+y)+\sin x \sin y \cos(x+y)$$

$$= \sin y \sin(2x+y). \quad ...(2)$$

Similarly $\frac{\partial u}{\partial y}= \sin x \sin(2y+x)$ ...(3)

For a maxima and minima, we must have

$$\frac{\partial u}{\partial x}= 0, \frac{\partial u}{\partial y}=0$$

So, $\frac{\partial u}{\partial x}= 0$

$\Rightarrow \sin y \sin(2x+y)=0$

$\Rightarrow \sin y=0$ or $\sin(2x+y)=0$

$\Rightarrow y=0$ or $\sin(x+x+y)=0$

$\Rightarrow y=0$

or $\sin x \cos(x+y)+\cos x \sin (x+y)=0$

$\Rightarrow \tan (x+y)= -\tan x$

$\Rightarrow \tan(x+y)= \tan(-x) = \tan(\pi-x)$ ...(4)

$\Rightarrow x+y=\pi-x$

$\Rightarrow 2x+y=\pi$ ...(5)

Similarly, from (3)

$x=0$

or $\tan(x+y)= -\tan y$ ...(6)

Now, by (4) and (6), we have

$\tan x=\tan y \Rightarrow x = y$.

Hence, by (5), we have

$$3y=\pi \quad \Rightarrow \quad y=\frac{\pi}{3} \text{ and } x=\frac{\pi}{3}$$

Therefore, the stationary points are

$\left(\frac{\pi}{3},\frac{\pi}{3}\right)$ and $(0, 0)$.

For (0,0): $u=0$.

For $\left(\frac{\pi}{3},\frac{\pi}{3}\right)$

$$r=\frac{\partial^2 u}{\partial x^2}=2\sin y\cos(2x+y)$$

$$=2\sin\frac{\pi}{3}\cos\left(\frac{2\pi}{3}+\frac{\pi}{3}\right)$$

$$=-\sqrt{3}<0$$

and $$s=\frac{\partial^2 u}{\partial x\partial y}$$

$$=\sin(2x+2y)$$

$$=\sin\left(\frac{2\pi}{3}+\frac{2\pi}{3}\right)$$

$$=\sin\left(\frac{4\pi}{3}\right)=-\frac{\sqrt{3}}{2}<0$$

$$t=\frac{\partial^2 u}{\partial y^2}=2\sin x\cos(x+2y)$$

$$=2\sin\frac{\pi}{3}\cos\pi=-\sqrt{3}<0$$

Now $rt-s^2$

$$=\left(-\sqrt{3}\right)\left(-\sqrt{3}\right)-\left(\frac{\sqrt{3}}{2}\right)^2=\frac{9}{4}>0$$

Thus $rt-s^2>0$ and $r<0$.

Hence, the function u will be maximum at $\left(\frac{\pi}{3},\frac{\pi}{3}\right)$.

Exercise-10.2

1. Prove that the function $u = x^2 + y^2 + x - 2z - xy$ is minimum at $\left(-\frac{2}{3},-\frac{1}{3},1\right)$.
2. Find the maximum and minimum values of $u = y^2+2z^2 - 5x^4 + 4x^5$.
3. Find the maximum or minimum values of the function u, where $u = axy^2z^3 - x^2y^2z^3 - xy^3z^3 - xy^2z^4$
4. Find the maximum value of $(ax+by+cz)\, e^{-\left(\alpha^2.x^2+\beta^2y^2+\gamma^2z^2\right)}$.
5. A rectangle box is placed on x-y plane. The one end of the box is at the origin. If the vertex opposite to the origin be on the plane $6x+4y+3z=24$, then find the maximum value of this box.
6. In a plane triangle xyz, find the maximum value of $\sin x \sin y \sin z$.
7. A rectangular box, open at the top is to have a given capacity. Show that the domain of the box requiring least material for its construction $x = y = (2v)^{1/3}$, where $v = xyz$.

ANSWERS

2. Minimum at (1,0,0), neither maximum nor minimum at (0,0,0).
3. Maximum at $\left(\frac{a}{7},\frac{2a}{7},\frac{3a}{7}\right)$, max. value$=\frac{108a^7}{7^7}$
4. Maximum at $\left(\frac{a}{2\alpha^2k},\frac{b}{2\beta^2k},\frac{c}{2\gamma^2k}\right)$ where $k=\sqrt{\left\{\frac{1}{2}\left(\frac{a^2}{\alpha^2}+\frac{b^2}{\beta^2}+\frac{c^2}{\gamma^2}\right)\right\}}$,

   Maximum value $=\sqrt{\left\{\frac{1}{2e}\left(\frac{a^2}{\alpha^2}+\frac{b^2}{\beta^2}+\frac{c^2}{\gamma^2}\right)\right\}}$
5. Maximum at $\left(\frac{4}{3},2\right)$. maximum value $=\frac{64}{9}$ cube units. Neither maximum nor minimum at (0,0).
6. Maximum at $\left(\frac{\pi}{3},\frac{\pi}{3},\frac{\pi}{3}\right)$, value$=\frac{3\sqrt{3}}{8}$

10.8 LAGRANGE'S METHOD OF UNDETERMINED MULTIPLIERS

Let $u=f(x_1, x_2, ..., x_n)$ be a function of n variables $x_1, x_2, ..., x_n$.

Let us suppose these variables $x_1,x_2,...,x_n$ are connected by k equations

$$g_1(x_1, x_2,..., x_n)= 0$$
$$g_2(x_1, x_2,..., x_n)= 0$$
$$\dots \quad \dots \quad \dots \quad \dots \quad \dots$$
$$g_k(x_1, x_2, ..., x_n)= 0$$

so, that there are $n-k$ independent variables out of these n variables. For the maxima and minima of u, we find

$$du = \frac{\partial u}{\partial x_1}dx_1 + \frac{\partial u}{\partial x_2}dx_2 + \ldots + \frac{\partial u}{\partial x_n}dx_n = 0 \qquad \ldots(1)$$

Also

$$dg_1 = \frac{\partial g_1}{\partial x_1}dx_1 + \frac{\partial g_1}{\partial x_2}dx_2 + \ldots + \frac{\partial g_1}{\partial x_n}dx_n = 0 \qquad \ldots(2)$$

$$dg_2 = \frac{\partial g_2}{\partial x_1}dx_1 + \frac{\partial g_2}{\partial x_2}dx_2 + \ldots + \frac{\partial g_2}{\partial x_n}dx_n = 0 \qquad \ldots(3)$$

$$\vdots \quad \vdots \quad \vdots \quad \vdots \quad \vdots \quad \vdots \quad \vdots \quad \vdots$$

$$dg_k = \frac{\partial g_k}{\partial x_1}dx_1 + \frac{\partial g_k}{\partial x_2}dx_2 + \ldots + \frac{\partial g_k}{\partial x_n}dx_n = 0 \qquad \ldots(k+1)$$

Multiplying equation (1),(2),(3)...(k+1) by $1, l_1, l_2, \ldots, k$ respectively and adding, we get the result, which can be written as

$$P_1dx_1+P_2dx_2+P_3dx_3+\ldots+P_ndx_n=0 \qquad \ldots(4)$$

where
$$P_k = \frac{\partial u}{\partial x_k} + l_1\frac{\partial g_1}{\partial x_k} + l_2\frac{\partial g_2}{\partial x_k} + \ldots + l_k\frac{\partial g_k}{\partial x_k}$$

Now we have at our choice k multiple *viz* $l_1, l_2, \ldots, l_k$ and can be chosen such that

$$P_1=0,\ P_2=0,\ \ldots,\ P_k=0$$

Then, the equation (4) reduces to

$$P_{k+1}dx_{k+1}+P_{k+2}dx_{k+2}+P_{k+3}dx_{k+3}+\ldots+P_ndx_n=0 \qquad \ldots(5)$$

Now, let us suppose that out of n variables, the $(n-k)$ variables $x_{k+1}, x_{k+2}, \ldots, x_n$ are independent.

Then, since $n-k$ quantities $dx_{k+1}, dx_{k+2}, \ldots, dx_n$ are independent so their coefficients must be separately zero. Hence, we have

$$P_{k+1}=0,\ P_{k+2}=0,\ \ldots,\ P_n=0$$

Thus, we have $k+n$ equations

$$P_1=0,\ P_2=0,\ \ldots,\ P_n=0$$

and
$$g_1=0,\ g_2=0,\ \ldots,\ g_k=0.$$

Hence, we get $(n+k)$ equations which determine the k multipliers $l_1, l_2, \ldots, l_k$ and get the possible value of u.

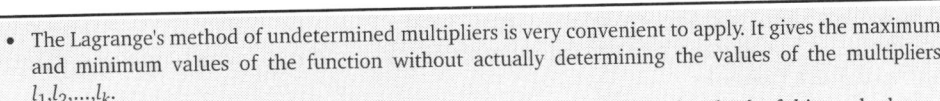

- The Lagrange's method of undetermined multipliers is very convenient to apply. It gives the maximum and minimum values of the function without actually determining the values of the multipliers $l_1, l_2, \ldots, l_k$.
- It does not determine the nature of stationary point, which is the only drawback of this method.

10.8.1 Applications of the Method of Undetermined Multipliers

The Lagrange's method of undetermined multipliers can be applied to determine the extreme values of the given functions, it does not detemine the nature of stationary point. Now, it is more convenient to find out the extreme values of a function F with the help of new function, given by

$$V = g + l_1f_1 + l_2f_2 + \ldots + l_mf_m$$

and use the following method. Here, we give the method for four variables x, y, u, v connected by the following two relations.

Let $F = g(x, y, u, v)$ be subjected to the conditions

$$f_1(x,y,u,v)=0 \qquad \ldots(1)$$

and
$$f_2(x,y,u,v)=0. \qquad \ldots(2)$$

For the maxima and minima of F, we have

$$dF = \frac{\partial g}{\partial x}dx + \frac{\partial g}{\partial y}dy + \frac{\partial g}{\partial u}du + \frac{\partial g}{\partial v}dv = 0 \qquad \ldots(3)$$

Now, from (1) and (2), we have

$$df_1 = \frac{\partial f_1}{\partial x}dx + \frac{\partial f_1}{\partial y}dy + \frac{\partial f_1}{\partial u}du + \frac{\partial f_1}{\partial v}dv = 0 \qquad \ldots(4)$$

and
$$df_2 = \frac{\partial f_2}{\partial x}dx + \frac{\partial f_2}{\partial y}dy + \frac{\partial f_2}{\partial u}du + \frac{\partial f_2}{\partial v}dv = 0 \qquad ...(5)$$

Multiplying (4) by l_1, (5) by l_2 and adding their sum to (3), we get

$$\left(\frac{\partial g}{\partial x} + l_1\frac{\partial f_1}{\partial x} + l_2\frac{\partial f_2}{\partial x}\right)dx + \left(\frac{\partial g}{\partial y} + l_1\frac{\partial f_1}{\partial y} + l_2\frac{\partial f_2}{\partial y}\right)dy$$
$$+\left(\frac{\partial g}{\partial u} + l_1\frac{\partial f_1}{\partial u} + l_2\frac{\partial f_2}{\partial u}\right)du + \left(\frac{\partial g}{\partial v} + l_1\frac{\partial f_1}{\partial v} + l_2\frac{\partial f_2}{\partial v}\right)dv = 0 \qquad ...(6)$$

Here, we have l_1 and l_2 are arbitrary, therefore we can choose them to satisfy the two linear equations

$$\frac{\partial g}{\partial x} + l_1\frac{\partial f_1}{\partial x} + l_2\frac{\partial f_2}{\partial x} = 0 \qquad ...(7)$$

and
$$\frac{\partial g}{\partial y} + l_1\frac{\partial f_1}{\partial y} + l_2\frac{\partial f_2}{\partial y} = 0 \qquad ...(8)$$

Using (7) and (8), equation (6) reduces to

$$\left(\frac{\partial g}{\partial u} + l_1\frac{\partial f_1}{\partial u} + l_2\frac{\partial f_2}{\partial u}\right)du + \left(\frac{\partial g}{\partial v} + l_1\frac{\partial f_1}{\partial v} + l_2\frac{\partial f_2}{\partial v}\right)dv = 0$$

Since, the given function contains four variables (namely x, y, u and v) and we are given two equations of conditions, therefore, only two of the variables are independent and it is immaterial which two of the four variables are regarded as independent. Let them be u and v then du and dv are also independent, therefore, their coefficients must be zero separately. Thus

$$\frac{\partial g}{\partial u} + l_1\frac{\partial f_1}{\partial u} + l_2\frac{\partial f_2}{\partial u} = 0 \qquad ...(9)$$
$$\frac{\partial g}{\partial v} + l_1\frac{\partial f_1}{\partial v} + l_2\frac{\partial f_2}{\partial v} = 0 \qquad ...(10)$$

Now, we have six equations namely (1),(2),(7),(8),(9) and (10) to determine the two multipliers l_1,l_2 and values of the four variables x,y,u and v for which maximum and minimum values of F are possible.

Now, defined a new function $V(x, y, u, v)$ such that

$$V(x,y,u,v) = g(x, y, u, v) + l_1 f_1(x, y, u, v) + l_2 f_2(x, y, u, v).$$

Assuming that x, y, u, v are now all independent variables. Hence, for the maxima and minima of V, we must have

$$\frac{\partial V}{\partial x} = \frac{\partial g}{\partial x} + l_1\frac{\partial f_1}{\partial x} + l_2\frac{\partial f_2}{\partial x} = 0 \qquad ...(11)$$
$$\frac{\partial V}{\partial y} = \frac{\partial g}{\partial y} + l_1\frac{\partial f_1}{\partial y} + l_2\frac{\partial f_2}{\partial y} = 0 \qquad ...(12)$$
$$\frac{\partial V}{\partial u} = \frac{\partial g}{\partial u} + l_1\frac{\partial f_1}{\partial u} + l_2\frac{\partial f_2}{\partial u} = 0 \qquad ...(13)$$

and
$$\frac{\partial V}{\partial v} = \frac{\partial g}{\partial v} + l_1\frac{\partial f_1}{\partial v} + l_2\frac{\partial f_2}{\partial v} = 0 \qquad ...(14)$$

Equations (11), (12), (13) and (14) are exactly the same as the equations (7). (8), (9) and (10). Hence, the maxima and minima of $V(x, y, u, v)$ are same as those of $F(x, y, u, v)$ assuming that $V(x, y, u, v)$ the variables x, y, u, v are now all independent.

Now, we proceed to find whether the values of F obtained with the help of above equations are maximum or minimum. For this, adopt the procedure, which is discussed ahead.

From (3), we get

$$d^2F = \left(\frac{\partial}{\partial x}dx + \frac{\partial}{\partial y}dy + \frac{\partial}{\partial u}du + \frac{\partial}{\partial y}dy\right)^2 g + \left(\frac{\partial g}{\partial x}d^2x + \frac{\partial g}{\partial y}d^2y + \frac{\partial g}{\partial u}d^2u + \frac{\partial g}{\partial y}d^2v\right)\ldots \quad \ldots(15)$$

Also

$$d^2f_1 = \left(\frac{\partial}{\partial x}dx + \frac{\partial}{\partial y}dy + \frac{\partial}{\partial u}du + \frac{\partial}{\partial v}dv\right)^2 f_1 + \frac{\partial f_1}{\partial x}d^2x + \frac{\partial f_1}{\partial y}d^2y + \frac{\partial f_1}{\partial u}d^2u + \frac{\partial f_1}{\partial v}d^2v = 0 \quad \ldots(16)$$

and $$d^2f_2 = \left(\frac{\partial}{\partial x}dx + \frac{\partial}{\partial y}dy + \frac{\partial}{\partial u}du + \frac{\partial}{\partial v}dv\right)^2 f_2 + \frac{\partial f_2}{\partial x}d^2x + \frac{\partial f_2}{\partial y}d^2y + \frac{\partial f_2}{\partial u}d^2u + \frac{\partial f_2}{\partial v}d^2v = 0 \quad \ldots(17)$$

Multiplying (16) by l_1 and (17) by l_2 and adding their sum to (15) and using the result (11), (12),(13) and (14), we have

$$d^2F = \left(\frac{\partial}{\partial x}dx + \frac{\partial}{\partial y}dy + \frac{\partial}{\partial u}du + \frac{\partial}{\partial v}dv\right)^2 (g + l_1f_1 + l_2f_2)$$

$$= \left(\frac{\partial}{\partial x}dx + \frac{\partial}{\partial y}dy + \frac{\partial}{\partial u}du + \frac{\partial}{\partial v}dv\right)^2 V = d^2V.$$

Hence d^2F is equal to d^2V, where d^2V is obtained by assuming all the variables x,y,u and v as independent. Therefore, it is clear that d^2F and d^2V have the same sign. Hence, F will be minimum or maximum according as V is minimum or maximum.

- This method has the advantage over the Lagrange's methods that it enables us to decide whether the values are maximum or minimum.

Solved Examples

EXAMPLE 1. *Find the maxima and minima of $x^2+y^2+z^2$ subject to the conditions : $ax^2+by^2+cz^2 = 1$ and $lx+my+nz = 0$* [UKTU–2011]

SOLUTION. Here, we have $u = x^2 + y^2 + z^2$ ...(1)

$$ax^2+by^2+cz^2=1 \quad \ldots(2)$$

and $$lx+my+nz=0 \quad \ldots(3)$$

For the maxima and minima of u, we must have

$$du=0$$

$$\Rightarrow 2xdx+2ydy+2zdz=0$$

$$\Rightarrow xdx+ydy+zdz=0 \quad \ldots(4)$$

From (2) and (3), we get

$$ax\,dx+by\,dy+cz\,dz=0 \quad \ldots(5)$$

$$ldx+mdy+ndz=0 \quad \ldots(6)$$

Now, multiplying (4) by 1, (5) by $l_1$and (6) by l_2 and adding, we get

$$(x\,dx+y\,dy+z\,dz) + l_1(ax\,dx+by\,dy+cz\,dz) + l_2(l\,dx+m\,dy+n\,dz)=0$$

$$\Rightarrow (x+al_1x+ll_2)dx+(y+bl_1y+ml_2)dy+(z+cl_1z+nl_2)dz = 0$$

Now equating the coefficient of dx, dy, dz to zero, we get

$$x+l_1ax+l_2l=0 \quad \ldots(7)$$

$$y+bl_1y+ml_2=0 \quad \ldots(8)$$

and $$z+cl_1z+nl_2=0 \quad \ldots(9)$$

Multiplying the equations (7), (8) and (9) by x, y and z respectively, and adding we get

$$x^2+y^2+z^2+l_1(ax^2+by^2+cz^2) + l_2(lx+my+nz)=0$$

or $u+l_1.1+l_2.0 = 0$

[By using (1), (2) and (3)]

$$\Rightarrow \quad l_1 = -u$$

Substituting for l_1 in the equations (7), (8) and (9), we get

$$x = \frac{l_2l}{au-1}, y = \frac{l_2m}{bu-1}, z = \frac{l_2n}{cu-1} \quad \ldots(10)$$

Now from (10) and (3), we get

$$\frac{l_2 l^2}{au-1}+\frac{l_2 m^2}{bu-1}+\frac{l_2 n^2}{cu-1}=0$$

or $$\frac{l^2}{au-1}+\frac{m^2}{bu-1}+\frac{n^2}{cu-1}=0 \quad ...(11)$$

which gives the maximum and minimum of $u = x^2 + y^2 + z^2$.

- Equation (11) is a quadratic in u. So it gives two stationary values of u.
- Geometrically, the surface $ax^2+by^2+cz^2=1$ represents an ellipsoid whose centre is origin, and $lx+my+nz=0$ represents a plane passing through the origin. The points (x, y, z) satisfying both the conditions (2) and (3) lies on the conic in which (2) and (3) intersect. $x^2+y^2+z^2$ gives the square of the distance (x, y, z) from the origin, which is also the centre of the conic of intersection. The maximum value of this distance is the major axis of this conic, and the minimum value of this distance is the minor axis of this conic. Hence, equation (11) gives the squares of the lengths of the semi-axis of the conic of intersection.

2. *Find the maxima and minima of $x^2+y^2+z^2$, where $ax^2 + by^2 + cz^2 + 2fyz + 2gzx + 2hxy = 1$.*

SOLUTION. Let $u= x^2+y^2+z^2$ ...(1)

where the relation between the variables x,y and z is

$$ax^2+by^2+cz^2+2fyz+2gzx+2hxy=1. \quad ...(2)$$

For a maximum or minima of u, we must have $du=0$

$$\Rightarrow \quad x\,dx+y\,dy+z\,dz=0. \quad ...(3)$$

From (2), we have

$$2ax\,dx+2by\,dy+2cz\,dz +2fy\,dz+2fz\,dy+2gz\,dx+2gx\,dz +2hx\,dy+2hy\,dx=0$$

$$\Rightarrow (ax+hy+gz)dx+(hx+by+fz)dy+(gx+fy+cz)dz=0. \quad ...(4)$$

Now, multiplying (3) by 1 and (4) by l_1, adding, and then equating the coefficient of dx, dy, dz to zero, we have

$$x+l_1(ax+hy+gz)=0. \quad ...(5)$$

$$y+l_1(hx+by+fz)=0. \quad ...(6)$$

$$z+l_1(gx+fy+cz)=0. \quad ...(7)$$

Multiplying (5) by x, (6) by y, (7) by z and adding, we get

$$x^2+y^2+z^2+l_1(ax^2+by^2+cz^2 +2fyz+2gzx+2hxy)=0$$

$$\Rightarrow \quad u+l_1.1=0 \quad \text{[From (1) and (2)]}$$

$$\therefore \quad l_1 =-u.$$

Hence, from (5), we have

$$x-u(ax+hy+gz)=0$$

$$\Rightarrow \left(a-\frac{1}{u}\right)x+hy+gz=0 \quad ...(8)$$

Similarly from (6) and (7), we get

$$hx+\left(b-\frac{1}{u}\right)y+fz=0 \quad ...(9)$$

and $$gx+fy+\left(c-\frac{1}{u}\right)z=0 \quad ...(10)$$

Eliminating x, y, z from (8), (9) and (10), we get

$$\begin{vmatrix} \left(a-\frac{1}{u}\right) & h & g \\ h & \left(b-\frac{1}{u}\right) & f \\ g & f & \left(c-\frac{1}{u}\right) \end{vmatrix}=0 \quad ...(11)$$

Hence, the maximum or minimum values of u are the roots of the equation (11).

3. *Find the maxima and minima of $u=x^2+y^2$ subject to the condition*

$$ax^2+2hxy+by^2=1.$$

SOLUTION. Here, we have

$$u = x^2+y^2 \quad ...(1)$$

where the relation between the variables x and y is

$$ax^2+2hxy+by^2 =1. \quad ...(2)$$

For the maxima and minima of u, we must have

$$du = 0$$

$$\Rightarrow \quad 2x\,dx+2y\,dy = 0$$

$$\Rightarrow \quad x\,dx+y\,dy = 0. \quad ...(3)$$

Now, from (2), we get

$$2ax\,dx+2hx\,dy+2hy\,dx+2by\,dy=0$$

$$\Rightarrow\quad (ax+hy)dx+(hx+by)dy=0 \qquad ...(4)$$

Now, multiplying (3) by 1, (4) by l_1, adding and then equating the coefficients of dx, dy to zero, we have

$$x+l_1(ax+hy)=0 \qquad ...(5)$$

and $$y+l_1(hx+by)=0 \qquad ..(6)$$

Multiplying (5) by x, (6) by y and adding, we get

$$x^2+y^2+l_1(ax^2+2hxy+by^2)=0$$

$$\Rightarrow\quad u+l_1.1=0 \qquad \text{[Using (1) and (2)]}$$

$$\Rightarrow\quad u=-l_1$$

Therefore, from (5), we have

$$x-u(ax+hy)=0$$

$$\Rightarrow\quad \left(a-\frac{1}{u}\right)x+hy=0 \qquad ...(7)$$

Similarly from (6), we have

$$hx+\left(b-\frac{1}{u}\right)y=0 \qquad ...(8)$$

Eliminating x and y from (7) and (8), we get

$$\begin{vmatrix} a-\dfrac{1}{u} & h \\ h & b-\dfrac{1}{u} \end{vmatrix}=0 \qquad ...(9)$$

Hence, the maximum or minimum values of u are the roots of the equation (9).

4. *Find the maximum value of $u=x^m y^n z^p$ subject to the condition $x+y+z=a$.* [ANNA–2009]

SOLUTION. Here, we have $\quad u=x^m y^n z^p \qquad ...(1)$

and x, y, z connected by the relation given by $\quad x+y+z=a \qquad ...(2)$

Taking log of both the sides of (1), we get

$$\log u = m\log x+n\log y+p\log z.$$

On differentiating, we get

$$\frac{1}{u}du=\frac{m}{x}dx+\frac{n}{y}dy+\frac{p}{z}dz$$

For the maxima and minima of u, we must have $du=0$

$$\Rightarrow\quad \frac{m}{x}dx+\frac{n}{y}dy+\frac{p}{z}dz=0 \qquad ...(3)$$

Now, differentiating (2), we get

$$dx+dy+dz=0. \qquad ...(4)$$

Now, multiplying (3) by 1 and (4) by l, and equating the coefficient of dx, dy, dz to zero (after adding), we get

$$\frac{m}{x}+l=0,\ \frac{n}{y}+l=0 \text{ and } \frac{p}{z}+l=0$$

which implies

$$x=-\frac{m}{l},\ y=-\frac{n}{l},\ z=-\frac{p}{l}$$

Putting the values of x, y and z in (2), we get $l=-\left(\dfrac{m+n+p}{a}\right)$ therefore, we can say that, u is stationary when

$$x=\frac{am}{m+n+p},\ y=\frac{an}{m+n+p},\ z=\frac{ap}{m+n+p}$$

Now, we find the nature of this stationary value of u.

Let us regard x and y as independent variable and z is a function of x and y given by (2) [It is justify, because the variables x, y and z are connected by the relation (2), any two of them may be regarded as independent].

Now from (1), we get

$$\log u = m\log x+n\log y+p\log z$$

$$\therefore\quad \frac{1}{u}\frac{\partial u}{\partial x}=\frac{m}{x}+\frac{p}{z}\frac{\partial z}{\partial x}$$

Now, differentiating (2) partially w.r.t x (treating y as constant), we get

$$1+\frac{\partial z}{\partial x}=0 \quad\Rightarrow\quad \frac{\partial z}{\partial x}=-1$$

Put this value in (5), we get

$$\frac{1}{u}\frac{\partial u}{\partial x}=\frac{m}{x}-\frac{p}{z}$$

$$\Rightarrow\quad \frac{1}{u}\frac{\partial^2 u}{\partial x^2}-\frac{1}{u^2}\left(\frac{\partial u}{\partial x}\right)^2$$

$$=-\frac{m}{x^2}+\frac{p}{z^2}\frac{\partial z}{\partial x}=-\frac{m}{x^2}-\frac{p}{z^2}$$

At stationary point, $\dfrac{\partial u}{\partial x}=0$

Therefore, $\frac{1}{u}\frac{\partial^2 u}{\partial x^2} = \frac{-m}{x^2} - \frac{p}{z^2}$

$$\Rightarrow \frac{\partial^2 u}{\partial x^2} = u\left[-\frac{m}{x^2} - \frac{p}{z^2}\right]$$

$$= -x^m y^n z^p\left[-\frac{m}{x^2} - \frac{p}{z^2}\right]$$

which is negative for the obtained values of x, y and z.

Hence, at the stationary point, u is maximum and maximum value is

$$= \left(\frac{am}{m+n+p}\right)^m\left(\frac{an}{m+n+p}\right)^n\left(\frac{ap}{m+n+p}\right)^p$$

Similar Problem

(1) Find the maximum and minimum value of $u = \frac{5xyz}{(x+2y+4z)}$ subject to the condition $xyz=8$.

5. *In a plane triangle ABC, find the maximum value of u = cosA cosB cosC.* [VTU–2010; ANNA–2006]

SOLUTION. Here, we have $u = \cos A \cos B \cos C$ ...(1)

Since, we know that the sum of the angles of a triangle is always 180°.

∴ The variables A, B and C are connected by the relation

$$A + B + C = \pi \quad ...(2)$$

From (1), we get

$$\log u = \log \cos A + \log \cos B + \log \cos C$$

$$\Rightarrow \frac{1}{u} du = -\tan A dA - \tan B dB - \tan C dC.$$

For the maxima and minima of u, we must have $du = 0$

$$\Rightarrow \tan A\, dA + \tan B\, dB + \tan C\, dC = 0 \quad ...(3)$$

Also from (2),

$$dA + dB + dC = 0 \quad ...(4)$$

Now, multiply (3) by 1, (4) by l, adding, and equating the coefficients of dA, dB and dC to zero, we get

$$\tan A + l = 0$$
$$\tan B + l = 0$$
$$\tan C + l = 0$$

$\Rightarrow l = -\tan A = -\tan B = -\tan C$

$\Rightarrow A = B = C.$

Now from (2), $A = B = C = \frac{\pi}{3}$ *i.e.*, the triangle is equilateral.

Now to show that the stationary value of u given by $A = B = C = \frac{\pi}{3}$ is maximum.

Let C be a function of A and B, regarding A and B as independent variables. From (1),

$$\log u = \log \cos A + \log \cos B + \log \cos C$$

$$\Rightarrow \frac{1}{u}\frac{\partial u}{\partial A} = -\tan A - \tan C\frac{\partial C}{\partial A}$$

Now, differentiating (2), partially w.r.t. A, we get

$$1 + \frac{dC}{dA} = 0 \Rightarrow \frac{\partial C}{\partial A} = -1$$

$$\therefore \frac{1}{u}\frac{\partial u}{\partial A} = -\tan A + \tan C$$

$$\Rightarrow \frac{1}{u}\frac{\partial^2 u}{\partial^2 A} - \frac{1}{u^2}\left(\frac{\partial u}{\partial A}\right)^2 = -\sec^2 A + \sec^2 C.\frac{\partial C}{\partial A}$$

$$= -(\sec^2 A + \sec^2 C)$$

At stationary point $\frac{\partial u}{\partial A} = 0$

$$\because \frac{\partial^2 u}{\partial^2 A} = -u\left(\sec^2 A + \sec^2 C\right) = -\text{ve}$$

for $A = B = C = \frac{\pi}{3}$.

Hence, u is maximum at $A = B = C = \frac{\pi}{3}$ and the maximum value is given by

$$u = \left(\cos\frac{\pi}{3}\right)^3 = \left(\frac{1}{2}\right)^3 = \frac{1}{8}.$$

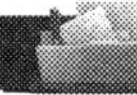

Exercise-10.3

Using Lagrange's method of undetermined multiplirers:

1. Find the maximum and minimum values of

$$\frac{x^2}{a^4}+\frac{y^2}{b^4}+\frac{z^2}{c^4}$$

where $lx+my+nz=0$ and $\frac{x^2}{a^2}+\frac{y^2}{b^2}+\frac{z^2}{c^2}=1$.

2. Find the maximum and minimum values of

$$f=a^2x^2+b^2y^2+c^2z^2$$

where $x^2+y^2+z^2=1$ and $lx+my+nz=0$.

3. Show that the maximum and minimum values of $u=x^2+y^2+z^2$ subject to the conditions

$$px+qy+rz = 0 \text{ and } \frac{x^2}{a^2}+\frac{y^2}{b^2}+\frac{z^2}{c^2}=1$$

are given by $\frac{a^2p^2}{u-a^2}+\frac{b^2q^2}{u-b^2}$.

4. Find the minimum value of $u=x+y+z$ subject to the condition $\frac{a}{x}+\frac{b}{y}+\frac{c}{z}=1$.

5. Find the minimum value of $u=x^2+y^2+z^2$, subject to the condition $ax+by+cz=p$.

(UKTU–2012, UPTU–2009)

6. Find the minimum value of $x+y+z$ where $xyz=c^3$.

7. Find the extreme values of $x^py^qz^r$ subject to the condition $\frac{a}{x}+\frac{b}{y}+\frac{c}{z}=1$.

8. Show that the maximum and minimum values of the radii vectors of the sections of the surface

$$(x^2+y^2+z^2)^2=\frac{x^2}{a^2}+\frac{y^2}{b^2}+\frac{z^2}{c^2}$$

by the plane $\lambda x+\mu y+\nu z=0$

are given by $\frac{a^2\lambda^2}{1-a^2r^2}+\frac{b^2\mu^2}{1-b^2r^2}+\frac{c^2\nu^2}{1-c^2r^2}=0$

9. Find the stationary points of the function $u=ax^p+by^q+cz^r$ subject to the condition

$$x^l+y^m+z^n=k.$$

10. If two variables x and y are connected by the relation $ax^2+by^2=ab$, show that the maximum and minimum values of the function $u=x^2+y^2+xy$ will be the roots of the equation $4(u-a)(u-b)=ab$.

11. Prove that of all rectangular parallelopipeds of the same volume, the cube has the least surface. [KURUKSHETRA–2006, UPTU–2004]

12. Prove that if $x+y+z=1$, $ayz+bzx+cxy$ has an extreme value equal to

$$\frac{abc}{2bc+2ca+2ab-a^2-b^2-c^2}$$

Also, prove if a, b, c are all positive and c lies between $a+b-2\sqrt{ab}$ and $a+b+2\sqrt{ab}$ this value is true maximum and that if a, b, c are all negative and c lies between $a+b\pm 2\sqrt{ab}$. It is true minimum.

13. Find the maximum value of u, when

$$u=\sin x \sin y \sin z$$

and x,y,z are the angles of a triangle.

14. Find the triangle of maximum area inscribed in a circle.

ANSWERS

1. The maximum and minimum values of the given function is given by the equation

$$\frac{l^2a^4}{a^2u-1}+\frac{m^2b^4}{b^2u-1}+\frac{n^2c^4}{c^2u-1}=0$$

2. The maximum and minimum values of the given function is given by the equation

$$\frac{l^2}{u-a^2}+\frac{m^2}{u-b^2}+\frac{m^2}{u-c^2}=0$$

4. Stationary points are $x=\sqrt{a}\left(\sqrt{a}+\sqrt{b}+\sqrt{c}\right), y=\sqrt{b}\left(\sqrt{a}+\sqrt{b}+\sqrt{c}\right), z=\sqrt{c}\left(\sqrt{a}+\sqrt{b}+\sqrt{c}\right)$, minimum value is $\left(\sqrt{a}+\sqrt{b}+\sqrt{c}\right)^2$.

5. Minimum value is $\frac{p^2}{\left(a^2+b^2+c^2\right)}$ **6.** u is minimum at the point $x=y=z=c$. Value is $=3c^4$.

7. u is stationary when $\frac{px}{a}=\frac{qy}{b}=\frac{rc}{c}=p+q+r$, Minimum value is $\frac{a^p b^q c^r}{p^p q^q r^r}(p+q+r)^{p+q+r}$.

9. Stationary points are given by $\frac{x^{p-1}}{l/pa}=\frac{y^{q-m}}{m/qb}=\frac{z^{r-n}}{n/rc}$ **13.** u is maximum, when $x=y=z=\frac{\pi}{3}$. Maximum value is $\frac{3\sqrt{3}}{8}$.

14. Equilateral.

❑❑❑❑❑❑

Chapter

11 Partial Differentiation and Change of Variables

11.1 INTRODUCTION

We know that the differential coefficient of $f(x)$ with respect to x is $\lim_{\delta x \to 0} \frac{f(x+\delta x)-f(x)}{\delta x}$, provided this limit exists, and it is denoted by

$$f'(x) \quad \text{or} \quad \frac{d}{dx}[f(x)]$$

If $u = f(x, y)$ be a continuous function of two independent variables x and y, then the differential coefficient of u w.r.t. x (regarding y as constant) is called the partial derivative or partial differential co-efficient of u w.r.t. x and is denoted by various symbols such as

$$\frac{\partial u}{\partial x}, \frac{\partial f}{\partial x}, f_x(x, y), f_x$$

Symbolically, if $u = f(x, y)$, then $\lim_{\delta x \to 0} \frac{f(x+\delta x, y)-f(x, y)}{\delta x}$

if it exists, is called the partial derivative or partial differential co-efficient of u w.r.t. x and is denoted by

$$\frac{\partial u}{\partial x} \quad \text{or} \quad \frac{\partial f}{\partial x} \quad \text{or} \quad f_x \quad \text{or} \quad u_x.$$

Similarly, by keeping x constant and allowing y alone to vary, we can define the partial derivative or partial differential coefficient of u w.r.t. y. It is denoted by any one of the symbols $\frac{\partial u}{\partial y}, \frac{\partial f}{\partial y}, f_y(x, y), f_y$.

Symbolically,
$$\frac{\partial u}{\partial y} = \lim_{\delta y \to 0} \frac{f(x, y+\delta y)-f(x, y)}{\delta y}$$

provided this limit exists.

For Example :

If $u = ax^2 + 2hxy + by^2$ then $\frac{\partial u}{\partial x} = 2ax + 2hy$ and $\frac{\partial u}{\partial y} = 2hx + 2by$.

11.2 RULES OF PARTIAL DIFFERENTIATION

Rule (1) :

(a) If u is a function of x, y and we are to differentiate partially w.r.t. x then, y is treated as constant.

(b) Similarly, if we are to differentiate u partially w.r.t. y then x is treated as constant.

(c) If u is a function of x, y, z and we are to differentiate partially w.r.t. x, then y and z are treated as constant.

Rule (2) : If $z = u \pm v$, where u and v are functions of x and y, then

$$\frac{\partial z}{\partial x} = \frac{\partial u}{\partial x} \pm \frac{\partial v}{\partial x} \text{ and } \frac{\partial z}{\partial y} = \frac{\partial u}{\partial y} \pm \frac{\partial v}{\partial y}.$$

Rule (3) : If $z = uv$, where u and v are functions of x and y, then

$$\frac{\partial z}{\partial x} = \frac{\partial}{\partial x}(uv) = u\frac{\partial v}{\partial x} + v\frac{\partial u}{\partial x} \text{ and } \frac{\partial z}{\partial y} = \frac{\partial}{\partial y}(uv) = u\frac{\partial v}{\partial y} + v\frac{\partial u}{\partial y}.$$

Rule (4) : If $z = \frac{u}{v}$, where u, v are functions of x and y, then

$$\frac{\partial z}{\partial x} = \frac{\partial}{\partial x}\left(\frac{u}{v}\right) = \frac{v\frac{\partial u}{\partial x} - u\frac{\partial v}{\partial x}}{v^2} \text{ and } \frac{\partial z}{\partial y} = \frac{\partial}{\partial y}\left(\frac{u}{v}\right) = \frac{v\frac{\partial u}{\partial y} - u\frac{\partial v}{\partial y}}{v^2}.$$

Rule (5) : If $z = f(u)$, where u is a function of x and y, then

$$\frac{\partial z}{\partial x} = \frac{\partial z}{\partial u}.\frac{\partial u}{\partial x} \text{ and } \frac{\partial z}{\partial y} = \frac{\partial z}{\partial u}.\frac{\partial u}{\partial y}.$$

- Partial means a 'part of'.
- If z is a function of one variable x, then $\frac{\partial z}{\partial x} = \frac{dz}{dx}$.
- If z is a function of two variables x_1 and x_2, we get $\frac{\partial z}{\partial x_1}$ and $\frac{\partial z}{\partial x_2}$.
- If z is a function of n variables $x_1, x_2, ..., x_n$ we can find $\frac{\partial z}{\partial x_1}, \frac{\partial z}{\partial x_2}, ..., \frac{\partial z}{\partial x_n}$.

11.2.1 Symmetric Function of x and y

A function $u = u(x, y)$ is said to be symmetric if, on interchanging x and y, u remains unchanged.

11.3 PARTIAL DERIVATIVES OF THE HIGHER ORDER

We can find partial derivative of $\frac{\partial u}{\partial x}$ and $\frac{\partial u}{\partial y}$ just as we found those of u for $\frac{\partial u}{\partial x}$ and $\frac{\partial u}{\partial y}$ are itself functions of x and y.

The four derivatives, thus obtained, called the second order partial derivatives of u or $f(x, y)$ are

$$\frac{\partial}{\partial x}\left(\frac{\partial u}{\partial x}\right), \frac{\partial}{\partial y}\left(\frac{\partial u}{\partial x}\right), \frac{\partial}{\partial x}\left(\frac{\partial u}{\partial y}\right), \frac{\partial}{\partial y}\left(\frac{\partial u}{\partial y}\right)$$

and are denoted as

$$\frac{\partial^2 u}{\partial x^2}, \frac{\partial^2 u}{\partial y \partial x}, \frac{\partial^2 u}{\partial x \partial y}, \frac{\partial^2 u}{\partial y^2}$$

or $\qquad f_{xx}, f_{yx}, f_{xy}, f_{yy}.$

- $\frac{\partial^2 u}{\partial x \partial y} = \frac{\partial}{\partial x}\left(\frac{\partial u}{\partial y}\right)$ and $\frac{\partial^2 u}{\partial y \partial x} = \frac{\partial}{\partial y}\left(\frac{\partial u}{\partial x}\right)$
- $\frac{\partial^2 u}{\partial x \partial y} \neq \frac{\partial u}{\partial x} \cdot \frac{\partial u}{\partial y}$
- The partial derivatives $\frac{\partial^2 u}{\partial x \partial y}$ and $\frac{\partial^2 u}{\partial y \partial x}$ are distinguished by the order in which u is successively differentiated by the order in which u is successively differntiated w.r.t. x and y, but it will be seen that, in general, that are equal.

Solved Examples

1. *Verify that* $\frac{\partial^2 u}{\partial x \partial y} = \frac{\partial^2 u}{\partial y \partial x}$, *where* $u = x \sin y + y \sin x$.

SOLUTION. We have $u = x \sin y + y \sin x$. ...(1)

Differentiating partially both sides of (1) *w.r.t.* x and y respectively, we get

$$\frac{\partial u}{\partial x} = \sin y + y \cos x \qquad ...(2)$$

and $$\frac{\partial u}{\partial y} = x \cos y + \sin x. \qquad ...(3)$$

Again differentiating (2) partially *w.r.t.* y and (3) *w.r.t.* x, we get

$$\frac{\partial^2 u}{\partial y \partial x} = \cos y + \cos x \qquad ...(4)$$

and $$\frac{\partial^2 u}{\partial x \partial y} = \cos y + \cos x. \qquad ...(5)$$

Form (4) and (5), we obtain

$$\frac{\partial^2 u}{\partial y \partial x} = \frac{\partial^2 u}{\partial x \partial y}.$$

2. *If* $u = x^2y + y^2z + z^2x$, *then show that*

$$\frac{\partial u}{\partial x} + \frac{\partial u}{\partial y} + \frac{\partial u}{\partial z} = (x+y+z)^2.$$

(UPTU(AG)–2006)

SOLUTION. Given that $u = x^2y + y^2z + z^2x$. ...(1)

Differentiating partially both sides of (1) *w.r.t.* x, y and z respectively, we get

$$\frac{\partial u}{\partial x} = 2xy + z^2 \qquad ...(2)$$

$$\frac{\partial u}{\partial y} = x^2 + 2yz \qquad ...(3)$$

and $$\frac{\partial u}{\partial z} = y^2 + 2zx. \qquad ...(4)$$

Adding (2), (3) and (4), we get

$$\frac{\partial u}{\partial x} + \frac{\partial u}{\partial y} + \frac{\partial u}{\partial z}$$
$$= 2xy + z^2 + x^2 + 2yz + y^2 + 2zx$$
$$= x^2 + y^2 + z^2 + 2xy + 2yz + 2zx$$
$$= (x+y+z)^2.$$

3. *If* $u = f\left(\frac{y}{x}\right)$, *show that*

$$x\frac{\partial u}{\partial x} + y\frac{\partial u}{\partial y} = 0.$$

SOLUTION. We have $u = f\left(\frac{y}{x}\right)$ ...(1)

Differentiating (1) partially w.r.t. x and y respectively, we get

$$\frac{\partial u}{\partial x} = f'\left(\frac{y}{x}\right).\left(-\frac{y}{x^2}\right)$$

$$\Rightarrow \qquad x\frac{\partial u}{\partial x} = -\frac{y}{x} f'\left(\frac{y}{x}\right) \qquad ...(2)$$

and $$\frac{\partial u}{\partial y} = f'\left(\frac{y}{x}\right).\frac{1}{x}$$

$$\Rightarrow \qquad y\frac{\partial u}{\partial y} = \frac{y}{x} f'\left(\frac{y}{x}\right) \qquad ...(3)$$

Adding (2) and (3), we get

$$x\frac{\partial u}{\partial x} + y\frac{\partial u}{\partial y} = 0.$$

4. *If* $z = f(x + ay) + \phi(x - ay)$, *prove that*

$$\frac{\partial^2 z}{\partial y^2} = a^2 \frac{\partial^2 z}{\partial x^2}.$$

(SRM–2006)

SOLUTION. Given that $z = f(x + ay) + \phi(x - ay)$. ...(1)

Differentiating partially both sides of (1) w.r.t. x and y respectively, we get

$$\frac{\partial z}{\partial x} = f'(x+ay) + \phi'(x-ay) \qquad ...(2)$$

and $$\frac{\partial z}{\partial y} = af'(x+ay) - a\phi'(x-ay). \qquad ...(3)$$

Again differentiating partially both

sides of (2) w.r.t. x and (3) *w.r.t.* y, we get

$$\frac{\partial^2 z}{\partial x^2} = f''(x+ay)+\phi''(x-ay) \quad \ldots(4)$$

and $$\frac{\partial^2 z}{\partial y^2}=a^2 f''(x+ay)+a^2\phi''(x-ay). \quad \ldots(5)$$

Form (4) and (5), we get

$$\frac{\partial^2 z}{\partial y^2} = a^2\frac{\partial^2 z}{\partial x^2}.$$

5. *If* $u=\log(x^3+y^3+z^3-3xyz)$, *show that* $\left(\frac{\partial}{\partial x}+\frac{\partial}{\partial y}+\frac{\partial}{\partial z}\right)^2 u=-\frac{9}{(x+y+z)^2}$.

[PTU–2010, ANNA–2007, BHOPAL–2008]

SOLUTION. We have $u=\log(x^3+y^3+z^3-3xyz)$

Differentiating partially with respect to x, we have

$$\frac{\partial u}{\partial x}=\frac{1}{x^3+y^3+z^3-3xyz}(3x^2-3yz)$$

$$\Rightarrow \frac{\partial u}{\partial x}=\frac{3(x^2-yz)}{x^3+y^3+z^3-3xyz}. \quad \ldots(1)$$

Similarly,

$$\frac{\partial u}{\partial y}=\frac{3(y^2-zx)}{x^3+y^3+z^3-3xyz} \quad \ldots(2)$$

and $$\frac{\partial u}{\partial z}=\frac{3(z^2-xy)}{x^3+y^3+z^3-3xyz} \quad \ldots(3)$$

Adding (1), (2) and (3), we get

$$\frac{\partial u}{\partial x}+\frac{\partial u}{\partial y}+\frac{\partial u}{\partial z}$$

$$=\frac{3(x^2+y^2+z^2-yz-zx-xy)}{x^3+y^3+z^3-3xyz}$$

$$=\frac{3(x^2+y^2+z^2-yz-zx-xy)}{(x+y+z)(x^2+y^2+z^2-yz-zx-xy)}$$

$$=\frac{3}{(x+y+z)}.$$

Also,

$$\left(\frac{\partial}{\partial x}+\frac{\partial}{\partial y}+\frac{\partial}{\partial z}\right)^2 u$$

$$=\left(\frac{\partial}{\partial x}+\frac{\partial}{\partial y}+\frac{\partial}{\partial z}\right)\left(\frac{\partial}{\partial x}+\frac{\partial}{\partial y}+\frac{\partial}{\partial z}\right)u$$

$$=\left(\frac{\partial}{\partial x}+\frac{\partial}{\partial y}+\frac{\partial}{\partial z}\right)\left(\frac{\partial u}{\partial x}+\frac{\partial u}{\partial y}+\frac{\partial u}{\partial z}\right)$$

$$=\left(\frac{\partial}{\partial x}+\frac{\partial}{\partial y}+\frac{\partial}{\partial z}\right)\left(\frac{3}{x+y+z}\right)$$

$$=3\left[\frac{\partial}{\partial x}\left(\frac{1}{x+y+z}\right)+\frac{\partial}{\partial y}\left(\frac{1}{x+y+z}\right)+\frac{\partial}{\partial z}\left(\frac{1}{x+y+z}\right)\right]$$

$$=3\left[-\frac{1}{(x+y+z)^2}-\frac{1}{(x+y+z)^2}-\frac{1}{(x+y+z)^2}\right]$$

$$=-\frac{9}{(x+y+z)^2}$$

6. *If* $u=\sin^{-1}\frac{x}{y}+\tan^{-1}\frac{y}{x}$, *show that* $x\frac{\partial u}{\partial x}+y\frac{\partial u}{\partial y}=0.$

SOLUTION. We have $u=\sin^{-1}\frac{x}{y}+\tan^{-1}\frac{y}{x}$

$$\Rightarrow \frac{\partial u}{\partial x}=\frac{1}{\sqrt{\left(1-\left(\frac{x}{y}\right)^2\right)}}.\frac{1}{y}+\frac{1}{1+\left(\frac{y}{x}\right)^2}.\left(-\frac{y}{x^2}\right)$$

$$=\frac{1}{\sqrt{y^2-x^2}}-\frac{y}{(x^2+y^2)}$$

$$\Rightarrow x\frac{\partial u}{\partial x}=\frac{x}{\sqrt{(y^2-x^2)}}-\frac{xy}{x^2+y^2} \quad \ldots(1)$$

Also, $$\frac{\partial u}{\partial y}=\frac{1}{\sqrt{\left(1-\left(\frac{x}{y}\right)^2\right)}}.\left(-\frac{x}{y^2}\right)+\frac{1}{1+\left(\frac{y}{x}\right)^2}.\left(\frac{1}{x}\right)$$

$$= -\frac{x}{y\sqrt{y^2 - x^2}} + \frac{x}{x^2 + y^2}$$

$$\Rightarrow \quad y\frac{\partial u}{\partial y} = -\frac{x}{\sqrt{(y^2 - x^2)}} + \frac{xy}{x^2 + y^2} \quad ..(2)$$

On adding (1) and (2), we get

$$x\frac{\partial u}{\partial x} + y\frac{\partial u}{\partial y} = 0.$$

7. *If* $u = f(r)$, *where* $r^2 = x^2 + y^2$, *show that* $\frac{\partial^2 u}{\partial x^2} + \frac{\partial^2 u}{\partial y^2} = f''(r) + \frac{1}{r}f'(r).$

(RAJASTHAN–2006)

SOLUTION. We have $r^2 = x^2 + y^2$

$$\left.\begin{aligned} &\Rightarrow \quad 2r\frac{\partial r}{\partial x} = 2x \text{ or } \frac{\partial r}{\partial x} = \frac{x}{r} \\ &\text{and} \quad 2r\frac{\partial r}{\partial y} = 2y \text{ or } \frac{\partial r}{\partial y} = \frac{y}{r} \end{aligned}\right] \quad ...(1)$$

Since, $u = f(r)$

$$\Rightarrow \quad \frac{\partial u}{\partial x} = [f'(r)].\frac{\partial r}{\partial x} = \frac{x}{r}f'(r)$$

$$\text{and} \quad \frac{\partial^2 u}{\partial x^2} = \frac{\partial}{\partial x}\left(\frac{\partial u}{\partial x}\right) = \frac{\partial}{\partial x}\left[x.\frac{1}{r}f'(r)\right]$$

$$= 1.\frac{1}{r}.f'(r) + [xf'(r)]\left[-\frac{1}{r^2}\frac{\partial r}{\partial x}\right] + \frac{x}{r}[f''(r)]\frac{\partial r}{\partial x}$$

$$= \frac{1}{r}.f'(r) - \frac{x}{r^2}.\frac{x}{r}f'(r) + \frac{x^2}{r^2}f''(r)$$

$$= \frac{1}{r}.f'(r) - \frac{x^2}{r^3}f'(r) + \frac{x^2}{r^2}f''(r). \quad ...(2)$$

Similarly, we may get

$$\frac{\partial^2 u}{\partial y^2} = \frac{1}{r}.f'(r) - \frac{y^2}{r^3}f'(r) + \frac{y^2}{r^2}f''(r) \quad ...(3)$$

Adding (2) and (3), we get

$$\frac{\partial^2 u}{\partial x^2} + \frac{\partial^2 u}{\partial y^2} = \frac{2}{r}.f'(r) - \frac{x^2 + y^2}{r^3}f'(r) + \frac{x^2 + y^2}{r^2}f''(r)$$

$$= \frac{2}{r}.f'(r) - \frac{r^2}{r^3}f'(r) + \frac{r^2}{r^2}f''(r)$$

$$= \frac{2}{r}.f'(r) - \frac{1}{r}f'(r) + f''(r)$$

$$= f''(r) + \frac{1}{r}.f'(r).$$

8. *If* $x^x y^y z^z = c$. *Show that at* $x = y = z$,

$$\frac{\partial^2 z}{\partial x \partial y} = -[x \log ex]^{-1}$$

(BHOPAL–2008)

SOLUTION. We have $\quad x^x y^y z^z = c. \quad ...(1)$

Here z can be regarding as a function of two independent variables x and y.

Taking log of both sides of (1), we have

$$x \log x + y \log y + z \log z = \log c. \quad ...(2)$$

Differentiating (2) partially w.r.t. x, we get

$$x.\frac{1}{x} + 1.\log x + \left[z.\frac{1}{z} + 1.\log z\right]\frac{\partial z}{\partial x} = 0$$

$$\Rightarrow \frac{\partial z}{\partial x} = -\frac{(1 + \log x)}{(1 + \log z)}. \quad ...(3)$$

Similarly differentiating (2), w.r.t. y, we get

$$\frac{\partial z}{\partial y} = -\frac{(1 + \log y)}{(1 + \log z)}. \quad ...(4)$$

$$\text{Also,} \quad \frac{\partial^2 z}{\partial x \partial y} = \frac{\partial}{\partial x}\left(\frac{\partial z}{\partial y}\right)$$

$$= \frac{\partial}{\partial x}\left[-\left(\frac{1 + \log y}{1 + \log z}\right)\right]$$

$$= -(1 + \log y)\frac{\partial}{\partial x}[(1 + \log z)^{-1}]$$

$$= -(1 + \log y).\left[-(1 + \log z)^{-2}\frac{1}{z}.\frac{\partial z}{\partial x}\right]$$

$$= \frac{(1 + \log y)}{z(1 + \log z)^2}.\left[-\left(\frac{1 + \log x}{1 + \log z}\right)\right].$$

For $x = y = z$, we have

$$\frac{\partial^2 z}{\partial x \partial y} = -\frac{(1 + \log x)^2}{x(1 + \log x)^3} = -\frac{1}{x(1 + \log x)}$$

$$= \frac{-1}{x[\log e + \log x]} \quad [\because \log e = 1]$$

$$= \frac{-1}{x \log(ex)} = -[x \log(ex)]^{-1}.$$

9. *If* $u = (1 - 2xy + y^2)^{-1/2}$, *prove that*

$$\frac{\partial}{\partial x}\left\{(1 - x^2)\frac{\partial u}{\partial x}\right\} + \frac{\partial}{\partial y}\left\{y^2\frac{\partial u}{\partial y}\right\} = 0.$$

(ROHTAK–2006)

SOLUTION. We have $u = (1-2xy+y^2)^{-1/2}$ ...(1)

Differentiating (1) partially with respect to x, we get

$$\frac{\partial u}{\partial x} = -\frac{1}{2}(1-2xy+y^2)^{-3/2}(-2y)$$

or $\frac{\partial u}{\partial x} = y(1-2xy+y^2)^{-3/2}$

$$\Rightarrow (1-x^2)\frac{\partial u}{\partial x} = y(1-x^2)(1-2xy+y^2)^{-\frac{3}{2}}$$

Again differentiating partially *w.r.t.* x, we get

$$\frac{\partial}{\partial x}\left\{(1-x^2)\frac{\partial u}{\partial x}\right\} = y\begin{bmatrix} -2x(1-2xy+y^2)^{-3/2} \\ +(1-x^2)\left(-\frac{3}{2}\right)(-2y) \\ (1-2xy+y^2)^{-5/2}\end{bmatrix}$$

$$= -2xy(1-2xy+y^2)^{-3/2} + 3y^2(1-x^2)(1-2xy+y^2)^{-5/2}$$

$$\therefore \frac{\partial}{\partial x}\left\{(1-x^2)\frac{\partial u}{\partial x}\right\} = -2xyu^3 + 3y^2(1-x^2)u^5$$

[Using (1)] ...(2)

Differentiating (1) partially *w.r.t.* y, we get

$$\frac{\partial u}{\partial y} = -\frac{1}{2}(1-2xy+y^2)^{-\frac{3}{2}}(-2x+2y)$$

or $\frac{\partial u}{\partial y} = (x-y)(1-2xy+y^2)^{-3/2}$

$$\Rightarrow y^2\frac{\partial u}{\partial y} = (x-y)y^2(1-2xy+y^2)^{-3/2}$$

Again differentiating partially *w.r.t.* y, we get

$$\frac{\partial}{\partial y}\left(y^2\frac{\partial u}{\partial y}\right) = (2xy-3y^2)(1-2xy+y^2)^{-\frac{3}{2}} + (xy^2-y^3)\left(-\frac{3}{2}\right)(-2x+2y)(1-2xy+y^2)^{-5/2}$$

$$= 2xy(1-2xy+y^2)^{-3/2} - 3y^2(1-2xy+y^2)^{-3/2} + 3y^2(x-y)^2(1-2xy+y^2)^{-5/2}$$

$$= 2xy(1-2xy+y^2)^{-3/2} - 3y^2(1-2xy+y^2)^{-5/2}\{(1-2xy+y^2)-(x-y)^2\}$$

$$= 2xy(1-2xy+y^2)^{-3/2} - 3y^2(1-x^2)(1-2xy+y^2)^{-5/2}$$

$$\therefore \frac{\partial}{\partial y}\left\{y^2\frac{\partial u}{\partial y}\right\} = 2xyu^3 - 3y^2(1-x^2)u^5$$

[Using (1)] ...(3)

Adding (2) and (3), we get

$$\frac{\partial}{\partial x}\left\{(1-x^2)\frac{\partial u}{\partial x}\right\} + \frac{\partial}{\partial y}\left\{y^2\frac{\partial u}{\partial y}\right\} = 0.$$

10. *If* $u = (x^2+y^2+z^2)^{-1/2}$, *show that*

(*i*) $x\frac{\partial u}{\partial x} + y\frac{\partial u}{\partial y} + z\frac{\partial u}{\partial z} = -u$

(*ii*) $\frac{\partial^2 u}{\partial x^2} + \frac{\partial^2 u}{\partial y^2} + \frac{\partial^2 u}{\partial z^2} = 0$

(GBTU–2011, VTU–2006, OSMANIA–2003)

SOLUTION. (i) We have $u = (x^2+y^2+z^2)^{-1/2}$ ...(1)

Differentiating (1) partially *w.r.t.* x, y and z respectively, we get

$$\frac{\partial u}{\partial x} = \left(-\frac{1}{2}\right)(x^2+y^2+z^2)^{-\frac{3}{2}}(2x)$$

or $\frac{\partial u}{\partial x} = \frac{-x}{(x^2+y^2+z^2)^{3/2}}$

$$\Rightarrow x\frac{\partial u}{\partial x} = \frac{-x^2}{(x^2+y^2+z^2)^{3/2}} \quad \text{...(2)}$$

Similarly, $y\frac{\partial u}{\partial y} = \frac{-y^2}{(x^2+y^2+z^2)^{3/2}}$ ...(3)

and $z\frac{\partial u}{\partial z} = \frac{-z^2}{(x^2+y^2+z^2)^{3/2}}$ ...(4)

Adding (2), (3) and (4), we get

$$x\frac{\partial u}{\partial x} + y\frac{\partial u}{\partial y} + z\frac{\partial u}{\partial z} = \frac{-(x^2+y^2+z^2)}{(x^2+y^2+z^2)^{3/2}} = -(x^2+y^2+z^2)^{-1/2}$$

$$\therefore x\frac{\partial u}{\partial x} + y\frac{\partial u}{\partial y} + z\frac{\partial u}{\partial z} = -u$$

(ii) We have $\frac{\partial^2 u}{\partial x^2} = \frac{\partial}{\partial x}\left(\frac{\partial u}{\partial x}\right)$

$$= \frac{\partial}{\partial x}\left\{\frac{-x}{(x^2+y^2+z^2)^{3/2}}\right\}$$

$$= -\left[\frac{1}{(x^2+y^2+z^2)^{3/2}} + x\left\{\frac{\left(-\frac{3}{2}\right)(2x)}{(x^2+y^2+z^2)^{-5/2}}\right\}\right]$$

$$= -\left[\frac{1}{(x^2+y^2+z^2)^{3/2}} - \frac{3x^2}{(x^2+y^2+z^2)^{5/2}}\right]$$

$$= -\frac{(y^2+z^2-2x^2)}{(x^2+y^2+z^2)^{5/2}}$$

$$\frac{\partial^2 u}{\partial x^2} = \frac{2x^2-y^2-z^2}{(x^2+y^2+z^2)^{5/2}} \quad \ldots(5)$$

Similarly,

$$\frac{\partial^2 u}{\partial y^2} = \frac{2y^2-x^2-z^2}{(x^2+y^2+z^2)^{5/2}} \quad \ldots(6)$$

and $$\frac{\partial^2 u}{\partial z^2} = \frac{2z^2-y^2-x^2}{(x^2+y^2+z^2)^{5/2}} \quad \ldots(7)$$

Adding (5), (6) and (7), we get

$$\frac{\partial^2 u}{\partial x^2} + \frac{\partial^2 u}{\partial y^2} + \frac{\partial^2 u}{\partial z^2} = 0$$

11. *If* $\theta = t^n e^{-r^2/4t}$, *find the value of n for which* $\frac{1}{r^2}\cdot\frac{\partial}{\partial r}\left(r^2\frac{\partial \theta}{\partial r}\right) = \frac{\partial \theta}{\partial t}$. (UPTU–2006, KURUKSHETRA–2006, NAGPUR–2009)

SOLUTION. We have $\theta = t^n e^{-r^2/4t}$ ...(1)

Then $$\frac{\partial \theta}{\partial r} = t^n\left[e^{-r^2/4t}\left(-\frac{2r}{4t}\right)\right]$$

$$= -\frac{r}{2}t^{n-1}e^{-r^2/4t}$$

$$\Rightarrow r^2\frac{\partial \theta}{\partial r} = -\frac{r^3}{2}t^{n-1}e^{-r^2/4t}$$

Now

$$\frac{\partial}{\partial r}\left(r^2\frac{\partial \theta}{\partial r}\right)$$

$$= -\frac{1}{2}t^{n-1}\left[3r^2e^{-r^2/4t} + r^3e^{-r^2/4t}\left(\frac{-2r}{4t}\right)\right]$$

$$= -\frac{3}{2}r^2t^{n-1}e^{-r^2/4t} + \frac{1}{4}r^4t^{n-2}e^{-r^2/4t}$$

$$\therefore \frac{1}{r^2}\cdot\frac{\partial}{\partial r}\left(r^2\frac{\partial \theta}{\partial r}\right)$$

$$= -\frac{3}{2}t^{n-1}e^{-r^2/4t} + \frac{1}{4}r^2t^{n-2}e^{-r^2/4t} \quad \ldots(2)$$

Again from (1), we get

$$\frac{\partial \theta}{\partial t} = nt^{n-1}e^{-r^2/4t} + t^n.e^{-r^2/4t}.\left(\frac{r^2}{4t^2}\right)$$

or $$\frac{\partial \theta}{\partial t} = nt^{n-1}e^{-r^2/4t} + \frac{1}{4}r^2t^{n-2}.e^{-r^2/4t} \quad \ldots(3)$$

Since, $$\frac{1}{r^2}\cdot\frac{\partial}{\partial r}\left(r^2\frac{\partial \theta}{\partial r}\right) = \frac{\partial \theta}{\partial t}$$

Then from (2) and (3), we have

$$-\frac{3}{2}t^{n-1}e^{-r^2/4t} + \frac{1}{4}r^2t^{n-2}e^{-r^2/4t}$$

$$= nt^{n-1}e^{-r^2/4t} + \frac{1}{4}r^2t^{n-2}.e^{-r^2/4t}$$

$$\Rightarrow n = -\frac{3}{2}.$$

Exercise-11.1

1. Find $\frac{\partial u}{\partial x}$ and $\frac{\partial u}{\partial y}$ when:

(i) $u = \log(x^2+y^2)$ (ii) $u = \cos^{-1}\left(\frac{x}{y}\right)$

(iii) $u = \frac{x^2}{a^2} + \frac{y^2}{b^2} - 1$

(iv) $u = \tan^{-1}\left(\frac{x^2+y^2}{x+y}\right)$

2. Find the second order partial derivatives of $\log(e^x + e^y)$.

3. Verify that $\frac{\partial^2 u}{\partial x\partial y} = \frac{\partial^2 u}{\partial y\partial x}$, where

(i) $u = \log(y \sin x + x \sin y)$

(ii) $u = \log\left(\frac{x^2+y^2}{xy}\right)$ (iii) $u = \log\left(\frac{x^2+y^2}{x+y}\right)$

(iv) $u = \sin^{-1}\frac{x}{y}$

(v) $u = x^y$ (ANNA–2009)

(vi) $u = \log\tan\left(\frac{y}{x}\right)$ (vii) $u = x^4 + x^2y^2 + y^4$

(viii) $u = \log\left(\frac{xy}{x^2+y^2}\right)$ (ix) $u = x \log y$

4. If $x = r\cos\theta$, $y = r\sin\theta$, show that

$$\frac{\partial r}{\partial x} = \frac{\partial x}{\partial r}, \frac{\partial x}{r\partial\theta} = r\frac{\partial\theta}{\partial x}.$$

5. If $u = \log(\tan x + \tan y)$, prove that

$$\sin 2x\frac{\partial u}{\partial x} + \sin 2y\frac{\partial u}{\partial y} = 2.$$

6. If $u = x^2\tan^{-1}\frac{y}{x} - y^2\tan^{-1}\frac{x}{y}$, prove that

$$\frac{\partial^2 u}{\partial x\partial y} = \frac{x^2-y^2}{x^2+y^2}.$$

(MUMBAI–2008, MADRAS–2000)

7. If $u = 2(ax+by)^2 - (x^2+y^2)$ and $a^2 + b^2 = 1$,

prove that $\frac{\partial^2 u}{\partial x^2} + \frac{\partial^2 u}{\partial y^2} = 0.$

8. If $u = \log(x^3 + y^3 - x^2y - xy^2)$, prove that

(i) $\frac{\partial u}{\partial x} + \frac{\partial u}{\partial y} = 2(x+y)^{-1}$

(ii) $\frac{\partial^2 u}{\partial x^2} + 2\frac{\partial^2 u}{\partial x\partial y} + \frac{\partial^2 u}{\partial y^2} = -4(x+y)^{-2}$

9. If $u = f(x+2y) + g(x-2y)$, show that

$$4\frac{\partial^2 u}{\partial x^2} = \frac{\partial^2 u}{\partial y^2}.$$

10. If $u = e^{xyz}$, show that

$$\frac{\partial^3 u}{\partial x\partial y\partial z} = (1 + 3xyz + x^2y^2z^2)e^{xyz}.$$

11. If $u(x+y) = x^2 + y^2$, show that

$$\left(\frac{\partial u}{\partial x} - \frac{\partial u}{\partial y}\right)^2 = 4\left(1 - \frac{\partial u}{\partial x} - \frac{\partial u}{\partial y}\right).$$

12. If $\tan u = \frac{\cos x}{\sinh y}$ and $\tanh v = \frac{\sinh x}{\cosh y}$ show that $\frac{\partial u}{\partial x} = \frac{\partial v}{\partial y}$ and $\frac{\partial u}{\partial y} = -\frac{\partial v}{\partial x}$.

13. Show that $\frac{\partial^2 u}{\partial x^2} + \frac{\partial^2 u}{\partial y^2} = 0$, if

(i) $u = e^{my}\cos mx$ (ii) $u = \tan^{-1}\frac{y}{x}$.

14. If $\frac{x^2}{a^2+u} + \frac{y^2}{b^2+u} + \frac{z^2}{c^2+u} = 1$, show that

$$\left(\frac{\partial u}{\partial x}\right)^2 + \left(\frac{\partial u}{\partial y}\right)^2 + \left(\frac{\partial u}{\partial z}\right)^2 = 2\left(x\frac{\partial u}{\partial x} + y\frac{\partial u}{\partial y} + z\frac{\partial u}{\partial z}\right)$$

15. Find the value of $\frac{1}{a^2}\frac{\partial^2 z}{\partial x^2} + \frac{1}{b^2}\frac{\partial^2 z}{\partial y^2}$, when

$$a^2x^2 + b^2y^2 - c^2z^2 = 0.$$

16. If $z = e^{ax+by}f(ax-by)$, show that

$$b\frac{\partial z}{\partial x} + a\frac{\partial z}{\partial y} = 2abz.$$

17. If $u = \sqrt{x^2+y^2+z^2}$, show that

$$\left(\frac{\partial u}{\partial x}\right)^2 + \left(\frac{\partial u}{\partial y}\right)^2 + \left(\frac{\partial u}{\partial z}\right)^2 = 1.$$

18. If $x = r\cos\theta$, $y = r\sin\theta$, prove that

(i) $\frac{\partial^2\theta}{\partial x^2} + \frac{\partial^2\theta}{\partial y^2} = 0$ except when $x = 0, y = 0$

(ii) $\left(\frac{\partial r}{\partial x}\right)^2 + \left(\frac{\partial r}{\partial y}\right)^2 = 1$ (BURDWAN–2003)

(iii) $\frac{\partial^2 r}{\partial x^2} + \frac{\partial^2 r}{\partial y^2} = \frac{2}{r}\left\{\left(\frac{\partial r}{\partial x}\right)^2 + \left(\frac{\partial r}{\partial y}\right)^2\right\}$.

19. If $u = \log(x^2 + y^2 + z^2)$, then prove that

$$x\frac{\partial^2 u}{\partial y\partial z} = y\frac{\partial^2 u}{\partial z\partial x} = z\frac{\partial^2 u}{\partial x\partial y}.$$

20. If $x^2(y-z) + y^2(z-x) + z^2(x-y)$, prove that

$$\frac{\partial u}{\partial x} + \frac{\partial u}{\partial y} + \frac{\partial u}{\partial z} = 0.$$

21. (i) If $u = \sqrt{x^2+y^2+z^2}$, then prove that

$$\frac{\partial^2 u}{\partial x^2} + \frac{\partial^2 u}{\partial y^2} + \frac{\partial^2 u}{\partial z^2} = \frac{2}{u}.$$

(ii) If $u = \log\sqrt{x^2+y^2+z^2}$, show that

$$(x^2+y^2+z^2)\left(\frac{\partial^2 u}{\partial x^2} + \frac{\partial^2 u}{\partial y^2} + \frac{\partial^2 u}{\partial z^2}\right) = 1.$$

22. (i) If $u = \sin^{-1}\left(\frac{x^{1/3}+y^{1/3}}{x^{1/2}-y^{1/2}}\right)^{1/2}$, show that

$$x\frac{\partial u}{\partial x} + y\frac{\partial u}{\partial y} = -\frac{1}{12}\tan u.$$

(ii) If $u = x\sin^{-1}\left(\frac{x}{y}\right) + y\sin^{-1}\left(\frac{y}{x}\right)$, show that

$$x^2\frac{\partial^2 u}{\partial x^2} + 2xy\frac{\partial^2 u}{\partial x\partial y} + y^2\frac{\partial^2 u}{\partial y^2} = 0.$$

(iii) If $u = x^2\tan^{-1}\left(\frac{y}{x}\right) - y^2\tan^{-1}\left(\frac{x}{y}\right)$, show that $x^2\frac{\partial^2 u}{\partial x^2} + 2xy\frac{\partial^2 u}{\partial x\partial y} + y^2\frac{\partial^2 u}{\partial y^2} = 2u.$

(HISAR–2003)

ANSWERS

1. (i) $\frac{2x}{x^2+y^2}, \frac{2y}{x^2+y^2}$ (ii) $-\frac{1}{\sqrt{y^2-x^2}}, \frac{x}{y\sqrt{y^2-x^2}}$ (iii) $\frac{2x}{a^2}, \frac{2y}{b^2}$

(iv) $\frac{(x^2+2xy-y^2)}{(x+y)^2+(x^2+y^2)^2}, \frac{(y^2+2xy-x^2)}{(x+y)^2+(x^2+y^2)^2}$

2. (i) $\frac{e^{x+y}}{(e^x+e^y)^2}, -\frac{e^{x+y}}{(e^x+e^y)^2}, \frac{e^{x+y}}{(e^x+e^y)^2}$ **15.** $\frac{1}{c^2z}$

11.4 HOMOGENEOUS FUNCTIONS

A function $f(x, y)$ is said to be homogeneous function of degree n, if the degree of each of its terms in x and y is equal to n. Thus

$$a_0x^n + a_1x^{n-1}y + a_2x^{n-2}y^2 + \ldots + a_{n-1}xy^{n-1} + a_ny^n \qquad \ldots(1)$$

is homogeneous function in x and y of order n.

- This definition of homogeneity applies to polynomial functions only. To widen the concept of homogeneity so as to bring even transcendental functions within its scope, we define u as a homogeneous function in x and y of order or degree n, if it can be expressed in the form of $x^n f\left(\frac{y}{x}\right)$.
- This definition also covers the polynomial function (1), which can be written as

$$x^n\left[a_0 + a_1\frac{y}{x} + a_2\left(\frac{y}{x}\right)^2 + \ldots + a_n\left(\frac{y}{x}\right)^n\right] = x^n f\left(\frac{y}{x}\right).$$

$\therefore$ It is a homogeneous function of order n.
- To test whether a given function $f(x, y)$, is homogeneous or not we put $x = hx$ and $y = hy$ in it. If we get $f(hx, hy) = h^n f(x, y)$, the function $f(x, y)$ is homogeneous of degree n, otherwise $f(x, y)$ is not a homogeneous function.
- A homogeneous function in x and y of degree n can also be written as $y^n f\left(\frac{x}{y}\right)$.
- A function u of three variables x, y, z is said to be homogeneous function of degree n, if it can be expressed in the form

$$u = x^n f_1\left(\frac{y}{x}, \frac{z}{x}\right) \quad \text{or} \quad y^n f_2\left(\frac{x}{y}, \frac{z}{y}\right) \quad \text{or} \quad z^n f_3\left(\frac{x}{z}, \frac{y}{z}\right).$$

In general, a function u of several variables $x_1, x_2, \ldots, x_n$ is said to be homogeneous function of degree m if it can be expressed in the form $u = x_1^m f_1\left(\frac{x_2}{x_1}, \frac{x_3}{x_1}, \ldots, \frac{x_n}{x_1}\right)$ or $x_2^m f_2\left(\frac{x_1}{x_2}, \frac{x_3}{x_2}, \ldots, \frac{x_n}{x_2}\right)$ or etc.

THEOREM 1. *If u is a homogeneous function of x and y of degree n, then $\frac{\partial u}{\partial x}$ and $\frac{\partial u}{\partial y}$ are homogeneous function of degree (n – 1) each.*

PROOF. Since, u is a homogeneous function of x and y of degree n therefore, u can be expressed as $u = x^n f\left(\frac{y}{x}\right)$. $\ldots(1)$

Now from (1)

$$\frac{\partial u}{\partial x} = nx^{n-1} f\left(\frac{y}{x}\right) + x^n f'\left(\frac{y}{x}\right)\left(-\frac{y}{x^2}\right) = x^{n-1}\left[nf\left(\frac{y}{x}\right) + f'\left(\frac{y}{x}\right)\left(-\frac{y}{x}\right)\right]$$

$$= x^{n-1} \times \text{a function of } \frac{y}{x} = x^{n-1} g\left(\frac{y}{x}\right) \text{ (say).}$$

which is a homogeneous function of degree $(n - 1)$.

Also, $$\frac{\partial u}{\partial y} = x^n f'\left(\frac{y}{x}\right).\left(\frac{1}{x}\right) = x^{n-1} f'\left(\frac{y}{x}\right) = x^{n-1} \times \text{a function of } \frac{y}{x}$$
$$= x^{n-1} g\left(\frac{y}{x}\right) \text{ (say).}$$

which is a homogeneous function of x and y of degree $(n - 1)$.

THEOREM 2. [Euler's Theorem on Homogeneous Functions].

If u be a homogeneous function of x and y of degree n, then $x\dfrac{\partial u}{\partial x} + y\dfrac{\partial u}{\partial y} = nu.$

PROOF. Since, u is a homogeneous function of x and y of degree n therefore, u can be expressed as

$$u = x^n f\left(\frac{y}{x}\right).$$

$$\therefore \quad \frac{\partial u}{\partial x} = nx^{n-1} f\left(\frac{y}{x}\right) + x^n f'\left(\frac{y}{x}\right)\left(-\frac{y}{x^2}\right) = nx^{n-1} f\left(\frac{y}{x}\right) - yx^{n-2} f'\left(\frac{y}{x}\right).$$

Also, $$\frac{\partial u}{\partial y} = x^n f'\left(\frac{y}{x}\right).\left(\frac{1}{x}\right) = x^{n-1} f'\left(\frac{y}{x}\right).$$

Now, $$\text{L.H.S.} = x\frac{\partial u}{\partial x} + y\frac{\partial u}{\partial y} = x\left[nx^{n-1} f\left(\frac{y}{x}\right) - yx^{n-2} f'\left(\frac{y}{x}\right)\right] + yx^{n-1} f'\left(\frac{y}{x}\right)$$
$$= nx^n f\left(\frac{y}{x}\right) - yx^{n-1} f'\left(\frac{y}{x}\right) + yx^{n-1} f'\left(\frac{y}{x}\right) = nx^n f\left(\frac{y}{x}\right) = nu = \text{R.H.S.}$$

- Euler's theorem can be extended to a homogeneous functions of several variables. Thus, if u be the function of m independent variables $x_1, x_2, ..., x_m$ of degree n then, Euler's theorem states that
$$x_1\frac{\partial u}{\partial x_1} + x_2\frac{\partial u}{\partial x_2} + ... + x_m\frac{\partial u}{\partial x_m} = nu.$$

THEOREM 3. *If u is a homogeneous function in x and y of degree n, then* $$x^2\frac{\partial^2 u}{\partial x^2} + 2xy\frac{\partial^2 u}{\partial x \partial y} + y^2\frac{\partial^2 u}{\partial y^2} = n(n-1)u.$$

PROOF. Since, u is a homogeneous function in x and y of degree n therefore, by Euler's theorem

$$x\frac{\partial u}{\partial x} + y\frac{\partial u}{\partial y} = nu \qquad ...(1)$$

Differentiating (1) partially *w.r.t.* x, we get

$$\frac{\partial}{\partial x}\left(x\frac{\partial u}{\partial x}\right) + \frac{\partial}{\partial x}\left(y\frac{\partial u}{\partial y}\right) = \frac{\partial}{\partial x}(nu)$$

$$\left(\because \text{ Each of } \frac{\partial u}{\partial x} \text{ and } \frac{\partial u}{\partial y} \text{ is a function of both } x \text{ and } y\right)$$

$$\Rightarrow \quad x\frac{\partial^2 u}{\partial x^2} + \frac{\partial u}{\partial x}.1 + y\frac{\partial^2 u}{\partial x \partial y} = n\frac{\partial u}{\partial x}$$

$$\Rightarrow \quad x\frac{\partial^2 u}{\partial x^2} + y\frac{\partial^2 u}{\partial x \partial y} = (n-1)\frac{\partial u}{\partial x} \qquad ...(2)$$

Again differentiating (2) partially w.r.t. y, we get

$$y\frac{\partial^2 u}{\partial y^2} + x\frac{\partial^2 u}{\partial x \partial y} = (n-1)\frac{\partial u}{\partial y} \qquad ...(3)$$

Now, multiply (2) by x, (3) by y and then adding, we get

$$x^2\frac{\partial^2 u}{\partial x^2}+2xy\frac{\partial^2 u}{\partial x\partial y}+y^2\frac{\partial^2 u}{\partial y^2}=(n-1)\left[x\frac{\partial u}{\partial y}+y\frac{\partial u}{\partial y}\right]=(n-1)nu=n(n-1)u.$$

- If z is a homogeneous function of x and y of degree n and if $z = f(u)$, then we have the following results :

  (i) $x\frac{\partial u}{\partial x}+y\frac{\partial u}{\partial y}=n\frac{f(u)}{f'(u)}=G(u)$

  (ii) $x^2\frac{\partial^2 u}{\partial x^2}+2xy\frac{\partial^2 u}{\partial x\partial y}+y^2\frac{\partial^2 u}{\partial y^2}=G(u)[G'(u)-1]$

Solved Examples

1. *Verify the Euler's theorem for the function* $u = axy + byz + czx$.

SOLUTION. We have $u = axy + byz + czx$. ...(1)

which is a homogeneous function of x, y and z of degree 2.

To verify the Euler's theorem, we must show $x\frac{\partial u}{\partial x}+y\frac{\partial u}{\partial y}+z\frac{\partial u}{\partial z}=2u$

Now, $\frac{\partial u}{\partial x}=ay+cz, \frac{\partial u}{\partial y}=ax+bz, \frac{\partial u}{\partial z}=by+cx.$

$$\therefore\ x\frac{\partial u}{\partial x}+y\frac{\partial u}{\partial y}+z\frac{\partial u}{\partial z}$$
$$=x(ay+cz)+y(ax+bz)+z(by+cx).$$
$$=2(axy+byz+czx)=2u.$$

Hence, Euler's theorem is verified.

2. *If* $u=\sin^{-1}\left[\frac{x^2+y^2}{x+y}\right]$, *show that*

$$x\frac{\partial u}{\partial x}+y\frac{\partial u}{\partial y}=\tan u.$$

(BHOPAL–2009)

SOLUTION. We have $\sin u=\left[\frac{x^2+y^2}{x+y}\right]$

Let $v=\frac{x^2+y^2}{x+y}$

$\Rightarrow v$ is a homogeneous of x and y of degree 1.

Then, by Euler's theorem, we have

$$x\frac{\partial v}{\partial x}+y\frac{\partial v}{\partial y}=v \qquad ...(1)$$

$$v=\sin u\Rightarrow\frac{\partial v}{\partial x}=\cos u\frac{\partial u}{\partial x}$$

and $$\frac{\partial v}{\partial y}=\cos u\frac{\partial u}{\partial y}.$$

Put these values in (1), we get

$$x\cos u\frac{\partial u}{\partial x}+y\cos u\frac{\partial u}{\partial y}=v$$
$$\Rightarrow x\frac{\partial u}{\partial x}+y\frac{\partial u}{\partial y}=\frac{v}{\cos u}=\frac{\sin u}{\cos u}=\tan u.$$

3. *If* $u=\tan^{-1}\frac{x^3+y^3}{x-y}$, *prove that*

$$x^2\frac{\partial^2 u}{\partial x^2}+2xy\frac{\partial^2 u}{\partial x\partial y}+y^2\frac{\partial^2 u}{\partial y^2}=(1-4\sin^2 u)\sin 2u.$$

SOLUTION. We have $u=\tan^{-1}\frac{x^3+y^3}{x-y}$

$$\therefore\ \tan u=\frac{x^3+y^3}{x-y}=\frac{x^3\left[1+\left(\frac{y}{x}\right)^3\right]}{x\left[1-\frac{y}{x}\right]}=x^2 f\left(\frac{y}{x}\right)$$

$\tan u$ is of the form $x^n f\left(\frac{y}{x}\right)$ with $n = 2$.

$\therefore$ $\tan u$ is a homogeneous function in x, y of degree 2. Then, by Euler's theorem

$$x\frac{\partial}{\partial x}(\tan u)+y\frac{\partial}{\partial y}(\tan u)=2\tan u$$

$$\Rightarrow x\sec^2 u\frac{\partial u}{\partial x}+y\sec^2 u\frac{\partial u}{\partial y}=2\tan u$$

$$\Rightarrow x\frac{\partial u}{\partial x}+y\frac{\partial u}{\partial y}=\frac{2\tan u}{\sec^2 u}$$

$$=2\sin u\cos u=\sin 2u \quad \ldots(1)$$

Differentiate (1) partially *w.r.t.* x, we get

$$\left(x\frac{\partial^2 u}{\partial x^2}+\frac{\partial u}{\partial x}\right)+y\frac{\partial^2 u}{\partial x\partial y}=2\cos 2u\frac{\partial u}{\partial x}$$

$$\therefore\ x\frac{\partial^2 u}{\partial x^2}+y\frac{\partial^2 u}{\partial x\partial y}=(2\cos 2u-1)\frac{\partial u}{\partial x} \quad \ldots(2)$$

Interchanging x and y in (2), we get

$$y\frac{\partial^2 u}{\partial y^2}+x\frac{\partial^2 u}{\partial x\partial y}=(2\cos 2u-1)\frac{\partial u}{\partial y} \quad \ldots(3)$$

Now multiplying (2) by x, (3) by y and then adding, we get

$$x^2\frac{\partial^2 u}{\partial x^2}+2xy\frac{\partial^2 u}{\partial x\partial y}+y^2\frac{\partial^2 u}{\partial y^2}$$

$$=(2\cos 2u-1)\left[x\frac{\partial u}{\partial x}+y\frac{\partial u}{\partial y}\right]$$

$$=(2\cos 2u-1).\sin 2u$$

$$=[2(1-2\sin^2 u)-1]\sin 2u$$

$$=(1-4\sin^2 u)\sin 2u.$$

4. *If* $u=\sin^{-1}\left(\frac{x}{y}\right)+\tan^{-1}\left(\frac{y}{x}\right)$, *show that*

$$x\frac{\partial u}{\partial x}+y\frac{\partial u}{\partial y}=0\times u=0$$

(HAZARIBAGH–2009, OSMANIA–2003)

SOLUTION. We have $u=\sin^{-1}\left(\frac{x}{y}\right)+\tan^{-1}\left(\frac{y}{x}\right)$

$$=x^0\left[\sin^{-1}\left(\frac{1}{y/x}\right)+\tan^{-1}\left(\frac{y}{x}\right)\right]$$

$\Rightarrow u$ is a homogeneous function of order 0.

Then, by Euler's theorem,we have

$$x\frac{\partial u}{\partial x}+y\frac{\partial u}{\partial y}=0\times u=0$$

5. *If* $u=\left(x^{1/4}+y^{1/4}\right)\left(x^{1/5}+y^{1/5}\right)$. *Apply Euler's theorem to find the value of* $x\frac{\partial u}{\partial x}+y\frac{\partial u}{\partial y}$.

SOLUTION. Here, we have

$$u(x,y)=\left(x^{1/4}+y^{1/4}\right)\left(x^{1/5}+y^{1/5}\right)$$

$$\Rightarrow u(tx,ty)=t^{\frac{1}{4}}(x^{\frac{1}{4}}+y^{\frac{1}{4}})t^{\frac{1}{5}}(x^{\frac{1}{5}}+y^{\frac{1}{5}})$$

$$=t^{9/20}\left(x^{1/4}+y^{1/4}\right)\left(x^{1/5}+y^{1/5}\right)$$

$$=t^{9/20}u(x,y)$$

Clearly, u is a homogeneous function of degree $\frac{9}{20}$.

Hence, by Euler's theorem we have

$$x\frac{\partial u}{\partial x}+y\frac{\partial u}{\partial y}=\frac{9}{20}u.$$

6. *Verify Euler's theoerm for* $f(x,y,z)=3x^2yz+5xy^2z+4z^4$. (JNTU–1999)

SOLUTION. Let $f(x, y, z) = 3x^2yz + 5xy^2z + 4z^4$.

$$\therefore \frac{\partial f}{\partial x}=6xyz+5y^2z;\frac{\partial f}{\partial y}=3x^2z+10xyz$$

and $\frac{\partial f}{\partial z}=3x^2y+5xy^2+16z^3$

$$\therefore\ x\frac{\partial f}{\partial x}+y\frac{\partial f}{\partial y}+z\frac{\partial f}{\partial z}=x(6xyz+5y^2z)$$

$$+y(3x^2z+10xyz)$$

$$z(3x^2y+5xy^2+16z^3)$$

$$=4(3x^2yz+5xy^2z+4z^4)=4f \quad \ldots(1)$$

Also,

$$f(x,y,z)$$

$$=x^4\left[3.\frac{y}{x}.\frac{z}{x}+5\left(\frac{y}{x}\right)^2\left(\frac{z}{x}\right)+4\left(\frac{z}{x}\right)^4\right]$$

is a homogeneous function of x, y, z of degree 4.

Hence, by Euler's theorem

$$x\frac{\partial f}{\partial x}+y\frac{\partial f}{\partial y}+z\frac{\partial f}{\partial z}=4f. \quad \ldots(2)$$

From (1) and (2) we conclude that Euler's theorem is verified.

7. *If* $u=f\left(\frac{y}{x}\right)+\sqrt{x^2+y^2}$, *show that*

$$x\frac{\partial u}{\partial x}+y\frac{\partial u}{\partial y}=\sqrt{x^2+y^2}.$$

(MUMBAI–2008)

SOLUTION. Let us write $u = v + w$

where $v = f\left(\frac{y}{x}\right) = x^0 f\left(\frac{y}{x}\right)$

and $w = \sqrt{x^2 + y^2} = x\sqrt{1+\left(\frac{y}{x}\right)^2}$

Therefore, v and w are homogeneous function of degree 0 and 1 in x and y respectively. Hence, by Euler's theorem

$$x\frac{\partial v}{\partial x} + y\frac{\partial v}{\partial y} = 0.v = 0 \quad \ldots(1)$$

and $x\frac{\partial w}{\partial x} + y\frac{\partial w}{\partial y} = 1.w = \sqrt{x^2+y^2}$ ...(2)

On adding (1) and (2), we get

$$x\left(\frac{\partial v}{\partial x} + \frac{\partial w}{\partial x}\right) + y\left(\frac{\partial v}{\partial y} + \frac{\partial w}{\partial y}\right) = \sqrt{x^2+y^2} \quad \ldots(3)$$

Now, since $u = v + w$, then using (3) we get $x\frac{\partial u}{\partial x} + y\frac{\partial u}{\partial y} = \sqrt{x^2+y^2}$.

8. *If* $z = x^n f_1\left(\frac{y}{x}\right) + y^{-n} f_2\left(\frac{x}{y}\right)$, *then show that*

$$x^2\frac{\partial^2 z}{\partial x^2} + 2xy\frac{\partial^2 z}{\partial x \partial y} + y^2\frac{\partial^2 z}{\partial y^2} + x\frac{\partial z}{\partial x} + y\frac{\partial z}{\partial y} = n^2 z$$

(ROHTAK(MDU)–2003, KURUKSHETRA–2009)

SOLUTION. Let $u = x^n f_1\left(\frac{y}{x}\right), v = y^{-n} f_2\left(\frac{x}{y}\right)$ ...(1)

$\therefore \quad z = u + v$ ...(2)

Clearly, u and v are homogeneous functions of degree n and $-n$ respectively. Then by Euler's theorem, we get

$$x\frac{\partial u}{\partial x} + y\frac{\partial u}{\partial y} = nu \quad \ldots(3)$$

$$x\frac{\partial v}{\partial x} + y\frac{\partial v}{\partial y} = (-n).v \quad \ldots(4)$$

$$x^2\frac{\partial^2 u}{\partial x^2} + 2xy\frac{\partial^2 u}{\partial x \partial y} + y^2\frac{\partial^2 u}{\partial y^2} = n(n-1)u \quad \ldots(5)$$

and $x^2\frac{\partial^2 v}{\partial x^2} + 2xy\frac{\partial^2 v}{\partial x \partial y} + y^2\frac{\partial^2 v}{\partial y^2} = (-n)(-n-1)v = n(n+1)v$ ...(6)

Since $z = u + v \Rightarrow \frac{\partial z}{\partial x} = \frac{\partial u}{\partial x} + \frac{\partial v}{\partial x}$

and $\frac{\partial z}{\partial y} = \frac{\partial u}{\partial y} + \frac{\partial v}{\partial y}$ ...(7)

Adding (3) and (4) and using (7) we get

$$x\frac{\partial z}{\partial x} + y\frac{\partial z}{\partial y} = n(u-v) \quad \ldots(8)$$

Similarly, adding (5) and (6) and using (7) we get

$$x^2\left[\frac{\partial^2 u}{\partial x^2} + \frac{\partial^2 v}{\partial x^2}\right] + 2xy\left[\frac{\partial^2 u}{\partial x \partial y} + \frac{\partial^2 v}{\partial x \partial y}\right] + y^2\left[\frac{\partial^2 u}{\partial y^2} + \frac{\partial^2 v}{\partial y^2}\right]$$

$$= n(n-1)u + n(n+1)v$$

$$\Rightarrow x^2\frac{\partial^2 z}{\partial x^2} + 2xy\frac{\partial^2 z}{\partial x \partial y} + y^2\frac{\partial^2 z}{\partial y^2} = n^2(u+v) - n(u-v)$$

$$= n^2 z - \left(x\frac{\partial z}{\partial x} + y\frac{\partial z}{\partial y}\right) \quad \text{(Using 8)}$$

$$\Rightarrow x^2\frac{\partial^2 z}{\partial x^2} + 2xy\frac{\partial^2 z}{\partial x \partial y} + y^2\frac{\partial^2 z}{\partial y^2} + x\frac{\partial z}{\partial x} + y\frac{\partial z}{\partial y} = n^2 z$$

9. *If* $u = \frac{x^3y^3z^3}{x^3+y^3+z^3} + \log\left(\frac{xy+yz+zx}{x^2+y^2+z^2}\right)$, *find the value of* $x\frac{\partial u}{\partial x} + y\frac{\partial u}{\partial y} + z\frac{\partial u}{\partial z}$.

(MUMBAI–2009)

SOLUTION. Let $v = \frac{x^3y^3z^3}{x^3+y^3+z^3}$

and $w = \log\left(\frac{xy+yz+zx}{x^2+y^2+z^2}\right)$

Clearly, $v = x^6\left[\frac{\left(\frac{y}{x}\right)^3\left(\frac{z}{x}\right)^3}{1+\left(\frac{y}{x}\right)^3+\left(\frac{z}{x}\right)^3}\right]$

is a homogeneous function of degree 6.

$\therefore$ By Euler's theorem

$$x\frac{\partial v}{\partial x}+y\frac{\partial v}{\partial y}+z\frac{\partial v}{\partial z}=6v \quad \ldots(1)$$

Further, $w=\log\left[\dfrac{\frac{y}{x}+\frac{y}{x}\cdot\frac{z}{x}+\frac{z}{x}}{1+\left(\frac{y}{x}\right)^2+\left(\frac{z}{x}\right)^2}\right]$

is a homogeneous function of degree zero.

Then, by Euler's theorem

$$x\frac{\partial w}{\partial x}+y\frac{\partial w}{\partial y}+z\frac{\partial w}{\partial z}=0 \quad \ldots(2)$$

Adding (1) and (2), we get

$$x\left(\frac{\partial v}{\partial x}+\frac{\partial w}{\partial x}\right)+y\left(\frac{\partial v}{\partial y}+\frac{\partial w}{\partial y}\right)+z\left(\frac{\partial v}{\partial z}+\frac{\partial w}{\partial z}\right)=6v$$

$$\Rightarrow x\left(\frac{\partial u}{\partial x}\right)+y\left(\frac{\partial u}{\partial y}\right)+z\left(\frac{\partial u}{\partial z}\right)=6.\frac{x^3y^3z^3}{x^3+y^3+z^3}$$

Exercise-11.2

1. Verify the Euler's theorem for the following functions :

(i) $u=\dfrac{x(x^3-y^3)}{x^3+y^3}$ (ii) $u=x^n\sin\left(\dfrac{y}{x}\right)$

(iii) $u=x^n\log\left(\dfrac{y}{x}\right)$ (iv) $u=\dfrac{1}{\sqrt{x^2+y^2}}$

(v) $u=x^n\sin\dfrac{y}{x}$ (vi) $x^4\log\dfrac{y}{x}$

(vii) $u=\log\left(\dfrac{x^2+y^2}{xy}\right)$

(viii) $u=\dfrac{x^{1/3}+y^{1/3}}{x^{1/2}+y^{1/2}}$ (GBTU–2010)

2. (i) If $u=xf\left(\dfrac{y}{x}\right)$, prove that $x\dfrac{\partial u}{\partial x}+y\dfrac{\partial u}{\partial y}=u.$

(ii) If $u=f\left(\dfrac{y}{x}\right)$, prove that $x\dfrac{\partial u}{\partial x}+y\dfrac{\partial u}{\partial y}=0.$

(iii) If $u=xyf\left(\dfrac{y}{x}\right)$, prove that

$$x\frac{\partial u}{\partial x}+y\frac{\partial u}{\partial y}=2u.$$

(iv) If $u=\log\left(\dfrac{x^2+y^2}{x+y}\right)$, show by Euler's theorem : $x\dfrac{\partial u}{\partial x}+y\dfrac{\partial u}{\partial y}=1.$

3. If $u=\tan^{-1}\left(\dfrac{x^3+y^3}{x+y}\right)$, show that

$$x\frac{\partial u}{\partial x}+y\frac{\partial u}{\partial y}=\sin 2u$$

and

$$x^2\frac{\partial^2 u}{\partial x^2}+2xy\frac{\partial^2 u}{\partial x\partial y}+y^2\frac{\partial^2 u}{\partial y^2}=2\cos 3u\sin u\,.$$

4. If $u=\tan^{-1}\dfrac{y}{x}$, show that(using Euler's theorem)

$$x\frac{\partial u}{\partial x}+y\frac{\partial u}{\partial y}=0.$$

5. If $u=\sin^{-1}\dfrac{x+y}{\sqrt{x}+\sqrt{y}}$, show that

(i) $x\dfrac{\partial u}{\partial x}+y\dfrac{\partial u}{\partial y}=\dfrac{1}{2}\tan u$

(RAJASTHAN–2006, CALICUT–2005)

(ii) $x^2\dfrac{\partial^2 u}{\partial x^2}+2xy\dfrac{\partial^2 u}{\partial x\partial y}+y^2\dfrac{\partial^2 u}{\partial y^2}=-\dfrac{\sin u\cos 2u}{4\cos^3 u}$

6. If $u=\sin^{-1}\dfrac{\sqrt{x}-\sqrt{y}}{\sqrt{x}+\sqrt{y}}$, show that

$$x\frac{\partial u}{\partial x}+y\frac{\partial u}{\partial y}=0.$$

7. (i) If $u=\log\dfrac{x^4+y^4}{x+y}$, show that

$$x\frac{\partial u}{\partial x}+y\frac{\partial u}{\partial y}=3.$$

(ii) If $u=\log\dfrac{x^3+y^3}{x+y}$, show that

$$x\frac{\partial u}{\partial x}+y\frac{\partial u}{\partial y}=2.$$

8. If $\sin u = \dfrac{x^2y^2}{x+y}$, show that

$$x\frac{\partial u}{\partial x} + y\frac{\partial u}{\partial y} = 3\tan u.$$

9. (i) If $u = \dfrac{x^2y^2}{x+y}$, show that

$$y\frac{\partial^2 u}{\partial y^2} + x\frac{\partial^2 u}{\partial x\partial y} = 2\frac{\partial u}{\partial y}.$$

(ii) If $u = \dfrac{xy}{x+y}$, show that

$$x\frac{\partial^2 u}{\partial x^2} + 2xy\frac{\partial^2 u}{\partial x\partial y} + y^2\frac{\partial^2 u}{\partial y^2} = 0.$$

(iii) If $u = \dfrac{x^2y^2}{x+y}$, show that

$$x\frac{\partial^2 u}{\partial x^2} + y\frac{\partial^2 u}{\partial y\partial x} = 2\frac{\partial u}{\partial x}.$$

10. If $u = xf_1\left(\dfrac{y}{x}\right) + f_2\left(\dfrac{y}{x}\right)$, show that

$$x^2\frac{\partial^2 u}{\partial x^2} + 2xy\frac{\partial^2 u}{\partial x\partial y} + y^2\frac{\partial^2 u}{\partial y^2} = 0.$$ (SVTU–2009)

11. (i) If $u = \log\left(\sqrt{x} + \sqrt{y}\right)$, show that

$$x\frac{\partial u}{\partial x} + y\frac{\partial u}{\partial y} = \frac{1}{2}.$$

(ii) If $u = \log\dfrac{x^4 + y^4 + x^2y^2}{x + y + \sqrt{xy}}$, show that

$$x\frac{\partial u}{\partial x} + y\frac{\partial u}{\partial y} = 3.$$

12. If z be a homogeneous function of degree n, show that $x\dfrac{\partial^2 z}{\partial x^2} + y\dfrac{\partial^2 z}{\partial x\partial y} = (n-1)\dfrac{\partial z}{\partial x}$.

13. If $u = \cos^{-1}\dfrac{x+y}{\sqrt{x}+\sqrt{y}}$, prove that

$$x\frac{\partial u}{\partial x} + y\frac{\partial u}{\partial y} = -\frac{1}{2}\cot u.$$

14. If $\sin u = \dfrac{x+2y+3z}{\sqrt{x^8+y^8+z^8}}$, show that

$$x\frac{\partial u}{\partial x} + y\frac{\partial u}{\partial y} + z\frac{\partial u}{\partial z} = -3\tan u.$$

15. If $u = \dfrac{x}{y+z} + \dfrac{y}{z+x} + \dfrac{z}{x+y}$, show that

$$x\frac{\partial u}{\partial x} + y\frac{\partial u}{\partial y} + z\frac{\partial u}{\partial z} = 0.$$ (VTU–2000)

16. If $u = \tan^{-1}\left(\dfrac{y^2}{x}\right)$, show that

$$x^2\frac{\partial^2 u}{\partial x^2} + 2xy\frac{\partial^2 u}{\partial x\partial y} + y^2\frac{\partial^2 u}{\partial y^2} = -\sin^2 u.\sin 2u.$$

(PTU–2005, BHILLAI–2005)

17. Show that $x\dfrac{\partial u}{\partial x} + y\dfrac{\partial u}{\partial y} = 2u\log u$ where $u = e^{x^2+y^2}$. (PTU–2010)

18. If $\log u = \dfrac{x^3+y^3}{3x+4y}$, show that

$$x\frac{\partial u}{\partial x} + y\frac{\partial u}{\partial y} = 2u\log u$$ (UKTU–2011)

19. If $u = x^3 + y^3 + z^3 + 3xyz$, show that

$$x\frac{\partial u}{\partial x} + y\frac{\partial u}{\partial y} + z\frac{\partial u}{\partial z} = 3u.$$ (GBTU–2010)

20. If $u = \sec^{-1}\left(\dfrac{x^3-y^3}{x+y}\right)$, show that

$$x\frac{\partial u}{\partial x} + y\frac{\partial u}{\partial y} = 2\cot u.$$

11.5 TOTAL DIFFERENTIAL

Let $u = f(x, y)$ ...(1)

be the given function of x and y, which have continuous partial derivatives of first order *w.r.t.* x and y.

Let δx and δy be the increments in x and y respectively and let δu be the consequent change in u, then we have

$$u + \delta u = f(x+\delta x, y+\delta y)$$

$$\therefore \quad \delta u = f(x+\delta x, y+\delta y) - f(x,y) \quad \text{...(2)}$$

$$= [f(x+\delta x, y+\delta y) - f(x, y+\delta y)] + [f(x, y+\delta y) - f(x,y)]$$

$$\Rightarrow \quad \frac{\delta u}{\delta t} = \frac{[f(x+\delta x, y+\delta y) - f(x, y+\delta y)]}{\delta t} + \frac{[f(x, y+\delta y) - f(x,y)]}{\delta t}$$

Now, $$\frac{du}{dt} = \lim_{\delta t \to 0} \frac{\delta u}{\delta t}$$

$$= \lim_{\delta t \to 0}\left[\frac{f(x+\delta x, y+\delta y) - f(x, y+\delta y)}{\delta x}\frac{\delta x}{\delta t} + \frac{f(x, y+\delta y) - f(x,y)}{\delta y}\frac{\delta y}{\delta t}\right] \quad ...(3)$$

Since δx and δy tends to zero, when $\delta t \to 0$ so we have

$$\lim_{\delta x \to 0} \frac{f(x+\delta x, y+\delta y) - f(x, y+\delta y)}{\delta x} = \frac{\partial f}{\partial x} = \frac{\partial u}{\partial x}.$$

Similarly, $$\lim_{\delta y \to 0} \frac{f(x, y+\delta y) - f(x,y)}{\delta y} = \frac{\partial f}{\partial y} = \frac{\partial u}{\partial y} \text{ and } \lim_{\delta t \to 0}\frac{\delta x}{\delta t} = \frac{dx}{dt}, \lim_{\delta t \to 0}\frac{\delta y}{\delta t} = \frac{dy}{dt}.$$

Therefore, from (3), we get $$\frac{du}{dt} = \frac{\partial u}{\partial x}.\frac{dx}{dt} + \frac{\partial u}{\partial y}.\frac{dy}{dt}.$$

- This result can be extended as follows :
  If $u = f(x_1, x_2, ..., x_m)$ and $x_1, x_2, ..., x_m$ all are functions of t, then
  $$\frac{du}{dt} = \frac{\partial u}{\partial x_1}.\frac{dx_1}{dt} + \frac{\partial u}{\partial x_2}.\frac{dx_2}{dt} + ... + \frac{\partial u}{\partial x_m}.\frac{dx_m}{dt}.$$
- The differentials dx and dy of the independent variables x and y are the actual changes δx and δy but the differential du of the dependent variable u is not the same as the change δu, it being the principal part of the increment δu.

11.6 IMPLICIT RELATION OF x AND y

In most of the cases, we are mainly concerned with the case in which y is expressed explicity *i.e.*, directly in terms of x. There are so many cases in which y is not expreesed directly in terms of x, but functionally it is implied by an algebraic relation $f(x, y) = 0$ connecting x and y.

The relation of the type $f(x, y) = c$, where y is not explicity in terms of x are called implicit function.

11.7 DIFFERENTIATION OF IMPLICIT FUNCTIONS

To find $\frac{dy}{dx}$ *for an implicit function* $f(x, y) = 0$ *or* $f(x, y) = c$:

Let $f(x, y)$ be a function of two variables x and y and y itself is a function of x *i.e.*, $f(x, y)$ may be consider as a composite function of x. Then, we have

$$\frac{df}{dx} = \frac{\partial f}{\partial x}.\frac{dx}{dx} + \frac{\partial f}{\partial y}.\frac{dy}{dx} \quad \Rightarrow \quad \frac{df}{dx} = \frac{\partial f}{\partial x} + \frac{\partial f}{\partial y}.\frac{dy}{dx} \quad ...(1)$$

Since $f(x, y) = 0$, therefore $\frac{df}{dx} = 0$.

Now from (1), we have $$\frac{\partial f}{\partial x} + \frac{\partial f}{\partial y}.\frac{dy}{dx} = 0$$

$$\Rightarrow \quad \frac{dy}{dx} = -\frac{\partial f}{\partial x} \Big/ \frac{\partial f}{\partial y} = -\frac{f_x}{f_y}, \text{ provided } f_y \neq 0.$$

Solved Examples

1. *If* $x^y + y^x = a^b$. *Find* $\frac{dy}{dx}$.

SOLUTION. Let $f(x, y) = x^y + y^x - a^b$

$\Rightarrow f(x, y) = 0$

Therefore

$$\frac{dy}{dx} = -\frac{\partial f/\partial x}{\partial f/\partial y} = -\frac{yx^{y-1} + y^x \log y}{x^y \log x + xy^{x-1}}.$$

2. *If* $u = \log[(x^2 + y^2)/xy]$, *find du.*

SOLUTION. Let $u = \log(x^2 + y^2) - \log x - \log y$.

$$\therefore \frac{\partial u}{\partial x} = \frac{2x}{x^2 + y^2} - \frac{1}{x}$$

$$= \frac{2x^2 - x^2 - y^2}{x(x^2 + y^2)} = \frac{x^2 - y^2}{x(x^2 + y^2)}$$

and $$\frac{\partial u}{\partial y} = \frac{2y}{x^2 + y^2} - \frac{1}{y}$$

$$= \frac{2y^2 - x^2 - y^2}{y(x^2 + y^2)} = \frac{y^2 - x^2}{y(x^2 + y^2)}$$

Now, $$du = \frac{\partial u}{\partial x}dx + \frac{\partial u}{\partial y}dy$$

$$= \frac{(x^2 - y^2)}{x(x^2 + y^2)}dx + \frac{(y^2 - x^2)}{y(x^2 + y^2)}dy$$

$$= \frac{(x^2 - y^2)}{xy(x^2 + y^2)}(ydx - xdy).$$

3. *If* $f(x, y) = 0$ *and* $g(y, z) = 0$, *show that*

$$\frac{\partial f}{\partial y}\cdot\frac{\partial g}{\partial z}\cdot\frac{dz}{dx} = \frac{\partial f}{\partial x}\cdot\frac{\partial g}{\partial y}.$$

SOLUTION. Let $f(x, y) = 0$, then we have

$$\frac{dy}{dx} = -\frac{\partial f/\partial x}{\partial f/\partial y}. \quad \ldots(1)$$

Also, let $g(y, z) = 0$

$$\Rightarrow \frac{dz}{dy} = -\frac{\partial g/\partial y}{\partial g/\partial z}. \quad \ldots(2)$$

Now, from (1) and (2), we have

$$\frac{dy}{dx}\cdot\frac{dz}{dy} = \left(\frac{\partial f}{\partial x}\cdot\frac{\partial g}{\partial y}\right) \bigg/ \left(\frac{\partial f}{\partial y}\cdot\frac{\partial g}{\partial z}\right)$$

$$\Rightarrow \frac{dz}{dx}\cdot\frac{\partial f}{\partial y}\cdot\frac{\partial g}{\partial z} = \frac{\partial f}{\partial x}\cdot\frac{\partial g}{\partial y}$$

4. *If* $u = x^2y$, *where* $x^2 + xy + y^2 = 1$. *Find* $\frac{du}{dx}$.

SOLUTION. We know that

$$\frac{du}{dx} = \frac{\partial u}{\partial x} + \frac{\partial u}{\partial y}\cdot\frac{dy}{dx}. \quad \ldots(1)$$

Given that $u = x^2y$

$$\frac{\partial u}{\partial x} = 2xy \text{ and } \frac{\partial u}{\partial y} = x^2$$

$$\therefore f(x, y) = x^2 + xy + y^2 - 1$$

Then $$\frac{dy}{dx} = -\frac{\partial f/\partial x}{\partial f/\partial y} = -\frac{2x + y}{x + 2y}$$

Putting all these values in (1), we get

$$\frac{du}{dx} = 2xy + x^2\cdot\left(-\frac{2x + y}{x + 2y}\right)$$

$$= 2xy - \frac{x^2(2x + y)}{x + 2y}$$

5. *If* $u = x \log(xy)$, *where* $x^3 + y^3 + 3xy = 1$. *Find* $\frac{du}{dx}$. (VTU–2009, UPTU–2006)

SOLUTION. We have $u = x \log(xy)$. ...(1)

$$\Rightarrow \frac{\partial u}{\partial x} = x\left(\frac{1}{xy}.y\right) + \log xy = 1 + \log xy$$

and $$\frac{\partial u}{\partial y} = x\left(\frac{1}{xy}.x\right) = \frac{x}{y}$$

Also it is given that

$$x^3 + y^3 + 3xy = 1 \quad \ldots(2)$$

Differentiating (2) we get

$$3x^2 + 3y^2\frac{dy}{dx} + 3\left(x\frac{dy}{dx} + y\right) = 0$$

$$\Rightarrow \frac{dy}{dx} = -\left(\frac{x^2 + y}{x + y^2}\right)$$

Now, $$\frac{du}{dx} = \frac{\partial u}{\partial x} + \frac{\partial u}{\partial y}\cdot\frac{dy}{dx}$$

$$= 1 + \log(xy) + \frac{x}{y}\left\{-\frac{(x^2 + y)}{(y^2 + x)}\right\}$$

$$= 1 + \log(xy) - \frac{x(x^2 + y)}{y(y^2 + x)}$$

Similar Problems

(1) If $u = \sin^{-1}(x-y), x = 3t, y = 4t^3$, show that $\dfrac{du}{dt} = \dfrac{3}{\sqrt{1-t^2}}$.

(2) Show that $\dfrac{\partial^2 z}{\partial u^2} + \dfrac{\partial^2 z}{\partial v^2} = \dfrac{\partial^2 z}{\partial u^2} + \dfrac{\partial^2 z}{\partial v^2}$ where $x = u\cos\alpha - v\sin\alpha, y = u\sin\alpha + v\cos\alpha$.

(UPTU–2008)

6. *If* $u = u\left(\dfrac{y-x}{xy}, \dfrac{z-x}{xz}\right)$, *show that*

$$x^2\frac{\partial u}{\partial x} + y^2\frac{\partial u}{\partial y} + z^2\frac{\partial u}{\partial z} = 0.$$

SOLUTION. Suppose $v = \dfrac{y-x}{xy} = \dfrac{1}{x} - \dfrac{1}{y}$

and $w = \dfrac{z-x}{xz} = \dfrac{1}{x} - \dfrac{1}{z}$ ...(1)

Then clearly, $u = u(v, w)$

$$\therefore \quad \frac{\partial u}{\partial x} = \frac{\partial u}{\partial v}.\frac{\partial v}{\partial x} + \frac{\partial u}{\partial w}.\frac{\partial w}{\partial x}$$

$$= \frac{\partial u}{\partial v}\left(-\frac{1}{x^2}\right) + \frac{\partial u}{\partial w}\left(-\frac{1}{x^2}\right)$$

$$\Rightarrow \quad x^2\frac{\partial u}{\partial x} = -\frac{\partial u}{\partial v} - \frac{\partial u}{\partial w} \quad ...(2)$$

Further, $\dfrac{\partial u}{\partial y} = \dfrac{\partial u}{\partial v}.\dfrac{\partial v}{\partial y} + \dfrac{\partial u}{\partial w}.\dfrac{\partial w}{\partial y}$

$$= \frac{\partial u}{\partial v}\left(\frac{1}{y^2}\right) + \frac{\partial u}{\partial w}(0)$$

$$\Rightarrow \quad y^2\frac{\partial u}{\partial y} = \frac{\partial u}{\partial v} \quad ...(3)$$

Similarly, $\dfrac{\partial u}{\partial z} = \dfrac{\partial u}{\partial v}.\dfrac{\partial v}{\partial z} + \dfrac{\partial u}{\partial w}.\dfrac{\partial w}{\partial z}$

$$= \frac{\partial u}{\partial v}(0) + \frac{\partial u}{\partial w}\left(\frac{1}{z^2}\right)$$

$$\Rightarrow \quad z^2\frac{\partial u}{\partial z} = \frac{\partial u}{\partial w} \quad ...(4)$$

Finally, adding (2), (3) and (4), we get

$$x^2\frac{\partial u}{\partial x} + y^2\frac{\partial u}{\partial y} + z^2\frac{\partial u}{\partial z} = 0.$$

7. *If* $f(x, y) = 0$, *show that*

$$\frac{\partial^2 y}{\partial x^2} = -\frac{q^2 r - 2pqs + p^2 t}{q^3}$$

(KURUKSHETRA–2006)

SOLUTION. We have $\dfrac{dy}{dx} = -\dfrac{\partial f/\partial x}{\partial f/\partial y} = \dfrac{-p}{q}$

$$\Rightarrow \quad \frac{d^2 y}{dx^2} = \frac{d}{dx}\left(\frac{dy}{dx}\right)$$

$$= -\frac{d}{dx}\left(\frac{p}{q}\right) = \frac{-q\dfrac{dp}{dx} + p\dfrac{dq}{dx}}{q^2} \quad ...(1)$$

Now, $\dfrac{dp}{dx} = \dfrac{\partial p}{\partial x} + \dfrac{\partial p}{\partial y}.\dfrac{dy}{dx}$

$$= r + s\left(-\frac{p}{q}\right) = \frac{qr - ps}{q}$$

and $\dfrac{dq}{dx} = \dfrac{\partial q}{\partial x} + \dfrac{\partial q}{\partial y}.\dfrac{dy}{dx}$

$$= s + t\left(-\frac{p}{q}\right) = \frac{qs - pt}{q}$$

Putting all these value in (1), we get

$$\frac{d^2 y}{dx^2} = -\frac{1}{q^2}\left[q\left(\frac{qr-ps}{q}\right) - p\left(\frac{qs-pt}{q}\right)\right]$$

$$= -\frac{q^2 r - 2pqs + p^2 t}{q^3}$$

Here, $p = \dfrac{\partial f}{\partial x}, q = \dfrac{\partial f}{\partial y}, \ r = \dfrac{\partial^2 f}{\partial x^2} = \dfrac{\partial p}{\partial x}$

$$s = \frac{\partial^2 f}{\partial x \partial y} = \frac{\partial q}{\partial x}, \ t = \frac{\partial^2 f}{\partial y^2} = \frac{\partial q}{\partial y}$$

8. *If* $u = f(r, s, t)$ *and* $r = \dfrac{x}{y}, s = \dfrac{y}{z}, t = \dfrac{z}{x}$,

prove that $x\dfrac{\partial u}{\partial x} + y\dfrac{\partial u}{\partial y} + z\dfrac{\partial u}{\partial z} = 0$.

(JNTU–1990, 2007)

SOLUTION. We have $u = f(r, s, t)$ ...(1)

then $\dfrac{\partial u}{\partial x} = \dfrac{\partial u}{\partial r}.\dfrac{\partial r}{\partial x} + \dfrac{\partial u}{\partial s}.\dfrac{\partial s}{\partial x} + \dfrac{\partial u}{\partial t}.\dfrac{\partial t}{\partial x}$

$$= \frac{1}{y}.\frac{\partial u}{\partial r} + 0.\frac{\partial u}{\partial s} - \frac{z}{x^2}.\frac{\partial u}{\partial t} \quad ...(2)$$

$$\frac{\partial u}{\partial y}=-\frac{x}{y^2}.\frac{\partial u}{\partial r}+\frac{1}{z}.\frac{\partial u}{\partial s}+0.\frac{\partial u}{\partial t} \quad \ldots(3)$$

and $$\frac{\partial u}{\partial z}=\frac{\partial u}{\partial r}.\frac{\partial r}{\partial z}+\frac{\partial u}{\partial s}.\frac{\partial s}{\partial z}+\frac{\partial u}{\partial t}.\frac{\partial t}{\partial z}$$

$$=0.\frac{\partial u}{\partial r}+\left(\frac{-y}{z^2}\right).\frac{\partial u}{\partial s}+\frac{1}{x}.\frac{\partial u}{\partial t} \quad \ldots(4)$$

Now multiplying (2) by x, (3) by y and (4) by z and then adding we get

$$x\frac{\partial u}{\partial x}+y\frac{\partial u}{\partial y}+z\frac{\partial u}{\partial z}=0$$

Exercise-11.3

1. If $(\tan x)^y + (y)^{\cot x} = a$. Find the value of $\frac{dy}{dx}$.
2. If $u = \sin(x^2 + y^2)$, where $a^2x^2 + b^2y^2 = c^2$. Find the value of $\frac{du}{dx}$.
3. If $u = f(y - z, z - x, x - y)$, prove that $\frac{\partial u}{\partial x}+\frac{\partial u}{\partial y}+\frac{\partial u}{\partial z}=0.$ (UKTU–2010, GBTU–2010)
4. If z is a function of x and y; where $x = e^u + e^{-v}$ and $y = e^{-u} - e^v$, show that $\frac{\partial z}{\partial u}-\frac{\partial z}{\partial v}=x\frac{\partial z}{\partial x}-y\frac{\partial z}{\partial y}$. (VTU–2003, 06)
5. Find the total derivative of u with respect to t, when
   (i) $u=\cosh\left(\frac{y}{x}\right)$, where $x = t^2, y = e^t$
   (ii) $u = e^x \sin y$, where $x = \log t, y = t^2$
6. If $u=\sqrt{(x^2+y^2)}$ and $x^3+y^3+3axy=5a^2$. Find the value of $\frac{du}{dx}$ at $x = a, y = a$.
7. Find $\frac{dy}{dx}$ and $\frac{d^2y}{dx^2}$ from the following implicit relations.
   (i) $x^2+y^2=a^2$ (ii) $x^{2/3}+y^{2/3}=a^{2/3}$
8. If $f(x, y, z) = 0$, show that $\left(\frac{\partial y}{\partial z}\right)_{x\text{ const.}}\left(\frac{\partial z}{\partial x}\right)_{y\text{ const.}}\left(\frac{\partial x}{\partial y}\right)_{z\text{ const.}}=-1.$
9. If $x+y=2e^{\theta}\cos\phi, x-y=2ie^{\theta}\sin\phi$, where $i=\sqrt{(-1)}$, show that $\frac{\partial^2 u}{\partial\theta^2}+\frac{\partial^2 u}{\partial\phi^2}=4xy\frac{\partial^2 u}{\partial x\partial y}$. (LUCKNOW–2005)

ANSWERS

1. $-\frac{y(\tan x)^{y-1}\sec^2 x - y^{\cot x}.\log y.\operatorname{cosec}^2 x}{(\tan x)^y \log\tan x + \cot x\, y^{\cot x-1}}$
2. $2x[\cos(x^2+y^2)]\left(1-\frac{a^2}{b^2}\right)$
5. (i) $\frac{du}{dt}=\frac{1}{x^2}(xe^t-2yt)\sinh\frac{y}{x}$ (ii) $\frac{du}{dt}=\frac{e^x}{t}(\sin y+2t^2\cos y)$, where $x = \log t, y = e^t$
6. 0
7. (i) $-\frac{x}{y}, \frac{-a^2}{y^3}$ (ii) $\frac{dy}{dx}=-\frac{y^{1/3}}{x^{1/3}}, \frac{d^2y}{dx^2}=\frac{a^{1/3}}{3x^{4/3}.y^{1/3}}$

11.8 CHANGE OF VARIABLES

11.8.1 CHANGE OF INDEPENDENT VARIABLE INTO DEPENDENT VARIABLE

Let $y = f(x)$ be a function with x independent and y is dependent variable. Then

$$\frac{dy}{dx}=1\Big/\left(\frac{dx}{dy}\right)=\left(\frac{dx}{dy}\right)^{-1} \quad \ldots(1)$$

$$\therefore \quad \frac{d^2y}{dx^2}=\frac{d}{dx}\left(\frac{dy}{dx}\right)=\frac{d}{dx}\left[\left(\frac{dx}{dy}\right)^{-1}\right]=\frac{d}{dy}\left[\left(\frac{dx}{dy}\right)^{-1}\right]\frac{dy}{dx}$$

$$=-\left(\frac{dx}{dy}\right)^{-2}.\frac{d^2x}{dy^2}.\frac{dy}{dx}=-\left(\frac{dx}{dy}\right)^{-2}.\frac{d^2x}{dy^2}\left(\frac{dx}{dy}\right)^{-1} \quad \text{[From (1)]}$$

or $$\frac{d^2y}{dx^2} = -\left(\frac{dx}{dy}\right)^{-3} \cdot \frac{d^2x}{dy^2} \qquad ...(2)$$

and $$\frac{d^3y}{dx^3} = \frac{d}{dx}\left(\frac{d^2y}{dx^2}\right) = \frac{d}{dx}\left[\left(-\frac{dx}{dy}\right)^{-3}\frac{d^2x}{dy^2}\right] \qquad \text{[From (2)]}$$

$$= \frac{d}{dy}\left[-\left(\frac{dx}{dy}\right)^{-3}\frac{d^2x}{dy^2}\right]\frac{dy}{dx} = \left\{3\left(\frac{dx}{dy}\right)^{-4}\frac{d^2x}{dy^2}\right\}\frac{d^2x}{dy^2}\cdot\frac{dy}{dx} - \left(\frac{dx}{dy}\right)^{-3}\frac{d^3x}{dy^3}\frac{dy}{dx}$$

$$= 3\left(\frac{dx}{dy}\right)^{-4}\left(\frac{d^2x}{dy^2}\right)^2\left(\frac{dx}{dy}\right)^{-1} - \left(\frac{dx}{dy}\right)^{-3}\frac{d^3x}{dy^3}\left(\frac{dx}{dy}\right)^{-1} \qquad \text{[From (1)]}$$

or $$\frac{d^3y}{dx^3} = 3\left(\frac{dx}{dy}\right)^{-5}\left(\frac{d^2x}{dy^2}\right)^2 - \left(\frac{dx}{dy}\right)^{-4}\frac{d^3x}{dy^3} \qquad ...(3)$$

Similarly, we can find $\frac{d^4y}{dx^4}, \frac{d^5y}{dx^5}$, etc.

Solved Examples

1. *Show that the equation* $\frac{dy}{dx}\cdot\frac{d^3y}{dx^3} - 3\left(\frac{d^2y}{dx^2}\right)^2 = 0$ *can be written in the form* $\frac{d^3x}{dy^3} = 0$.

SOLUTION. Here, we have

$$\frac{dy}{dx} = \left(\frac{dx}{dy}\right)^{-1}, \frac{d^2y}{dx^2} = -\left(\frac{dx}{dy}\right)^{-3}\frac{d^2x}{dy^2}$$

and

$$\frac{d^3y}{dx^3} = 3\left(\frac{dx}{dy}\right)^{-5}\left(\frac{d^2x}{dy^2}\right)^2 - \left(\frac{d^3x}{dy^3}\right)\left(\frac{dx}{dy}\right)^{-4}$$

Making these substitutions in the given equation, we have

$$\left(\frac{dx}{dy}\right)^{-1}\left[3\left(\frac{dx}{dy}\right)^{-5}\left(\frac{d^2x}{dy^2}\right)^2 - \left(\frac{d^3x}{dy^3}\right)\left(\frac{dx}{dy}\right)^{-4}\right] - 3\left[-\left(\frac{dx}{dy}\right)^{-3}\frac{d^2x}{dy^2}\right]^2 = 0$$

$$\Rightarrow -\frac{d^3x}{dy^3}\left(\frac{dx}{dy}\right)^{-3} = 0$$

$$\Rightarrow \frac{d^3x}{dy^3} = 0 \text{ since } \frac{dx}{dy} \neq 0.$$

11.8.2 CHANGE OF INDEPENDENT VARIABLE INTO ANOTHER VARIABLE z, GIVEN $x = f(z)$

We have $$\frac{dy}{dx} = \frac{dy}{dz}\cdot\frac{dz}{dx} = \frac{dy}{dz}\left(\frac{dx}{dz}\right)^{-1} \qquad ...(1)$$

or $$\frac{d}{dx}(y) = \left(\frac{dx}{dz}\right)^{-1}\frac{d}{dz}(y) \qquad ...(2)$$

i.e., the operator $\frac{d}{dx}$ is equivalent to the operator $\left(\frac{dx}{dz}\right)^{-1}\frac{d}{dz}$ or $\frac{d}{dx} \equiv \left(\frac{dx}{dz}\right)^{-1}\frac{d}{dz}$.

Therefore, $$\frac{d^2y}{dx^2} = \frac{d}{dx}\left(\frac{dy}{dx}\right) = \left(\frac{dx}{dz}\right)^{-1}\frac{d}{dz}\left(\frac{dy}{dx}\right), \text{ with the help of (2)}$$

$$= \left(\frac{dx}{dz}\right)^{-1} \frac{d}{dz}\left[\frac{dy}{dz}\left(\frac{dx}{dz}\right)^{-1}\right] \qquad \text{[From (1)]}$$

$$= \left(\frac{dx}{dz}\right)^{-1}\left[\frac{dy}{dz}\left\{-\left(\frac{dx}{dz}\right)^{-2} \cdot \frac{d^2x}{dz^2}\right\} + \left(\frac{dx}{dz}\right)^{-1}\frac{d^2y}{dz^2}\right]$$

or
$$\frac{d^2y}{dx^2} = \left(\frac{dx}{dz}\right)^{-3}\left[\frac{dx}{dz}\cdot\frac{d^2y}{dz^2} - \frac{dy}{dz}\cdot\frac{d^2x}{dz^2}\right] = \frac{\frac{dx}{dz}\cdot\frac{d^2y}{dz^2} - \frac{dy}{dz}\cdot\frac{d^2x}{dz^2}}{\left(\frac{dx}{dz}\right)^3} \qquad \ldots(3)$$

and
$$\frac{d^3y}{dx^3} = \frac{d}{dx}\left[\frac{d^2y}{dx^2}\right] = \left(\frac{dx}{dz}\right)^{-1}\frac{d}{dz}\left(\frac{d^2y}{dx^2}\right), \qquad \text{[From (2)]}$$

$$= \left(\frac{dx}{dz}\right)^{-1}\frac{d}{dz}\left[\frac{\frac{dx}{dz}\cdot\frac{d^2y}{dz^2} - \frac{dy}{dz}\cdot\frac{d^2x}{dz^2}}{\left(\frac{dx}{dz}\right)^3}\right], \qquad \text{[From (3)]}$$

$$= \frac{\left(\frac{dx}{dz}\right)^{-1}\left[\left(\frac{dx}{dz}\right)^3\left\{\frac{dx}{dz}\cdot\frac{d^3y}{dz^3} + \frac{d^2x}{dz^2}\cdot\frac{d^2y}{dz^2} - \frac{d^2y}{dz^2}\cdot\frac{d^2x}{dz^2} - \frac{dy}{dz}\cdot\frac{d^3x}{dz^3}\right\} - 3\left(\frac{dx}{dz}\right)^2\cdot\frac{d^2x}{dz^2}.N_r z\right]}{\left(\frac{dx}{dz}\right)^6}$$

where
$$N_r = \frac{dx}{dz}\cdot\frac{d^2y}{dz^2} - \frac{dy}{dz}\cdot\frac{d^2x}{dz^2}$$

or
$$\frac{d^3y}{dx^3} = \left(\frac{dx}{dz}\right)^{-5}\left[\left(\frac{dx}{dz}\frac{d^3y}{dz^3} - \frac{dy}{dz}\frac{d^3x}{dz^3}\right)\frac{dx}{dz} - 3\frac{d^2x}{dz^2}\left(\frac{dx}{dz}\frac{d^2y}{dz^2} - \frac{dy}{dz}\frac{d^2x}{dz^2}\right)\right]$$

Solved Examples

1. *Transform the equation*

$$\frac{d}{dx}\left\{(1-x^2)\frac{dy}{dx}\right\} + n(n+1)y = 0,$$

by the substitution $x = \frac{1}{2}[z + (1/z)]$.

SOLUTION. Given $\quad x = \frac{1}{2}[z + (1/z)]$

$$\therefore \quad \frac{dx}{dz} = \frac{1}{2}\left(1 - \frac{1}{z^2}\right) = \frac{z^2-1}{2z^2} \qquad \ldots(1)$$

$$\therefore \quad \frac{dy}{dx} = \frac{dy}{dz}\cdot\frac{dz}{dx} = \frac{2z^2}{z^2-1}\cdot\frac{dy}{dz}$$

[From (1)]

or

$$(1-x^2)\frac{dy}{dx} = \left[1 - \frac{1}{4}\left(z + \frac{1}{z}\right)^2\right]\frac{2z^2}{z^2-1}\frac{dy}{dz},$$

(substituting value of x)

$$= \left[1 - \frac{1}{4}z^2 - \frac{1}{4z^2} - \frac{1}{2}\right]\frac{2z^2}{z^2-1}\frac{dy}{dz}$$

$$= \frac{2z^2 - z^4 - 1}{4z^2}\cdot\frac{2z^2}{z^2-1}\frac{dy}{dz} = -\frac{1}{2}(z^2-1)\frac{dy}{dz}$$

$\therefore$ Putting this value of $(1-x^2)\frac{dy}{dx}$ in given equation, we get

$$\frac{d}{dx}\left\{-\frac{1}{2}(z^2-1)\frac{dy}{dz}\right\} + n(n+1)y = 0$$

or $-\frac{1}{2}\frac{d}{dz}\left\{(z^2-1)\frac{dy}{dz}\right\}.\frac{dz}{dx}+n(n+1)y=0$

or $-\frac{1}{2}\left[(z^2-1)\frac{d^2y}{dz^2}+2z.\frac{dy}{dz}\right].\frac{2z^2}{z^2-1}$
$+n(n+1)y=0$

or $z^2(z^2-1)\frac{d^2y}{dz^2}+2z^3\frac{dy}{dz}$
$-n(n+1)(z^2-1)y=0.$

2. *Transform the equation*

$$(1+x^2)^2y_2+2x(1+x^2)y_1+y=0$$

by the substitution $x=\tan z$.

SOLUTION. Given $x=\tan z.$ ...(1)

$\therefore \quad \frac{dx}{dz}=\sec^2 z$

or $\quad \frac{dz}{dx}=\cos^2 z$ ...(2)

Now $y_1=\frac{dy}{dx}=\frac{dy}{dz}.\frac{dz}{dx}=\cos^2 z.\frac{dy}{dz}$ [From (1)]

$y_2=\frac{d^2y}{dx^2}=\frac{d}{dx}\left(\frac{dy}{dx}\right)=\frac{d}{dx}\left[\cos^2 z\frac{dy}{dz}\right]$ [From (2)]

$=\frac{d}{dz}\left[\cos^2 z\frac{dy}{dz}\right]\frac{dz}{dx}$

$=\left[\cos^2 z\frac{d^2y}{dz^2}+2\cos z(-\sin z)\frac{dy}{dz}\right]\cos^2 z$ [From (1)]

or $\frac{d^2y}{dx^2}=\cos^4 z\frac{d^2y}{dz^2}-2\sin z\cos^3 z\frac{dy}{dz}$ ...(3)

Substituting the value of x, y_1 and y_2 in the given equation, we get

$(1+\tan^2 z)^2\left[\cos^4 z\frac{d^2y}{dz^2}-2\sin z\cos^3 z\frac{dy}{dz}\right]$
$+2\tan z(1+\tan^2 z)\cos^2 z\frac{dy}{dz}+y=0$

or $\frac{d^2y}{dz^2}-2\tan z\frac{dy}{dz}+2\tan z\frac{dy}{dz}+y=0$

or $\frac{d^2y}{dz^2}+y=0.$

3. *Transform the equation*

$$y_2+[1-(1/x)]y_1+4x^2ye^{-2x}=4(x^2+x^3)e^{-3x}$$

by the substitution $z=(1+x)e^{-x}$.

SOLUTION. Given $z=(1+x)e^{-x}$

$\therefore \frac{dz}{dx}=(1+x)(-e^{-x})+e^{-x}=-xe^{-x}$ ...(1)

Now, $\frac{dy}{dx}=\frac{dy}{dz}.\frac{dz}{dx}=-xe^{-x}\frac{dy}{dz}$ [From (1)] ...(2)

and $\frac{d^2y}{dx^2}=\frac{d}{dx}\left(\frac{dy}{dx}\right)=\frac{d}{dx}\left[-xe^{-x}\frac{dy}{dz}\right]$ [From (2)]

$=-\left[e^{-x}\frac{dy}{dz}+x(-e^{-x})\frac{dy}{dz}+xe^{-x}\frac{d}{dx}\left(\frac{dy}{dz}\right)\right]$

$=-e^{-x}\left[\frac{dy}{dz}-x\frac{dy}{dz}+x\frac{d^2y}{dz^2}\frac{dz}{dx}\right]$

$\left[\because \frac{d}{dx}\left(\frac{dy}{dz}\right)=\frac{d^2y}{dz^2}\frac{dz}{dx}\right]$

$=-e^{-x}\left[\frac{dy}{dz}-x\frac{dy}{dz}-x^2e^{-x}\frac{d^2y}{dz^2}\right]$ [From (1)]

Substituting these values of dy/dx, d^2y/dx^2 in the given equation, we get

$-e^{-x}\left[\frac{dy}{dz}-x\frac{dy}{dz}-x^2e^{-x}\frac{d^2y}{dz^2}\right]$
$+\left(1-\frac{1}{x}\right)\left(-xe^{-x}\frac{dy}{dz}\right)+4x^2ye^{-2x}$
$=4x^2(1+x)e^{-3x}$

or $x^2e^{-2x}\frac{d^2y}{dz^2}+(x-1-x+1)e^{-x}\frac{dy}{dx}$
$+4x^2ye^{-2x}$
$=4x^2(1+x)e^{-3x}$

or $(d^2y/dz^2)+4y=4(1+x)e^{-x}=4z$ $[\because z=(1+x)e^{-x}]$

or $\left(d^2y/dz^2\right)+4y=4z$

which is the required equation.

11.8.3 TRANSFORMATION INVOLVING CHANGE OF DEPENDENT AS WELL AS INDEPENDENT VARIABLES

Such transformations will be clear from the examples given below.

1. *Transform into cartesian the polar formula* $\tan\phi = \dfrac{r d\theta}{dr}$.

SOLUTION. We know $x = r\cos\theta, y = r\sin\theta$.

Hence we get $r^2 = x^2 + y^2$ and $\theta = \tan^{-1}(y/x)$.

$$\therefore \quad 2r\frac{dr}{dx} = 2x + 2y\frac{dy}{dx}$$

$$\text{or} \quad r\frac{dr}{dx} = x + y\frac{dy}{dx} \quad \ldots(1)$$

$$\text{and} \quad \frac{d\theta}{dx} = \frac{1}{1+(y/x)^2}\cdot\frac{x(dy/dx) - y.1}{x^2}$$

$$= \frac{1}{x^2+y^2}\left(x\frac{dy}{dx} - y\right) \quad \ldots(2)$$

$$\text{Now, } \tan\phi = r\frac{d\theta}{dr} = \frac{r\dfrac{d\theta}{dx}}{\dfrac{dr}{dx}}$$

$$= \frac{r\left[1/(x^2+y^2)\right]\left(x\dfrac{dy}{dx} - y\right)}{(1/r)\left(x + y\dfrac{dy}{dx}\right)}$$

[From (1) and (2)]

$$\text{or } \tan\phi = \frac{x(dy/dx) - y}{x + y(dy/dx)},$$

using $r^2 = x^2 + y^2$.

This is the required formula in cartesian form.

2. *Transform cartesian formula*

$$\rho = \frac{\left[1 + (dy/dx)^2\right]^{3/2}}{d^2y/dx^2}$$

into polar form.

SOLUTION. We know $x = r\cos\theta, y = r\sin\theta$.

$$\therefore \quad \frac{dx}{d\theta} = r(-\sin\theta) + \cos\theta.\frac{dr}{d\theta} \quad \ldots(1)$$

$$\text{and} \quad \frac{dy}{d\theta} = r\cos\theta + \sin\theta\frac{dr}{d\theta} \quad \ldots(2)$$

$$\text{Now } \frac{dy}{dx} = \frac{dy/d\theta}{dx/d\theta}$$

$$= \frac{r\cos\theta + \sin\theta(dr/d\theta)}{\cos\theta(dr/d\theta) - r\sin\theta} \quad \ldots(3)$$

$$\text{Again } \frac{d^2y}{dx^2} = \frac{d}{dx}\left(\frac{dy}{dx}\right) = \frac{d}{d\theta}\left(\frac{dy}{dx}\right)\frac{d\theta}{dx}$$

$$= \frac{d}{d\theta}\left[\frac{\left(r\cos\theta + \sin\theta.\dfrac{dr}{d\theta}\right)}{\cos\theta(dr/d\theta) - r\sin\theta}\right]\frac{1}{dx/d\theta}.$$

[From (3)]

$$= \frac{\left\{\dfrac{dr}{d\theta}\cos\theta - r\sin\theta\right\}\left\{\dfrac{dr}{d\theta}\cos\theta - r\sin\theta + \dfrac{dr}{d\theta}\cos\theta + \sin\theta\dfrac{d^2r}{d\theta^2}\right\} - \left\{r\cos\theta + \sin\theta.\dfrac{dr}{d\theta}\right\}\times\left\{\cos\theta\dfrac{d^2r}{d\theta^2} - \sin\theta\dfrac{dr}{d\theta} - \dfrac{dr}{d\theta}\sin\theta - r\cos\theta\right\}}{\left[(dr/d\theta)\cos\theta - r\sin\theta\right]^3}$$

$$= \frac{\left\{\dfrac{dr}{d\theta}\cos\theta - r\sin\theta\right\}\left\{\sin\theta\dfrac{d^2r}{d\theta^2} + 2\dfrac{dr}{d\theta}\cos\theta - r\sin\theta\right\} - \left\{r\cos\theta + \sin\theta.\dfrac{dr}{d\theta}\right\}\times\left\{\cos\theta\dfrac{d^2r}{d\theta^2} - 2\sin\theta\dfrac{dr}{d\theta} - r\cos\theta\right\}}{\left[(dr/d\theta)\cos\theta - r\sin\theta\right]^3}$$

$$= \frac{\left[2\left(\dfrac{dr}{d\theta}\right)^2 - r\dfrac{d^2r}{d\theta^2} + r^2\right]}{\left[\dfrac{dr}{d\theta}\cos\theta - r\sin\theta\right]^3}.$$

After simplification putting these values in cartesian formula, we get

$$\rho = \frac{\left[1 + (dy/dx)^2\right]^{3/2}}{d^2y/dx^2}$$

$$= \frac{\dfrac{\left[1+\left\{\dfrac{r\cos\theta+\sin\theta(dr/d\theta)}{\cos\theta(dr/d\theta)-r\sin\theta}\right\}^2\right]^{3/2}}{\left[2\left(\dfrac{dr}{d\theta}\right)^2-r\dfrac{d^2r}{d\theta^2}+r^2\right]}}{\left[\dfrac{dr}{d\theta}\cos\theta-r\sin\theta\right]^3} \qquad = \frac{\left[\left(\dfrac{dr}{d\theta}\right)^2+r^2\right]^{3/2}}{\left[2\left(\dfrac{dr}{d\theta}\right)^2-r\dfrac{d^2r}{d\theta^2}+r^2\right]}$$

which is required polar form.

11.8.4 TRANSFORMATION IN THE CASE OF TWO INDEPENDENT VARIABLES

Here we use the following important results :

1. If $z = f(x, y)$, then $dz = \frac{\partial z}{\partial x}dx + \frac{\partial z}{\partial y}dy$. ...(1)
2. If $z = f(x, y)$, where $x = \phi(t)$ and $y = \psi(t)$, then $\frac{dz}{dt} = \frac{\partial z}{\partial x}\frac{dx}{dt} + \frac{\partial z}{\partial y}\frac{dy}{dt}$. ...(2)
3. If $z = f(x, y)$, where $x = \phi(t_1, t_2)$ and $y = \psi(t_1, t_2)$, then $\frac{\partial z}{\partial t_1} = \frac{\partial z}{\partial x}\frac{\partial x}{\partial t_1} + \frac{\partial z}{\partial y}\frac{\partial y}{\partial t_1}$ and $\frac{\partial z}{\partial t_2} = \frac{\partial z}{\partial x}\frac{\partial x}{\partial t_2} + \frac{\partial z}{\partial y}\frac{\partial y}{\partial t_2}$ ...(3)
4. In case $x = \phi(t_1, t_2)$ and $y = \psi(t_1, t_2)$ can easily be solved for t_1 and t_2 in terms of x and y, say $t_1 = F_1(x,y)$ and $t_2 = F_2(x,y)$, then the following formulae are used $\frac{\partial z}{\partial x} = \frac{\partial z}{\partial t_1}\frac{\partial t_1}{\partial x} + \frac{\partial x}{\partial t_2}\frac{\partial t_2}{\partial x}$ and $\frac{\partial z}{\partial y} = \frac{\partial z}{\partial t_1}\frac{\partial t_1}{\partial y} + \frac{\partial z}{\partial t_2}\frac{\partial t_2}{\partial y}$. ...(4)

Solved Examples

1. *If $z = f(x,y), x^2 = uv$ and $y^2 = u/v$, change the independent variables to u, v in the equation*

$$x^2\frac{\partial^2 z}{\partial x^2} - 2xy\frac{\partial^2 z}{\partial x\partial y} + y^2\frac{\partial^2 z}{\partial y^2} + 2y\frac{\partial z}{\partial y} = 0.$$

SOLUTION. Solving $x^2 = uv$ and $y^2 = u/v$, we get

$$u = xy \text{ and } v = x/y. \qquad \text{...(1)}$$

$$\therefore \quad \frac{\partial u}{\partial x} = y, \frac{\partial u}{\partial y} = x, \frac{\partial v}{\partial x} = \frac{1}{y}, \frac{\partial v}{\partial y} = -\frac{x}{y^2}. \qquad \text{...(2)}$$

Now, $\frac{\partial z}{\partial x} = \frac{\partial z}{\partial u}.\frac{\partial u}{\partial x} + \frac{\partial z}{\partial v}.\frac{\partial v}{\partial x}$

$$= \frac{\partial z}{\partial u}(y) + \frac{\partial z}{\partial v}\left(\frac{1}{y}\right) \text{[From (2)]}$$

or $x\frac{\partial z}{\partial x} = (xy)\frac{\partial z}{\partial u} + \left(\frac{x}{y}\right)\frac{\partial z}{\partial v} = u\frac{\partial z}{\partial u} + v\frac{\partial z}{\partial v}$ [From (1)]

$$\therefore \quad x\frac{\partial}{\partial x} \equiv u\frac{\partial}{\partial u} + v\frac{\partial}{\partial v} \qquad \text{...(3)}$$

and similarly $y\frac{\partial}{\partial y} \equiv u\frac{\partial}{\partial u} - v\frac{\partial}{\partial v}$ ...(4)

Now $\left(x\frac{\partial}{\partial x} - y\frac{\partial}{\partial y}\right)^2 z$

$$= \left(x\frac{\partial}{\partial x} - y\frac{\partial}{\partial y}\right)\left(x\frac{\partial z}{\partial x} - y\frac{\partial z}{\partial y}\right)z$$

$$= x\frac{\partial}{\partial x}\left(x\frac{\partial z}{\partial x} - y\frac{\partial z}{\partial y}\right)z$$

$$- y\frac{\partial}{\partial y}\left(x\frac{\partial z}{\partial x} - y\frac{\partial z}{\partial y}\right)z$$

$$= x\left[x\frac{\partial^2 z}{\partial x^2} + \frac{\partial z}{\partial x} - y\frac{\partial^2 z}{\partial x\partial y}\right]z$$

$$- y\left[x\frac{\partial^2 z}{\partial x\partial y} - y\frac{\partial^2 z}{\partial y^2} - \frac{\partial z}{\partial y}\right]z$$

or $\left(x\frac{\partial}{\partial x}-y\frac{\partial}{\partial y}\right)^2 z$

$$= x^2\frac{\partial^2 z}{\partial x^2}-2xy\frac{\partial^2 z}{\partial x\partial y}+y^2\frac{\partial^2 z}{\partial y^2}+x\frac{\partial z}{\partial x}+y\frac{\partial z}{\partial y}.$$

$\therefore$ The given equation

$$\left(x\frac{\partial}{\partial x}-y\frac{\partial}{\partial y}\right)^2 z+\left(y\frac{\partial z}{\partial y}-x\frac{\partial z}{\partial x}\right)=0$$

which with the help of (3) and (4) reduces to

$$\left[\left(u\frac{\partial}{\partial u}+v\frac{\partial}{\partial v}\right)-\left(u\frac{\partial}{\partial u}-v\frac{\partial}{\partial v}\right)\right]^2 z+\left[\left(u\frac{\partial z}{\partial u}-v\frac{\partial z}{\partial v}\right)-\left(u\frac{\partial z}{\partial u}+v\frac{\partial z}{\partial v}\right)\right]=0$$

or $4\left(v\frac{\partial}{\partial v}\right)^2 z-2v\frac{\partial z}{\partial v}=0$

or $2v\frac{\partial}{\partial v}\left(v\frac{\partial z}{\partial v}\right)-v\frac{\partial z}{\partial v}=0$

or $2\left[v\frac{\partial^2 z}{\partial v^2}+\frac{\partial z}{\partial v}\right]-\frac{\partial z}{\partial v}=0$

or $2v\frac{\partial^2 z}{\partial v^2}+\frac{\partial z}{\partial v}=0$

11.8.5 Transformation from Cartesian to Polar Co-ordinates and Vice-versa

Transform the Laplace equation $\frac{\partial^2 u}{\partial x^2}+\frac{\partial^2 u}{\partial y^2}=0$ *to polars.*

We know $x = r\cos\theta,\ y = r\sin\theta.$ ...(1)

$\therefore$ $r^2 = x^2+y^2.$ ...(2)

and $\theta=\tan^{-1}(y/x)$ ...(3)

From (2), we get $2r\frac{\partial r}{\partial x}=2x$ or $\frac{\partial r}{\partial x}=\frac{x}{r}=\frac{r\cos\theta}{r}$ [From (1)]

or $\frac{\partial r}{\partial x}=\cos\theta$ ...(4)

Similarly, $\frac{\partial r}{\partial y}=\frac{y}{r}=\frac{r\sin\theta}{r}=\sin\theta$ ...(5)

Also, from (3), $\frac{\partial\theta}{\partial x}=\frac{1}{1+(y/x)^2}\left(-\frac{y}{x^2}\right)=-\frac{y}{x^2+y^2}=-\frac{r\sin\theta}{r^2}$ or $\frac{\partial\theta}{\partial x}=-\frac{\sin\theta}{r}$ ...(6)

and $\frac{\partial\theta}{\partial y}=\frac{1}{1+(y/x)^2}\left(\frac{1}{x}\right)=\frac{x}{x^2+y^2}=\frac{r\cos\theta}{r^2}=\frac{\cos\theta}{r}$ ...(7)

Now $\frac{\partial u}{\partial x}=\frac{\partial u}{\partial r}.\frac{\partial r}{\partial x}+\frac{\partial u}{\partial\theta}.\frac{\partial\theta}{\partial x}$ ...(8)

$=\frac{\partial u}{\partial r}.(\cos\theta)+\frac{\partial u}{\partial\theta}\left(-\frac{\sin\theta}{r}\right)$ [From (4) and (6)]

or $\frac{\partial}{\partial x}(u)=\cos\theta\frac{\partial}{\partial r}(u)-\frac{\sin\theta}{r}\frac{\partial}{\partial\theta}(u)$ ...(9)

Again $\frac{\partial u}{\partial y}=\frac{\partial u}{\partial r}.\frac{\partial r}{\partial y}+\frac{\partial u}{\partial\theta}.\frac{\partial\theta}{\partial y}$ [From (5) and (7)]

or $\frac{\partial}{\partial y}(u)=\sin\theta\frac{\partial}{\partial r}(u)+\frac{\cos\theta}{r}\frac{\partial}{\partial\theta}(u)$ ...(10)

$\therefore$ $\frac{\partial^2 u}{\partial x^2}=\frac{\partial}{\partial x}\left(\frac{\partial u}{\partial x}\right)=\cos\theta\frac{\partial}{\partial r}\left(\frac{\partial u}{\partial x}\right)-\frac{\sin\theta}{r}\frac{\partial}{\partial\theta}\left(\frac{\partial u}{\partial x}\right)$ replacing u by $\frac{\partial u}{\partial x}$ in (9)

$$= \cos\theta \frac{\partial}{\partial r}\left[\cos\theta \frac{\partial u}{\partial r} - \frac{\sin\theta}{r}\frac{\partial u}{\partial \theta}\right] - \frac{\sin\theta}{r}\frac{\partial}{\partial \theta}\left[\cos\theta \frac{\partial u}{\partial r} - \frac{\sin\theta}{r}\frac{\partial u}{\partial \theta}\right]$$

substituting from (9) the polar equivalent of $\frac{\partial u}{\partial x}$

$$= \cos\theta\left[\cos\theta \frac{\partial^2 u}{\partial r^2} - \sin\theta \frac{\partial}{\partial r}\left(\frac{1}{r}\frac{\partial u}{\partial \theta}\right)\right]$$

$$-\frac{\sin\theta}{r}\left[\left(\cos\theta \frac{\partial^2 u}{\partial \theta \partial r} - \sin\theta \frac{\partial u}{\partial r}\right) - \frac{1}{r}\frac{\partial}{\partial \theta}\left(\sin\theta \frac{\partial u}{\partial \theta}\right)\right]$$

$$= \cos\theta\left[\cos\theta \frac{\partial^2 u}{\partial r^2} - \sin\theta\left\{\frac{1}{r}\frac{\partial^2 u}{\partial r \partial \theta} - \frac{1}{r^2}\frac{\partial u}{\partial \theta}\right\}\right]$$

$$-\frac{\sin\theta}{r}\left[\left(\cos\theta \frac{\partial^2 u}{\partial r \partial \theta} - \sin\theta \frac{\partial u}{\partial r}\right) - \frac{1}{r}\left(\sin\theta \frac{\partial^2 u}{\partial \theta^2} + \cos\theta \frac{\partial u}{\partial \theta}\right)\right]$$

or
$$\frac{\partial^2 u}{\partial x^2} = \cos^2\theta \frac{\partial^2 u}{\partial r^2} - \frac{2\sin\theta\cos\theta}{r}\frac{\partial^2 u}{\partial r \partial \theta} + \frac{\sin^2\theta}{r^2}\frac{\partial^2 u}{\partial \theta^2}$$

$$+\frac{\sin^2\theta}{r}\frac{\partial u}{\partial r} + \frac{2\cos\theta\sin\theta}{r^2}\frac{\partial u}{\partial \theta} \quad \ldots(11)$$

Similarly, from $\frac{\partial^2 u}{\partial y^2} = \frac{\partial}{\partial y}\left(\frac{\partial u}{\partial y}\right) = \sin\theta \frac{\partial}{\partial r}\left(\frac{\partial u}{\partial y}\right) + \frac{\cos\theta}{r}\frac{\partial}{\partial \theta}\left(\frac{\partial u}{\partial y}\right)$, from (10), we get

$$\frac{\partial^2 u}{\partial y^2} = \sin^2\theta \frac{\partial^2 u}{\partial r^2} + \frac{2\sin\theta\cos\theta}{r}\frac{\partial^2 u}{\partial r \partial \theta} + \frac{\cos^2\theta}{r^2}\frac{\partial^2 u}{\partial \theta^2}$$

$$+\frac{\cos^2\theta}{r}\frac{\partial u}{\partial r} - \frac{2\cos\theta\sin\theta}{r^2}\frac{\partial u}{\partial \theta}. \quad \ldots(12)$$

Adding (11) and (12), we get

$$\frac{\partial^2 u}{\partial x^2} + \frac{\partial^2 u}{\partial y^2} = (\cos^2\theta + \sin^2\theta)\frac{\partial^2 u}{\partial r^2} + \frac{1}{r^2}(\sin^2\theta + \cos^2\theta)\frac{\partial^2 u}{\partial \theta^2}$$

$$+\frac{1}{r}(\sin^2\theta + \cos^2\theta)\frac{\partial u}{\partial r} = \frac{\partial^2 u}{\partial r^2} + \frac{1}{r^2}\frac{\partial^2 u}{\partial \theta^2} + \frac{1}{r}\frac{\partial u}{\partial r}.$$

Hence, the given differential equation

$$\frac{\partial^2 u}{\partial x^2} + \frac{\partial^2 u}{\partial y^2} = 0 \text{ transforms into } \frac{\partial^2 u}{\partial r^2} + \frac{1}{r^2}\frac{\partial^2 u}{\partial \theta^2} + \frac{1}{r}\frac{\partial u}{\partial r} = 0.$$

Case II. Transformation from Polar to Cartesian.

Now let us consider the converse of Case I, *i.e.*, let us transform the polar differential equation $\frac{\partial^2 u}{\partial r^2} + \frac{1}{r^2}\frac{\partial^2 u}{\partial \theta^2} + \frac{1}{r}\frac{\partial u}{\partial r} = 0$ to cartesian.

As before, $x = r\cos\theta,\ y = r\sin\theta$. ...(1)

Then, $$\frac{\partial u}{\partial r} = \frac{\partial u}{\partial x}\cdot\frac{\partial x}{\partial r} + \frac{\partial u}{\partial y}\cdot\frac{\partial y}{\partial r} \quad \ldots(2)$$

Now, from (1) $$\left.\begin{aligned}\frac{\partial x}{\partial r} &= \cos\theta = \frac{x}{r}; \frac{\partial x}{\partial \theta} = -r\sin\theta = -y\\ \frac{\partial y}{\partial r} &= \sin\theta = \frac{y}{r}; \frac{\partial y}{\partial \theta} = r\cos\theta = x\end{aligned}\right] \quad \ldots(3)$$

Hence, from (2), we get $$\frac{\partial u}{\partial r} = \frac{\partial u}{\partial x}\left(\frac{x}{r}\right) + \frac{\partial u}{\partial y}\left(\frac{y}{r}\right) \quad \text{[Using (3)]}$$

or $$r\frac{\partial}{\partial r}(u) = x\frac{\partial}{\partial x}(u) + y\frac{\partial}{\partial y}(u) \quad \ldots(4)$$

Also we have $$\frac{\partial u}{\partial \theta} = \frac{\partial u}{\partial x}\frac{\partial x}{\partial \theta} + \frac{\partial u}{\partial y}\frac{\partial y}{\partial \theta} = \frac{\partial u}{\partial x}(-y) + \frac{\partial u}{\partial y}(x) \quad \text{[From (3)]}$$

or $$\frac{\partial}{\partial \theta}(u) = x\frac{\partial}{\partial y}(u) - y\frac{\partial}{\partial x}(u). \quad \ldots(5)$$

Now $$r\frac{\partial}{\partial r}\left(r\frac{\partial u}{\partial r}\right) = x\frac{\partial}{\partial x}\left(r\frac{\partial u}{\partial r}\right) + y\frac{\partial}{\partial y}\left(r\frac{\partial u}{\partial r}\right) \quad \left(\text{Replacing } u \text{ by } r\frac{\partial u}{\partial r} \text{ in (4)}\right)$$

$$= x\frac{\partial}{\partial x}\left[x\frac{\partial u}{\partial x} + y\frac{\partial u}{\partial y}\right] + y\frac{\partial}{\partial y}\left(x\frac{\partial u}{\partial x} + y\frac{\partial u}{\partial y}\right)$$

Substituting the value of $r\frac{\partial u}{\partial r}$ from (4)

or $$r\left[r\frac{\partial^2 u}{\partial r^2} + \frac{\partial u}{\partial r}\right] = x\left[x\frac{\partial^2 u}{\partial x^2} + \frac{\partial u}{\partial x} + y\frac{\partial^2 u}{\partial x \partial y}\right] + y\left[x\frac{\partial^2 u}{\partial y \partial x} + y\frac{\partial^2 u}{\partial y^2} + \frac{\partial u}{\partial y}\right]$$

or $$r^2\frac{\partial^2 u}{\partial r^2} + r\frac{\partial u}{\partial r} = x^2\frac{\partial^2 u}{\partial x^2} + 2xy\frac{\partial^2 u}{\partial x \partial y} + y^2\frac{\partial^2 u}{\partial y^2} + x\frac{\partial u}{\partial x} + y\frac{\partial u}{\partial y}$$

or $$r^2\frac{\partial^2 u}{\partial r^2} = x^2\frac{\partial^2 u}{\partial x^2} + 2xy\frac{\partial^2 u}{\partial x \partial y} + y^2\frac{\partial^2 u}{\partial y^2} \quad \ldots(6)$$

Since $r\frac{\partial u}{\partial r} = x\frac{\partial u}{\partial x} + y\frac{\partial u}{\partial y}$, (from (4))

and $$\frac{\partial^2 u}{\partial \theta^2} = \frac{\partial}{\partial \theta}\left(\frac{\partial u}{\partial \theta}\right) = x\frac{\partial}{\partial y}\left(\frac{\partial u}{\partial \theta}\right) - y\frac{\partial}{\partial x}\left(\frac{\partial u}{\partial \theta}\right) \text{ replacing } u \text{ by } \frac{\partial u}{\partial \theta} \text{ in (5)}$$

$$= x\frac{\partial}{\partial y}\left(x\frac{\partial u}{\partial y} - y\frac{\partial u}{\partial x}\right) - y\frac{\partial}{\partial x}\left(x\frac{\partial u}{\partial y} - y\frac{\partial u}{\partial x}\right)$$

(Substituting the value of $\frac{\partial u}{\partial \theta}$ from (5))

$$= x\left(x\frac{\partial^2 u}{\partial y^2} - y\frac{\partial^2 u}{\partial x \partial y} - \frac{\partial u}{\partial x}\right) - y\left(x\frac{\partial^2 u}{\partial x \partial y} + \frac{\partial u}{\partial y} - y\frac{\partial^2 u}{\partial x^2}\right)$$

$$= x^2\frac{\partial^2 u}{\partial y^2} - 2xy\frac{\partial^2 u}{\partial x \partial y} + y^2\frac{\partial^2 u}{\partial x^2} - \left(x\frac{\partial u}{\partial x} + y\frac{\partial u}{\partial y}\right)$$

or $$\frac{\partial^2 u}{\partial \theta^2} + r\frac{\partial u}{\partial r} = x^2\frac{\partial^2 u}{\partial y^2} - 2xy\frac{\partial^2 u}{\partial x \partial y} + y^2\frac{\partial^2 u}{\partial x^2} \quad \ldots(7)$$

Adding (6) and (7), we get

$$r^2\frac{\partial^2 u}{\partial r^2}+\frac{\partial^2 u}{\partial \theta^2}+r\frac{\partial u}{\partial r}=(x^2+y^2)\frac{\partial^2 u}{\partial x^2}+(x^2+y^2)\frac{\partial^2 u}{\partial y^2}=r^2\left(\frac{\partial^2 u}{\partial x^2}+\frac{\partial^2 u}{\partial y^2}\right)$$

$[\because r^2 = x^2 + y^2]$

or $$\frac{\partial^2 u}{\partial r^2}+\frac{1}{r^2}\frac{\partial^2 u}{\partial \theta^2}+\frac{1}{r}\frac{\partial u}{\partial r}=\frac{\partial^2 u}{\partial x^2}+\frac{\partial^2 u}{\partial y^2}$$

Hence, the given differential equation

$$\frac{\partial^2 u}{\partial r^2}+\frac{1}{r^2}\frac{\partial^2 u}{\partial \theta^2}+\frac{1}{r^2}\frac{\partial u}{\partial r}=0 \text{ transforms into } \frac{\partial^2 u}{\partial x^2}+\frac{\partial^2 u}{\partial y^2}=0.$$

Solved Examples

1. *If $x = r\cos\theta$, $y = r\sin\theta$, prove that*

$$\frac{\partial^2 r}{\partial x^2}\frac{\partial^2 r}{\partial y^2}=\left(\frac{\partial^2 r}{\partial x\partial y}\right)^2.$$

SOLUTION. We know that $\frac{\partial r}{\partial x}=\frac{x}{r}, \frac{\partial r}{\partial y}=\frac{y}{r}$.

Now $$\frac{\partial^2 r}{\partial x^2}=\frac{\partial}{\partial x}\left(\frac{\partial r}{\partial x}\right)=\frac{\partial}{\partial x}\left(\frac{x}{r}\right)$$

$$=\frac{r.1-x(\partial r/\partial x)}{r^2}$$

$$=\frac{r-x(x/r)}{r^2}=\frac{r^2-x^2}{r^3}=\frac{y^2}{r^3}.$$

$[\because x^2+y^2=r^2]$ ...(1)

Similarly, we can get

$$\frac{\partial^2 r}{\partial y^2}=\frac{x^2}{r^3} \quad ...(2)$$

Also, $$\frac{\partial^2 r}{\partial x\partial y}=\frac{\partial}{\partial x}\left(\frac{\partial r}{\partial y}\right)=\frac{\partial}{\partial x}\left(\frac{y}{r}\right)$$

$$=\frac{r.0-y(\partial r/\partial x)}{r^2}$$

$$=-\frac{y(x/r)}{r^2}=-\frac{xy}{r^3}.$$

$$\therefore \left(\frac{\partial^2 r}{\partial x\partial y}\right)^2=\left(-\frac{xy}{r^3}\right)^2=\frac{x^2}{r^3}.\frac{y^2}{r^3}$$

$$=\frac{\partial^2 r}{\partial y^2}.\frac{\partial^2 r}{\partial x^2}.$$

[From (1) an d (2)]

2. *If $x = r\cos\theta$, $y = r\sin\theta$, prove that*

$$\frac{\partial^2 r}{\partial x^2}+\frac{\partial^2 r}{\partial y^2}=\frac{1}{r}\left\{\left(\frac{\partial r}{\partial x}\right)^2+\left(\frac{\partial r}{\partial y}\right)^2\right\}.$$

SOLUTION. As in example 1 above, we can get

$$\frac{\partial^2 r}{\partial x^2}+\frac{\partial^2 r}{\partial y^2}=\frac{y^2}{r^3}+\frac{x^2}{r^3}=\frac{x^2+y^2}{r^3}$$

$$=\frac{r^2}{r^3}=\frac{1}{r}$$

$[\because x^2+y^2=r^2]$ ...(1)

Also, we can get $\frac{\partial r}{\partial x}=\frac{x}{r}, \frac{\partial r}{\partial y}=\frac{y}{r}$.

$$\therefore \frac{1}{r}\left\{\left(\frac{\partial r}{\partial x}\right)^2+\left(\frac{\partial r}{\partial y}\right)^2\right\}$$

$$=\frac{1}{r}\left\{\frac{x^2}{r^2}+\frac{y^2}{r^2}\right\}$$

$$=\frac{1}{r}\left\{\frac{x^2+y^2}{r^2}\right\}=\frac{1}{r}\left\{\frac{r^2}{r^2}\right\}. \quad ...(2)$$

Hence, from (1) and (2), we get

$$\frac{\partial^2 r}{\partial x^2}+\frac{\partial^2 r}{\partial y^2}=\frac{1}{r}\left\{\left(\frac{\partial r}{\partial x}\right)^2+\left(\frac{\partial r}{\partial y}\right)^2\right\}.$$

3. *Transform $\frac{\partial^2 u}{\partial x^2}+\frac{\partial^2 u}{\partial y^2}=0$ into polars and show that $u=\left(Ar^n+Br^{-n}\right)\sin n\theta$ satisfies the above equation.*

SOLUTION. We can transform the given equation

$$\frac{\partial^2 u}{\partial x^2}+\frac{\partial^2 u}{\partial y^2}=0 \text{ into } \frac{\partial^2 u}{\partial r^2}+\frac{1}{r^2}\frac{\partial^2 u}{\partial \theta^2}+\frac{1}{r}\frac{\partial u}{\partial r}=0$$

Now $u=\left(Ar^n+Br^{-n}\right)\sin n\theta$

$$\therefore \quad \frac{\partial u}{\partial r}=\left(nAr^{n-1}-Bnr^{-n-1}\right)\sin n\theta$$

$$\frac{\partial^2 u}{\partial r^2} = n[(n-1)Ar^{n-2} + Bn(n+1)r^{-n-2}]\sin n\theta$$

$$\frac{\partial u}{\partial \theta} = n[Ar^n + Br^{-n}]\cos n\theta;$$

$$\frac{\partial^2 u}{\partial \theta^2} = -n^2[Ar^n + Br^{-n}]\sin n\theta.$$

$$\therefore \frac{\partial^2 u}{\partial r^2} + \frac{1}{r^2}\frac{\partial^2 u}{\partial \theta^2} + \frac{1}{r}\frac{\partial u}{\partial r}$$

$$= n[(n-1)Ar^{n-2} + B(n+1)r^{-n-2}]\sin n\theta + \frac{1}{r^2}[-n^2(Ar^n + Br^{-n})\sin n\theta]$$

$$+\frac{1}{r}n(Ar^{n-1} - Br^{-n-1})\sin n\theta$$

$$= [A\{n(n-1) - n^2 + n\}r^{n-2} + \{Bn(n+1) - n^2 - n\}r^{-n-2}]\sin n\theta = 0$$

Hence, the equation

$$\frac{\partial^2 u}{\partial r^2} + \frac{1}{r^2}\frac{\partial^2 u}{\partial \theta^2} + \frac{1}{r}\frac{\partial u}{\partial r} = 0 \quad \text{i.e.,}$$

$\dfrac{\partial^2 u}{\partial x^2} + \dfrac{\partial^2 u}{\partial y^2} = 0$ is satisfied by

$$(Ar^n + Br^{-n})\sin n\theta.$$

11.8.6 To Transform $\nabla^2 V$ into Polar Co-ordinates, where the Operator ∇^2 stands for $\dfrac{\partial^2}{\partial x^2} + \dfrac{\partial^2}{\partial y^2} + \dfrac{\partial^2}{\partial z^2}$

For polar transformation (in three dimensions), we have $x = r\sin\theta\cos\phi$, $y = r\sin\theta\sin\phi$, $z = r\cos\theta$.

Let $r\sin\theta = u$, then $x = u\cos\phi$, $y = u\sin\phi$.

Then, as in § 11.8.5 Case I, we can have

$$\frac{\partial^2 V}{\partial x^2} + \frac{\partial^2 V}{\partial y^2} = \frac{\partial^2 V}{\partial u^2} + \frac{1}{u}\cdot\frac{\partial V}{\partial u} + \frac{1}{u^2}\cdot\frac{\partial^2 V}{\partial \phi^2} \quad \ldots(1)$$

Again, we have $z = r\cos\theta$, $u = r\sin\theta$.

$$\therefore \quad \frac{\partial^2 V}{\partial z^2} + \frac{\partial^2 V}{\partial u^2} = \frac{\partial^2 V}{\partial r^2} + \frac{1}{r}\cdot\frac{\partial V}{\partial r} + \frac{1}{r^2}\cdot\frac{\partial^2 V}{\partial \theta^2} \quad \ldots(2)$$

Also,
$$\frac{\partial V}{\partial u} = \frac{\partial V}{\partial r}\cdot\frac{\partial r}{\partial u} + \frac{\partial V}{\partial \theta}\cdot\frac{\partial \theta}{\partial u} \quad \ldots(3)$$

Now $u = r\sin\theta$, $z = r\cos\theta$, wherence we get

$$r^2 = u^2 + z^2 \quad \text{and} \quad \theta = \tan^{-1}(u/z).$$

$$\therefore \quad 2r\frac{\partial r}{\partial u} = 2u \quad \text{or} \quad \frac{\partial r}{\partial u} = \frac{u}{r} = \frac{r\sin\theta}{r} = \sin\theta$$

and
$$\frac{\partial \theta}{\partial u} = \frac{1}{1+(x/z)^2}\cdot\frac{1}{z} = \frac{z}{u^2+z^2} = \frac{r\cos\theta}{r^2} = \frac{\cos\theta}{r}$$

Substituting these values of $\partial r/\partial u$ and $\partial\theta/\partial u$ in (3), we get

$$\frac{\partial V}{\partial u} = \frac{\partial V}{\partial r}(\sin\theta) + \frac{\partial V}{\partial \theta}\left(\frac{\cos\theta}{r}\right)$$

or
$$\frac{1}{u}\left(\frac{\partial V}{\partial u}\right) = \frac{1}{r\sin\theta}\left(\frac{\partial V}{\partial u}\right) = \frac{1}{r\sin\theta}\left[\sin\theta\frac{\partial V}{\partial r} + \frac{\cos\theta}{r}\frac{\partial V}{\partial \theta}\right] \text{ or } \frac{1}{u}\frac{\partial V}{\partial u} = \frac{1}{r}\frac{\partial V}{\partial r} + \frac{\cot\theta}{r^2}\frac{\partial V}{\partial \theta}. \quad \ldots(4)$$

Now adding (1) and (2), we get

$$\nabla^2 V = \frac{\partial^2 V}{\partial x^2} + \frac{\partial^2 V}{\partial y^2} + \frac{\partial^2 V}{\partial z^2} = \frac{1}{u}\frac{\partial V}{\partial u} + \frac{1}{u^2}\frac{\partial^2 V}{\partial \phi^2} + \frac{\partial^2 V}{\partial r^2} + \frac{1}{r}\frac{\partial V}{\partial r} + \frac{1}{r^2}\frac{\partial^2 V}{\partial \theta^2}$$

$$= \frac{1}{r}\frac{\partial V}{\partial r} + \frac{\cot\theta}{r^2}\frac{\partial V}{\partial \theta} + \frac{1}{r^2\sin^2\theta}\cdot\frac{\partial^2 V}{\partial \phi^2} + \frac{\partial^2 V}{\partial r^2} + \frac{1}{r}\frac{\partial V}{\partial r} + \frac{1}{r^2}\frac{\partial^2 V}{\partial \theta^2}$$

i.e.,
$$\nabla^2 V = \frac{\partial^2 V}{\partial r^2} + \frac{2}{r}\frac{\partial V}{\partial r} + \frac{1}{r^2}\frac{\partial^2 V}{\partial \theta^2} + \frac{\cot\theta}{r^2}\frac{\partial V}{\partial \theta} + \frac{1}{r^2\sin^2\theta}\cdot\frac{\partial^2 V}{\partial \phi^2}$$

Solved Examples

1. *If $x = r\cos\theta$, $y = r\sin\theta$ and $r = e^t$, prove that*

$$x^2\frac{\partial^2 u}{\partial x^2} + 2xy\frac{\partial^2 u}{\partial y\partial x} + y^2\frac{\partial^2 u}{\partial y^2} = r\frac{\partial}{\partial r}\left(r\frac{\partial}{\partial r} - 1\right)u = \frac{\partial}{\partial z}\left(\frac{\partial}{\partial z} - 1\right)u$$

and $$x^2\frac{\partial^2 u}{\partial y^2} - 2xy\frac{\partial^2 u}{\partial x\partial y} + y^2\frac{\partial^2 u}{\partial x^2} = \frac{\partial^2 u}{\partial \theta^2} + r\frac{\partial u}{\partial r} = \frac{\partial^2 u}{\partial \theta^2} + \frac{\partial u}{\partial z}$$

SOLUTION. As in § 11.8.5 Case II, we can show that

$$r\frac{\partial u}{\partial r} = x\frac{\partial u}{\partial x} + y\frac{\partial u}{\partial y}$$

Therefore,

$$r\frac{\partial}{\partial r}\left(r\frac{\partial}{\partial r} - 1\right)u = \left(x\frac{\partial}{\partial x} + y\frac{\partial}{\partial y}\right)\left[x\frac{\partial u}{\partial x} + y\frac{\partial u}{\partial y} - u\right]$$

$$= x\left[x\frac{\partial^2 u}{\partial x^2} + \frac{\partial u}{\partial x} + y\frac{\partial^2 u}{\partial x\partial y} - \frac{\partial u}{\partial x}\right] + y\left[x\frac{\partial^2 u}{\partial y\partial x} + y\frac{\partial^2 u}{\partial y^2} + \frac{\partial u}{\partial y} - \frac{\partial u}{\partial y}\right]$$

$$= x^2\frac{\partial^2 u}{\partial x^2} + 2xy\frac{\partial^2 u}{\partial x\partial y} + y^2\frac{\partial^2 u}{\partial y^2}.$$

Also as $r = e^z$ or $z = \log r$.

$\therefore$ Using $\frac{\partial u}{\partial r} = \frac{\partial u}{\partial z}\cdot\frac{\partial z}{\partial r} = \frac{\partial u}{\partial z}\cdot\frac{1}{r}$

$$\therefore \quad r\frac{\partial u}{\partial r} = \frac{\partial u}{\partial z}$$

or $$r\frac{\partial}{\partial r} \equiv \frac{\partial}{\partial z} \qquad \ldots(1)$$

$$\therefore \quad r\frac{\partial}{\partial r}\left(r\frac{\partial}{\partial r} - 1\right)u = \frac{\partial}{\partial z}\left(\frac{\partial}{\partial z} - 1\right)u.$$

Again, as in § 11.8.6 Case I, we can prove that $\frac{\partial u}{\partial \theta} = x\frac{\partial u}{\partial y} - y\frac{\partial u}{\partial x}$.

$$\therefore \frac{\partial^2 u}{\partial \theta^2} = \frac{\partial}{\partial \theta}\left(\frac{\partial u}{\partial \theta}\right) = \left(x\frac{\partial}{\partial y} - y\frac{\partial}{\partial x}\right)\left(x\frac{\partial u}{\partial y} - y\frac{\partial u}{\partial x}\right)$$

$$= x\frac{\partial}{\partial y}\left(x\frac{\partial u}{\partial y} - y\frac{\partial u}{\partial x}\right) - y\frac{\partial}{\partial x}\left(x\frac{\partial u}{\partial y} - y\frac{\partial u}{\partial x}\right)$$

$$= x\left[x\frac{\partial^2 u}{\partial y^2} - \frac{\partial u}{\partial x} - y\frac{\partial^2 u}{\partial y\partial x}\right] - y\left[x\frac{\partial^2 u}{\partial x\partial y} + \frac{\partial u}{\partial y} - y\frac{\partial^2 u}{\partial x^2}\right]$$

$$= x^2\frac{\partial^2 u}{\partial y^2} - 2xy\frac{\partial^2 u}{\partial x\partial y} + y^2\frac{\partial^2 u}{\partial x^2} - \left(x\frac{\partial u}{\partial x} + y\frac{\partial u}{\partial y}\right)$$

or $$\frac{\partial^2 u}{\partial \theta^2} + r\frac{\partial u}{\partial r} = x^2\frac{\partial^2 u}{\partial y^2} - 2xy\frac{\partial^2 u}{\partial x\partial y} + y^2\frac{\partial^2 u}{\partial x^2}.$$ [From (1)]

Also, from (1), we get

$$\frac{\partial^2 u}{\partial \theta^2} + r\frac{\partial u}{\partial r} = \frac{\partial^2 u}{\partial \theta^2} + \frac{\partial u}{\partial z}.$$

2. *If V be a function of r along where $r^2 = x^2 + y^2 + z^2$, show that*

$$\frac{\partial^2 V}{\partial x^2}+\frac{\partial^2 V}{\partial y^2}+\frac{\partial^2 V}{\partial z^2}=\frac{\partial^2 V}{\partial r^2}+\frac{2}{r}\frac{dV}{dr}.$$

SOLUTION. As V is given to be a function of r alone,

so we have $\frac{\partial V}{\partial x}=\frac{dV}{dr}\frac{\partial r}{\partial x}$ ...(1)

Also, from $r^2 = x^2 + y^2 + z^2$,

we get $2r\frac{\partial r}{\partial x} = 2x$.

$\therefore$ From (1), $\frac{\partial V}{\partial x}=\frac{dV}{dr}\frac{x}{r}$

$$\therefore \frac{\partial^2 V}{\partial x^2}=\frac{\partial}{\partial x}\left(\frac{\partial V}{\partial x}\right)=\frac{\partial}{\partial x}\left[\frac{dV}{dr}\frac{x}{r}\right]$$

$$=\frac{dV}{dr}\frac{\partial}{\partial x}\left(\frac{x}{r}\right)+\frac{x}{r}\frac{\partial}{\partial x}\left(\frac{dV}{dr}\right)$$

$$=\frac{dV}{dr}\left[\frac{1}{r}+x\left(-\frac{1}{r^2}\frac{\partial r}{\partial x}\right)\right]+\frac{x}{r}\left(\frac{d^2V}{dr^2}\frac{\partial r}{\partial x}\right)$$

$$=\frac{1}{r}\frac{dV}{dr}-\frac{x}{r^2}\frac{dV}{dr}\left(\frac{x}{r}\right)+\frac{x}{r}\frac{d^2V}{dr^2}\left(\frac{x}{r}\right)$$

$$\left(\because \frac{\partial r}{\partial x}=\frac{x}{r}\right)$$

or $$\frac{\partial^2 V}{\partial x^2}=\frac{1}{r}\frac{dV}{dr}-\frac{x^2}{r^3}\frac{dV}{dr}+\frac{x^2}{r^2}\frac{d^2V}{dr^2}$$

Similarly,

$$\frac{\partial^2 V}{\partial y^2}=\frac{1}{r}\frac{dV}{dr}-\frac{y^2}{r^3}\frac{dV}{dr}+\frac{y^2}{r^2}\frac{d^2V}{dr^2}$$

and $$\frac{\partial^2 V}{\partial z^2}=\frac{1}{r}\frac{dV}{dr}-\frac{z^2}{r^3}\frac{dV}{dr}+\frac{z^2}{r^2}\frac{d^2V}{dr^2}$$

On adding, we get

$$\frac{\partial^2 V}{\partial x^2}+\frac{\partial^2 V}{\partial y^2}+\frac{\partial^2 V}{\partial z^2}$$

$$=\frac{3}{r}\frac{dV}{dr}-\frac{1}{r}\frac{dV}{dr}+\frac{d^2V}{dr^2}$$

$$=\frac{2}{r}\frac{dV}{dr}+\frac{d^2V}{dr^2}$$

Exercise-11.4

1. Reduce the equation $\frac{d^2x}{dy^2}=a$ to the form $\frac{d^2y}{dx^2}+a\left(\frac{dy}{dx}\right)^3=0.$

2. Transform the equation $x^4\left(\frac{d^2y}{dx^2}\right)+a^2y=0$ by the substitution $x = 1/z$.

3. Transform the equation

$$\sin^2 2z\frac{d^2y}{dz^2}+\sin 4z\frac{dy}{dz}+4y=0$$

the substitution $\tan z = e^z$.

4. If $x^2 + z^2 = 1$, show that the equation

$$\frac{d}{dx}\left\{(1-x^2)\frac{dy}{dx}\right\}+n(n+1)y=0 \text{ becomes}$$

$$z(z^2-1)\frac{d^2y}{dz^2}+(2z^2-1)\frac{dy}{dz}-n(n+1)zy=0.$$

5. Show that the equation $x^2\frac{d^2y}{dx^2}+x\frac{dy}{dx}+y=0$ becomes $\frac{d^2y}{dz^2}+y=0$ by substituting e^z for x.

6. Transform $\frac{d^2y}{dx^2}$ to new variables u and v by taking u as independent variable such that $y = uv, xy = 1$.

7. Show that $\frac{\partial^2 u}{\partial x^2}+\frac{\partial^2 u}{\partial y^2}=\frac{\partial^2 u}{\partial \xi^2}+\frac{\partial^2 u}{\partial \eta^2}$ where $x = \xi\cos\alpha - \eta\sin\alpha,\ y = \xi\sin\alpha + \eta\cos\alpha$.

8. If $x = e^\theta, y = e^\phi$, show that

$$e^{2\theta}\frac{\partial^2 v}{\partial x^2}+e^{2\phi}\frac{\partial^2 v}{\partial y^2}+e^\theta\frac{\partial v}{\partial x}+e^\phi\frac{\partial v}{\partial y}=\frac{\partial^2 v}{\partial \theta^2}+\frac{\partial^2 v}{\partial \phi^2}.$$

9. If $f(x, y)$ has continuous partial derivatives of first two orders and $x + y = (u + v)^3$,

$(x-y) = (u-v)^3$, then show that

$$9(x^2-y^2)\left(\frac{\partial^2 f}{\partial x^2}-\frac{\partial^2 f}{\partial y^2}\right)=(u^2-v^2)\left\{\frac{\partial^2 f}{\partial u^2}-\frac{\partial^2 f}{\partial v^2}\right\}.$$

10. If z is a function of u and v, where $u = x^2 - y^2 - 2xy$ and $v = y$, show that the equation $(x+y)\frac{\partial z}{\partial x}+(x-y)\left(\frac{\partial z}{\partial y}\right)=0$ is transformed into $\frac{\partial v}{\partial z}=0$.

11. Show that the equation $xy\left(\frac{\partial^2 u}{\partial x^2}-\frac{\partial^2 u}{\partial y^2}\right)-(x^2-y^2)\frac{\partial^2 u}{\partial x \partial y}=0$ becomes $r.\frac{\partial^2 u}{\partial r \partial \theta}-\frac{\partial u}{\partial \theta}=0$, when transformed to polar.

12. If $x = r\cos\theta$, $y = r\sin\theta$ and $z = f(x, y)$, show that $\frac{\partial z}{\partial x}=\frac{\partial z}{\partial r}\cos\theta-\frac{1}{r}\frac{\partial z}{\partial \theta}\sin\theta$. Also show that

$$\frac{\partial^2(r^n\cos n\theta)}{\partial x \partial y}=-n(n-1)r^{n-2}\sin(n-2)\theta.$$

13. If $x + y = 2e^{\theta}\cos\phi$ and $x - y = 2e^{\theta}\sin\phi$, show that $\frac{\partial^2 V}{\partial \theta^2}+\frac{\partial^2 V}{\partial \phi^2}=4xy\frac{\partial^2 V}{\partial x \partial y}$.

ANSWERS

2. $\frac{d^2y}{dz^2}+\frac{2}{z}\frac{dy}{dz}+a^2y=0$ **3.** $\frac{d^2y}{dx^2}+y=0$ **6.** $4v^4\left(\frac{dv}{du}\right)^{-1}+2uv^3-v^5\left(\frac{d^2v}{du^2}\right)\left(\frac{dv}{du}\right)^{-3}$

❑❑❑❑❑❑

Chapter

12 Tangent and Normal

12.1 INTRODUCTION

Let P be a given point and Q be any other point on it. Let Q travel towards P along the curve.

Let Q travel towards P along the curve. Then, the limiting position PT of the secant PQ is known as the tangent to the curve.

The line PS through P which is perpendicular to the tangent PT is called the normal of the curve.

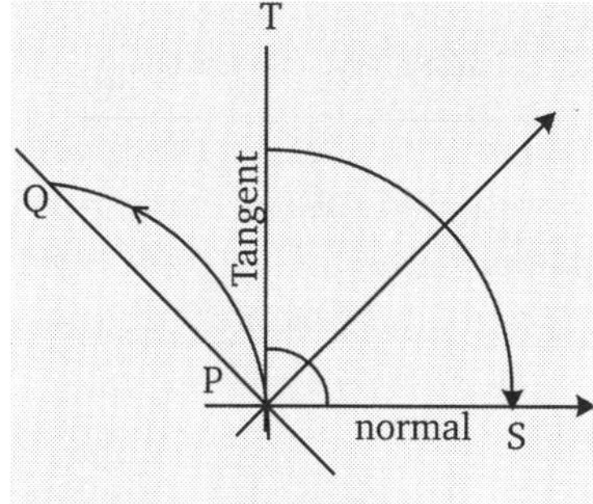

Fig. 1

12.1.1 SOME FUNDAMENTAL CONCEPTS

(i) Slope of a line, $m = \tan\theta$, where θ is the angle which the line makes with the positive direction of x-axis.

(ii) Slope of the line $ax + by + c = 0$ is given by $m = -\dfrac{a}{b}$

(iii) Slope of the line joining the points (x_1, y_1) and (x_2, y_2) is $= \dfrac{y_2 - y_1}{x_2 - x_1}$

(iv) Slope of x-axis $= 0$, Slope of y-axis $= \infty$

(v) Two lines are parallel iff $m_1 = m_2$.

(vi) Two lines are perpendicular iff $m_1 m_2 = -1$.

(vii) Angle between two lines having slopes m_1 and m_2 is given by $\theta = \tan^{-1}\left(\dfrac{m_1 - m_2}{1 + m_1 m_2}\right)$

(viii) Equation of the line (one point form)

$$y - y_1 = m(x - x_1)$$

passing through the point (x_1, y_1).

(ix) Perpendicular distance formula $= \dfrac{|ax_1 + by_1 + c|}{\sqrt{a^2 + b^2}}$

12.1.2 EQUATION OF THE TANGENT

Let $y = f(x)$ be the equation of the curve, and $P(x_1, y_1)$ be any given point on this curve.

Let $Q = Q(x + \delta x, y + \delta y)$ be any neighbouring point of P. Let PT be the tangent at the point (x_1, y_1).

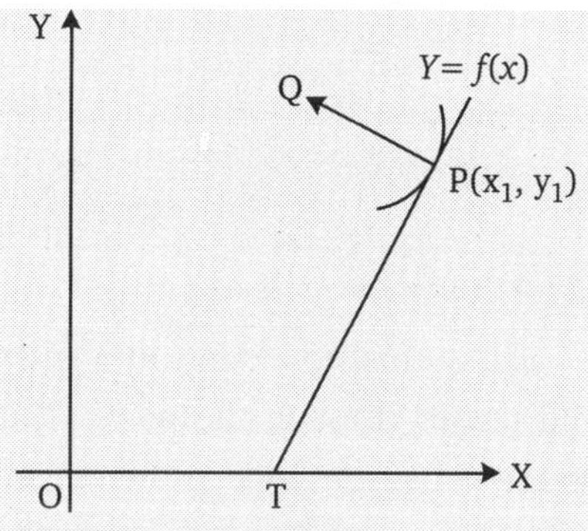

Fig. 2.

The slope of the tangent at $(x_1, y_1) = \frac{dy_1}{dx_1}$.

Now, tangent is a line through the point $P(x_1, y_1)$ and its slope $m = \frac{dy_1}{dx_1}$.

Hence, by Co-ordinate Geometry, the equation of the tangent is $y - y_1 = \frac{dy_1}{dx_1}(x - x_1)$.

- It should be clearly understood that by $\frac{dy_1}{dx_1}$ we mean the value of $\frac{dy}{dx}$ at (x_1, y_1) and not as derivative of y_1 with respect to x_1.
- The equation of the tangent at a point t_1 to the curve $x = f(t), y = g(t)$ is given by

$$y - g(t_1) = \frac{g'(t_1)}{f'(t_1)}[x - f(t_1)].$$

12.1.2 GEOMETRICAL MEANING OF $\frac{dy}{dx}$

Let $y = f(x)$ be the given function and let it be represented by the curve AB. Take two neighbouring points $P(x, y)$ and $Q(x+\delta x, y+\delta y)$ on the curve AB. Join PQ and let PQ be produced to meet OX at the point R.

Slope of the secant PQ

$$= \frac{y + \delta y - y}{x + \delta x - x} = \frac{\delta y}{\delta x}. \quad \ldots(1)$$

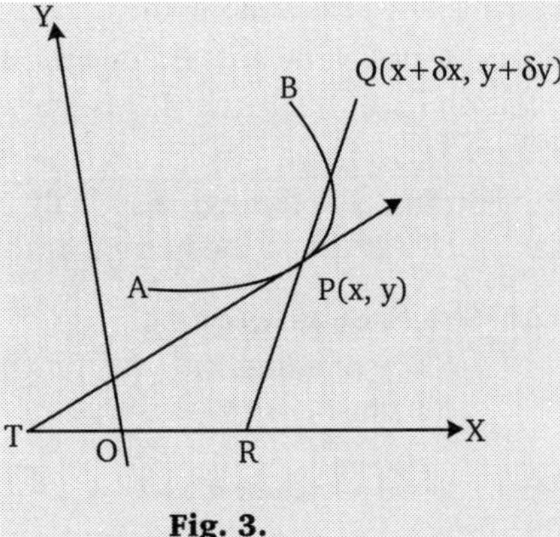

Fig. 3.

Now, let the point Q move along the curve and approach the point P in the limiting position. $\delta x \to 0$, $\delta y \to 0$ and the secant PQ becomes the tangent PT at P.

Therefore, from (1)

Slope of the tangent PT at $(x, y) = \lim_{\substack{\delta x \to 0 \\ \delta y \to 0}} \frac{\delta y}{\delta x} = \frac{dy}{dx}$

i.e., the value of the derivative at a point P of the curve is equal to the slope of tangent at that point to the curve.

- If the tangent at a point on the curve $y = f(x)$ is parallel to x-axis, its slope is zero *i.e.*, $\frac{dy}{dx}$ at the point $= 0$.
- If the tangent at a point on the curve is perpendicular to x-axis, *i.e.*, parallel to y-axis. Its slope is ∞, *i.e.*, $\frac{dy}{dx}$ at the point $= \infty$.

12.1.3 EQUATION OF THE NORMAL

The normal to a curve at a given point is a line perpendicular to the tangent at that point and passes through the point. The slope of the normal at point $P(x_1, y_1)$ will be negative reciprocal of the slope of the tangent.

Hence, the slope of the normal at $(x_1, y_1) = -\frac{1}{dy_1 / dx_1}$

$\therefore$ The equation of the normal at $P(x_1, y_1)$ is

$$y - y_1 = -\frac{1}{dy_1 / dx_1}(x - x_1)$$

Solved Examples

1. *Find the point on the curve $y = x^2 - x - 8$ at which the tangent is parallel to x-axis.*

SOLUTION. Let the required point be (x_1, y_1), then

$$y_1 = x_1^2 - x_1 - 8 \quad ...(i)$$

Given curve $y = x^2 - x - 8$

$$\therefore \quad \frac{dy}{dx} = 2x - 1$$

$\therefore$ The slope of the tangent at point

$$(x_1, y_1) = \left(\frac{dy}{dx}\right)_{(x_1, y_1)} = 2x_1 - 1 \quad ...(ii)$$

Since the tangent is parallel to x-axis, therefore

$$m = \frac{dy}{dx} = 0$$

$\therefore$ From eqn. (ii),

$$2x_1 - 1 = 0 \Rightarrow x_1 = \frac{1}{2}$$

Putting $x_1 = \frac{1}{2}$ in eqn. (i), we get

$$y_1 = \left(\frac{1}{2}\right)^2 - \left(\frac{1}{2}\right) - 8 = \frac{1}{4} - \frac{1}{2} - 8$$

$$\therefore \quad y_1 = -\frac{33}{4}$$

Hence, required point is $\left(\frac{1}{2}, -\frac{33}{4}\right)$.

2. *Prove that the straight line $\frac{x}{a} + \frac{y}{b} = 1$ touches the curve $y = be^{-x/a}$ at the point where the curve cut y-axis.*

SOLUTION. Equation of the tangent

$$\frac{x}{a} + \frac{y}{b} = 1 \quad ...(i)$$

Equation of the curve

$$y = be^{-x/a} \quad ...(ii)$$

Since, curve cut y-axis. So, at the point where curve cut y-axis, $x = 0$. Putting in eqn. (ii), we get $y = b$

$\therefore$ Required point = $(0, b)$

We have to prove that the tangent at point $(0, b)$ on the curve is eqn. (i). From eqn. (ii);

$$\frac{dy}{dx} = -\frac{b}{a}e^{-x/a}$$

$$\therefore \quad \left(\frac{dy}{dx}\right)_{(0,b)} = -\frac{b}{a}$$

Equation of the tangent at point $(0, b)$ is

$$y - b = -\frac{b}{a}(x - 0)$$

$$\Rightarrow \quad \frac{y - b}{b} = -\frac{x}{a}$$

$$\Rightarrow \quad \frac{x}{a} + \frac{y}{b} = 1$$

3. *Find the equation of the normal to the parabola $y^2 = 4ax$ at (x_1, y_1).*

SOLUTION. The given curve $y^2 = 4ax$

Differentiating w.r.t. x, we get

$$2y\frac{dy}{dx} = 4a$$

$$\Rightarrow \quad \frac{dy}{dx} = \frac{2a}{y}$$

$$\therefore \quad \left(\frac{dy}{dx}\right)_{(x_1, y_1)} = \frac{2a}{y_1}$$

$\therefore$ The slope of the normal of the parabola $= \dfrac{-1}{\left(\frac{dy}{dx}\right)_{(x_1, y_1)}} = -\dfrac{y_1}{2a}$

$\therefore$ The equation of the normal of the parabola at the point (x_1, y_1) is

$$y - y_1 = \frac{-y_1}{2a}(x - x_1)$$

$$\Rightarrow \quad \frac{y - y_1}{-y_1} = \frac{(x - x_1)}{2a}$$

4. *Find the point on the curve $9x^2+4y^2=36$ at which the equation of the normal is (i) parallel to x-axis (ii) parallel to y-axis.*

SOLUTION. The given curve $9x^2 + 4y^2 = 36$ ...(i)

Let (x_1, y_1) be the required point on the curve, therefore

$$9x_1^2 + 4y_1^2 = 36 \qquad \text{...(ii)}$$

Differentiating eqn. (i) w.r.t. x, we get

$$18x + 8y\frac{dy}{dx} = 0$$

$$\Rightarrow \quad \left(\frac{dy}{dx}\right) = \frac{-9x}{4y}$$

$$\therefore \quad \left(\frac{dy}{dx}\right)_{(x_1,y_1)} = -\frac{9x_1}{4y_1}$$

$$\therefore \text{ Slope of the normal } = \frac{-1}{\left(\frac{dy}{dx}\right)_{(x_1,y_1)}}$$

$$= \frac{4y_1}{9x_1}$$

(i) Since normal is parallel to x-axis, therefore

$$\frac{4y_1}{9x_1} = 0 \quad \Rightarrow \quad y_1 = 0$$

From eqn. (ii)

$$9x_1^2 = 36 \quad \Rightarrow \quad x_1 = \pm 2$$

$\therefore$ Required point is $(\pm 2, 0)$

(ii) Since normal is parallel to y-axis

$$\therefore \quad \frac{4y_1}{9x_1} = \infty \quad \Rightarrow \quad \frac{9x_1}{4y_1} = 0$$

$$\therefore \quad x_1 = 0$$

From eqn. (ii)

$$4y_1^2 = 36 \quad \Rightarrow \quad y_1^2 = 9$$

$$\therefore \quad y_1 = \pm 3$$

$\therefore$ Required point is $(0, \pm 3)$.

12.2 POLAR CO-ORDINATES

Let OX be a fixed straight line through fixed point O. The fixed point O is called the pole, or the origin and the fixed straight line OX is called initial line or the polar axis.

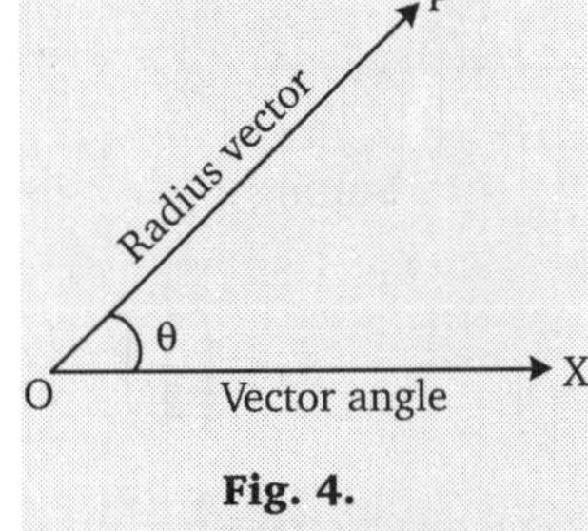

Fig. 4.

Let P be any point in the plane through the line OX. Join OP, then

(i) The length OP is called the radius vector of the point P and is denoted by r.

(ii) The angle XOP is called the vectorial angle of the point P and denoted by θ.

(iii) The number r and θ taken together in this order and called p, the polar-co-ordinates of the point P and we write it as $P(r, \theta)$.

(iv) If (x, y) are the co-ordinates of P referred to cartesian system, then it can be easily found that $x = r\cos\theta$, $y = r\sin\theta$.

12.3 ANGLE BETWEEN RADIUS VECTOR AND TANGENT

Let (r, θ) be the co-ordinate of any point P' on the curve $r = f(\theta)$. Let the tangent at P makes an angle ψ with OX.

Let ϕ be the angle between the radius vector and the tangent at P, *i.e.*, $\angle MPN = \phi$ is the angle between the radius vector OP and the tangent at P to the curve $r = f(\theta)$.

To show that for any point (r, θ) of the curve $r = f(\theta)$, the angle ϕ between the radius vector and tangent is given by $\tan\phi = r\dfrac{d\theta}{dr}$.

Let $P(r, \theta)$ be any point on the given curve

$$r = f(\theta) \text{ or } f(r, \theta) = 0.$$

Let us suppose $Q(r + \delta r, \theta + \delta\theta)$ be the point in the neighbourhood of P on the curve.

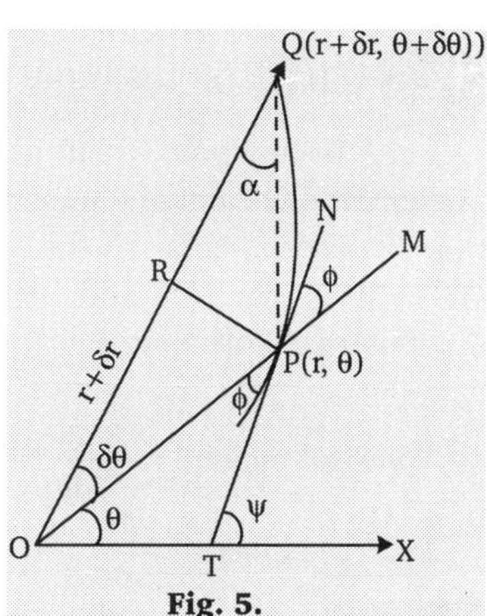

Fig. 5.

Join OP, OQ, PQ, then

$$OP = r,\ OQ = r + \delta r$$

$\angle XOP = \theta$, $\angle XOQ = \theta + \delta\theta$ and $\angle POQ = \delta\theta$.

Draw $PR \perp OQ$ and $\angle PQR = \alpha$.

Now, let the angle between the radius vector OP and the tangent PT is ϕ *i.e.*,

$$\angle OPT = \phi$$

Also, we have

$$\frac{PR}{OP} = \sin\delta\theta \quad \Rightarrow PR = r\sin\delta\theta$$

$$RQ = OQ - OR = (r + \delta r) - OP\cos\delta\theta$$

$$= r + \delta r - r\cos\delta\theta$$

$$= \delta r + r(1 - \cos\delta\theta) = \delta r + 2r\sin^2\frac{\delta\theta}{2}.$$

$$\tan\alpha = \frac{PR}{QR} = \frac{r\sin\delta\theta}{\delta r + 2r\sin^2\delta\theta/2}$$

Dividing the numerator and denominator by $\delta\theta$, we get

$$\tan\alpha = \frac{r.\dfrac{\sin\delta\theta}{\delta\theta}}{\dfrac{\delta r}{\delta\theta} + r.\dfrac{\sin\delta\theta/2}{\delta\theta/2}\sin\dfrac{\delta\theta}{2}}$$

when $Q \to P$ along the curve $\alpha \to \phi$ ($\because$ PQ becomes the tangent PT and OQ coincides with OP).

$$\tan\phi = \lim_{Q\to P}\tan\alpha = \lim_{\delta\theta\to 0}\frac{r.\dfrac{\sin\delta\theta}{\delta\theta}}{\dfrac{\delta r}{\delta\theta} + r.\dfrac{\sin\delta\theta/2}{\delta\theta/2}\sin\dfrac{\delta\theta}{2}} = \frac{r.1}{dr/d\theta + r.1.0} = \frac{r}{dr/d\theta}$$

Hence, $$\tan\phi = r\frac{d\theta}{dr}.$$

- ϕ is the angle between the radius vector and tangent and taken to be positive when measured in the anticlockwise direction.
- Relation between θ, ϕ and ψ is $\psi = \theta + \phi$.

12.4 ANGLE OF INTERSECTION OF TWO CURVES

If the tangent to the two curves make angle ϕ_1 and ϕ_2 with the common radius vector to their point of intersection, then angle between the curves.

$$= \text{angle between tangents} = |\phi_1 - \phi_2|.$$

- The two curves intersect orthogonally if $\tan\phi_1 \tan\phi_2 = -1$.
- If $\dfrac{\tan\phi_1 - \tan\phi_2}{1 + \tan\phi_1.\tan\phi_2}$ is positive, we shall get acute angle of intersection at P and if $\dfrac{\tan\phi_1 - \tan\phi_2}{1 + \tan\phi_1.\tan\phi_2}$ is negative, we get the obtuse angle of intersection at P.

12.5 LENGTH OF SUBTANGENT AND SUBNORMAL

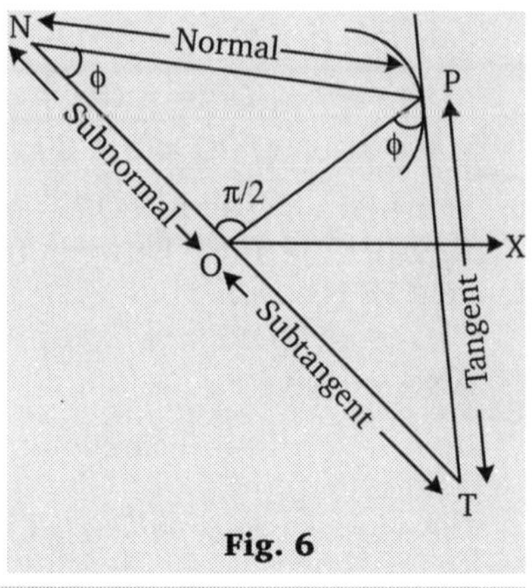

Fig. 6

Let P be any point (r, θ) on a curve $f(r, \theta) = 0$. Let the tangent and normal at P meet the straight line through the pole O perpendicular to the radius vector OP in T and N respectively. Then OT and ON are called polar subtangent and polar subnormal at P.

Hence,

Polar subtangent $= r^2 \dfrac{d\theta}{dr}$

Polar subnormal $= \dfrac{dr}{d\theta}$

12.6 LENGTH OF THE PERPENDICULAR FROM POLE TO THE TANGENT

Let p be the length of the perpendicular from the pole to the tangent at any point (r, θ) of a curve $r = f(\theta)$, then

(i) $p = r \sin \phi$

(ii) $\dfrac{1}{p^2} = \dfrac{1}{r^2} + \dfrac{1}{r^4} \cdot \left(\dfrac{dr}{d\theta}\right)^2$

(iii) $\dfrac{1}{p^2} = u^2 + \left(\dfrac{du}{d\theta}\right)^2$ where $u = \dfrac{1}{r}$

PROOF. (i) Let PT be the tangent at any point $P(r, \theta)$ on the curve $r = f(\theta)$ making an angle ψ with the initial line OX.

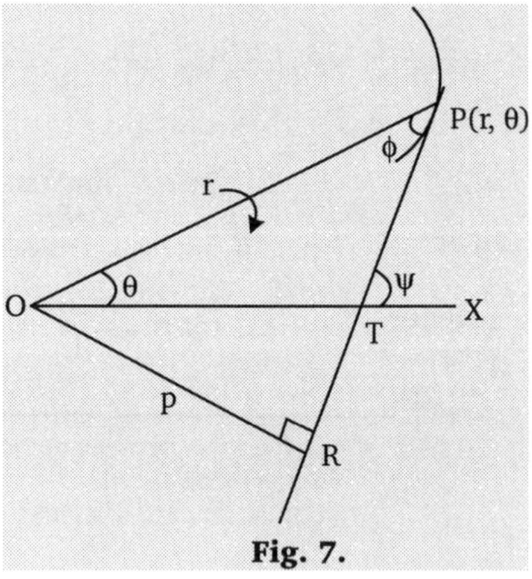

Fig. 7.

From the pole O, draw $OR \perp$ to the tangent PT.

$\therefore \quad OR = p.$

Joint OP, also, $\angle OPT = \phi$.

Now from figure, we have

$$\frac{OR}{OP} = \sin\phi \quad \Rightarrow \quad \frac{p}{r} = \sin\phi$$

$$\Rightarrow \quad p = r\sin\phi$$

(ii) From (i), we have

$$\frac{1}{p^2} = \frac{1}{r^2 \sin^2\phi} = \frac{1}{r^2}\text{cosec}^2\,\phi \qquad \ldots(1)$$

Also, $\tan\phi = r\dfrac{d\theta}{dr}$.

$$\therefore \ \text{cosec}^2\,\phi = 1 + \cot^2\phi = 1 + \frac{1}{r^2}\left(\frac{dr}{d\theta}\right)^2$$

Substitute it in (1), we get

$$\frac{1}{p^2} = \frac{1}{r^2}\left[1 + \frac{1}{r^2}\left(\frac{dr}{d\theta}\right)^2\right] \quad \Rightarrow \quad \frac{1}{p^2} = \frac{1}{r^2} + \frac{1}{r^4}\left(\frac{dr}{d\theta}\right)^2$$

(iii) Put $r = \dfrac{1}{u}$ in (ii),

$$\frac{1}{p^2} = \frac{1}{r^2} + \frac{1}{r^4}\left(\frac{dr}{d\theta}\right)^2 \Rightarrow u^2 + u^4 . \frac{1}{u^4}\left(\frac{du}{d\theta}\right)^2 \qquad \left(\because r = \frac{1}{u} \Rightarrow \frac{dr}{d\theta} = -\frac{1}{u^2}.\frac{du}{d\theta}\right)$$

$$\Rightarrow \quad \frac{1}{p^2} = u^2 + \left(\frac{du}{d\theta}\right)^2$$

12.7 THE PEDAL EQUATION

Let r be the distance of any point on the curve from the origin (or pole), and p, is the length prependicular from the origin to the tangent at that point, then

The relation between p and r, where r is the distance of any point on the curve from the origin (or pole) and p is perpendicular from origin (or pole) to the tangent at that point is called the Pedal equation of the curve.

12.7.1 Pedal Equation of a Curve whose Cartesian Equation is given

Let the equation of the curve is

$$f(x, y) = 0 \qquad \ldots(1)$$

Then, the equation of the tangent at any point (x, y) is

$$Y - y = \frac{dy}{dx}(X - x) = y_1(X - x) \text{ where } y_1 = \frac{dy}{dx}$$

$$\Rightarrow \quad Xy_1 - Y + y - xy_1 = 0.$$

If p be the length prependicular from the origin to this tangent, then

$$p = \frac{y - xy_1}{\sqrt{1 + y_1^2}} \qquad \ldots(2)$$

Also, $\qquad r^2 = x^2 + y^2 \qquad \ldots(3)$

Eliminating x, y from the equation (1), (2) and (3), we get the required pedal equation of the curve (1).

12.7.2 Pedal Equation of a Curve whose Polar Equation is Given

Let $\quad r = f(\theta) \ldots(1)$ be the polar curve. Find ϕ in terms of θ.

Eliminating θ and ϕ from both the above equations and $p = r \sin \phi$, we get the required pedal equation of curve (1).

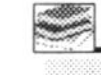

- The pedal equation is sometimes more conveniently obtained by eliminating θ between (1) and the equation $\dfrac{1}{p^2} = \dfrac{1}{r^2} + \dfrac{1}{r^4}\left(\dfrac{dr}{d\theta}\right)^2$.

12.8 DIFFERENTIAL COEFFICIENT OF ARC LENGTH (CARTESIAN FORM)

Let $y = f(x)$ be the given curve and s denote the length of the arc, then

$$\frac{ds}{dx} = \pm\sqrt{\left[1 + \left(\frac{dy}{dx}\right)^2\right]}$$

- If the equation of the curve is $x = f(y)$, then $\frac{ds}{dy} = \pm\sqrt{\left[1+\left(\frac{dx}{dy}\right)^2\right]}$
- If the given equation is in parametric form *i.e.*, $x = f_1(t), y = f_2(t)$, then $\frac{ds}{dt} = \pm\sqrt{\left[\left(\frac{dx}{dt}\right)^2+\left(\frac{dy}{dt}\right)^2\right]}$

12.9 DIFFERENTIAL COEFFICIENT OF ARC LENGTH (POLAR FORM)

To prove that $\frac{ds}{d\theta} = \sqrt{r^2+\left(\frac{dr}{d\theta}\right)^2}$ *where* $r = f(\theta)$ *is the polar form of curve* :

Let $r = f(\theta)$ be the equation of the curve and s denote the length of arc AP. Obviously s is a function of θ. Let Q be the neighbouring point of P such that

$AQ = s + \delta s \quad \Rightarrow \quad PQ = \delta s.$

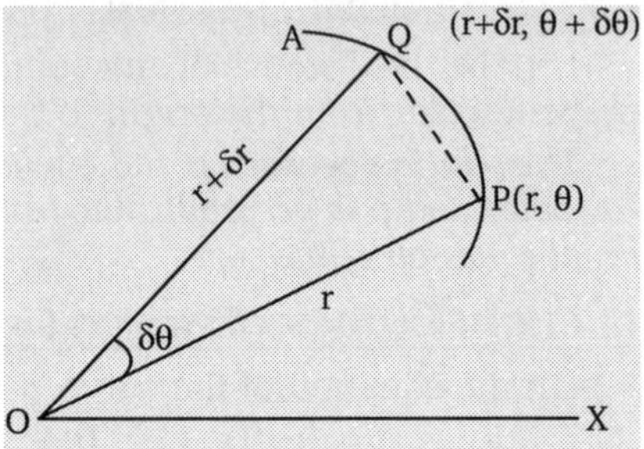

Fig. 8

As $Q \to P$, $\delta\theta \to \theta$ and $\delta r \to 0$

From ΔOPQ, we have

$$(\text{chord } PQ)^2 = OP^2 + OQ^2 - 2OP.OQ\cos(\angle QOP)$$
$$= r^2 + (r+\delta r)^2 - 2r(r+\delta r)\cos\delta\theta$$
$$= (\delta r)^2 + 2r\delta r(1-\cos\delta\theta) + 2r^2(1-\cos\delta\theta)$$

Dividing by $(\delta\theta)^2$, we get

$$\left(\frac{\text{chord } PQ}{\delta\theta}\right)^2 = \left(\frac{\delta r}{\delta\theta}\right)^2 + r\left(\frac{\sin\frac{\delta\theta}{2}}{\frac{\delta\theta}{2}}\right)^2.\delta r + r^2\left(\frac{\sin\frac{\delta\theta}{2}}{\frac{\delta\theta}{2}}\right)^2$$

and $$\left(\frac{\text{chord } PQ}{\delta s}\right)^2 = \left(\frac{\delta r}{\delta\theta}\right)^2 + r\left(\frac{\sin\frac{\delta\theta}{2}}{\frac{\delta\theta}{2}}\right)^2.\delta r + r^2\left(\frac{\sin\frac{\delta\theta}{2}}{\frac{\delta\theta}{2}}\right)^2$$

Taking limit as $Q \to P$, we have

$$\left(\frac{ds}{d\theta}\right)^2 = \left(\frac{dr}{d\theta}\right)^2 + r.1.0 + r^2.1 \qquad \left[\because \lim_{Q\to P}\frac{\text{chord } PQ}{PQ(=\delta s)} = 1 \text{ and } \lim_{\delta\theta\to\theta}\frac{\delta r}{\delta\theta} = \frac{dr}{d\theta}\right]$$

$$\Rightarrow \quad \left(\frac{ds}{d\theta}\right)^2 = r^2 + \left(\frac{dr}{d\theta}\right)^2 \Rightarrow \frac{ds}{d\theta} = \pm\sqrt{\left\{r^2+\left(\frac{dr}{d\theta}\right)^2\right]}$$

- Here + or – sign is to be taken according as s increases or decreases as θ increases, we have

$$\frac{ds}{d\theta} = \pm\sqrt{\left\{r^2 + \left(\frac{dr}{d\theta}\right)^2\right\}}$$

- If $\theta = f(r)$ is the given equation of the curve, then

$$\frac{ds}{dr} = \pm\sqrt{\left\{1 + r^2\left(\frac{d\theta}{dr}\right)^2\right\}}$$

- The result $\cos\phi = \frac{dr}{ds}$ and $\sin\phi = r\frac{d\theta}{ds}$ can be remember with the help of adjoining figure(9).

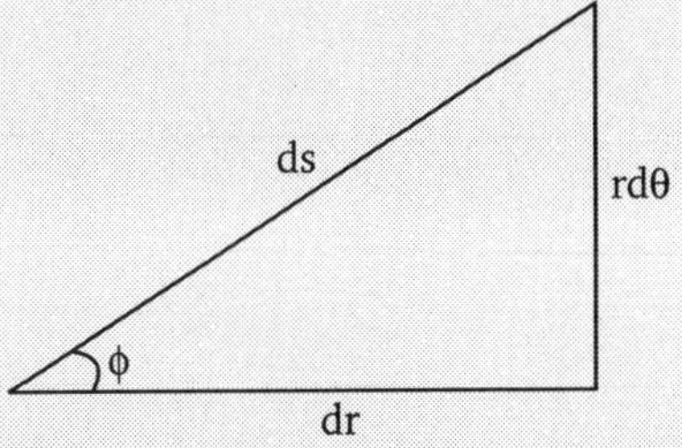

Fig. 9.

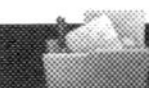

Solved Examples

1. *Find the equation on the tangent at the point t to the cycloid $x = a(t + \sin t)$, $y = a(1 - \cos t)$.*

SOLUTION. We have

$$x = a(t + \sin t) \Rightarrow \frac{dx}{dt} = a(1 + \cos t)$$

and $y = a(1 - \cos t) \Rightarrow \frac{dy}{dt} = a\sin t$

Therefore,

$$\frac{dy}{dx} = \frac{dy/dt}{dx/dt} = \frac{a\sin t}{a(1+\cos t)}$$

$$= \frac{2\sin t/2 \cdot \cos t/2}{2\cos^2 t/2} = \tan\frac{t}{2}$$

Now, the equation of the tangent at 't' is

$$y - a(1 - \cos t) = \tan\frac{t}{2}[x - a(t + \sin t)]$$

$$\Rightarrow y - 2a\sin^2\frac{t}{2} = (x - at)\tan\frac{t}{2} - a\sin t.\tan\frac{t}{2}$$

$$\Rightarrow y - 2a\sin^2\frac{t}{2} = (x - at)\tan\frac{t}{2} - 2a\sin^2\frac{t}{2}$$

$$\Rightarrow \quad y = (x - at)\tan t/2.$$

2. *Show that the parabolas*

$$r = \frac{a}{(1+\cos\theta)} \text{ and } r = \frac{b}{(1-\cos\theta)}$$

intersect orthogonally.

SOLUTION. Here we have $r = \frac{a}{(1+\cos\theta)}$ ...(1)

and $r = \frac{b}{(1-\cos\theta)}$ ...(2)

Taking log of both sides of (1), we get

$$\log r = \log a - \log(1 + \cos\theta)$$

Differentiating with respect to θ, we get

$$\frac{1}{r}.\frac{dr}{d\theta} = \frac{-(-\sin\theta)}{(1+\cos\theta)} = \frac{2\sin\frac{\theta}{2}\cos\frac{\theta}{2}}{2\cos^2\frac{\theta}{2}}$$

$$= \tan\frac{\theta}{2}$$

$$\Rightarrow \quad \cot\phi = \tan\frac{\theta}{2} = \cot\left(\frac{\pi}{2} - \frac{\theta}{2}\right)$$

$$\Rightarrow \quad \phi_1 = \frac{\pi}{2} - \frac{\theta}{2}$$

Now, from (2), we get

$$\log r = \log b - \log(1 - \cos\theta)$$

Differentiating with respect to θ, we get

$$\frac{1}{r}.\frac{dr}{d\theta} = \frac{-\sin\theta}{1-\cos\theta} = -\frac{2\sin\frac{\theta}{2}\cdot\cos\frac{\theta}{2}}{2\sin^2\frac{\theta}{2}}$$

$$= -\cot\frac{\theta}{2}$$

$$\therefore \cot\phi = -\cot\frac{1}{2}\theta = \cot\left(\pi - \frac{1}{2}\theta\right)$$

$$\Rightarrow \quad \phi = \pi - \frac{1}{2}\theta \quad \Rightarrow \quad \phi_2 = \pi - \frac{1}{2}\theta$$

Now, the angle of intersection $= \phi_1 \sim \phi_2$

$$= \left(\pi - \frac{1}{2}\theta\right) - \left(\frac{1}{2}\pi - \frac{1}{2}\theta\right) = \frac{\pi}{2}$$

Both curves intersect orthogonally.

3. *Show that the pedal equation of the ellipse* $\frac{x^2}{a^2}+\frac{y^2}{b^2}=1$ *is* $\frac{1}{p^2}=\frac{1}{a^2}+\frac{1}{b^2}-\frac{r^2}{a^2b^2}$.

SOLUTION. Here, the equation of the curve is

$$\frac{x^2}{a^2}+\frac{y^2}{b^2}=1.$$

Let $x = a\cos t, y = b\sin t$.

$$\therefore \quad \frac{dx}{dt}=-a\sin t, \frac{dy}{dt}=b\cos t$$

$$\Rightarrow \quad \frac{dy}{dx}=-\frac{b\cos t}{a\sin t}$$

Therefore, the equation of the tangent at 't' is

$$Y-b\sin t=-\frac{b\cos t}{a\sin t}(X-a\cos t)$$

$$\Rightarrow ab-b\cos t.X-a\sin t.Y=0 \quad \ldots(1)$$

Since p denote the length prependicular from (0, 0) to (1), therefore

$$p=\frac{ab}{\sqrt{a^2\sin^2 t+b^2\cos^2 t}}$$

$$\frac{1}{p^2}=\frac{a^2\sin^2 t+b^2\cos^2 t}{a^2b^2} \quad \ldots(2)$$

$$\text{Now, } r^2=x^2+y^2=a^2\cos^2 t+b^2\sin^2 t$$

$$=a^2+b^2-a^2\sin^2 t-b^2\cos^2 t \ldots(3)$$

From (3) $a^2\sin^2 t+b^2\cos^2 t=(a^2+b^2)-r^2$.

Therefore, from (3), we get

$$\frac{1}{p^2}=\frac{(a^2+b^2)-r^2}{a^2b^2}=\frac{1}{a^2}+\frac{1}{b^2}-\frac{r^2}{a^2b^2}.$$

4. *Find the pedal equation of* $r^n = a^n \sin n\theta$.

SOLUTION. Here, the given curve is

$$r^n = a^n \sin n\theta \quad \ldots(1)$$

Taking logarithm of both the sides of (1), we get

$$n\log r = n\log a + \log\sin n\theta. \quad \ldots(2)$$

Differentiating w.r.t. θ, we get

$$\frac{n}{r}.\frac{dr}{d\theta}=n\frac{\cos n\theta}{\sin n\theta}=n\cot n\theta$$

$$\Rightarrow \quad \cot\phi=\frac{1}{r}.\frac{dr}{d\theta}=\cot n\theta$$

$$\therefore \quad \phi=n\theta$$

Also, $p = r\sin\phi \Rightarrow p = r\sin n\theta \quad \ldots(3)$

Now from (1) and (3), we have

$$\sin n\theta=\frac{p}{r}$$

Putting the value in (1), we get

$$pa^n = r^{n+1}.$$

5. *Find the angle at which the radius vector cuts the curves* $\frac{l}{r}=1+e\cos\theta$.

SOLUTION. Here, the given equation of the curve is

$$\frac{l}{r}=1+e\cos\theta$$

$$\Rightarrow \quad \log l-\log r=\log(1+e\cos\theta).$$

Diff. w.r.t. θ, we get

$$-\frac{1}{r}.\frac{dr}{d\theta}=\frac{1}{(1+e\cos\theta)}(-e\sin\theta)$$

$$\therefore \quad \cot\phi=\frac{1}{r}.\frac{dr}{d\theta}=\frac{e\sin\theta}{1+e\cos\theta}$$

$$\Rightarrow \quad \tan\phi=\frac{1+e\cos\theta}{e\sin\theta}$$

$$\Rightarrow \quad \phi=\tan^{-1}\left[\frac{1+e\cos\theta}{e\sin\theta}\right].$$

6. *For the cardiod* $r = a(1-\cos\theta)$, *prove that*

(*i*) $\phi=\frac{1}{2}\theta$ (VTU–2004)

(*ii*) $2ap^2 = r^3$

SOLUTION. Here the given curve is

$$r = a(1-\cos\theta) \quad \ldots(1)$$

$$\Rightarrow \quad \frac{dr}{d\theta}=a\sin\theta$$

(i) Since, we have

$$\tan\phi=r\frac{d\theta}{dr}=\frac{a(1-\cos\theta)}{a\sin\theta}$$

$$=\frac{2a\sin^2\frac{\theta}{2}}{2a\sin\frac{\theta}{2}\cdot\cos\frac{\theta}{2}}=\tan\frac{\theta}{2}$$

$\Rightarrow \ \phi = \dfrac{\theta}{2}$

(ii) Since, we have $p = r\sin\phi = r\sin\theta/2$

$$\Rightarrow \quad r = 2a\sin^2\frac{\theta}{2} = 2a\frac{p^2}{r^2}$$

$\therefore \ 2ap^2 = r^3$

7. *Find the pedal equation of the curve* $x^{2/3} + y^{2/3} = a^{2/3}$.

SOLUTION. Here, the given curve is

$$x^{2/3} + y^{2/3} = a^{2/3} \quad \ldots(1)$$

Let $x = a\cos^3 t, y = a\sin^3 t$

$$\Rightarrow \frac{dy}{dx} = \frac{dy/dt}{dx/dt} = \frac{3a\sin^2 t\cos t}{-3a\cos^2 t\sin t} = -\frac{\sin t}{\cos t}.$$

Hence, the equation of tangent of (1) is

$$y - a\sin^3 t = -\frac{\sin t}{\cos t}(x - a\cos^3 t)$$

$$\Rightarrow x\sin t + y\cos t = a\sin t\cos t(\cos^2 t + \sin^2 t)$$

$$= a\sin t\cos t \quad \ldots(2)$$

p = the length of the prependicular from (0, 0) to (2)

$$= \frac{a\sin t\cos t}{\sqrt{\sin^2 t + \cos^2 t}} = a\sin t\cos t.$$

Now,

$$r^2 = x^2 + y^2 = a^2\cos^6 t + a^2\sin^6 t$$

$$= a^2[(\cos^2 t)^3 + (\sin^2 t)^3]$$

$$= a^2[(\cos^2 t + \sin^2 t)^3 - 3\cos^2 t\sin^2 t(\cos^2 t + \sin^2 t)]$$

$$= a^2[1 - 3(p^2/a^2).1] = a^2 - 3p^2.$$

8. *Show that for any curve*

$$\sin^2\phi\left(\frac{d\phi}{d\theta}\right) + r\left(\frac{d^2r}{ds^2}\right) = 0.$$

SOLUTION. We have $\dfrac{dr}{ds} = \cos\phi$

$$\Rightarrow \quad \frac{d^2r}{ds^2} = -\sin\phi\left(\frac{d\phi}{ds}\right)$$

$$= -\sin\phi\left(\frac{d\phi}{d\theta}\right)\left(\frac{d\theta}{ds}\right)$$

$$\Rightarrow \quad r\left(\frac{d^2r}{ds^2}\right) = -\sin\phi\left(\frac{d\phi}{d\theta}\right).r\left(\frac{d\theta}{ds}\right)$$

$$\Rightarrow \quad r\left(\frac{d^2r}{ds^2}\right) = -\sin\phi\left(\frac{d\phi}{d\theta}\right).\sin\phi$$

$$\left(\because r\frac{d\theta}{ds} = \sin\phi\right)$$

$$\therefore \ r\left(\frac{d^2r}{ds^2}\right) + \sin^2\phi\left(\frac{d\phi}{d\theta}\right) = 0.$$

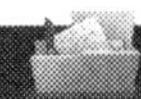

Exercise-12.1

1. Find the angle of intersection of the curve $r^2 = 16\sin 2\theta$ and $r^2\sin 2\theta = 4$.
2. Show that in the curve $r = a\theta$, the polar subnormal is constant and in the curve $r\theta = a$, the polar subtangent is constant.
3. Show that the curves $r = a(1 + \cos\theta)$ and $r = b(1 - \cos\theta)$ intersect at right angles. (VTU–2011)
4. Show that the spiral $r^n = a^n\cos n\theta$ and $r^n = b^n\sin n\theta$ intersect orthogonally. (VTU–2010)
5. Find the angle ϕ for the curve $a\theta = (r^2 - a^2)^{1/2} - a\cos^{-1} a/r$.
6. Show that the curves $r = (1 + \sin\theta)$ and $r = a(1 - \sin\theta)$ cut orthogonally.
7. Show that the curves $r = 2\sin\theta$ and $r = 2\cos\theta$ intersect at right angles.
8. Find the angle of intersection between the pair of curves $r = 6\cos\theta$ and $r = 2(1 + \cos\theta)$.
9. Show that the pedal equation of the
   (i) conic $\dfrac{l}{r} = 1 + e\cos\theta$ is $\dfrac{1}{p^2} = \dfrac{1}{l^2}\left(\dfrac{2l}{r} - 1 + e^2\right)$
   (ii) curve $r = a\theta$ is $p^2 = \dfrac{r^4}{r^2 + a^2}$
   (iii) cardiod $r = a(1 + \cos\theta)$ is $r^3 = 2ap^2$.

(iv) spiral $r = a \operatorname{sech} n\theta$ is $\frac{1}{p^2} = \frac{A}{r^2} + B$.

(v) hyperbola $r^2\cos 2\theta = a^2$ is $pr = a^2$.

(vi) lemniscate $r^2 = a^2\cos 2\theta$ is $r^3 = a^2 p$.

10. Show that the normal at any point (r, θ) to the curve $r^n = a^n \cos n\theta$ makes an angle $(n + 1)\theta$ with the initial line.

11. Show that in the equiangular spiral $r = ae^{\theta\cot\alpha}$, the tangent is inclined at a constant angle α to the radius vector.

12. For the curve $r = ae^{\theta\cot a}$, prove that $\frac{s}{r} =$ constant, s being measured from the pole.

13. Show that

(i) $\frac{ds}{d\theta} = \frac{r^2}{p}$ (ii) $\frac{ds}{dr} = \frac{r}{\sqrt{r^2 - p^2}}$

14. For the ellipse $x = a\cos t$, $y = b\sin t$, prove that $\frac{ds}{dt} = a(1 - e^2\cos^2 t)^{1/2}$.

15. For the curve $r^n = a^n \cos n\theta$, show that

$$a^{2n}\frac{d^2r}{ds^2} + nr^{2n-1} = 0.$$

16. For the cycloid $x = a(1 - \cos t), y = a(t + \sin t)$, show that

(i) $\frac{ds}{dt} = 2a\cos\frac{t}{2}$ (ii) $\frac{ds}{dx} = \operatorname{cosec}\frac{t}{2}$

(iii) $\frac{ds}{dy} = \sec\frac{t}{2}$

17. Show that for the curve $r^m = a^m \cos m\theta$, $\frac{ds}{d\theta} = \frac{a^m}{r^{m-1}}$.

18. Show that the pedal equation of the parabola $y^2 = 4a(x + a)$ is $p^2 = ar$.

19. Prove that for the ellipse $\frac{x^2}{a^2} + \frac{y^2}{b^2} = 1, f = \frac{a^2b^2}{p^3}$, p being the perpendicular from centre upon the tangent (x, y).

ANSWERS

1. $\frac{2\pi}{3}$ **5.** $\cos^{-1}\frac{a}{r}$ **8.** $\frac{\pi}{6}$

❑❑❑❑❑❑

Chapter

13 Curvature

13.1 INTRODUCTION

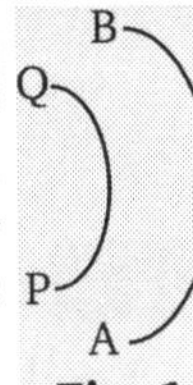

Fig. 1.

The measure of the sharpness of the bending of a curve at a particular point is called curvature of the curve at the point. In figure (1), curve *PQ* bends more sharply than the curve *AB*. In this chapter, we shall find mathematical expressions for the curvature of a curve at a given point.

13.2 CURVATURE

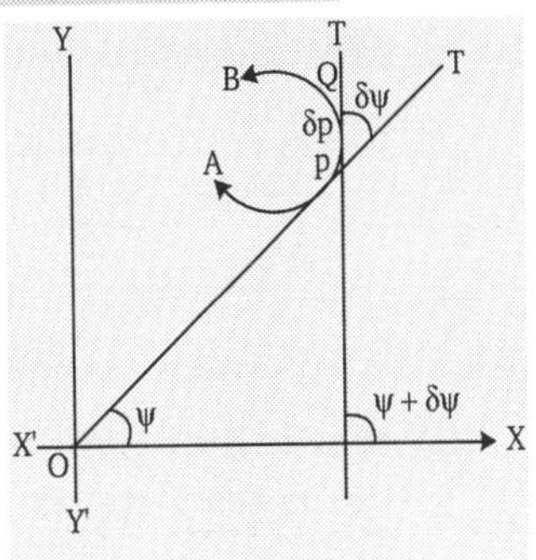

Fig. 2.

Let *P*, *Q* be two neighbouring points on a curve *AB*.

Also, let *AP* = *s*, arc *AQ* = *s* + δ*s* and arc *PQ* = δs.

Let the tangent to the curve at points *P* and *Q* makes angle ψ and ψ + δψ respectively with a fixed line say *X*-axis, then

(i) The angle δψ through which the tangent turns as its points of contact travels along the arc *PQ* is called the total bending or total curvature of arc *PQ*.

(ii) The ratio $\frac{\delta\psi}{\delta s}$ is called the mean or average curvature of arc *PQ*.

(iii) The limiting value of the mean curvature when *Q* tends to *P* is called the curvature of the curve at the point *P*. Therefore, the curvature *K* at point *P* is

$$\lim_{Q\to P}\frac{\delta\psi}{\delta s}=\lim_{\delta s\to 0}\frac{\delta\psi}{\delta s}=\frac{d\psi}{ds}$$

(iv) The reciprocal of the curvature of the given curve at *P*. (provided this curvature is not equal to zero), is called the radius of curvature of the curve at *P*. This is denoted by ρ.

$$\rho=\frac{1}{K}=\frac{ds}{d\psi}$$

13.3 FORMULA FOR RADIUS OF CURVATURE (CARTESIAN FORM)

Let $y = f(x)$ be the equation of curve. Then the slope of the tangent at any point $= \tan\psi=\frac{dy}{dx}$

Differentiating both sides, w.r.t. *s*, we get

$$\sec^2\psi\frac{d\psi}{ds}=\frac{d}{ds}\left(\frac{dy}{dx}\right)\quad\Rightarrow\quad\sec^2\psi.\frac{1}{\rho}=\frac{d}{dx}\left(\frac{dy}{dx}\right)\frac{dx}{ds}$$

$$\Rightarrow\qquad \sec^2\psi.\frac{1}{\rho}=\frac{d^2y}{dx^2}.\cos\psi \qquad\qquad \left(\because\ \frac{dx}{ds}=\cos\psi\right)$$

Therefore

$$\rho=\frac{\sec^2\psi}{\cos\psi\frac{d^2y}{dx^2}}=\frac{\sec^3\psi}{\frac{d^2y}{dx^2}}=\frac{(1+\tan^2\psi)^{3/2}}{\frac{d^2y}{dx^2}}\Rightarrow\qquad \rho=\frac{\left[1+\left(\frac{dy}{dx}\right)^2\right]^{3/2}}{\frac{d^2y}{dx^2}}$$

- The positive root is taken in numerator of above formula, therefore, radius of curvature r, will be positive when $\frac{d^2y}{dx^2}$ is positive (*i.e.*, when the curve is concave upward) and negative when $\frac{d^2y}{dx^2}$ is negative (*i.e.*, when the curve is concave downward).
- At a point of inflexion, the curvature of a curve is not defined. $\left(\because \text{ at the point of inflexion } \frac{d^2y}{dx^2} = 0\right)$
- When the equation of the curve is given in the form $x = f(y)$ then by interchanging x and y (It is justify because curvature is a length, and its value is independent of the choice of axis), we get

$$\rho = \frac{\left[1 + (dx/dy)^2\right]^{3/2}}{d^2x/dy^2}$$

- When the equation of curve is given in parametric form, *i.e.*, $x = f(t)$ and $y = g(t)$, then radius of curvature is given by $\rho = \frac{(x'^2 + y'^2)^{3/2}}{x'y'' - y'x''}$, where dash (') denote the derivative w.r.t., 't'.

$$\frac{1}{\rho^2} = \left(\frac{d^2x}{ds^2}\right)^2 + \left(\frac{d^2y}{ds^2}\right)^2$$

13.4 RADIUS OF CURVATURE AT THE ORIGIN

Let the curve $y = f(x)$ passes through the origin. Then, we may use the following methods, to find the radius of curvature.

(i) Method of direct substitution. Since $y = f(x)$ be given. Calculate the values of $\frac{dy}{dx}$ and $\frac{d^2y}{dx^2}$ at origin and then use the following formula

$$\rho = \frac{\left[1 + \left(\frac{dy}{dx}\right)^2\right]^{3/2}}{d^2y/dx^2}$$

(ii) Method of Expansion. Let $y = f(x)$ be the equation of curve. Since, it passes through the origin, therefore $f(0) = 0$.

Therefore, by Maclaurin's series expansion, we have

$$y = f(0) + xf'(0) + \frac{x^2}{2!}f''(0) + \frac{x^3}{3!}f'''(0) + \ldots$$

$$\Rightarrow \quad y = xf'(0) + \frac{x^2}{2!}f''(0) + \frac{x^3}{3!}f'''(0) + \ldots \qquad [\because f(0) = 0]$$

$$\Rightarrow y = p_1x + \frac{1}{2!}p_2x^2 + \frac{1}{3!}p_3x^3 + \ldots (1)$$

where $p_1 = f'(0) = y_1(0), p_2 = f''(0) = y_2(0)$, etc.

Now, differentiating (1) with respect to x, we get

$$y_1 = p_1 + \frac{2p_2x}{2!} + \frac{3p_3x^2}{3!} + \ldots$$

Again differentiating w.r.t. x. we get

$$y_2 = \frac{2p_2}{2!} + \frac{6p_3x}{3!} + \ldots$$

At the origin (*i.e.*, $x = 0$), we have

$$y_1 = p_1 \text{ and } y_2 = \frac{2p_2}{2!} = p_2$$

Now putting these values of y_1 and y_2 in the formula $\rho = \frac{(1+y_1^2)^{3/2}}{y_2}$, We get $\rho = \frac{(1+p_1^2)^{3/2}}{p_2}$

- We can find the values of p and q in the following manner:
  Put the value of $y = p_1x + \frac{p_2x^2}{2!} + \frac{p_3x^3}{3!} + \ldots$ in the given equation of the curve and equating the coefficients of the powers of x.

(iii) Newton's Method. If a curve passes through the origin, and axis of x is the tangent at the origin, then radius of curvature ρ at origin

$$= \lim_{\substack{x\to 0\\ y\to 0}} \frac{x^2}{2y}$$

Since the axis of x is the tangent at the origin, therefore, we have

$$y_1(0) = \left(\frac{dy}{dx}\right)_{(0,0)} = 0$$

Here, we observed that $\frac{x^2}{2y}$ is of the indeterminate form $\left(\frac{0}{0}\right)$ as $x \to 0, y \to 0$.

Using L' Hospital rule, we have

$$\lim_{\substack{x\to 0\\ y\to 0}} \frac{x^2}{2y} = \lim_{\substack{x\to 0\\ y\to 0}} \frac{2x}{2y_1} = \lim_{\substack{x\to 0\\ y\to 0}} \frac{x}{y_1} = \lim_{\substack{x\to 0\\ y\to 0}} \frac{1}{y_2} = \frac{1}{y_2(0)} \quad \ldots(1)$$

Now, ρ at origin $= \frac{[1+y_1^2(0)]^{3/2}}{y_2(0)} = \frac{(1+0)^{3/2}}{y_2(0)} = \frac{1}{y_2(0)}$ ...(2)

From (1) and (2), we have

$$\rho_{(\text{at origin})} = \lim_{\substack{x\to 0\\ y\to 0}} \frac{x^2}{2y}$$

- If a curve passes through the origin and axis of y is the tangent, then radius of curvature at the origin is given by $\lim_{\substack{x\to 0\\ y\to 0}} \frac{y^2}{2x}$.

Solved Examples

1. *For $x = a(t + \sin t)$, $y = a(1 - \cos t)$, prove that $\rho = 4a\cos\frac{t}{2}$.* (SRM-2010)

SOLUTION. We have

$$x = a(t+\sin t) \Rightarrow \frac{dx}{dt} = a(1+\cos t)$$

and $y = a(1-\cos t) \Rightarrow \frac{dy}{dt} = a\sin t$

$$\Rightarrow \frac{dy}{dx} = \frac{dy/dt}{dx/dt} = \frac{a\sin t}{a(1+\cos t)}$$

$$= \frac{2\sin t/2 \cos t/2}{2\cos^2 t/2} = \tan\frac{t}{2}$$

Also $\frac{d^2y}{dx^2} = \frac{d}{dx}\left(\frac{dy}{dx}\right) = \frac{d}{dx}\left(\tan\frac{t}{2}\right)$

$$= \frac{1}{2}\sec^2\frac{t}{2}.\frac{dt}{dx}$$

$$= \frac{1}{2}\sec^2\frac{t}{2}.\frac{1}{a(1+\cos t)} = \frac{1}{4a}\sec^4\frac{t}{2}$$

Now, putting the values of $\frac{dy}{dx}$ and $\frac{d^2y}{dx^2}$

in $\rho = \frac{\left[1+\left(\frac{dy}{dx}\right)^2\right]^{3/2}}{\frac{d^2y}{dx^2}}$

We get $\rho = \frac{[1+\tan^2 t/2]^{3/2}}{\frac{1}{4a}\sec^4 t/2}$

$$= \frac{4a\sec^3 t/2}{\sec^4 t/2} = 4a\cos t/2$$

2. *Find the curvature of the curve $x^3+y^3=3axy$ at the point (3a/2, 3a/2).* (ANNA–2009, VTU–2008, KURUKSHATRA–2009, KERELA–2005)

SOLUTION. The equation of the curve is

$$x^3+y^3=3axy \quad \ldots(1)$$

Differentiating w.r.t. x, we get

$$3x^2+3y^2\frac{dy}{dx}=3ay+3ax\frac{dy}{dx}$$

$$\Rightarrow x^2+y^2\frac{dy}{dx}=ay+ax\frac{dy}{dx}$$

$$\Rightarrow \frac{dy}{dx}=\frac{x^2-ay}{ax-y^2} \quad \ldots(2)$$

$$\Rightarrow \left(\frac{dy}{dx}\right)_{at\left(\frac{3}{2}a,\frac{3}{2}a\right)}=-1$$

From (2), we have

$$2x+2y\left(\frac{dy}{dx}\right)^2+y^2\frac{d^2y}{dx^2}$$

$$=a\frac{dy}{dx}+a\frac{dy}{dx}+ax\frac{d^2y}{dx^2}$$

$$\Rightarrow (ax-y^2)\frac{d^2y}{dx^2}=2x+2y\left(\frac{dy}{dx}\right)^2-2a\frac{dy}{dx} \quad \ldots(3)$$

Putting $x=\frac{3a}{2}, y=\frac{3a}{2}$

and $\left(\frac{dy}{dx}\right)_{\left(\frac{3a}{2},\frac{3a}{2}\right)}=-1,$

We get $\left[\frac{d^2y}{dx^2}\right]_{\left(\frac{3a}{2},\frac{3a}{2}\right)}=-\frac{32}{3}.\frac{1}{a}$

Hence, the radius of curvature ρ at $\left(\frac{3a}{2},\frac{3a}{2}\right)$, we get

$$\rho=\left[\frac{\left[1+\left(\frac{dy}{dx}\right)^2\right]^{3/2}}{\frac{d^2y}{dx^2}}\right]_{at\left(\frac{3a}{2},\frac{3a}{2}\right)}$$

$$=\frac{(1+1)^{3/2}}{-\frac{32}{3}.\frac{1}{a}}=-\frac{3a}{8\sqrt{2}}$$

Therefore, the curvature $\frac{1}{\rho}=+\frac{8\sqrt{2}}{3a}$.

(By ignoring the negative sign)

3. *Show that the radii of curvature of the curve $y^2=x^2\left(\frac{a+x}{a-x}\right)$ at the origin are $a\sqrt{2}$.*

SOLUTION. The equation of the curve is

$$y^2=x^2\left(\frac{a+x}{a-x}\right)$$

$$\Rightarrow y=\pm\frac{x(a+x)^{1/2}}{(a-x)^{1/2}}$$

$$=\pm x\frac{a^{1/2}\left(1+\frac{x}{a}\right)^{1/2}}{a^{1/2}\left(1-\frac{x}{a}\right)^{1/2}}$$

$$\Rightarrow y=\pm x\left(1+\frac{x}{a}\right)^{1/2}\left(1-\frac{x}{a}\right)^{-1/2}$$

$$\Rightarrow y=\pm x\left(1+\frac{x}{2a}+\ldots\right)\left(1+\frac{x}{2a}+\ldots\right)$$

(Expanding by Binomial Expansions)

$$\text{or } y=\pm x\left(1+\frac{x}{2a}+\frac{x}{2a}+\frac{x^2}{4a^2}+\ldots\right)$$

$$\Rightarrow y=\pm\left(x+\frac{x^2}{a}+\frac{x^3}{4a^2}+\ldots\right)$$

Therefore,

$$\frac{dy}{dx} = y_1 = \pm\left(1+\frac{2x}{a}+\frac{3x^2}{4a^2}+\ldots\right)$$

and $\dfrac{d^2y}{dx^2} = y_2 = \pm\left(\dfrac{2}{a}+\dfrac{6x}{4a^2}+\ldots\right)$

At(0, 0) $y_1 = \pm 1$ and $y_2 = \pm\dfrac{2}{a}$

$$\therefore \rho = \frac{(1+y_1^2)^{3/2}}{y_2} = \frac{(1+1)^{3/2}}{\pm 2/a}$$

$$= \pm 2\sqrt{2}.\frac{a}{2}$$

$\Rightarrow \rho = \pm\sqrt{2}\cdot a = \sqrt{2}\cdot a$. (Numerically)

4. *Apply Netwon's formula, find the radius of curvature at the origin for the curve*

$$x^3 - 2x^2y + 3xy^2 - 4y^3 + 5x^2 - 6xy + 7y^2 - 8y = 0.$$

SOLUTION. Since, the curve passes through the origin. Equating to zero, the lowest degree terms, we may find $y = 0$

$\Rightarrow$ x axis is the tangent at the origin.

Therefore, by Newton's formula, ρ at (0, 0)

$$= \lim_{\substack{x\to 0\\ y\to 0}} \frac{x^2}{2y}$$

Dividing the equation of the curve by $2y$, we get

$$x.\frac{x^2}{2y} - x^2 + \frac{3}{2}xy - 2y^2 + 5.\frac{x^2}{2y} - 3x + \frac{7}{2}y - 4 = 0$$

Taking lim $x \to 0$ and $y \to 0$, we get

$$\lim_{\substack{x\to 0\\ y\to 0}} \frac{x^2}{2y} - 4 = 0 \Rightarrow 5\rho - 4 = 0 \Rightarrow \rho = \frac{4}{5}.$$

5. *For the curve* $y = \dfrac{ax}{a+x}$, *if* ρ *is the radius of curvature at any point* (x, y), *show that* $\left(\dfrac{2\rho}{a}\right)^{2/3} = \left(\dfrac{y}{x}\right)^2 + \left(\dfrac{x}{y}\right)^2$.

(VTU–2008)

SOLUTION. Let $\quad y = \dfrac{ax}{a+x}$ ...(1)

Therefore, $\dfrac{dy}{dx} = a\dfrac{a+x-x}{(a+x)^2}$

$$= a^2(a+x)^{-2}$$

Now, again

$$\frac{d^2y}{dx^2} = \frac{d}{dx}\left(\frac{dy}{dx}\right)$$

$$= -2a^2(a+x)^{-3} = \frac{-2a^2}{\left(\dfrac{ax}{y}\right)^3}$$

$$\Rightarrow \frac{d^2y}{dx^2} = \frac{-2y^3}{ax^3}$$

$$\therefore 1+\left(\frac{dy}{dx}\right)^2 = 1+\frac{a^4}{(a+x)^4}$$

$$= 1+\frac{a^4}{\left(\dfrac{ax}{y}\right)^4} = 1+\frac{y^4}{x^4}$$

$$\therefore \rho = \frac{\left[1+\left(\dfrac{dy}{dx}\right)^2\right]^{3/2}}{d^2y/dx^2}$$

$$= \frac{[(x^4+y^4)/x^4]^{3/2}}{(-2y^3/ax^3)}$$

$$= -\frac{a(x^4+y^4)^{3/2}}{2x^6(y^3/x^3)} = -\frac{a}{2}\frac{(x^4+y^4)^{3/2}}{x^3y^3}$$

Hence,

$$\left(\frac{2\rho}{a}\right)^{2/3} = \frac{x^4+y^4}{x^2y^2} = \frac{x^2}{y^2}+\frac{y^2}{x^2}$$

$$\Rightarrow \left(\frac{2\rho}{a}\right)^{2/3} = \left(\frac{x}{y}\right)^2 + \left(\frac{y}{x}\right)^2.$$

6. *Find the radius of curvature at origin for the curve* $x^3 + y^3 - 2x^2 + 6y = 0$.

(BURDWAN 2003)

SOLUTION. The curve passes through origin. Equating to zero the lowest degree terms we get $y=0$ *i.e.*, x axis as tangent to the curve at origin.

$\therefore$ By Newtons method, ρ (at origin)

$$= \lim_{x\to 0} \frac{x^2}{2y}$$

Dividing by 2y, the equation of the curve can be written as

$$x.\frac{x^2}{2y} + \frac{1}{2}y^2 - 2.\frac{x^2}{2y} + 3 = 0$$

Taking limit as $x \to 0, y \to 0$ and

$\lim_{x\to 0} \frac{y^2}{2x} = \rho$, we get

$$0.\rho + 0 - 2\rho + 3 = 0 \quad i.e., \quad \rho = 3/2.$$

7. *If ρ_1 and ρ_2 be the radii of curvature of the extremities of two conjugate diameters of an ellipse prove that*

$$(\rho_1^{2/3} + \rho_2^{2/3})(ab)^{2/3} = a^2 + b^2.$$

SOLUTION. Let the equation of an ellipse be

$$\frac{x^2}{a^2} + \frac{y^2}{b^2} = 1. \qquad \ldots(1)$$

Let

$P(a\cos\theta, b\sin\theta)$ and $Q(-a\sin\theta, b\cos\theta)$

be the extremities of two conjugate diameters of (1).

Differentiating both sides of (1) w.r.t x we get

$$\frac{2x}{a^2} + \frac{2y}{b^2}.\frac{dy}{dx} = 0$$

or

$$\frac{dy}{dx} = -\frac{b^2x}{a^2y} \qquad ..(2)$$

Again differentiating, we get

$$\frac{d^2y}{dx^2} = -\frac{b^2}{a^2}\left[\frac{y - x\frac{dy}{dx}}{y^2}\right]$$

$$= -\frac{b^2}{a^2}\left[\frac{y - x\left(-\frac{b^2x}{a^2y}\right)}{y^2}\right]$$

$$= -\frac{b^2}{a^2}\left[\frac{\left(\frac{y^2}{b^2} + \frac{x^2}{a^2}\right)}{y^3}\right]b^2$$

$$= -\frac{b^4}{a^2y^3} \qquad \text{[Using (1)]}$$

We know that

$$\rho = \frac{\left[1 + \left(\frac{dy}{dx}\right)^2\right]^{3/2}}{\frac{d^2y}{dx^2}} = \frac{\left[1 + \left(-\frac{b^2x}{a^2y}\right)^2\right]^{3/2}}{-b^4/a^2y^3}$$

$$\rho = \frac{(a^4y^2 + b^4x^2)^{3/2}}{-a^4b^4}$$

At $P(a\cos\theta, b\sin\theta)$, $\quad \rho = \rho_1$

$$\therefore \rho_1 = \frac{(a^4.b^2\sin^2\theta + b^4a^2\cos^2\theta)^{3/2}}{-a^4b^4}$$

or $\rho_1 = \dfrac{(a^2\sin^2\theta + b^2\cos^2\theta)^{3/2}}{-ab}$

or $\rho_1(-ab) = (a^2\sin^2\theta + b^2\cos^2\theta)^{3/2}$

or $\rho_1^{2/3}(ab)^{2/3} = a^2\sin^2\theta + b^2\cos^2\theta \qquad \ldots(3)$

At $Q(-a\sin\theta, b\cos\theta), \rho = \rho_2$

$\therefore \ \rho_2^{2/3}(ab)^{2/3} = a^2\cos^2\theta + b^2\sin^2\theta \qquad \ldots(4)$

Adding (3) and (4), we get

$$(\rho_1^{2/3} + \rho_2^{2/3})(ab)^{2/3} = a^2 + b^2$$

8. *Prove that for the ellipse $\frac{x^2}{a^2} + \frac{y^2}{b^2} = 1$, $\rho = \frac{a^2b^2}{p^3}$; p being the perpendicular from centre upon the tangent at (x, y).*

(JNTU–2002)

SOLUTION. We have $\frac{x^2}{a^2} + \frac{y^2}{b^2} = 1 \Rightarrow \frac{dy}{dx} = -\frac{b^2x}{a^2y}$

and $\dfrac{d^2y}{dx^2} = -\dfrac{b^2}{a^2}\left[\dfrac{y - x\frac{dy}{dx}}{y^2}\right] = -\dfrac{b^4}{a^2y^3}$

Let $(a\cos\theta, b\sin\theta)$ be any point on the ellipse. The equation of the tangent at this point is

$$y - b\sin\theta = \frac{-b\cos\theta}{a\sin\theta}(x - a\cos\theta)$$

or $bx\cos\theta + ay\sin\theta - ab = 0$ ...(2)

We are given that

p = Perpendicular from (0, 0) to the tangent (2)

or $p = \dfrac{-ab}{\sqrt{b^2\cos^2\theta + a^2\sin^2\theta}}$ ...(3)

Now the radius of curvature ρ is

$$\rho = \frac{\left[1+\left(\frac{dy}{dx}\right)^2\right]^{3/2}}{\frac{d^2y}{dx^2}} = \frac{a^2y^3\left(1+\frac{b^4x^2}{a^4y^2}\right)^{3/2}}{-b^4}$$

$$= \frac{(a^4y^2+b^4x^2)^{3/2}}{-a^4b^4}$$

The ρ at $(a\cos\theta, b\sin\theta)$ is given by

$$\rho = -\frac{(a^4b^2\sin^2\theta + b^4a^2\cos^2\theta)^{3/2}}{a^4b^4}$$

$$= -\frac{(a^2\sin^2\theta + b^2\cos^2\theta)^{3/2}}{ab}$$

$$= -\frac{(-ab/p)^3}{ab} \quad \text{[Using (3)]}$$

$$\rho = \frac{a^2b^2}{p^3}.$$

9. *If ρ_1 and ρ_2 be the radii of curvature at the ends of a focal chord of the parabola $y^2 = 4ax$, then show that $\rho_1^{-2/3} + \rho_2^{-2/3} = (2a)^{-2/3}$.*

(KURUKSHETRA–2005, ROHTAK–2006)

SOLUTION. We have $y^2 = 4ax$ ...(1)

Parametric form of (1) is given by

$$x = at^2, y = 2at$$

$\therefore$ $x' = 2at, y' = 2a$

and $x'' = 2a, y'' = 0$

Therefore, radius of curvature ρ at $(at^2, 2at)$ is given by

$$\rho = \frac{(x'^2+y'^2)^{3/2}}{x'y''-x''y'}$$

$$= \frac{(4a^2t^2+4a^2)^{3/2}}{0-4a^2} = 2a(1+t^2)^{3/2}$$

(Ignore –ve sign)

If $P(t_1)$ and $Q(t_2)$ be the extremities of the focal chord of the parabola, then

$$t_1t_2 = -1 \Rightarrow t_2 = -\frac{1}{t_1}$$

So, ρ_1 at $P(t_1) = 2a(1+t_1^2)^{3/2}$

ρ_2 at $Q(t_2) = 2a(1+t_2^2)^{3/2}$

$\therefore \rho_1^{-2/3} + \rho_2^{-2/3}$

$$= (2a)^{-2/3}.[(1+t_1^2)^{-1} + (1+t_2^2)^{-1}]$$

$$= (2a)^{-2/3}.\left[\frac{1}{1+t_1^2} + \frac{t_1^2}{1+t_1^2}\right]$$

$$= (2a)^{-2/3}.$$

Exercise-13.1

1. Find the radius of curvature of the following curves:

(i) $x^{1/2} + y^{1/2} = a^{1/2}$ (ii) $a^2y = x^3 - a^3$

(iii) $x^{2/3} + y^{2/3} = a^{2/3}$ (JNTU-2005)

(iv) $x^m + y^m = 1$

(v) $\sqrt{x} + \sqrt{y} = 1$ at $\left(\frac{1}{4}, \frac{1}{4}\right)$ (JNTU-2006)

(vi) $s = 4a\sin\psi$ at (s, ψ) (vii) $ay^2 = x^3$

(viii) $y = e^x$ at the point where it cuts the y-axis.

(ix) $x^{2/3} + y^{2/3} = a^{2/3}$ at $(a\cos^3\theta, a\sin^3\theta)$ (ANNA–2009)

(x) $y = 4\sin x - \sin 2x$ at $x = \frac{\pi}{2}$ (VTU–2009)

(xi) $y = x^3(x-a)$ at $(a, 0)$ (VTU–2010)

2. Find the radius of curvature at the origin of the following curves :

(i) $x^3 + y^3 = 3axy$ (ii) $y = x^3 + 5x^2 + 6x$

(iii) $5x^3+7y^3+4x^2y+xy^2+2x^2+3xy+y^2+4x=0$

(iv) $a(y^2 - x^2) = x^3$

(v) $y - x = x^2 + 2xy + y^2$

(vi) $2x^4+4x^3+xy^2+6y^3-3x^2-2xy+y^2-4x=0$

(vii) $\sqrt{x} + \sqrt{y} = a$ at $\left(\frac{a}{4}, \frac{a}{4}\right)$ (JNTU–2006)

3. Show that the curvature at a point of the curve $y = f(x)$ is given by $\frac{d^2y}{dx^2}\cos^3\psi$, where ψ is the inclination of the tangent at the point to the axis of x.

4. Show that for the curve $s = ae^{x/a}$, $a\rho = s(s^2 - a^2)^{1/2}$.

5. Show that if ρ be the radius of curvature at any point P on the parabola $y^2 = 4ax$ and S be its focus, then ρ varies as $(SP)^2$.
(KURUKSHETRA–2006)

6. Show that for any curve $\frac{1}{\rho} = \frac{d}{dx}\left(\frac{dy}{dx}\right)$.

Hints to the Selected Problems

1. (i) Differentiating two times the given equation w.r.t. x, we get $\frac{d^2y}{dx^2} = \frac{x^{1/2}+y^{1/2}}{2x^{3/2}} = \frac{a^{1/2}}{2x^{3/2}}$.
Then put this value in the formula.

2. (i) The given curve is passes through the origin. Therefore, equating the lowest degree term equal to zero, *i.e.*, $x = 0$ and $y = 0$ are the required trangent.
Then use $\rho = \lim_{x\to 0}\left(\frac{y^2}{x^2}\right)$.

3. We have $\tan\psi = \left(\frac{dy}{dx}\right)$. Put this value in the formula of radius of curvature.

4. Find $\frac{dy}{dx}$ and $\frac{d^2y}{dx^2}$ by using $\frac{ds}{dx} = \sqrt{1+\left(\frac{dy}{dx}\right)^2}$.
$\therefore \frac{d^2y}{dx^2} = \frac{s^2}{a^2\sqrt{s^2-a^2}}$.
Then use the formula of radius of curvature.

5. Let $P(at^2, 2at)$ be any point on $y^2 = 4ax$ and $S = (a, 0)$ be the coordinate of its focus. Then
$SP = \sqrt{(at-a)^2+(2at)^2} = \sqrt{(at^2+a)^2} = t^2+1$
Now find $\frac{d^2y}{dx^2}$ by the equation of the parabola.
Then find the relation between ρ and SP, by using formula of radius of curvature.

6. Since we have
$$\frac{ds}{dy} = \sqrt{1+\left(\frac{dx}{dy}\right)^2} \Rightarrow \frac{dy}{ds} = \frac{ds/dx}{\sqrt{1+\left(\frac{dy}{dx}\right)^2}}$$
$$\therefore \frac{d}{dx}\left(\frac{dy}{ds}\right) = \frac{\left(\frac{d^2y}{dx^2}\right)}{\left[1+\left(\frac{dy}{dx}\right)^2\right]^{3/2}} = \frac{1}{\rho}.$$

ANSWERS

1. (i) $\frac{2(x+y)^{3/2}}{\sqrt{y}}$ (ii) $\frac{(a^4+9x^4)^{3/2}}{6a^4x}$ (iii) $3a^{1/3}x^{1/3}y^{1/3}$ (iv) $\frac{(x^{2m-2}+y^{2m-2})^{3/2}}{(1-m)x^{m-2}y^{m-2}}$ (v) $\frac{1}{\sqrt{2}}$ (vi) $4a\cos\psi$ (vii) $\frac{1}{6a}(4a+9x)^{3/2}x^{1/2}$ (viii) $\sqrt{8}$ (ix) $3a\sin\theta\cos\theta$ (x) $\frac{5\sqrt{5}}{4}$ (xi) $(1+a^3)^{3b}/6a^2$

2. (i) $\frac{3a}{2}$ (ii) $\frac{37\sqrt{37}}{10}$ (iii) –2 (iv) $2a\sqrt{2}$ (v) $\frac{1}{2\sqrt{2}}$ (vi) 2 (vii) $\frac{a}{\sqrt{2}}$

13.5 RADIUS OF CURVATURE FOR PEDAL EQUATIONS

To prove that $\rho = r\frac{dr}{dp}$

Proof. Let the pedal equation of the curve be
$p = f(r)$.
Form the adjoining figure, we have
$$\psi = \theta + \phi$$
$$\Rightarrow \frac{d\psi}{ds} = \frac{d\theta}{ds} + \frac{d\phi}{ds} \Rightarrow \frac{1}{\rho} = \frac{d\theta}{ds} + \frac{d\phi}{ds} \quad \ldots(1)$$
Since, we know that $p = r\sin\phi$
$$\therefore \frac{dp}{dr} = \sin\phi + r\cos\phi\frac{d\phi}{dr}$$

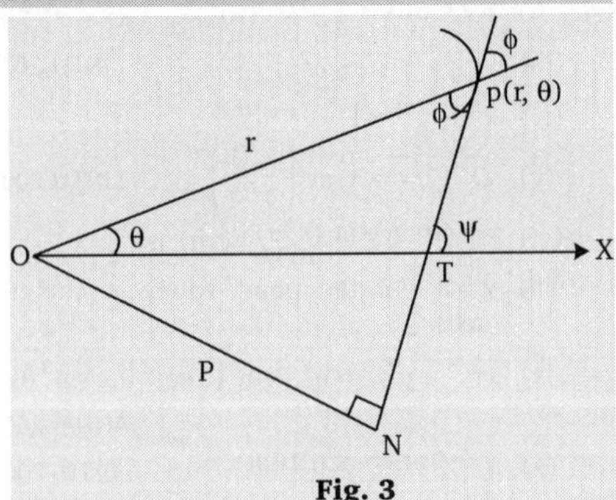

Fig. 3

$$= r.\frac{d\theta}{ds} + r\frac{dr}{ds}.\frac{d\phi}{dr} \qquad \left[\because \sin\phi = r.\frac{d\theta}{ds} \text{ and } \cos\phi = \frac{dr}{ds}\right]$$

$$= r\left[\frac{d\theta}{ds} + \frac{d\phi}{ds}\right] = r\frac{1}{\rho}$$

or $\frac{dp}{dr} = r\frac{1}{\rho}$ $\qquad \therefore \rho = \frac{r}{dp/dr} = r.\frac{dr}{dp} \Rightarrow \rho = r\frac{dr}{dp}$.

13.6 RADIUS OF CURVATURE FOR TANGENTIAL POLAR EQUATIONS $p = f(\psi)$

To prove that $\rho = p + \frac{d^2p}{d\psi^2}$

Proof. Let p be the length of the perpendicular drawn from the origin on the tangent to curve at the point $P(x, y)$. Also, let ψ be the angle which the tangent makes with X-axis.

Here we observe that OL makes an angle $\psi - \frac{\pi}{2}$ with the positive direction of X-axis.

$\therefore$ Equation of the tangent PT is

$$p = X\cos\left(\psi - \frac{\pi}{2}\right) + Y\sin\left(\psi - \frac{\pi}{2}\right)$$

[Normal form: $x\cos\alpha + y\sin\alpha = p$]

$\Rightarrow \quad p = X\sin\psi - Y\cos\psi$

where X and Y are cartesian co-ordinates of any point on the tangent PT.

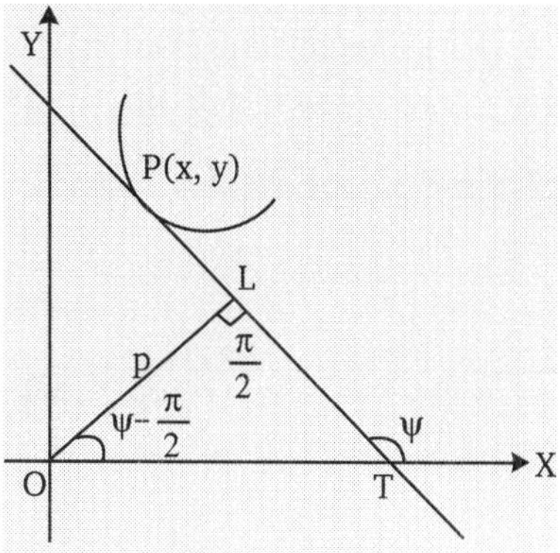

Since, $P(x, y)$ lies on PT, therefore

$$p = x\sin\psi - y\cos\psi \qquad \ldots(1)$$

Y
P(x, y)
L
p
$\frac{\pi}{2}$
$\psi - \frac{\pi}{2}$
ψ
O
T
X

Fig. 4.

$$\Rightarrow \frac{dp}{d\psi} = x\cos\psi + \sin\psi\frac{dx}{d\psi} + y\sin\psi - \cos\psi.\frac{dy}{d\psi}$$

$$= x\cos\psi + y\sin\psi + \sin\psi\frac{dx}{ds}.\frac{ds}{d\psi} - \cos\psi.\frac{dy}{ds}.\frac{ds}{d\psi}$$

$$= x\cos\psi + y\sin\psi + \sin\psi.\rho.\cos\psi - \cos\psi.\rho.\sin\psi \qquad \left(\because \frac{dx}{ds} = \cos\psi \text{ and } \frac{dy}{ds} = \sin\psi\right)$$

$$= x\cos\psi + y\sin\psi$$

Differentiating again w.r.t. ψ, we get

$$\frac{d^2p}{d\psi^2} = -x\sin\psi + \cos\psi.\frac{dx}{d\psi} + y\cos\psi + \sin\psi.\frac{dy}{d\psi}$$

$$= -x\sin\psi + y\cos\psi + \cos\psi.\frac{dx}{ds}.\frac{ds}{d\psi} + \sin\psi.\frac{dy}{ds}.\frac{ds}{d\psi}$$

$$= (-x\sin\psi + y\cos\psi) + \cos\psi.\cos\psi.\rho + \sin\psi.\sin\psi.\rho$$

$$= -p + \rho[\cos^2\psi + \sin^2\psi] \qquad \text{(Using (1))}$$

$$\Rightarrow \qquad \rho = p + \frac{d^2p}{d\psi^2}.$$

WORKING PROCEDURE

To transform polar equation to pedal equation, proceed as follows :

STEP 1. Find ϕ, using formula $\tan\phi = \dfrac{r}{dr/d\theta}$.

STEP 2. Substittute the value of ϕ in $p = r\sin\phi$.

STEP 3. Eliminate θ.

13.7 RADIUS OF CURVATURE IN POLAR FORM

To prove that $\rho = \dfrac{\left[r^2 + \left(\dfrac{dr}{d\theta}\right)^2\right]^{3/2}}{r^2 + 2\left(\dfrac{dr}{d\theta}\right)^2 - r\dfrac{d^2r}{d\theta^2}}$

Proof. We know that $\dfrac{1}{p^2} = \dfrac{1}{r^2} + \dfrac{1}{r^4}\left(\dfrac{dr}{d\theta}\right)^2$. ...(1)

Differentiating (1) w.r.t. r, we get

$$-\frac{2}{p^3}\frac{dp}{dr} = -\frac{2}{r^3} - \frac{4}{r^5}\left(\frac{dr}{d\theta}\right)^2 + \frac{1}{r^4}\left\{\frac{d}{dr}\left(\frac{dr}{d\theta}\right)^2\right\}$$

$$= -\frac{2}{r^3} - \frac{4}{r^5}\left(\frac{dr}{d\theta}\right)^2 + \frac{1}{r^4}\left[\frac{d}{d\theta}\left(\frac{dr}{d\theta}\right)^2\right].\frac{d\theta}{dr} = -\frac{2}{r^3} - \frac{4}{r^5}\left(\frac{dr}{d\theta}\right)^2 + \frac{2}{r^4}\frac{d^2r}{d\theta^4}$$

$$\frac{1}{p^3}.\frac{dp}{dr} = \frac{1}{r^5}\left[r^2 + 2\left(\frac{dr}{d\theta}\right)^2 - r\frac{d^2r}{d\theta^2}\right]$$

Now $$\rho = r\frac{dr}{dp} = \frac{r.\dfrac{1}{p^3}}{\dfrac{1}{r^5}\left[r^2 + 2\left(\dfrac{dr}{d\theta}\right)^2 - r\dfrac{d^2r}{d\theta^2}\right]}$$

Form (1), we have

$$\frac{1}{p^3} = \left[\frac{1}{r^2} + \frac{1}{r^4}\left(\frac{dr}{d\theta}\right)^2\right]^{3/2} = \frac{1}{r^6}\left[r^2 + \left(\frac{dr}{d\theta}\right)^2\right]^{3/2}$$

Hence, $$\rho = \frac{r^6.\dfrac{1}{r^6}\left[r^2 + \left(\dfrac{dr}{d\theta}\right)^2\right]^{3/2}}{r^2 + 2\left(\dfrac{dr}{d\theta}\right)^2 - r\dfrac{d^2r}{d\theta^2}} \Rightarrow \rho = \frac{\left[r^2 + \left(\dfrac{dr}{d\theta}\right)^2\right]^{3/2}}{r^2 + 2\left(\dfrac{dr}{d\theta}\right)^2 - r\dfrac{d^2r}{d\theta^2}}.$$

Solved Examples

1. *Find the radius of curvature for the curve* $r^n = a^n \cos n\theta$.

(JNTU–2006, PTU–2010)

SOLUTION. We have $r^n = a^n \cos n\theta$

$\Rightarrow$ $n \log r = n \log a + \log \cos n\theta$.

Now differentiating w.r.t. θ, we get

$$\frac{n}{r}.\frac{dr}{d\theta} = 0 + \frac{1}{\cos n\theta}(-n\sin n\theta) = -n\tan n\theta \quad ...(1)$$

$\Rightarrow$ $r_1 = -r\tan n\theta$

Again diiferentiating, we get

$$r_2 = -r.n.\sec^2 n\theta - r_1.\tan n\theta$$
$$= -rn\sec^2 n\theta + r\tan^2 n\theta. \quad \ldots(2)$$

Putting all these values in

$$\rho = \frac{[r^2+r_1^2]^{3/2}}{r^2+2r_1^2-rr_2}$$
$$= \frac{(r^2+r^2\tan^2 n\theta)^{3/2}}{r^2+2r^2\tan^2 n\theta+r^2.n\sec^2 n\theta - r^2\tan^2 n\theta}$$
$$= \frac{r^3\sec^3 n\theta}{(n+1)r^2\sec^2 n\theta} = \frac{r\sec n\theta}{(n+1)}$$
$$= \frac{r}{n+1}.\frac{1}{\cos n\theta}$$
$$= \frac{r}{(n+1)\frac{r^n}{a^n}} = \frac{a^n}{(n+1)r^{n-1}}$$

2. *Show that in the rectangular hyperbola $r^2 \cos 2\theta = a^2$, the radius of curvature $\rho = \frac{r^3}{a^2}$.*

SOLUTION. The given curve is

$$r^2 \cos 2\theta = a^2 \quad \ldots(1)$$

$\Rightarrow 2\log r + \log\cos 2\theta = 2\log a$

Differentiating w.r.t. θ, we get

$$\frac{2}{r}\frac{dr}{d\theta} + \frac{1}{\cos 2\theta}(-2\sin 2\theta) = 0$$
$$\Rightarrow \frac{1}{r}\frac{dr}{d\theta} = \cot\phi = \tan 2\theta = \cot\left(\frac{\pi}{2} - 2\theta\right)$$
$$\Rightarrow \phi = \frac{\pi}{2} - 2\theta$$

Now $p = r\sin\phi = r\sin\left(\frac{\pi}{2} - 2\theta\right)$

$$= r\cos 2\theta = r.\frac{a^2}{r^2} = \frac{a^2}{r}$$
$$\Rightarrow \frac{dp}{dr} = -\frac{a^2}{r^2}$$

Hence, $\rho = r\frac{dr}{dp} = -\frac{r^3}{a^2} = \frac{r^3}{a^2}$.

(By neglecting the negative sign)

Similar Problems

(1) Show that for the hypercycloid P = A sin Bψ, ρ varies as P.

(2) Find the radius of curvature at the point (p, r) on the spiral $p^2 = r^4/(r^2+a^2)$.

Ans. $\rho = \frac{(r^2+a^2)^{3/2}}{r^2+2a^2}$

(3) Prove that for any curve $\frac{r}{\rho} = \sin\phi\left(1+\frac{d\phi}{d\theta}\right)$, where ρ is the radius of curvature and $\tan\phi = r\frac{d\theta}{dr}$.

3. *Show that at any point on the equiangular spiral $r = ae^{\theta\cot\alpha}$, $\rho = r\,\mathrm{cosec}\,\alpha$ and that it subtends a right angle at the pole.*

SOLUTION. The given equation is $r = ae^{\theta\cot\alpha}$. ...(1)

Differentiating (1) w.r.t. θ, we have

$$\frac{dr}{d\theta} = ae^{\theta\cot\alpha}.\cot\alpha = r\cot\alpha.$$
$$\therefore (1/r)\frac{dr}{d\theta} = \cot\alpha$$

or $\cot\phi = \cot\alpha \Rightarrow \phi = \alpha$.

Now, $p = r\sin\phi$, thus the pedal equation of (1) is $p = r\sin\alpha$.

Therefore, $\frac{dp}{dr} = \sin\alpha$.

Now $\rho = r\frac{dr}{dp} = \frac{r}{\sin\alpha} = r\,\mathrm{cosec}\,\alpha$.

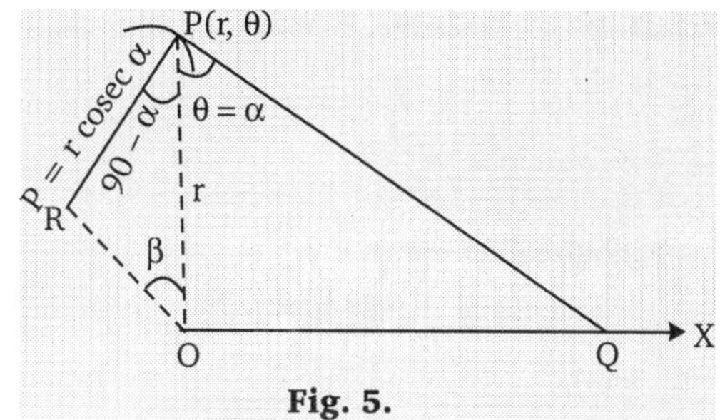

Fig. 5.

Second part. Let $P(r, \theta)$ be any point on the given curve. PQ is the tangent and PR is the normal to the curve at P. Let R be center of curvatrure of the point P of the curve. Then PR = the radius of curvature of the curve at $P = r \operatorname{cosec} \alpha$.

Intersect OP and OR, where O is the pole.

Let $\angle POR = \beta$. Then to show that $\beta = 90°$.

We have $\angle OPQ = \phi = \alpha$

$\angle OPR = 90° - \alpha$, (since PR is normal at P) i.e., perpendicular to the tangent PQ.

Now in ΔOPR, we have

$\angle ORP = 180° - (90° - \alpha + \beta) = 90° + \alpha - \beta$.

Therefore, applying the sine theorem for ΔOPR, we get

$$\frac{OP}{\sin \angle ORP} = \frac{PR}{\sin\beta} \text{ or } \frac{r}{\sin(90+\alpha-\beta)} = \frac{\rho}{\sin\beta}$$

$$\text{or } \frac{r}{\cos(\alpha-\beta)} = \frac{r\operatorname{cosec}\alpha}{\sin\beta} \quad (\because \rho = r\operatorname{cosec}\alpha)$$

$\sin\alpha \sin\beta = \cos(\alpha - \beta)$

or $\sin\alpha\sin\beta = \cos\alpha\cos\beta + \sin\alpha\sin\beta$

or $\cos\alpha\cos\beta = 0$ or $\cos\beta = 0$.

Hence, $\beta = 90°$.

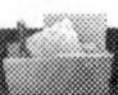

Exercise-13.2

1. FInd the radius of curvature in polar form on each of the following curves :
   (i) $r = a(1 - \cos\theta)$ (VTU–2003)
   (ii) $r(1 + \cos\theta) = 2a$ (iii) $r^2 = a^2 \cos 2\theta$
2. Find the radius of curvature at any point (p,r) on the following curves :
   (i) $p^2 = ar$
   (ii) $r^2 = a^2 - b^2 + \dfrac{a^2b^2}{p^2}$
   (iii) $2ap^2 = r^3$ (iv) $pa^2 = r^3$
3. Show that the radius of curvature of the cardoid $r = a(1 + \cos\theta)$ at the origin is 0.
4. Show that the radius of curvature at any point on the curve $r = a(1 \pm \cos\theta)$ varies as square root of the radius vector.
5. If ρ_1, ρ_2 be the radii of curvature at the extrimities of any chord of the cardoid $r = a(1 + \cos\theta)$, which passes through the pole, then ${\rho_1}^2 + {\rho_2}^2 = 16a^2/9$.
6. Show that the radius of curvature at the point (p, r) of the ellipse $\dfrac{1}{p^2} = \dfrac{1}{a^2} + \dfrac{1}{b^2} - \dfrac{r^2}{a^2b^2}$ is $\dfrac{a^2b^2}{p^3}$. (VTU–2010)
7. Show that the radius of curvature for the hyperbola
   $$p^2 = a^2\cos^2\psi + b^2\sin^2\psi \text{ is } \frac{a^2b^2}{p^3}.$$
8. Show that the curvature of the curves $r = a\theta$ and $r\theta = a$ at their common point are in the ratio 3 : 1.
9. By Newton's method, show that the radius of curvature of the curve $r = a \sin n\theta$ at the origin is $\dfrac{na}{2}$.
10. Show that the radius of curvature at each point of the curve $x = a\left(\cos t + \log\tan\dfrac{t}{2}\right), y = a\sin t$ is inversely proportional to the length of the normal intercepted between the point on the curve and the x-axis. (JNTU–2003)

Hint to Selected Problems

1. (i) Find $\dfrac{d^2r}{d\theta^2} (= -a\cos\theta)$ to the given equation and use the formula $\rho = \dfrac{\left[r^2 + \left(\dfrac{dr}{d\theta}\right)^2\right]^{3/2}}{r^2 + 2\left(\dfrac{dr}{d\theta}\right)^2 - r\dfrac{d^2r}{d\theta^2}}$.
2. For the curve of the type $r = f(p)$, the radius of curvature is $\rho = r\dfrac{dr}{dp}$.
5. Let $P(r, \theta)$ and $Q(r, \pi + \theta)$ be the extremities of any chord of the cardoid $r = a(1 + \cos\theta)$
   Then for ρ_1, use $r = a(1 + \cos\theta)$
   $$\Rightarrow \frac{dr}{d\theta} = -a\sin\theta \text{ and } \frac{d^2r}{d\theta^2} = -a\cos\theta$$
   and for ρ_2, use $r = a[1 + \cos(\pi + \theta)] = a(1 - \cos\theta)$
   $$\Rightarrow \frac{dr}{d\theta} = a\sin\theta \text{ and } \frac{d^2r}{d\theta^2} = a\cos\theta$$

Then find ρ_1 and ρ_2 and form a relation between ρ_1 and ρ_2.

6. Find $r\dfrac{dr}{dp}$ from the given equation *i.e.*, $r\dfrac{dr}{dp} = \dfrac{a^2b^2}{p^3}$. Then use the formula $\rho = r\dfrac{dr}{dp}$.

7. If the curve is $p = f(\psi)$, then the radius of curvature is $\rho = p + \dfrac{d^2p}{d\psi^2}$. ...(1)

Obtain the value of $\dfrac{d^2p}{d\psi^2}$ form the given equation and substitute in (1).

8. Clearly, $(a, 1)$ and $(a, -1)$ are the common points. Now find the radius of curvature for both the above points.

9. $r = a \sin n\theta$ is the equation of the given curve. At $r = 0 \Rightarrow \theta = 0$. Then, use the formula given below

$$\rho_{\text{at origin}} = \lim_{x \to 0} \frac{x^2}{2y}.$$

ANSWERS

1. (i) $\dfrac{2}{3}\sqrt{2ar}$ (ii) $2\sqrt{(r^3/a)}$ (iii) $\dfrac{a^2}{3r}$ **2.** (i) $\dfrac{2r^{3/2}}{\sqrt{a}}$ (ii) $\dfrac{a^2b^2}{p^3}$ (iii) $\dfrac{2}{3}\sqrt{2ar}$ (iv) $\dfrac{a^2}{3r}$

13.8 CENTRE OF CURVATURE

For any point P of a curve, the centre of curvature is the point on the positive direction of the normal at P, at a distance ρ from it.

Let PD be the normal curve at P and C be a point on it such that $PC = \rho$, then C is said to be the center of curvature at P.

Fig. 6.

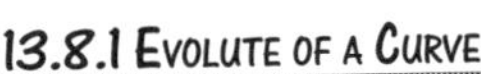

13.8.1 Evolute of a Curve

The locus of the center of curvature of the given curve is called the evolute of the curve.

13.8.2 Circle of Curvature

The circle with its center at the center of curvature C and radius equal to ρ is called the circle of curvature.

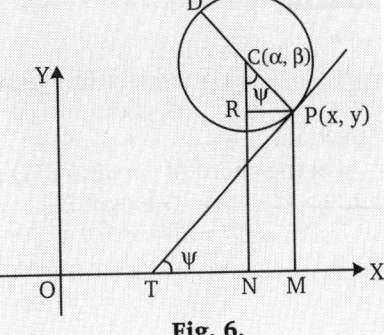

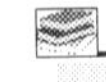

- The circle of curvature touches the curve at P and both the curve and the circle of curvature have the same curvature at this point.

13.9 CO-ORDINATES OF THE CENTRE OF CURVATURE

Let $y = f(x)$ be the given curve and $P(x, y)$ be any given point.

Let $C(\alpha, \beta)$ be the center of curvature corresponding to any point $P(x, y)$ on the given curve, then from above fig. (7), we have $PC = \rho$.

Suppose, the tangent TP makes an angle ψ with positive direction of x-axis. Draw PM and CN perpendicular to x-axis and draw perpendicular to CN. Then

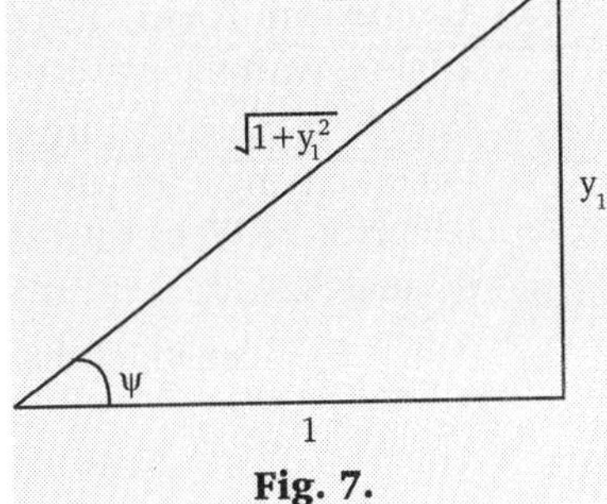

Fig. 7.

$$\angle PCN = 90^\circ - \angle CPR = 90^\circ - (90^\circ - \angle RPT)$$
$$= \angle RPT = \angle PTX = \psi$$
$$\therefore \quad \alpha = ON = OM - NM = OM - RP = x - CP \sin\psi = x - \rho \sin\psi \quad ...(1)$$

Also, $\beta = NC = NR + RC = MP + RC = y + CP \cos \psi = y + \rho \cos \psi$ ...(2)

Since, we know that $y_1 = \tan \psi$

$$\Rightarrow \quad \sin \psi = \frac{y_1}{\sqrt{1+y_1^2}} \text{ and } \cos \psi = \frac{1}{\sqrt{1+y_1^2}}.$$

Also, $$\rho = \frac{(1+y_1^2)^{3/2}}{y_2}$$

Putting all these values in (1) and (2), we get

$$\alpha = x - \frac{y_1(1+y_1^2)}{y_2} \text{ and } \beta = y + \frac{(1+y_1^2)}{y_2}.$$

- From (1) and (2) we have $\alpha = x - \rho \sin \psi$ and $\beta = y + \rho \cos \psi$. Since x, y, ρ, ψ depends upon s, therefore the above equations may be treated as parametric equations of the evolute.
- The equation of the circle of curvature at the given point is $(x-\alpha)^2 + (y-\beta)^2 = \rho^2$.

13.10 CHORD OF CURVATURE

The length intercepted by the circle of curvature of the curve at P, on a straight line drawn through P in any given direction is called chord of curvature through P in that direction.

Let the chord of curvature PQ makes an angle α, with the normal PD, then its length PQ is given by

$PQ = PD \cos \alpha$

($\because \angle DQP$, being a semicircle is a right angle.)

$= 2 \rho \cos \alpha$, which is the chord of curvature perpendicular to radius vector

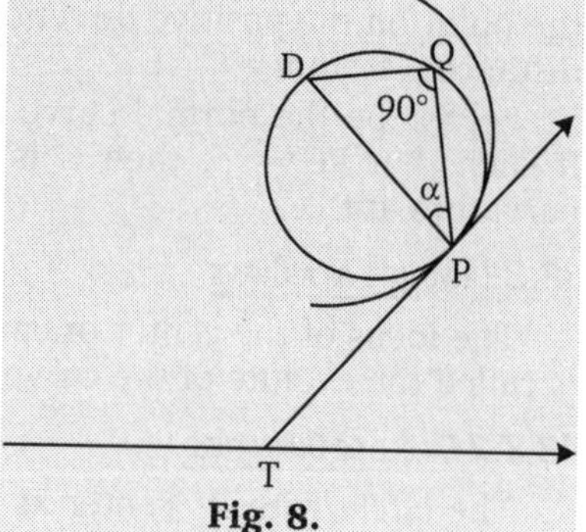

Fig. 8.

- The chord of curvature through pole is given by $2\rho \sin \alpha$.

13.11 LENGTH OF THE CHORD OF CURVATURE

(1) Cartesian form. Since, the tangent at P makes an angle ψ with the x-axis therefore,

the chord of curvature PA is parallel to x-axis, which makes an angle $90 - \psi$ with the normal PCD and chord of curvature PB parallel to y-axis makes angle ψ with the normal PCD.

$\therefore$ C_x = length of the chord of curvature PA, parallel to x-axis.

$$= PD \cos(90 - \psi) = 2\rho \sin \psi$$

$$= \frac{2(1+y_1^2)^{3/2}}{y_2} \cdot \frac{y_1}{\sqrt{1+y_1^2}} = \frac{2y_1(1+y_1^2)}{y_2}$$

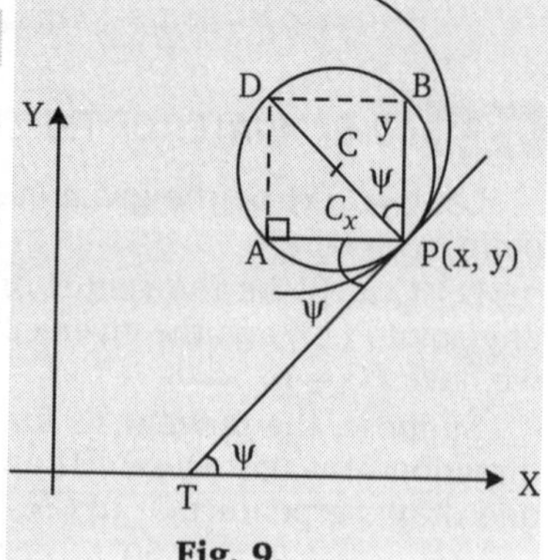

Fig. 9.

Similarly, $C_y = \dfrac{2(1+y_1^2)^{3/2}}{y_2}$.

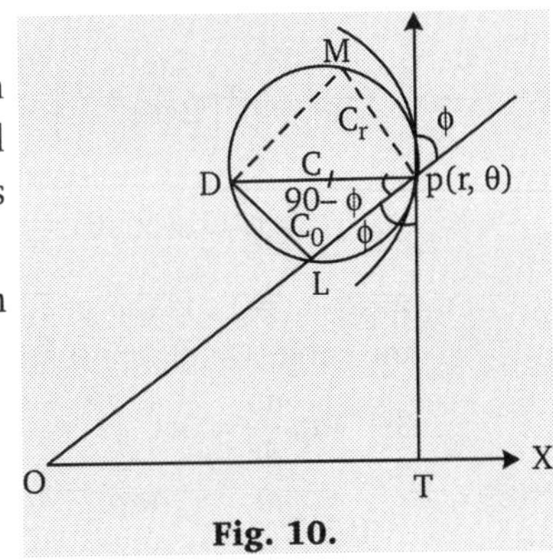

Fig. 10.

(2) Polar form. Let the chord of curvature *PL* makes an angle $90 - \phi$ with *PCD*, the normal of the curve at *P*, and *PM*, the chord of curvature perpendicular to the radius vector *OP*, makes an angle ϕ with the normal *PCD*.

$\therefore \quad C_o$ = Length of the chord of curvature *PL* through origin (or pole)

$$= PD(\cos 90 - \phi)$$

$$= 2\rho \sin\phi = \frac{2(r^2 + r_1^2)^{3/2}}{r^2 + 2r_1^2 - rr_2} \cdot \frac{r}{\sqrt{r^2 + r_1^2}}$$

$$= \frac{2r(r^2 + r_1^2)}{r^2 + 2r_1^2 - rr_2}$$

and $\quad C_p$ = length of the chord of curvature *PM* perpendicular to radius vector.

$$= PD \cos\phi = 2\rho\cos\phi = \frac{2(r^2 + r_1^2)^{3/2}}{r^2 + 2r_1^2 - rr_2} \cdot \frac{r}{\sqrt{r^2 + r_1^2}} = \frac{2r(r^2 + r_1^2)}{r^2 + 2r_1^2 - rr_2}$$

(3) Pedal form. Let $p = f(r)$ be the given equation of the curve.

Let $\quad C_o$ = length of the chord of curvature through pole along radius vector

$$= PD \cos(90 - \phi) = 2\rho \sin\phi \qquad \ldots(1)$$

Now using $\quad \rho = r\dfrac{dr}{dp}$ and $\sin\phi = \dfrac{p}{r}$ in (1), we get $C_o = 2r\dfrac{dr}{dp}.\dfrac{p}{r} = 2p.\dfrac{dr}{dp} \qquad \ldots(2)$

Now $\quad p = f(r) \Rightarrow \dfrac{dp}{dr} = f'(r)$ and $\sin\phi = \dfrac{p}{r} = \dfrac{f(r)}{r}$

$\therefore$ From (1), $\quad C_o = 2\rho\sin\phi = 2.r.\dfrac{dr}{dp}.\sin\phi = 2r.\dfrac{1}{f'(r)}.\dfrac{f(r)}{r} = \dfrac{2f(r)}{f'(r)}$

Also $\quad C_p$ = length of the chord perpendicular to the radius vector

$$= DP\cos\phi = 2\rho\cos\phi$$

$$= 2.r.\frac{dr}{dp}\frac{\sqrt{r^2 - p^2}}{r} \qquad \left[\because \sin\phi = \frac{p}{r} \text{ and } \cos\phi = \frac{\sqrt{r^2-p^2}}{r}\right]$$

$$= 2.\sqrt{r^2 - p^2}.\frac{dr}{dp}.$$

Solved Examples

1. *Find the chord of curvature through the pole of the cardioid* $r = a(1 + \cos\theta)$.

SOLUTION. We have $r = a(1 + \cos\theta)$

$$\Rightarrow \frac{dr}{d\theta} = -a\sin\theta$$

$$\therefore \tan\phi = r\frac{d\theta}{dr} = \frac{a(1+\cos\theta)}{-a\sin\theta}$$

$$= -\cot\frac{1}{2}\theta = \tan\left(\frac{\pi}{2} + \frac{\theta}{2}\right)$$

Now $p = r\sin\phi$

$$= r\sin\left(\frac{\pi}{2}+\frac{\theta}{2}\right) = r\cos\frac{\theta}{2}$$

$$\therefore\ 2p^2 = r^2\left(2\cos^2\frac{\theta}{2}\right)$$

$$= r^2(1+\cos\theta) = r^2 - \frac{r}{a} = \frac{r^3}{a}$$

$\Rightarrow 2p^2a = r^3$ is the pedal equation of the curve. On differentiating w.r.t. r we get $4ap\frac{dp}{dr} = 3r^2$

$$\therefore\ \rho = r\frac{dr}{dp} = r.\frac{4ap}{3r^2} = \frac{4ap}{3r}$$

Therefore, the chord of curvature through the pole

$$= 2\rho\sin\phi = 2.\frac{4ap}{3r}.\frac{p}{r}\ [\because p = r\sin\phi]$$

$$= \frac{8ap^2}{3r^2} = \frac{8}{3r^2}.\frac{r^3}{2} = \frac{4r}{3}$$

$[\because 2ap^2 = r^3]$

2. *Show that the chord of curvature through the pole of the curve $r^n = a^n \cos n\theta$ is $\frac{2r}{n+1}$.*

SOLUTION. The given curve is

$$r^n = a^n \cos n\theta$$

$\Rightarrow n \log r = n \log a + \log \cos n\theta$

Differentiating w.r.t. θ, we have

$$\frac{n}{r}\frac{dr}{d\theta} = -\frac{n}{\cos n\theta}.\sin n\theta$$

$$\Rightarrow\quad \cot\phi = -\tan n\theta = \cot\left(\frac{\pi}{2}+n\theta\right)$$

$$\therefore\quad \phi = \frac{\pi}{2}+n\theta$$

Now

$$p = r\sin\phi = r\sin\left(\frac{\pi}{2}+n\theta\right) = r\cos n\theta$$

$\because$ Pedal equation of the curve is $p = \frac{r^{n+1}}{a^n}$.

$$\therefore\quad \frac{dp}{dr} = \frac{(n+1)r^n}{a^n}$$

Also, $\rho = r\frac{dr}{dp} = \frac{a^n}{(n+1)r^{n-1}}$

Therefore, the chord of curvature through pole is

$$= 2\rho\sin\phi = 2\rho\sin\left(\frac{\pi}{2}+n\theta\right) = 2\rho\cos n\theta$$

$$= 2\frac{a^n}{(n+1)r^{n-1}}.\frac{r^n}{a^n} = \frac{2r}{(n+1)}.$$

3. *Find the co-ordinate of the centre of curvature at any point of the parabola $y^2 = 4ax$. Hence, show that its evolute is $27ay^2 = 4(x-2a)^3$.* (VTU–2000)

SOLUTION. We have $y^2 = 4ax$

$$\Rightarrow\quad 2yy_1 = 4a \text{ i.e., } y_1 = \frac{2a}{y}$$

and $y_2 = -\frac{2a}{y^2}.y_1 = -\frac{4a^2}{y^3}$

If $(\bar{x},\bar{y})$ be the centre of curvature, then

$$\bar{x} = x - \frac{y_1(1+y_1^2)}{y_2} = x - \frac{\frac{2a}{y}\left(1+\frac{4a^2}{y^2}\right)}{-4a^2/y^3}$$

$$= x + \frac{y^2+4a^2}{2a}$$

$$= x + \frac{4ax+4a^2}{2a} = 3x+2a \quad \ldots(1)$$

and

$$\bar{y} = y + \frac{1+y_1^2}{y_2} = y + \frac{1+4a^2/y^2}{-4a^2/y^3}$$

$$= y - \frac{y(y^2+4a^2)}{4a^2} = \frac{-y^3}{4a^2} = -\frac{2x^{3/2}}{\sqrt{a}} \quad \ldots(2)$$

Therefore, the required centre of curvature is $\left\{(3x+2a), -2x\sqrt{\frac{x}{a}}\right\}$. To find the required evolute, eliminate x from (1) and (2), we have

$$(\bar{y})^2 = \frac{4x^3}{a} = \frac{4}{a}\left(\frac{\bar{x}-2a}{3}\right)^3$$

$$\Rightarrow\quad 27a(\bar{y})^2 = 4(\bar{x}-2a)^3 \quad \ldots(3)$$

Now, locus of $(\bar{x},\bar{y})$ is $27ay^2 = 4(x-2a)^3$ which is the required equation of evolute.

4. *Show that the evolute of the cycloid $x = a(\theta - \sin\theta)$, $y = a(1-\cos\theta)$ is another equal cycloid.* (MADRAS–2006)

SOLUTION. We have $x = a(\theta - \sin\theta)$ and $y = a(1-\cos\theta)$

$$\Rightarrow\ y_1 = \frac{dy}{d\theta}.\frac{d\theta}{dx} = \frac{a\sin\theta}{a(1-\cos\theta)} = \cot\frac{\theta}{2}$$

Now $y_2 = \frac{d}{dx}(y_1) = \frac{d}{d\theta}\left(\cot\frac{\theta}{2}\right).\frac{d\theta}{dx}$

$$= -\operatorname{cosec}^2\frac{\theta}{2}.\frac{1}{2}.\frac{1}{a(1-\cos\theta)}$$

$$= -\frac{1}{4a\sin^4\theta/2}$$

If $(\bar{x},\bar{y})$ be the center of curvature, then

$$\bar{x} = x - \frac{y_1(1+y_1^2)}{y_2}$$

$$= a(\theta-\sin\theta) + \cot\frac{\theta}{2}(4a\sin^4\frac{\theta}{2})(1+\cot^2\frac{\theta}{2})$$

$$= a(\theta-\sin\theta) + \frac{\cos\theta/2}{\sin\theta/2}.4a\sin^4\frac{\theta}{2}.\operatorname{cosec}^2\frac{\theta}{2}$$

$$= a(\theta-\sin\theta) + 4a\sin\frac{\theta}{2}.\cos\frac{\theta}{2}$$

$$= a(\theta-\sin\theta) + 2a\sin\theta$$

$$= a(\theta + \sin\theta)$$

and $\bar{y} = y + \frac{1+y_1^2}{y_2}$

$$= a(1-\cos\theta) + (1+\cot^2\frac{\theta}{2})(-4a\sin^4\frac{\theta}{2})$$

$$= a(1-\cos\theta) - 4a\sin^4\theta/2.\operatorname{cosec}^2\theta/2$$

$$= a(1-\cos\theta) - 4a\sin^2\frac{\theta}{2}$$

$$= a(1-\cos\theta) - 2a(1-\cos\theta)$$

$$= -a(1-\cos\theta)$$

Hence, the required evolute is given by

$$x = a(\theta+\sin\theta), y = -a(1-\cos\theta)$$

which is another equal cycloid.

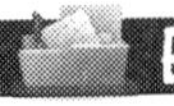

Exercise-13.3

1. In the curve $y=a\log\sec\left(\frac{x}{a}\right)$, show that the chord of curvature parallel to the axis of y is of constant length.
2. Prove that the centre of curvature (α, β) for the curve
$$x = 3t, y = t^2 - 6 \text{ is } \alpha = -\frac{4}{3}t^3, \beta = 3t^2 - \frac{3}{2}.$$
3. If C_x and C_y be the chords of curvature parallel to the axis at any point of the curve $y = ae^{x/a}$, show that
$$\frac{1}{{C_x}^2} + \frac{1}{{C_y}^2} = \frac{1}{2aC_x}.$$
4. Show that the centre of curvature (α, β) at the point determined by t on the ellipse $x = a\cos t, y = b\sin t$, is given by
$$\alpha = \frac{a^2-b^2}{a}\cos^3 t, \beta = -\left(\frac{a^2-b^2}{b}\right)\sin^3 t.$$
5. Show that in any curve the chord of curvature perpendicular to the radius vector is $2\rho\sqrt{(r^2-p^2)}/r$.
6. Show that the chord of curvature through the pole of the equiangular spiral $r = ae^{m\theta}$ is $2r$.
7. Find the coordinates of the centre of curvature of ellipse $\frac{x^2}{a^2} + \frac{y^2}{b^2} = 1$ or $x = a\cos\theta$, $y = b\sin\theta$. Hence, show that the equation of its evolute is $(ax)^{2/3} + (by)^{2/3} = (a^2 - b^2)^{2/3}$.
8. Find the chord of curvature through the pole of the curve $a\theta = \sqrt{r^2 - a^2} - a\cos^{-1}(a/r)$.
9. If C_r and C_θ be the chords of curvature of the curve $r = a(1+\cos\theta)$ through the pole and perpendicular to the radius vector, then prove that $3({C_r}^2 + {C_\theta}^2) = 8rC_r$.

Hint to Selected Problems

1. Given that $y = a\log\sec\frac{x}{a}$
$$\Rightarrow \frac{dy}{dx} = \tan\frac{x}{a} \text{ and } \frac{d^2y}{dx^2} = \frac{1}{a}\sec^2\frac{2}{a}$$
Put all these values in the radius of curvature, we get $\rho = a\sec\frac{x}{a}$.
Then, chord of curvature parallel to y-axis is $= 2\rho\cos\psi$.
2. $$\frac{dx}{dt} = 3, \frac{dy}{dt} = 2t \Rightarrow \frac{dy}{dx} = \frac{2t}{3}$$
and $\frac{d^2y}{dx^2} = \frac{2}{3}\frac{dt}{dx} = \frac{2}{3}.\frac{1}{3} = \frac{2}{9}$.
Putting these values in the formula of centre of curvature.
3. Since $C_x = 2\rho\sin\psi$, $C_y = 2\rho\cos\psi$.

Then, find the value of ρ using the given curve and by putting the value of ρ in the above expression, find a relation betwen C_x and C_y.

4. $x = a \cos t, y = b \sin t$

$$\Rightarrow \frac{dx}{dt} = -a\sin t, \frac{dy}{dt} = b\cos t \Rightarrow \frac{dy}{dx} = -\frac{b}{a}\cot t$$

$$\therefore \frac{d^2y}{dx^2} = -\frac{b}{a}(-\text{cosec}^2 t)\frac{dt}{dx} = -\frac{b}{a^2}\text{cosec}^3 t$$

Then use the formulae for the centre of curvature.

5. The chord of curvature perpendicular to the radius vector is $2\rho \cos \phi$.

Since $p = r\sin\phi \Rightarrow \frac{dp}{dr} = \sin\phi$

$$\therefore \rho = r\frac{dr}{dp} = \frac{r^2}{p}$$

Now $\cos \phi = \sqrt{1-\sin^2\phi} = \sqrt{1-\frac{p^2}{n}}$. Put this value in $2\rho \cos \phi$.

6. Here, $\frac{dr}{d\theta} = mr, \frac{d^2r}{d\theta^2} = m^2r$.

Then we may get $\rho = r(1 + m^2)^{1/2}$.

To find the chord of curvature through the pole is given by $2\rho \sin \phi$.

where value of $\sin \phi$ can be obtained by using $r\frac{d\theta}{dr} = \tan\phi$.

7. $x = a \cos \theta, y = b \sin \theta$

$$\Rightarrow \frac{dx}{d\theta} = -a\sin\theta, \frac{dy}{d\theta} = b\cos\theta.$$

Therefore, $\frac{dy}{dx} = -\left(\frac{b}{a}\right)\cot\theta$ and $\frac{d^2y}{dx^2} = -\frac{b}{a^2}\text{cosec}^3\theta$

Put these values in the formulae of centre of curvature (α, β). Also, to find the equation of evolute, find the locus of α and β.

ANSWERS

7. $\left(\frac{a^2-b^2}{a}\cos^3\theta, -\frac{a^2-b^2}{b}\sin^3\theta\right)$ **8.** $\frac{2(r^2-a^2)}{r}$

□□□□□□

Chapter

14

Asymptotes

14.1 INTRODUCTION

In calculus, there are some curves whose branches seem to go to infinity. It is not necessary that there always exists a definite straight line for all such curves which seems to touch the branch of the curves at infinite but more or less there are some certain curves for which this type of definite straight line exists, this straight line is therefore known as asymptote.

Definition. *A definite straight line whose distance from branch of the curve continuously decreases as we move away from the origin along the branch of the curve and seems to touch the branch at infinity, provided the distance of this line from origin should be finite initially, is called an asymptote of the curve.*

Suppose in the equalion of a curve, two or more than two values of y exists for every value of x, then we obtain different branches of the curve corresponding to these distinct values of y. If each branch have its own separate asymptote, then we can say that a curve may have more than one asymptote.

14.2 DETERMINATION OF ASYMPTOTES

Consider a curve $$f(x, y) = 0 \qquad ...(1)$$

and also consider that there are no asymptotes parallel to y-axis. Thus we shall take the equation which is not parallel to y-axis. in the form of

$$y = mx + c \qquad ...(2)$$

Let us take a point $P(x, y)$ on the curve (1), therefore this point as tends to infinity along the straight line (2), x must tend to infinity. Now find the tangent to the curve $f(x, y) = 0$ at the point $P(x, y)$.

$\therefore$ The equation of tangent at $P(x, y)$ is

$$Y - y = \frac{dy}{dx}(X - x) \quad \text{or} \quad Y = \frac{dy}{dx}X + \left(y - x\frac{dy}{dx}\right). \qquad ...(3)$$

The equation (3) is of the form $y = mx + c$, so in order to exist the asymptote of the curve there must both $\frac{dy}{dx}$ and $\left(y - x\frac{dy}{dx}\right)$ tend to finite limits as x tends to infinity. Therefore, if the equation (3) tends to the straight line given in (2) as x tends to infinity, then the line (2) will be an asymptote of the curve $f(x, y) = 0$ and also we have

$$m = \lim_{x\to\infty} \frac{dy}{dx} \quad \text{and} \quad c = \lim_{x\to\infty}\left(y - x\frac{dy}{dx}\right)$$

Since c is finite, then we have

$$\lim_{x\to\infty}\left(\frac{y - x\frac{dy}{dx}}{x}\right) = \lim_{x\to\infty}\frac{c}{x} = 0 \quad \text{or} \quad \lim_{x\to\infty}\left(\frac{y}{x} - \frac{dy}{dx}\right) = 0$$

or $$\lim_{x\to\infty}\left(\frac{y}{x}\right)=\lim_{x\to\infty}\frac{dy}{dx} \quad \text{or} \quad \lim_{x\to\infty}\frac{y}{x}=m.$$

Also $$c=\lim_{x\to\infty}\left(y-x\frac{dy}{xx}\right) \quad \text{or} \quad c=\lim_{x\to\infty}(y-mx).$$

Hence, if $y = mx + c$ is an asymptote to the curve $f(x, y) = 0$, then we obtain

$$m=\lim_{x\to\infty}\frac{dy}{dx}=\lim_{x\to\infty}\frac{y}{x} \text{ and } \quad c=\lim_{x\to\infty}(y-mx).$$

14.3 ASYMPTOTES OF GENERAL EQUATION

Let the general rational algebraic equation of a curve be

$$\{a_0y^n+a_1y^{n-1}x+a_2y^{n-2}x^2+\ldots+a_{n-1}yx^{n-1}+a_nx^n\}$$
$$+\{b_1y^{n-1}+b_2y^{n-2}x+\ldots+b_{n-1}yx^{n-2}+b_nx^{n-1}\}$$
$$+\{c_2y^{n-2}+c_3y^{n-3}+\ldots+c_{n-1}yx^{n-3}+c_nx^{n-2}\}+\ldots=0 \qquad \ldots(1)$$

or $$x^n\left\{a_0\left(\frac{y}{x}\right)^n+a_1\left(\frac{y}{x}\right)^{n-1}+a_2\left(\frac{y}{x}\right)^{n-2}+\ldots+a_{n-1}\left(\frac{y}{x}\right)+a_n\right\}+x^{n-1}\left\{b_1\left(\frac{y}{x}\right)^{n-1}+b_2\left(\frac{y}{x}\right)^{n-2}+\ldots+b_n\right\}$$
$$+x^{n-2}\left\{c_2\left(\frac{y}{x}\right)^{n-2}+c_3\left(\frac{y}{x}\right)^{n-3}+\ldots+c_n\right\}+\ldots=0$$

or $$x^n\phi_n\left(\frac{y}{x}\right)+x^{n-1}\phi_{n-1}\left(\frac{y}{x}\right)+x^{n-2}\phi_{n-2}\left(\frac{y}{x}\right)+\ldots+x\phi_1\left(\frac{y}{x}\right)+\phi_0\left(\frac{y}{x}\right)=0 \qquad \ldots(2)$$

where $\phi_k\left(\frac{y}{x}\right)$ is a polynomial of degree k in $\left(\frac{y}{x}\right)$.

Divide (2) by x^n, we get

$$\phi_n\left(\frac{y}{x}\right)+\frac{1}{x}\phi_{n-1}\left(\frac{y}{x}\right)+\frac{1}{x^2}\phi_{n-2}\left(\frac{y}{x}\right)+\ldots+\frac{1}{x^{n-1}}\phi_1\left(\frac{y}{x}\right)+\frac{1}{x^n}\phi_0\left(\frac{y}{x}\right)=0$$

Now taking limit as $x \to \infty$, and assuming there is no asymptote parallel to y-axis then $m=\lim_{x\to\infty}\left(\frac{y}{x}\right)$, we get $\phi_n(m) = 0$. ...(3)

This equation (3) is of degree n in m so it has at most n roots, real as well as imaginary. Out of these n roots some roots may be identical. Thus we get n values of m corresponding to the n branches of the curve (1). Since, we will have only real values of m so ignore all imaginary roots of (3) if they exists. Further if $y = mx+ c$ is an asymptote of (1), then we have

$$c=\lim_{x\to\infty}(y-mx), \text{ for each specified value of } m.$$

Determination of c. For the determination of c corresponding to each distinct value of m, we put $y = mx + p$

in the equation of curve (2), where $p \to c$ as $x \to \infty$.

Now putting $y = mx + p$ *i.e.*, $\frac{y}{x}=m+\frac{p}{x}$, in the (2), we get

$$x^n\phi_n\left(m+\frac{p}{x}\right)+x^{n-1}\phi_{n-1}\left(m+\frac{p}{x}\right)+x^{n-2}\phi_{n-2}\left(m+\frac{p}{x}\right)+\ldots+x\phi_1\left(m+\frac{p}{x}\right)+\phi_0\left(m+\frac{p}{x}\right)=0.$$

Expand each term by Taylor's expansion, we get

$$x^n\left[\phi_n(m)+\frac{p}{x}\phi_n'(m)+\frac{p^2}{2!x^2}\phi_n''(m)+\ldots\right]+x^{n-1}\left[\phi_{n-1}(m)+\frac{p}{x}\phi_{n-1}'(m)+\ldots\right]$$
$$+x^{n-2}\left[\phi_{n-2}(m)+\frac{p}{x}\phi_{n-2}'(m)+\ldots\right]+\ldots=0$$

or $\quad x^n\phi_n(m)+x^{n-1}[p\phi_n'(m)+\phi_{n-1}(m)]+x^{n-2}\left[\frac{p^2}{2!}\phi_n''(m)+\frac{p}{1!}\phi_{n-1}'(m)+\phi_{n-2}(m)\right]+\ldots=0$

Since we know that $\phi_n(m) = 0$, then

$$x^{n-1}[p\phi_n'(m)+\phi_{n-1}(m)]+x^{n-2}\left[\frac{p^2}{2!}\phi_n''(m)+\frac{p}{1!}\phi_{n-1}'(m)+\phi_{n-2}(m)\right]+\ldots=0$$

Dividing by x^{n-1} and taking limit as $x \to \infty$, we get

$$\lim_{x\to\infty}[p\phi_n'(m)+\phi_{n-1}(m)]=0 \quad \text{or} \quad \left(\lim_{x\to\infty} p\right)\phi_n'(m)+\phi_{n-1}(m)=0$$

or $\quad c\phi_n'(m)+\phi_{n-1}(m)=0 \qquad \left(\because \lim_{x\to\infty} p = c\right)$

Hence, from above relation we can determine the value of c for each distinct value of m.

- To find the polynomial $\phi_n(m)$. We should put $y = m$ and $x = 1$ in the nth degree terms of the curve. Similarly to get $\phi_{n-1}(m)$ we put $y = m$ and $x = 1$ in the $(n-1)^{\text{th}}$ degree terms of the curve. Therefore in general, to get $\phi_k(m)$ we should put $y = m$ and $x = 1$ in the kth degree terms of the curves.

14.4 EXISTENCE OF ASYMPTOTES

From the equation $\phi_n(m) = 0$, if we obtain one or more than one values of m such that $\phi_n'(m)=0$ and $\phi_{n-1}(m) \neq 0$, then from the equation for the determining of c. we obtain $0.c + \phi_{n-1}(m) = 0$.

Thus we get c is either, $+\infty$ or $-\infty$. Hence, we can say that corresponding to such values of m no asymptotes will exists.

14.5 DETERMINATION OF C CORRESPONDING TO SOME IDENTICAL VALUES OF M

Let us suppose some of the roots of the equation $\phi_n(m) = 0$ are identical and let these identical values be r in number which will make $\phi_n'(m), \phi_n''(m), \ldots \phi_m^{r-1}(m)$ equal to zero. Now for the existence of the asymptotes $\phi_{n-1}(m)$ must be zero corresponding to the identical values of m. Also , if it will make $\phi_{n-1}'(m), \phi_{n-1}''(m), \ldots \phi_{n-1}^{r-2}(m); \phi_{n-2}(m), \phi_{n-2}'(m), \ldots \phi_{n-2}^{r-3}(m); \phi_{n-3}'(m), \phi_{n-3}'(m), \ldots \phi_{n-3}^{r-4}(m) \ldots;$ $\phi_{n-r+2}(m), \phi_{n-r+2}'(m)$ and $\phi_{n-r+1}(m)$ equal to zero, then the equation to determine c will become

$$0.c^{r-1}+0.c^{r-2}+\ldots+0.c+0=0$$

and thus we cannot find the value of c in this way.

So to determine c let us put $\phi_n(m), \phi'(m), \ldots, \phi_n^{r-1}(m); \phi_{n-1}(m), \phi_{n-1}'(m), \ldots \phi_{n-1}^{r-2}(m); \phi_{n-2}(m),$ $\phi_{n-2}'(m), \ldots \phi_{n-2}^{r-3}(m); \phi_{n-3}(m), (\phi_{n-3}'(m), \ldots \phi_{n-3}^{r-4}(m) \ldots \phi_{n-r+2}(m), \phi_{n-r+2}'(m)$ and $\phi_{n-r+1}(m)$ equal to zero in the following equation

$$x^n\phi_n(m)+x^{n-1}[p\phi_n'(m)+\phi_{n-1}(m)]+x^{n-2}\left[\frac{p^2}{2!}\phi_n''(m)+\frac{p}{1!}\phi_{n-1}'(m)+\phi_{n-2}(m)\right]+\ldots$$

$$+x^{n-r+1}\left[\frac{p^{r-1}}{r-1!}\phi_n^{r-1}(m)+\frac{p^{r-2}}{r-2!}\phi_{n-1}^{r-2}(m)+\ldots+\frac{p}{1!}\phi_{n-r+2}'(m)+\phi_{n+r+1}'(m)\right]$$

$$+x^{n-r}\left[\frac{p^r}{r!}\phi_n^r(m)+\frac{p^{r-1}}{r-1!}\phi_{n-1}^{r-1}(m)+\frac{p^{r-2}}{r-2!}\phi_{n-2}^{r-2}(m)+\ldots+\frac{p}{1!}\phi_{n-r+1}'(m)+\phi_{n-r}(m)\right]=0$$

Now dividing above equation by x^{n-r} and taking the limit as $x \to \infty$, we get

$$\frac{c^r}{r!}\phi_n^r(m) + \frac{c^{r-1}}{r-1!}\phi_{n-1}^{r-1}(m) + \ldots + \frac{c}{1!}\phi'_{n-r+1}(m) + \phi_{n-r}(m) = 0 \text{ where } c = \lim_{x\to\infty} p.$$

Therefore this equation gives r values of c corresponding to the identical values of m. Hence, we obtain r parallel asymptotes.

14.6 NUMBER OF ASYMPTOTES OF A CURVE

Suppose the degree of an algebraic curve is n, then we find a polynomial $\phi_n(m)$ by putting $y = m$ and $x = 1$ in the nth degree terms of the curve. Thus the equation $\phi_n(m) = 0$ is of degree n in m and which gives atmost n values of m real as well as imaginary. These n values of m are nothing but the slopes of the asymptotes, which are not parallel to y axis. If there are some asymptotes, parallel to y-axis, then the degree of $\phi_n(m)$ will be smaller than n by the same number of parallel asymptotes. Suppose all the roots of $\phi_n(m) = 0$ are distinct and real, then to each value of m we obtain one value of c. Hence, we obtain n asymptotes. In case, there some roots say r (out of n) of $\phi_n(m) = 0$ are same, then we can find the values of c for these same roots the following equation

$$\frac{c^r}{r!}\phi_n^r(m) + \frac{c^{r-1}}{r-1!}\phi_{n-1}^{r-1}(m) + \ldots + \phi_{n-r}(m) = 0$$

This equation in c is of degree r so we get r distinct values of c for the same roots, hence, again we obtain n asymptotes. Therefore we can say that the total number of asymptotes of a curve are equal to the degree of the curve. These asymptotes are real as well as imaginary but we have required only real asymptotes so we ignore all the imaginary asymptotes.

14.7 ASYMPTOTES PARALLEL TO CO-ORDINATES AXES

(a) Asymptotes parallel to x-axis. Let the general equation of an algebraic curve in decreasing powers of x be

$$x^n\phi(y) + x^{n-1}\phi_1(y) + x^{n-2}\phi_2(y) + \ldots = 0 \qquad \ldots(1)$$

where $\phi(y), \phi_1(y), \phi_2(y), \ldots$ are the function of y only.

Now divide (1) by x^n, we get

$$\phi(y) + \frac{1}{x}\phi_1(y) + \frac{1}{x^2}\phi_2(y) + \ldots = 0. \qquad \ldots(2)$$

If $y = k$ is an asymptote parallel to x-axis, then we can say that x alone tends to infinity as a point $P(x, y)$ on the curve tends to infinity along the line $y = k$ and also we have $k = \lim_{x\to\infty} y$.

Now taking the limit of both sides of (2) as $x \to \infty$ and $y \to k$, we get $\phi(k) = 0$.

Thus k is a root of the equation $\phi(y) = 0$. If k_1, k_2, etc. are the roots of $\phi(y) = 0$, then the asymptotes parallel to x-axis are given by $y = k_1, y = k_2$, etc. Since k is a root of the equation $\phi(y) = 0$, then $(y - k)$ is a factor of the equation $\phi(y) = 0$. Also $\phi(y)$ is the coefficient of the highest power of x *i.e.*, x^n in the equation of the curve. Hence, we obtain the asymptotes parallel to x-axis by taking the coefficient of highest power of x in the equation of the curve equal to zero.

(b) Asymptotes parallel to y-axis. Similarly, we may obtain the asymptotes parallel to y-axis by taking the coefficient of highest power of y in the equation of the curve equal to zero.

- If the coefficient of highest power of x or y or both are constant, then no asymptotes parallel to either x or y or both axes exists respectively.

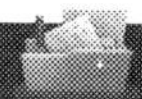

Solved Examples

1. *Find the asymptotes of the curve $x^3+y^3-3axy=0$.*

SOLUTION. Obviously, the degree of the curve is 3, so it will have 3 asymptotes real as well as imaginary. Here the coefficient of highest degree in x and y are constant so no asymptote parallel to co-ordinate axis exist. Let

$$y = mx + c \qquad \ldots(1)$$

be the asymptote of the curve.

So putting $y = m$ and $x = 1$ in the highest degree terms of the curve, we get

$$\phi_3(m) = 1 + m^3.$$

Solving the equation

$$\phi_3(m) = 0$$

i.e., $\quad 1 + m^3 = 0$

or $\quad (1+m)(m^2 - m + 1) = 0$

or $\quad m = -1$

is only real root and other two roots are imaginary so ignore them.

Next, putting $y = m$ and $x = 1$ is second degree terms in the equation of the curve (1), we get

$$\phi_2(m) = -3am.$$

Now we find value of c by the following equation

$$c\phi_n'(m) + \phi_{n-1}(m) = 0$$

or $\quad c\phi_3'(m) + \phi_2(m) = 0$

or $\quad c(3m^2) + (-3am) = 0$

$[\because \phi_3(m) = 1 + m^3 \Rightarrow \phi_3'(m) = 3m^2]$

If $m = -1$, then

$$c[3(-1)^2] + [-3a(-1)] = 0$$

$$3c + 3a = 0$$

or $\quad c = -a.$

Hence, the asymptote is $\quad y = -x - a$

or $\quad x + y + a = 0.$

2. *Find all the asymptotes of the curve $x^3 + x^2y - xy^2 - y^3 - 3x - y - 1 = 0$.*

SOLUTION. The degree of the curve is 3 so it has 3 asymptotes which are real as well as imaginary. Since the coefficients of highest degree *i.e.*, 3rd degree of x and y are constant so there are no asymptotes parallel to co-ordinate axes. Thus there are oblique asymptotes of the form $y = mx + c$.

Now putting $y = m$ and $x = 1$ in the third degree terms of the curve, we get

$$\phi_3(m) = 1 + m - m^2 - m^3.$$

Solving the equation

$$\phi_3(m) = 0 \text{ i.e, } 1 + m - m^2 - m^3 = 0,$$

we get $\quad (1+m)(1-m^2) = 0$

or $\quad m = -1, -1, 1.$

Determination of c. For $m = 1$, we use the following equation

$$c\phi_n'(m) + \phi_{n-1}(m) = 0$$

or $\quad c\phi_3'(m) + \phi_2(m) = 0 \qquad \ldots(1)$

Putting $y = m$ and $x = 1$ in the second degree terms of the equation we get

$$\phi_2(m) = 0.$$

From (1), we get

$$c(1-2m-3m^2)+0=0$$

at $m = 1$

$$c(1 - 2 - 3) + 0 = 0$$

or $\quad -4c = 0$

or $\quad c = 0$

Thus one of the asymptote is $y = x$

Determination of c for $m = -1, -1$. Since two out of three roots of the equation $\phi_3(m) = 0$ are same, then we use the following formula to determine c

$$\frac{c^2}{2!}\phi_3''(m) + \frac{c}{1!}\phi_2'(m) + \phi_1(m) = 0. \qquad \ldots(2)$$

Putting $y = m$ and $x = 1$ in the first degree terms of the equation we obtain $\phi_1(m) = -3 - m$.

From (2), we have

$$\frac{c^2}{2!}(-2 - 6m) + \frac{c}{1!}.0 + (-3 - m) = 0$$

at $m = -1$

$$\frac{c^2}{2}(-2+6) - 3 + 1 = 0$$

or $\quad 2c^2 - 2 = 0$

or $\quad c = \pm 1$

Thus other two asymptotes are

$$y = -x + 1, \; y = -x - 1.$$

Hence, all the asymptotes of the given curve are

$$y = x, x + y - 1 = 0, x + y + 1 = 0.$$

3. *Find all the asymptotes of the curve $(x - 2y)^2 (x - y) - 4y(x - 2y) - (8x + 7y) = 0$.*

SOLUTION. Simplifying the equation of curve

$(x^2+4y^2-4xy)(x-y)-4xy+8y^2-8x-7y=0$

or $x^3+8xy^2-5x^2y-4y^3-4xy+8y^2-8x-7y=0$. ...(1)

The degree of the curve (1) is 3 so it has 3 asymptotes which are real as well as imaginary. Obviously there are no asymptotes parallel to co-ordinate axis. Thus there are only oblique asymptotes of the form $y = mx + c$.

Putting $y = m$ and $x = 1$ in the highest degree *i.e.*, third degree terms of the curve (1), we obtain

$$\phi_3(m) = 1 - 5m + 8m^2 - 4m^3.$$

Solving the equation $\phi_3(m) = 0$

i.e., $1 - 5m + 8m^2 - 4m^3 = 0$

or $(1-m)(1-2m)^2 = 0$

or $m = \frac{1}{2}, \frac{1}{2}, 1.$

Determination of c for $m = 1$:

Putting $y = m$ and $x = 1$ in the second degree terms of the curve (1), we obtain

$$\phi_2(m) = -4m + 8m^2.$$

Applying the formula

$$c.\phi_3'(m) + \phi_2(m) = 0$$

or $c(-5+16m-12m^2) - 4m + 8m^2 = 0.$

Substitute $m = 1$, we get

$$c(-5+16-12) - 4 + 8 = 0$$

or $-c + 4 = 0$

or $c = 4.$

Thus the asymptote is $y = x + 4$

or $x - y + 4 = 0.$

Determination of c for $m = \frac{1}{2}, \frac{1}{2}$:

Putting $y = m$ and $x = 1$ in the first degree terms of the curve (1) we obtain

$$\phi_1(m) = -8 - 7m.$$

Since $m = \frac{1}{2}, \frac{1}{2}$ are two repeated roots of $\phi_3(m) = 0$, then apply the following formula to determine c,

$$\frac{c^2}{2!}[\phi_3''(m)] + \frac{c}{1!}\phi_2'(m) + \phi_1(m) = 0$$

or $\frac{c^2}{2!}(16-24m)+c(-4+16m)-8-7m=0$

At $m = \frac{1}{2}$

$$\frac{c^2}{2}(16-12) + c(-4+8) - 8 - \frac{7}{2} = 0$$

or $2c^2 + 4c - \frac{23}{2} = 0$

or $4c^2 + 8c - 23 = 0 \Rightarrow c = \frac{-2 \pm 3\sqrt{3}}{2}.$

Thus the other asymptotes are

$$y = \frac{1}{2}x + \frac{-2 \pm 3\sqrt{3}}{2}$$

or $2y = x - 2 \pm 3\sqrt{3}.$

Hence, all the three asymptotes of the curve are

$$x - y + 4 = 0,\ 2y = x - 2 \pm 3\sqrt{3}.$$

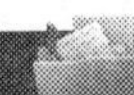

Similar Problems

(1) Find all the asymptotes of the curve $y^2(x^2 - a^2) = x^2(x^2 - 4a^2)$. **Ans.** $x = \pm a, y = \pm x$

(2) Find all the asymptotes of the curve $y^3 - xy^2 - x^2y + x^3 + x^2 - y^2 - 1 = 0$.

Ans. $y + x = 0, y - x = 0$ and $y - x - 1 = 0$

4. *Find asymptotes of the curve* $x^2y^2 - x^2y - xy^2 + x + y + 1 = 0$

SOLUTION. Degree of the given curve is 4, so it has at most 4 asymptotes (Real and imaginary).

Asymptote parallel to x-axis :

Equating the coefficient of highest degree term of x (*i.e.*, x^2) to zero, we get

$$y^2 - y = 0 \quad \Rightarrow \quad y(y-1) = 0$$

$\Rightarrow$ $y = 0$ and $y = 1$

Thus, $y = 0$ and $y = 1$ are two asymptotes parallel to x-axis.

Asymptote parallel to y-axis :

Equating the coefficient of highest degree term of y (*i.e.*, y^2) to zero, we get

$$x^2 - x = 0 \quad \Rightarrow \quad x(x-1) = 0$$

$\Rightarrow$ $x = 0$ and $x = 1$

Thus, $y = 0$ and $x = 1$ are two asymptotes parallel to x-axis.

Hence, $x=0$, $y = 0$, $x = 1$ and $y = 1$ are the required asymptotes.

5. *Find asymptotes parallel to axes for the curve $y^2(x^2 - a^2) = x$.*

SOLUTION. The given curve is a degree 4, so it cannot have more than four asymptotes. Now, equating to zero the coefficient of the highest power of y (*i.e.*, of y^2), the asymptotes parallel to y-axis are given by

$$x^2 - a^2 = 0 \Rightarrow x = \pm a.$$

Again equating to zero the coefficient of the highest power of x (*i.e.*, of x^2), the asymptotes parallel to x-axis are given by

$$y^2 = 0 \Rightarrow y = 0, y = 0.$$

Hence, all the four asymptotes are given by $x = \pm a, y = 0, y = 0$.

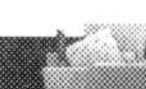

Exercise-14.1

Find all the asymptotes of the following curves:

1. $a^2/x^2 - b^2/y^2 = 1$
2. $a^2/x^2 + b^2/y^2 = 1$
3. $y^2(a^2 - x^2) = x^4$
4. $x^2y^2 = a^2(x^2 + y^2)$
5. $x^2y^2 - x^2y - xy^2 - y + 1 = 0$
6. $3x^3 + 2x^2y - 7xy^2 + 2y^3 + 14xy + 7y^2 + 4x + 5y = 0$
7. $2x^3 - x^2y - 2xy^2 + y^3 - 4x^2 + 8xy - 4x + 1 = 0$
8. $x^3 + 2x^2y + xy^2 - x^2 - xy + 2 = 0$
9. $y^3 - 5xy^2 + 8x^2y - 4x^3 - 3y^2 + 9xy - 6x^2 + 2y - 2x + 1 = 0$
10. $y^3 - x^2y - 2xy^2 + 2x^3 - 7xy + 3y^2 + 2x^2 + 2x + 2y + 1 = 0$ (MTU–2012)
11. $y^3 - xy^2 - x^2y + x^3 + x^2 - y^2 - 1 = 0$
12. $(x^2 - y^2)(y^2 - 4x^2) - 6x^3 + 5yx^2 + 3xy^2 - 2y^3 - x^2 + 3xy - 1 = 0$
13. $y^3 = x^3 + ax^2$
14. $x^2y^3 + x^3y^2 = x^3 + y^3$.
15. $(y - x)(y - 2x)^2 + (y + 3x)(y - 2x) + 2x + 2y - 1 = 0$.
16. $x^3 + 2x^2y - xy^2 - 2y^3 + 4y^2 + 2xy + y - 1 = 0$.
17. $(x + y)^2(x + 2y + 2) = x + 9y + 2$ (MDU–2005)
18. $x^2(x - y)^2 + a^2(x^2 - y^2) - a^2xy = 0$
19. $y^3 - 2y^2x - yx^2 + 2x^3 + y^2 - 6xy + 5x^2 - 2y + 2x + 1 = 0$
20. $x^3 + 3x^2y - 4y^3 - x + y + 3 = 0$
21. $x^3 - 5x^2y + 8xy^2 - 4y^3 + x^2 - 3xy + 2y^2 - 1 = 0$
22. $xy^2 = 4a^2(2a + x)$.
23. $x^3 + 2x^2y - xy^2 - 2y^3 + xy - y^2 - 1 = 0$
24. $y^3 + x^2y + 2xy^2 - y + 1 = 0$
25. $(2x - 3y + 1)^2(x + y) - 8x + 2y - 9 = 0$
26. $(x^2 - y^2)^2 - 4y^2 + y = 0$
27. $y^2(x - 2a) = x^3 - a^3$
28. $(x^3 + a^3)y = bx^3$

ANSWERS

1. $x = \pm a$ **2.** $x = \pm a, y = \pm b$ **3.** $x = \pm a$ **4.** $x = \pm a, y = \pm a$ **5.** $y = 0; y = 1; x = 0; x = 1$
6. $x + 2y = 1, 2x - 2y = -7, 6x - 2y = 15$ **7.** $x + y - 2 = 0; x - y + 2 = 0; 2x - y - 4 = 0$
8. $x = 0; x + y = 0; x + y - 1 = 0$ **9.** $x - y = 0; 2x - y + 2 = 0; 2x - y + 1 = 0$
10. $x - y - 1 = 0; x + y + 2 = 0; 2x - y = 0$ **11.** $x + y = 0; x - y = 0; x - y + 1 = 0$
12. $x - y = 0; 2x - y = 0; x + y + 1 = 0; 2x + y + 1 = 0$ **13.** $3x - 3y + a = 0$
14. $y = \pm 1; x = \pm 1; x + y = 0$ **15.** $2x - y - 2 = 0; 2x - y - 3 = 0; x - y + 4 = 0$
16. $x - y + 1 = 0; x + y - 1 = 0; x + 2y = 0$ **17.** $x + 2y + 2 = 0;\ x + y \pm 2\sqrt{2} = 0$
18. $y = \pm a; x - y = \pm a$ **19.** $x - y = 0; 2x - y + 1 = 0; x + y + 2 = 0$
20. $x - y = 0; x + 2y - 1 = 0; x + 2y + 1 = 0$ **21.** $x - y = 0; x - 2y = 0; x - 2y + 1 = 0$
22. $x = 0, y = \pm 2a$ **23.** $x + 2y - 1 = 0; x - y = 0; x + y + 1 = 0$
24. $y = 0; x + y - 1 = 0; x + y + 1 = 0$ **25.** $x + y = 0; 2x - 3y + 3 = 0; 2x - 3y - 1 = 0$
26. $x + y = \pm 1; x - y = \pm 1$ **27.** $x = 2a, y = x + a, y = -x - a$
28. $x + a = 0, y - b = 0$

14.8 OTHER METHODS FOR FINDING THE ASYMPTOTE OF AN ALGEBRAIC CURVE

THEOREM 1. *The asymptotes of an algebraic curve are parallel to the lines which obtained by equating to zero the linear factors of the highest degree terms of the equation of curve.*

PROOF. Let us suppose the equation of the curve is of degree n and let $y - mx$ be a linear factor of the

n^{th} degree term in the equation of the curve. Since $\phi_n(m)$ is a polynomial of degree n in m and obtained by putting $y = m$ and $x = 1$ in the nth degree terms of the curve, then $(m - m_1)$ is a factor of $\phi_n(m)$. Thus m_1 is a root of the equation $\phi_n(m) = 0$ which gives the slope of the asymptote. Hence, there is an asymptote parallel to the line $y = m_1 x = 0$.

Conversely, let m_1 be a root of the equation $\phi_n(m) = 0$ so that there is an asymptote which is parallel to the line $y - m_1 x = 0$, then $(m_1 - m)$ must be a factor of $\phi_n(m)$ and therefore, $(y/x - m_1)$ will be a linear factor of $\phi_n(y/x)$. Hence $(y - m_1 x)$ is a linear factor of $x^n\,\phi_n(y/x)$ which is the highest degree terms in the equation of the curve.

Hence the theorem is proved.

Since we know that if $y = mx + c$ is an asymptote of the curve $f(x, y) = 0$, then we have

$$\left. m = \lim_{x\to\infty} \frac{y}{x} \text{ and } c = \lim_{x\to\infty} (y - mx) = \lim_{x\to\infty,\, \frac{y}{x}\to\infty} (y - mx) \right\} \qquad \ldots(1)$$

With the help of (1) and above theorem we may find the asymptotes of an algebraic curves.

WORKING PROCEDURE

STEP 1. First we collect all the highest degree terms in the equation of the curve and then resolve into linear factors.

STEP 2. After getting linear factors there may arise following cases.

CASE I. If the linear factor $(y - m_1 x)$ of the highest degree *i.e.*, n^{th} degree terms in the equation of the curve is simple (non-repeated). Then the given equation of the curve can be written as

$$(y - m_1 x)F_{n-1} + P_{n-1} = 0. \qquad \ldots(2)$$

where F_{n-1} contains only terms of degree $n - 1$ and P_{n-1} contains the terms of various degree not exceeding $n - 1$. Therefore $y - m_1 x = c$ is an asymptote of the curve where c is to be determined. Let us take a point (x, y) on the curve (1), then we have

$$y - m_1 x = -\frac{P_{n-1}}{F_{n-1}}.$$

Now taking the limit as $x \to \infty$, $y/x \to m_1$, then we have

$$\lim_{x\to\infty,\, \frac{y}{x}\to m_1} (y - m_1 x) = \lim_{x\to\infty,\, \frac{y}{x}\to m_1} \left(-\frac{P_{n-1}}{F_{n-1}}\right) \text{ or } c = \lim_{x\to\infty,\, \frac{y}{x}\to m_1} \left(-\frac{P_{n-1}}{F_{n-1}}\right).$$

Now substitute this value of c in the equation $y = m_1 x + c$

We obtained the asymptote which is parallel to the line $y - m_1 x = 0$ corresponding to the linear factor $(y - m_1 x)$. Similarly we may obtain other asymptotes.

CASE II. If $(y - m_1 x)$ is a linear factor of the nth degree terms of order two but $(y - m_1 x)$ is not a factor of the $(n - 1)^{th}$ degree terms of the curve, then we have $\phi'_n(m_1) = 0$ and $\phi'_{n-1}(m_1) \neq 0$. Therefore, no asymptotes corresponding to $(y - m_1 x)^2$ will exist. On the other hand if there are no terms of $(n - 1)^{th}$ degree in the equation of the curve, then make them by adding with zero coefficient and thus we can say that $(y - m_1 x)$ is now a factor of $(n - 1)^{th}$ degree terms, then we have the case III.

CASE III. If $(y - m_1x)^2$ is a linear factor of nth degree terms and $(y - m_1x)$ is a factor of $(n - 1)^{th}$ degree terms, then the equation of the curve can be written as

$$(y - m_1x)^2 F_{n-2} + (y - m_1x)G_{n-2} + P_{n-2} = 0 \qquad \ldots(3)$$

where F_{n-2} and G_{n-2} contain only the terms of degree $n - 2$, and P_{n-2} contains various degree terms not exceeding $n - 2$. Now divide (2) by F_{n-2} and taking the limit as $x \to \infty$ and $y/x \to m_1$, we get

$$\lim_{x\to\infty,(y/x)\to m_1} (y - m_1x)^2 + \lim_{x\to\infty,(y/x)\to m_1} (y - m_1x)\left(\frac{G_{n-2}}{F_{n-2}}\right) + \lim_{x\to\infty,(y/x)\to m_1} \left(\frac{P_{n-2}}{F_{n-2}}\right) \qquad \ldots(4)$$

Since we know that $c = \lim_{x\to\infty,(y/x)\to m_1} (y - m_1x)$

and $A = \lim_{x\to\infty,(y/x)\to m_1} \left(\frac{G_{n-2}}{F_{n-2}}\right)$ and $B = \lim_{x\to\infty,(y/x)\to m_1} \left(\frac{P_{n-2}}{F_{n-2}}\right)$

then (4) becomes $c^2 + Ac + B = 0.$

This is a quadratic equation in c so it has two roots let c_1 and c_2 be these two roots. Then we obtain two asymptotes $y - m_1x = c_1$ and $y - m_1x = c_2$ corresponding to m_1.

- As a consequence we can say that the two asymptotes corresponding to the factor $(y - m_1x)^2$ may obtain by solving the quadratic equation $(y - m_1x)^2 + A(y - m_1x) + B = 0$.
  Similarly, we can also find the asymptotes corresponding to the factor $(y - m_1x)^3$, etc. of the nth degree terms in the equation of the curve.

CASE IV. Suppose the equation of the curve is of the form

$$(ax + by + c)P_{n-1} + Q_{n-1} = 0 \qquad \ldots(5)$$

where P_{n-1} and Q_{n-1} contain various degree term not exceeding the degree $(n - 1)^{th}$, and P_{n-1} contains atleast one term of degree $(n - 1)$ such that (5) becomes of degree n. Therefore, we can say that $(ax + by)$ is a linear factor of nth degree terms in the equation (5). Thus (5) can also be written as

$$(ax + by) P_{n-1} + cP_{n-1} + Q_{n-1} = 0.$$

Divide this equation by P_{n-1} and taking the limit as $x \to \infty$ and $y/x \to -a/b$, we obtain

$$(ax + by + c) + \lim_{x\to\infty, y/x\to(-a/b)} (Q_{n-1} / P_{n-1}) = 0$$

This the required equation of the asymptote.

CASE V. Let the equation of the curve of nth degree be of the form

$$F_n + P = 0 \qquad \ldots(1)$$

where F_n is of degree n and P is of degree $n - 2$ or lower and if $F_n = 0$ can be expressed as the product of n linear factors which give n straight lines such that no two of them are parallel or coincident, then all the asymptotes of the curve (1) are obtained by equating to zero the linear factors of F_n.

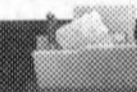

Solved Examples

1. *Find the asymptotes of* $(x-y)^2(x^2+y^2)-10(x-y)x^2+12y^2+2x+y=0.$

SOLUTION. We have

$$(x-y)^2-10(x-y)\lim_{x\to\infty\ y/x\to 1}\frac{x^2}{x^2+y^2}+12\lim_{x\to\infty\ y/x\to 1}\frac{y^2}{x^2+y^2}=0$$

or $(x-y)^2-5(x-y)+6=0$

which gives parallel asymptotes $x-y=2$ and $x-y=3$.

The other two asymptotes are imaginary. Since the remaining linear factors of the four degree terms in the equation to the curve are imaginary.

2. *Find the asymptotes of* $(x-y-1)^2(x^2+y^2+2)+6(x-y-1)(xy+7)-8x^2-2x-1=0.$

SOLUTION. Dividing by the coefficient of $(x-y-1)^2$ and taking limits, we see that the asymptotes parallel to $x-y-1=0$ are

$$(x-y-1)^2+6(x-y-1)\lim_{x\to\infty\ \frac{y}{x}\to 1}\frac{xy+7}{x^2+y^2+2}+\lim_{x\to\infty\ \frac{y}{x}\to 1}\frac{-8x^2-2x-1}{x^2+y^2+2}=0$$

$$\Rightarrow (x-y-1)^2+3(x-y-1)-4=0$$

$$\Rightarrow x-y-1=\frac{-3\pm\sqrt{9+16}}{2}=1,-4.$$

Hence, the two asymptotes are $x-y-2=0$ and $x-y+3=0$ the remaining two asymptotes are imaginary.

14.9 ASYMPTOTES BY EXPANSION

THEOREM. *Let the equation of the curve be of the form* $y=mx+c+\dfrac{A_1}{x}+\dfrac{A_2}{x^2}+\dfrac{A_3}{x^3}+\ldots$ ...(1) *then* $y=mx+c$ *is the asymptote of* (1).

PROOF. Since the equation of the curve is

$$y=mx+c+\frac{A_1}{x}+\frac{A_2}{x^2}+\frac{A_3}{x^3}+\ldots;\ \text{where}\ \frac{A_1}{x}+\frac{A_2}{x^2}+\frac{A_3}{x^3}+\ldots\ \text{is convergent}$$

for sufficiently large values of x.

Differentiating (1) w.r.t. 'x', we get $\dfrac{dy}{dx}=m-\dfrac{A_1}{x^2}-\dfrac{2A_2}{x^3}-\dfrac{3A_3}{x^4}-\ldots$

Now the equation of the tangent to (1) at the point $P(x, y)$ is

$$Y-y=\left(m-\frac{A_1}{x^2}-\frac{2A_2}{x^3}-\frac{3A_3}{x^4}-\ldots\right)(X-x)$$

or

$$Y=\left(m-\frac{A_1}{x^2}-\frac{2A_2}{x^3}-\frac{3A_3}{x^4}-\ldots\right)X+c+\frac{2A_1}{x}+\frac{3A_2}{x^2}+\ldots \qquad \text{[Using(1)]}$$

Now taking the limit as $x\to\infty$, we get

$$Y=mX+c.$$

Hence $y=mx+c$ is an asymptote of the curve $y=mx+c+\dfrac{A_1}{x}+\dfrac{A_2}{x^2}+\dfrac{A_3}{x^3}+\ldots$

Solved Examples

1. *Find the asymptotes of the hyperbola* $\dfrac{x^2}{a^2}-\dfrac{y^2}{b^2}=1.$

SOLUTION. The equation of the curve can be written as

$$y^2=b^2\left(-1+\frac{x^2}{a^2}\right)$$

or $y=\pm b\sqrt{\left(-1+\dfrac{x^2}{a^2}\right)}=\pm\dfrac{b}{a}x\sqrt{\left(1-\dfrac{a^2}{x^2}\right)}$

$$y = \pm\frac{b}{a}x\left[1-\frac{1}{2}\frac{a^2}{x^2}-\frac{1}{8}\frac{a^4}{x^4}+\ldots\right]$$

[Using binomial expansion]

Since we know that $y = mx + c$ is an asymptote of the curve

$$y = mx + c + \frac{A_1}{x}+\frac{A_2}{x^2}+\ldots$$

Hence, $y = \pm\frac{b}{a}x$ are the asymptotes of the given curve.

2. *Find all the asymptotes of the curve* $(y^2 - x^2)(y - 2x) - 7xy + 3y^2 + 2x^2 + 2x + 2y + 1 = 0$.

SOLUTION. The given equation can be written as

$(y - x)(y + x)(y - 2x) - 7xy + 3y^2 + 2x^2 + 2x + 2y + 1 = 0$. ...(1)

The slope of the asymptote corresponding to the factor $y - x$ is 1. Thus the asymptote corresponding to this factor is

$$y-x = \lim_{x\to\infty,\frac{y}{x}\to 1}\frac{7xy-3y^2-2x^2-2x-2y-1}{(y+x)(y-2x)}$$

$$= \lim_{x\to\infty,\frac{y}{x}\to 1}\frac{7\left(\frac{y}{x}\right)-3\left(\frac{y}{x}\right)^2-2-\frac{2}{x}-2\frac{y}{x}\left(\frac{1}{x}\right)-\frac{1}{x^2}}{\left(\frac{y}{x}+1\right)\left(\frac{y}{x}-2\right)}$$

$$=\frac{7-3-2}{2(1-2)}=\frac{2}{-2}=-1.$$

$\therefore y - x + 1 = 0$

Similarly the second asymptote corresponding to the factor $(y + x)$ is

$$x+y = \lim_{x\to\infty,\frac{y}{x}\to -1}\frac{7xy-3y^2-2x^2-2x-2y-1}{(y-x)(y-2x)}$$

$$= \lim_{x\to\infty,\frac{y}{x}\to -1}\frac{7\left(\frac{y}{x}\right)-3\left(\frac{y}{x}\right)^2-2-\frac{2}{x}-2\left(\frac{y}{x}\right)\left(\frac{1}{x}\right)-\frac{1}{x^2}}{\left(\frac{y}{x}-1\right)\left(\frac{y}{x}-2\right)}$$

$$=\frac{7(-1)-3(-1)^2-2}{(-1-1)(-1-2)}$$

$$=\frac{-7-3-2}{(-2)(-3)}=-2$$

$\therefore\quad x + y + 2 = 0$

and the third asymptote corresponding to the factor $y - 2x$ is

$$y-2x = \lim_{x\to\infty,\frac{y}{x}\to 2}\frac{7xy-3y^2-2x^2-2x-2y-1}{(y-x)(y+x)}$$

$$= \lim_{x\to\infty,\frac{y}{x}\to 2}\frac{7\left(\frac{y}{x}\right)-3\left(\frac{y}{x}\right)^2-2-2\left(\frac{1}{x}\right)-2\left(\frac{y}{x}\right)\left(\frac{1}{x}\right)-\frac{1}{x^2}}{\left(\frac{y}{x}-1\right)\left(\frac{y}{x}+1\right)}$$

$$=\frac{7(2)-3(2)^2-2}{(2-1)(2+1)}=\frac{14-12-2}{3}=0.$$

$\Rightarrow y - 2x = 0$

Hence, all the asymptotes are $y - x + 1 = 0$, $x + y + 2 = 0$ and $y - 2x = 0$.

3. *Find all the asymptotes of the curve* $(y-x)(y-2x)^2+(y+3x)(y-2x)+2x+2y-1=0$.

SOLUTION. The equation of the curve is

$(y-x)(y-2x)^2+(y+3x)(y-2x)+2x+2y-1 = 0$

The asymptotes corresponding to the factor $(y - 2x)^2$ are

$$(y-2x)^2+(y-2x)\lim_{x\to\infty,\ y/x\to 2}\frac{y+3x}{y-x}+\lim_{x\to\infty,y/x\to 2}\frac{2x+2y-1}{(y-x)}=0$$

or $$(y-2x)^2+(y-2x)\lim_{x\to\infty,\ y/x\to 2}\left(\frac{\frac{y}{x}+3}{\frac{y}{x}-1}\right)+\lim_{x\to\infty,\ y/x\to 2}\frac{2+2(y/x)-1/x}{(y/x-1)}=0$$

or $(y-2x)^2+5(y-2x)+6=0$

or $$(y-2x)=\frac{-5\pm\sqrt{(25-24)}}{2}=\frac{-5\pm 1}{2}$$

or $y - 2x = -2$ and $y - 2x = -3$

or $y - 2x + 2 = 0$ and $y - 2x + 3 = 0$

And the asymptote corresponding to the factor $(y - x)$ is

$$(y-x)+\lim_{x\to\infty,\ y/x\to 1}\frac{(y+3x)(y-2x)}{(y-2x)^2}+\lim_{x\to\infty,y/x\to 1}\frac{2x+2y-1}{(y-2x)^2}=0$$

or $(y-x)+\lim_{\substack{x\to\infty,\\ y/x\to 1}} \dfrac{(y/x+3)(y/x-2)}{(y/x-2)^2}$

$+\lim_{\substack{x\to\infty,\\ y/x\to 1}} \dfrac{2+2(y/x)-1/x}{x(y/x-2)^2}=0$

or $(y-x)+\dfrac{(1+3)(1-2)}{(1-2)^2}+0=0$

or $y-x-4=0$

Hence, all the asymptotes of the given curve are $y-2x+2=0$, $y-2x+3=0$ and $y-x-4=0$.

Exercise-14.2

Find all the asymptotes of the following curves:

1. $(x^2-y^2)(x+2y+1)+x+y+1=0$
2. $x^5-y^5=a^3xy$
3. $(x^2-y^2)(y^2-4x^2)-6x^3+5x^2y+3xy^2-2y^3-x^2+3xy-1=0$
4. $x^2(x^2-y^2)(x-y)+2x^3(x-y)-4y^3=0$
5. $xy(x^2-y^2)(x^2-4y^2)+xy(x^2-y^2)+x^2+y^2-7=0$
6. $(x-2y)^2(x-y)-4y(x-2y)-(8x+7y)=0$
7. $(x-y)^2(x^2+y^2)-10(x-y)x^2+12y^2+2x+y=0$
8. $(x-y-1)^2(x^2+y^2+2)+6(x-y-1)(xy+7)-8x^2-2x-1=0$
9. $(\alpha_1x+\beta_1y+\gamma_1)(\alpha_2x+\beta_2y+\gamma_2)+\gamma_3=0$
10. $(x-y+2)(2x-3y+4)(4x-5y+6)+5x-6y+7=0$
11. $(x-y+1)(x-y-2)(x+y)=8x-1$
12. $(x^2-3x+2)(x+y-2)+1=0$
13. $x(y-3)^3-4y(x-1)^3=0$
14. $x^2(x+y)(x-y)^2+ax^3(x-y)-a^2y^3=0$
15. $(y-a)^2(x^2-a^2)=x^4+a^4$

Hints to the Selected Problems

1. Asymptotes corresponding to the factor $(x-y)$ is

$$(x-y)+\lim_{\substack{x\to\infty\\ y/x\to 1}} \frac{(x+y+1)}{(x+y)(x+2y+1)}=0$$

which gives $x-y=0$.

Similarly, asymptotes corresponding to the factor $(x+y)$ is given by $x+y=0$ and so on.

Note. Apply the same procedure to all other questions.

ANSWERS

1. $x-y=0, x+y=0, x+2y+1=0$
2. $y-x=0$
3. $x-y=0, 2x-y=0, x+y+1=0, 2x+y+1=0$
4. $x-y+2=0, x-y-1=0, x+y+1=0, x+2=0$
5. $x=0, y=0, x-y=0, x+y=0, x-2y=0$ and $x+2y=0$
6. $x-y+4=0, x-2y=2\pm 3\sqrt{3}$
7. $x-y-2=0, x-y-3=0$
8. $x-y-2=0, x-y+3=0$
9. $\alpha_1x+\beta_1x+\gamma_1=0, \alpha_2x+\beta_2y+\gamma_2=0$
10. $x-y+2=0, 2x-3y+4=0, 4x-5y+6=0$
11. $y+x=0, x-y-2=0, x-y+1=0$
12. $x=1, x=2, x+y-2=0$
13. $x=0, y=0, 4x-2y+3=0, 4x+2y-15=0$
14. $x\pm a=0, x-y+a=0, y=\pm x-\frac{1}{2}a$
15. $x\pm a=0, x-y+a=0, x+y-a=0$

14.10 INTERSECTION OF A CURVE WITH ITS ASYMPTOTES

Let the equation $y=mx+c$ ...(1)

be an asymptote of the curve

$$x^n\phi_n\left(\frac{y}{x}\right)+x^{n-1}\phi_{n-1}\left(\frac{y}{x}\right)+x^{n-2}\phi_{n-2}\left(\frac{y}{x}\right)+\ldots=0. \quad \ldots(2)$$

Solving (1) and (2) to find the intersection points so eliminating y between (1) and (2), we get

$$x^n\phi_n\left(m+\frac{c}{x}\right)+x^{n-1}\phi_{n-1}\left(m+\frac{c}{x}\right)+x^{n-2}\phi_{n-2}\left(m+\frac{c}{x}\right)+\ldots=0.$$

Now expand each term of above equation by Taylor's theorem, we have

$$x^n\left[\phi_n(m)+\frac{c}{x}\phi_n'(m)+\frac{c^2}{x^2}\cdot\frac{1}{2!}\phi_n''(m)+\ldots\right]+x^{n-1}\left[\phi_{n-1}(m)+\frac{c}{x}\phi_{n-1}'(m)+\ldots\right]$$
$$+x^{n-2}\left[\phi_{n-2}(m)+\frac{c}{x}\phi_{n-2}'(m)+\ldots\right]=0$$

or $$x^n\phi_n(m)+[c\phi_n'(m)+\phi_{n-1}(m)]x^{n-1}+\left[\frac{c^2}{2!}\phi_n''(m)+\frac{c}{1!}\phi_{n-1}'(m)+\phi_{n-2}(m)\right]x^{n-2}+\ldots=0. \quad \ldots(3)$$

Since $y = mx + c$ is an asymptotes of the curve (2), then we have $\phi_n(m) = 0$ and $c\phi_n'(m)+\phi_{n-1}(m)=0$.

Thus (3) becomes $$\left[\frac{c^2}{2!}\phi_n''(m)+\frac{c}{1!}\phi_{n-1}'(m)+\phi_{n-2}(m)\right]x^{n-2}+\ldots=0. \quad \ldots(4)$$

This is a equation of degree $n-2$ in x so it will have atmost $n-2$ values of x provided there is no asymptote parallel to $y = mx + c$ of the given curve.

Hence, in general we can say that any asymptote of a curve of the nth degree cuts the curve in $(n-2)$ points.

- Since one asymptote of the curve of nth degree cuts the curve in $(n-2)$ points so n asymptotes of that curve will cut in $n(n-2)$ points.
- If the equation of the curve of degree n can be written as $F_n + P = 0$, where F_n contains n non-repeated linear factors and P contains the terms almost of degree $n-2$, then $n(n-2)$ points of intersection of the curve will lie on the curve $P = 0$.

Solved Examples

1. *Show that the four asymptotes of the curve* $(x^2-y^2)(y^2-4x^2)+6x^3-5x^2y-3xy^2+2y^3-x^2+3xy-1=0.$ *cut the curve in eight points which lie on the circle* $x^2+y^2=1$.

SOLUTION. The given equation of the curve can be written as

$$(x-y)(x+y)(y-2x)(y+2x)+6x^3-5x^2y-3xy^2+2y^3-x^2+3xy-1=0 \quad \ldots(1)$$

The asymptote corresponding to the factor $x-y$ is

$$x-y+\lim_{\substack{x\to\infty,\\ y/x\to 1}}\frac{6x^3-5x^2y-3xy^2+2y^3-x^2+3xy-1}{(x+y)(y-2x)(y+2x)}=0$$

or $$x-y+\lim_{\substack{x\to\infty,\\ \frac{y}{x}\to 1}}\frac{6-5\left(\frac{y}{x}\right)-3\left(\frac{y}{x}\right)^2+2\left(\frac{y}{x}\right)^3-\frac{1}{x}+3\left(\frac{y}{x}\right)\left(\frac{1}{x}\right)-\frac{1}{x^3}}{\left(1+\frac{y}{x}\right)\left(\frac{y}{x}-2\right)\left(\frac{y}{x}+2\right)}=0$$

or $$x-y+\lim_{\substack{x\to\infty,\\ \frac{y}{x}\to 1}}\frac{6-5-3+2}{(1+1)(1-2)(1+2)}=0$$

or $$x-y=0.$$

The asymptote corresponding to the factor $x+y$ is

$$x+y+\lim_{\substack{x\to\infty,\\ y/x\to -1}}\frac{6x^3-5x^2y-3xy^2+2y^3-x^2+3xy-1}{(x-y)(y-2x)(y+2x)}=0$$

or $$x+y+\lim_{\substack{x\to\infty,\\ y/x\to -1}}\frac{6-5(y/x)-3(y/x)^2+2(y/x)^3-(1/x)+3(y/x)(1/x)-(1/x^3)}{(1-y/x)(y/x-2)(y/x+2)}=0$$

or $$x+y+\frac{6-5(-1)-3(-1)^2+2(-1)^3}{(1+1)(-1-2)(-1+2)}=0$$

or $$x+y-1=0.$$

Now the asymptote corresponding to the factor $y-2x$ is

$$y-2x+\lim_{\substack{x\to\infty,\\ y/x\to 2}}\frac{\{6x^3-5x^2y-3xy^2+2y^3-x^2+3xy-1\}}{(x-y)(x+y)(y+2x)}=0$$

or

$$y-2x+\lim_{\substack{x\to\infty,\\ y/x\to 2}}\frac{\{6-5(y/x)-3(y/x)^2+2(y/x)^3-(1/x)+3(y/x)(1/x)-(1/x^3)\}}{(1-y/x)(1+y/x)(y/x+2)}=0$$

or $$y-2x+\frac{6-5(2)-3(2)^2+2(2)^3}{(1-2)(1+2)(2+2)}=0$$

or $$y-2x=0.$$

The asymptote corresponding to the factor $y+2x$ is

$$y+2x+\lim_{\substack{x\to\infty,\\ y/x\to -2}}\frac{\{6x^3-5x^2y-3xy^2+2y^3-x^2+3xy-1\}}{(x-y)(x+y)(y-2x)}=0$$

or

$$y+2x+\lim_{\substack{x\to\infty,\\ y/x\to -2}}\frac{\{6-5(y/x)-3(y/x)^2+2(y/x)^3-(1/x)+3(y/x)(1/x)-(1/x^3)\}}{(1-y/x)(1+y/x)(y/x-2)}=0$$

or $$y+2x+\frac{6-5(-2)-3(-2)^2+2(-2)^3}{(1+2)(1-2)(-2-2)}=0$$

or $$y+2x-1=0.$$

Hence, all the four asymptotes are $x-y=0$, $x+y-1=0$, $y-2x=0$ and $y+2x-1=0$.

Since one asymptote cuts the curve in $(4-2)=2$ points so all the four asymptotes cut the curve in $4\times 2=8$ points. Now combine all the asymptotes, we get

$$(x-y)(x+y-1)(y-2x)(y+2x-1)=0$$

or $$[x^2-y^2-(x-y)][y^2-4x^2-(y-2x)]=0$$

or $$(x^2-y^2)(y^2-4x^2)-(x^2-y^2)(y-2x)-(x-y)(y^2-4x^2)+(x-y)(y-2x)=0$$

or $$(x^2-y^2)(y^2-4x^2)-(x^2y-2x^3-y^3+2xy^2)-(xy^2-4x^3-y^3+4x^2y)+xy-2x^2-y^2-2xy=0$$

or $$(x^2-y^2)(y^2-4x^2)+6x^3-5x^2y-3xy^2+2y^3-2x^2-y^2+3xy=0. \quad \text{...(2)}$$

Now subtract (2) from (1), we get

$$x^2+y^2=1.$$

Hence, all the eight points of intersection lie on the circle $x^2+y^2=1$.

Exercise-14.3

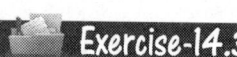

1. Show that the asymptotes of the curve
$$4(x^4+y^4)-17x^2y^2-4x(4y^2-x^2)+2(x^2-2)=0$$
cut the curve in eight points which lie on the ellipse $x^2+4y^2=4$.
2. Find the asymptotes of the curve $x^2y-xy^2+xy+y^2+x-y=0$ and show that they cut the curve again in three points which lie on the straight line $x+y=0$.
3. Show that the eight points of intersection of the curve
$$x^4-5x^2y^2+4y^4+x^2-y^2+x+y+1=0$$
and its asymptotes lie on a rectangular hyperbola.
4. Show that the asymptotes of the cubic
$$x^3-2y^3+xy(2x-y)+y(x-y)+1=0$$
cut the curve in three points which lie on the straight line $x-y+1=0$.
5. Find the equation of the cubic which has the same asymptotes as the curve
$$x^3-6x^2y+11xy^2-6y^3+x+y+1=0$$
and which passes through the points (0, 0), (1, 0) and (0,1).
6. Show that the asymptotes of the curve $y^2(x^2-a^2)=x^2(x^2-4a^2)$ form two right angle triangles with the x-axis. ($y>0$).

ANSWERS

2. $y=0, x=1, x-y+2=0$ **5.** $x^3-6x^2y+11xy^2-6y^3-x+6y=0$.

14.11 ASYMPTOTES OF NON-ALGEBRAIC CURVES

Definition. *A curve in which there are some terms involving cosine, sine, etc. is called non-algebraic curve.*

The method for finding the asymptotes of non-algebraic curves can be explained by following example.

Example. Let the equation of the curve be $y = \sec x$, then differentiating this w.r.t. 'x', we get

$$\frac{dy}{dx} = \sec x \tan x.$$

Therefore, the tangent at $P(x, y)$ on the curve is

$$Y - \sec x = \frac{dy}{dx}(X - x)$$

or
$$Y - \sec x = \sec x \tan x(X - x)$$

or
$$Y \cos^2 x - \cos x = (X - x)\sin x. \quad \ldots(1)$$

Now taking the distance of $P(x, y)$ from $(0, 0)$ infinity as $x \to \pi/2$ and $y \to \infty$, we get

$$Y.0 - 0 = (X - \pi/2).1 \quad \text{or} \quad X = \pi/2.$$

This is one asymptote and the other asymptotes are $X = -\pi/2, \pm 3/2\pi, \ldots$

14.12 ASYMPTOTES OF POLAR CURVES

(i) Equation of a line in polar form. Let O be the pole and OX the initial line and let $P(r, \theta)$ be any point on the line whose equation is to be required as shown in Fig. 1.

Draw a perpendicular OM from O to the line such that $OM = p$ and $\angle MOX = \alpha$ (say).

$\therefore$ In ΔOPM

$$\angle POM = \theta - \alpha$$

then,
$$\frac{OM}{OP} = \cos \angle POM$$

or
$$\frac{p}{r} = \cos(\theta - \alpha)$$

or
$$p = r\cos(\theta - \alpha).$$

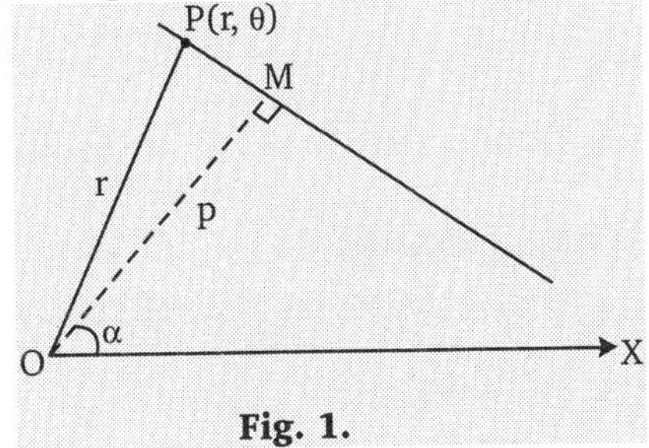

Fig. 1.

This is the equation of line in polar form, where p is the perpendicular length from pole to this line and α is an angle which the perpendicular makes with initial line.

(ii) Asymptotes of polar curves.

THEOREM 1. *If $\theta = \alpha$ is a root of the equation $f(\theta) = 0$, then $r\sin(\theta - \alpha) = 1/f'(\alpha)$ is an asymptote of the curve $1/r = f(\theta)$.*

PROOF. Since the equation of a curve in polar form is $\frac{1}{r} = f(\theta)$. ...(1)

Let $P(r, \theta)$ be any point on this curve and draw a line through O perpendicular to OP, then radius vector which meets the tangent at P in T as show in Fig. 2.

Then OT is a polar subtangent of the curve at P.

$$OT = r^2 \frac{d\theta}{dr} \qquad \text{(From calculus)}$$

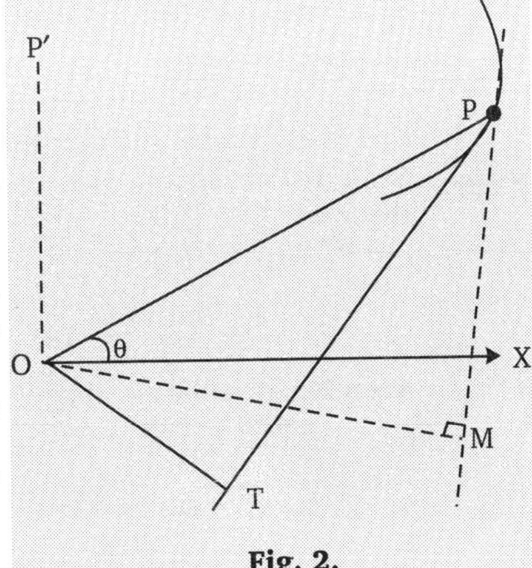

Fig. 2.

Now differentiating (1) w.r.t. 'θ', we get

$$-\frac{1}{r^2}\frac{dr}{d\theta} = f'(\theta).$$

$$\therefore \qquad OT = r^2 \frac{d\theta}{dr} = -\frac{1}{f'(\theta)}.$$

Since α is a root of $f(\theta) = 0$ as $\theta \to \alpha$, then $r \to \infty$ from (1) and the tangent PT tends to the asymptote and $OT \to \left[-\frac{1}{f'(\theta)}\right]_{\theta=\alpha}, f'(\alpha) \neq 0.$

And OP, PT will become parallel to lines shown dotted in the figure 2. Thus $\angle OTP \to \pi/2$ and $OT \to OM$, where OM is a perpendicular distance from O to the asymptote.

$$\therefore \qquad OM = -\frac{1}{f'(\alpha)}$$

when $\theta \to \alpha$ *i.e.*, $OP \to OP'$. Then $\angle XOP' = \alpha$

$$\therefore \qquad \angle MOX = -\left(\frac{\pi}{2} - \alpha\right) \qquad \text{(In the clockwise direction)}$$

Therefore the equation of the asymptote is

$$r\cos\left[\theta - \left\{-\left(\frac{\pi}{2} - \alpha\right)\right\}\right] = -\frac{1}{f'(\alpha)} \qquad [\text{using } p = r\cos(1 - \alpha)]$$

$$\text{or} \quad r\cos\left(\frac{\pi}{2} + \theta - \alpha\right) = -\frac{1}{f'(\alpha)} \qquad \text{or} \qquad -r\sin(\theta - \alpha) = -\frac{1}{f'(\alpha)}$$

$$\text{or} \quad r\sin(\theta - \alpha) = \frac{1}{f'(\alpha)}$$

WORKING PROCEDURE

To find the asymptotes of polar curves, we use the follows steps :

STEP 1. Convert the equation of the given curve in the form $\frac{1}{r} = f(\theta)$.

STEP 2. Find the roots of the equation $f(\theta) = 0$ *i.e.*, values of θ. Suppose α, β, etc. are the roots of $f(\theta) = 0$.

STEP 3. Now the asymptote corresponding to $\theta = \alpha$ is

$$r \sin\, (\theta - \alpha) = \frac{1}{f'(\alpha)}$$

where $f'(\alpha)$ = value of $f'(\theta)$ at $\theta = \alpha$.

Solved Examples

1. *Find the asymptotes of the curve $r \sin n\theta = a$.*

SOLUTION. **Step I.** Convert the given curve into the form

$$\frac{1}{r} = f(\theta).$$

$$\therefore \qquad \frac{1}{r} = \frac{\sin n\theta}{a} = f(\theta). \qquad \ldots(1)$$

Step II. Solve the equation $f(\theta) = 0$.

$$\textit{i.e.,} \qquad \frac{\sin n\theta}{a} = 0.$$

or $\quad \sin n\theta = \sin r\pi,\ r = 0, 1, 2, \ldots,$

or $\quad n\theta = r\pi$ or $\theta = \frac{r\pi}{n}, r = 0, 1, 2, 3, \ldots.$

Let $\quad \alpha = \frac{r\pi}{n}$.

Now differentiating (1) w.r.t. 'θ', we get

$$f'(\theta) = +\frac{n\cos n\theta}{a}.$$

$$\therefore\ f'(\alpha) = \frac{n\cos n\alpha}{a} = \frac{n}{a}\cos r\pi = \frac{n}{a}(-1)^r.$$

Step III. Therefore, the asymptotes of the curve are

$$r\sin(\theta - \alpha) = \frac{1}{f'(\alpha)}$$

$$\text{or} \quad r\sin\left(\theta - \frac{r\pi}{n}\right) = \frac{a}{n(-1)^r},$$

where r is any integer.

2. *Find the asymptotes of the curve $r \sin \theta = a \cos 2\theta$.*

SOLUTION. First put the equation in the form of $\frac{1}{r} = f(\theta)$.

i.e., $\frac{1}{r} = \frac{\sin\theta}{a\cos 2\theta}$.

$\therefore\ f(\theta) = \frac{\sin\theta}{a\cos 2\theta}$. ...(1)

Now solve the equation $f(\theta) = 0$. Then

$$\frac{\sin\theta}{a\cos 2\theta} = 0$$

or $\sin\theta = \sin n\pi$ or $\theta = n\pi$.

Let $\alpha = n\pi$ be the root of the equation $f(\theta) = 0$.

Now differentiating (1) w.r.t. 'θ', we get

$$f'(\theta) = \frac{1}{a}\left[\frac{\cos 2\theta.\cos\theta + 2\sin 2\theta \sin\theta}{\cos^2 2\theta}\right]$$

$$\therefore\ f'(\alpha) = \frac{1}{a}\left[\frac{\cos 2\alpha.\cos\alpha + 2\sin 2\alpha \sin\alpha}{\cos^2 2\alpha}\right]$$

$$= \frac{1}{2a}\left[\frac{\cos 2n\pi.\cos n\pi + 2\sin 2n\pi \sin n\pi}{\cos^2 2n\pi}\right]$$

($\because\ \alpha = n\pi$)

$$= \frac{1}{a}\cos n\pi.$$

The asymptote corresponding to $\alpha = n\pi$ is $r\sin(\theta - n\pi) = \frac{1}{f'(\alpha)} = \frac{a}{\cos n\pi}$

or $r(\sin\theta\cos n\pi - \cos\theta\sin n\pi) = \frac{a}{\cos n\pi}$

or $r\sin\theta\cos n\pi = \frac{a}{\cos n\pi}$

($\because\ \sin n\pi = 0$)

or $r\sin\theta\cos^2 n\pi = a$

or $r\sin\theta = a$ ($\because\ \cos n\pi = 1$)

3. *Find the asymptotes of the curve $r\theta = a$.*

SOLUTION. First putting the equation of curve in the form $\frac{1}{r} = f(\theta)$ so we have

$$\frac{1}{r} = \frac{\theta}{a}.$$

$$\therefore\quad f(\theta) = \frac{\theta}{a}. \quad ...(1)$$

Putting $f(\theta) = 0$, we get $\theta = 0$.

Then $\alpha = 0$ is the root of $f(\theta) = 0$.

Now differentiating (1) w.r.t. 'θ', we get

$$f'(\theta) = \frac{1}{a}. \Rightarrow\ f'(\alpha) = \frac{1}{a}.$$

Thus the asymptote corresponding to $\theta = \alpha$ is

$$r\sin(\theta - \alpha) = \frac{1}{f'(\alpha)}.$$

$$\therefore\quad r\sin(\theta - 0) = \frac{1}{(1/a)}$$

or $\quad r\sin\theta = a.$

4. *Find the circular asymptotes of the curve $r = a.\frac{\theta}{\theta - 1}$.*

SOLUTION. The circular asymptote is given by

$$r = a\lim_{\theta\to\infty}\frac{\theta}{\theta - 1} = a\,.$$

Thus $r = a$ is the circular asymptote.

Exercise-14.4

Find the asymptotes of the following curves:

1. $y = \tan x$.
2. $r = a \operatorname{cosec}\theta + b$
3. $r\sin 2\theta = a$
4. $r\sin\theta = 2\cos 2\theta$
5. $r\sin\theta = 2\cos\theta$
6. $r\theta\cos\theta = a\cos 2\theta$
7. $r(1 - 2\cos\theta) = 2a$
8. $r = 4(\sec\theta + \tan\theta)$
9. $r\cos\theta = 4\sin^2\theta$
10. $r(e^\theta - 1) = a(e^\theta + 1)$
11. $r\cos\theta = a\sin\theta$
12. $r(1 + 2\sin\theta) = 2$
13. $r\sin\theta = 2\theta$

Hint to Selected Problems

1. (i) $y = \tan x \Rightarrow \frac{dy}{dx} = \sec^2 x$

Tangent at (x, y)

$$Y - \tan x = \sec^2 x(Y - x)$$

$\Rightarrow Y\cos^2 x - \sin x\cos x = (X - x)$.

Now as $x \to \pi/2, y \to \infty$ and the distance of (x, y) from $(0, 0) \to \infty$.

$\therefore\ Y.0 - 0 = (X - \pi/2) \Rightarrow X = \pi/2$.

2. $\frac{1}{r} = f(\theta) = \frac{\sin\theta}{a + b\sin\theta}$. Solving, $f(0) = 0$. we get

$\theta = n\pi = \alpha$ (say)

$\Rightarrow\ f'(\alpha) = \frac{1}{a}\cos n\pi.$

Now required asymptotes are given by

$$r\sin(\theta-\alpha)=\frac{1}{f'(\alpha)}.$$

3. $\frac{1}{r}=f(\theta)=\frac{\sin 2\theta}{a}.$

Now on solving $f(0)=0$ we get $\theta=\frac{n\pi}{2}=\alpha$ (say).

Also, $f'(\alpha)=\frac{2\cos n\pi}{a}.$

Therefore, the asymptotes of the given curve is

$$r\sin(\theta-\alpha)=\frac{1}{f'(\alpha)}.$$

4. $\frac{1}{r}=f(\theta)=\frac{\sin\theta}{2\cos 2\theta}$

Now, $f'(\alpha)=\frac{\cos n\pi}{2}.$ Therefore, the asymptotes of the given curve is given by $r\sin(\theta-\alpha)=\frac{1}{f'(\alpha)}.$

5. Here $\theta=n\pi=\alpha$, $f'(\alpha)=\frac{1}{2}$. Then use the required formula.

6. $\theta=0, \left(k\pi+\frac{\pi}{2}\right),\quad f'(\alpha)=\frac{1}{a}$

7. $\theta=\pm\frac{\pi}{3}, f'(\theta_1)=\frac{-\sqrt{3}}{2a},\quad f'(\theta_2)=\frac{\sqrt{3}}{2a}$

8. $\theta=\left(2n\pi+\frac{\pi}{2}\right)=\alpha(\text{say}),\quad f'(\alpha)=-\frac{1}{8}$

9. $\theta=\left(2n\pi+\frac{\pi}{2}\right)=\alpha(\text{say}),\quad f'(\alpha)=-\frac{1}{4}$

10. $\theta=2n\pi=\alpha,\quad f'(\alpha)=\frac{1}{2a}$

11. $\theta=\left(n\pi+\frac{\pi}{2}\right)=\alpha,\quad f'(\alpha)=\frac{-1}{a}$

12. $\theta=\frac{-\pi}{6}=\alpha,\quad f'(\alpha)=\frac{\sqrt{3}}{2}$

13. $\theta=n\pi=\alpha,\quad f'(\alpha)=\frac{1}{2}\left(\frac{\cos n\pi}{n\pi}\right)$

ANSWERS

1. $x=\pm\pi/2, \pm 3\pi/2\ldots$ **2.** $r\sin\theta=a$ **3.** $r\sin\theta=\pm\frac{1}{2}a, r\cos\theta=\pm\frac{1}{2}a$

4. $r\sin\theta=2$ **5.** $r\sin\theta=\pm 2$ **6.** $r\sin\theta=a, r\cos\theta=\frac{a}{\left(k+\frac{1}{2}\right)\pi}$, k is any integer

7. $r\sin\left(\theta-\frac{\pi}{3}\right)=\frac{2a}{\sqrt{3}}, r\sin\left(\theta+\frac{\pi}{3}\right)=-\frac{2a}{\sqrt{3}}$ **8.** $r\cos\theta=8$ **9.** $r\cos\theta=4$

10. $r\sin\theta=2a$ **11.** $r\cos\theta=\pm a$ **12.** $r\sin\left(\theta\pm\frac{\pi}{6}\right)=\frac{2}{\sqrt{3}}$ **13.** $r\sin\theta=2n\pi, n=\pm1,\pm2,\ldots$

❑❑❑❑❑❑

Chapter

15 Singular Points and Curve Tracing

15.1 INTRODUCTION

If P is any point on a curve and CD is any given line which does not passes through this point P. Then the curve is said to be concave at P with respect to the line CD if the small arc of the curve containing P lies entirely within the acute angle between the tangent at P to the curve and the line CD and the curve is said to be convex at P if the arc of the curve containing P lies wholly outside the acute angle between that tangent at P and the line CD which are shown in figures below :

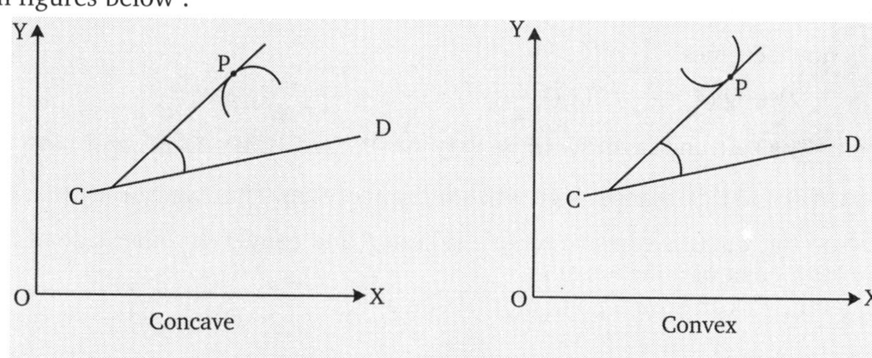

Fig. 1.

15.2 POINT OF INFLEXION

A point P on the curve is said to be the point of inflexion, if the curve in one side of P is concave and other side of P is convex with respect to the line CD which does not passes through the point P as shown in fig. 2.

15.2.1 Inflexion Tangent

The tangent at the point of inflexion of a curve is said to be inflexion tangent. In the fig. 2 the line PQ is the inflexion tangent.

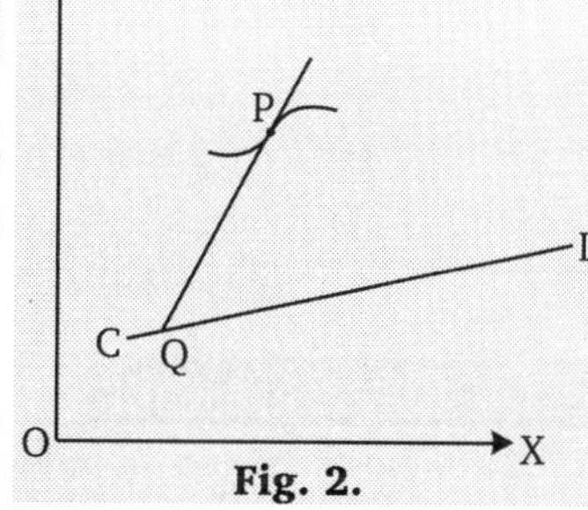

Fig. 2.

15.3 DETERMINATION OF THE POINTS OF INFLEXION

Let $y = f(x)$ be the equation of a curve and let $P(x, y)$ be any point on the curve and assuming that the tangent at P is not parallel to y-axis as shown in fig. 3.

Since the tangent is taken not to be parallel to y-axis, then $\frac{dy}{dx} = f'(x)$ must be finite. Let $Q(x + h, y + k)$ be any point on the curve in the neighbourhood of P. We may take this point

Q either side of P. Suppose the ordinate OM of Q intersects the tangent line at Q'.

$$Y - y = f'(x)(X - x) \qquad \ldots(1)$$

Since at point $Q(x + h, x + k)$ we have $X = x + h$ so putting $X = x + h$ in (1), we get

$$Q'M - y = f'(x)(x + h - x) \qquad [\because Y = Q'M]$$

or $$Q'M = y + hf'(x)$$

or $$Q'M = f(x) + hf'(x). \qquad [\because y = f(x)]$$

But we know that

$$QM = f(x+h) = f(x) + hf'(x) + \frac{h^2}{2!}f''(x) + \frac{h^3}{3!}f'''(x) + \ldots$$

(Using Taylor's theorem)

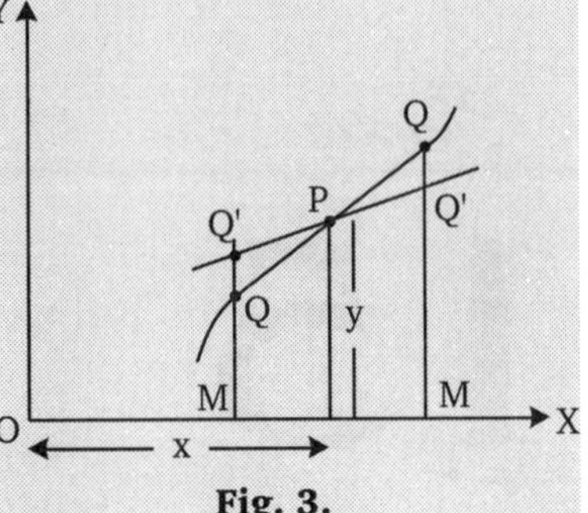

Fig. 3.

$$\therefore \quad QM - Q'M = \frac{h^2}{2!}f''(x) + \frac{h^3}{3!}f'''(x) + \ldots + \frac{h^n}{n!}f^{(n)}(x + \theta h) \text{ where } 0<\theta<1. \qquad \ldots(2)$$

Let us suppose $f''(x) \neq 0$ and taking h sufficiently small, then $(QM - Q'M)$ will have the same sign as $\frac{h^2}{2!}f''(x)$. But $\frac{h^2}{2!}f''(x)$ will have invariable sign because h^2 will always be positive. This means that on both sides of P the curve will be either concave or convex. Hence, we can say that the necessary condition for the existence of a point of inflexion at P is given by

$$f''(x) = 0 \text{ or } \frac{d^2y}{dx^2} = 0.$$

Thus (2) now becomes

$$QM - Q'M = \frac{h^3}{3!}f'''(x) + \frac{h^4}{4!}f^{iv}(x) + \ldots + \frac{h^n}{n!}f^{(n)}(x + \theta h) \qquad \ldots(3)$$

Further, if $f'''(x) \neq 0$ and taking h to be very small, then $(QM - Q'M)$ will have the same sign as $\frac{h^3}{3!}f'''(x)$ and this changes sign when h changes sign. Thus we can say that the curve with respect to the x-axis is concave on one side of P and convex on other side of P. Hence, there will exist a point of inflexion at P.

Consequently, we can have a point of inflexion at P, if $\frac{d^2y}{dx^2} = 0$ but $\frac{d^3y}{dx^3} \neq 0$.

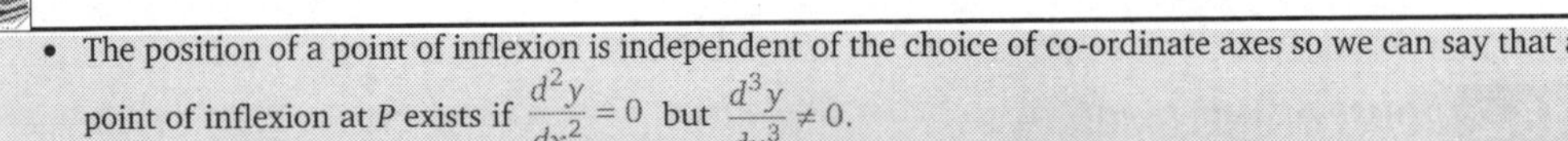

- The position of a point of inflexion is independent of the choice of co-ordinate axes so we can say that a point of inflexion at P exists if $\frac{d^2y}{dx^2} = 0$ but $\frac{d^3y}{dx^3} \neq 0$.
- If $f''(x) = 0 = f'''(x) = \ldots = f^{(n-1)}(x)$ and $f^{(n)}(x) \neq 0$, then there will be a point of inflexion if n is odd and if n is even and greater than 2, then the point is called point of undulation.
- If the tangent at P is parallel to y-axis, then $\frac{dy}{dx}$ will be infinite at P so change the curve to the form $x = f(y)$ and then find the point of inflexion.

Solved Examples

1. *Find the points of inflexion of the curve* $x = (\log y)^3$.

SOLUTION. The equation of the curve is

$$x = (\log y)^3 \qquad \ldots(1)$$

Differentiating (1) with respect to 'y', we get

$$\frac{dx}{dy} = 3(\log y)^2 . \frac{1}{y}$$

Again differentiating *w.r.t.* y

$$\frac{d^2x}{dy^2} = 3\left[\frac{2\log y}{y^2} - \frac{(\log y)^2}{y^2}\right]. \qquad \ldots(2)$$

Again differentiating w.r.t. 'y', we get

$$\frac{d^3x}{dy^3} = 3\left[\frac{2}{y^3} - \frac{4\log y}{y^3} - \frac{2\log y}{y^3} - \frac{2(\log y)^2}{y^2}\right]. \qquad \ldots(3)$$

For the point of inflexion, we have

$$\frac{d^2x}{dy^2} = 0.$$

$$\therefore \quad 3\left[\frac{2\log y - (\log y)^2}{y^2}\right] = 0$$

or $\quad 3(\log y)(2 - \log y) = 0$

or $\quad \log y = 0, \log y = 2$

or $\quad y = 1, y = e^2$

From (3) it is obvious that at $y = 1$, $y = e^2$, $\dfrac{d^3x}{dy^3} \neq 0.$

Hence, the points of inflexion are (0, 1) (8, e^2).

2. *Find the points of inflexion of the curve*

$$y^2 = x(x + 1)^2.$$

SOLUTION. The equation of the curve can be written as $y = (x+1)\sqrt{x}$. ...(1)

Differentiating (1) w.r.t. 'x', we get

$$\frac{dy}{dx} = \frac{3}{2}.x^{1/2} + \frac{1}{2\sqrt{x}}.$$

Again differentiating w.r.t. 'x'

$$\frac{d^2y}{dx^2} = \frac{3}{4\sqrt{x}} - \frac{1}{4x^{3/2}}. \quad ...(2)$$

and again differentiating w.r.t. 'x', we get

$$\frac{d^3y}{dx^3} = -\frac{3}{8x^{3/2}} + \frac{3}{8x^{5/2}}. \quad ...(3)$$

For the point of inflexion, we have

$$\frac{d^2y}{dx^2} = 0.$$

$$\therefore \quad \frac{3}{4\sqrt{x}} - \frac{1}{4x\sqrt{x}} = 0$$

or $\quad \left(3 - \dfrac{1}{x}\right) = 0 \quad$ or $x = 1/3$.

From (3) it is obvious that at $x = 1/3$,

$$\frac{d^3y}{dx^3} \neq 0.$$

Thus, the point of inflexion are given by $(1/3, \pm 4/3\sqrt{3})$.

Exercise-15.1

1. Find the points of inflexion of the curve $x = \log(y/x)$.
2. Find the points of inflexion of the curve $y(a^2 + x^2) = x^3$.
3. Find the points of inflexion of the curve $y = (x-1)^4(x-2)^3$.
4. Find the points of inflexion of the curve $xy = a^2\log(y/a)$.
5. Show that the points of inflexion of the curve
$$y^2 = (x-a)^2(x-b)$$
lie on the line $3x + a = 4b$.
6. Show that the origin is a point of inflexion of the curve $a^{m-1}.y = x^m$, if m is odd and greater than 2.
7. Show that the points of inflexion of the curve $x^2y = a^2(x - y)$ are given by $x = 0, x = \pm a\sqrt{3}$.
8. Prove that the curve $y = (1 - x)/(1 + x^2)$ has three points of inflexion which lie on a straight line.
9. Show that the abscissae of the points of inflexion on the curve $y^2 = f(x)$ satisfy the equation $[f'(x)]^2 = 2f(x)f''(x)$.
10. Show that the points of inflexion on the curve $y = be^{-(x/a)^2}$ are given by $x = \pm a/\sqrt{2}$.
11. Find the points of inflexion on the curve $r(\theta^2 - 1) = a\theta^2$.
12. Show that the points of inflexion of the curve $r = b\theta^n$ are given by $r = b\{-n(n+1)\}^{n/2}$.
13. Find the points of inflexion of the curve
$$x = a(2\theta - \sin\theta), y = a(2 - \cos\theta).$$
14. Find the points of inflexion of the curve $y = 3x^4 - 4x^3 + 1$.

Hints to the Selected Problems

1. Given that $x = \log\left(\dfrac{y}{x}\right) \Rightarrow y = xe^x$

$$\Rightarrow \frac{dy}{dx} = xe^x + e^x, \frac{d^2y}{dx^2} = xe^x + 2e^x$$

and $\quad \dfrac{d^3y}{dx^3} = xe^x + 3e^x$

For the point of inflexion, putting $\dfrac{d^2y}{dx^2} = 0$ and $\dfrac{d^3y}{dx^3} \neq 0$.

5. $y = (x-a)\sqrt{x-b}$

$$\Rightarrow \frac{dy}{dx} = \frac{3x - a - 2b}{2\sqrt{x-b}} \text{ and } \frac{d^2y}{dx^2} = \frac{3x + a - 4b}{4(x-b)^{3/2}}$$

Also, $\dfrac{d^3y}{dx^3} = \dfrac{-3x-3a+6b}{4(x-b)^{5/2}}$

By putting $\dfrac{d^2y}{dx^2} = 0$, we get $3x + a = 4b$ at which $\dfrac{d^3y}{dx^3} \neq 0$.

9. $y^2 = f(x) \Rightarrow \dfrac{dy}{dx} = \dfrac{f'(x)}{2y} = \dfrac{f'(x)}{2\sqrt{f(x)}}$

$$\frac{d^2y}{dx^2} = \frac{2f(x).f''(x)-[f'(x)]^2}{4[f(x)]^{3/2}}$$

and $$\frac{d^3y}{dx^3} = \frac{4[f(x)]^2.f'''(x)-6f(x)f'(x)f''(x) + 3[f'(x)]^3}{8[f(x)]^{5/2}}.$$

For point of inflexion, put $\dfrac{d^2y}{dx^2} = 0$.

11. Given that $r(\theta^2-1) = a\theta^2$

$\Rightarrow \dfrac{dr}{d\theta} = -\dfrac{2a\theta}{(\theta^2-1)^2}$ and $\dfrac{d^2r}{d\theta^2} = \dfrac{2a(1+3\theta^2)}{(\theta^2-1)^3}$.

At the point of inflexion, use

$$r^2 + 2\left(\frac{dr}{d\theta}\right)^2 - r\frac{d^2r}{d\theta^2} = 0.$$

ANSWERS

1. $(-2, -2/e^2)$ **2.** $(0,0), \left(\sqrt{3}a, \dfrac{3\sqrt{3}}{4}a\right), \left(-\sqrt{3}a, \dfrac{-3\sqrt{3}}{4}a\right)$

3. Point of inflection at $x = 2$, $(11 \pm \sqrt{2})/7$ **4.** $\left(\dfrac{3}{2}ae^{-3/2}, ae^{3/2}\right)$ **11.** $\theta = \pm\sqrt{3}$

13. $\left[\left(4n\pi \pm \dfrac{2\pi}{3} \mp \dfrac{\sqrt{3}}{2}\right)a, \dfrac{3a}{2}\right]$ **14.** $\left(\dfrac{2}{3}, \dfrac{11}{27}\right), (0,1)$

15.4 MULTIPLE AND SINGULAR POINTS

Definition 1. *A point on the curve is said to be multiple point if through this point more than one branches of a curve passes.*

Definition 2. *A point on the curve is called a double point if through it two branches of the curve passes.*

Definition 3. *If three branches of the curve passes through a point, then this point is called triple point.*

Definition 4. *If n branches passes through a point on the curve, then this point is called a multiple point of nth order.*

Definition 5. *The points of inflexion and multiple points are also called the singular points. Or An unusual point on the curve is basically called a singular point.*

15.5 TYPES OF DOUBLE POINT

15.5.1 NODE

A double point on a curve is said to be a node, if through this double point two branches of the curve passes which are real and having two different tangents at that point (Fig. 4).

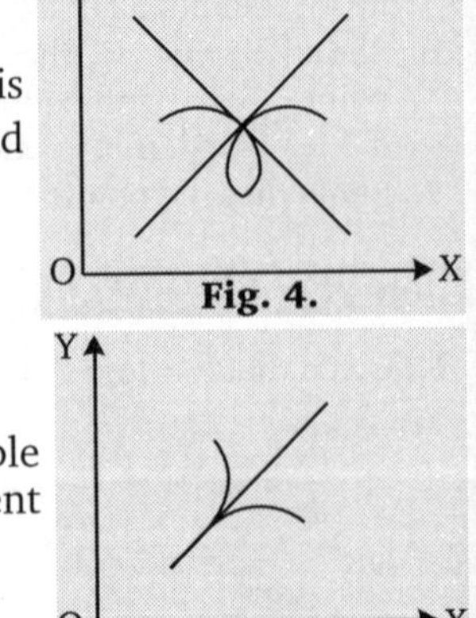

Fig. 4.

Fig. 5.

15.5.2 CUSP

A double point on a curve is called a cusp if through this double point two real branches of the curve passes and have real coincident tangents at that point (Fig. 5).

15.5.3 CONJUGATE POINT

A point P on the curve is said to be conjugate point if there are no real points on the curve in the neighbourhood of that point and having no real tangent at that point (Fig. 6).

Fig. 6.

15.6 SPECIES OF CUSP

Definition. *A cusp is said to be single if the curve lies entirely on one side of the common tangent* (Fig. 7(ii)).

Definition. *A cusp is said to be double if the curve lies on both sides of the common tangent* (Fig. 7(i)).

Definition. *A cusp is said to be of first species if the two branches of the curve lie on opposite sides of common tangent* (Fig. 7(iii)).

Definition. *A cusp is said to be of second species if the two branches of the curve lie on same side of the common tangent* (Fig. 7(ii)).

There are five different types of cusp :

(i) Single cusp of first species
(ii) Single cusp of second species
(iii) Double cusp of first species
(iv) Double cusp of second species
(v) Double cusp with change of species.

These all five types of cusp are shown below respectively :

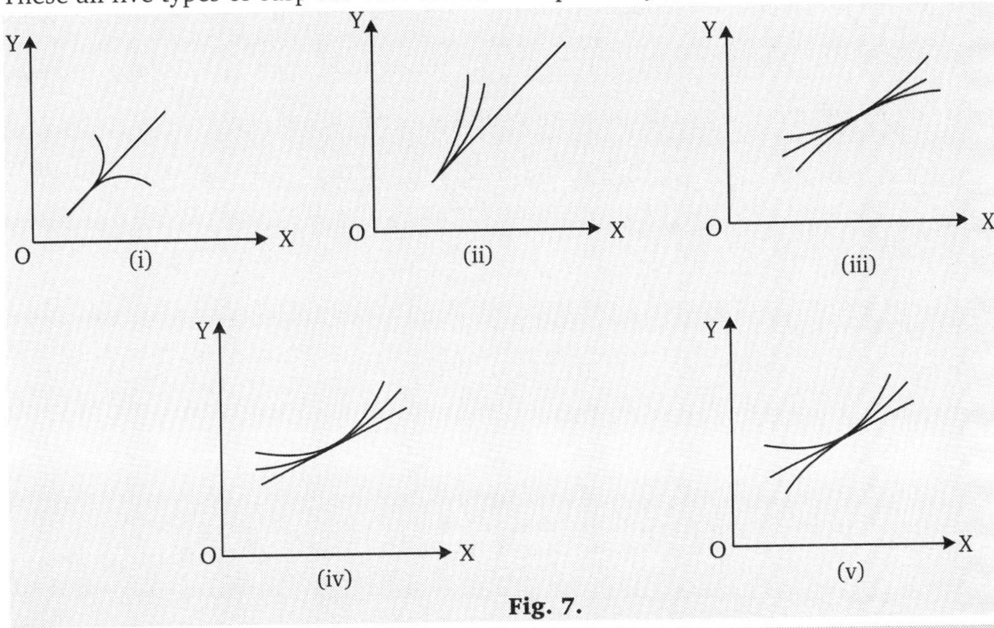

Fig. 7.

15.7 TANGENTS AT THE ORIGIN

The nature of a double point depends on the tangents so we find the tangent or tangents there. If a curve passes through the origin, then the equation of the tangent or tangents at the origin are obtained by equating to zero the lowest degree terms in the equation of the curve.

15.8 CHANGE OF ORIGIN (SHIFT OF ORIGIN)

Let $P(x, y)$ be any point with respect to the co-ordinate axes OX and OY and let $O'(h, k)$ be any other point with respect to the same co-ordinate system with origin O'.

Now draw $O'X$ and $O'Y$ parallel to the OX and OY axis respectively through $O'(h, k)$ and let co-ordinates of P with respect to the axes OX and OY be (X, Y). Then

$$M'P = PM - M'M.$$

$\therefore$ $$Y = y - k \text{ or } y = Y + k$$

and $$N'P = PN - NN'.$$

$\therefore$ $$X = x - h \text{ or } x = X + h.$$

Thus using the transformations $x = X + h$, and $y = Y + k$, the origin O is shifted to $O'(h, k)$.

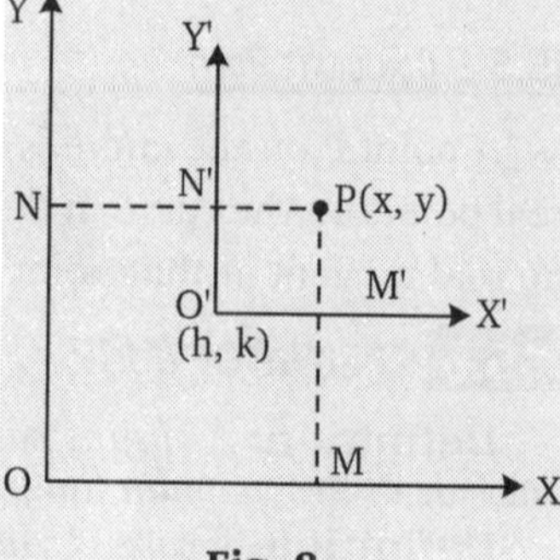

Fig. 8.

15.9 TANGENT AT THE POINT (h, k) TO A CURVE

In order to find the tangent at (h, k) to the given curve, we first shift the origin at (h, k) and then find the tangent at the origin to the transformed curve by equating to zero the lowest degree terms.

15.10 POSITION AND NATURE OF DOUBLE POINTS

Let $P(x, y)$ be any point on the curve $f(x, y) = 0$, we have

$$\frac{dy}{dx} = -\frac{\partial f/\partial x}{\partial f/\partial y} \quad \text{or} \quad \frac{\partial f}{\partial x} + \frac{\partial f}{\partial y}\frac{dy}{dx} = 0. \qquad \ldots(1)$$

Therefore, the slope of the tangent at $P(x, y)$ is equal to dy/dx which is given above.

Since by the definition of a multiple point we know that the curve has atleast two tangents so $\frac{dy}{dx}$ has atleast two values at a multiple point. But the equation (1) is of first degree in dy/dx. Therefore dy/dx will have two values or more than one value, if and only if

$$\frac{\partial f}{\partial x} = 0, \frac{\partial f}{\partial y} = 0$$

Thus the necessary and sufficient condition for any point of the curve $f(x, y) = 0$ to be a multiple point are that $\frac{\partial f}{\partial x} = 0 = \frac{\partial f}{\partial y}$.

Hence, to find the multiple point of the curve $f(x, y) = 0$ we shall simultaneously solve the following equations

$$f(x,y) = 0, \frac{\partial f}{\partial x} = 0, \frac{\partial f}{\partial y} = 0.$$

Next, differentiating (1) w.r.t. 'x', we get

$$\frac{d}{dx}\left(\frac{\partial f}{\partial x}\right) + \frac{d}{dx}\left(\frac{\partial f}{\partial y}\cdot\frac{dy}{dx}\right) = 0$$

$$\frac{\partial}{\partial x}\left(\frac{\partial f}{\partial x}\right) + \frac{\partial}{\partial y}\left(\frac{\partial f}{\partial x}\right)\frac{dy}{dx} + \frac{d}{dx}\left(\frac{\partial f}{\partial y}\right)\frac{dy}{dx} + \frac{\partial f}{\partial y}\cdot\frac{d^2y}{dx^2} = 0$$

or $$\frac{\partial^2 f}{\partial x^2} + \frac{\partial}{\partial y}\left(\frac{\partial f}{\partial x}\right)\frac{dy}{dx} + \left[\frac{\partial}{\partial x}\left(\frac{\partial f}{\partial y}\right) + \frac{\partial}{\partial y}\left(\frac{\partial f}{\partial y}\right)\cdot\frac{dy}{dx}\right]\frac{dy}{dx} + \frac{\partial f}{\partial y}\cdot\frac{d^2y}{dx^2} = 0.$$

Since at the multiple point $\frac{\partial f}{\partial y} = 0$. Therefore, $\frac{\partial^2 f}{\partial x^2} + \frac{\partial^2 f}{\partial y\partial x}\cdot\frac{dy}{dx} + \frac{\partial^2 f}{\partial x\partial y}\frac{dy}{dx} + \frac{\partial^2 f}{\partial y^2}\left(\frac{dy}{dx}\right)^2 = 0$

or $$\frac{\partial^2 f}{\partial x^2} + 2\frac{\partial^2 f}{\partial x\partial y}\frac{dy}{dx} + \frac{\partial^2 f}{\partial y^2}\left(\frac{dy}{dx}\right)^2 = 0 \qquad \ldots(2)$$

$$\left(\because \frac{\partial^2 f}{\partial x\partial y} = \frac{\partial^2 f}{\partial y\partial x}\right)$$

This is a quadratic equation in $\frac{dy}{dx}$ and the multiple point will be double point if the equation (2) will remain quadratic in $\frac{dy}{dx}$, and for the quadratic in $\frac{dy}{dx}$ it is assumed that $\frac{\partial^2 f}{\partial x^2}, \frac{\partial^2 f}{\partial x \partial y}, \frac{\partial^2 f}{\partial y^2}$ are not all zero. From the equation (2) it is obvious that the two values of dy/dx will be real and distinct, coincident, or imaginary according as

$$\left[\left(\frac{\partial^2 f}{\partial x \partial y}\right)^2 - \frac{\partial^2 f}{\partial x^2}\frac{\partial^2 f}{\partial y^2}\right] >, = \text{or} < 0.$$

Therefore, the two tangents will be real and distinct, coincident or imaginary according as

$$\left[\left(\frac{\partial^2 f}{\partial x \partial y}\right)^2 - \frac{\partial^2 f}{\partial x^2}\frac{\partial^2 f}{\partial y^2}\right] >, = \text{or} < 0.$$

Hence we obtained that the double point will be node, cusp or conjugate point according as

$$\left(\frac{\partial^2 f}{\partial x \partial y}\right)^2 > \text{or} = \text{or} < \frac{\partial^2 f}{\partial x^2} \cdot \frac{\partial^2 f}{\partial y^2}.$$

- If $\frac{\partial^2 f}{\partial x^2}, \frac{\partial^2 f}{\partial x \partial y}, \frac{\partial^2 f}{\partial y^2}$ are all zero, then the point $P(x, y)$ will be a multiple point of order greater than two.

15.11 NATURE OF A CUSP AT THE ORIGIN

Let (0, 0) be a cusp of the curve. Then there will be two coincident tangents at (0, 0). Therefore, the curve will be of the form

$$(ax + by)^2 + \text{terms of degree greater then two} = 0 \quad ...(1)$$

Thus the common tangent to the curve (1) at the origin is

$$ax + by = 0. \quad ...(2)$$

Let us suppose p is perpendicular from any point $P(x, y)$ to the equation (2), then

$$p = \frac{ax + by}{\sqrt{a^2 + b^2}} \quad ...(3)$$

where $P(x, y)$ is any point in the neighbourhood of (0,0).

From the equation (3) it is obvious that p is proportional to $ax + by$ so let us take

$$p = ax + by. \quad ...(4)$$

Now eliminating either x or y between (1) and (4), we get the equation involving p and x. Since p is small and there are two branches of the curve passes through the origin, therefore, neglecting all those terms having the degree of p greater than two. Thus we obtain a quadratic in p of the form

$$Ap^2 + Bp + C = 0 \quad ...(5)$$

where A, B, C are the functions of x only.

Now solving (5), we get $p = -\frac{B \pm \sqrt{(B^2 - 4AC)}}{2A}$ also $p_1 p_2 = C/A$

where p_1 and p_2 are the roots of (5).

Now there arises following cases :

Case I. If for all numerically small values of x either negative or positive, the values of p obtained from (5) are imaginary, then the origin will be a conjugate point.

Case II. If the values of p are real for all numerically small values of x, then there will be a double cusp at origin.

Case III. If the reality of p depends on the sign of x, then origin will be a single cusp.

Case IV. If p is real for numerically small values of x and if $p_1p_2 > 0$, then p_1 and p_2 will have same sign. Therefore the origin will be a cusp of second species because the two perpendiculars p_1 and p_2 lie on the same side of the common tangent. On the other hand if $p_1p_2 < 0$,then p_1 and p_2 are of opposite signs. Then the origin will be a cusp of the first species because the two perpendicular line on the opposite sides of the common tangent.

15.12 NATURE OF A CUSP AT ANY POINT

In order to find the nature of the cusp at any point (h, k). We first shift the origin at (h, k) and then apply above process discussed in § 15.11.

Solved Examples

1. *Show that the origin is a node on the curve $x^3 + y^3 - 3axy = 0$.*

SOLUTION. The tangent at the origin are obtained by equating to zero the lowest degree terms *i.e.*, second degree term in the given equation of the curve.

$\therefore \quad -3axy = 0$ or $x = 0, y = 0$.

Thus at the origin there are two real and distinct tangents. Hence (0, 0) is a node.

2. *Find the double point of the curve $(x-2)^2 = y(y-1)^2$.*

SOLUTION. Let $f(x, y) \equiv (x-2)^2 - y(y-1)^2 = 0 \quad \ldots(1)$

Differentiating (1) partially w.r.t. x and y, we get

$$\frac{\partial f}{\partial x} = 2(x-2) \quad \ldots(2)$$

and $$\frac{\partial f}{\partial y} = -(y-1)^2 - 2y(y-1). \quad \ldots(3)$$

Since the necessary and sufficient condition for a double points are

$$\frac{\partial f}{\partial x} = 0, \frac{\partial f}{\partial y} = 0, \Rightarrow 2(x-2) = 0 \quad \ldots(4)$$

$$-(y-1)^2 - 2y(y-1) = 0. \quad \ldots(5)$$

Now solving $f(x, y) = 0$, $\frac{\partial f}{\partial x} = 0$ and $\frac{\partial f}{\partial y} = 0$ simultaneously.

From (4), we get $x = 2$ and from (5), we get

$$-(y-1)(y-1+2y) = 0$$

or $-(y-1)(3y-1) = 0$ or $y = 1$ and $y = 1/3$.

$\therefore$ Possible double points are (2, 1) and (2, 1/3)

But (2, 1/3) does not satisfy $f(x, y) = 0$.

Hence only double point is (2, 1).

3. *Examine the nature of the origin on the following curve : $y^2 = a^2x^2 + bx^3 + cxy^2$.*

SOLUTION. The given curve is

$$f(x, y) \equiv y^2 - a^2x^2 - bx^3 - cxy^2 = 0. \quad \ldots(1)$$

Equating to zero the lowest degree terms in the equtaion of curve (1), we get $y^2 - a^2x^2 = 0$ or $y = \pm ax$.

Thus we have obtained two real and distinct tangents at (0, 0). Hence (0, 0) is a node.

4. *Find the position and nature of the double points on the curve $x^2y^2 = (a+y)^2(b^2 - y^2)$ if*

(i) $b > a$ *(ii)* $b = a$ *(iii)* $b < a$.

SOLUTION. Let $f(x, y) \equiv x^2y^2 - (a+y)^2(b^2 - y^2) = 0. \quad \ldots(1)$

Differentiating (1) partially w.r.t. 'x' and 'y' respectively, we get

$$\frac{\partial f}{\partial x} = 2xy^2 \quad \ldots(2)$$

and

$$\frac{\partial f}{\partial y} = 2x^2y - 2(a+y)(b^2-y^2) + 2y(a+y)^2. \quad \ldots(3)$$

Again differentiating, we get

$$\frac{\partial^2 f}{\partial x^2} = 2y^2 \; ; \; \frac{\partial^2 f}{\partial x \partial y} = 4xy$$

and $$\frac{\partial^2 f}{\partial y^2} = 2x^2 - 2(b^2 - y^2) + 4(a+y)y + 2(a+y)^2 + 4y(a+y)$$

For double point, we have

$$\frac{\partial f}{\partial x}=0,\frac{\partial f}{\partial y}=0,\therefore 2xy^2=0 \qquad \ldots(4)$$

$$2x^2y-2(a+y)(b^2-y^2)+2y(a+y)^2=0 \qquad \ldots(5)$$

From (4) we get $x = 0, y = 0$
From (5) and $x = 0$, we get

$$2(a + y)[-(b^2 - y^2) + y(a + y)] = 0$$

or $\quad 2(a+y)(2y^2+ay-b^2)=0$

or $y = -a$ and $y=\dfrac{-a\pm\sqrt{(a^2+8b^2)}}{4}$

Thus we obtain $(0, -a)$ and $\left(0,\dfrac{-a\pm\sqrt{(a^2+8b^2)}}{4}\right)$ and from (5), we get two points.

Hence, $(0, -a)$ and $\left(0,\dfrac{-a\pm\sqrt{(a^2+8b^2)}}{4}\right)$ are possible double points. But only $(0, -a)$ satisfies the equation $f(x, y) = 0$. Hence, $(0, -a)$ is only the double point.

$$\left(\frac{\partial^2 f}{\partial x^2}\right)_{(0,-a)}=(2y^2)_{(0,-a)}=2a^2$$

$$\left(\frac{\partial^2 f}{\partial x\partial y}\right)_{(0,-a)}=(4xy)_{(0,-a)}=0$$

$$\left(\frac{\partial^2 f}{\partial y^2}\right)_{(0,-a)}$$

$$=[2x^2-2(b^2-y^2)+4y(a+y)+2(a+y)^2+4y(a+y)]_{(0,-a)}$$

$$=2(a^2-b^2)$$

Then $\left(\dfrac{\partial^2 f}{\partial x\partial y}\right)^2-\dfrac{\partial^2 f}{\partial x^2}\cdot\dfrac{\partial^2 f}{\partial y^2}$

$$=0-2a^2[2(a^2-b^2)]$$

$$=+4a^2(b^2-a^2).$$

(i) If $b>a$, then $\left(\dfrac{\partial^2 f}{\partial x\partial y}\right)^2>\dfrac{\partial^2 f}{\partial x^2}\cdot\dfrac{\partial^2 f}{\partial y^2}$

and thus $(0, -a)$ is a node.

(ii) If $b = a$, then $\left(\dfrac{\partial^2 f}{\partial x\partial y}\right)^2=\dfrac{\partial^2 f}{\partial x^2}\cdot\dfrac{\partial^2 f}{\partial y^2}$

and thus $(0, -a)$ is a cusp.

(iii) If $b< a$, then $\left(\dfrac{\partial^2 f}{\partial x\partial y}\right)^2<\dfrac{\partial^2 f}{\partial x^2}\cdot\dfrac{\partial^2 f}{\partial y^2}$

and thus $(0, -a)$ is a conjugate point.

5. *Find the nature of origin on the curve* $x^4 + y^3 + 2x^2 + 3y^2 = 0$.

SOLUTION. Let $f(x, y) = x^4 + y^3 + 2x^2 + 3y^2 = 0$

Then $\dfrac{\partial f}{\partial x}=4x^3+4x,\ \dfrac{\partial f}{\partial y}=3y^2+6y$

$$\frac{\partial^2 f}{\partial x^2}=12x^2+4,\ \frac{\partial^2 f}{\partial y^2}=6y+6$$

and $\dfrac{\partial^2 f}{\partial x\partial y}=0.$

At $(0,0)$ $\dfrac{\partial^2 f}{\partial x^2}=4,\ \dfrac{\partial^2 f}{\partial y^2}=6,\ \dfrac{\partial^2 f}{\partial x\partial y}=0.$

$$\therefore \left(\frac{\partial^2 f}{\partial x\partial y}\right)^2=0<\left(\frac{\partial^2 f}{\partial x^2}\right)\left(\frac{\partial^2 f}{\partial y^2}\right).$$

Hence, the origin is a conjugate point.

Exercise-15.2

1. Find the equation of the tangents at the origin to the following curves :
   (a) $(x^2 + y^2)(2a - x) = b^2x$
   (b) $a^4y^2 = x^4(x^2 - a^2)$
   (c) $x^4 + 3x^3y + 2xy - y^2 = 0$
   (d) $x^3 + y^3 = 3axy$
2. Examine the nature of the origin on the curve $(2x + y)^2 - 6xy(2x + y) - 7x^3 = 0$.
3. Show that the origin is a conjugate point on the curve $a^2x^2 + b^2y^2 = (x^2 + y^2)^2$.
4. Show that the origin is a conjugate point on the curve $y^2 = 2x^2y + x^4y - 2x^4$.
5. Find the position and nature of double points of the curve $y^3 = x^3 + ax^2$.
6. Examine the nature of the double points of the curve $2(x^3 + y^3) - 3(3x^2 + y^2) + 12x = 4$.
7. Find the position and nature of the double points of the curve $a^4y^2 = x^4(2x^2 - 3a^2)$.
8. Find the position and nature of the double points of the curve $x^4 - 2y^3 - 3y^2 - 2x^2 + 1 = 0$.
9. Determine the existence and nature of the double points on the curve $y^2 = (x - 2)^2(x - 1)$.

10. Prove that the curve $ay^2 = (x - a)^2(x - b)$ has at $x = a$, a conjugate point if $a < b$, a node if $a > b$ and a cusp if $a = b$.

11. Examine the curve $x^3 + 2x^2 + 2xy - y^2 + 5x - 2y = 0$ for singular points and show that it has a cusp of the first kind at the point $(-1, -2)$.

12. Show that the curve $y^2 = bx \tan(x/a)$ has a node or a conjugate point at the origin according as a and b have like or unlike signs.

13. Determine the position and nature of the double points of the curves :

(a) $y(y-1)^2 = (x-2)^2$.

(b) $x^3 - y^2 - 7x^2 + 4y + 15x - 13 = 0$.

(c) $y^2 = x(x-a)^2, a > 0$ (d) $y^2 = x^2(a - x^2)$

(e) $y(y-6) = x^2(x-2)^3 - 9$.

14. Discuss the nature of the double points of the curve $(x + y)^3 - \sqrt{2}(y - x + 2)^2 = 0$.

15. Show that the origin is a conjugate point on the curve $x^4 - ax^2y + axy^2 + a^2y^2 = 0$.

16. Show that curve $(xy + 1)^2 + (x - 1)^3(x - 2) = 0$ has a single cusp of the first species at the point $(1, -1)$.

17. Show that the curve $y^3 = (x - a)^2(2x - a)$ has a single cusp of the first species at the point $(a, 0)$.

18. Find the nature and position of double points of the curve $a^4y^2 = x^4(a^2 - x^2)$.

ANSWERS

1. (a)$x = 0$(b)$y = 0, y = 0$ (c) $y = 0, 2x - y = 0$ (d) $x = 0, y = 0$
2. Origin is a single cusp of first species **5.** A cusp at (0, 0) **6.** Node at (2, 0)
7. Cusp at (0, 0) **8.** Double points (0, –1), (1, 0) and (–1, 0) are nodes
9. Node at (2, 0) **13.** (a) Node at (2, 1) (b) Node at (3, 2) (c) Node at $(a, 0)$ (d) Node at (0, 0) (e) Conjugate at (0, 3) and a single cusp of the first species at (2, 3)
14. A single cusp of first species at (–1, 1) **18.** Double cusp of the first species at (0, 0).

15.13 CURVE TRACING : CARTESIAN FORM

To trace any curve of cartesian form we should apply following procedure :

(a) Symmetricity. In order to find the symmetry of the curve we should apply following rules :

(i) If the powers of y in the equation of the curve are all even, then curve is symmetrical about x-axis.

(ii) If the powers of x in the equation of the curve are all even, then the curve is symmetrical about y-axis.

(iii) If the powers of x as well as y in the equation of the curve are all even, the curve is symmetrical about both axes.

(iv) If the equation of curve remains unchanged when x is replaced by $-x$ and y is replaced by $-y$, then the curve is symmetrical in opposite quadrants.

(v) If the equation of the curve remains unchanged when x and y are interchanged, then the curve is symmetrical about the line $y = x$.

(b) Nature of the origin on the curve. If the curve passes through the origin, then find the tangent at (0, 0) by equating to zero the lowest degree terms of the curve. If we obtain two tangent at the origin, then origin will be a double point and then find the nature of this double point.

(c) Intersection of curve with co-ordinate axes. We should check whether the curve cuts the co-ordinate axes or not, for this put $y = 0$ in the equation of the curve and find the values of x, then we get the points at which the curve cuts the x-axis. Similarly if the curve cuts the y-axis, then put $x = 0$ in the equation of the curve and obtain the points on the y-axis. Hence in this way we obtain the points of intersection of the curve with co-ordinate axis. Thereafter we should find the tangents at these points of intersection. For this first we shift the origin at these points and then obtain the tangent at these new origin by equating to zero the lowest degree terms in the new equation of the curve. On the other hand the value of dy/dx at these points of intersection can also be used to find the slope of the tangent at that point.

(d) Nature of y or x in the curve. We should now solve the equation of the curve either for y or for x whichever is convenient. Suppose we solve for y and see that nature of y as

x increases from 0 to $+\infty$. Similarly see the nature of y as x decreases from 0 to $-\infty$ and finally collect those values of x for which $y = 0$ or $y \to \infty$ or $-\infty$.

- If the curve is symmetrical about x-axis in opposite quadrants then there is no need to take the values of x of both positive and negative. We can take only positive values of x to see the variation in y.

(e) Regions in which curve does not exist. In order to find the regions where the curve does not exist we should solve the equation of curve for one variable in terms of the other. Therefore, the curve will not exist for those values of one variable which make the other variable imaginary.

(f) Asymptotes. Next, we should find all the asymptotes of the curve because the branches of the curve approach to the asymptotes if they exist.

(g) Sign of dy/dx. Next, we should find the value of dy/dx from the equation of the curve and find the points on the curve at which $dy/dx = 0$ or $dy/dx = \infty$. Therefore at these points we obtain the nature of tangents. Suppose in any region $a < x < b$, dy/dx remains positive throughout, then in this region y increase continuously as x increases. On the other hand if dy/dx remains negative, then y decreases continuously as x increases.

(h) Special points. If necessary, we should find the some special point on the curve.

(i) Points of inflexion. If necessary, we should find the point of inflexion to know the position of the curves at that point.

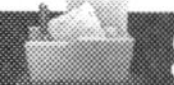

Solved Examples

1. *Trace the curve* $y^2(2a - x) = x^3$.

SOLUTION. (i) Obviously the given curve is symmetrical about x-axis.

(ii) The curve passes through the origin and the tangents at the origin are obtained by equating to zero the lowest degree terms *i.e.*, $2ay^2$ in the equation of the curve.

$\therefore\ 2ay^2 = 0$ or $y = 0, y = 0$.

Thus at the origin we obtained two coincident tangents $y = 0$, $y = 0$ *i.e.*, x-axis. Therefore (0, 0) is a cusp.

(iii) From the equation of the curve it is obvious that the curve does not cut the co-ordinate axes.

(iv) Now solving the equation of the curve for y, we get $y^2 = x^3/(2a - x)$ when $x = 0, y^2 = 0$ and when $x = 2a$, thus $y^2 \to \infty$ thus $x = 2a$ is an asymptote of the curve.

It is observed that y increases as x increases from 0 to $2a$.

(v) When x lies between 0 and $2a$, y^2 will be positive and the curve will exist in this region. When $x > 2a$, y^2 will be negative so the curve will not exist beyond the line $x = 2a$. When $x < 0$ again y^2 will be negative and thus the curve will also not exist for $x < 0$. Hence we can say that the curve only exists in the region $0 < x < 2a$.

(vi) In order to find the asymptotes, putting $y = m$ and $x = 1$ in the third degree terms in the equation of the curve, we get

$$\phi_3(m) = m^2 + 1.$$

Therefore the equation $\phi_3(m) = 0$ gives both its roots imaginary so ignore them. Consequently $x = 2a$ is only the asymptote of the curve.

(vii) Differentiating the equation of the curve

$$y = \frac{x^{3/2}}{\sqrt{(2a - x)}}$$

We get $\dfrac{dy}{dx} = \dfrac{(3a - x)x^{1/2}}{(2a - x)^{3/2}}$.

In the region $0 < x < 2a$, $\dfrac{dy}{dx}$ will be positive, so therefore in this region y increase continuously as x increases.

Now taking all above points of consideration in the mind and draw the curve whose shape is shown in fig. 9.

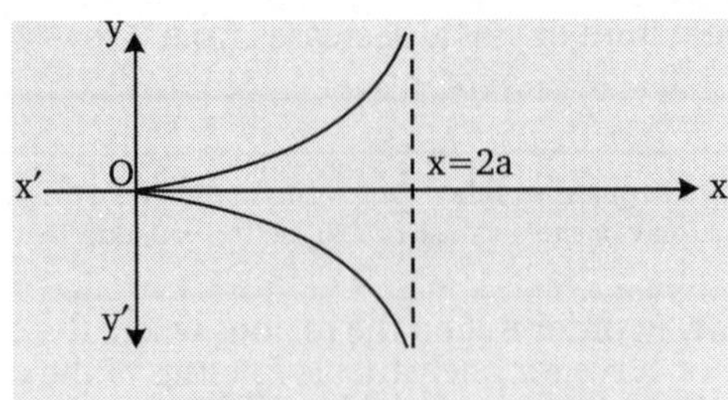

Fig. 9.

2. *Trace the curve* $y^2(1-x^2) = x^2(1+x^2)$.

SOLUTION. (i) In the equation of the curve the powers of both x and y are all even so the curve is symmetrical about both axes.

(ii) The curve passes through the origin. The tangents at the origin are obtained by equating to zero the lowest degree terms in the equation of the curve.

$\therefore \quad y^2 - x^2 = 0$ or $y = \pm x$.

Thus there are two real and distinct tangent at the origin so (0, 0) is a node.

(iii) From the equation of the curve it is clear that curve does not cut any co-ordinate axes.

(iv) Solving the equation of the curve for y, we get

$$y^2 = \frac{x^2(1+x^2)}{(1-x^2)}.$$

When $x = 0, y = 0$ and when $x = \pm 1$, $y \to \infty$ so $x = \pm 1$ are two asymptotes parallel to y-axis.

(v) When $-1 < x < 1$, y^2 is positive, so the curve exists in this region. When $x > 1$, y will be negative thus curve will not exist beyond the line $x = 1$. Also when $x < -1$, y^2 will be negative so that curve will not exist for $x < -1$.

(vi) In order to find the asymptotes, putting $y = m$ and $x = 1$ in the fourth degree terms of the curve, we get $\phi^4(m) = m^2 + 1$.

Solving $\phi^4(m) = 0$, we get both values of m imaginary so ignore them. Consequently $x = \pm 1$ are only two real asymptotes.

(vii) Since, we have

$$y = x\sqrt{\left(\frac{1+x^2}{1-x^2}\right)}.$$

$$\therefore \frac{dy}{dx} = \frac{\sqrt{1-x^2}\left(\sqrt{1+x^2}+\dfrac{x^2}{\sqrt{1+x^2}}\right) - x\sqrt{(1+x^2)}\left[\dfrac{-x}{\sqrt{1-x^2}}\right]}{(1-x^2)}$$

$$= \frac{(1-x^2)(1+x^2+x^2) - x(1+x^2)(-x)}{(1-x^2)^{3/2}(1+x^2)^{1/2}}$$

$$= \frac{2x^2+1-x^4}{(1-x^2)^{3/2}(1+x^2)^{1/2}}.$$

When $-1 < x < 0$, $\frac{dy}{dx}$ is negative this means that when x decreases from -1 to 0, y decreases. When $0 < x < 1$; $\frac{dy}{dx}$ is positive this implies that when x increases from 0 to 1, y increases.

Now taking all the above facts in mind and draw the shape of the curve we get the following figure:

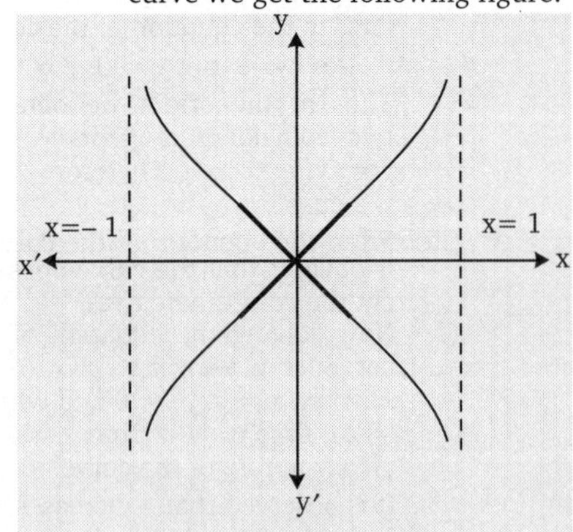

Fig. 10.

3. *Trace the curve* $ay^2 = x^2(a-x)$.

(SVTU–2004, KURUKSHETRA–2009)

SOLUTION. (i) The curve is symmetrical about x-axis because the powers of y are all even.

(ii) This curve passes through the origin. The tangents at the origin are obtained by equating to zero the lowest degree terms in the equation of the curve, we get $ay^2 - ax^2 = 0$ or $y = \pm x$.

Thus there are two real and distinct tangents at (0, 0). Therefore (0, 0) is a node.

(iii) The curve cuts the x-axis only at the point where $y = 0$.

$\therefore x^2(a - x) = 0$ or $x = 0, x = a$.

Thus the curve cuts the x-axis at $(a, 0)$.

Now $y = x\sqrt{\dfrac{a-x}{a}}$

$$\therefore \frac{dy}{dx} = \frac{1}{\sqrt{a}}\left[\sqrt{a-x} - \frac{x}{2\sqrt{a-x}}\right]$$

$$= \frac{2(a-x)-x}{2\sqrt{a(a-x)}} = \frac{2a-3x}{2\sqrt{a(a-x)}}.$$

At $(a, 0)$, $\dfrac{dy}{dx} = \infty$. Therefore the tangent at $(a, 0)$ is perpendicular to x-axis.

(iv) Since we have

$$y = x\sqrt{\frac{a-x}{a}}$$

when $x = 0$, $y^2 = 0$ and when $x = a$, y^2 also equals zero. Also when x increases from 0 to $a/2$ y increases and when x increases from $a/2$ to a, y decreases.

(v) When $0 < x < a$, y^2 is always positive so the curve will exist in this region. When $x < 0$, y^2 is also positive so that the curve will also exist for $x < 0$. When $x > a$, y^2 will be negative and therefore in this region the curve will not exist.

Taking all above facts into consideration and draw the shape of the curve we obtain as shown below.

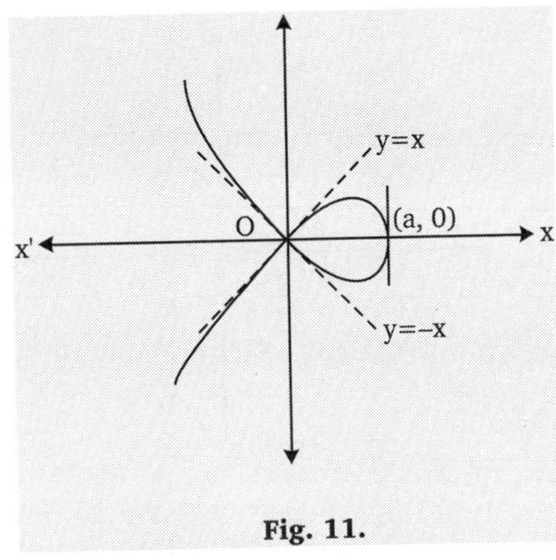

Fig. 11.

4. *Trace the curve* $x^3 + y^3 = 3axy$.

SOLUTION. (i) The given curve is symmetrical about the line $y = x$.

(ii) Curve is passing through the origin so the trangents at (0, 0) are $xy = 0 \Rightarrow x = 0$ and $y = 0$. Thus (0, 0) is a node.

(iii) The curve does not intersect the axes.

(iv) If x is replaced by $-x$ and that of y by $-y$, the equation of the curve is changed. Thus the curve does not exist in third quadrant.

(v) The given curve has only one real asymptote which is $x + y + a = 0$.

(vi) The curve cuts the line $y = x$ at the point $\left(\dfrac{3a}{2}, \dfrac{3a}{2}\right)$.

From the curve, $\dfrac{dy}{dx} = \dfrac{ay - x^2}{y^2 - ax}$.

so at $\left(\dfrac{3a}{2}, \dfrac{3a}{2}\right)$ $\dfrac{dy}{dx} = -1$

Thus, the tangent at $\left(\dfrac{3a}{2}, \dfrac{3a}{2}\right)$ makes an angle 135° with the positive axis of x.

Now taking all above facts into consideration and draw the curve, we get figure (12).

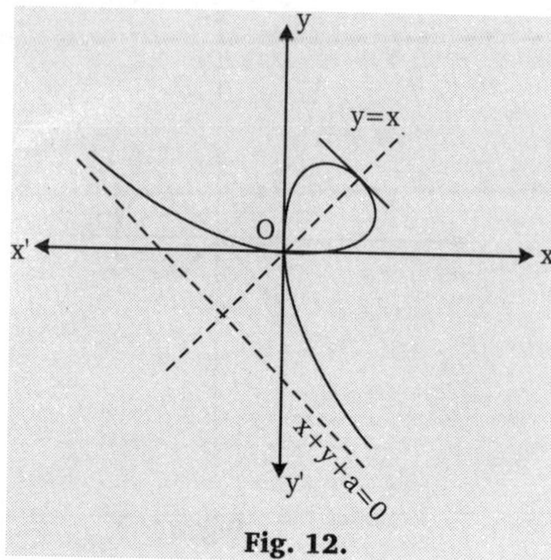

Fig. 12.

5. *Trace the curve* $y = 1 - \dfrac{1}{1+x^2}$.

SOLUTION. The given curve is

$$y = 1 - \frac{1}{1+x^2}. \qquad \ldots(1)$$

(i) Clearly, the curve is symmetric about y-axis.

(ii) The curve passes through the origin, because (0, 0) satisfies (1).

(iii) Tangent at origin is given by $y = 0$.

(iv) Asymptotes parallel to x-axis is $y - 1 = 0 \Rightarrow y = 1$.

(v) Clearly the given curve meets the axes only at the origin.

Special points

x	–2	–1	0	1	2
y	4/5	1/2	0	1/2	4/5

Now taking all the above facts in find, we draw the curve as in figure (13).

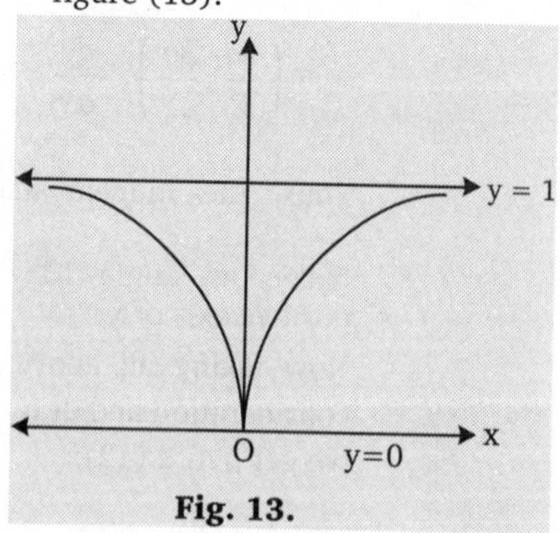

Fig. 13.

6. *Trace the curve* $x^{2/3} + y^{2/3} = a^{2/3}$.

SOLUTION. The given curve is $x^{2/3} + y^{2/3} = a^{2/3}$ ...(1)

(i) The curve is symmetric about both the axes. Also, the curve is symmetric about the line $y = x$ and $y = -x$.

(ii) The curve does not passes through the origin.

(iii) The curve meets x-axis at $(a, 0)$ and $(-a, 0)$. Also, the curve meets y-axis at $(0, a)$ and $(0, -a)$.

(iv) The curve has no asymptotes.

(v) From (1) $\dfrac{dy}{dx} = -\dfrac{y^{1/3}}{x^{1/3}}$

$\dfrac{dy}{dx} = 0$, when $y = 0$

Again from (1) $x = \pm a$, when $y = 0$

Thus, the tangents to the curve are parallel to x-axis at the points $(\pm a, 0)$. Further, $\dfrac{dy}{dx} \to 0$ when $x = 0$.

From (1) when $x = 0, y = \pm a$.

Therefore, the tangents to the curve are parallel to y-axis at the points $(0, \pm a)$

(vi) From (1) we can write $y^{2/3} = a^{2/3} - x^{2/3}$.

If $|x| > a, y^{2/3}$ is negative $\Rightarrow y^2$ is negative.

$\Rightarrow$ y is imaginary.

$\Rightarrow$ Curve does not lie beyond the lines $x = \pm a$.

Similarly, the curve does not lie beyond the lines $y = \pm a$.

Further, when $x = 0, y = a$. As x-increases from 0 to a, y decreases from a to 0.

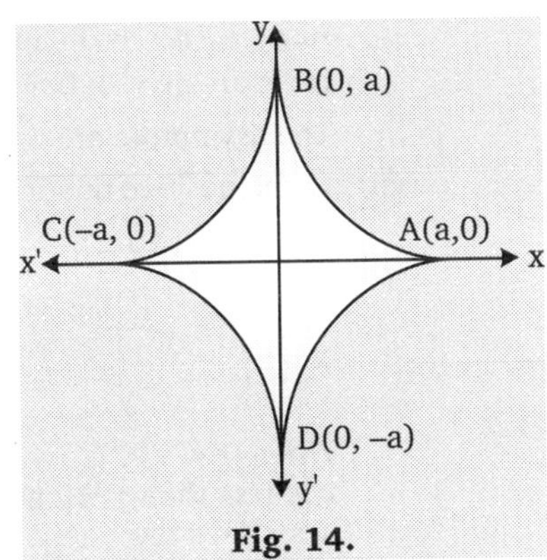

Fig. 14.

7. *Trace the curve* $y = x^3 - 12x - 16$.

(PTU–2008)

SOLUTION. (i) The curve has no symmetry.

(ii) The curve does not passes through the origin.

(iii) The curve has no asymptotes.

(iv) The curve cuts x-axis at (–2, 0), (4, 0) and y-axis at (0, –16).

(v) We have $\frac{dy}{dx} = 3x^2 - 12$.

At (–2, 0), $\frac{dy}{dx} = 0 \Rightarrow$ tangent is parallel to x-axis at (–2, 0)

At (4, 0), $\frac{dy}{dx} = 36 \Rightarrow$ tangent makes an acute angle $\tan^{-1}36$ with x-axis at (4, 0)

Also, $\frac{dy}{dx} = 0 \Rightarrow 3x^2 - 12 = 0$

$\Rightarrow x = \pm 2$

$\Rightarrow$ tangent is parallel to x-axis at (2, –32).

(vi) $y \to \infty$ as $x \to \infty$ and $y \to -\infty$ as $x \to -\infty$: y is positive for $x > 4$ and y is –ve for $x < 4$.

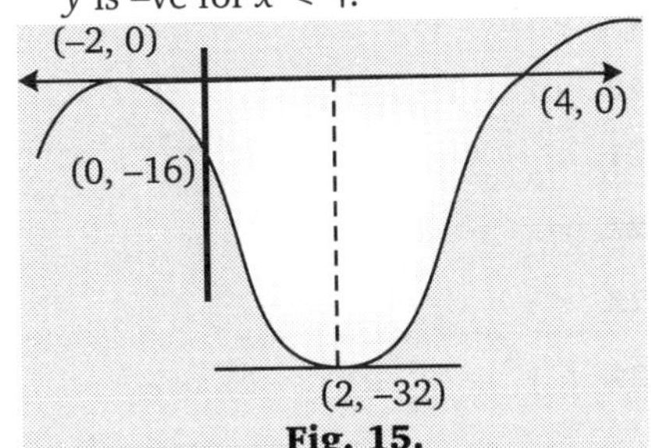

Fig. 15.

8. *Trace the curve* $9ay^2 = (x - 2a)(x - 5a)^2$.

(JNTU–2008)

SOLUTION. (i) The curve is symmetric about x-axis.

(ii) The curve does not passes through the origin.

(iii) The curve has no asymptotes.

(iv) The curve cuts the x-axis at $x = 2a$ and $x = 5a$ *i.e.*, at $A(2a, 0)$ and $B(5a, 0)$. It cuts the y-axis at

$$y^2 = -50\frac{a^2}{9}$$

$\Rightarrow y$ is imaginary. Therefore curve does not cut the x-axis

(v) $$y = \frac{(x-5a)\sqrt{x-2a}}{3\sqrt{a}}$$

$\Rightarrow$ y is imaginary for $x < 2a$.

$\Rightarrow$ curve exists only for $x \geq 2a$.

and $\frac{dy}{dx} = \pm\frac{(x-3a)}{2\sqrt{a}\sqrt{x-2a}}$

At $A(2a, 0)$, $\frac{dy}{dx} = \infty$ *i.e.*, tangent is parallel to y-axis.

At $B(5a, 0)$, $\frac{dy}{dx} = \pm\frac{1}{\sqrt{3}}$ *i.e.*, there are two distinct tangents.

$\Rightarrow$ There is a node at $B(5a, 0)$.

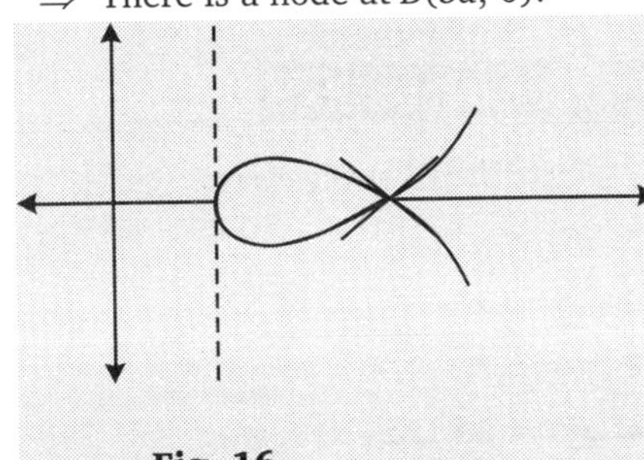
Fig. 16.

9. *Trace the curve* : $y^2(x^2 + y^2) + a^2(x^2 - y^2) = 0$ or $x^2(y^2 + a^2) + y^2(y^2 - a^2) = 0$

SOLUTION. (i) The curve is symmetric about both the axes.

(ii) The curve passes through the origin and $a^2(x^2 - y^2) = 0$ *i.e.*, $y = \pm x$ are two tangents at origin. So, origin is a node.

(iii) The curve intersects the x-axis only at origin. It intersects the y-axis at (0, 0), (0, a) and (0, –a).

(iv) Shifting the origin at (0, a) the equation of the curve becomes

$$(y+a)^2\{x^2 + (y+a)^2\} + a^2\{x^2 - (y+a)^2\} = 0$$

$$\Rightarrow (y^2 + 2ay + a^2)(x^2 + y^2 + 2ay + a^2) + a^2(x^2 - y^2 - 2ay - a^2) = 0$$

Equating to zero the the lowest degree terms, we get

$2a^3y + 2a^3y - 2a^3y = 0 \Rightarrow y = 0$, which is the tangent at new origin. Here we need not find the tangent at (0, $-a$) as the curve is symmetric about x-axis.

(v) On solving the given equation for x, we get $x^2 = y^2(a^2 - y^2)/(a^2 + y^2)$ when $y = 0$, $x^2 = 0$ and when $y = a$, $x^2 = 0$.

When $0 < y < a$, x^2 is positive. Therefore, the curve exists in the region $0 < y < a$. When $y > a$, x^2 is negative, so the curve does not exist in the region $y > a$.

(vi) The asymptotes parallel to x-axis are given by $a^2 + y^2 = 0$ *i.e.*, $y = \pm ai$.

Also, $\phi_4(m) = m^2(1 + m^2)$. Its roots are $m = 0, 0, i, -i$.

The asymptote are imaginary.

(vii) In the positive quadrant we have

$$x = y(a^2 - y^2)^{1/2}/(a^2 + y^2)^{1/2}, y > 0$$

$$x = y\left(1 - \frac{y^2}{a^2}\right)^{1/2} \Big/ \left(1 + \frac{y^2}{a^2}\right)^{1/2}$$

When $0 < y < a$, we observe that x is less than y. Hence, the curve lies above the line $y = x$ which is tangent at origin.

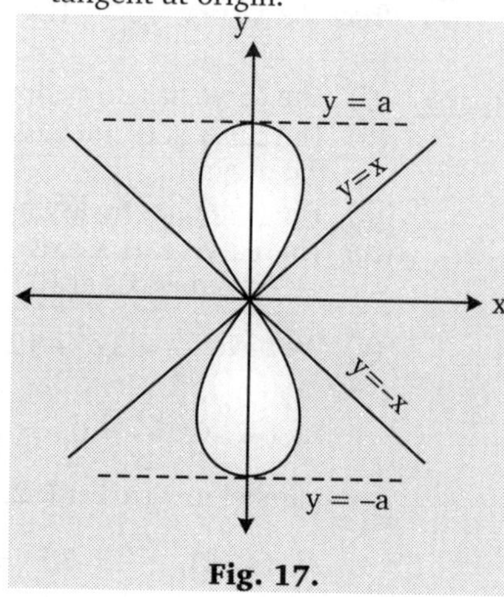

Fig. 17.

Exercise-15.3

Trace the following curves:

1. $ay^2 = x^3$
2. $a^2y = x^3$
3. $y = x(x^2 - 1)$
4. $xy^2 = 4a^2(2a - x)$
5. $y^2(a + x) = x^2(a - x)$ (VTU–2004, SVTU–2008)
6. $x^2(x^2 - 4a^2) = y^2(x^2 - a^2)$. (UPTU–2009)
7. $x^3 + y^3 = x$
8. $x^2y^2 = a^2(x^2 + y^2)$
9. $y^2(a^2 + x^2) = x^2(a^2 - x^2)$ (VTU–2010)
10. $y^2(x + 3a) = x(x - a)(x - 2a)$
11. $y^2(x^2 + y^2) + a^2(x^2 - y^2) = 0$
12. $a^2y^2 = x^3(2a - x)$
13. $9ay^2 = x(x - 3a)^2$
14. $x^2y^2 = (1 + y)^2 (4 - y^2)$
15. $y^3 + x^3 = a^2x$
16. $x^4 + y^4 = 4a^2xy$
17. $y^2 = (x - a)(x - b)(x - c)$, $a > b > c$
18. $y^2(x - a) = x^2(x + a)$ (VTU–2010, BPTU–2005)
19. $y^2(x^2 - 1) = x$
20. $y(x^2 - 1) = (x^2 + 1)$
21. $a^2y^2 = x^2(a^2 - x^2)$ (PTU–2009)
22. $y(x^2 + 4a^2) = 8a^3$
23. $x^3y = x + 1$
24. $a^3y^2 = (x - a)^4(x - b)$, $a > b$

ANSWERS

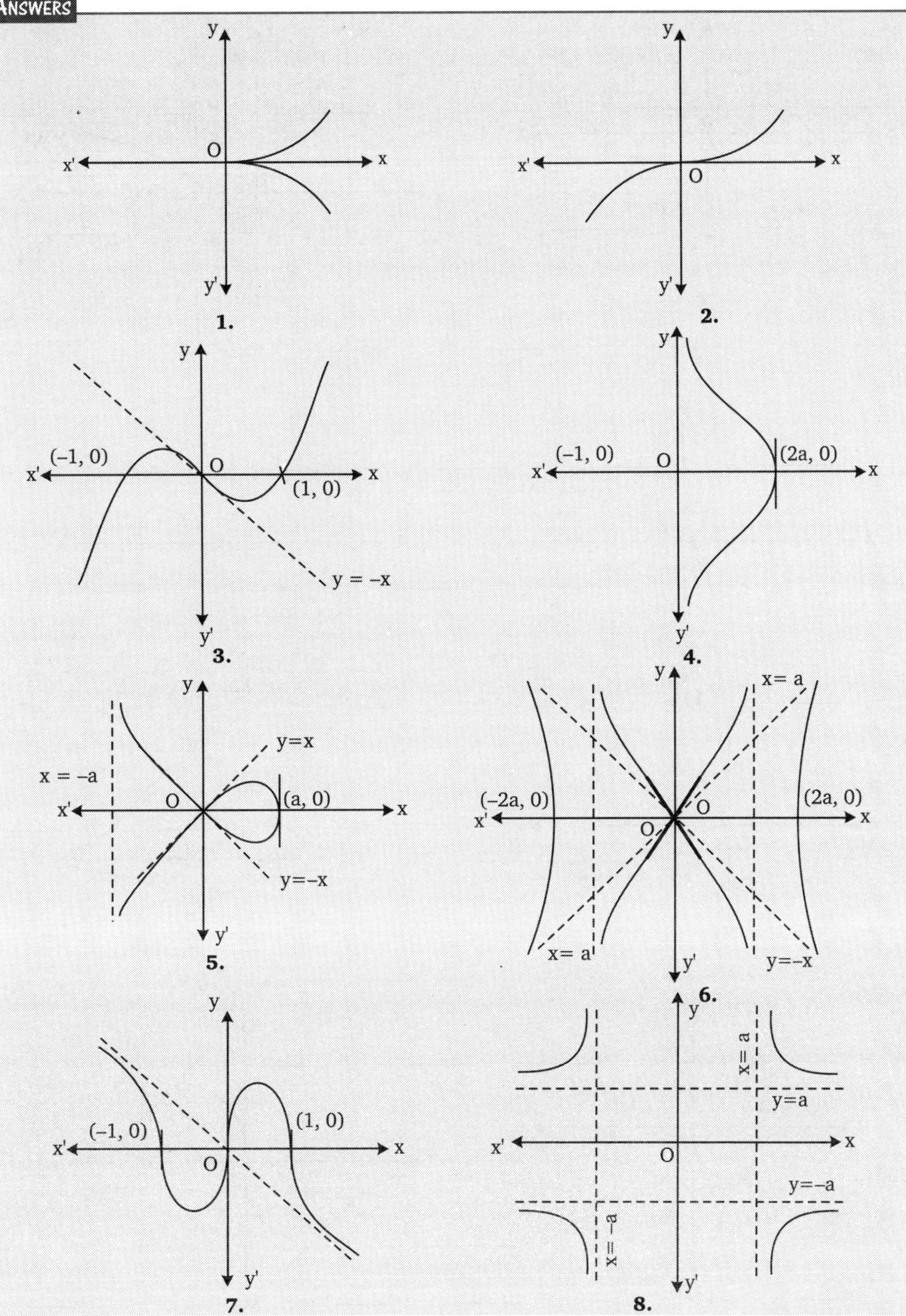
y
x'
O
x
y'
1.
y
x'
O
x
y'
2.
y
(–1, 0)
x'
O
x
(1, 0)
y = –x
y'
3.
y
(–1, 0)
O
(2a, 0)
x'
x
y'
4.
y
x = –a
y=x
x'
O
(a, 0)
x
y=–x
y'
5.
y
x= a
(–2a, 0)
(2a, 0)
x'
O
O
x
x= a
y'
y=–x
6.
y
(–1, 0)
(1, 0)
x'
O
x
y'
7.
y
x = a
y=a
x'
O
x
y=–a
x = –a
y'
8.

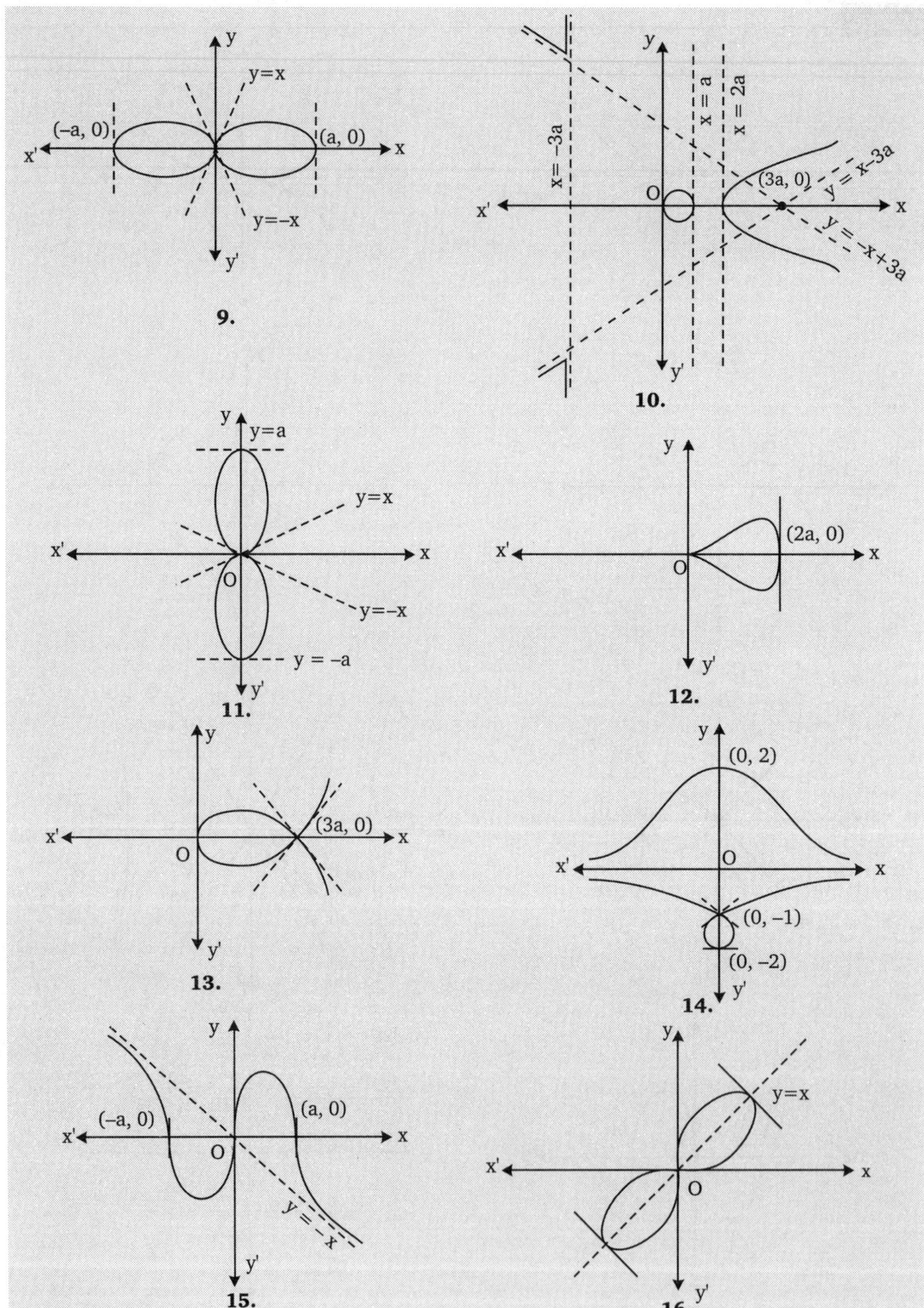

y
y=x
(–a, 0)
(a, 0)
x'
x
y=–x
y'
9.
y
x = –3a
x = a
x = 2a
y = x–3a
(3a, 0)
O
x'
x
y = –x+3a
y'
10.
y
y=a
y=x
x'
x
O
y=–x
y = –a
y'
11.
y
(2a, 0)
x'
x
O
y'
12.
y
(3a, 0)
x'
x
O
y'
13.
y
(0, 2)
O
x'
x
(0, –1)
(0, –2)
y'
14.
y
(–a, 0)
(a, 0)
x'
x
O
y = –x
y'
15.
y
y=x
x'
x
O
y'
16.

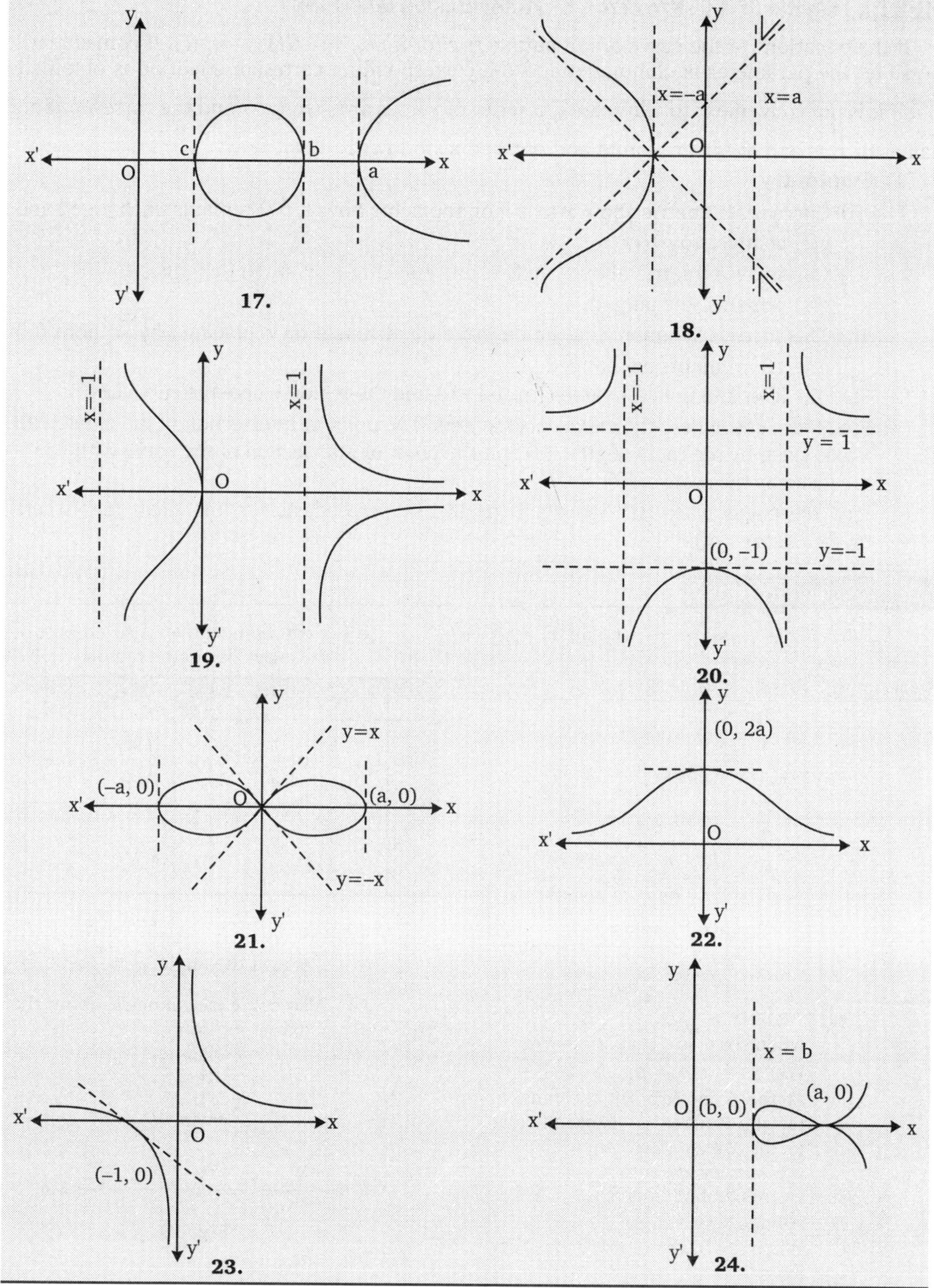
y
x'
x
O
c
b
a
y'
17.
y
x=–a
x=a
x'
O
x
y'
18.
y
x=–1
x=1
x'
O
x
y'
19.
y
x=–1
x=1
y = 1
x'
x
O
(0, –1)
y=–1
y'
20.
y
y=x
(–a, 0)
x'
O
(a, 0)
x
y=–x
y'
21.
y
(0, 2a)
x'
O
x
y'
22.
y
x'
x
O
(–1, 0)
y'
23.
y
x = b
(a, 0)
O
(b, 0)
x'
x
y'
24.

15.14 TRACING OF A CURVE GIVEN BY PARAMETRIC EQUATIONS

If the equations of the curve are in parametric form *i.e.*, $x = f(t), y = g(t)$. If conveniently possible, the parameter is eliminated and the corresponding cartesian equation is obtained. But if it is not convenient to eliminate t, a series of values are given to t and the corresponding values of x, y, and dy/dx are found and proceed as follows :

(1) Symmetry

(i) Curve is symmetric about x-axis if on replacing t by $-t$, $f(t)$ remains unchanged and $g(t)$ changes to $-g(t)$.

(ii) Curve is symmetric about y-axis if on replacing t by $-t$, $f(t)$ changes to $-f(t)$ and $g(t)$ remains unchanged.

(iii) The curve is symmetric in the opposite quadrants if on replacing t by $-t$, both $f(t)$ and $g(t)$ remains unchanged.

(2) Find the least and greatest value of x and y to find the region where the curve lies.

(3) Find the points where the curve cuts the axes. The point of intersection of the curve with x-axis given by the roots of $g(t) = 0$ and the point of intersection of the curve with y-axis are given by the roots of $f(t) = 0$.

(4) Find the points where the tangent is parallel or perpendicular to the x-axis (*i.e.*, where $dy/dx = 0$ or $\to \infty$)

Solved Examples

1. *Trace the curve* $x = a(t+\sin t)$ *and* $y=a(1+ \cos t)$

SOLUTION. (i) Given $x = a(t+\sin t)$

$$\Rightarrow \frac{dx}{dt} = a(1+\cos t)$$

$$y = a(1 + \cos t)$$

$$\Rightarrow \frac{dy}{dt} = -a\sin t$$

$$\therefore \frac{dy}{dx} = \frac{dy/dt}{dx/dt} = \frac{-a\sin t}{a(1+\cos t)}$$

$$= \frac{-2a\sin t/2\cos t/2}{2a\cos^2\frac{t}{2}} = -\tan\frac{t}{2}$$

(ii) We have $y = 0$,
when $\cos t = -1$, *i.e*, $t = -\pi, \pi$
When $t = \pi$, $x = a\pi$, $dy/dx = -\infty$
At the point $(a\pi, 0)$, the tangent to the curve is perpendicular to the x-axis. Also when $t = -\pi$, $x = -a\pi$, $dy/dx = \infty$

(iii) y is maximum when $\cos t = 1$, *i.e.*, when $t = 0$
When $t = 0$, $x = 0$, $y = 2a$ and $dy/dx = 0$.
So at the point $(0, 2a)$, the tangent to the curve is parallel to x-axis.

(iv) y can be negative. Also no part of the curve lies in the region $y > 2a$.

t	$-\pi$	$-\pi/2$	0	$\pi/2$	π
x	$-a\pi$	$-a\left(\frac{\pi}{2}+1\right)$	0	$a\left(\frac{\pi}{2}+1\right)$	$a\pi$
y	0	a	$2a$	a	0
$\frac{dy}{dx}$	∞	1	0	-1	$-\infty$

At $(-a\pi, 0)$ the tangent inclined to x-axis at the angle $\psi = \frac{\pi}{2}$

Also curve is symmetric about the y-axis.

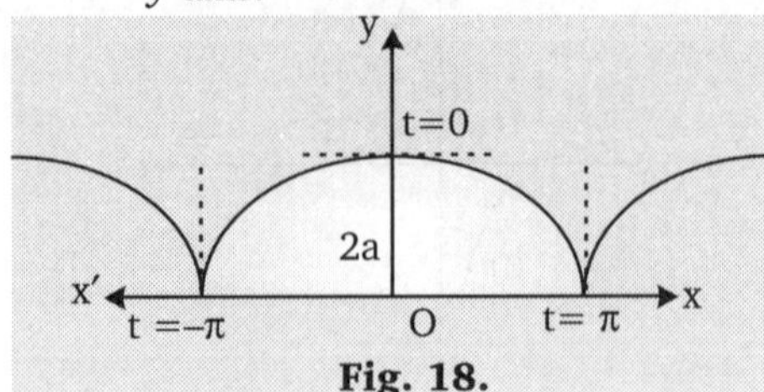

Fig. 18.

2. *Trace the curve*

$$x = a\cos t + \frac{1}{2}a\log\tan^2\frac{t}{2}, y = a\sin t$$

SOLUTION. (i) Put $-t$ for t in the given equation of the curve, we get

$$x = a\cos t + \frac{1}{2}a\log\tan^2\frac{t}{2}$$

and $y = -a\sin t$

Therefore, for every value of x there are two equal and opposite value of $y \Rightarrow$ curve is summetric about x-axis.

Further, put $\pi - t$ for t in the given equation of the curve, we get

$$x = -a\cos t + \frac{1}{2}a\log\cot^2\frac{t}{2}$$

$$= -a\cos t - \frac{1}{2}a\log\tan^2\frac{t}{2}$$

and $y = a\sin t$

$\Rightarrow$ For every value of y, there are two equal and opposite values of x, so curve is symmetric about y-axis.

(ii) Differentiating the given equation w.r.t. t we get

$$\frac{dx}{dt} = -a\sin t + \frac{1}{2}a\frac{1}{\tan^2\frac{t}{2}}$$

$$(2\tan\frac{t}{2}\sec^2\frac{t}{2}).\frac{1}{2}$$

$$= -a\sin t + \frac{a}{2\sin\frac{t}{2}\cos\frac{t}{2}}$$

$$= -a\sin t + \frac{a}{\sin t}$$

$$= \frac{a(1-\sin^2 t)}{\sin t} = \frac{a\cos^2 t}{\sin t}$$

and $\quad \dfrac{dy}{dt} = a\cos t$

$$\therefore \frac{dy}{dx} = \frac{dy/dt}{dx/dt} = \frac{a\cos t.\sin t}{a\cos^2 t} = \tan t$$

(iii) We have $y = 0$ when $\sin t = 0$, *i.e.*, $t = 0$, when $t \to 0$, $x \to -\infty$. Therefore, $x \to -\infty$ when $y \to 0$ showing that the line $y = 0$ is an asymptote of the curve.

(iv) Clearly y is maximum when $\sin t = 1$ *i.e.*, $t = \pi/2$. When $t = \pi/2$,

$x = 0, y = a$ and $\dfrac{dy}{dx} = \tan\dfrac{\pi}{2} = \infty$

$\Rightarrow$ Curve passes through the point $(0, a)$ and the tangent at this point is the x-axis.

(v) Clearly, the numerical value of y cannot be greater than a. Therefore, curve does exist in the region $y > a$ and $y < -a$.

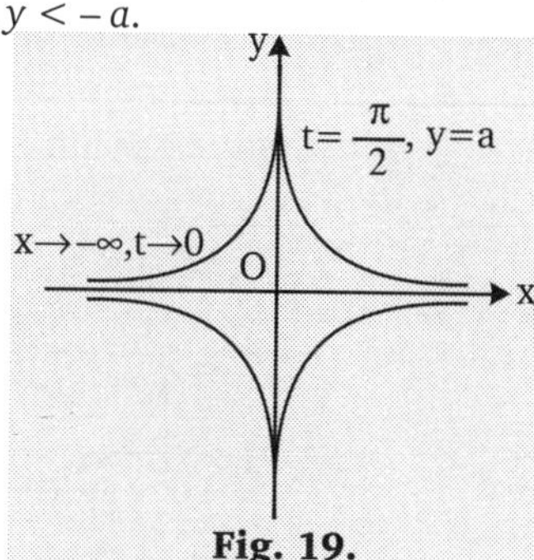

Fig. 19.

3. *Trace the curve $x = a(t + \sin t)$, $y = a(1 - \cos t)$ when $-\pi \le t \le \pi$.*

SOLUTION. We have $x = a(t + \sin t)$

$$\Rightarrow \frac{dx}{dt} = a(1+\cos t)$$

$$y = a(1 - \cos t) \Rightarrow \frac{dy}{dt} = a\sin t$$

$$\therefore \frac{dy}{dx} = \frac{dy/dt}{dx/dt} = \frac{a\sin t}{a(1+\cos t)} = \tan\frac{t}{2}$$

(i) Clearly, $y = 0$ when $\cos t = 0$ *i.e.*, $t = 0$

When $t = 0, x = 0, \dfrac{dy}{dx} = \tan 0 = 0$

$\Rightarrow$ Curve passes through the origin and the axis of x is tangent at the origin.

(ii) y is maximum when $\cos t = -1$ *i.e.*, $t = \pi$ and $-\pi$. When $t = \pi$, $x = a\pi$, $y = 2a$ and $\dfrac{dy}{dx} = \infty$. So at the point $t = \pi$, whose coordinates are $(a\pi, 2a)$, the tangent is perpendicular to the x-axis. When $t = -\pi$, $x = -a\pi$, $y = 2a$, $\dfrac{dy}{dx} = -\infty$.

(iii) Here y can not be negative, so curve lies entirely above the axis of x and no portion of the curve lies in the region $y > 2a$.

(iv)

t	$-\pi$	$-\pi/2$	0	$\pi/2$	π
x	$-a\pi$	$-a\left(\frac{\pi}{2}+1\right)$	0	$a\left(\frac{\pi}{2}+1\right)$	$a\pi$
y	$2a$	a	0	a	$2a$
dy/dx	$-\infty$	-1	0	1	∞

Replace t by $-t$ in the given curve, we get $x = -a(t + \sin t)$ and $y = a(1 - \cos t)$. Therefore, for every value of y, there are two equal and opposite value of x. So, curve is symmetric about y-axis.

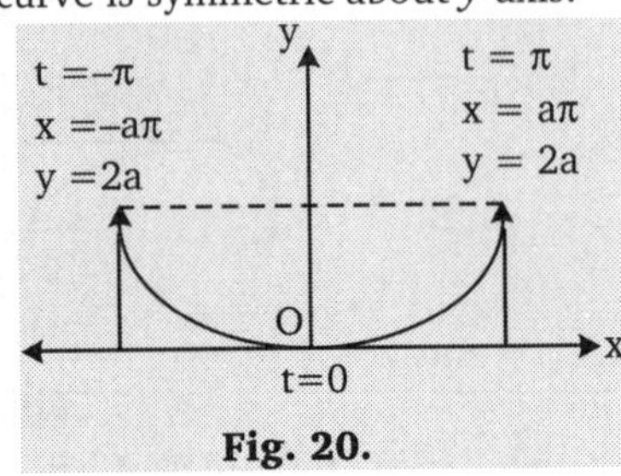

Fig. 20.

4. *Trace the curve* $x = a(t - \sin t)$, $y = a(t - \cos t)$.

SOLUTION. We have $x = a(t - \sin t)$

$$\Rightarrow \frac{dx}{dt} = a(1 - \cos t)$$

$$y = a(t - \cos t) \Rightarrow \frac{dy}{dt} = a\sin t$$

$$\therefore \frac{dy}{dx} = \frac{dy/dt}{dx/dt} = \frac{a\sin t}{a(1-\cos t)}$$

$$= \frac{2\sin t/2 \cos t/2}{2\sin^2 t/2} = \cot t/2$$

Here, $y = 0$ when $\cos t = 1$ *i.e.*, $t = 0$, 2π. When $t = 0$, $x = 0$, $y = 0$ and $\frac{dy}{dx} = \cot 0 = \infty$. Therefore, the curve passes through the origin and axis of y is tangent to the curve at this point.

Also, y is maximum when $\cos t = -1$ *i.e.*, $t = \pi$

When $t = \pi$, $x = a(\pi - \sin \pi) = a\pi$, $y = 2a$, $\frac{dy}{dx} = \cot\frac{\pi}{2} = 0$

Therefore, at $t = \pi$, whose cartesian coordinates are $(a\pi, 2a)$ the tangent to the curve is parallel to x-axis and curve does not lie in the region $y > 2a$.

In this curve y cannot be negative because cos$t$ cannot be greater than 1. Hence, one complete arc of the given cycloid lying between $0 \le t \le 2\pi$.

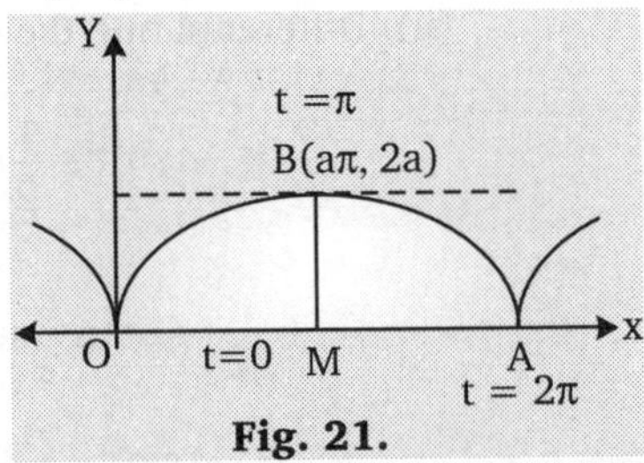

Fig. 21.

Some Standard Transformations

- If $x = a \cos t$, $y = b \sin t$ then $\frac{x^2}{a^2} + \frac{y^2}{b^2} = 1$ **(Ellipse)**
- If $x = a \cos t$, $y = b \sin t$ Then $x^2 + y^2 = a^2$ **(Circle)**
- If $x = a \cos^3 t$, $y = b \sin^3 t$ Then $\left(\frac{x}{a}\right)^{2/3} + \left(\frac{y}{b}\right)^{2/3} = 1$ **(Hypo-Cycloid)**
- If $x = a \cos^3 t$, $y = a \sin^3 t$ Then $x^{2/3} + y^{2/3} = a^{2/3}$ **(Astroid)**
- If $x = t^2$, $y = t - \frac{t^3}{3}$, $y^2 = x(1 - x/3)^2$
- If $x = a \sin^3 t$, $y = a\frac{\sin^3 t}{\cos t}$ Then $y^2(a - x) = x^3$ **(Cissoid)**
- If $x = \frac{1-t^2}{1+t^2}$, $y = \frac{2t}{1+t^2}$ Then $x^2 + y^2 = 1$ **(Circle)**
- If $x = \frac{3at}{1+t^3}$, $y = \frac{3at^2}{1+t^3}$ Then $x^3 + y^3 = 3axy$ **(Follium of Descarte's)**

15.15 TRACING OF EQUATION IN POLAR FROM

To trace the curve in polar form, we use the following procedure :

(a) Symmetry. In order to find the symmetry we use the following rules :

(i) If the curve $r = f(\theta)$ remains unchanged when θ is replaced by $-\theta$, then the curve is symmetrical about the initial line.

(ii) If the curve $r = f(\theta)$ remains unchanged when r is replaced by $-r$ then the curve is symmetrical about the pole. (origin).

(b) Special points on the curve. If r becomes zero for some values of θ, then the curve will pass through the pole. Therefore, if $r = 0$ when $\theta = \alpha$ (say), then $\theta = \alpha$ is the tangent to the curve at the pole.

Next we should find the maximum and minimum values of r which will exist for some values of θ.

(c) Solve these equations for r and observe the variation of r as θ varies from 0 to $+\infty$ and also we have to observe the variation as θ decreases from 0 to $-\infty$.

Therefore, we should form the table for the values of r corresponding to the values of θ.

(d) Regions where curve does not exist. If we obtain the values of r, imaginary for $\alpha < \theta < \beta$ then the curve will not exist in this region.

(e) Asymptotes. Next we should find the asymptotes if exist. For this if $r \to \infty$ for $\theta = \alpha$, then $\theta = \alpha$ is an asymptotes of the curve.

(f) Direction of tangents. Find $r\dfrac{d\theta}{dr}$ from $r = f(\theta)$. But we have $\tan\phi = r\dfrac{d\theta}{dr}$. If for some $\theta = \alpha$, ϕ comes to be zero at any point then the line $\theta = \alpha$ will be the tangent at that point.

Therefore, if ϕ comes out to be zero, $\theta = \pi/2$ then $\theta = \pi/2$ is the tangent perpendicular to the radius vector $\theta = \alpha$.

Now taking all above facts into consideration and draw the shape of the curve.

- Sometimes we face some problem to trace the curve of the form $r = f(\theta)$. Then for conveniently change the polar form of the curve into cartesian form by the following transformation : $x = r\cos\theta$, $y = r\sin\theta$ and then trace the curve.

Solved Examples

1. *Trace the following curve* $r^2 = a^2\cos 2\theta$.

(VTU-2007, GBTU-2012, KURUKSHETRA-2006)

SOLUTION. (i) The curve is symmetrical about both the initial line and the pole.

(ii) $r=0$ when $\cos 2\theta=0$ *i.e.*, when $\theta=\pm\pi/4$. Thus $\theta = -\pi/4$ and $\theta = \pi/4$ are two real and distinct tangent at the pole so that the pole is a node.

(iii) The maximum value of r is a when $\cos 2\theta = 1$ *i.e.*, when $\theta = 0$ and π.

(iv) $\tan\phi = r\dfrac{d\theta}{dr} = -\cot 2\theta$

$$\tan\phi = \tan\left(\frac{\pi}{2} + 2\theta\right).$$

$$\therefore \quad \phi = \frac{\pi}{2} + 2\theta.$$

At the points $(a, 0)$ and (a, π), ϕ comes out to be $\pi/2$ and $2\pi+\pi/2$.

Thus at these points tangents the perpendicular to the initial line.

(v) The following table gives the corresponding values of r and θ.

θ	0	$\pi/6$	$\pi/4$	$\pi/3$	$3\pi/4$	π
r	a	$a/\sqrt{2}$	0	imag.	0	$-a$

(vi) **Region.** When $-\pi/4 < \theta < \pi/4$, r^2 is negative so the curve will not exist in this region and when $\frac{5\pi}{4} < \theta < \frac{7\pi}{4}$, r^2 is negative. Also the curve will not exist in this region.

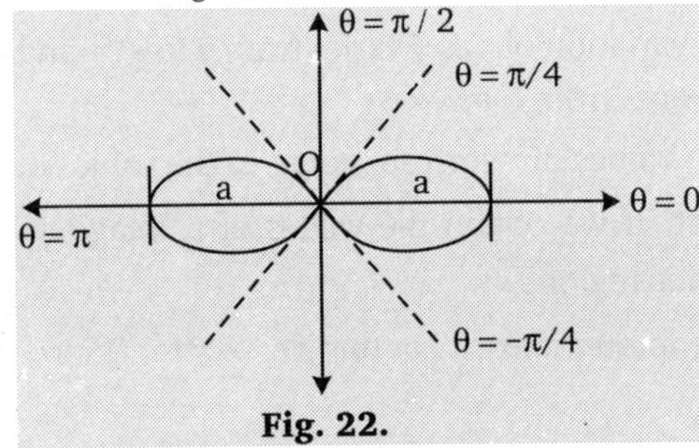

Fig. 22.

2. *Trace the curve $r = a \sin 4\theta$.*

SOLUTION. (i) The curve is symmetrical about the initial line, since on putting $(\pi - \theta)$ in place of θ and $-r$ in place of r, the equation of the curve remains unchanged.

(ii) The curve is symmetrical about the pole because on replacing θ by $(\pi + \theta)$ the equation of the curves remains unchanged.

(iii) Since the curve is finite, there are no asymptotes.

(iv) Draw a table for values of r and θ.

It is evident that the greatest numerical value of r is a. Hence, the curve, between $\theta = 0$ and $\theta = \pi$, is as shown in fig. 23.

If θ increases from π to 2π, the corresponding branches of the curve are known because of symmetry about the pole. Since the curve is periodic, the values of θ outside the range $(0, 2\pi)$ need not be considered.

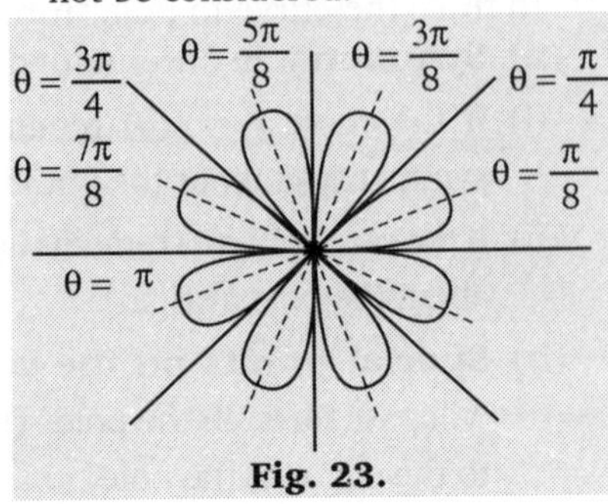

Fig. 23.

3. *Trace the curve $r = a + b \cos \theta$, $a < b$.*

SOLUTION. (i) The curve is symmetrical about the initial line.

(ii) $r=0$, when $a+b \cos \theta = 0$ *i.e.*,

$\cos \theta = \left(-\frac{a}{b}\right)$ or $\theta = \cos{-1}\left(-\frac{a}{b}\right)$

but $a < b$ *i.e.*, $\frac{a}{b} < 1$, therefore $\cos^{-1}\left(-\frac{a}{b}\right)$ comes out to be real so that $\theta = \cos{-1}\left(-\frac{a}{b}\right)$ is the trangent at the pole.

(iii) r is maximum when $\cos \theta = 1$ *i.e.*, $\theta = 0$. Then the maximum value of $r = a + b$ and the minimum value of $r = a - b$ when $\cos \theta = -1$ *i.e.*, $\theta = \pi$.

(iv) Since we have

$$r = a + b \cos \theta.$$

$$\therefore \qquad \frac{dr}{d\theta} = -b \sin \theta$$

then $\tan \phi = r\frac{d\theta}{dr} = -\frac{(a + b\cos\theta)}{b\sin\theta}$.

Now if $\theta = 0$ and π, $\phi = 90°$, thus at the points $(a + b, 0)$, $(a - b, \pi)$ the tangents are perpendicular to the initial line.

(v) The following table gives the corresponding value of r and θ

θ	0	$\pi/2$	$\cos^{-1}\left(-\frac{a}{b}\right)$
r	$a+b$	a	0
θ	$\cos\left(-\frac{a}{b}\right) < \theta < \pi$	π	
r	r is negative	$a-b$	

Thus from above facts the shape of the curve is shown below :

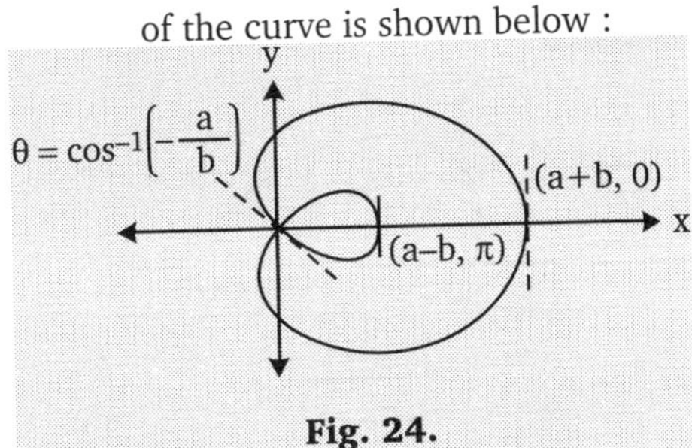

Fig. 24.

15.16 SOME STANDARD FIGURES AND THEIR EQUATIONS

S. No.	Name	Equation	S. No.	Name	Equation
1.	Cubical Parabola	$y = x^3$	**9.**	Cycloid	$x = a(t + \sin t)$ $y = a(t + \cos t)$
2.	Semi cubical parabola	$ay^2 = x^3$	**10.**	Tractrix	$x = a\cos t + \frac{1}{2}a\log\tan^2\frac{t}{2}$ $y = a\sin t$
3.	Cissoid	$y^2(2a - x) = x^3$	**11.**	Astroid	$x^{2/3} + y^{2/3} = a^{2/3}$
4.	Folium of Descartes	$x^3 + y^3 = 3axy$	**12.**	Inverted Cycloid	$x = a(t + \sin t)$ $y = a(1 - \cos t)$
5.	Circle	$x^2 + y^2 = a^2$ $r = 2a\cos\theta$	**13.**	Strophoid	$y^2(a - x) = x^2(a + x)$
6.	Cardioid	$r = a(1 - \cos\theta)$ $r = a(1 + \cos\theta)$	**14.**	Four leaved rose	$r = a\sin 2\theta$
7.	Limacon	$r = a + b\cos\theta$	**15.**	Spiral of Archimedes	$r\theta = a$
8.	Equiangular spiral	$r = ae^{m\theta}$			

Exercise-15.4

Trace the following curves :

1. $r = a(1 + \cos\theta)$

2. $r = 2a\cos\theta$

3. $r = a + b\cos\theta,\ a > b$

4. $r = a(\sec\theta + \cos\theta)$

5. $r\cos\theta = 2a\sin^2\theta$

6. $r^2 = a^2\sin 2\theta$

7. $r = a\sin 3\theta$

8. $r = ae^{m\theta}$

9. $2a/r = 1 + \cos\theta$.

10. $r = a\cos 3\theta$.

11. $r = a(1 - \cos\theta)$.

12. $r = a\sin 2\theta$.

13. $2r = 1 + 2\cos 2\theta$.

14. $x = a(\theta - \sin\theta),\ y = a(1 - \cos\theta)$. (SRM-2008)

15. $x = a\cos\theta + \frac{1}{2}a\log\tan^2\frac{\theta}{2},\ y = a\sin\theta$.

16. $x = a(\theta + \sin\theta),\ y = a(1 - \cos\theta)$. (JNTU–2009)

17. $r = a\cos 2\theta$.

18. $x = a(t - \sin t),\ y = a(1 - \cos t)$.

ANSWERS

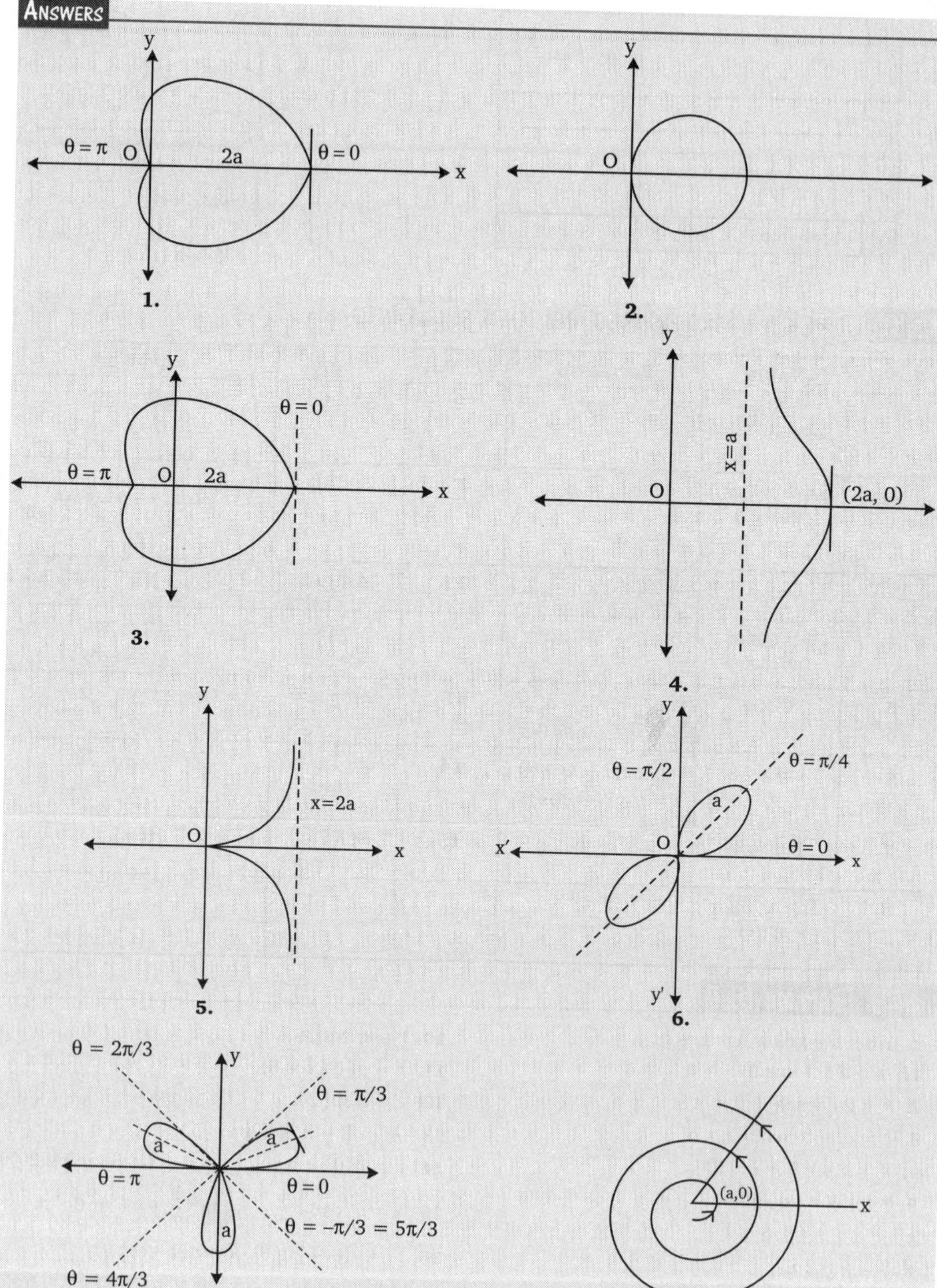
y
θ = π
O
2a
θ = 0
x
1.
y
O
x
2.
y
θ = 0
θ = π
O
2a
x
3.
y
x = a
O
(2a, 0)
x
4.
y
x=2a
O
x
5.
y
θ = π/2
θ = π/4
a
x′
O
θ = 0
x
y′
6.
θ = 2π/3
y
θ = π/3
a
a
θ = π
θ = 0
a
θ = −π/3 = 5π/3
θ = 4π/3
7.
(a,0)
x
8.

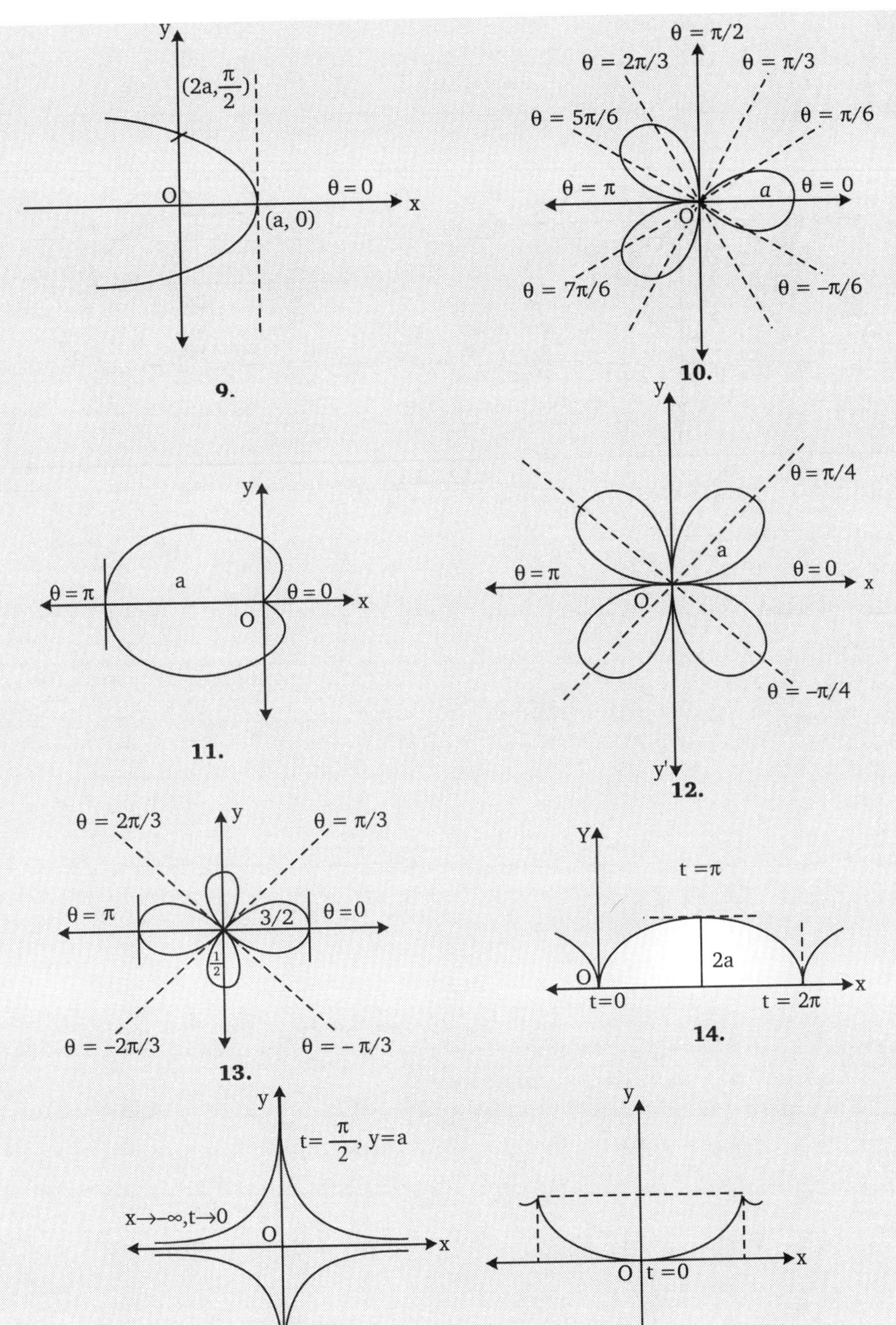

y
(2a, π/2)
O
θ = 0
x
(a, 0)
9.
θ = π/2
θ = 2π/3
θ = π/3
θ = 5π/6
θ = π/6
θ = π
a
θ = 0
O
θ = 7π/6
θ = −π/6
10.
y
θ = π
a
θ = 0
x
O
11.
y
θ = π/4
a
θ = π
θ = 0
x
O
θ = −π/4
y'
12.
θ = 2π/3
y
θ = π/3
θ = π
3/2
θ = 0
1/2
θ = −2π/3
θ = − π/3
13.
Y
t = π
2a
O
t=0
t = 2π
X
14.
y
t= π/2, y=a
x→−∞, t→0
O
x
15.
y
O
t = 0
x
16.

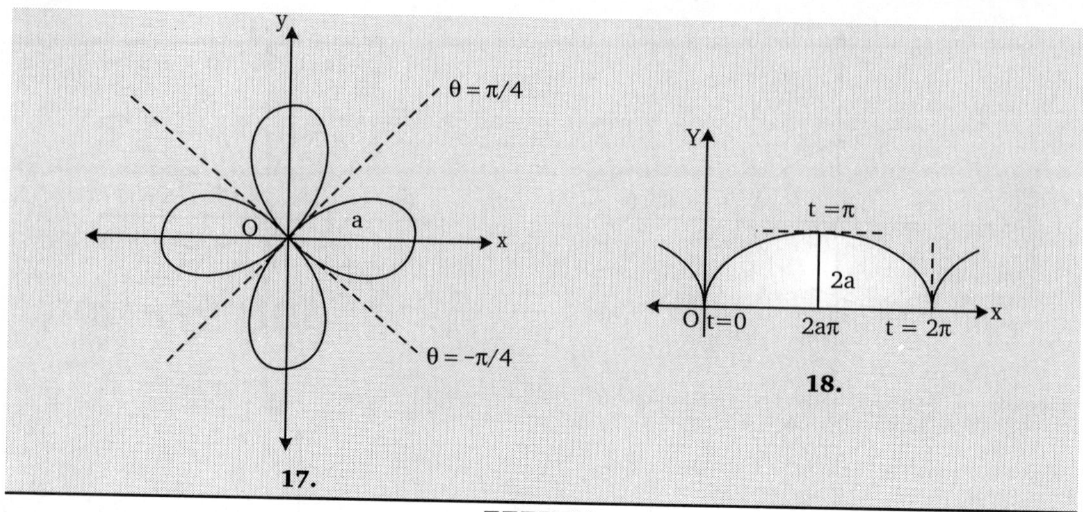
y
θ = π/4
O
a
x
θ = −π/4
17.
Y
t = π
2a
O
t=0
2aπ
t = 2π
X
18.

❑❑❑❑❑❑

Chapter

16 Integration

16.1 INTRODUCTION

We have already discuss the methods of finding the derivatives of a function $f(x)$. We have notice that the derivative of a function is also a function (may be the function of independent variable or constant). In this chapter we dealt with the converse of the derivative.

Consider the following questions :

(i) What is the function, whose derivative is $8x^7$.

(ii) What is the function, whose derivative is 8.

Obviously, x^8 and $8x$ be the functions, whose derivative is $8x^7$ and 8 respectively, which are called the integrals of the given functions. Further, integral is the inverse operation of differentiation.

For example: If the derivative of tan x is $\sec^2 x$ then integration of $\sec^2 x$ is tan x. Now if $f(x)$ is the function of x which is differentiable, such that $\frac{d}{dx}[F(x)] = f(x)$. Then $F(x)$ is known as the integral of $f(x)$ and denoted by $F(x) = \int f(x)\, dx$ and the function $f(x)$ is called the integrand of $\int f(x)\, dx$ and the function $\int f(x)\, dx$ is read as the integral of $f(x)$ w.r.t. x".

Thus, integration is the process of finding the integral of a given function.

- Integral is also known as primitive or antiderivative or an indefinite integral.
- The symbol $\int ...dx$, is stands for integral and taking separately the symbols is meaningless.
- In general, integral is defined as the sum of the certain infinite terms of a function at very small interval.

16.2 INDEFINITE INTEGRAL

To define the indefinite integral, let $F(x)$ be a function and C be a constant.

So, $\frac{d}{dx}[F(x) + C] = \frac{d}{dx}[F(x)] + \frac{dC}{dx} = f(x)$

[$\because$ derivative of a constant function is always zero]

Hence, $\int f(x)dx = F(x) + C$, where, the symbol '$\int$' is an integral sign, and C is the constant of integration. The constant C may have any value, but in general C is omitted and the function $F(x)$ is called the indefinite integral of integrand $f(x)$.

SOME STANDARD RESULTS

(i) $\int x^n dx = \frac{x^{n+1}}{n+1} + c, (\text{if } n \neq -1)$	(ii) $\int e^x dx = e^x + c,$
(iii) $\int \frac{1}{x} dx = \frac{\log_a x}{\log_a e} + c$	(iv) $\int \frac{1}{x} dx = \log_e x + c$
(v) $\int a^x dx = \frac{a^x}{\log_e a} + c$	(vi) $\int \cos x\, dx = \sin x + c$
(vii) $\int \sin x\, dx = -\cos x + c$	(viii) $\int \operatorname{cosec}^2 x dx = -\cot x + c$
(ix) $\int \sec^2 x\, dx = \tan x + c$	(x) $\int \sec x \tan x\, dx = \sec x + c$
(xi) $\int \operatorname{cosec} x \cdot \cot x\, dx = -\operatorname{cosec} x + c$	(xii) $\int \frac{dx}{\sqrt{(1-x^2)}} = \sin^{-1} x + c$
(xiii) $\int \frac{(-1)dx}{\sqrt{(1-x^2)}} = \cos^{-1} x + c$	(xiv) $\int \frac{dx}{x\sqrt{(x^2-1)}} = \sec^{-1} x + c$
(xv) $\int -\frac{dx}{x\sqrt{(x^2-1)}} = \operatorname{cosec}^{-1} x + c$	(xvi) $\int \frac{dx}{1+x^2} = \tan^{-1} x + c$
(xvii) $\int \frac{-dx}{1+x^2} = \cot^{-1} x + c$	(xviii) $\int c\, dx = cx + d$, where c is a constant

SOME RESULTS

(1) The integral of the product of a function with a constant is equal to the product of the constant and integral of that function.

(2) The integral of the sum or difference of two functions is equal to the sum or difference of their integral.

i.e., $\int \{f_1(x) \pm f_2(x)\} dx = \int f_1(x) dx \pm \int f_2(x) dx$

- From the above discussion, we can write
$$\int [f_1(x) \pm f_2(x) \pm \ldots] dx = \int f_1(x) dx \pm \int f_2(x) dx \pm \ldots.$$

Solved Examples

1. *Evaluate the following integrals.*

(i) $\int 5x^4\, dx$ (ii) $\int x^7\, dx$

(iii) $\int x^{-n}\, dx;\ n \neq 1$

(iv) $\int (ax^5 + bx^3 + cx + d)\, dx$

(v) $\int \frac{1}{\sqrt{1-x^2}} dx$

(vi) $\int \left(\sqrt{x} + \frac{1}{\sqrt{x}}\right)^2 dx$

(vii) $\int \frac{1}{t\sqrt{t^2-1}} dt.$

SOLUTION. (i) Here, $\int 5x^4 dx = 5\int x^4 dx = 5\frac{x^{4+1}}{4+1}$

$$= 5 \cdot \frac{x^5}{5} = x^5 + C.$$

(ii) $\int x^7 dx = \frac{x^{7+1}}{7+1} = \frac{x^8}{8} + C$

(iii) $\int x^{-n} dx = \frac{x^{-n+1}}{-n+1} + C;\ n \neq 1$

(iv) $\int (ax^5 + bx^3 + cx + d)\,dx$

$= a\int x^5 dx + b\int x^3 dx + c\int x\,dx + \int d\,dx$

$= a\cdot\frac{x^{5+1}}{5+1} + b\cdot\frac{x^{3+1}}{3+1} + c\frac{x^{1+1}}{1+1} + d\cdot x + C$

$= a\frac{x^6}{6} + b\frac{x^4}{4} + c\frac{x^2}{2} + d\cdot x + C$

(v) $\int \frac{1}{\sqrt{(1-x^2)}}dx = \sin^{-1} x + C$

(vi) $\int\left(\sqrt{x} + \frac{1}{\sqrt{x}}\right)^2 dx$

$= \int\left(x + \frac{1}{x} + 2\right)dx$

$= \int x\,dx + \int\frac{1}{x}dx + \int 2\,dx$

$= \frac{x^{1+1}}{1+1} + \log x + 2x + C$

$= \frac{x^2}{2} + \log x + 2x + C$

(vi) $\int \frac{1}{t\sqrt{t^2-1}}dt = \sec^{-1} t + C.$

2. *Evaluate the following integrals.*

(i) $\int(\operatorname{cosec} x \cot x - 3\sec^2 x)dx$

(ii) $\int\left(\sqrt{bx} + \frac{1}{\sqrt{bx}}\right)dx$

(iii) $\int \tan^2 x\,dx$

(iv) $\int \frac{(x+a)^3}{2\sqrt{x}}dx$

(v) $\int \sqrt{(1+\cos 2x)}\,dx$

(vi) $\int\left(\frac{4\sin x}{5\cos^2 x} + \frac{3}{5\sin^2 x}\right)dx.$

SOLUTION. (i) Here, we have

$\int(\operatorname{cosec} x \cot x - 3\sec^2 x)dx$

$= \int \operatorname{cosec} x.\cot x\,dx - 3\int \sec^2 x\,dx$

$= -\operatorname{cosec} x - 3\tan x + C.$

(ii) We have

$I = \int\left(\sqrt{bx} + \frac{1}{\sqrt{bx}}\right)dx$

$= \sqrt{b}\int x^{1/2}dx + \frac{1}{\sqrt{b}}\int x^{-1/2}dx$

$= \sqrt{b}\,\frac{x^{1/2+1}}{\frac{1}{2}+1} + \frac{1}{\sqrt{b}}\,\frac{x^{-1/2+1}}{-\frac{1}{2}+1} + C$

$= \frac{2\sqrt{b}x^{3/2}}{3} + \frac{2x^{1/2}}{\sqrt{b}} + C.$

(iii) We have

$I = \int \tan^2 x\,dx = \int(\sec^2 x - 1)dx$

$= \int \sec^2 x\,dx - \int dx = \tan x - x + C.$

(iv) We have

$I = \int\frac{(x+a)^3}{2\sqrt{x}}dx$

$= \frac{1}{2}\int\left(\frac{x^3 + 3ax^2 + 3a^2x + a^3}{\sqrt{x}}\right)dx$

$= \frac{1}{2}\int\frac{x^3}{\sqrt{x}}dx + \frac{3}{2}a\int\frac{x^2}{\sqrt{x}}dx + \frac{3}{2}a^2\int\frac{x}{\sqrt{x}}dx + \frac{1}{2}a^3\int\frac{dx}{\sqrt{x}}$

$= \frac{1}{2}\int x^{5/2}dx + \frac{3}{2}a\int x^{3/2}dx + \frac{3}{2}a^2\int x^{1/2}dx + \frac{1}{2}a^3\int x^{-1/2}dx$

$= \frac{1}{2}\frac{x^{5/2+1}}{\frac{5}{2}+1} + \frac{3}{2}a\cdot\frac{x^{3/2+1}}{\frac{3}{2}+1} + \frac{3}{2}a^2\frac{x^{1/2+1}}{\frac{1}{2}+1} + \frac{1}{2}a^3\frac{x^{-1/2+1}}{-\frac{1}{2}+1} + C$

$= \frac{1}{7}x^{7/2} + \frac{3a}{5}x^{5/2} + a^2x^{3/2} + a^3x^{1/2} + C$

(v) We have,

$\int\sqrt{1+\cos 2x}\,dx = \int\sqrt{(1+2\cos^2 x - 1)}dx$

$(\because \cos 2x = 2\cos^2 x - 1)$

$= \int\sqrt{(2\cos^2 x)}dx = \sqrt{2}\int \cos x\,dx$

$= \sqrt{2}\sin x + C$

(vi) We have

$I = \int\left(\frac{4\sin x}{5\cos^2 x} + \frac{3}{5\sin^2 x}\right)dx$

$= \frac{4}{5}\int\frac{\tan x}{\cos x}dx + \frac{3}{5}\int \operatorname{cosec}^2 x\,dx$

$= \frac{4}{5}\int \tan x.\sec x\,dx + \frac{3}{5}\int \operatorname{cosec}^2 x\,dx$

$= \frac{4}{5}\sec x + \frac{3}{5}(-\cot x) + c$

$= \frac{4}{5}\sec x - \frac{3}{5}\cot x + C.$

3. *If* $\frac{d}{dx}[f(x)] = 3x^2 + 2x + 1$, *then find* $f(x)$.

SOLUTION. Since $\frac{d}{dx}f(x) = 3x^2 + 2x + 1$

then $f(x) = \int (3x^2 + 2x + 1)\,dx$

$$= 3\int x^2 dx + 2\int x\,dx + \int 1.dx$$

$$= 3\frac{x^{2+1}}{2+1} + \frac{2\cdot x^{1+1}}{1+1} + x + C$$

$$= x^3 + x^2 + x + C$$

4. *Evaluate the following integrals.*

(i) $\int (ae^x + x^3)\,dx$

(ii) $\int (1+x)(2-5x)\,dx$

(iii) $\int \left(\frac{x^3 + 5x - 6}{x^2}\right) dx$

(iv) $\int (x-a)^2 dx$

(v) $\int \left(\frac{ax^3 + bx^2 + cx + d}{x}\right) dx$

(vi) $\int \left(\frac{4 + 3\sin x}{\cos^2 x}\right) dx.$

SOLUTION. (i) We have

$$I = \int (ae^x + x^3)\,dx = a\int e^x dx + \int x^3 dx$$

$$= ae^x + \frac{x^{3+1}}{3+1} = ae^x + \frac{x^4}{4} + C.$$

(ii) We have

$$I = \int (1+x)(2-5x)dx$$

$$= \int (2 - 3x - 5x^2)dx$$

$$= 2\int dx - 3\int x\,dx - 5\int x^2 dx$$

$$= 2x - \frac{3x^{1+1}}{1+1} - \frac{5x^{2+1}}{2+1}$$

$$= 2x - \frac{3}{2}x^2 - \frac{5}{3}x^3 + C$$

(iii) We have

$$I = \int \left(\frac{x^3 + 5x - 6}{x^2}\right) dx$$

$$= \int \left(x + \frac{5}{x} - \frac{6}{x^2}\right) dx$$

$$= \int x\,dx + 5\int \frac{1}{x} - 6\int x^{-2} dx$$

$$= \frac{x^{1+1}}{1+1} + 5\cdot\log_e x - 6\frac{x^{-2+1}}{-2+1}$$

$$= \frac{x^2}{2} + 5\log_e x + \frac{6}{x} + C.$$

(iv) We have

$$I = \int (x-a)^2 dx$$

$$= \int (x^2 + a^2 - 2ax)dx$$

$$= \int x^2 dx + a^2\int dx - 2a\int x\,dx$$

$$= \frac{x^{2+1}}{2+1} + a^2 x - 2a\cdot\frac{x^{1+1}}{1+1} + C$$

$$= \frac{x^3}{3} + a^2 x - ax^2 + C.$$

(v) We have

$$I = \int \left(\frac{ax^3 + bx^2 + cx + d}{x}\right) dx$$

$$= \int \left(ax^2 + bx + c + \frac{d}{x}\right) dx$$

$$= a\int x^2 dx + b\int x\,dx$$

$$+ c\int 1.dx + d\int \frac{1}{x}dx$$

$$= a\frac{x^{2+1}}{2+1} + b\frac{x^{1+1}}{1+1} + cx$$

$$+ d\log_e x + C$$

$$= \frac{ax^3}{3} + \frac{bx^2}{2} + cx + d\log_e x + C$$

(vi) We have

$$I = \int \left(\frac{4 + 3\sin x}{\cos^2 x}\right) dx$$

$$= \int \left(\frac{4}{\cos^2 x} + \frac{3\sin x}{\cos^2 x}\right) dx$$

$$= \int (4\sec^2 x + 3\tan x \cdot \sec x)\,dx$$

$$= 4\int \sec^2 x\,dx + 3\int \tan x.\sec x\,dx$$

$$= 4\tan x + 3\sec x + C$$

5. *Evaluate* $\int \frac{x^4}{x^2+1} dx.$

(MEERUT(BCA)–2007, 11)

SOLUTION. Consider $I = \int \frac{x^4}{x^2+1} dx$

$$= \int \frac{(x^4 - 1) + 1}{x^2 + 1} dx$$

$$= \int \frac{x^4 - 1}{x^2+1} dx + \int \frac{dx}{x^2+1}$$

$$= \int \frac{(x^2-1)(x^2+1)}{x^2+1}dx + \int \frac{dx}{x^2+1}$$

$$= \int (x^2-1)dx + \int \frac{dx}{x^2+1}$$

$$= \frac{x^3}{3} - x + \tan^{-1} x + C$$

16.3 METHOD OF INTEGRATION

16.3.1 INTEGRATION BY SUBSTITUTION

In this method, we transform the given integral into the another standard integral of some other independent variable. The method of changing the variable is called substitution method. To explain the method of substitution,

Consider the integral $\int f\{\phi(x)\}\phi'(x)dx$.

Put $\phi(x) = t$ so $\phi'(x)dx = dt$.

So, $\int f\{\phi(x)\}\cdot\phi'(x)dx = \int f(t)dt$

Now, $\int f(t)dt$ can be easily evaluated, then substitute $t = \phi(x)$ and get the required result.

16.3.2 SOME IMPORTANT SUBSTITUTION

Expression	Substitution
(i) $a^2 + x^2$	$x = a\tan\theta$ or $a\cot\theta$
(ii) $a^2 - x^2$	$x = a\sin\theta$ or $a\cos\theta$
(iii) $x^2 - a^2$	$x = a\sec\theta$ or $a\,\mathrm{cosec}\,\theta$
(iv) $\sqrt{\frac{a-x}{a+x}}$ or $\sqrt{\frac{a+x}{a-x}}$	$x = a\cos 2\theta$
(v) $\sqrt{\frac{x-a}{x-b}}$ or $\sqrt{(x-a)(x-b)}$	$x = a\cos^2\theta + b\sin^2\theta$

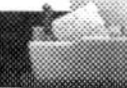

Solved Examples

1. *Obtain the following integrals*

(i) $\int x^2 \sin x^3 dx$

(ii) $\int (4x+5)^6 dx$

(iii) $\int x(x^2+4)^5 dx$

(iv) $\int 2x^3\sqrt{(x^2+4)}\, dx$.

SOLUTION. (i) The given integral is $\int x^2 \sin x^3 dx$.

Put $x^3 = t$ so $3x^2 dx = dt$.

So,

$$\int x^2 \sin x^3 dx = \frac{1}{3}\int \sin t \cdot dt$$

$$= \frac{1}{3}(-\cos t) = -\frac{\cos t}{3} + C$$

$$= -\frac{1}{3}\cos x^3 + C \qquad (\because\ t = x^3)$$

(ii) The given integral is $\int (4x+5)^6 dx$.

Put $4x+5 = t \Rightarrow 4dx = dt$

So, $\int t^6 \frac{dt}{4} = \frac{1}{4}\int t^6 dt = \frac{1}{4}\frac{t^7}{7} + C$

$$= \frac{1}{4}\frac{(4x+5)^7}{7} + C$$

(On putting $t = 4x+5$)

(iii) The given integral is

$$\int x(x^2+4)^5 dx.$$

Put $x^2 + 4 = t$ so, $2x\,dx = dt$

So, $\int t^5 \frac{dt}{2} = \frac{1}{2}\int t^5 dt$

$= \frac{1}{2}\frac{t^{5+1}}{5+1} = \frac{1}{12}t^6 + C$

$= \frac{1}{2}(x^2+4)^6 + C$

(On putting $t = x^2 + 4$)

(iv) The given integral is

$\int 2x^3\sqrt{x^2+4}\,dx.$

Put $(x^2+4) = t$ so $2x\,dx = dt$

and $x^2 = t - 4$.

So, $\int 2x^2 \cdot x\sqrt{x^2+4}dx$

$= \int (t-4)\sqrt{t}dt$

$= \int t^{3/2}dt - 4\int t^{1/2}dt$

$= \frac{t^{3/2+1}}{\frac{3}{2}+1} - 4\frac{t^{1/2+1}}{\frac{1}{2}+1} + C$

$= \frac{2}{5}t^{5/2} - \frac{8}{3}t^{3/2} + C$

$= \frac{2}{5}(x^2+4)^{5/2} - \frac{8}{3}(x^2+4)^{3/2} + C$

(On putting $t = x^2 + 4$)

16.3.3 SOME SPECIAL CASES OF METHOD OF SUBSTITUTION

Case 1. Functions of linear function of x, *i.e.*, $(ax + b)$

If the integrand is a function of the form $(ax+b)$, then the integral of the same form of the function is obtained by dividing the integral of function by the coefficient of x in the $ax+b$, *i.e.*, if, $\int f(x)dx = \phi(x)$, then we have $\int f(ax+b)dx = \frac{\phi(ax+b)}{a}$.

2. *Obtain the integral* $\int \frac{dx}{\sqrt{1-(cx+d)^2}}$.

SOLUTION. Here, the given integral is

$\int \frac{dx}{\sqrt{1-(cx+d)^2}}$

Put $cx + d = t$, so $c\,dx = dt$ or $dx = \frac{dt}{c}$

So, $\int \frac{dx}{\sqrt{1-(cx+d)^2}} = \frac{1}{c}\int \frac{dt}{\sqrt{1-t^2}}$

$= \frac{1}{c}\sin^{-1} t$

$= \frac{1}{c}\sin^{-1}(cx+d) + K$

(On putting $t = cx + d$)

3. *Obtain* $\int 10^{6x}\,dx$.

SOLUTION. Put $6x = t$ so $6\,dx = dt$ or $dx = \frac{dt}{6}$

So, $\int 10^{6x}dx = \int 10^t \frac{dt}{6} = \frac{1}{6}\int 10^t dt$

$= \frac{1}{6}\frac{10^t}{\log_e 10} = \frac{1}{6}\frac{10^{6x}}{\log_e 10} + C$

(On putting $t = 6x$)

16.3.4 SOME IMPORTANT RESULTS

(i) $\int (ax+b)^n dx = \frac{1}{a}\frac{(ax+b)^{n+1}}{n+1} + c, n \neq -1$

(ii) $\int e^{ax}dx = \frac{1}{a}e^{ax} + c, a \neq 0$

(iii) $\int \frac{dx}{ax+b} = \frac{1}{a}\log_e(ax+b) + c, a \neq 0$

(iv) $\int e^{ax+b}dx = \frac{e^{ax+b}}{a} + c, a \neq 0$

(v) $\int \frac{1}{(ax+b)^n}dx = -\frac{1}{a(n-1)(ax+b)^{n-1}} + c, a \neq 0, n \neq 1$

(vi) $\int \cos(ax+b)dx = \frac{\sin(ax+b)}{a} + c \quad a \neq 0$

(vii) $\int \sin(ax+b)dx = -\frac{1}{a}\cos(ax+b)+c, a \neq 0$

(viii) $\int \sec(ax+b)\tan(ax+b)dx = \frac{1}{a}\sec(ax+b)+c, a \neq 0$

(ix) $\int \operatorname{cosec}^2(ax+b)dx = -\frac{1}{a}\cot(ax+b)+c, a \neq 0$

(x) $\int a^{cx+d}dx = \frac{1}{c}\frac{a^{cx+d}}{\log_e a}+e, c \neq 0$ (xi) $\int -\operatorname{cosec}(ax+b)\cot(ax+b)dx = \frac{1}{a}\operatorname{cosec}(ax+b)+c$

Case II. Integral of the type $\int [\phi(x)]^n \phi'(x)\, dx$:

In this case, we put $\phi(x) = t$. So, $\phi'(x)dx = dt$, then we get,

$$f(x) = \int t^n dt = \frac{t^{n+1}}{n+1}+c, (n \neq 1)$$

Now, put $t = \phi(x)$ in above result, we get

$$\int [\phi(x)]^n \phi'(x)dx = \frac{[\phi(x)]^{n+1}}{n+1}+c.$$

4. *Evaluate the integral* $\int \tan^3 x \sec^2 x\, dx$.

SOLUTION. Here, the given integral is

$$\int \tan^3 x \cdot \sec^2 x\, dx.$$

Put $\tan x = t$, so $\sec^2 x\, dx = dt$

So, we get

$$\int \tan^3 x \sec^2 x\, dx$$

$$= \int t^3 dt = \frac{t^{3+1}}{3+1}+c = \frac{t^4}{4}+c$$

$$= \frac{\tan^4 x}{4}+c \qquad \text{(Putting } t = \tan x\text{)}$$

Case III. Function of the type $(a^2 \pm x^2)$

In this case, put $x = at$ so, $dx = a\,dt$ and then substitute these values in given integral and then integrate. After integration, put, $t = \frac{x}{a}$, we get the required result.

5. *Evaluate* $\int \frac{1}{a^2+x^2}dx$.

SOLUTION. The given integral is $\int \frac{1}{a^2+x^2}dx$.

Put $x = at \Rightarrow dx \Rightarrow a\,dt$

So, $\int \frac{1}{a^2+x^2}dx = \int \frac{a\,dt}{a^2+a^2t^2} = \int \frac{a\,dt}{a^2(1+t^2)}$

$$= \frac{1}{a}\int \frac{dt}{1+t^2} = \frac{1}{a}\tan^{-1} t$$

Now, put $t = \frac{x}{a}$, we get

$$\int \frac{1}{a^2+x^2}dx = \frac{1}{a}\tan^{-1}\left(\frac{x}{a}\right).$$

Similarly, we can obtain the following results:

(i) $\int \frac{1}{\sqrt{a^2-x^2}}dx = \sin^{-1}\frac{x}{a} + c$

(ii) $\int \frac{-1}{\sqrt{a^2-x^2}}dx = \cos^{-1}\left(\frac{x}{a}\right) + c$

(iii) $\int \frac{1}{x\sqrt{x^2-a^2}}dx = \frac{1}{a}\sec^{-1}\left(\frac{x}{a}\right) + c$

(iv) $\int \frac{-dx}{x\sqrt{x^2-a^2}} = \frac{1}{a}\operatorname{cosec}^{-1}\left(\frac{x}{a}\right) + c$

(v) $\int \frac{-dx}{a^2+x^2} = \frac{1}{a}\cot^{-1}\left(\frac{x}{a}\right) + c$

Case IV. Integral of the type $\int x^{n-1} f(x^n)\,dx$.

In this case, put $x^n = t \Rightarrow nx^{n-1}\,dx = dt$, substitute these values in given integral and then integrate and after integration, put $t = x^n$, to get the required result.

6. *Evaluate the integral $\int x^4 \tan x^5 dx$.*

SOLUTION. The given integral is $\int x^4 \tan x^5 dx$.
Put $x^5 = t$ so,

$$5x^4 dx = dt \Rightarrow x^4 dx = \frac{dt}{5}.$$

So, we get

$$\int x^4 \tan x^5 dx = \frac{1}{5}\int \tan t\,dt = -\frac{1}{5}\log\cos t + C$$

$$= -\frac{1}{5}\log\cos x^5 + C \text{ (On putting } t = x^5\text{)}$$

7. *Evaluate the integral $\int x^3 \sin x^4 dx$.*

SOLUTION. The given integral is $\int x^3 \sin x^4 = dx$.
Put $x^4 = t \Rightarrow 4x^3 dx = dt$

or $x^3 dx = \frac{dt}{4}$

So, we get

$$\int x^3 \sin x^4 dx = \frac{1}{4}\int \sin t\,dt = \frac{1}{4}(-\cos t) + C$$

$$= -\frac{1}{4}\cos x^4 + C \text{ (On putting } t = x^4\text{)}$$

Case V. Integral of the type $\int \frac{f'(x)}{f(x)}\,dx$.

In this case, put $f(x) = t$. So, $f'(x)dx = dt$

So, we get $\int \frac{f'(x)}{f(x)} dx = \int \frac{dt}{t} = \log t = \log f(x)$ [On putting $t = f(x)$]

For example, Evaluate the integral $\int \frac{nx^{n-1}}{x^n} dx$.

Solution. Put $x^n = t$ so $nx^{n-1}dx = dt$

So, $\int \frac{nx^{n-1}}{x^n} dx = \int \frac{dt}{t} = \log t + C = \log x^n + C$ (On putting $t = x^n$)

MORE IMPORTANT RESULTS

(i) $\int \cot x\,dx = \log\sin x + c$

(ii) $\int \sec x\,dx = \log(\sec x + \tan x) = \log\tan\left(\frac{\pi}{4} + \frac{x}{2}\right) + c$

(iii) $\int \tan x\,dx = -\log\cos x = \log\sec x + c$

(iv) $\int \operatorname{cosec} x\,dx = -\log(\operatorname{cosec} x + \cot x) = \log\tan\left(\frac{x}{2}\right) + c$

8. *Evaluate the integral $\int \frac{e^x + e^{-x}}{e^x - e^{-x}} dx$.*

[MEERUT(BCA)–2008]

SOLUTION. Put $e^x - e^{-x} = t$ so, $(e^x + e^{-x})dx = dt$
Therefore,

$$\int \frac{e^x + e^{-x}}{e^x - e^{-x}} dx = \int \frac{dt}{t} = \log t + C$$

$$= \log(e^x - e^{-x}) + C$$

(On putting $t = e^x - e^{-x}$)

9. *Evaluate $\int \frac{3x^2 + 2x}{x^3 + x^2 + 1} dx$.*

[MEERUT(BCA)–2007; ROHILKHAND(BCA)–2013]

SOLUTION. Let $I = \int \frac{3x^2 + 2x}{x^3 + x^2 + 1} dx$

Put $x^3 + x^2 + 1 = t$, differentiating w.r.t. x. We get $(3x^2 + 2x)dx = dt$

Then $I = \int \frac{dt}{t} = \log t + C$

$$= \log(x^3 + x^2 + 1) + C$$

10. *Evaluate the following integrals.*

(*i*) $\int \frac{2x\sin x^2}{\cos x^2} dx$

(*ii*) $\int \left(\frac{e^{2\log x} - 1}{e^{2\log x} + 1}\right)\frac{1}{x} dx$

SOLUTION. (i) Here, the given integral is

$$\int \frac{2x\sin x^2}{\cos x^2}dx.$$

Put $x^2 = t$ so $2x\,dx = dt$

Therefore,

$$\int \frac{2x\sin x^2}{\cos x^2}dx = \int \frac{\sin t}{\cos t}dt.$$

Again put $\cos t = v$, so

$$-\sin t\,dt = dv$$

Therefore,

$$\int \frac{\sin t}{\cos t}dt = \int \frac{-dv}{v} = -\log v$$

$$= -\log\cos t + C$$

(On putting $v = \cos t$)

$$= -\log\cos x^2 + C$$

(On putting $t = x^2$)

$$= \log\sec x^2 + C$$

(ii) The given integral is

$$\int \left(\frac{e^{2\log x}-1}{e^{2\log x}+1}\right)\frac{1}{x}dx$$

Put $\log x = t$ so, $1/x dx = dt$

Therefore,

$$\int \left(\frac{e^{2\log x}-1}{e^{2\log x}+1}\right)\frac{1}{x}dx = \int \frac{e^{2t}-1}{e^{2t}+1}dt$$

$$= \int \frac{e^t - e^{-t}}{e^t + e^{-t}}dt$$

(Dividing numerator and denominator by e^t)

$$= \log(e^t + e^{-t}) + C$$

$$= \log(e^{\log x} + e^{-\log x}) + C$$

(On putting $t = \log x$)

$$= \log(x + x^{-1}) + C$$

Similar Problems

(1) Evaluate the following integrals :

(i) $\int \frac{dx}{\tan^{-1}x(1+x^2)}$ (ii) $\int \frac{\cos^2 x}{\sin^4 x}dx$ (iii) $\int \frac{nx^{n-1}}{\sqrt{(1-x^{2n})}}dx.$

Ans. (i) $\log(\tan^{-1}x) + C$ (ii) $-\frac{t^3}{3} + C = -\frac{\cot^3 x}{3} + C$ (iii) $\sin^{-1}(x^n) + C$

11. *Find*

(*i*) $\int \frac{1+x^2}{1+x^4}dx$ (MEERUT(BCA)–2008)

(*ii*) $\int \frac{x+\sin x}{1+\cos x}dx$

SOLUTION. (i) Consider

$$I = \int \frac{1+x^2}{1+x^4}dx = \int \frac{1+\frac{1}{x^2}}{x^2+\frac{1}{x^2}}dx$$

$$= \int \frac{\left(1+\frac{1}{x^2}\right)}{\left(x-\frac{1}{x}\right)^2 + (\sqrt{2})^2}dx \cdot$$

Let $x - \frac{1}{x} = t.$

Then $\left(1+\frac{1}{x^2}\right)dx = dt$

$$I = \int \frac{dt}{t^2 + (\sqrt{2})^2}$$

$$= \frac{1}{\sqrt{2}}\tan^{-1}\frac{t}{\sqrt{2}} + C$$

$$I = \frac{1}{\sqrt{2}}\tan^{-1}\left(\frac{x^2-1}{\sqrt{2}x}\right) + C$$

(ii) We have $I = \int \frac{x+\sin x}{1+\cos x}dx$

$$I = \int \frac{x}{1+\cos x}dx + \int \frac{\sin x}{1+\cos x}dx$$

$$= \int \frac{x}{2\cos^2 x/2}dx + \int \frac{\sin x}{1+\cos x}dx$$

$$= \frac{1}{2}\int x\sec^2 x/2\,dx + \int\left(-\frac{1}{t}\right)dt$$

where $1+\cos x = t \Rightarrow -\sin x dx = dt$

$$= \frac{1}{2}\left[x\cdot\tan\frac{x}{2}\times 2 - \int 1\cdot\tan\frac{x}{2}\cdot 2\right] - \log t$$

$$= x \cdot \tan\frac{x}{2} - \log\left(\sec\frac{x}{2}\right) \times 2 - \log(1+\cos x) + C$$

$$= x\tan\frac{x}{2} - 2\log\sec\frac{x}{2} - \log(1+\cos x) + C$$

12. *Evaluate the following integral.*

(i) $\int \frac{\log x}{x} dx$

(ii) $\int \frac{\sin x \cos x}{1+\sin^2 x} dx$

SOLUTION. (i) Here, the given integral is

$$\int \frac{\log x}{x} dx.$$

Put $\log x = t$, so $\frac{1}{x}\, dx = dt$

So, $\int \frac{\log x}{x} dx$

$$= \int t\, dt = \frac{t^2}{2} + C$$

$$= \frac{(\log x)^2}{2} + C$$

(On putting $t = \log x$)

(ii) Here, put $1 + \sin^2 x = t$

$\Rightarrow$ $2\sin x.\cos x dx = dt$

Therefore,

$$\int \frac{\sin x \cos x}{1+\sin^2 x} dx = \frac{1}{2}\int \frac{dt}{t} = \frac{1}{2}\log t$$

$$= \frac{1}{2}\log(1+\sin^2 x)$$

13. *Evaluate* $\int \frac{f(x)}{(x+1)^2} dx$ *where* $f(x)$ *is a polynomial of degree 2 in x such that* $f(0) = 1, f(1) = 3$ *and* $f(-1) = 5$.

[MEERUT(BCA)–2003, HIMACHAL(BCA)–2009, CHENNAI–2011]

SOLUTION. Consider a second degree polynomial

$$f(x) = ax^2 + bx + c$$

Now, $f(0) = 1 \Rightarrow c = 1$

$f(1) = 3 \Rightarrow a + b + c = 3$

$f(-1) = 5 \Rightarrow a - b + c = 5$

On solving we get $a = 3, b = -1, c = 1$

$\therefore$ $f(x) = 3x^2 - x + 1$

$\therefore$ Consider

$$\int \frac{3x^2 - x + 1}{(x+1)^2} dx$$

$$= \int \frac{3(x+1)^2 - 7x - 2}{(x+1)^2} dx$$

$$= \int 3\, dx - \int \frac{7x+2}{(x+1)^2} dx$$

$$= \int 3\, dx - \int \left\{\frac{7(x+1) - 5}{(x+1)^2}\right\} dx$$

$$= \int 3\, dx - \int \frac{7}{x+1} dx + 5\int \frac{1}{(x+1)^2} dx$$

$$= 3x - 7\log(x+1) + \frac{5(-1)}{(x+1)} + C$$

$$= 3x - 7\log(x+1) - \frac{5}{(x+1)} + C$$

16.4 INTEGRATION BY PARTS

The method of 'integration by parts' is very powerful method of finding the integral. If the integrand is the product of two different functions, then the method of "integration by parts" can be used.

If $f(x)$ and $g(x)$ are two functions of x, then

$$\int f(x)g(x)dx = f(x)\int g(x)dx - \int \frac{d}{dx} f(x)\left\{\int g(x)dx\right\} dx$$

Proof. Let $f(x)$ and $g(x)$ be two functions of x, then

$$\frac{d}{dx}[f(x)g(x)] = f(x)\frac{d}{dx}g(x) + g(x)\cdot\frac{d}{dx}f(x).$$

Now integrating both the sides w.r.t x, we get

$$f(x)\,g(x) = \int\left\{f(x)\frac{d}{dx}g(x)\right\}dx + \int\left\{\frac{d}{dx}f(x).g(x)\right\}dx$$

So,
$$\int\left\{f(x)\cdot\frac{d}{dx}g(x)\right\}dx = f(x)\cdot g(x) - \int\left\{\frac{d}{dx}f(x)\cdot g(x)\right\}dx$$

or $\int f(x)g(x)\,dx = f(x)\int g(x)\,dx - \int\left\{\frac{d}{dx}f(x)\left(\int g(x)\,dx\right)\right\}dx$

The method of 'integration by parts, can be written into words as follows:
The integral of the product of two functions
= First function × integral of the second function
– integral of (the derivative of first function × integral of the second function)

WORKING PROCEDURE

There is no general rule to choose the first and second function, but remember the following points:

STEP 1. If the second function is not given then unity may be taken as the second function.

STEP 2. The integral of second function must be known.

STEP 3. If necessary, then the above formula can be applied more than once.

STEP 4. If the integral is of the form $\int x^n f(x)dx$ where n is positive integer, then x^n must be taken as the first function.

STEP 5. Trick using here is ILATE which stands for

$I \to$ Inverse Trigonometric function $L \to$ Logarithmic function
$A \to$ Algebraic function $T \to$ Trigonometric function
$E \to$ Exponential function

Solved Examples

1. *Evaluate the following integrals.*
(i) $\int x^2 \sin x\,dx$
(ii) $\int \log x\,dx$ (iii) $\int x^2 e^{3x}\,dx$.

SOLUTION. (i) Here, the given integral is

$$\int x^2 \sin x\,dx.$$

Now, integrating by parts, taking x^2 as first function, we get

$$\int x^2 \sin x dx = x^2 \int \sin x dx - \int\left\{\frac{d}{dx}x^2 \int \sin x dx\right\}dx$$

$$= -x^2 \cos x - \int\{2x.(-\cos x)\}dx$$

$$= -x^2 \cos x + 2\int x.\cos x\,dx$$

$$= -x^2 \cos x + 2\left[x.\int \cos x\,dx - \int\left\{\frac{d}{dx}(x).\int \cos x\,dx\right\}dx\right]$$

$$= -x^2 \cos x + 2[x \sin x - \int \sin x dx]$$

$$= -x^2 \cos x + 2x \sin x + 2\cos x + C,$$

where C the constant of integration.

(ii) Here, the given integral is

$$\int \log x\,dx.$$

Since the second function is not given, therefore we take the second function as unity (*i.e.*, 1).

$$\int \log x.1\,dx = \log x \int 1.dx - \int\left\{\frac{d}{dx}\log x \int 1\,.\,dx\right\}dx$$

$$= x \log x - \int \frac{1}{x} x\,dx = x(\log x - 1) + C$$

$$= x \log x - x + C$$

(iii) Here, the given integral is

$$\int x^2 e^{3x}\,dx.$$

Now, integrating by parts, taking x^2 as the first function, we get

$$\int x^2 e^{3x} dx = x^2 \int e^{3x} dx - \int\left\{\frac{d}{dx}x^2 \int e^{3x} dx\right\}dx$$

$$= \frac{x^2 e^{3x}}{3} - \int 2x \frac{e^{3x}}{3} dx$$

$$= \frac{x^2 e^{3x}}{3} - \frac{2}{3}\int x \cdot e^{3x} dx.$$

Again integrating by parts, taking x as the first function, we get

$$\int x^2 e^{3x}\,dx = \frac{x^2 e^{3x}}{3} - \frac{2}{3}\left[x.\int e^{3x} dx - \int\left\{1.\int e^{3x} dx\right\}dx\right]$$

$$=\frac{x^2e^{3x}}{3}-\frac{2}{3}\left[x\cdot\frac{e^{3x}}{3}-\frac{1}{3}\int e^{3x}dx\right]$$

$$=\frac{x^2e^{3x}}{3}-\frac{2}{3}\left[x.\frac{e^{3x}}{3}-\frac{e^{3x}}{9}\right]+C$$

$$=\frac{x^2e^{3x}}{3}-\frac{2xe^{3x}}{9}+\frac{2e^{3x}}{27}+C$$

2. *Evaluate the following integrals.*

(i) $\int\frac{1}{(a^2-x^2)^{3/2}}dx$

(ii) $\int(\log_e x)^2 dx$

(iii) $\int x^2e^x dx$ (iv) $\int x^n \log x\, dx.$

SOLUTION. (i) The given integral is

$$\int\frac{1}{(a^2-x^2)^{3/2}}dx.$$

Put $x = a\sin\theta \Rightarrow dx = a\cos\theta\, d\theta$

So,

$$\int\frac{1}{(a^2-x^2)^{3/2}}dx=\int\frac{a\cos\theta\, d\theta}{(a^2-a^2\sin^2\theta)^{3/2}}$$

$$=\frac{1}{a^2}\int\frac{\cos\theta\, d\theta}{(1-\sin^2\theta)^{3/2}}=\frac{1}{a^2}\int\sec^2\theta\, d\theta$$

$$=\frac{1}{a^2}\tan\theta+C=\frac{1}{a^2}\left\{\frac{x}{\sqrt{a^2-x^2}}\right\}+C$$

(ii) The given integral is $\int(\log_e x)^2dx.$ Here, the second function is not given so, we take second function as unity.

Therefore,

$$\int(\log_e x)^2\cdot 1\,dx=(\log_e x)^2\int 1\,dx-\int\left\{\frac{d}{dx}(\log_e x)^2\int 1\cdot dx\right\}dx$$

$$=x(\log_e x)^2-\int 2\log_e x\frac{1}{x}.\,x\quad dx$$

$$=x\left(\log_e x\right)^2-2\int\log_e x\,.\,1dx$$

$$=x(\log_e x)^2-2\left[\log_e x\int 1dx-\int\left\{\frac{d}{dx}\log_e x\int 1dx\right\}dx\right]$$

$$=x(\log_e x)^2-2x\log_e x+2\int\frac{1}{x}x\,dx$$

$$=x(\log_e x)^2-2x\log_e x+2x+C$$

(iii) The given integral is $\int x^2e^xdx.$ Integrating by parts, taking x^2 as the first function, we get

$$\int x^2e^xdx=x^2\int e^xdx-\int\left\{\frac{d}{dx}x^2\int e^xdx\right\}dx$$

$$=x^2e^x-2\int x\,.\,e^xdx$$

$$=x^2e^x-2\left[x\int e^xdx-\int\left\{\frac{d}{dx}x\int e^xdx\right\}dx\right].$$

$$=x^2e^x-2xe^x+2\int e^x\cdot dx$$

$$=x^2e^x-2xe^x+2e^x+C$$

$$=e^x(x^2-2x+2)+C$$

(iv) Here, given integral is $\int x^n\log x\,dx.$ Now, integrating by parts, taking $\log x$ as the first function, we get

$$\int x^n\log x\,dx=\log x\int x^ndx-\int\left\{\frac{d}{dx}\log x\int x^ndx\right\}dx$$

$$=\log x\frac{x^{n+1}}{n+1}-\int\frac{1}{x}\frac{x^{n+1}}{n+1}dx$$

$$=\log x\frac{x^{n+1}}{n+1}-\int\frac{x^n}{n+1}dx$$

$$=\log x\frac{x^{n+1}}{n+1}-\frac{1}{n+1}\frac{x^{n+1}}{(n+1)}+C$$

$$=\frac{1}{n+1}\left(x^{n+1}\log x-\frac{x^{n+1}}{n+1}\right)+C$$

3. *Evaluate the following integrals :*

(i) $\int\cos^{-1}\left(\frac{1-x^2}{1+x^2}\right)dx$

(ii) $\int x\sin x dx$

SOLUTION. (i) Here, given integral is

$$\int\cos^{-1}\left(\frac{1-x^2}{1+x^2}\right)dx$$

Put $x=\tan\theta\Rightarrow dx=\sec^2\theta\, d\theta$

So, $\int\cos^{-1}\left(\frac{1-x^2}{1+x^2}\right)dx$

$$=\int\cos^{-1}\left(\frac{1-\tan^2\theta}{1+\tan^2\theta}\right)\sec^2\theta\, d\theta$$

$= \int \cos^{-1}(\cos 2\theta) \sec^2 \theta \, d\theta$

$= 2\int \theta \sec^2 \theta d\theta$

$= 2\left[\theta \int \sec^2 \theta d\theta - \int \left\{\frac{d}{d\theta}\theta \int \sec^2 \theta \, d\theta\right\} d\theta\right]$

$= 2\theta \tan\theta - 2\int 1 \cdot \tan\theta \cdot d\theta + C$

$= 2\theta \tan\theta - 2\log \sec\theta + C$

$= 2x \tan^{-1} x - 2\log \sqrt{1+x^2} + C$

(Putting the value of θ)

(ii) Here, given integral is $\int x \sin x \, dx$. Integrating by parts, talking x as the first function.

We get

$\int x \sin x \, dx = x\int \sin x \, dx - \int \left(\frac{d}{dx} x \int \sin x \, dx\right) dx$

$= -x \cos x + \int \cos x \, dx + C$

$= -x \cos x + \sin x + C$

TWO IMPORTANT FORMULAE

(i) $\int e^{ax} \cos bx \, dx = \frac{e^{ax}}{a^2+b^2}(a \cos bx + b \sin bx) + C$

(ii) $\int e^{ax} \sin bx \, dx = \frac{e^{ax}}{a^2+b^2}(a \sin bx - b \cos bx) + C$

4. *Evaluate the following integrals :*

(*i*) $\int x^2 \cos x dx$ (*ii*) $\int x^3 \cos x dx$

(*iii*) $\int x^2 \sin x dx$ (*iv*) $\int e^x \cos x dx$

SOLUTION. (i) Here, the given integral is $\int x^2 \cos x \, dx$. Integrating by parts, taking x^2 as the first function, we get

$\int x^2 \cos x \, dx = x^2 \int \cos x \, dx - \int \left[\frac{d}{dx}(x^2) . \int \cos x \, dx\right] dx$

$= x^2 \sin x - 2\int x \sin x dx$

$= x^2 \sin x - 2\left[x(-\cos x) - \int \left\{\frac{d}{dx}(x) \int \sin x \, dx\right\} dx\right]$

$= x^2 \sin x - 2[-x \cos x + \int \cos x \, dx]$

$= x^2 \sin x + 2x \cos x - 2\sin x + C$

(ii) Here, the given integral is $\int x^3 \cos x \, dx$.

Integrating by parts, taking x^3 as the first function, we get

$\int x^3 \cos x \, dx = x^3 \int \cos x \, dx - \int \left[\frac{d}{dx}(x)^3 \int \cos x \, dx\right] dx$

$= x^3 \sin x - 3\int x^2 \sin x \, dx$

$= x^3 \sin x - 3[x^2 \int \sin x \, dx - \int \{2x . \int \sin x \, dx\} dx]$

$= x^3 \sin x + 3x^2 \cos x - 6[x . \sin x - \int \sin x \, dx]$

$= x^3 \sin x + 3x^2 \cos x - 6x \sin x - 6\cos x + C,$

where C is the constant of integration.

$= (x^3 - 6x) \sin x + (3x^2 - 6) \cos x + C$

(iii) Here, the given integral is $\int x^2 \sin x \, dx$.

Integrating by parts, taking x^2 as the first function, we get

$\int x^2 \sin x \, dx = x^2 \int \sin x \, dx - \int (2x \int \sin x \, dx) dx$

$= -x^2 \cos x + 2\int x \cos x \, dx$

$= -x^2 \cos x + 2[x \sin x - \int \sin x \, dx]$

$= -x^2 \cos x + 2x \sin x + 2\cos x + C$

(iv) Here, the given integral is $\int e^x . \cos x \, dx$

Let $I = \int e^x . \cos x \, dx$.

Integrating by parts, taking $\cos x$ as the first function, we get

$\int e^x \cos x \, dx = \cos x . e^x + \int \sin x . e^x \, dx.$

Again integrating by parts, we get

$\int e^x \cos x \, dx = e^x \cos x + \sin x e^x - \int \cos x e^x dx$

$$I = e^x \cos x + e^x \sin x - I$$

$$\text{or } 2I = e^x \cos x + e^x \sin x$$

$$I = \frac{1}{2}(e^x \cos x + e^x \sin x)$$

$$= \frac{e^x}{2}(\cos x + \sin x) + C$$

5. *Evaluate* $\int \frac{x}{1+\sin x} dx$

SOLUTION. Consider

$$\int \frac{x}{1+\sin x} dx = \int \frac{x(1-\sin x)}{\cos^2 x} dx$$

$$= \int x(\sec^2 x - \tan x \sec x) dx$$

$$= \int \underset{\text{I}}{x} \underset{\text{II}}{\sec^2 x} - \int \underset{\text{I}}{x} \underset{\text{II}}{\tan x \sec x}\, dx$$

$$= x \tan x - \int \tan x\, dx - x \sec x + \int \sec x\, dx$$

$$= x \tan x + \log \cos x - x \sec x + \log(\sec x + \tan x) + c$$

$$= x(\tan x - \sec x) + \log \cos x(\sec x + \tan x) + c$$

$$= x(\tan x - \sec x) + \log(1 + \sin x) + c$$

16.5 INTEGRATION BY PARTIAL FRACTIONS

If the given function is of the type $\frac{f(x)}{g(x)}$, where $f(x)$ and $g(x)$ both are polynomials, then we may assume that the numerator $f(x)$ and denominator $g(x)$ have no common polynomial factor and that the degree of $f(x)$ is less than the degree of $g(x)$. If the degree of numerator $f(x)$ is greater than or equal to the degree of denominator $g(x)$, then we have to divide $f(x)$ by $g(x)$ so that $\frac{f(x)}{g(x)} = h(x) + \frac{R(x)}{g(x)}$, where $h(x)$ is the quotient (a polynomial) and $R(x)$ is the remainder whose degree is less than the degree of $g(x)$. The method in which we change the $\frac{f(x)}{g(x)}$ into partial fractions, depends on factors of the denominator. We know that every polynomial can be expressed as a product of linear and irreducible quadratic factors with real coefficient. So, we have the following cases :

(i) If all the factor of denominator are linear and non repeated, then for each linear non-repeated factor $(ax + b)$, there corresponds a fraction of the form $\frac{A}{ax+b}$, where A is a constant, is to be obtained.

(ii) If all the factors in the denominator are linear but some of them are repeated, then for each linear factor $(ax+b)^n$ repeating n times, there correspond the sum of r partial fractions as:

$$\frac{A_1}{ax+b} + \frac{A_2}{(ax+b)^2} + \ldots + \frac{A_n}{(ax+b)^n}, \text{ where } A_1, A_2, \ldots, A_n \text{ are constants.}$$

(iii) If the factor in the denominator are linear and irreduciable but quadratic factor and are non repeated, then for each irreduciable quadratic $ax^2 + bx + c$, which occurs only one in the denominator, there correspond a partial fraction of the form $\frac{Ax+B}{ax^2+bx+c}$.

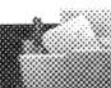

Solved Examples

1. *Evaluate the integral* $\int \frac{x+4}{3+2x-x^2}dx.$.

SOLUTION. Here, the given integral is

$$\int \frac{x+4}{3+2x-x^2}dx.$$

Consider

$$\frac{x+4}{3+2x-x^2} = \frac{x+4}{(3-x)(1+x)}$$

$$= \frac{A}{3-x} + \frac{B}{1+x}.$$

So, $x+4 = (1+x)A + (3-x)B$

Putting $x = 3$, we get $A = \frac{7}{4}$ and putting, $x = -1$, we get $B = \frac{3}{4}$

So, we have

$$\frac{x+4}{3+2x-x^2} = \frac{7}{4(3-x)} + \frac{3}{4(1+x)}$$

Hence,

$$\int \frac{x+4}{3+2x-x^2}dx = \frac{7}{4}\int \frac{1}{3-x}dx + \frac{3}{4}\int \frac{1}{1+x}dx;$$

Integrating

$$= -\frac{7}{4}\log(x-3) + \frac{3}{4}\log(1+x) + C$$

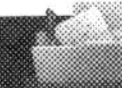

Similar Problems

(1) Show that $\int \frac{3x+2}{(x-2)(x+1)^2}dx = \frac{8}{9}\log\left(\frac{x-2}{x+1}\right) - \frac{1}{3(x+1)} + C$

(2) Show that $\int \frac{1}{x(1-x^2)}dx = \frac{1}{2}\log\left\{\frac{x^2}{1-x^2}\right\} + C$

2. *Evaluate the integral* $\int \frac{7x^2+3x+1}{x(x+1)}dx.$

SOLUTION. Here, the given integral is

$$\int \frac{7x^2+3x+1}{x(x+1)}.$$

To change the integrand into partial fraction, first we divide $(7x^2+3x+1)$ by (x^2+x), because the degree of numerator must be less than the degree of denominator. So, we get

$$\frac{7x^2+3x+1}{x^2+x} = 7 + \frac{1-4x}{x^2+x}$$

So, $\int \frac{7x^2+3x+1}{x^2+x}dx$

$$= 7\int dx + \int \frac{1-4x}{x^2+x}dx$$

$$= 7x + \int \frac{1-4x}{x^2+x}dx \qquad \ldots(1)$$

Now, to find $\int \frac{1-4x}{x^2+x}dx.$

Let $\frac{1-4x}{x^2+x} = \frac{A}{x} + \frac{B}{x+1}$

$$\Rightarrow 1-4x = A(x+1) + Bx \qquad \ldots(2)$$

Now, putting $x = -1 \Rightarrow B = -5$ and putting $x = 0 \Rightarrow A = 1$

Thus, $\frac{1-4x}{x^2+x} = \frac{1}{x} - \frac{5}{x+1}$

So, $\int \frac{1-4x}{x^2+x}dx = \int \frac{1}{x}dx - 5\int \frac{1}{x+1}dx$

$$= \log x - 5\log(x+1) + C$$

Hence, by equation (1), we get

$$\int \frac{7x^2+3x+1}{x^2+x}dx$$

$$= 7x + \log x - 5\log(x+1) + C.$$

3. *Evaluate the integral*

$$\int \frac{x}{(x-1)(2x+1)}dx.$$

SOLUTION. Here, the given integral is

$$\int \frac{x}{(x-1)(2x+1)}dx.$$

Consider, $\frac{x}{(x-1)(2x+1)}$

$$= \frac{A}{(x-1)} + \frac{B}{(2x+1)}$$

$$\Rightarrow x = (2x+1)A + (x-1)B.$$

Now, putting $x = 1$, we get $A = \frac{1}{3}$, and

putting $x = -\frac{1}{2}$, we get $B = \frac{1}{3}$

Thus, $\frac{x}{(x-1)(2x+1)}$

$$= \frac{1}{3(x-1)} + \frac{1}{3(2x+1)}$$

Hence, $\int \frac{x}{(x-1)(2x+1)} dx$

$$= \frac{1}{3}\int \frac{1}{x-1} dx + \frac{1}{3}\int \frac{1}{2x+1} dx$$

$$= \frac{1}{3}\log(x-1) + \frac{1}{3}\cdot\frac{1}{2}\log(2x+1) + C$$

$$= \frac{1}{3}\log(x-1) + \frac{1}{6}\log(2x+1) + C$$

4. *Evaluate the integral*

$$\int \frac{1}{x[(\log x)^2 - 5\log x + 6]} dx.$$

SOLUTION. Here, the given integral is

$$\int \frac{1}{x[(\log x)^2 - 5\log x + 6]} dx.$$

Let $\log x = u \Rightarrow \frac{1}{x} dx = du$

So, $\int \frac{1}{x[(\log x)^2 - 5\log x + 6]} dx$

$$= \int \frac{1}{u^2 - 5u + 6} du$$

$$= \int \frac{1}{(u-2)(u-3)} du$$

Now let

$$\frac{1}{(u-2)(u-3)} = \frac{A}{(u-2)} + \frac{B}{(u-3)}$$

$\Rightarrow 1 = (u-3)A + (u-2)B.$

Now, putting $u = 3$, we get $B = 1$ and putting $u = 2$, we get $A = -1$

Thus, $\frac{1}{(u-2)(u-3)} = \frac{1}{u-3} - \frac{1}{u-2}$

So, $\int \frac{1}{x[(\log x)^2 - 5\log x + 6]} dx$

$$= \int \frac{1}{(u-2)(u-3)} du$$

$$= \int \frac{1}{u-3} du - \int \frac{1}{u-2} du$$

$$= \log(u-3) - \log(u-2) + C$$

$$= \log\left(\frac{u-3}{u-2}\right) + C$$

Now, put $u = \log x$, we get

$$\int \frac{1}{x[(\log x)^2 - 5\log x + 6]} dx = \log\left(\frac{\log x - 3}{\log x - 2}\right) + C$$

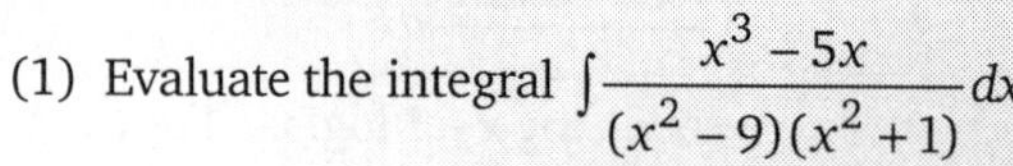

(1) Evaluate the integral $\int \frac{x^3 - 5x}{(x^2-9)(x^2+1)} dx.$ **Ans.** $\frac{1}{5}\log(x^2-9) + \frac{3}{10}\log(x^2+1) + C.$

5. *Evaluate the integral* $\int \frac{1-\cos x}{\cos x(1+\cos x)} dx$

SOLUTION. Here, the given integral is

$$\int \frac{1-\cos x}{\cos x(1+\cos x)} dx.$$

Let $\cos x = t$, then we have

$$\frac{1-\cos x}{\cos x(1+\cos x)} = \frac{1-t}{t(1+t)} = \frac{A}{t} + \frac{B}{(1+t)}$$

$\Rightarrow (1-t) = (1+t)A + tB.$

Putting $t = 0$, we get $A = 1$ and putting $t = -1$, we get $B = -2$ thus, we have

$$\frac{1-t}{t(1+t)} = \frac{1}{t} - \frac{2}{(1+t)}$$

$$\therefore \frac{1-\cos x}{\cos x(1+\cos x)} = \frac{1}{\cos x} - \frac{2}{(1+\cos x)}$$

$$= \sec x - \frac{2}{2\cos^2\frac{x}{2}} = \sec x - \sec^2\frac{x}{2}$$

Hence, $\int \frac{1-\cos x}{\cos x(1+\cos x)} dx$

$$= \int \sec x\, dx - \int \sec^2\frac{x}{2} dx$$

$$= \log(\sec x + \tan x) - 2\tan\frac{x}{2} + C$$

6. *Evaluate* $I = \int \frac{dx}{\sin(x-a)\sin(x-b)} dx$

SOLUTION. We have $I = \int \frac{dx}{\sin(x-a)\sin(x-b)}$

$$= \int \frac{\sin(a-b)}{\sin(a-b)\sin(x-a)\sin(x-b)} dx$$

$$= \int \frac{\sin\{(a-x)-(b-x)\}}{\sin(a-b)\sin(x-a)\sin(x-b)} dx$$

$$= \int \frac{\sin(a-x)\cos(b-x) - \cos(a-x)\sin(b-x)}{\sin(a-b)\sin(x-a)\sin(x-b)} dx$$

$$= \frac{1}{\sin(a-b)} \int \frac{-\sin(x-a)\cos(x-b) + \sin(x-b)\cos(x-a)}{\sin(x-a)\sin(x-b)} dx$$

$$= \frac{1}{\sin(a-b)} \int \{-\cot(x-b) + \cot(x-a)\} dx$$

$$= \frac{1}{\sin(a-b)} \{-\log\sin(x-b) + \log\sin(x-a)\} + C$$

$$= \frac{1}{\sin(a-b)} \log\left\{\frac{\sin(x-a)}{\sin(x-b)}\right\} + C$$

7. *Evaluate the integral*

$$\int \frac{1+x}{(1+x^2)(1-x+x^2)} dx.$$

SOLUTION. Here, the given integral is

$$\int \frac{1+x}{(1+x^2)(1-x+x^2)} dx.$$

Let $\frac{1+x}{(1+x^2)(1-x+x^2)} = \frac{Ax+B}{1+x^2} + \frac{Cx+D}{1-x+x^2}$

$$\Rightarrow 1+x = (1-x+x^2)(Ax+B) + (1+x^2)(Cx+D) \quad \ldots(1)$$

Here, to find the four constants A, B, C and D, the method of comparing the coefficient is lengthy. So, we equate each quadratic factor equal to zero and find the value of x^2 and put this value of x^2 in both sides of (1).

So, $1+x^2 = 0 \Rightarrow x^2 = -1$.

Then, from (1), we get

$$1+x = (Ax+B)(1-x-1) = -(Ax^2+Bx).$$

Again put $x^2 = -1$. Now, comparing x and constant, we get

$$B = -1, A = 1$$

Again, $1-x+x^2 = 0 \Rightarrow x^2 = x-1$

Then from (1), we get

$$1+x = C(x-1) + D(x) = (C+D)x - C$$

Comparing x and constants, we get

$$C = -1 \text{ and } D+C = 1 \Rightarrow D = 2.$$

So, $\frac{1+x}{(1+x^2)(1-x+x^2)} = \left\{\frac{x-1}{(1+x^2)} + \frac{(-x+2)}{1-x+x^2}\right\}$

Hence,

$$\int \frac{1+x}{(1+x^2)(1-x+x^2)} dx$$

$$= \int \left(\frac{x-1}{1+x^2} - \frac{(x-2)}{1-x+x^2}\right) dx$$

$$= \int \left(\frac{1}{2}\cdot\frac{2(x-1)}{1+x^2} - \frac{1}{2}\frac{(2x-1)-3}{1-x+x^2}\right) dx$$

$$= \frac{1}{2}\int \frac{2x}{1+x^2} dx - \int \frac{1}{1+x^2} dx - \frac{1}{2}\int \frac{(2x-1)-3}{1-x+x^2} dx$$

$$= \frac{1}{2}\log(1+x^2) - \tan^{-1} x - \frac{1}{2}\log(1-x+x^2) + \frac{3}{2}\int \frac{dx}{\left(x-\frac{1}{2}\right)^2 + \left(\frac{\sqrt{3}}{2}\right)^2}$$

$$= \frac{1}{2}\log(1+x^2) - \tan^{-1} x - \frac{1}{2}\log(1-x+x^2) + \frac{3}{2}\cdot\frac{2}{\sqrt{3}}\tan^{-1}\frac{x-\frac{1}{2}}{\sqrt{3}/2} + C$$

$$= \frac{1}{2}\log\left(\frac{1+x^2}{1-x+x^2}\right) - \tan^{-1} x + \sqrt{3}\tan^{-1}\left(\frac{2x-1}{\sqrt{3}}\right) + C$$

8. *Evaluate the integral* $\int \frac{x^2}{(x-1)^3(x-2)} dx.$

SOLUTION. Here, the given integral is

$$\int \frac{x^2}{(x-1)^3(x-2)}dx.$$

Let $\frac{x^2}{(x-1)^3(x-2)} = \frac{A}{x-1} + \frac{B}{(x-1)^2} + \frac{C}{(x-1)^3} + \frac{D}{x-2}$

$\Rightarrow x^2 = (x-1)^2(x-2)A + (x-1)(x-2)B + (x-2)C + (x-1)^3 D$ ...(1)

Put $x = 1 \Rightarrow C = -1$

Put $x = 2 \Rightarrow D = 4$

Now, we want to find the coefficient A and B.

On comparing the coefficient of x^3 in (1), we get

$A + D = 0$

Now comparing the constant terms in (1), we get

$-2A + 2B - 2C - D = 0$

Putting the value of C and D, we get

$A = -4, B = -3$

Thus, $\frac{x^2}{(x-1)^3(x-2)} = -\frac{4}{x-1} - \frac{3}{(x-1)^2} - \frac{1}{(x-1)^3} + \frac{4}{x-2}.$

Hence, $\int \frac{x^2}{(x-1)^3(x-2)}dx$

$$= -4\int \frac{1}{x-1}dx - 3\int \frac{1}{(x-1)^2}dx - \int \frac{1}{(x-1)^3}dx + 4\int \frac{1}{x-2}dx$$

$$= -4\log(x-1) + \frac{3}{x-1} + \frac{1}{2(x-1)^2} + 4\log(x-2) + C$$

$$= 4\log\left(\frac{x-2}{x-1}\right) + \frac{3}{x-1} + \frac{1}{2(x-1)^2} + C.$$

More Solved Examples Based on Integral by Substitution

1. *Evaluate* $\int \frac{1}{1+e^{-x}}dx.$

SOLUTION. $I = \int \frac{1}{1+e^{-x}}dx = \int \frac{1}{1+\frac{1}{e^x}}dx = \int \frac{e^x}{1+e^x}dx$

Putting $1 + e^x = t \Rightarrow e^x dx = dt$

$$I = \int \frac{dt}{t} = \log|t| + C = \log\left|1 + e^x\right| + C$$

2. *Evaluate* $\int \frac{\sin 2x}{a^2\sin^2 x + b^2\cos^2 x}dx$

SOLUTION. We have $I = \int \frac{\sin 2x\,dx}{a^2\sin^2 x + b^2\cos^2 x}$ ...(1)

Let $a^2\sin^2 x + b^2\cos^2 x = t$

$\Rightarrow (2a^2\sin x\cos x - 2b^2\sin x\cos x)dx = dt$

$\Rightarrow (a^2\sin 2x - b^2\sin 2x)dx = dt$

$\Rightarrow \sin 2x dx = \frac{dt}{a^2 - b^2}$

Putting in (1), we get

$$I = \int \frac{dt}{t(a^2-b^2)} = \frac{1}{a^2-b^2}\log|t| + C$$

$$= \frac{1}{a^2-b^2}\log\left|a^2\sin^2 x + b^2\cos^2 x\right| + C$$

3. *Find* $\int \frac{dx}{x(1+x^n)}$ (MEERUT(BCA)–2002)

SOLUTION. Let $I = \int \frac{dx}{x(1+x^n)} = \int \frac{x^{n-1}dx}{x^n(1+x^n)}$

(Multiply by x^{n-1} into Nr. and Dr.)

Put $(1+x^n) = t \Rightarrow x^n = t - 1$

$\Rightarrow nx^{n-1}dx = dt \Rightarrow x^{n-1}dx = \frac{dt}{n}$

Therefore, $I = \frac{1}{n}\int \frac{dt}{(t-1)t}$

$$= \frac{1}{n}\int\left(\frac{1}{t-1} - \frac{1}{t}\right)dt$$

(By partial fraction)

Integrating

$$I = \frac{1}{n}\{\log|t-1| - \log|t|\} + C$$

$$= \frac{1}{n}\log\left|\frac{t-1}{t}\right| + C$$

$$= \frac{1}{n}\log\left|\frac{x^n}{x^n+1}\right| + C$$

(By putting the value of t)

4. *Evaluate* $\int \frac{(2x+5)}{\sqrt{x^2+3x+1}}dx$

(MEERUT(BCA)–2002, 05, 13)

SOLUTION. Let $I=\int \frac{(2x+5)}{\sqrt{x^2+3x+1}}dx=\int \frac{(2x+3)+2}{\sqrt{x^2+3x+1}}dx$

$$= \underbrace{\int \frac{(2x+3)}{\sqrt{x^2+3x+1}}dx}_{I_1} + \underbrace{\int \frac{2}{\sqrt{x^2+3x+1}}dx}_{I_2} \quad ...(1)$$

Suppose $I_1 = \int \frac{(2x+3)}{\sqrt{x^2+3x+1}}dx$

Put $x^2 + 3x + 1 = t \Rightarrow (2x+3)dx = dt$

Now $I_1 = \int \frac{dt}{\sqrt{t}} = \int t^{-1/2}dt = \frac{t^{-1/2+1}}{-\frac{1}{2}+1}+C_1$

$$= 2t^{1/2}+C_1 = 2\sqrt{x^2+3x+1}+C_1$$

$$I_2 = \int \frac{2dx}{\sqrt{x^2+3x+1}}$$

$$= 2\int \frac{dx}{\left(x^2+3x+\frac{9}{4}-\frac{9}{4}+1\right)^{1/2}}$$

$$= 2\int \frac{dx}{\left\{\left(x+\frac{3}{2}\right)^2-\left(\frac{\sqrt{5}}{2}\right)^2\right\}^{1/2}}$$

$$= 2\log\left|\left(x+\frac{3}{2}\right)+\sqrt{x^2+3x+1}\right|+C_2$$

Putting the value of I_1 and I_2 in (1), we get

$$I = 2\sqrt{x^2+3x+1}+C_1 + 2\log\left|\left(x+\frac{3}{2}\right)+\sqrt{x^2+3x+1}\right|+C_2$$

$$= 2\sqrt{x^2+3x+1} + 2\log\left|\left(x+\frac{3}{2}\right)+\sqrt{x^2+3x+1}\right|+C$$

where, $C = C_1 + C_2$

5. *Evaluate* $\int \frac{\cot x}{\log \sin x}dx.$

SOLUTION. Let $I = \int \frac{\cot x}{\log \sin x}dx$

Putting $\log \sin x = t$

$$\Rightarrow \frac{1}{\sin x}\cos x\,dx = dt$$

$$\Rightarrow \cot x\,dx = dt$$

Then $I = \int \frac{dt}{t} = \log|t|+C$

$$= \log|\log \sin x|+C$$

6. *Evaluate* $\int \frac{1}{\sqrt{x}(\sqrt{x}+1)}dx$

SOLUTION. Let $I = \int \frac{1}{\sqrt{x}(\sqrt{x}+1)}dx$

Putting $\sqrt{x}+1 = t$, differentiating w.r.t. x $\frac{1}{2\sqrt{x}}dx = dt$

$$\frac{dx}{\sqrt{x}} = 2dt$$

Then $I = \int \frac{2dt}{t} = 2\log|t|+C$

$$= 2\log\left|\sqrt{x}+1\right|+C$$

7. *Evaluate* $\int \cot x\, e^{m\log(\sin x)}dx$

[MEERUT(BCA)–2003, 04; AGRA(BCA)–2011; PURVANCHAL(BCA)–2009]

SOLUTION. Let $I = \int \cot x e^{m\log(\sin x)}dx$

Putting $\log \sin x = t$ and diff. w.r.t. x, we get

$$\frac{\cos x}{\sin x}dx = dt \quad \Rightarrow \quad \cot x\,dx = dt$$

Then $I = \int e^{mt}dt.$

Integrating

$$I = \frac{e^{mt}}{m}+C = \frac{e^{m\log(\sin x)}}{m}+C$$

(Putting value of t)

Similar Problem

(1) Evaluate $\int \frac{3x^2+1}{x(x^2+1)}dx$ **Ans.** $\log\left|x^3+x\right|+C$

8. *Evaluate* $\int \frac{\sin x}{\sin(x-a)} dx.$

SOLUTION. Let $I = \int \frac{\sin x}{\sin(x-a)} dx$

Putting $x - a = t$, *i.e.*, $dx = dt$ we get

$$I = \int \frac{\sin(a+t)}{\sin t} dt$$
$$= \int \frac{\sin a \cos t + \cos a \sin t}{\sin t} dt$$
$$= \sin a \int \cot t\, dt + \cos a \int 1\, dt$$
$$= \sin a \log \sin t + t \cos a + C.$$

Putting the value of t, we have

$$I = \sin a \log \sin(x-a) + (x-a)\cos a + C.$$

9. *Evaluate* $\int x^5 \sqrt{a^3 + x^3}\, dx$

SOLUTION. Let $I = \int x^5 \sqrt{a^3 + x^3}\, dx$

$$= \int x^3 x^2 \sqrt{a^3 + x^3}\, dx$$

Putting $a^3 + x^3 = t$, differentiating w.r.t. x,

$$3x^2 dx = dt$$
$$x^2 dx = \frac{dt}{3}$$

Then, $I = \frac{1}{3} \int (t - a^3)\sqrt{t}\, dt$

$$= \frac{1}{3} \int (t^{3/2} - a^3 t^{1/2})\, dt,$$

(On integrating)

$$= \frac{1}{3} \cdot \frac{t^{5/2}}{5/2} - \frac{a^3}{3} \frac{t^{3/2}}{3/2} + C$$

Putting the value of t, we have

$$I = \frac{2}{15}(a^3 + x^3)^{5/2} - \frac{2}{9} a^3 (a^3 + x^3)^{3/2} + C$$

10. *Evaluate* $\int \frac{\log \tan x/2}{\sin x} dx.$

SOLUTION. Let $I = \int \frac{\log \tan \frac{x}{2}}{\sin x} dx$

Putting, $\log \tan \frac{x}{2} = t$, and differentiating, we get

$$\frac{1}{\tan x/2} \sec^2 x/2 \cdot \frac{1}{2} dx = dt$$

$$\Rightarrow \frac{1}{2 \frac{\sin x/2}{\cos x/2} \cdot \cos^2 x/2} dx = dt$$

$$\Rightarrow \frac{1}{2 \sin x/2 \cos x/2} dx = dt$$

$$\Rightarrow \frac{1}{\sin x} dx = dt$$

Then $I = \int t\, dt = \frac{t^2}{2} + C$

$$= \frac{(\log \tan x/2)^2}{2} + C$$

11. *Evaluate* $\int \sec^3 x \tan x\, dx.$

SOLUTION. Let $I = \int \sec^3 x \tan x\, dx$

$$I = \int \sec^2 x (\sec x \tan x)\, dx$$

Putting, $\sec x = t$, differentiating w.r.t. x, we get

$$\sec x \tan x\, dx = dt$$

Then $I = \int t^2 dt = \frac{t^3}{3} + C,$

Now, putting the value of t, we have

$$I = \frac{\sec^3 x}{3} + C$$

12. *Evaluate* $\int \frac{1}{\sin x \cos^3 x} dx$

SOLUTION. Let $I = \int \frac{dx}{\frac{\sin x}{\cos x} \cos^4 x} = \int \frac{dx}{\tan x \cos^4 x}$

$$= \int \frac{\sec^4 x\, dx}{\tan x}$$
$$= \int \frac{\sec^2 x \sec^2 x}{\tan x} dx$$
$$= \int \frac{(1 + \tan^2 x)\sec^2 x}{\tan x} dx$$

Putting, $\tan x = t$

$$\Rightarrow \sec^2 x\, dx = dt$$

Then $I = \int \frac{1+t^2}{t} dt = \int \left(\frac{1}{t} + t\right) dt,$

Integrating and putting the value of t, we get

$$I = \log|t| + \frac{t^2}{2} + C$$
$$= \log|\tan x| + \frac{\tan^2 x}{2} + C$$

13. *Evaluate* $\int \frac{\log x^2}{x} dx.$

SOLUTION. Let $I = \int \frac{\log x^2}{x} dx$

$$I = \int \frac{\log x^2}{x} dx = \int \frac{2\log x}{x} dx$$

Putting $\log x = t$, differentiating

$$\frac{1}{x} dx = dt$$

Then $I = 2\int t\, dt = \frac{2t^2}{2} + C = t^2 + C$

After putting the value of t, we have

$$I = (\log x)^2 + C$$

14. *Evaluate* $\int \frac{x^2 \tan^{-1} x^3}{1+x^6} dx$

SOLUTION. Let $I = \int \frac{x^2 \tan^{-1} x^3}{1+x^6} dx$

Let us put $\tan^{-1} x^3 = t$, differentiating

$$\frac{1}{1+(x^3)^2} \cdot 3x^2 dx = dt$$

$$\Rightarrow \quad \frac{x^2}{1+x^6} dx = \frac{dt}{3}$$

Then $I = \frac{1}{3}\int t\, dt = \frac{t^2}{6} + C$

On integrating and putting the value of t, we get $I = \frac{(\tan^{-1} x^3)^2}{6} + C$

15. *Evaluate* $\int \tan x \sec^2 x \sqrt{1-\tan^2 x}\, dx$

SOLUTION. Let $I = \int \tan x \sec^2 x \sqrt{1-\tan^2 x}\, dx$

Putting $1 - \tan^2 x = t$

$$\Rightarrow -2\tan x \sec^2 x\, dx = dt$$

$$\tan x \sec^2 x\, dx = -\frac{dt}{2}$$

Then $I = -\frac{1}{2}\int \sqrt{t} dt = -\frac{1}{2}\frac{t^{3/2}}{3/2} + C$

$$= -\frac{1}{3}(1-\tan^2 x)^{3/2} + C$$

(After putting the value of t)

16. *Evaluate* $\int \frac{e^{m\sin^{-1} x}}{\sqrt{1-x^2}} dx.$

SOLUTION. Let $I = \int \frac{e^{m\sin^{-1} x}}{\sqrt{1-x^2}} dx$

Putting, $\sin^{-1} x = t$, differentiating w.r.t. x, we get

$$\frac{1}{\sqrt{1-x^2}} dx = dt$$

Then $I = \int e^{mt} dt = \frac{e^{mt}}{m} + C = \frac{e^{m\sin^{-1} x}}{m} + C$

(After putting the value of t)

17. *Evaluate* $\int \frac{\cos^9 x}{\sin x} dx$

SOLUTION. Let $I = \int \frac{\cos^9 x}{\sin x} dx = \int \frac{\cos^8 x \cos x}{\sin x} dx$

$$= \int \frac{(\cos^2 x)^4 \cos x\, dx}{\sin x}$$

$$= \int \frac{(1-\sin^2 x)^4 \cos x}{\sin x} dx$$

Put $\sin x = t \quad \Rightarrow \quad \cos x\, dx = dt$

Then $I = \int \frac{(1-t^2)^4 dt}{t}$

$$= \int \frac{1 - 4t^2 + 6t^4 - 4t^6 + t^8}{t} dt$$

$$= \int \left(\frac{1}{t} - 4t + 6t^3 - 4t^5 + t^7\right) dt$$

$$= \log|t| - 2t^2 + \frac{3}{2}t^4 - \frac{2}{3}t^6 + \frac{1}{8}t^8 + C,$$

(On integrating)

$$= \log|\sin x| - 2\sin^2 x + \frac{3}{2}\sin^4 x - \frac{2}{3}\sin^6 x + \frac{1}{8}\sin^8 x + C$$

(After putting the value of t)

18. *Evaluate* $\int \sec^4 x\, dx$

SOLUTION. Let $I = \int \sec^4 x\, dx = \int \sec^2 x \sec^2 x\, dx$

$$= \int \sec^2 x (1+\tan^2 x) dx$$

$$= \int (\sec^2 x + \sec^2 x \tan^2 x)\, dx$$

$$= \int \sec^2 x\, dx + \int \sec^2 x \tan^2 x\, dx$$

$$= \tan x + \int \sec^2 x \tan^2 x\, dx$$

Put $\tan x = t$, in 2nd integral, we have

$$\sec^2 x\, dx = dt$$

Then $I = \tan x + \int t^2 dt + C$

$= \tan x + \frac{t^3}{3} + C$

$= \tan x + \frac{\tan^3 x}{3} + C$

19. *Evaluate* $\int \frac{x^2}{\sqrt{1+x}} dx$

SOLUTION. Let $I = \int \frac{x^2}{\sqrt{1+x}} dx$

put $1 + x = t^2 \Rightarrow x = t^2 - 1$, $dx = 2t\,dt$

Then $I = \int \frac{(t^2-1)^2 . 2t\,dt}{\sqrt{t^2}} = 2\int \frac{(t^2-1)^2 t\,dt}{t}$

$= 2\int (t^2-1)^2 dt = 2\int (t^4 - 2t^2 + 1) dt$

$= 2\left[\frac{t^5}{5} - \frac{2t^3}{3} + t\right] + C;$

$= \frac{2}{5}(1+x)^{5/2} - \frac{4}{3}(1+x)^{3/2} + 2\sqrt{1+x} + C$

20. *Evaluate* $\int \cos^3 \sqrt{x}\, dx$

[MEERUT(BCA)–2009; MUMBAI–2013]

SOLUTION. Consider $\int \cos^3 \sqrt{x}\, dx$

Putting $\sqrt{x} = t \Rightarrow x = t^2$

$\Rightarrow dx = 2t\,dt$

$\therefore \int \cos^3 \sqrt{x}\, dx = 2\int \cos^3 t . t\, dt$

Now using $\cos 3x = 4\cos^3 x - 3\cos x$, we have

$= 2\int t\left[\frac{\cos 3t + 3\cos t}{4}\right] dt$

$= \frac{1}{2}\int t\cos 3t\, dt + \frac{3}{2}\int t\cos t\, dt$

$= \frac{1}{2}\left[t\frac{\sin 3t}{3} + \frac{1}{9}\cos 3t\right] + \frac{3}{2}[t\sin t + \cos t] + c$

$= \frac{1}{6}\left[t\sin 3t + \frac{1}{3}\cos 3t\right] + \frac{3}{2}[t\sin t + \cos t] + c$

$= \frac{1}{6}\left[\sqrt{x}\sin 3\sqrt{x} + \frac{1}{3}\cos 3\sqrt{x}\right] + \frac{3}{2}(\sqrt{x}\sin\sqrt{x} + \cos\sqrt{x}) + C$ $(\because \sqrt{x} = t)$

Exercise-16.1

Evaluate the following Integrals:

1. $\int \frac{\sin\sqrt{x}}{\sqrt{x}} dx$

2. $\int \frac{1}{x^2}\cos^2\left(\frac{1}{x}\right) dx$

3. $\int (4x+2)\sqrt{x^2+x+1} dx$

4. $\int \operatorname{cosec} x \cdot \log(\operatorname{cosec} x - \cot x) dx$

5. $\int \frac{\sec^2(2\tan^{-1} x)}{1+x^2} dx$

6. $\int \frac{1-\sin 2x}{x+\cos^2 x} dx$

7. $\int \frac{\operatorname{cosec} x}{\log \tan \frac{x}{2}} dx$

8. $\int \frac{1-\cot x}{1+\cot x} dx$

9. $\int 4x^3\sqrt{5-x^2} dx$

10. $\int \frac{(x+1)e^x}{\cos^2(xe^x)} dx$

11. $\int \frac{dx}{\sin\frac{x}{2} + \tan\frac{x}{2}}$ [MEERUT(BCA)–2001, 09]

Hint to the Selected Problems

1. $I = \int \frac{\sin\sqrt{x}}{\sqrt{x}} dx$

Put $\sqrt{x} = t \Rightarrow \frac{1}{2\sqrt{x}} dx = dt \Rightarrow \frac{dx}{\sqrt{x}} = 2\,dt$

$\therefore I = 2\int \sin t\, dt = -2\cos t + C = -2\cos\sqrt{x} + C$

2. $I = \int \frac{1}{x^2}\cos^2\left(\frac{1}{x}\right) dx$

Put $\frac{1}{x} = t \Rightarrow \frac{dt}{dx} = -\frac{1}{x^2} \Rightarrow \frac{dx}{x^2} = -dt$

$I = -\int \cos^2 t\, dt = -\int\left(\frac{1+\cos 2t}{2}\right) dt$ $\left(\because \cos^2 x = \frac{1+\cos 2x}{2}\right)$

$= -\frac{1}{2}\int (1+\cos 2t) dt,$

Integrating

$= -\frac{1}{2}\left(t + \frac{\sin 2t}{2}\right) + C = -\frac{1}{2x} - \frac{1}{4}\sin\frac{2}{x} + C$

3. $I = \int (4x+2)\sqrt{x^2+x+1}\,dx$

Put $x^2 + x + 1 = t$

$\Rightarrow \quad (2x+1)\,dx = dt$

$I = 2\int \sqrt{t}\,dt$

$= 2\dfrac{t^{3/2}}{3/2} + C = \dfrac{4}{3}t^{3/2} + C$

4. $I = \int \text{cosec}\,x \cdot \log(\text{cosec}\,x - \cot x)dx$

Put $\log(\text{cosec}\,x - \cot x) = t$

$$\frac{1}{\text{cosec}\,x - \cot x}(-\text{cosec}\,x\cot^2 x + \text{cosec}^2 x)dx = dt$$

$\Rightarrow \quad \text{cosec}\,x\,dx = dt$

$I = \int t\,dt = \dfrac{t^2}{2} + C$

$= \dfrac{1}{2}\{\log(\text{cosec}\,x - \cot x)\}^2 + C$

5. $I = \int \dfrac{\sec^2(2\tan^{-1}x)}{1+x^2}dx$

Put $\tan^{-1}x = t$

$\dfrac{1}{1+x^2}dx = dt$

$I = \int \sec^2(2t)\,dt$. Integrating

$= \dfrac{\tan 2t}{2} + C$

6. $I = \int \dfrac{1-\sin 2x}{x+\cos^2 x}dx$

Put $x + \cos^2 x = t$

$(1 - 2\sin x\cos x)\,dx = dt$

$(1 - \sin 2x)\,dx = dt$

$I = \int \dfrac{dt}{t}$,

Integrating $= \log t + C = \log\left|x + \cos^2 x\right| + C$

7. $I = \int \dfrac{\text{cosec}\,x}{\log\tan\dfrac{x}{2}}dx$

put $\log\tan\dfrac{x}{2} = t$, differentiating

We get $\dfrac{1}{\tan\dfrac{x}{2}}\left(\sec^2\dfrac{x}{2}\right)\dfrac{1}{2}dx = dt$

$\Rightarrow \quad \dfrac{1}{2\sin x/2\cos x/2}dx = dt$

$\Rightarrow \quad \text{cosec}\,x\,dx = dt$

$I = \int \dfrac{dt}{t}$, Integrating

$= \log t + C$

8. $I = \int \dfrac{1-\cot x}{1+\cot x}dx = \int \dfrac{\sin x - \cos x}{\sin x + \cos x}dx$

Put $\cos x + \sin x = t \quad \Rightarrow -(\sin x - \cos x)\,dx = dt$

$I = -\int \dfrac{dt}{t} = -\log t + C,$

9. $I = \int 4x^3\sqrt{5-x^2}dx = \int 4x^2 \cdot x\sqrt{5-x^2}dx;$

Put $5 - x^2 = t \quad \Rightarrow \quad -x\,dx = \dfrac{dt}{2}$

$I = 4\int (5-t)\sqrt{t}\left(-\dfrac{dt}{2}\right)$

$= -2\int (5\sqrt{t} - t^{3/2})dt$, Integrating

$= -2\left\{5\dfrac{t^{3/2}}{3/2} - \dfrac{2}{5}t^{5/2}\right\} + C$

$= \dfrac{-20}{3}t^{3/2} + \dfrac{4}{5}t^{5/2} + C,$

10. $I = \int \dfrac{(x+1)e^x}{\cos^2(xe^x)}dx$

Put $xe^x = t \quad \Rightarrow \quad (e^x + xe^x)\,dx = dt$

$\Rightarrow \quad e^x(x+1)dx = dt$

$I = \int \dfrac{dt}{\cos^2 t} = \int \sec^2 t\,dt$; Integrating

ANSWERS

1. $-2\cos\sqrt{x} + C$ **2.** $-\dfrac{1}{2x} - \dfrac{1}{4}\sin\dfrac{2}{x} + C$ **3.** $\dfrac{4}{3}(x^2+x+1)^{3/2} + C$

4. $\dfrac{1}{2}\{\log|\text{cosec}\,x - \cot x|\}^2 + C$ **5.** $\dfrac{1}{2}\tan(2\tan^{-1}x) + C$ **6.** $\log|x + \cos^2 x| + C$

7. $\log\left|\log\tan\frac{x}{2}\right|+C$ **8.** $-\log|\cos x+\sin x|+C$ **9.** $\frac{4}{5}(5-x^2)^{5/2}-\frac{20}{3}(5-x^2)^{3/2}+C$

10. $\tan(xe^x)+C$ **11.** $\log\tan\frac{x}{4}-\frac{\left(\sec\frac{x}{4}\right)^2}{2}+C$

16.6 DEFINITE INTEGRAL

If $f(x)$ is a continuous and non-negative function over a closed interval $[a,b]$, then $\int_a^b f(x)dx$ is called the definite integral of $f(x)$ between the limits a and $b(b > a)$..

If $\int f(x)dx = F(x)+c$, then $\int_a^b f(x)dx = [F(x)+c]_a^b = F(b)-F(a)$ is a definite value.

Here, a is called the lower limit and b is called the upper limit and the interval $[a,b]$ is called the range of integration.

- $\int_a^b f(x)dx$ represents the area bounded by the lines $x = a$ and $x = b$.
- If $F(b) - F(a)$ is not a definite value, then the integral $\int_a^b f(x)dx$ is indefinite.

16.7 PROPERTIES OF DEFINITE INTEGRALS

1. $\int_a^a f(x)dx = 0$.

Proof. Let $\int f(x)dx = F(x)$,

then $\int_a^a f(x)dx = [F(x)]_a^a = F(a)-F(a)=0$

2. *The value of definite integral is independent of the variable of integration.*

i.e., $\int_a^b f(x)dx = \int_a^b f(u)du$.

Proof. Let $\int f(x)dx = F(x)$,

then $\int_a^b f(x)dx = [F(x)]_a^b = F(b)-F(a) = \int_a^b f(u)du$

3. $\int_a^b f(x)dx = -\int_b^a f(x)dx$.

Proof. Let $\int f(x)dx = F(x)$,

then $\int_a^b f(x)dx = [F(x)]_a^b = F(b)-F(a) = -[F(x)]_b^a = \int_b^a f(x)dx$

4. $\int_a^c f(x)dx + \int_c^b f(x)dx = \int_a^b f(x)dx$ *where* $a < c < b$.

Proof. Let $\int f(x)dx = F(x)$,

then $\int_a^c f(x)dx + \int_c^b f(x)dx = [F(x)]_a^c + [F(x)]_c^b = [F(c)-F(a)]+[F(b)-F(c)]$

$= F(b)-F(a) = [F(x)]_a^b = \int_a^b f(x)dx$.

5. $\int_0^a f(a-x)dx = \int_0^a f(x)dx$

Proof. We have $\int_0^a f(a-x)dx$

Let $a-x=t$, then $-dx = dt$. If $x=0 \Rightarrow t=a$ and $x=a, t=0$.

So, $\int_0^a f(a-x)dx = -\int_a^0 f(t)dt = \int_0^a f(x)dx$ (By property 2)

6. *If f(x) is an even function of x, then* $\int_{-a}^{a} f(x)\,dx = 2\int_0^a f(x)\,dx$ *and if f(x) is an odd function then* $\int_{-a}^{a} f(x)\,dx = 0$.

Proof. Consider $\int_{-a}^{a} f(x)\,dx$.

Then, $\int_{-a}^{a} f(x)\,dx = \int_{-a}^{0} f(x)\,dx + \int_0^a f(x)\,dx.$

Now let $I = \int_{-a}^{0} f(x)\,dx$

Put $x = -t$, so $x = -a \Rightarrow t = a$ and $x = 0 \Rightarrow t = 0$.

So, $\int_{-a}^{0} f(x)\,dx = -\int_a^0 f(-t)\,dt = \int_0^a f(-t)\,dt = \int_0^a f(-x)\,dx$ (By 2)

Thus, we have $\int_{-a}^{a} f(x)\,dx = \int_0^a f(-x)\,dx + \int_0^a f(x)\,dx = \int_0^a [f(-x) + f(x)]\,dx.$

Now, if $f(x)$ is an even function, *i.e.*, $f(-x) = f(x)$, then we get

$$\int_{-a}^{a} f(x)\,dx = \int_0^a [f(x) + f(x)]\,dx = 2\int_0^a f(x)dx$$

and, if $f(x)$ an odd function, *i.e.*, $f(-x) = -f(x)$, then we get

$$\int_{-a}^{a} f(x)\,dx = \int_0^a [-f(x) + f(x)]\,dx = 0.$$

7. $\int_0^{2a} f(x)\,dx = 2\int_0^a f(x)\,dx$ *if* $f(2a - x) = f(x)$ *and* $\int_0^{2a} f(x)dx = 0$ *if* $f(2a - x) = -f(x)$.

Proof. This integral can be written as

$$\int_0^{2a} f(x)dx = \int_0^a f(x)dx + \int_a^{2a} f(x)dx \quad \text{...(1)}$$

Now, consider the integral $\int_a^{2a} f(x)\,dx$

Put $x = 2a - t$, then $dx = -dt$

And if $x = a$ then $t = a$ and if $x = 2a$ then $t = 0$.

So, $\int_a^{2a} f(x)\,dx = -\int_a^0 f(2a - t)\,dt = \int_0^a f(2a - t)dt = \int_0^a f(2a - x)\,dx$ (By 2)

Therefore, from (1), we have

$$\int_0^{2a} f(x)dx = \int_0^a f(x)\,dx + \int_0^a f(2a - x)\,dx = \int_0^a [f(x) + f(2a - x)]\,dx. \quad \text{...(2)}$$

Now, if $f(2a - x) = f(x)$ then from (2), we get

$$\int_0^{2a} f(x)\,dx = 2\int_0^a f(x)\,dx$$

and if $f(2a - x) = -f(x)$, then from (2), we get

$$\int_0^{2a} f(x)\,dx = \int_0^a [f(x) - f(x)]\,dx = 0.$$

8. $\int_0^{na} f(x)\,dx = n\int_0^a f(x)\,dx$, *if* $f(x + ma) = f(x)$ *for all integral values of m and n is a positive integer.*

Proof. The given integral can be written as

$$\int_0^{na} f(x)\,dx = \int_0^a f(x)\,dx + \int_0^{2a} f(x)\,dx + ... + \int_{(m-1)a}^{ma} f(x)\,dx + ... + \int_{(n-1)a}^{na} f(x)dx \quad \text{...(1)}$$

Now, consider the integral $\int_{(m-1)a}^{ma} f(x)\,dx$,

Put $x = y + ma \Rightarrow dx = dy$

So, $\int_{(m-1)a}^{ma} f(x)dx = \int_0^a f(y+ma)dy.$

But $f(y+ma) = f(y)$ is given, so we have

$$\int_{(m-1)a}^{ma} f(x)\,dx = \int_0^a f(y)\,dy = \int_0^a f(x)\,dx.$$

Now from (1) we have

$$\int_0^{na} f(x)\,dx = \int_0^a f(x)\,dx + \int_0^a f(x)\,dx + \ldots + \int_0^a f(x)\,dx = n\int_0^a f(x)\,dx.$$

Hence, $\int_0^{na} f(x)\,dx = n\int_0^a f(x)\,dx$ if $f(x+ma) = f(x)$ for all integral value of m.

Solved Examples

1. *Evaluate the following integrals*

(i) $\int_0^{\pi/2} \log\tan x\,dx$

(ii) $\int_0^{\pi/4} \log(1+\tan\theta)\,d\theta$ [MEERUT(BCA)–2005, 09, 13,16]

(iii) $\int_0^{\pi} \frac{x\sin x}{1+\sin x}dx$

(iv) $\int_0^{\pi/2} \log\sin x\,dx$ [KANPUR(BCA)–2001, MEERUT(BCA)-2002, RAJASTHAN-2007]

SOLUTION. (i) Consider, $I = \int_0^{\pi/2} \log\tan x\,dx.$

Now, $I = \int_0^{\pi/2} \log\tan\left(\frac{\pi}{2} - x\right)dx$

$\left(\because \int_0^a f(x)dx = \int_0^a f(a-x)\,dx\right)$

$I = \int_0^{\pi/2} \log\cot x\,dx$

On adding, we get

$$2I = \int_0^{\pi/2} \log\tan x\,dx + \int_0^{\pi/2} \log\cot x\,dx$$
$$= \int_0^{\pi/2} \log(\tan x\cot x)\,dx$$
$$= \int_0^{\pi/2} \log 1 = 0$$

Hence, $2I = 0 \Rightarrow I = 0.$

(ii) Consider $I = \int_0^{\pi/4} \log(1+\tan\theta)d\theta$

$$I = \int_0^{\pi/4} \log\left[1+\tan\left(\frac{\pi}{4} - \theta\right)\right]d\theta$$

$\left[\because \int_0^a f(x)\,dx = \int_0^a f(a-x)\,dx\right]$

$$= \int_0^{\pi/4} \log\left[1+\frac{1-\tan\theta}{1+\tan\theta}\right]d\theta$$
$$= \int_0^{\pi/4} \log\left(\frac{2}{1+\tan\theta}\right)d\theta$$
$$= \int_0^{\pi/4} [\log 2 - \log(1+\tan\theta)]\,d\theta$$
$$= \int_0^{\pi/4} \log 2\,d\theta - \int_0^{\pi/4} \log(1+\tan\theta)d\theta$$
$$= \frac{\pi}{4}\log 2 - I$$

So, $2I = \frac{\pi}{4}\log 2$

Hence $I = \frac{\pi}{8}\log 2$

(iii) Here $I = \int_0^{\pi} \frac{x\sin x}{1+\sin x}dx$

Now $I = \int_0^{\pi} \frac{(\pi-x)\sin(\pi-x)}{1+\sin(\pi-x)}dx$

$\left(\because \int_0^a f(x)\,dx = \int_0^a f(a-x)\,dx\right)$

$$= \int_0^{\pi} \frac{(\pi-x)\sin x}{1+\sin x}dx$$
$$= \int_0^{\pi} \frac{\pi\sin x}{1+\sin x}dx - \int_0^{\pi} \frac{x\sin x}{1+\sin x}dx$$
$$= \int_0^{\pi} \frac{\pi\sin x}{1+\sin x}dx - I$$

So, $2I = \int_0^{\pi} \frac{\pi\sin x}{1+\sin x}dx = \pi\int_0^{\pi} \frac{\sin x}{1+\sin x}$

$$= \pi\cdot\int_0^{\pi}\left(1 - \frac{1}{1+\sin x}\right)dx$$
$$= \pi\int_0^{\pi}\left(1 - \frac{1-\sin x}{\cos^2 x}\right)dx$$
$$= \pi\int_0^{\pi}[1 - \sec^2 x + \sec x\tan x]\,dx$$
$$= \pi[x - \tan x + \sec x]_0^{\pi} = \pi(\pi-2)$$

$\therefore\ 2I = \pi(\pi-2)$

Hence, $I = \pi\left(\frac{\pi}{2} - 1\right)$

(iv) Here $I = \int_0^{\pi/2} \log \sin x \, dx$.

Also, $I = \int_0^{\pi/2} \log \sin\left(\frac{\pi}{2} - x\right) dx$

$\left(\because \int_0^a f(x)dx = \int_0^a f(a-x)dx\right)$

$\therefore \quad I = \int_0^{\pi/2} \log \cos x \, dx.$

On adding, we get

$$2I = \int_0^{\pi/2} (\log \sin x) dx + \int_0^{\pi/2} \log \cos x \, dx$$

$$= \int_0^{\pi/2} \log\left(\frac{\sin 2x}{2}\right) dx$$

$$= \int_0^{\pi/2} \log \sin 2x \, dx - \int_0^{\pi/2} \log 2 dx$$

Let $2x = t$ for first integral, then on differentiating, we get $2dx = dt$

Now $2I = \frac{1}{2}\int_0^{\pi} \log \sin t \, dt - [(x \log 2)]_0^{\pi/2}$

$$= \frac{1}{2}\int_0^{\pi} \log \sin t \, dt - \frac{\pi}{2}\log 2$$

$$= \int_0^{\pi/2} \log \sin t \, dt - \frac{\pi}{2}\log 2$$

$\therefore \quad 2I = I - \frac{\pi}{2}\log 2$

Hence, $I = -\frac{\pi}{2}\log 2.$

2. *Evaluate the following integral :*

(*i*) $\int_0^3 |3x-1| dx$ (*ii*) $\int_0^{\pi} |\cos x| dx$

(*iii*) $\int_0^6 |x+2| dx$

SOLUTION. (i) Given integral is $\int_0^3 |3x-1| dx$.

Now,

$$|3x-1| = \begin{cases} 3x-1; \text{when } x \geq \frac{1}{3} \\ -(3x-1) \text{ when } x < \frac{1}{3} \end{cases}$$

So, $\int_0^3 |3x-1| dx = \int_0^{1/3} -(3x-1) dx + \int_{1/3}^3 (3x-1) dx$

$$= \left[-\frac{3x^2}{2} + x\right]_0^{1/3} + \left[\frac{3x^2}{2} - x\right]_{1/3}^3$$

$$= \frac{65}{6}.$$

(ii) Here, the given integral is

$$\int_0^{\pi} |\cos x| dx.$$

Now $|\cos x| = \begin{cases} \cos x, 0 \leq x \leq \frac{\pi}{2} \\ -\cos x, \frac{\pi}{2} \leq x \leq \pi \end{cases}$

So, $\int_0^{\pi} |\cos x| dx$

$$= \int_0^{\pi/2} \cos x \, dx + \int_{\pi/2}^{\pi} (-\cos x) dx$$

$$= \int_0^{\pi/2} \cos x \, dx - \int_{\pi/2}^{\pi} \cos x \, dx$$

$$= [\sin x]_0^{\pi/2} - [\sin x]_{\pi/2}^{\pi} = 2$$

(iii) Let $\int_0^6 |x+2| dx = \int_0^6 (x+2) dx$

$$= \int_0^6 x \, dx + \int_0^6 2 dx$$

$$= \left(\frac{x^2}{2}\right)_0^6 + (2x)_0^6 = \frac{36}{2} - 0 + 2 \times 6$$

$$= 18 + 12 = 30$$

3. *Evaluate the integral*

$$\int_0^{\pi} \log(1 + \cos x) dx.$$

SOLUTION. We have, $I = \int_0^{\pi} \log(1 + \cos x) dx$

Now, $I = \int_0^{\pi} \log\{1 + \cos(\pi - x)\} dx$

$$= \int_0^{\pi} \log(1 - \cos x) dx$$

On adding,

$$2I = \int_0^{\pi} \log(1 + \cos x) dx + \int_0^{\pi} \log(1 - \cos x) dx$$

$$= \int_0^{\pi} \log(1 + \cos x)(1 - \cos x) dx$$

$$= \int_0^{\pi} \log \sin^2 x \, dx = 2\int_0^{\pi} \log \sin x \, dx$$

$= 4\int_0^{\pi/2} \log \sin x \, dx$ (Using property 7)

$\therefore \; 2I = 4\left(-\frac{\pi}{2}\log 2\right)$ So, $I = -\pi \log 2.$

Hence, $I = \pi \log\left(\frac{1}{2}\right)$

4. *Evaluate the integral* $\int_0^1 \frac{\sin^{-1} x}{x} dx.$

SOLUTION. We have, $I = \int_0^1 \frac{\sin^{-1} x}{x} dx.$

Putting $x = \sin\theta \;\Rightarrow\; dx = \cos\theta \; d\theta.$

So, $I = \int_0^{\pi/2} \theta \cot\theta \; d\theta.$

Now, integrating by parts w.r.t. θ, we get

$$I = [\theta.\log\sin\theta]_0^{\pi/2} - \int_0^{\pi/2}\log\sin\theta\,d\theta$$

$$= 0 - \left[-\frac{\pi}{2}\log 2\right] = \frac{\pi}{2}\log 2.$$

5. *Evaluate the integral*

$$\int_0^{\infty}\log\left(\frac{1+x^2}{x}\right)\frac{dx}{1+x^2}.$$

SOLUTION. We have, $I = \int_0^{\infty}\log\left(\frac{1+x^2}{x}\right)\frac{dx}{1+x^2}.$

Now, putting $x = \tan\theta$

$$\Rightarrow \theta = \tan^{-1}x,\ d\theta = \frac{dx}{1+x^2}.$$

So, $I = \int_0^{\pi/2}\log\left(\frac{\sec^2\theta}{\tan\theta}\right).d\theta$

$$= \int_0^{\pi/2}\log\left(\frac{1}{\sin\theta\,.\,\cos\theta}\right)d\theta$$

$$= \int_0^{\pi/2}\log\left(\frac{2}{2\sin\theta\cos\theta}\right)d\theta$$

$$= \int_0^{\pi/2}\log 2\,d\theta - \int_0^{\pi/2}\log\sin 2\theta\,d\theta$$

$$= \frac{\pi}{2}.\log 2 - \int_0^{\pi/2}\log\sin 2\theta\,d\theta$$

Let $2\theta = t \Rightarrow 2d\theta = dt.$

Then $I = \frac{\pi}{2}\log 2 - \frac{1}{2}\int_0^{\pi}\log\sin t\,dt$

$$= \frac{\pi}{2}.\log 2 - \int_0^{\pi/2}\log\sin x\,dx$$

(Using property 7)

$$= \frac{\pi}{2}.\log 2 - \left(-\frac{\pi}{2}\log 2\right) = \pi\log 2.$$

$$\left(\because \int_0^{\pi/2}\log\sin x\,dx = -\frac{\pi}{2}\log 2\right)$$

6. *Evaluate the integral* $\int_{-1}^{1}f(x)\,dx,$ *where*

$$f(x) = \begin{cases} e^x, & -1 \le x \le 0 \\ 1, & 0 \le x \le \frac{1}{2} \\ 3^x, & \frac{1}{2} \le x \le 1 \end{cases}$$

SOLUTION. We can write

$$\int_{-1}^{1}f(x)dx = \int_{-1}^{0}f(x)dx + \int_0^{1/2}f(x)dx + \int_{1/2}^{1}f(x)dx$$

$$= \int_{-1}^{0}e^x dx + \int_0^{1/2}1dx + \int_{1/2}^{1}3^x dx$$

$$= [e^x]_{-1}^{0} + [x]_0^{1/2} + \left[\frac{3^x}{\log 3}\right]_{1/2}^{1}$$

$$= (e^0 - e^{-1}) + \frac{1}{2} + \frac{1}{\log 3}(3-\sqrt{3})$$

$$= 1 - \frac{1}{e} + \frac{1}{2} + \frac{1}{\log 3}(3-\sqrt{3})$$

7. *Evaluate the integral* $\int_0^{\pi}\frac{x\tan x}{\sec x + \tan x}dx.$

SOLUTION. Here, $I = \int_0^{\pi}\frac{x\tan x}{\sec x+\tan x}dx$ ...(1)

Now, $I = \int_0^{\pi}\frac{(\pi-x)\tan(\pi-x)}{\sec(\pi-x)+\tan(\pi-x)}dx$

$$\left(\because \int_0^a f(x)dx = \int_0^a f(a-x)dx\right)$$

$$= \int_0^{\pi}\frac{(\pi-x)\tan x}{\sec x+\tan x}. \quad \text{...(2)}$$

On adding, (1) and (2) we get

$$2I = \int_0^{\pi}\frac{x\tan x}{\sec x+\tan x}dx + \int_0^{\pi}\frac{(\pi-x)\tan x}{\sec x\tan x}dx$$

$$= \int_0^{\pi}\frac{\pi\tan x}{\sec x+\tan x}dx$$

$$= \int_0^{\pi}\frac{\pi\tan x(\sec x-\tan x)}{\sec^2 x-\tan^2 x}dx$$

$$(\because\ \sec^2\theta - \tan^2\theta = 1)$$

$$= \pi\int_0^{\pi}[\sec x\tan x - \sec^2 x + 1]dx$$

$$= \pi[\sec x - \tan x + x]_0^{\pi}$$

$$= \pi[\{\sec\pi - \tan\pi + \pi\} - \{\sec 0 - \tan 0 + 0\}]$$

$$= \pi(-1+\pi-1) = \pi(\pi-2)$$

So, $I = \pi\left(\frac{\pi}{2}-1\right).$

8. *Evaluate* $\int_0^{\pi/2}\frac{dx}{5+4\sin x}.$

[MEERUT(BCA)–2006, 12]

SOLUTION. Let $I = \int_0^{\pi/2} \frac{dx}{5 + 8\sin x/2 \cdot \cos x/2}$

Divide Nr and Dr by $\cos^2 x/2$ we have

$$I = \int_0^{\pi/2} \frac{\sec^2 x/2 dx}{5\sec^2 \frac{x}{2} + 8\tan\frac{x}{2}}$$

$$= \int_0^{\pi/2} \frac{\sec^2 x/2 dx}{5\left(1 + \tan^2\frac{x}{2}\right) + 8\tan x/2}$$

Put $\tan\frac{x}{2} = t \Rightarrow \frac{1}{2}\sec^2\frac{x}{2}dx = dt$

$\Rightarrow \sec^2\frac{x}{2}dx = 2dt$

When $x = 0 \Rightarrow t = 0$

$x = \frac{\pi}{2} \Rightarrow t = 1$

Then $I = \int_0^1 \frac{2dt}{5t^2 + 8t + 5}$

$$= \frac{2}{5}\int_0^1 \frac{dt}{t^2 + \frac{8}{5}t + 1}$$

$$= \frac{2}{5}\int_0^1 \frac{dt}{\left(t + \frac{4}{5}\right)^2 + \left(\frac{3}{4}\right)^2}$$

$$= \frac{2}{5}\cdot\frac{4}{3}\left[\tan^{-1}\left(\frac{t + \frac{4}{5}}{3/4}\right)\right]_0^1$$

$$= \frac{8}{15}\left[\tan^{-1}\frac{36}{15} - \tan^{-1}\frac{16}{15}\right]$$

9. *Evaluate* $\int_0^1 \sin^{-1} x\, dx$.

[MEERUT(BCA)–2006, 13]

SOLUTION. Let $I = \int_0^1 \sin^{-1} x\, dx$

Putting $x = \sin\theta \Rightarrow dx = \cos\theta\, d\theta$

When $x = 0 \Rightarrow \theta = 0$

and $x = 1 \Rightarrow \theta = \frac{\pi}{2}$

Then $I = \int_0^{\pi/2} \theta\cos\theta\, d\theta$;

Integrating by parts, we get

$$I = (\theta\sin\theta)_0^{\pi/2} - \int_0^{\pi/2} \sin\theta\, d\theta$$

$$= \frac{\pi}{2} + [\cos\theta]_0^{\pi/2} = \frac{\pi}{2} - 1 = \frac{\pi - 2}{2}$$

10. *Evaluate* $\int_0^a \frac{x^4.dx}{\sqrt{a^2 - x^2}}$

SOLUTION. Let $I = \int_0^a \frac{x^4.dx}{\sqrt{a^2 - x^2}}$

Put $x = a\sin\theta \Rightarrow dx = a\cos\theta\, d\theta$

When $x = 0 \Rightarrow \theta = 0$

and $x = a \Rightarrow \theta = \pi/2$

Then $I = \int_0^{\pi/2} \frac{a^4\sin^4\theta \cdot a\cos\theta d\theta}{\sqrt{a^2 - a^2\sin^2\theta}}$

$$= a^4\int_0^{\pi/2} \sin^4\theta d\theta$$

$$= a^4 \cdot \frac{3.1}{4.2}\frac{\pi}{2} \quad \text{By Walli's formula}$$

$$= \frac{3\pi}{16}a^4.$$

11. *Evaluate* $\int_2^3 \frac{dx}{\sqrt{5x - 6 - x^2}}$.

[MEERUT(BCA)–2006]

SOLUTION. Let $I = \int_2^3 \frac{dx}{\sqrt{5x - 6 - x^2}}$

$$= \int_2^3 \frac{dx}{2\sqrt{-(x^2 - 5x + 6)}}$$

$$= \int_2^3 \frac{dx}{\sqrt{-\left\{\left(x - \frac{5}{2}\right)^2 - \frac{1}{4}\right\}}}$$

$$= \int_2^3 \frac{dx}{\sqrt{\left(\frac{1}{2}\right)^2 - \left(x - \frac{5}{2}\right)^2}}$$

$$= \left[\sin^{-1}\left(\frac{x - 5/2}{1/2}\right)\right]_2^3$$

$$= [\sin^{-1}(2x - 5)]_2^3$$

$$= [\sin^{-1}1 - \sin^{-1}(-1)]$$

$$= [\sin^{-1}1 + \sin^{-1}1] = 2\sin^{-1}1$$

$$= 2\cdot\frac{\pi}{2} = \pi$$

12. *Evaluate* $\int_0^\infty \frac{dx}{(x^2 + a^2)(x^2 + b^2)}$

[MEERUT(BCA)–2002]

SOLUTION. Let $\frac{1}{(x^2+a^2)(x^2+b^2)} = \frac{Ax+B}{(x^2+a^2)} + \frac{Cx+D}{x^2+b^2}$

$$\Rightarrow 1=(Ax+B)(x^2+b^2) + (Cx+D)(x^2+a^2) \qquad \ldots(1)$$

Equating like powers of x on both the sides of (1) we get

$$0=A+C,\ 0=B+D$$
$$0 = b^2A + a^2C$$
$$1=b^2B+a^2D$$

Solving these equations we get

$A=C=0$ and $B=-D=\dfrac{1}{b^2-a^2}$

Thus, we can write

$$\int_0^\infty \frac{dx}{(x^2+a^2)(x^2+b^2)} = \frac{1}{b^2-a^2}\int_0^\infty \frac{dx}{x^2+a^2} + \frac{1}{a^2-b^2}\int_0^\infty \frac{dx}{x^2+b^2}$$

$$= \frac{1}{a(b^2-a^2)}\left[\tan^{-1}\frac{x}{a}\right]_0^\infty + \frac{1}{b(a^2-b^2)}\left[\tan^{-1}\frac{x}{b}\right]_0^\infty$$

$$= \frac{1}{a(b^2-a^2)}\left(\tan^{-1}\frac{\infty}{a} - \tan^{-1}\frac{0}{a}\right) + \frac{1}{b(a^2-b^2)}\left(\tan^{-1}\frac{\infty}{b} + \tan^{-1}\frac{0}{b}\right)$$

$$= \frac{1}{a(b^2-a^2)}\left[\frac{\pi}{2}-0\right] + \frac{1}{b(a^2-b^2)}\left(\frac{\pi}{2}-0\right)$$

$$= \frac{\pi}{2ab(a+b)}$$

13. *Evaluate* $\int_{-1}^{1}\log\left(\dfrac{2-x}{2+x}\right)dx$.

[MEERUT(BCA)–2009, 11, 16]

SOLUTION. Let $I=\int_{-1}^{1}\log\left(\dfrac{2-x}{2+x}\right)dx$

Clearly $f(x)=\log\left(\dfrac{2-x}{2+x}\right)$ is an odd function because

$$f(-x)=-f(x)$$

Therefore, $\int_{-1}^{1}\log\left(\dfrac{2-x}{2+x}\right)dx=0$

Exercise-16.2

1. Evaluate the integral $\int_0^{\pi/2}\dfrac{\sin^4 x\,dx}{\sin^4 x+\cos^4 x}$.
2. Evaluate the integral $\int_0^{\pi/2}\dfrac{\sin x-\cos x}{1+\sin x\cos x}dx$.
3. Evaluate the integral $\int_0^4 f(x)\,dx$, where
$$f(x)=\begin{cases}2x+3, & 0\le x\le 3\\ 3x, & 3\le x\le 4\end{cases}$$
4. Evaluate $\int_0^{\pi/2}\dfrac{x\sin x\cos x}{\cos^4 x+\sin^4 x}dx$
5. Evaluate the integral $\int_0^{\pi}\dfrac{x\sin x}{1+\cos^2 x}dx$.
6. Show that $\int_0^{\pi}\dfrac{x\,dx}{a^2\cos^2 x+b^2\sin^2 x}=\dfrac{\pi^2}{2ab}$.
7. Evaluate the integral $\int_0^{\pi/2}\log(\tan x+\cot x)dx$.
8. Evaluate $\int_0^1 e^{\sin^{-1}x}dx$. [MEERUT(BCA)–2002]

Hint to Selected Problems

1. $$I=\int_0^{\pi/2}\frac{\sin^4 x\,dx}{\sin^4 x+\cos^4 x} \qquad \ldots(1)$$

$$=\int_0^{\pi/2}\frac{\sin^4\left(\frac{\pi}{2}-x\right)}{\sin^4\left(\frac{\pi}{2}-x\right)+\cos^4\left(\frac{\pi}{2}-x\right)}dx$$

$$I=\int_0^{\pi/2}\frac{\cos^4 x}{\sin^4 x+\cos^4 x}dx \qquad \ldots(2)$$

Adding (1) and (2), we get

$$2I=\int_0^{\pi/2}dx=\frac{\pi}{2} \quad\Rightarrow\quad I=\frac{\pi}{4}$$

2. $$I=\int_0^{\pi/2}\frac{\sin x-\cos x}{1+\cos x\sin x} \qquad \ldots(1)$$

$$=\int_0^{\pi/2}\frac{\sin\left(\frac{\pi}{2}-x\right)-\cos\left(\frac{\pi}{2}-x\right)}{1+\cos\left(\frac{\pi}{2}-x\right)\sin\left(\frac{\pi}{2}-x\right)}dx$$

$$= \int_0^{\pi/2} \frac{\cos x - \sin x}{1 + \sin x \cos x} dx \qquad \ldots(2)$$

Adding (1) and (2)

$$2I = 0 \quad \Rightarrow \quad I = 0$$

3. $I = \int_0^4 f(x)\,dx = \int_0^3 (2x+3)dx + \int_3^4 3x\,dx$

$$= [x^2 + 3x]_0^3 + \left[\frac{3x^2}{2}\right]_3^4 = \frac{57}{2}$$

4. $I = \int_0^{\pi/2} \frac{x \sin x \cos x\,dx}{\cos^4 x + \sin^4 x}$

$$= \int_0^{\pi/2} \frac{\left(\frac{\pi}{2} - x\right)\sin\left(\frac{\pi}{2} - x\right)\cos\left(\frac{\pi}{2} - x\right)}{\cos^4\left(\frac{\pi}{2} - x\right) + \sin^4\left(\frac{\pi}{2} - x\right)} dx$$

$$= \int_0^{\pi/2} \frac{\pi}{2} \frac{\sin x \cos x}{\sin^4 x + \cos^4 x} dx - \int_0^{\pi/2} \frac{x \sin x \cos x\,dx}{\sin^4 x + \cos^4 x}$$

$$\Rightarrow 2I = \frac{\pi}{2} \int_0^{\pi/2} \frac{\sin x \cos x\,dx}{\sin^4 x + \cos^4 x}$$

divide Nr and Dr by $\cos^4 x$

$$2I = \frac{\pi}{2} \int_0^{\pi/2} \frac{\tan x \sec^2 x}{1 + \tan^4 x} dx$$

Put $\tan^2 x = t \Rightarrow 2 \tan x \sec^2 x\,dx = dt$

$$\Rightarrow \tan x \sec^2 x\,dx = \frac{dt}{2}$$

$$= \frac{\pi}{2} \int_0^\infty \frac{1}{2} \frac{dt}{1+t^2} \quad \text{When } x = 0 \Rightarrow t = 0$$

When $x = \pi/2 \Rightarrow t = \infty$

$$= \frac{\pi}{4}[\tan^{-1} t]_0^\infty = \frac{\pi}{4}\left(\frac{\pi}{2} - 0\right) = \frac{\pi^2}{8}$$

So, $I = \frac{\pi^2}{16}$

5. $I = \int_0^\pi \frac{x \sin x}{1 + \cos^2 x} dx \qquad \ldots(1)$

$$= \int_0^\pi \frac{(\pi - x)\sin(\pi - x)}{1 + \cos^2(\pi - x)} dx \qquad \ldots(2)$$

Adding (1) and (2)

$$2I = \int_0^\pi \frac{(x + \pi - x)\sin x}{1 + \cos^2 x} dx = \pi \int_0^\pi \frac{\sin x}{1 + \cos^2 x} dx$$

Let $\cos x = t$

$$\Rightarrow \quad \sin x\,dx = -dt$$

$$x = 0 \Rightarrow t = 1$$

$$x = \pi \Rightarrow t = -1$$

Now $2I = -\pi \int_1^{-1} \frac{dt}{1+t^2} = -\pi[\tan^{-1} t]_1^{-1}$

$$= -\pi\left[-\frac{\pi}{4} - \frac{\pi}{4}\right]$$

$$2I = \frac{\pi^2}{2} \quad \Rightarrow \quad I = \frac{\pi^2}{4}$$

6. $I = \int_0^\pi \frac{x\,dx}{a^2 \cos^2 x + b^2 \sin^2 x} \qquad \ldots(1)$

$$= \int_0^\pi \frac{(\pi - x)\,dx}{a^2 \cos^2(\pi - x) + b^2 \sin^2(\pi - x)}$$

$$= \int_0^\pi \frac{(\pi - x)}{a^2 \cos^2 x + b^2 \sin^2 x} dx \qquad \ldots(2)$$

Adding (1) and (2) we get

$$2I = \int_0^\pi \frac{(x + \pi - x)\,dx}{a^2 \cos^2 x + b^2 \sin^2 x}$$

$$= \pi \int_0^\pi \frac{dx}{a^2 \cos^2 x + b^2 \sin^2 x} dx$$

$$= 2\pi \int_0^{\pi/2} \frac{dx}{a^2 \cos^2 x + b^2 \sin^2 x}$$

$$\left[\int_0^{2a} f(x)dx = 2\int_0^a f(x)\,dx; f(2a - x) = f(x)\right]$$

Divide Nr and Dr by $\cos^2 x$

$$I = \pi \int_0^{\pi/2} \frac{\sec^2 x\,dx}{a^2 + b^2 \tan^2 x}$$

Put $\tan x = t$

$$\sec^2 x\,dx = dt$$

When $x = 0 \Rightarrow t = 0$

$$x = \frac{\pi}{2} \Rightarrow t = \infty$$

7. $I = \int_0^{\pi/2} \log(\tan x + \cot x)dx$

$$= \int_0^{\pi/2} \log\left(\frac{\sin^2 x + \cos^2 x}{\sin x \cos x}\right) dx$$

$$= \int_0^{\pi/2} \log\left(\frac{1}{\sin x \cos x}\right) dx$$

$$= \int_0^{\pi/2} -(\log\cos x + \log \sin x)dx$$

$$= -\left[\int_0^{\pi/2} \log \sin x\,dx + \int_0^{\pi/2} \log \cos x\,dx\right]$$

$$= -2\int_0^{\pi/2} \log \sin x\, dx$$

$$\left[\because \int_0^{\pi/2} \log \sin x\, dx = \int_0^{\pi/2} \log \cos x\, dx = -\frac{\pi}{2}\log 2\right]$$

$$= -2\left(-\frac{\pi}{2}\log 2\right) = \pi \log 2$$

8. $I = \int_0^1 e^{\sin^{-1} x} dx$

Put $\sin^{-1} x = t \Rightarrow \sin t = x \Rightarrow \cos t\, dt = dx$

When $x = 0 \Rightarrow t = 0$

$x = 1 \Rightarrow t = \pi/2$

$$I = \int_0^{\pi/2} e^t \cos t\, dt = \left[\frac{1}{1^2+1^2}[e^t \cos t + e^t \sin t]\right]_0^{\pi/2}$$

$$= \frac{1}{2}[e^{\pi/2}(0+1) - 1]$$

$$\left[\text{Since } \int_0^{\pi/2} e^{ax} \cos bx\, dx = \frac{1}{a^2+b^2}[a\,e^{ax} \cos bx + be^{ax} \sin bx]\right]$$

$$= \frac{1}{2}(e^{\pi/2} - 1)$$

Answers

1. $\frac{\pi}{4}$ **2.** 0 **3.** $\frac{57}{2}$ **4.** $\frac{\pi^2}{16}$ **5.** $\frac{\pi^2}{4}$ **7.** $\pi \log 2$ **8.** $\frac{e^{\pi/2}-1}{2}$

Some More Solved Problems Related to Definite Integrals

1. *Evaluate* $\int_0^{\pi} x \sin^6 x \cos^4 x dx$.

Solution. Here $I = \int_0^{\pi} x \sin^6 x \cos^4 x\, dx$

$$= \int_0^{\pi} (\pi - x) \sin^6 (\pi - x) \cos^4 (\pi - x)\, dx$$

$$= \int_0^{\pi} (\pi - x) \sin^6 x \cos^4 x\, dx$$

$$= \int_0^{\pi} \pi \sin^6 x \cos^4 x\, dx - \int_0^{\pi} x \sin^6 x \cos^4 x\, dx$$

$$= \pi \int_0^{\pi} \sin^6 x \cos^4 x\, dx - I$$

Hence, $2I = \pi \int_0^{\pi} \sin^6 x \cos^4 x\, dx$

$$= 2\pi \int_0^{\pi/2} \sin^6 x \cos^4 x\, dx$$

$$I = \pi \int_0^{\pi/2} \sin^6 x \cos^4 x\, dx$$

$$= \pi \cdot \frac{5\cdot 3\cdot 1\cdot 3\cdot 1}{10\cdot 8\cdot 6\cdot 4\cdot 2} \cdot \frac{\pi}{2} = \frac{3\pi^2}{512}.$$

(By Walli's formula)

2. *Evaluate*

$$\int_0^{\pi} \sin^3 \theta (1 + 2\cos\theta)(1+\cos\theta)^2 d\theta$$

Solution. Let $I = \int_0^{\pi} \sin^3 \theta (1 + 2\cos\theta)(1+\cos\theta)^2 d\theta$

$$= \int_0^{\pi} \sin^3 \theta (1 + 2\cos\theta)(1+2\cos\theta+\cos^2\theta) d\theta$$

$$= \int_0^{\pi} (\sin^3 \theta + 4\sin^3 \theta \cos\theta + 5\sin^3 \theta \cos^2 \theta + 2\sin^3 \theta \cos^3 \theta)\, d\theta.$$

Now $\int_0^{\pi} \sin^m \theta \cos^n \theta\, d\theta$

$$= 2\int_0^{\pi/2} \sin^m \theta \cos^n \theta\, d\theta, \text{ if } n \text{ is even}$$

$= 0$, if n is odd.

Hence, $I = 2 \cdot \frac{2}{3\cdot 1} + 10 \cdot \frac{2\cdot 1}{5\cdot 3\cdot 1}$

$$= \frac{4}{3} + \frac{4}{3} = \frac{8}{3}$$

3. *Evaluate* $\int_0^{\pi/2} \log \sin 2x\, dx.$

[MEERUT(BCA)–2002, 06, 11]

Solution. Let $I = \int_0^{\pi/2} \log \sin 2x\, dx.$ ...(1)

Put $2x = t \Rightarrow 2dx = dt$, we get

$$I = \frac{1}{2}\int_0^{\pi} \log \sin t\, dt = \frac{1}{2}.2\int_0^{\pi/2} \log \sin t\, dt$$

$$= \int_0^{\pi/2} \log \sin t\, dt = \int_0^{\pi/2} \log \sin\left(\frac{\pi}{2} - t\right) dt$$

$$= \int_0^{\pi/2} \log \cos t\, dt. \quad ...(2)$$

Adding (1) and (2), we get

$$\Rightarrow 2I = \int_0^{\pi/2} (\log \sin t) dt + \int_0^{\pi/2} \log \cos t\, dt$$

$$= \int_0^{\pi/2} \log\left(\frac{\sin 2t}{2}\right) dt$$

$$= \int_0^{\pi/2} \log \sin 2t\, dt - \int_0^{\pi/2} \log 2 dt$$

$$= I - \frac{\pi}{2}\log 2$$

Hence, $I = -\frac{\pi}{2}\log 2$

4. *Show that*

$$\int_0^{\pi/2} \frac{\sqrt{\sin x}}{\sqrt{\sin x} + \sqrt{\cos x}} dx = \frac{\pi}{4}.$$

SOLUTION. Let $I = \int_0^{\pi/2} \frac{\sqrt{\sin x}}{\sqrt{\sin x} + \sqrt{\cos x}} dx$ ...(1)

$$= \int_0^{\pi/2} \frac{\sqrt{\sin\left(\frac{\pi}{2} - x\right)}}{\sqrt{\sin\left(\frac{\pi}{2} - x\right)} + \sqrt{\cos\left(\frac{\pi}{2} - x\right)}} dx$$

$$= \int_0^{\pi/2} \frac{\sqrt{\cos x}}{\sqrt{\cos x} + \sqrt{\sin x}} dx. \quad ...(2)$$

Adding (1) and (2), we get

$$2I = \int_0^{\pi/2} \left[\frac{\sqrt{\sin x} + \sqrt{\cos x}}{\sqrt{\sin x} + \sqrt{\cos x}}\right] dx$$

$$= \int_0^{\pi/2} 1.dx = \frac{\pi}{2}$$

Hence, $I = \frac{\pi}{4}$.

5. *Show that*

$$\int_0^{\pi/2} \frac{\sin^2 x}{(\sin x + \cos x)} dx = \frac{1}{\sqrt{2}} \log(\sqrt{2} + 1).$$

SOLUTION. Let $I = \int_0^{\pi/2} \frac{\sin^2 x}{(\sin x + \cos x)} dx$ ...(1)

$$= \int_0^{\pi/2} \frac{\sin^2\left(\frac{\pi}{2} - x\right)}{\sin\left(\frac{\pi}{2} - x\right) + \cos\left(\frac{\pi}{2} - x\right)} dx$$

$$= \int_0^{\pi/2} \frac{\cos^2 x}{\cos x + \sin x} dx \quad ...(2)$$

Adding (1) and (2), we get

$$2I = \int_0^{\pi/2} \frac{\sin^2 x}{\sin x + \cos x} dx + \int_0^{\pi/2} \frac{\cos^2 x}{\cos x + \sin x} dx$$

$$= \int_0^{\pi/2} \frac{dx}{\sin x + \cos x}$$

$$= \int_0^{\pi/2} \frac{(1/\sqrt{2})dx}{\left(\frac{1}{\sqrt{2}} \sin x + \frac{1}{\sqrt{2}} \cos x\right)}$$

$$= \frac{1}{\sqrt{2}} \int_0^{\pi/2} \frac{dx}{\cos(x - \pi/4)}$$

$$= \frac{1}{\sqrt{2}} \int_0^{\pi/2} \sec\left(x - \frac{\pi}{4}\right) dx$$

$$= \frac{1}{\sqrt{2}} \log\left[\sec\left(x - \frac{\pi}{4}\right) + \tan\left(x - \frac{\pi}{4}\right)\right]_0^{\pi/2}$$

$$= \frac{1}{\sqrt{2}}\left[\log\left(\sec\frac{\pi}{4} + \tan\frac{\pi}{4}\right) - \log\left\{\sec\left(-\frac{\pi}{4}\right) + \tan\left(-\frac{\pi}{4}\right)\right\}\right]$$

$$= \frac{1}{\sqrt{2}} \log\left[\frac{(\sqrt{2}+1)(\sqrt{2}+1)}{(\sqrt{2}-1)(\sqrt{2}+1)}\right]$$

$$= \frac{1}{\sqrt{2}} \log(\sqrt{2}+1)^2$$

$$= \frac{1}{\sqrt{2}} \cdot 2\log(\sqrt{2}+1)$$

Hence, $I = \frac{1}{\sqrt{2}} \log(\sqrt{2}+1)$

Exercise-16.3

Prove the following:

1. $\int_0^{\pi} x \log \sin x \, dx = \frac{1}{2}\pi^2 \log\frac{1}{2}$.
2. $\int_0^{\pi/2} x \cot x \, dx = \frac{\pi}{2} \log 2$.
3. $\int_0^{\pi/2} \left[\frac{\theta}{\sin\theta}\right]^2 d\theta = \pi \log 2$.
4. $\int_0^{1} \frac{\sin^{-1} x}{x} dx = \frac{\pi}{2} \log 2$.
5. $\int_0^{\pi/4} \log(1 + \tan\theta) d\theta = \frac{\pi}{8} \log 2$.
6. $\int_0^{\infty} \frac{x\,dx}{(1+x)(1+x^2)} = \frac{\pi}{4}$.
7. $\int_0^{\pi/2} \frac{\sqrt{\tan x}}{\sqrt{\tan x} + \sqrt{\cot x}} dx = \frac{\pi}{4}$.
8. $\int_0^{\pi/2} \frac{\cos^2 x\,dx}{(\sin x + \cos x)} = \frac{1}{\sqrt{2}} \log(\sqrt{2}+1)$.
9. $\int_0^{\pi} \sin^m x \cos^{2m+1} x \, dx = 0$.
10. $\int_0^{\pi} \frac{x^2 \sin 2x \sin\left(\frac{\pi}{2}\cos x\right)}{2x - \pi} = \frac{8}{\pi}$.

Hint to Selected Problems

1. $I = \int_0^\pi x \log\sin x\, dx = \int_0^\pi (\pi - x)\log\sin(\pi - x)dx$

$= \int_0^\pi \pi \log\sin x\, dx - \int_0^\pi x\log\sin x\, dx$

$\Rightarrow 2I = \pi\int_0^\pi \log\sin x\, dx = 2\pi\int_0^{\pi/2}\log\sin x\, dx$

$(\because \int_a^{2a} f(x)dx = 2\int_0^a f(x)dx$ if $f(2a-x) = f(x)$

$= 2\pi\left(-\frac{\pi}{2}\log 2\right) = \pi^2\log\frac{1}{2}$

$I = \frac{\pi^2}{2}\log\frac{1}{2}$

3. $I = \int_0^{\pi/2}\left(\frac{\theta}{\sin\theta}\right)^2 d\theta = \int_0^{\pi/2}\theta^2\,\text{cosec}^2\theta\, d\theta$

$= (-\theta^2\cot\theta)_0^{\pi/2} - \int_0^{\pi/2} -2\theta\cot\theta\, d\theta$

$= (-0+0) - 2\int_0^{\pi/2} -\theta\cot\theta\, d\theta$

$= +2\left[(\theta\log\sin\theta)_0^{\pi/2} - \int_0^{\pi/2}\log\sin\theta\, d\theta\right]$

$= +2\left[(0-0) - \int_0^{\pi/2}\log\sin\theta\, d\theta\right]$

$= +2\left(\frac{\pi}{2}\log 2\right)$

[Since $\int_0^{\pi/2}\log\sin\theta d\theta = -\frac{\pi}{2}\log 2$]

$= \pi\log 2$

5. $I = \int_0^{\pi/4}\log(1+\tan\theta)\, d\theta$

$= \int_0^{\pi/4}\log\left\{1+\tan\left(\frac{\pi}{4}-\theta\right)\right\}d\theta$

$= \int_0^{\pi/4}\log\left\{1+\frac{\tan\pi/4 - \tan\theta}{1+\tan\pi/4\cdot\tan\theta}\right\}d\theta$

$= \int_0^{\pi/4}\log\left\{1+\frac{1-\tan\theta}{1+\tan\theta}\right\}d\theta$

$= \int_0^{\pi/4}\log\left\{\frac{2}{1+\tan\theta}\right\}d\theta$

$= \int_0^{\pi/4}\log 2dx - \int_0^{\pi/4}\log(1+\tan\theta)\, d\theta$

$2I = \log 2[x]_0^{\pi/4} = \frac{\pi}{4}\log 2$

$I = \frac{\pi}{8}\log 2$

7. $I = \int_0^{\pi/2}\frac{\sqrt{\tan x}}{\sqrt{\tan x}+\sqrt{\cot x}}dx \quad \ldots(1)$

$= \int_0^{\pi/2}\frac{\sqrt{\tan\left(\frac{\pi}{2}-x\right)}}{\sqrt{\tan\left(\frac{\pi}{2}-x\right)}+\sqrt{\cot\left(\frac{\pi}{2}-x\right)}}dx$

$= \int_0^{\pi/2}\frac{\sqrt{\cot x}}{\sqrt{\cot x}+\sqrt{\tan x}} \quad \ldots(2)$

Adding (1) and (2)

$2I = \int_0^{\pi/2}dx = \frac{\pi}{2}$

$I = \frac{\pi}{4}$

8. $I = \int_0^{\pi/2}\frac{\cos^2 x\, dx}{\sin x+\cos x} \quad \ldots(1)$

$= \int_0^{\pi/2}\frac{\cos^2\left(\frac{\pi}{2}-x\right)}{\sin\left(\frac{\pi}{2}-x\right)+\cos\left(\frac{\pi}{2}-x\right)}dx$

$= \int_0^{\pi/2}\frac{\sin^2 x}{\cos x+\sin x}dx \quad \ldots(2)$

Adding (1) and (2)

$2I = \int_0^{\pi/2}\frac{\cos^2 x+\sin^2 x}{\cos x+\sin x}dx$

$= \int_0^{\pi/2}\frac{dx}{\cos x+\sin x}$

$= \int_0^{\pi/2}\frac{dx}{1-2\sin^2\frac{x}{2}+2\sin\frac{x}{2}\cos\frac{x}{2}}$

Divide Nr and Dr by $\cos^2\frac{x}{2}$

$2I = \int_0^{\pi/2}\frac{\sec^2 x/2\, dx}{1+2\tan\frac{x}{2}-\tan^2\frac{x}{2}}$

Let $\tan\frac{x}{2} = t \Rightarrow \sec^2\frac{x}{2}dx = 2dt$

Also when $x = 0 \Rightarrow t = 0$

$x = \frac{\pi}{2} \Rightarrow t = 1$

$2I = \int_0^1\frac{2dt}{2t+1-t^2} = 2\int_0^1\frac{dt}{(\sqrt{2})^2-(t-1)^2}$

$= 2\times\frac{1}{2\sqrt{2}}\left[\log\left|\frac{\sqrt{2}+t-1}{\sqrt{2}-t+1}\right|\right]_0^1$

$= \frac{1}{\sqrt{2}}\left[\log\left(\frac{\sqrt{2}}{\sqrt{2}}\right)-\log\left(\frac{\sqrt{2}-1}{\sqrt{2}+1}\right)\right]$

$= -\frac{1}{\sqrt{2}}\log\left\{\frac{\sqrt{2}-1}{\sqrt{2}+1}\right\} = \frac{1}{\sqrt{2}}\log\frac{\sqrt{2}+1}{\sqrt{2}-1}$

$= \frac{1}{\sqrt{2}}\log\left\{\frac{(\sqrt{2}+1)(\sqrt{2}+1)}{(\sqrt{2}-1)(\sqrt{2}+1)}\right\}$

$$= \frac{1}{\sqrt{2}}\log(\sqrt{2}+1)^2 = \frac{2}{\sqrt{2}}\log(\sqrt{2}+1)$$

So, $I = \frac{1}{\sqrt{2}}\log(\sqrt{2}+1)$

9. $I = \int_0^{\pi} \sin^m x \cos^{2m+1} x\, dx = f(x)$, say

Here $f(x) = \sin^m x \cos^{2m+1} x$

$$f(\pi - x) = \sin^m(\pi - x)\cos^{(2m+1)}(\pi - x)$$
$$= -\sin^m x \cos^{2m+1} x = f(-x)$$

So, $I = 0$

Since, $\int_0^{2a} f(x) = 0$ if $f(2a - x) = -f(x)$

16.8 DEFINITE INTEGRAL AS THE LIMIT OF THE SUM

It is always possible to regard a definite integral as the limit of the sum of certain number of terms, when the number of terms tends to infinity and each term tends to zero.

Here, we define the definite integral as follows:

$$\int_a^b f(x)\,dx = \lim h[f(a) + f(a+h) + f(a+2h) + \ldots + f\{a+(n-1)h\}]$$

when $n \to \infty$, $h \to 0$ and $nh \to b - a$.

Solved Examples

1. *Evaluate $\int_a^b x^2 dx$, directly from the definition of integral as the limit of a sum.*

SOLUTION. We know that

$$\int_a^b f(x)\,dx = \lim_{n\to\infty} h[f(a) + f(a+h) + f(a+2h) + \ldots + f\{a+(n-1)h\}] \quad \ldots(1)$$

Here $f(x) = x^2$

$$f(a) = a^2$$
$$f(a+h) = (a+h)^2$$

... ... and so on.

Put all these values in (1), we get

$$\int_a^b x^2 dx = \lim_{n\to\infty} h[a^2 + (a+h)^2 + (a+2h)^2 + \ldots + \{a+(n-1)h\}^2]$$

where $h \to 0$ as $n \to \infty$ and $nh \to b - a$

$$= \lim_{n\to\infty} h[na^2 + 2ah\{1+2+3+\ldots+(n-1)\}] + h^2[1^2 + 2^2 + \ldots + (n-1)^2]$$

Using $\sum n = \frac{n(n+1)}{2}$ and

$$\sum n^2 = \frac{n(n+1)(2n+1)}{6}$$

$$\therefore \int_a^b x^2 dx = \lim_{n\to\infty} h\left[na^2 + 2ah\frac{(n-1)n}{2} + \frac{h^2}{6}(n-1)n(2n-1)\right]$$

$$= \lim_{n\to\infty} [(nh)a^2 + a(nh)(n-1)h + \frac{1}{6}(nh)(n-1)h(2n-1)h]$$

$$= \lim_{n\to\infty}\left[(nh)a^2 + a(nh)^2\left(1 - \frac{1}{n}\right) + \frac{1}{6}2(nh)^3\left(1-\frac{1}{n}\right)\left(1-\frac{1}{2n}\right)\right]$$

$$= (b-a)a^2 + a(b-a)^2 + \frac{1}{3}(b-a)^3$$

$(\because$ as $n \to \infty, h \to 0, nh \to b - a)$

$$= \frac{1}{3}(b-a)[3a^2 + 3(b-a)a + b^2 - 2ab + a^2]$$

$$= \frac{1}{3}(b-a)(a^2 + ab + b^2) = \frac{1}{3}(b^3 - a^3)$$

2. *From the definition of a definite integral as the limit of a sum, evaluate $\int_a^b e^x dx$.*

SOLUTION. Here, we have $f(x) = e^x$.

Therefore $f(a) = e^a$

$$f(a+h) = e^{a+h}$$

... ... etc.

Now $\int_a^b e^x dx = \lim_{h\to 0} h[e^a + e^{a+h} + e^{a+2h} + \ldots + e^{a+(n-1)h}]$

where, $nh = b - a$ and $n \to \infty$ as $h \to 0$

$$= \lim_{h\to 0} he^a[1 + e^h + e^{2h} + \ldots + e^{(n-1).h}]$$

$$= \lim_{h\to 0} he^a \left\{\frac{(e^h)^n - 1}{e^h - 1}\right\} = \lim_{h\to 0} he^a \left\{\frac{e^{nh} - 1}{e^h - 1}\right\}$$

$$= \lim_{h\to 0} he^a \left[\frac{e^{b-a} - 1}{e^h - 1}\right] \quad [\because nh = b - a]$$

$$= \lim_{h\to 0} e^a \left[\frac{e^{b-a} - 1}{\frac{e^h - 1}{h}}\right] = e^b - e^a$$

$$\left(\because \lim_{h\to 0} \frac{e^h - 1}{h} = 1\right)$$

16.9 SUMMATION OF SERIES WITH THE HELP OF DEFINITE INTEGRAL

We know that $\int_a^b f(x)\,dx = \lim_{n\to\infty} h[f(a) + f(a+h) + \ldots + f\{a + (n-1)h\}]$

$$= \lim_{n\to\infty} h \sum_{r=0}^{n-1} f(a + rh), \qquad \text{where } nh = b - a$$

Now putting $a = 0$ and $b = 1$ so that $h = 1/n$, we get

$$\int_0^1 f(x)dx = \lim_{n\to\infty} \frac{1}{n} \sum_{r=0}^{n-1} f\left(\frac{r}{n}\right).$$

WORKING PROCEDURE

STEP 1. Write the rth term of the series.

STEP 2. Write the rth term in the form of $\frac{1}{n} f\left(\frac{r}{n}\right)$

STEP 3. Replace $\frac{r}{n}$ by x, $\frac{1}{n}$ by dx and $\lim_{x\to\infty}$ by f.

Then, lower limit of the definite integral will be value of $\frac{r}{n}$ for the first term as $n \to \infty$ and the upper limit will be the value of $\frac{r}{n}$ for the last term as $n \to \infty$.

Solved Examples

1. *Evaluate the following :*

$$\lim_{n\to\infty} \left[\frac{1}{n+1} + \frac{1}{n+2} + \ldots + \frac{1}{2n}\right].$$

SOLUTION. The general term is given by (r^{th} term)

$$= \frac{1}{n+r}$$

We have to find

$$\lim_{n\to\infty} \sum_{r=1}^{n} \frac{1}{n+r} = \lim_{n\to\infty} \sum_{r=1}^{n} \frac{1}{n[1 + r/n]}$$

$$= \lim_{n\to\infty} \frac{1}{n} \sum_{r=1}^{n} \frac{1}{[1 + r/n]}$$

Since the limit of r in the summation is 1 to n, therefore the lower limit of integration $= \lim_{n\to\infty} \frac{1}{n} = 0$.

Also, the upper limit of integration

$$= \lim_{n\to\infty} \frac{n}{n} = 1.$$

Hence, the required limit

$$\int_0^1 \frac{1}{1+x} dx = \left[\log(1+x)\right]_0^1 = \log 2$$

2. *Evaluate :*

$$\lim_{n\to\infty} n\left[\frac{1}{(n+1)(n+2)} + \frac{1}{(n+2)(n+4)} + \ldots + \frac{1}{6n^2}\right]$$

SOLUTION. The given limit

$$= \lim_{n\to\infty} n \sum_{r=1}^{n} \frac{1}{(n+r)(n+2r)}$$

$$= \lim_{n\to\infty} \frac{n}{n^2} \sum_{r=1}^{n} \frac{1}{(1 + r/n)(1 + 2r/n)}$$

$$= \lim_{n\to\infty} \frac{1}{n} \sum_{r=1}^{n} \frac{1}{\left(1+\frac{r}{n}\right)\left(1+\frac{2r}{n}\right)}$$

$$= \int_0^1 \frac{1}{(1+x)(1+2x)} dx$$

$$= \int_0^1 \left[\frac{-1}{1+x} + \frac{2}{1+2x}\right] dx$$

(Resolving into partial fraction)

$$= \left[-\log(1+x) + \log(1+2x)\right]_0^1$$

$$= \log\left[\frac{(1+2x)}{(1+x)}\right]_0^1$$

$$= \log\frac{3}{2} - \log 1 = \log\frac{3}{2}.$$

3. *Evaluate:*

$$\lim_{n\to\infty}\left[\left(1+\frac{1}{n^2}\right)\left(1+\frac{2^2}{n^2}\right)\left(1+\frac{3^2}{n^2}\right)\ldots\left(1+\frac{n^2}{n^2}\right)\right]^{1/n}$$

SOLUTION. Let

$$A = \lim_{n\to\infty}\left[\left(1+\frac{1}{n^2}\right)\left(1+\frac{2^2}{n^2}\right)\left(1+\frac{3^2}{n^2}\right)\ldots\left(1+\frac{n^2}{n^2}\right)\right]^{1/n}$$

$$\Rightarrow \quad \log A$$

$$= \lim_{n\to\infty}\frac{1}{n}\left[\log\left(1+\frac{1}{n^2}\right)+\log\left(1+\frac{2^2}{n^2}\right) + \log\left(1+\frac{3^2}{n^2}\right)+\ldots+\log\left(1+\frac{n^2}{n^2}\right)\right]$$

$$= \lim_{n\to\infty}\frac{1}{n}\sum_{r=1}^{n}\log\left(1+\frac{r^2}{n^2}\right) = \int_0^1 \log(1+x^2)dx$$

$$= \int_0^1 \log(1+x^2).1dx$$

$$= [x\log(1+x^2)]_0^1 - \int_0^1 \frac{2x.x\,dx}{1+x^2}$$

$$= \log 2 - 2\int_0^1 \frac{(1+x^2)-1}{1+x^2}dx$$

$$= \log 2 - 2\int_0^1\left[1-\frac{1}{(1+x^2)}\right]dx$$

$$= \log 2 - 2\left[x - \tan^{-1} x\right]_0^1$$

$$= \log 2 - 2\left(1-\frac{\pi}{4}\right)$$

Therefore, $\log A = \log 2 + \frac{1}{2}(\pi - 4)$

$$\Rightarrow \quad \log\frac{A}{2} = \frac{1}{2}(\pi-4)$$

$$\Rightarrow \quad A = 2e^{(\pi-4)/2}$$

4. *Find the limit of* $\left[\frac{n!}{n^n}\right]^{1/n}$ *when* $n\to\infty$.

SOLUTION. Let $A = \lim_{n\to\infty}\left[\frac{n!}{n^n}\right]^{1/n}$

$$= \lim_{n\to\infty}\left[\frac{1\cdot2\cdot3\cdot4\ldots n}{n\cdot n\cdot n\ldots n}\right]^{1/n}$$

$$\Rightarrow \log A = \lim_{n\to\infty}\frac{1}{n}\left[\log\left(\frac{1}{n}\right)+\log\left(\frac{2}{n}\right) + \log\left(\frac{3}{n}\right)+\ldots+\log\left(\frac{n}{n}\right)\right]$$

$$= \lim_{n\to\infty}\sum_{r=1}^{n}\frac{1}{n}\log\left(\frac{r}{n}\right)$$

$$= \int_0^1 \log x\,dx = \int_0^1 \log x.1\,dx$$

$$= \left[(\log x)\cdot x\right]_0^1 - \int_0^1 \frac{1}{x}\cdot x\,dx$$

$$= 0 - [x]_0^1 = -1$$

Hence, $A = e^{-1} = \frac{1}{e}$.

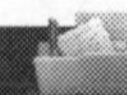

Exercise-16.4

1. Show that the limit of the sum

$$\frac{1}{n}+\frac{1}{n+1}+\frac{1}{n+2}+\ldots+\frac{1}{6n}$$

when n is indefinitely increased is log 6.

[MEERUT(BCA)–2001]

2. Evaluate $\int_a^b x^2 dx$ directly from the definition of the integral as the limit of the sum.

3. Evaluate by summation $\int_1^2 x\,dx$.

4. Evaluate by summation $\int_a^b \sin x\,dx$.

5. Evaluate by summation $\int_0^{\pi/2} \sin x\,dx$.

6. Show that the limit (when $n \to \infty$) of the series $\frac{n}{(n+1)^2}+\frac{n}{(n+2)^2}+\ldots+\frac{n}{(n+n)^2}$ is $\frac{1}{2}$.

7. Show that $\lim_{n\to\infty}\left[\frac{n}{n^2}+\frac{n}{n^2+1^2}+\frac{n}{n^2+n^2}+\ldots+\frac{n}{n^2+(n+1)^2}\right]=\frac{\pi}{4}$.

8. Show that

$$\lim_{n\to\infty}\left[\frac{n}{n^2+1^2}+\frac{n}{n^2+2^2}+\ldots+\frac{n}{2n}\right]=\frac{\pi}{4}.$$

9. Show that $\lim_{n\to\infty}\left[\frac{1}{n^3}(1+4+9+\ldots+n^2)\right]=\frac{1}{3}$.

10. Show that

$$\lim_{n\to\infty}\left[\frac{1}{n}+\frac{n^2}{(n+1)^3}+\frac{n^2}{(n+2)^2}+\ldots+\frac{1}{8n}\right]=\frac{3}{8}.$$

11. Show that

$$\lim_{n\to\infty}\left[\frac{1}{n}+\frac{1}{\sqrt{n^2-1^2}}+\frac{1}{\sqrt{n^2-2^2}}+\ldots+\frac{1}{\sqrt{n^2-(n-1)^2}}\right]=\frac{\pi}{2}.$$

12. Show that

$$\lim_{n\to\infty}\left[\frac{1}{n^2}\sec^2\frac{1}{n^2}+\frac{2}{n^2}\sec^4\frac{4}{n^2}+\frac{3}{n^2}\sec^2\frac{9}{n^2}+\ldots+\frac{1}{n}\sec^2 1\right]=\frac{1}{2}\tan 1.$$

13. Show that

$$\lim_{n\to\infty}\left[\frac{1}{\sqrt{n^2-1^2}}+\frac{1}{\sqrt{n^2-2^2}}+\ldots+\frac{1}{\sqrt{n^2-(n-1)^2}}\right]=\frac{\pi}{2}.$$

14. Show that

$$\lim_{n\to\infty}\left[\frac{n^{1/2}}{n^{3/2}}+\frac{n^{1/2}}{(n+3)^{3/2}}+\frac{n^{1/2}}{(n+6)^{3/2}}+\ldots+\frac{n^{1/2}}{\{n+3(n+1)\}^{3/2}}\right]=\frac{1}{3}.$$

Hint to Selected Problems

1. $\lim_{n\to\infty}\left[\frac{1}{n}+\frac{1}{n+1}+\frac{1}{n+2}+\ldots+\frac{1}{6n}\right]$

$$= \lim_{n\to\infty}\sum_{r=0}^{5n}\left[\frac{1}{n+r}\right]$$

$$= \lim_{n\to\infty}\frac{1}{n}\sum_{r=0}^{5n}\left[\frac{1}{1+\frac{r}{n}}\right]=\int_0^5\frac{1}{1+x}dx$$

$$= [\log(1+x)]_0^5 = \log 6 - \log 1 = \log 6$$

4. Let $I=\int_a^b \sin x\,dx$ Here $f(x)=\sin x$

Let $h=\frac{b-a}{n}, n\in \mathbf{N}$

$$I=\lim_{n\to\infty} h[f(a)+f(a+h)+\ldots+f(a+(n-1)h]$$

$$=\lim_{n\to\infty} h[\sin a+\sin(a+h)+\ldots+\sin(a+(n-1)h)]$$

Now $\sin a+\sin(a+h)+\ldots+\sin(a+(n-1)h)$

$$=\frac{1}{2\sin\frac{h}{2}}\left[2\sin a\sin\frac{h}{2}+2\sin(a+h).\sin\frac{h}{2}+\ldots+2\sin(a+(n-1)\sin\frac{h}{2}\right]$$

$$=\frac{1}{2\sin h/2}\left[\left\{\cos\left(a-\frac{h}{2}\right)-\cos\left(a+\frac{h}{2}\right)\right\}+\left\{\cos\left(a+\frac{h}{2}\right)-\cos\left(a+\frac{3h}{2}\right)\right\}+\ldots+\left\{\cos\left(a+\left(n-\frac{3}{2}\right)h\right)-\cos\left(a+\left(n-\frac{1}{2}\right)h\right)\right\}\right]$$

$$=\frac{1}{2\sinh/2}\left[\cos\left(a-\frac{h}{2}\right)-\cos\left(a+\left(n-\frac{1}{2}\right)h\right)\right]$$

$$=\frac{1}{2\sin h/2}\left[\cos\left(a-\frac{h}{2}\right)-\cos\left(b-\frac{h}{2}\right)\right]$$

$b = a + nh$

$$I = \lim_{h\to 0} h.\frac{1}{2\sin h/2}\left[\cos\left(a-\frac{h}{2}\right)-\cos\left(b-\frac{h}{2}\right)\right]$$

$$= \lim_{h\to 0}\frac{h/2}{\sin h/2}\lim_{h\to 0}\left[\cos\left(a-\frac{h}{2}\right)-\cos\left(b-\frac{h}{2}\right)\right]$$

$$= 1.[\cos(a-0-\cos(b-0)] = \cos a - \cos b$$

6. $$\lim_{n\to\infty}\left[\frac{n}{(n+1)^2}+\frac{n}{(n+2)^2}+\frac{n}{(n+3)^2}+\ldots+\frac{n}{(n+n)^2}\right]$$

$$= \lim_{n\to\infty}\sum_{r=0}^{n+1}\frac{n}{(n+r)^2}$$

$$= \lim_{n\to\infty}\frac{1}{n}\sum_{r=0}^{n+1}\frac{1}{\left(1+\frac{r}{n}\right)^2} = \int_0^1\frac{1}{(1+x)^2}dx$$

$$= \left[-\frac{1}{(1+x)}\right]_0^1 = \frac{1}{2}$$

7. $$\lim_{n\to\infty}\left[\frac{n}{n^2}+\frac{n}{n^2+1^2}+\frac{n}{n^2+2^2}+\ldots+\frac{n}{n^2+(n+1)^2}\right]$$

$$= \lim_{n\to\infty}\sum_{r=0}^{n}\frac{n}{n^2+r^2} = \lim_{n\to\infty}\frac{1}{n}\sum_{r=0}^{n+1}\frac{1}{1+\left(\frac{r}{n}\right)^2}$$

$$= \int_0^1\frac{1}{1+x^2}dx = (\tan^{-1}x)_0^1 = \tan^{-1}1-\tan^{-1}0$$

$$= \pi/4$$

9. $$\lim_{n\to\infty}\left[\frac{1}{n^3}(1+4+9+\ldots+n^2)\right]$$

$$= \lim_{n\to\infty}\frac{1}{n^3}[1^2+2^2+3^2+\ldots+n^2]$$

$$= \lim_{n\to\infty}\sum_{r=0}^{n}\frac{1}{n^3}r^2 = \lim_{n\to\infty}\frac{1}{n}\sum_{r=0}^{n}\left(\frac{r}{n}\right)^2$$

$$= \int_0^1 x^2dx = \left(\frac{x^3}{3}\right)_0^1 = \frac{1}{3}$$

11. $$\lim_{n\to\infty}\left[\frac{1}{n}+\frac{1}{\sqrt{n^2-1^2}}+\frac{1}{\sqrt{n^2-2^2}}+\ldots+\frac{1}{\sqrt{n^2-(n-1)^2}}\right]$$

$$= \lim_{n\to\infty}\sum_{r=0}^{n-1}\frac{1}{\sqrt{n^2-r^2}}$$

$$= \lim_{n\to\infty}\frac{1}{n}\sum_{r=0}^{n-1}\frac{1}{\sqrt{1-\left(\frac{r}{n}\right)^2}}$$

$$= \int_0^1\frac{1}{\sqrt{1-x^2}} = (\sin^{-1}x)_0^1$$

$$= \sin^{-1}(1)-\sin^{-1}(0) = \pi/2$$

12. $$\lim_{n\to\infty}\left[\frac{1}{n^2}\sec^2\frac{1}{n^2}+\frac{2}{n^2}\sec^2\frac{4}{n^2}+\frac{3}{n^2}\sec^2\frac{9}{n^2}+\ldots+\frac{1}{n}\sec^2 1\right]$$

$$= \lim_{n\to\infty}\sum_{r=0}^{n}\frac{r}{n^2}\sec^2\frac{r^2}{n^2}$$

$$= \lim_{n\to\infty}\frac{1}{n}\sum_{r=0}^{n}\left(\frac{r}{n}\right)\sec^2\left(\frac{r}{n}\right)^2$$

$$= \int_0^1 x\cdot\sec^2 x^2dx$$

Let $x^2 = t \Rightarrow 2x\,dx = dt$

$$= \frac{1}{2}\int_0^1\sec^2 t\,dt = \frac{1}{2}.(\tan t)_0^1 = \frac{1}{2}\tan 1$$

14. $$\lim_{n\to\infty}\frac{n^{1/2}}{n^{3/2}}+\frac{n^{1/2}}{(n+3)^{3/2}}+\frac{n^{1/2}}{(n+6)^{3/2}}+\ldots+\frac{n^{1/2}}{\{n+3(n+1)\}^{3/2}}$$

$$= \lim_{n\to\infty}\sum_{r=0}^{n}\frac{n^{1/2}}{(n+3r)^{3/2}}$$

$$= \lim_{n\to\infty}\frac{1}{n}\sum_{r=0}^{n}\frac{1}{\left(1+\frac{3r}{n}\right)^{\frac{3}{2}}} = \int_0^1\frac{1}{(1+3x)^{3/2}}dx$$

$$= \int_0^1(1+3x)^{-3/2}dx = \left[\frac{(1+3x)^{-1/2}}{-1/2\times 3}\right]_0^1$$

$$= -\frac{2}{3}[(1+3x)^{-1/2}]_0^1 = -\frac{2}{3}[4^{-1/2}-1^{-1/2}]$$

$$= -\frac{2}{3}\left[\frac{1}{2}-1\right] = -\frac{2}{3}\left[-\frac{1}{2}\right] = \frac{1}{3}.$$

ANSWERS

2. $\frac{1}{3}(b^3-a^3)$ **3.** $\frac{3}{2}$ **4.** $\cos b-\cos a$ **5.** 1

16.10 REDUCTION FORMULA

The process relating one integral to one or more integrals of the same type but simpler is called a reduction and this relation between integrals is called a reduction formula.

The reduction formula is derived by two different methods; one is integration by parts and other is differentiation of a suitable function, says $P(x)$. Here the function $P(x)$ is chosen in such a way that $\frac{dP}{dx}$ has atleast one function, which is the integral of the given integral, whose reduction formula is required. It consists of the following steps :

(i) Selection of $P(x)$ (ii) Differentiation of $P(x)$ (iii) Integral of (ii).

16.11 REDUCTION FORMULAE FOR $\int \sin^m x \cos^n x dx$

(i) $I_{m,n} = \int \sin^m x \cos^n x dx = \frac{\cos^{n-1} x \sin^{m+1} x}{m+n} + \frac{n-1}{m+n} I_{m,n-2}$ $(m + n \neq 0)$

(ii) $I_{m,n} = \int \sin^m x \cos^n x dx = -\frac{\sin^{m-1} x \cos^{n+1} x}{m+n} + \frac{m-1}{m+n} I_{m-2,n}$ $(m + n \neq 0)$

PROOF. (i) Here $I_{m,n} = \int \sin^m x \cos^n x dx$

$$= \cos^{n-1} x \int \sin^m x \cos x dx - \int \left[\frac{d}{dx}(\cos^{n-1} x) \int \sin^m x \cos x dx \right] .dx$$

$$= \frac{\cos^{n-1} x \sin^{m+1} x}{m+1} + \frac{n-1}{m+1} \int \cos^{n-2} x \sin^{m+2} x dx$$

$$= \frac{\cos^{n-1} x \sin^{m+1} x}{m+1} + \frac{n-1}{m+1} \int \cos^{n-2} x \sin^m x (1 - \cos^2 x) dx$$

$$= \frac{\cos^{n-1} x \sin^{m+1} x}{m+1} + \frac{n-1}{m+1} .I_{m,n-2} - \frac{n-1}{m+1} .I_{m,n}$$

or $$\left(1 + \frac{n-1}{m+1}\right) I_{m,n} = \frac{\cos^{n-1} x \sin^{m+1} x}{m+1} + \frac{n-1}{m+1} .I_{m,n-2}$$

$\Rightarrow$ $$I_{m,n} = \frac{\cos^{n-1} x \sin^{m+1} x}{m+n} + \frac{n-1}{m+n} I_{m,n-2}, m + n \neq 0.$$

- The above formula reduces the power or exponent m of cosine in each successive steps by 2. So, to establish the relation, one cosine is separated from the product so that $\sin^m x \cos x$ can be integrated.
- Here, one sine is separated from the product, so that $\cos^n x \sin x$ can be integrated and can be treated as a second function of the integration by parts. Therefore, following the same procedure as above, we can easily find

$$I_{m,n} = -\frac{\sin^{m-1} x \cos^{n+1} x}{m+n} + \frac{m-1}{m+n} I_{m-2,n}, m + n \neq 0.$$

- Put $m = 0$ in reduction formula (i), we may find

$$I_n = \int \cos^n x dx = \frac{\sin x \cos^{n-1} x}{n} + \frac{n-1}{n} I_{n-2}, n \neq 0.$$

- Put $n = 0$ in (ii), we may get

$$I_m = \int \sin^m x dx = -\frac{\sin^{m-1} x \cos x}{m} + \frac{m-1}{m} I_{m-2}, m \neq 0.$$

16.12 REDUCTION FORMULA FOR $\int \frac{dx}{\sin^m x \cos^n x} = \int \operatorname{cosec}^m x \sec^n x dx$

Replace n by $n + 2$ in § 16.11 (i), we get

$$I_{m,n+2} = \int \sin^m x \cos^{n+2} x dx = \frac{\sin^{m+1} x \cos^{n+1} x}{m+n+2} + \frac{n+1}{m+n+2} I_{m,n}$$

Let us replace m by $-m$ and n by $-n$, we get

$$I_{-m,-n+2} = \int \frac{dx}{\sin^m x \cos^{n-2} x} = -\frac{1}{m+n-2} \cdot \frac{1}{\sin^{m-1} x \cos^{n-1} x} + \frac{n-1}{m+n-2} I_{-m,-n}$$

or $$I_{-m,-n} = \int \frac{dx}{\sin^m x \cos^n x} = \frac{1}{(n-1)\sin^{m-1} x \cos^{n-1} x} + \frac{m+n-2}{n-1} I_{-m,-n+2}, n \neq 1 \quad ...(1)$$

Similarly from § 16.11 (ii), we get

$$I_{-m,-n} = \int \frac{dx}{\sin^m x \cos^n x} = \frac{1}{(m-1)\sin^{m-1} x \cos^{n-1} x} + \frac{m+n-2}{m-1} I_{-m+2,-n}, m \neq 1 \quad ...(2)$$

Here, from (1) and (2), we observed that powers of cosines and sines are respectively reduced by 2 in each step of reduction.

Now, putting $m = 0$ in (1), and n = 0 in (2), we can obtain

$$I_{-n} = \int \frac{1}{\cos^n x} dx = \int \sec^n x dx = \frac{\sin x}{(n-1)\cos^{n-1} x} + \frac{n-2}{n-1} I_{-n+2}, n \neq 1 \quad ...(3)$$

and $$I_{-m} = \int \frac{1}{\sin^m x} dx = \int \operatorname{cosec}^m x dx = -\frac{\cos x}{(m-1)\sin^{m-1} x} + \frac{m-2}{m-1} I_{-m+2}, m \neq 1 \quad ...(4)$$

From equations (1), (2), (3) and (4), we may get

$$I_{m,n} = \int \operatorname{cosec}^m x \sec^n x dx = \frac{\operatorname{cosec}^{m-1} x \sec^{n-1} x}{n-1} + \frac{m+n-2}{n-1} I_{m,n-2}, n \neq 1$$

$$I_{m,n} = \int \operatorname{cosec}^m x \sec^n x dx = \frac{\operatorname{cosec}^{m-1} x \sec^{n-1} x}{m-1} + \frac{m+n-2}{m-1} I_{m-2n}, m \neq 1$$

$$I_n = \int \sec^n x dx = \frac{\tan x \sec^{n-2} x}{n-1} + \frac{n-2}{n-1} I_{n-2}, n \neq 1$$

and $$I_m = \int \operatorname{cosec}^m x dx = -\frac{\cot x \operatorname{cosec}^{m-2} x}{m-1} + \frac{m-2}{m-1} I_{m-2}, m \neq 1$$

16.13 REDUCTION FORMULA FOR $\int \sin^m x \sec^n x dx$ AND $\int \cos^n x \operatorname{cosec}^m x dx$

Let $$I_{m,-n} = \int \frac{\sin^m x}{\cos^n x} dx = \int \frac{\sin^{m-1} x \sin x}{\cos^n x} dx = \frac{\sin^{m-1} x}{(n-1)\cos^{n-1} x} - \frac{m-1}{n-1} \int \frac{\sin^{m-2} x}{\cos^{n-2} x} dx$$

$$= \frac{\sin^{m-1} x}{(n-1)\cos^{n-1} x} - \frac{m-1}{n-1} I_{m-2,-n+2}, n \neq 1$$

$$\Rightarrow \quad \int \sin^m x \sec^n x dx = \frac{\sin^{m-1} x}{(n-1)\cos^{n-1} x} - \frac{m-1}{n-1} I_{m-2,-n+2}, n \neq 1 \quad ...(1)$$

Similarly we can find

$$I_{-m,n} = \int \frac{\cos^n x}{\sin^m x} dx = -\frac{\cos^{m-1} x}{(m-1)\sin^{m-1} x} - \frac{n-1}{m-1} I_{-m+2,n-2}, m \neq 1 \quad ...(2)$$

Here, we observed that, in the above two cases powers of the numerator have been reduced. In the former case, a sine and in the latter case a cosine of the numerator has been separated and integrated separately. Finally, the powers of both numerator and denominator have been reduced by two in both cases.

The formuale (1) and (2) can also be written as

$$I_{m,n} = \int \sin^m x \sec^n x dx = \frac{\sin^{m-1} x \sec^{n-1} x}{n-1} - \frac{m-1}{n-1} I_{m-2,n-2}, n \neq 1 \quad \ldots(3)$$

and $$I_{m,n} = \int \text{cosec}^m x \cos^n x dx = -\frac{\text{cosec}^{m-1} x \cos^{n-1} x}{m-1} - \frac{n-1}{m-1} I_{m-2,n-2}, m \neq 1 \quad \ldots(4)$$

16.14 REDUCTION FORMULAE FOR $\int \tan^n xdx$ AND $\int \cot^n xdx$

(i) $$I_n = \int \tan^n xdx = \int \tan^{n-2} x \tan^2 xdx = \int \tan^{n-2} x(\sec^2 x - 1)dx$$

$$= \int \tan^{n-2} x \sec^2 xdx - \int \tan^{n-2} x\, dx \quad \ldots(1)$$

Now $\int \tan^{n-2} x \sec^2 xdx = \int t^{n-2} dt$, putting $\tan x = t$ and $\sec^2 t\, dt = dx$

$$\int \tan^{n-2} x \sec^2 xdx = \frac{t^{n-1}}{n-1} = \frac{\tan^{n-1} x}{n-1} \quad \ldots(2)$$

From equations (1) and (2), we get the reduction formula :

$$\therefore \quad \int \tan^n xdx = \frac{\tan^{n-1} x}{n-1} - \int \tan^{n-2} xdx, n \neq 1$$

(ii) Similarly, $$I_n = \int \cot^n xdx = \int \cot^{n-2} x \cot^2 xdx = \int \cot^{n-2} x(\text{cosec}^2 x - 1)dx$$

$$= \int \cot^{n-2} x\, \text{cosec}^2 x\, dx - \int \cot^{n-2} x\, dx$$

$$\therefore \quad \int \cot^n xdx = -\frac{\cot^{n-1} x}{n-1} - \int \cot^{n-2} xdx.$$

16.15 REDUCTION FORMULAE FOR $\int \sec^n xdx$ AND $\int \text{cosec}^n xdx$

(i) Let $$I_n = \int \sec^n xdx = \int \sec^{n-2} x \sec^2 xdx$$

$$= \sec^{n-2} x \int \sec^2 xdx - \int \left\{ \frac{d}{dx}(\sec^{n-2} x) \int \sec^2 xdx \right\} dx$$

$$= \tan x \sec^{n-2} x - (n-2) \int \sec^{n-2} x \tan^2 xdx$$

$$= \tan x \sec^{n-2} x - (n-2) \int \sec^{n-2} x(\sec^2 x - 1)dx$$

or $$I_n = \tan x \sec^{n-2} x - (n-2) \int \sec^n xdx + (n-2) \int \sec^{n-2} xdx$$

or $$I_n = \tan x \sec^{n-2} x - (n-2) I_n + (n-2) I_{n-2}$$

or $$I_n (1 + n - 2) = \tan x \sec^{n-2} x + (n-2) I_{n-2}$$

$$\therefore \quad I_n = \frac{1}{n-1} \tan x \sec^{n-2} x + \frac{n-2}{n-1} I_{n-2}, n \neq 1$$

Hence $$\int \sec^n xdx = \frac{\sec^{n-2} x \tan x}{n-1} + \frac{n-2}{n-1} \int \sec^{n-2} xdx$$

Similarly, we obtain $$\int \text{cosec}^n xdx = -\frac{\text{cosec}^{n-2} x \cot x}{n-1} + \frac{n-2}{n-1} \int \text{cosec}^{n-2} xdx$$

16.16 REDUCTION FORMULAE FOR $\int \tan^m x \sec^n x dx$ AND $\int \cot^m x \operatorname{cosec}^n x dx$

(i) Let $I_{m,n} = \int \tan^m x \sec^n x dx = \int \tan^{m-1} x(\sec^{n-1} x \sec x \tan x)dx$

$$= \tan^{m-1} x \frac{\sec^n x}{n} - \frac{m-1}{n} \int \tan^{m-2} x \sec^2 x \sec^n x dx$$

$$= \frac{\tan^{m-1} x \sec^n x}{n} - \frac{m-1}{n} I_{m-2,n} - \frac{m-1}{m+n-1} I_{m,n}$$

$$\Rightarrow \quad I_{m,n} = \int \tan^m x \sec^n x dx = \frac{\tan^{m-1} x \sec^n x}{m+n-1} - \frac{m-1}{m+n-1} I_{m-2,n}, \; m+n \neq 1$$

(ii) Similarly, the power of $\sec x$ is reduced by two during integrating $\int \tan^m x \sec^n x dx$ by parts and then, we get

$$I_{m,n} = \int \tan^m x \sec^n x dx = \frac{\tan^{m+1} x \sec^{n-2} x}{m+n-1} - \frac{n-2}{m+n-1} I_{m,n-2}, (m+n \neq 1)$$

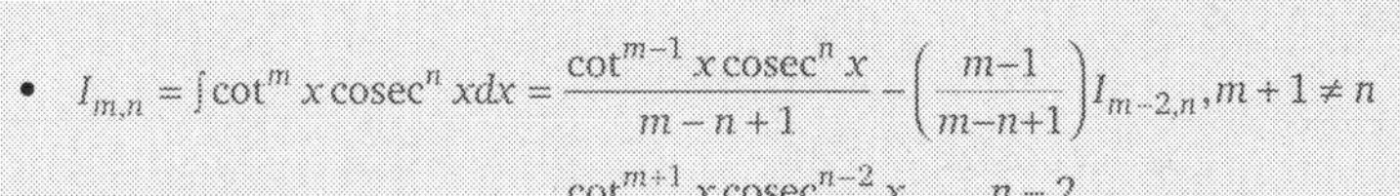

- $I_{m,n} = \int \cot^m x \operatorname{cosec}^n x dx = \dfrac{\cot^{m-1} x \operatorname{cosec}^n x}{m-n+1} - \left(\dfrac{m-1}{m-n+1}\right) I_{m-2,n}, m+1 \neq n$
- $I_{m,n} = \int \cot^m x \operatorname{cosec}^n x dx = \dfrac{\cot^{m+1} x \operatorname{cosec}^{n-2} x}{n-m+1} - \dfrac{n-2}{n-m+1} I_{m,n-2}, n+1 \neq m$

16.17 REDUCTION FORMULAE FOR $\int \cos^m x \cos nx dx$, $\int \cos^m x \sin nx dx$, $\int \sin^m x \cos nx dx$ ETC.

(i) Let $I_{m,n} = \int \cos^m x \cos nx dx = \cos^m x \frac{\sin nx}{n} + \frac{m}{n} \int \cos^{m-1} x \sin x \sin nx dx$ ...(1)

$$= \frac{\cos^m x \sin nx}{n} + \frac{m}{n} \int \cos^{m-1} x \{\cos(n-1)x - \cos nx \cos x\} dx$$

$[\because \cos(n-1)x = \cos nx \cos x + \sin nx \sin x]$

$$= \frac{\cos^m x \sin nx}{n} + \frac{m}{n} I_{m-1,n-1} - \frac{m}{n} I_{m,n}$$

$$\Rightarrow \quad \left(1+\frac{m}{n}\right) I_{m,n} = \frac{\cos^m x \sin nx}{n} + \frac{m}{n} I_{m-1,n-1}$$

$$\Rightarrow \quad I_{m,n} = \frac{\cos^m x \sin nx}{n} + \frac{m}{n} I_{m-1,n-1}, m+n \neq 0 \qquad \text{...(2)}$$

Intetgrate (1) by parts and using (2), we get

$$I_{m,n} = \frac{\cos^m x \sin nx}{n} + \frac{m}{n} \left\{ \cos^{m-1} x \sin x \left(-\frac{\cos nx}{n} \right) + \int [\cos^m x - (m-1)\cos^{m-2} x \sin^2 x] \frac{\cos nx}{n} dx \right\}$$

$$= \frac{\cos^m x \sin nx}{n} - \frac{m}{n^2} \cos^{m-1} x \sin x \cos nx + \frac{m^2}{n^2} I_{m,n} - \frac{m(m-1)}{n^2} I_{m-2,n}$$

$$\Rightarrow \quad \left(1-\frac{m^2}{n^2}\right) I_{m,n} = \frac{\cos^m x \sin nx}{n} - \frac{m}{n^2} \cos^{m-1} x \sin x \cos nx - \frac{m(m-1)}{n^2} I_{m-2,n}$$

$$\Rightarrow \quad I_{m,n} = -\frac{n \cos^m x \sin nx}{m^2-n^2} + \frac{m}{m^2-n^2} \cos^{m-1} x \sin x \cos nx + \frac{m(m-1)}{m^2-n^2} I_{m-2,n}$$

$$= -\frac{\cos^{m-1} x}{m^2-n^2} [n \cos x \sin nx - m \sin x \cos nx] + \frac{m(m-1)}{m^2-n^2} I_{m-2,n}$$

$$\Rightarrow \quad I_{m,n} = -\frac{\cos^2 nx}{m^2 - n^2}\frac{d}{dx}\left(\frac{\cos^m x}{\cos nx}\right) + \frac{m(m-1)}{m^2 - n^2} I_{m-2,n}$$

- Here the power of cosine is reduced by two only.

(ii) Let $I_{m,n} = \int \cos^m x \sin nx dx = \cos^m x\left(-\frac{\cos nx}{n}\right) - \int m\cos^{m-1} x(-\sin x)\left(-\frac{\cos nx}{n}\right)dx$

$$= -\frac{\cos^m x \cos nx}{n} - \frac{m}{n}\int \cos^{m-1} x \sin x \cos nx\, dx \qquad \ldots(1)$$

$$= -\frac{\cos^m x \cos nx}{n} - \frac{m}{n}\int \cos^{m-1} x[\sin nx \cos x - \sin(n-1)x]dx$$

$[\because \sin(n-1)x = \sin nx \cos x - \cos nx \sin x]$

$$= -\frac{\cos^m x \cos nx}{n} - \frac{m}{n} I_{m,n} + \frac{m}{n} I_{m-1,n-1}$$

$$\Rightarrow \quad \left(1+\frac{m}{n}\right) I_{m,n} = -\frac{\cos^m x \cos nx}{m+n} + \frac{m}{m+n} I_{m-1,n-1}$$

$$\Rightarrow \quad I_{m,n} = -\frac{\cos^m x \cos nx}{m+n} + \frac{m}{m+n} I_{m-1,n-1}, m+n \neq 0$$

On intetgrating by parts the right hand integral of (1), we get

$$I_{m,n} = -\frac{\cos^m x \cos nx}{n} - \frac{m}{n}\left[(\cos^{m-1} x \sin x)\frac{\sin nx}{n} - \int\{(m-1)\cos^{m-2} x(-\sin^2 x) + \cos^m x\}\frac{\sin nx}{n}dx\right]$$

$$= -\frac{\cos^m x \cos nx}{n} - \frac{m}{n^2}\cos^{m-1} x \sin x \sin nx + \frac{m}{n^2}\int\{-(m-1)\cos^{m-2} x(1-\cos^2 x) + \cos^m x\}\sin nx dx$$

$$= -\frac{\cos^m x \cos nx}{n} - \frac{m}{n^2}\cos^{m-1} x \sin x \sin nx - \frac{m(m-1)}{n^2} I_{m-2,n} + \frac{m^2}{n^2} I_{m,n}$$

$$\Rightarrow \left(1-\frac{m^2}{n^2}\right) I_{m,n} = -\frac{\cos^m x \cos nx}{n} - \frac{m}{n^2}\cos^{m-1} x \sin x \sin nx - \frac{m(m-1)}{n^2} I_{m-2,n}$$

$$\Rightarrow \quad I_{m,n} = \frac{n\cos^m x \cos nx}{m^2 - n^2} + \frac{m\cos^{m-1} x \sin x \sin nx}{m^2 - n^2} - \frac{m(m-1)}{m^2 - n^2} I_{m-2,n}$$

(iii) Here, let $I_{m,n} = \int \sin^m x \cos nx dx = \sin^m x \frac{\sin nx}{n} - \int m\sin^{m-1} x \cos x \frac{\sin nx}{n} dx$

$$= \frac{\sin^m x \sin nx}{n} - \frac{m}{n}\int \sin^{m-1} x \cos x \sin nx dx$$

$$= \frac{\sin^m x \sin nx}{n} - \frac{m}{n}\left[(\sin^{m-1} x \cos x)\left(-\frac{\cos nx}{n}\right) - \int\{(m-1)\sin^{m-2} x \cos^2 x - \sin^m x\}\left(-\frac{\cos nx}{n}\right)dx\right]$$

[Integrating by parts]

$$= \frac{\sin^m x \sin nx}{n} + \frac{m}{n^2}\sin^{m-1} x \cos x \cos nx - \frac{m}{n^2}\int\{(m-1)\sin^{m-2} x(1-\sin^2 x) - \sin^m x\}\cos nx dx$$

$$= \frac{\sin^m x \sin nx}{n} + \frac{m}{n^2}\sin^{m-1} x \cos x \cos nx - \frac{m(m-1)}{n^2} I_{m-2,n} + \frac{m^2}{n^2} I_{m,n}$$

$$\Rightarrow \quad I_{m,n} = -\frac{n\sin^m x \sin nx}{m^2-n^2} - \frac{m\sin^{m-1} x \cos x \cos nx}{m^2-n^2} + \frac{m(m-1)}{m^2-n^2} I_{m-2,n}$$

(iv) Let $I_{m,n} = \int \sin^m x \sin nx dx$

Proceed as above, we may easily get

$$\Rightarrow \quad I_{m,n} = -\frac{n\sin^m x \cos nx}{m^2-n^2} - \frac{m\sin^{m-1} x \cos x \sin nx}{m^2-n^2} + \frac{m(m+1)}{m^2-n^2} I_{m-2,n}.$$

16.18 REDUCTION FORMULAE FOR $\int x^n \sin mx dx$ AND $\int x^n \cos mx dx$

(i) Let $I(m,n) = \int x^n \sin mx dx = x^n \int \sin mx\, dx - \int\left\{\frac{d}{dx}(x^n)\int \sin mx\, dx\right\}dx$ (KANPUR–2002)

$$= -\frac{x^n \cos mx}{m} + \frac{n}{m}\int x^{n-1}\cos mx\, dx$$

$$= -\frac{x^n \cos mx}{m} + \frac{n}{m}\left[\frac{x^{n-1}\sin mx}{m} - \frac{n-1}{m}\int x^{n-2}\sin mx\, dx\right]$$

or $$I(m,n) = -\frac{x^n \cos mx}{m} + \frac{nx^{n-1}\sin mx}{m^2} - \frac{n(n-1)}{m^2}\int x^{n-2}\sin mx\, dx$$

Hence, $$\int x^n \sin mx\, dx = -\frac{x^n \cos mx}{m} + \frac{nx^{n-1}\sin mx}{m^2} - \frac{n(n-1)}{m^2}\int x^{n-2}\sin mx\, dx$$

Similarly, $$\int x^n \cos mx\, dx = \frac{x^n \sin mx}{m} + \frac{nx^{n-1}\cos mx}{m^2} - \frac{n(n-1)}{m^2}\int x^{n-2}\cos mx\, dx \cdot$$

16.19 REDUCTION FORMULAE FOR $\int x \sin^n x dx$ AND $\int x \cos^n x dx$

(i) Let $I_n = \int x \sin^n x dx$

$I_n = \int (x \sin^{n-1} x)\sin x dx$ (Integrating by part)

$$= x\sin^{n-1} x \int \sin x dx - \int\{\sin^{n-1} x + x(n-1)\sin^{n-2} x \cos x\}(-\cos x)dx$$

$$= -x\sin^{n-1} x \cos x + \int \sin^{n-1} x \cos x dx + (n-1)\int x\sin^{n-2} x \cos^2 x dx$$

$$= -x\sin^{n-1} x \cos x + \int \sin^{n-1} x \cos x dx + (n-1)\int x\sin^{n-2} x(1-\sin^2 x)dx$$

$\therefore$ $$I_n = -x\sin^{n-1} x \cos x + \frac{\sin^n x}{n} + (n-1)\int x\sin^{n-2} x dx - (n-1)\int x \sin^n x dx$$

or $$I_n = -x\sin^{n-1} x \cos x + \frac{\sin^n x}{n} + (n-1)\int x\sin^{n-2} x dx - (n-1)I_n$$

or $$I_n(1+n-1) = -x\sin^{n-1} x \cos x + \frac{\sin^n x}{n} + (n-1)\int x\sin^{n-2} x dx$$

Hence, $$\int x\sin^n x\,dx = \frac{-x\sin^{n-1}x\cos x}{n} + \frac{\sin^n x}{n^2} + \frac{n-1}{n}\int x\sin^{n-2}x\,dx$$

Similarly, $$\int x\cos^n x\,dx = \frac{x\cos^{n-1}x\sin x}{n} + \frac{\cos^n x}{n^2} + \frac{n-1}{n}\int x\cos^{n-2}x\,dx \cdot$$

16.20 REDUCTION FORMULAE FOR $\int e^{ax}\cos^n x\,dx$ AND $\int e^{ax}\sin^n x\,dx$

(i) Let $$I_n = \int e^{ax}\cos^n x\,dx = \frac{e^{ax}}{a}\cos^n x + \frac{n}{a}\int e^{ax}\cos^{n-1}x\sin x\,dx$$

$$= \frac{e^{ax}}{a}\cos^n x + \frac{n}{a}\left\{\frac{e^{ax}}{a}\cos^{n-1}x\sin x - \int\frac{e^{ax}}{a}[\cos^n x-(n-1)\cos^{n-2}x\sin^2 x]dx\right\}$$

$$= \frac{e^{ax}}{a}\cos^n x + \frac{n}{a^2}e^{ax}\cos^{n-1}x\sin x - \frac{n}{a^2}I_n + \frac{n(n-1)}{a^2}\int e^{ax}\cos^{n-2}x(1-\cos^2 x)dx$$

$$= \frac{e^{ax}}{a}\cos^n x + \frac{n}{a^2}e^{ax}\cos^{n-1}x\sin x - \frac{n}{a^2}I_n + \frac{n(n-1)}{a^2}I_{n-2} - \frac{n(n-1)}{a^2}I_n$$

$$\Rightarrow \left(1+\frac{n}{a^2}+\frac{n(n-1)}{a^2}\right)I_n = e^{ax}\cos^{n-1}x\,\frac{(a\cos x+n\sin x)}{a^2} + \frac{n(n-1)}{a^2}I_{n-2}$$

$$\Rightarrow \quad I_n = \frac{e^{ax}\cos^{n-1}x(a\cos x+n\sin x)}{(n^2+a^2)} + \frac{n(n-1)}{n^2+a^2}I_{n-2}.$$

(ii) Similarly, we can find that

$$I_n = \int e^{ax}\sin^n x\,dx = \frac{e^{ax}\sin^{n-1}x}{n^2+a^2}(a\sin x - n\cos x) + \frac{n(n-1)}{n^2+a^2}I_{n-2}.$$

16.21 REDUCTION FORMULAE FOR $\int \cos nx \operatorname{cosec} x\,dx$ AND $\int \sin nx \sec x\,dx$

(i) Let $$I_n = \int \cos nx \operatorname{cosec} x\,dx = \frac{\sin nx}{n}\operatorname{cosec} x + \int\frac{\sin nx}{n}\operatorname{cosec} x\cot x\,dx$$

$$= \frac{\sin nx}{n}\operatorname{cosec} x + \int\frac{1}{n}\frac{\sin nx\cos x}{\sin^2 x}dx$$

$$= \frac{\sin nx}{n}\operatorname{cosec} x + \int\frac{1}{n}\frac{\sin(n-1)x+\cos nx\sin x}{\sin^2 x}dx$$

$$= \frac{\sin nx\operatorname{cosec} x}{n} + \frac{1}{n}\int\sin(n-1)x\operatorname{cosec}^2 x\,dx + \frac{1}{n}I_n$$

$$\Rightarrow \quad \left(1-\frac{1}{n}\right)I_n = \frac{\sin nx\operatorname{cosec} x}{n} + \frac{1}{n}[\sin(n-1)x(-\cot x) - (n-1)\int\cos(n-1)x(-\cot x)dx]$$

$$\Rightarrow \quad \frac{n-1}{n}I_n = \frac{\sin nx\operatorname{cosec} x}{n} - \frac{\sin(n-1)x\cot x}{n} + \frac{(n-1)}{n}\int\frac{\cos(n-1)x\cos x}{\sin x}dx.$$

$$\Rightarrow \quad I_n = \frac{\sin nx\operatorname{cosec} x}{n-1} - \frac{\sin(n-1)x\cot x}{n-1} + \int\frac{\cos(n-2)x-\sin(n-1)x\sin x}{\sin x}dx$$

$$= \frac{\sin nx\operatorname{cosec} x}{n-1} - \frac{\sin(n-1)x\cot x}{n-1} + I_{n-2} - \int\sin(n-1)x\,dx$$

$$= \frac{\sin nx \operatorname{cosec} x}{n-1} - \frac{\sin(n-1)x \cot x}{n-1} + I_{n-2} + \frac{1}{n-1}\cos(n-1)x$$

$$I_n - I_{n-2} = \frac{1}{n-1}\left[\frac{\sin nx}{\sin x} - \frac{\sin(n-1)x\cos x}{\sin x} + \cos(n-1)x\right]$$

$$= \frac{1}{n-1}\left[\frac{\sin nx - \sin(n-1)x\cos x}{\sin x} + \cos(n-1)x\right]$$

$$= \frac{1}{n-1}\left[\frac{\sin[(n-1)+1]x - \sin(n-1)x\cos x}{\sin x} + \cos(n-1)x\right]$$

$$= \frac{2\cos(n-1)x}{n-1}$$

$$I_n = \frac{2\cos(n-1)x}{n-1} + I_{n-2}$$

(ii) Similarly, $I_n = \int \sin nx \sec x dx = -\frac{2\cos(n-1)x}{n-1} - I_{n-2}$.

16.22 REDUCTION FORMULAE FOR $\int(\sin^{-1}x)^n dx$ AND $\int(\cos^{-1}x)^n dx$

(i) Let $I_n = \int(\cos^{-1}x)^n dx = x(\cos^{-1}x)^n - \int n(\cos^{-1}x)^{n-1}\left(\frac{-1}{\sqrt{1-x^2}}\right)x dx$

$$= x(\cos^{-1}x)^n + n\int(\cos^{-1}x)^{n-1}\frac{x}{\sqrt{1-x^2}}dx$$

$$= x(\cos^{-1}x)^n - n(\cos^{-1}x)^{n-1}\sqrt{1-x^2}$$

$$- n\int(n-1)(\cos^{-1}x)^{n-2}\left(-\frac{1}{\sqrt{1-x^2}}\right)\sqrt{1-x^2}dx$$

$\Rightarrow$ $I_n = x(\cos^{-1}x)^n - n(\cos^{-1}x)^{n-1}\sqrt{1-x^2} + n(n-1)I_{n-2}$

(ii) Proceeding as same manner we get

$$I_n = \int(\sin^{-1}x)^n dx = x(\sin^{-1}x)^n + n(\sin^{-1}x)^{n-1}\sqrt{1-x^2} - n(n-1)I_{n-2}.$$

16.23 REDUCTION FORMULA FOR $\int\frac{dx}{(a+b\cos x)^n}$ AND $\int\frac{dx}{(a+b\sin x)^n}$

(i) Let $I_n = \int\frac{dx}{(a+b\cos x)^n}$

Also, let $P(x) = \frac{\sin x}{(a+b\cos x)^{n-1}} = \frac{\sin x}{t^{n-1}}$, where $t = a + b\cos x$

$\Rightarrow$ $\cos x = \frac{t-a}{b}$

Differentiating with respect to x, we get

$$\frac{dP(x)}{dx} = \frac{\cos x}{t^{n-1}} - (n-1)\frac{\sin x}{t^n}\frac{dt}{dx} = \frac{\cos x}{t^{n-1}} - (n-1)\frac{\sin x}{t^n}(-b\sin x)$$

$$= \frac{t-a}{bt^{n-1}} + \frac{b(n-1)}{t^n}(1-\cos^2 x) = \frac{t-a}{bt^{n-1}} + \frac{b(n-1)}{t^n}\left[1-\left(\frac{t-a}{b}\right)^2\right]$$

$$= \frac{t-a}{bt^{n-1}} + \frac{b(n-1)}{t^n}\left[1-\frac{t^2-2at+a^2}{b^2}\right] = \frac{(n-1)(b^2-a^2)}{bt^n} + \frac{a(2n-3)}{bt^{n-1}} - \frac{n-2}{bt^{n-2}}$$

$$= \frac{(n-1)(b^2-a^2)}{b}\cdot\frac{1}{(a+b\cos x)^n} + \frac{a(2n-3)}{b}\cdot\frac{1}{(a+b\cos x)^{n-1}} - \frac{n-2}{b}\cdot\frac{1}{(a+b\cos x)^{n-2}}$$

On integrating *w.r.t.* x, we get

$$P(x) = \frac{(n-1)(b^2-a^2)}{b}I_n + \frac{a(2n-3)}{b}I_{n-1} - \frac{n-2}{b}I_{n-2}$$

$$\Rightarrow \quad I_n = \frac{b\sin x}{(n-1)(b^2-a^2)(a+b\cos x)^{n-1}} - \frac{a(2n-3)}{(n-1)(b^2-a^2)}I_{n-1} + \frac{n-2}{(n-1)(b^2-a^2)}I_{n-2}$$

(ii) Similarly, by setting $P(x) = \frac{\cos x}{(a+b\sin x)^{n-1}}$, we may easily get

$$I_n = \int\frac{dx}{(a+b\sin x)^n} = \frac{b}{(n-1)(a^2-b^2)}\cdot\frac{\cos x}{(a+b\sin x)^{n-1}} + \frac{(2n-3)a}{(n-1)(a^2-b^2)}I_{n-1} - \frac{n-2}{(n-1)(a^2-b^2)}I_{n-2}.$$

16.24 REDUCTION FORMULA FOR $\int x^m (\log x)^n dx$

Let $\quad I(m,n) = \int x^m (\log x)^n dx$ (Integrating by part)

$$= (\log x)^n \int x^m dx - \int\left\{\frac{n(\log x)^{n-1}}{x}\cdot\frac{x^{m+1}dx}{m+1}\right\}$$

$$= \frac{x^{m+1}(\log x)^n}{m+1} - \frac{n}{m+1}\int x^m (\log x)^{n-1} dx$$

Hence, $\int x^m (\log x)^n dx = \frac{x^{m+1}(\log x)^n}{m+1} - \frac{n}{m+1}\int x^m (\log x)^{n-1} dx$.

16.25 REDUCTION FORMULA FOR $\int \frac{x^n}{\sqrt{ax^2+bx+c}}dx$

Let

$$I_n = \int\frac{x^n}{\sqrt{ax^2+bx+c}}dx = \frac{1}{2a}\int\frac{[(2ax+b)-b]x^{n-1}}{\sqrt{ax^2+bx+c}}dx$$

$$= \frac{1}{2a}\int\frac{(2ax+b)x^{n-1}}{\sqrt{ax^2+bx+c}}dx - \frac{b}{2a}\int\frac{x^{n-1}}{\sqrt{ax^2+bx+c}}dx$$

$$= \frac{1}{2a}\left[x^{n-1}.2\sqrt{ax^2+bx+c} - \int(n-1)x^{n-2}2\sqrt{ax^2+bx+c}dx\right] - \frac{b}{2a}I_{n-1}$$

$$= \frac{1}{a}x^{n-1}\sqrt{ax^2+bx+c} - \frac{(n-1)}{a}\int \frac{x^{n-2}(ax^2+bx+c)}{\sqrt{ax^2+bx+c}}dx - \frac{b}{2a}I_{n-1}$$

$$= \frac{1}{a}x^{n-1}\sqrt{ax^2+bx+c} - (n-1)I_n - \frac{b(n-1)}{a}I_{n-1} - \frac{(n-1)}{a}I_{n-2} - \frac{b}{2a}I_{n-1}$$

$$\Rightarrow \quad I_n = \frac{1}{na}x^{n-1}\sqrt{ax^2+bx+c} - \frac{b(2n-1)}{2an}I_{n-1} - \frac{c(n-1)}{an}I_{n-2}.$$

16.26 REDUCTION FORMULA FOR $\int \frac{px+q}{(ax^2+bx+c)^n}dx$

Let
$$I_n = \int \frac{px+q}{(ax^2+bx+c)}dx = \frac{p}{2a}\int \frac{2ax}{(ax^2+bx+c)^n}dx + \left(q - \frac{bp}{2a}\right)\int \frac{dx}{(ax^2+bx+c)^n}$$

$$= -\frac{p}{2a(n-1)}\frac{1}{(ax^2+bx+c)^{n-1}} + \left(q - \frac{bp}{2a}\right).\frac{1}{a^n}\int \frac{dx}{\left[\left(x+\frac{b}{2a}\right)^2 + \frac{4ac-b^2}{4a^2}\right]^n}$$

$$= -\frac{p}{2a(n-1)}.\frac{1}{(ax^2+bx+c)^{n-1}} + \frac{2qa-pb}{2a^{n+1}}\int \frac{dt}{(t^2+r)^n} \qquad ...(1)$$

where $t = x + \frac{b}{2a}$ and $r = \frac{4ac-b^2}{4a^2}$

Integrating right hand integral of (1), by parts, we have

$$P_n = \int -\frac{dt}{(t^2+r)^n} = \frac{t}{(t^2+r)^n} + \int \frac{2t^2}{(t^2+r)^{n+1}}dt = \frac{t}{(t^2+r)^n} + 2n\int \frac{(t^2+r)-r}{(t^2+r)^{n+1}}dt$$

$$= \frac{t}{(t^2+r)^n} + 2n\int \frac{dt}{(t^2+r)^n} - 2nr\int \frac{dt}{(t^2+r)^{n+1}}$$

Now, replacing n by $n-1$ in this relation and solving for $\int \frac{dt}{(t^2+r)^n}$, we get

$$\int \frac{dt}{(t^2+r)^n} = \frac{1}{2(n-r)r}\cdot\frac{t}{(t^2+r)^{n-1}} + \frac{2n-3}{2(n-1)r}\int \frac{dt}{(t^2+r)^{n-1}} \qquad ...(2)$$

From (1) and (2), we conclude that

$$I_n = -\frac{p}{2a(n-1)}\cdot\frac{1}{(ax^2+bx+c)^{n-1}} + \frac{2aq-pb}{2a^{n+1}}\left[\frac{1}{2(n-r)r}\cdot\frac{1}{(t^2+r)^{n-1}} + \frac{2n-3}{2(n-1)r}P_{n-1}\right]$$

$$\Rightarrow \quad I_n = \frac{-p}{2a(n-1)}\cdot\frac{1}{(ax^2+bx+c)^{n-1}} + \frac{2aq-qb}{4(n-1)r}\left[\frac{1}{(t^2+r)^{n-1}} + (2n-3)P_{n-1}\right]$$

where $P_n = \int \frac{dt}{(t^2+r)^n}, t = x + \frac{b}{2a}$ and $r = \frac{4ac-b^2}{4a^2}$.

16.27 SOME MORE IMPORTANT REDUCTION FORMULAE

The reduction formulae for $I_{m,p} = \int x^m (a+bx^n)^p dx$ are :

(i) $I_{m,p} = \dfrac{x^{m-n+1}.(a+bx^n)^{p+1}}{(np+m+1)^b} - \dfrac{(m-n+1)}{(np+m+1)^b} I_{m-n,p}, (np+m+1 \neq 0)$

(ii) $I_{m,p} = \dfrac{x^{m+1}(a+bx^n)^p}{np+m+1} + \dfrac{anp}{np+m+1} I_{m,p-1}, (np+m+1 \neq 0)$

(iii) $I_{m,p} = \dfrac{x^{m+1}(a+bx^n)^{p+1}}{(m+1)a} - \dfrac{(np+n+m+1)b}{(m+1)a} I_{m+n,p}, (m+1 \neq 0)$

(iv) $I_{m,p} = \dfrac{-x^{m+1}(a+bx^n)^{p+1}}{n(p+1)a} + \dfrac{(np+n+m+1)}{n(p+1)a} I_{m,p+1}, (n, p+1 \neq 0)$

Solved Examples

1. *Use reduction formula to integrate* $\sin^{1/2} x \cos^{7/2} x$.

SOLUTION. Since, we have

$$I_{m,n} = \int \sin^m x \cos^n x dx$$

$$= \frac{\cos^{n-1} x \sin^{m+1} x}{m+n} + \frac{n-1}{m+n} I_{m,n-2},$$

$$m + n \neq 0$$

Put $m = 1/2$, $n = 7/2$, we get

$$I_{\frac{1}{2},\frac{7}{2}} = \int \sin^{1/2} x \cos^{7/2} x dx$$

$$= \frac{\cos^{5/2} x \sin^{3/2} x}{4} + \frac{5}{8} I_{1/2,3/2}.$$

Also,

$$I_{\frac{1}{2},\frac{3}{2}} = \frac{\cos^{1/2} x \sin^{3/2} x}{2} + \frac{1}{4} I_{1/2,-1/2}$$

$$I_{\frac{1}{2},\frac{7}{2}} = \frac{\cos^{5/2} x \sin^{3/2} x}{4} + \frac{5}{16} \cos^{1/2} x \sin^{3/2} x + \frac{5}{32} I_{1/2,-1/2}.$$

Here, further reduction is not possible because

$$m + n = \frac{1}{2} - \frac{1}{2} = 0.$$

But $I_{\frac{1}{2},-\frac{1}{2}} = \int \frac{\sqrt{\sin x}}{\sqrt{\cos x}} dx = \int \sqrt{\tan x} dx$

$$= \frac{1}{2} \tan^{-1}\left(\frac{\tan x - 1}{\sqrt{2 \tan x}}\right) + \frac{1}{2\sqrt{2}} \log \frac{\tan x - \sqrt{2 \tan x}}{\tan x + \sqrt{2 \tan x}}$$

Therefore,

$$I_{\frac{1}{2},\frac{7}{2}} = \frac{1}{4} \sqrt{\cos x \sin^{3/2} x} \left(\cos^2 x + \frac{5}{4}\right) + \frac{5}{32}\left[\frac{1}{2} \tan^{-1}\left(\frac{\tan x - 1}{\sqrt{2 \tan x}}\right) + \frac{1}{2\sqrt{2}} \log \frac{\tan x - \sqrt{2 \tan x}}{\tan x + \sqrt{2 \tan x}}\right] + c$$

2. *Compute* $\int \sin^4 x \cos^5 x dx$. (COCHIN–2005)

SOLUTION. We know that

$$I_{m,n} = \int \sin^m x \cos^n x dx$$

$$= -\frac{\sin^{m-1} x \cos^{n+1} x}{m+n} + \frac{m-1}{m+n} I_{m-2,n}, m + n \neq 0.$$

Put $m = 4$, $n = 5$, we get

$$I_{4,5} = \int \sin^4 x \cos^5 x dx$$

$$= -\frac{\sin^3 x \cos^6 x}{9} + \frac{1}{3} I_{2,5}$$

Now $I_{2,5} = \int \sin^2 x \cos^5 x dx$

$$= -\frac{\sin x \cos^6 x}{5} + \frac{1}{7} I_{0,5}$$

Here, $I_{0,5} = I_5 = \int \cos^5 x dx$

$$= \frac{\sin x \cos^4 x}{5} + \frac{4}{5} I_3$$

and $I_3 = \int \cos^3 x dx$

$$= \frac{\sin x \cos^2 x}{3} + \frac{2}{3} I_1$$

$$I_1 = \int \cos x dx = \sin x$$

Therefore,

$$I_{4,5} = -\frac{\sin^3 x \cos^6 x}{9} - \frac{1}{21} \sin x \cos^6 x + \frac{1}{105} \sin x \cos^4 x + \frac{4}{315} \sin x \cos^2 x + \frac{8}{315} \sin x + c$$

$$= \frac{\sin x}{315} [35 \cos^8 x - 50 \cos^6 x + 3 \cos^4 x + 4 \cos^2 x + 8] + c$$

3. *If n is a positive integer, prove that*

$$\int_0^{\pi/2} \cos^n x \cos nx dx = \frac{\pi}{2^{n+1}}.$$

SOLUTION. We know that

$$I(m,n) = \int \cos^m x \cos nx dx$$

$$= \frac{\cos^m x \sin nx}{m+n} + \frac{m}{m+n} \int \cos^{m-1} x \cos(n-1) x \, dx$$

Then

$$\int_0^{\pi/2} \cos^n x \cos nx dx$$

$$= \left[\frac{\cos^m x \sin nx}{m+n} \right]_0^{\pi/2} + \frac{m}{m+n} \int_0^{\pi/2} \cos^{m-1} x \cos(n-1) x dx$$

$$= \frac{m}{m+n} \int_0^{\pi/2} \cos^{m-1} x \cos(n-1) x dx$$

i.e., $I(m,n) = \frac{m}{m+n} I(m-1, n-1)$

Now putting $m = n$, we get

$$I(n,n) = \frac{n}{n+n} I(n-1, n-1)$$

or $I(n,n) = \frac{1}{2} I(n-1, n-1) \quad \ldots(1)$

Now replacing n by $n - 1$ on both sides of (1), we get

$$I(n-1, n-1) = \frac{1}{2} I(n-2, n-2) \quad \ldots(2)$$

Putting the value of $I(n - 1, n - 1)$ in (1), we get

$$I(n,n) = \frac{1}{2} \cdot \frac{1}{2} I(n-2, n-2)$$

$$= \frac{1}{2^2} I(n-2, n-2)$$

Continuing in the same way, we get

$$I(n,n) = \frac{1}{2^n} I(0,0)$$

Now $I(0,0) = \int_0^{\pi/2} \cos^0 x \cos 0x dx$

$$= \int_0^{\pi/2} dx$$

$$= [x]_0^{\pi/2} = \frac{\pi}{2}$$

$$\therefore \quad I(n,n) = \frac{\pi}{2^{n+1}}$$

Hence $\int_0^{\pi/2} \cos^n x \cos nx dx = \frac{\pi}{2^{n+1}}.$

4. *If* $I_n = \int_0^{\pi/4} \tan^n x dx$, *show that* $I_n + I_{n-2} = \frac{1}{n-1}$. *Hence, deduce the value of* I_5.

SOLUTION. We know that

$$\int \tan^n x dx = \frac{\tan^{n-1} x}{n-1} - \int \tan^{n-2} x dx$$

Then

$$I_n = \int_0^{\pi/4} \tan^n x dx$$

$$= \left[\frac{\tan^{n-1} x}{n-1} \right]_0^{\pi/4} - \int_0^{\pi/4} \tan^{n-2} x dx$$

or $I_n = \frac{1}{n-1} - I_{n-2}$

$$\therefore \quad I_n + I_{n-2} = \frac{1}{n-1} \quad \ldots(1)$$

Next, putting $n = 3$ and 5 successively, we get

$$I_3 + I_1 = \frac{1}{2}, \; I_5 + I_3 = \frac{1}{4}$$

Form these equations, we get

$$I_5 = \frac{1}{4} - I_3 = \frac{1}{4} - \left(\frac{1}{2} - I_1 \right)$$

or $I_5 = -\frac{1}{4} + I_1$

or $$I_5 = -\frac{1}{4} + \int_0^{\pi/4} \tan x dx$$

$$= -\frac{1}{4} + \left[\log \sec x\right]_0^{\pi/4}$$

$$= -\frac{1}{4} + \left[\log \sec\frac{\pi}{4} - \log\sec 0\right]$$

$$= -\frac{1}{4} + \left[\log\sqrt{2} - \log 1\right]$$

$$= -\frac{1}{4} + \log\sqrt{2} - 0$$

Hence, $I_5 = \frac{1}{2}\left[\log 2 - \frac{1}{2}\right]$.

5. *If* $u_n = \int_0^{\pi/2} x^n \sin x dx$ *and* $n > 1$, *prove that*

$$u_n + n(n-1)u_{n-2} = n\left(\frac{\pi}{2}\right)^{n-1}$$

Hence evaluate $\int_0^{\pi/2} x^5 \sin x dx$.

(MADRAS–2000)

SOLUTION. By reduction formula, we have

$$\int x^n \sin mx dx = -\frac{x^n \cos mx}{m} + \frac{nx^{n-1}\sin mx}{m^2} - \frac{n(n-1)}{m^2}\int x^{n-2}\sin mx dx$$

Putting $m = 1$ in both sides, we get

$$\int x^n \sin x dx = -x^n \cos x + nx^{n-1}\sin x - n(n-1)\int x^{n-2}\sin x dx$$

Then $u_n = \int_0^{\pi/2} x^n \sin nx dx$

$$= \left[-x^n \cos x + nx^{n-1}\sin x\right]_0^{\pi/2} - n(n-1)\int_0^{\pi/2} x^{n-2}\sin x dx$$

or $$u_n = \left[u\left(\frac{\pi}{2}\right)^{n-1}\right] - n(n-1)u_{n-2}$$

$$\therefore u_n + n(n-1)u_{n-2} = n\left(\frac{\pi}{2}\right)^{n-1} \quad \ldots(1)$$

Next, putting $n = 3$ and 5 successively in (1), we get

$$u_5 + 5(5-1)u_3 = 5\left(\frac{\pi}{2}\right)^4$$

and $$u_3 + 3(3-1)u_1 = 3\left(\frac{\pi}{2}\right)^2$$

From these equations, we get

$$u_5 + 20\left[3\left(\frac{\pi}{2}\right)^2 - 6u_1\right] = 5\left(\frac{\pi}{2}\right)^4$$

Now, $u_1 = \int_0^{\pi/2} x \sin x dx$

$$= \left[-x\cos x\right]_0^{\pi/2} - \int_0^{\pi/2}(-\cos x)dx$$

$$= 1$$

$$= [0] + \left[\sin x\right]_0^{\pi/2}$$

$$\therefore u_5 + 20\left[3\left(\frac{\pi}{2}\right)^2 - 6(1)\right] = 5\left(\frac{\pi}{2}\right)^4$$

or $$u_5 = \frac{5}{16}\pi^4 - 15\pi^2 + 120$$

6. *Evaluate* $\int_0^1 x^m (\log x)^n dx$, *when* $m \geq 0$ *and n is positive integer.*

(SVTU–2009, BHILLAI–2005)

SOLUTION. We know by reduction formula

$$\int x^m (\log x)^n dx = \frac{x^{m+1}(\log x)^n}{m+1} - \frac{n}{m+1}\int x^m (\log x)^{n-1} dx$$

Let $I(m,n) = \int_0^1 x^m (\log x)^n dx$,

then we have

$$I(m,n) = \left[\frac{x^{m+1}(\log x)^n}{m+1}\right]_0^1 - \frac{n}{m+1} I(m,n-1)$$

or $$I(m,n) = [0-0] - \frac{n}{m+1} I(m,n-1)$$

or $$I(m,n) = -\frac{n}{m+1} I(m,n-1) \quad \ldots(1)$$

Replace n by $n-1$ in (1), we get

$$I(m,n-1) = -\frac{n-1}{m+1} I(m,n-2) \quad \ldots(2)$$

From (2) and (1), we get

$$I(m,n) = (-1)^2\left(\frac{n}{m+1}\right)\left(\frac{n-1}{m+1}\right) I(m,n-2) \quad \ldots(3)$$

Again by repeated application of (1), we get

$$I(m,n) = (-1)^n \left(\frac{n}{m+1}\right)\left(\frac{n-1}{m+1}\right)\left(\frac{n-2}{m+1}\right) \cdots \left(\frac{1}{m+1}\right) I(m,0)$$

or $$I(m,n) = (-1)^n \frac{n!}{(m+1)^n} I(m,0)$$

Now

$$I(m,0) = \int_0^1 x^m dx = \left[\frac{x^{m+1}}{m+1}\right]_0^1 = \frac{1}{m+1}$$

$$\therefore \quad I(m,n) = (-1)^n \frac{n!}{(m+1)^n}\cdot\frac{1}{m+1} = \frac{(-1)^n n!}{(m+1)^{n+1}}$$

Hence, $\int_0^1 x^m (\log x)^n dx = \dfrac{(-1)^n n!}{(m+1)^{n+1}}$.

Exercise-16.5

Use reduction formulae, compute the following:

1. $\int \cos^3 x \operatorname{cosec}^2 x dx$
2. $\int \sqrt{\cos\theta}.\sin^3\theta d\theta$
3. $\int \cos^{-3}\theta \sin^{-1}\theta d\theta$
4. $\int \dfrac{x^4}{\sqrt{1-x^2}} dx$
5. $\int (1+x^2)^{3/2} dx$
6. $\int \dfrac{x^4}{(a^2+x^2)^2} dx$
7. $\int \dfrac{x^2}{\sqrt{2ax-x^2}} dx$ (MADRAS–2000)
8. $\int \dfrac{x^5}{(a+bx^2)^4} dx$
9. $\int \dfrac{dx}{x^{1/2}(1+x^2)^{5/4}}$
10. $\int \dfrac{x^3}{\sqrt{4x-x^2}} dx$
11. $\int \dfrac{x^3+5x^2-3x+4}{\sqrt{x^2+x+1}} dx$
12. $\int x^3 \cos 3x dx$
13. $\int x^3 e^{ax} dx$
14. Prove that : $I_n = \int x^n e^{-x} dx = -x^n e^{-x} + nI_{n-1}$.
15. Find the following integrals using reduction formula

    (i) $\int \dfrac{x+1}{(x^2+1)^3} dx$ (ii) $\int \dfrac{x^2-a^2}{(x^2+a^2)^3} dx$

16. (i) If $I_n = \int \dfrac{dx}{(x^2+a^2)^n}$, then show that

    $$I_{n+1} = \frac{1}{2na^2}\cdot\frac{x}{(x^2+a^2)^n} + \frac{2n-1}{2n}\cdot\frac{1}{a^2} I_n .$$

    (ii) If $I_n = \int (\log x)^n dx$, then show that

    $$I_n = x(\log x)^n - nI_{n-1} .$$

    (iii) If $I_n = \int x^n e^x dx$, then show that

    $$I_n = x^n e^x - nI_{n-1} .$$ (MADRAS–2000)

    (iv) If $I_n = \int e^{ax}\sin^n x dx$, then show that

    $$I_n = \frac{e^{ax}}{a^2+n^2}\sin^{n-1} x(a\sin x - n\cos x) + \frac{n(n-1)}{a^2+n^2} I_{n-2}$$

    (GORAKHPUR–1999)

17. Evaluate the following integrals :

    (i) $\int_0^{\pi/4} \tan^5\theta d\theta$ (ii) $\int_0^{\pi/4} \tan^7 x dx$

18. If $I_n = \int_0^{\pi/4} \tan^n x dx$, prove that

    $$n(I_{n-1} + I_{n+1}) = 1.$$ (VTU–2009)

19. If $I_n = \int_0^{\pi/3} \tan^n x dx$, prove that

    $$(n-1)(I_n + I_{n-2}) = \left(\sqrt{3}\right)^{n-1}.$$

20. Evaluate $\int \dfrac{d\theta}{\sin^4 \dfrac{\theta}{2}}$
21. Prove that

    $$\int_0^{\pi/4} \sec^3 x dx = \frac{1}{3}\left\{\sqrt{2} + \log(\sqrt{2}+1)\right\}.$$

22. Prove that

    $$\int_0^{\pi} \sin^m x \sin nx dx = \frac{m(m-1)}{m^2-n^2}\int_0^{\pi} \sin^{m-2} x \sin nx dx .$$

23. If n is a positive integer greater than 1, prove that $\int_0^{\pi/2} \cos^{n-2} x \sin nx dx = \dfrac{1}{n-1}$.
24. If $u_n = \int_0^{\pi/2} x^n \sin mx\, dx$, prove that

    $$u_n = \frac{n}{m^2}\left(\frac{\pi}{2}\right)^{n-1} - \frac{n(n-1)}{m^2} u_{n-2}$$

    where m is of the form $4r+1$.

    (MARATHWADA–2008)

25. Evaluate the following integrals :

(i) $\int_0^{\pi/2} x^3 \sin 3x dx$ (ii) $\int_0^{\pi} x \sin^3 x dx$ (iii) $\int_0^{\pi/2} x^5 \sin x dx$ (iv) $\int_0^{\pi} \theta \sin^2 \theta \cos \theta d\theta$

ANSWERS

1. $-\frac{1}{3}\sin x[\cot^2 x + 2\cos^2 x + 4] + c$ **2.** $\frac{2}{7}\cos^{7/2}\theta - \frac{2}{3}\cos^{3/2}\theta + c$ **3.** $\frac{1}{2}\tan^2\theta + \log\tan\theta + c$

4. $\frac{1.3}{2.4}\sin^{-1}x - \frac{x\sqrt{1-x^2}}{8}(3+2x^2) + c$ **5.** $\frac{\sin\theta}{4\cos^4\theta} + \frac{3\sin\theta}{8\cos^2\theta} + \frac{3}{8}\log(\sec\theta + \tan\theta) + c \ (x = \tan\theta)$

6. $c - \frac{x^3}{2(a^2+x^4)} + \frac{3}{2}\left(x - a\tan^{-1}\frac{x}{a}\right)$ **7.** $c - \sqrt{2ax - x^2}\left(\frac{x}{2} + \frac{3a}{2}\right) + 3a^2\sin^{-1}\frac{x-a}{a}$

8. $\frac{1}{6a}\cdot\frac{x^4}{(a+bx^2)^3} + \frac{1}{12a^2}\cdot\frac{x^4}{(a+bx^2)^2} + c$ **9.** $2\sqrt{x}(1+x^2)^{-1/4} + c$

10. $c - \frac{1}{3}(x^2+5x+30)\sqrt{4x-x^2} + 10\cos^{-1}\left(1 - \frac{x-2}{2}\right)$

11. $\left(\frac{1}{3}x^3 + \frac{25}{12}x - \frac{163}{24}\right)\sqrt{x^2+x+1} + \frac{85}{16}\sin^{-1}\left(\frac{2x+1}{\sqrt{3}}\right) + c$

12. $\frac{1}{27}(9x^2-2)\cos 3x + \frac{1}{9}(3x^2-2x)\sin 3x + c$

13. $\frac{e^{ax}}{a^4}(a^3x^3 - 3a^2x^2 + 6ax - 6) + c$ **15.** (i) $\frac{x-1}{4(x^2+1)^2} + \frac{3x}{8(x^2+1)} + \frac{3}{8}\tan^{-1}x + c$

(ii) $-\frac{x}{4a^2(x^2+a^2)} - \frac{x}{2(x^2+a^2)^2} - \frac{1}{4a^3}\tan^{-1}\frac{x}{a} + c$

17. (i) $\frac{1}{2}\left(\log 2 - \frac{1}{2}\right)$ (ii) $\frac{5}{12} - \frac{1}{2}\log 2$ **20.** $-\frac{2}{3}\left[\operatorname{cosec}^2\frac{\theta}{2}\cot\frac{\theta}{2} + 2\cot\frac{\theta}{2}\right]$

25. (i) $\frac{2}{27} - \frac{\pi^2}{12}$ (ii) $\frac{2\pi}{3}$ (iii) $\frac{5}{16}\pi^4 - 15\pi^2 + 120$ (iv) $-\frac{4}{9}$

□□□□□□

Chapter

17 Multiple Integrals

17.1 INTRODUCTION

Double integral is an extension of a definite integral in two-dimensional space.

Let (x, y) be a single valued function of x and y, bounded and defined in the region R of XY-plane, and A be the area of region R and let R be divided in any manner into n-sub regions $\alpha_1, \alpha_2, \ldots, \alpha_n$, whose areas are $\delta s_1, \delta s_2, \ldots \delta s_n$ respectively. Suppose $P_r(\xi_r, \eta_r)$ is any point inside the given region.

Let $B_n = \sum_{r=1}^{n} f(\xi_r, \eta_r)\delta s_r$ then the limits of B_n which is assumed to exists as $n \to \infty$ such that every $\alpha_r \to 0$ in all its dimensions is known as double integral of $f(x, y)$ over the region R and is denoted by

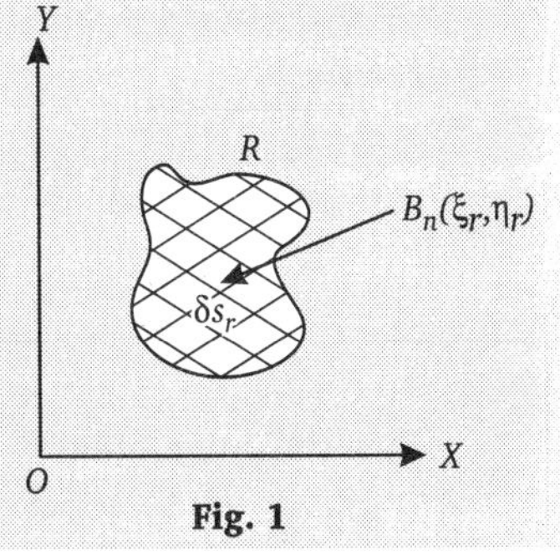

Fig. 1

$$\iint f(x,y)ds \quad \text{or} \quad \iint_R f(x,y)dx\,dy.$$

Hence, the area R is called the region or field of integration for the double integral and ds is called element of area.

- Let the region A be divided into the rectangular partitions and dx be the length of a sub-rectangular and dy be its width, so that the $dx\,dy$ is an element of area in cartesian co-ordinates, then the integral $\iint f(x,y)\,ds$ is written as $\iint_A f(x,y)dx\,dy$ and is called the double integral of $f(x, y)$ over the region R.

17.2 PROPERTIES OF DOUBLE INTEGRAL

(1) When the region R is partitioned into two parts say R_1 and R_2 then

$$\iint_R f(x,y)dx\,dy = \iint_{R_1} f(x,y)dx\,dy + \iint_{R_2} f(x,y)dx\,dy$$

Similarly, we divide the region into three or more parts.

(2) The double integral of a algebraic sum of a fixed number of functions is equal to the algebraic sum of double integrals taken for each term separately. Thus

$$\iint_R [f_1,(x,y) + f_2(x,y) + f_3(x,y) + \ldots]dx\,dy$$
$$= \iint_R f_1(x,y)dx\,dy + \iint_R f_2(x,y)dx\,dy + \iint_R f_3(x,y)dx\,dy + \ldots$$

(3) A constant factor may be taken outside the integral sign. Thus

$$\iint_R mf(x,y)dx\,dy = m\iint_R f(x,y)dx\,dy \text{ where } m \text{ is a constant.}$$

17.3 EVALUATION OF DOUBLE INTEGRALS

(i) *Over a rectangular region R.* If the region R be given by the inequalities $a \le x \le b$, $c \le y \le d$, then the double integral

$$\iint_R f(x,y)dx\,dy = \int_a^b \int_c^d f(x,y)dx\,dy$$

$$= \int_a^b \left[\int_c^d f(x,y)dy\right]dx \cdot \qquad ...(1)$$

We first evaluate $\int_c^d f(x,y)dy$ i.e., integrate f(x, y) with respect to y regarding x as constant and then resulting function of x is to be integrated with respect to x between the limits a and b

or $$\iint_R f(x,y)dx\,dy = \int_c^d \int_a^b f(x,y)\,dx\,dy$$

$$= \int_c^d \left[\int_a^b f(x,y)dx\right]dy \cdot \qquad ...(2)$$

Now, we integrate $\int_a^b f(x,y)dx$ first and then integrate with respect to y.

(ii) *Over the regions which are not rectangular.* Let the region R be described by $a \le x \le b$ and $\phi_1(x) \le y \le \phi_2(x)$ so that $y = \phi_1(x)$ and $y = \phi_2(x)$ respectively, the boundary of R then

$$\iint_R f(x,y)dx\,dy = \int_a^b \left[\int_{\phi_1(x)}^{\phi_2(x)} f(x,y)dy\right]dx$$

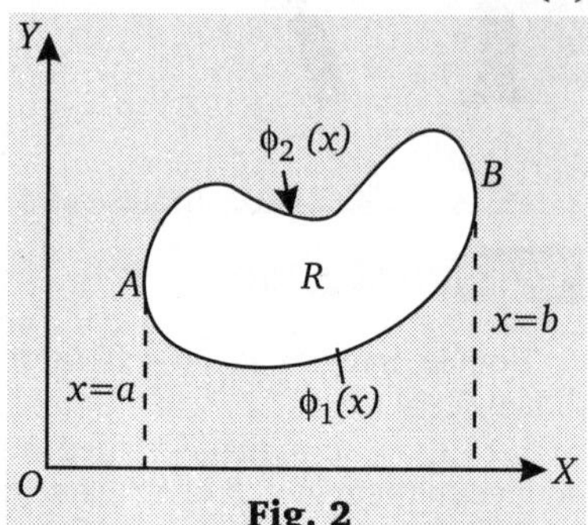

Fig. 2

Here, the inner integral $\int_{\phi_1(x)}^{\phi_2(x)} f(x,y)dy$ is integrated first and in this integral the result of integration is a function of x, say $\phi_1(x)$. Then $\phi_1(x)$ is integrated with respect to x between the limits a and b to obtain the value of double integral.

Fig. 3

In a similar way, if R can be described by

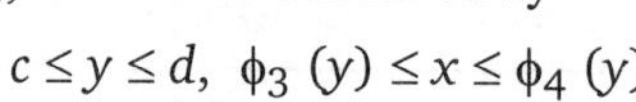

$$c \le y \le d, \;\; \phi_3(y) \le x \le \phi_4(y)$$

then we get

$$\iint_R f(x,y)dx\,dy = \int_c^d \left[\int_{\phi_3(y)}^{\phi_4(y)} f(x,y)dx\right]dy\,.$$

Here, the result of integration

$$\int_{\phi_3(y)}^{\phi_4(y)} f(x,y)dx\,.$$

which is evaluated first, is a function of y say $\phi_2(y)$, then $\phi_2(y)$ is integrated with respect to y between the limits c to d.

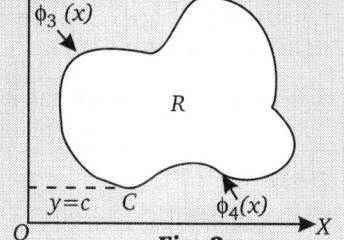

WORKING PROCEDURE

- While evaluating double integrals, first integrate with respect to variable having variable limits and treating the other variable as constant and then integrate with respect to variable with constant limits.

17.3.1 CONVERSION OF CARTESIAN TO POLAR CO-ORDINATES

The transformation formula required is $x = r\cos\theta$, $y = r\sin\theta$ and elementary area $\delta A = r\delta\theta.\,\delta r$ so that

$$\iint f(x,y)dx\;dy = \iint f(x,y)dA = \iint f(r,\theta)r\,d\theta\,dr.$$

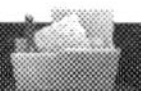

Solved Examples

1. *Evaluate* $\int_1^2 \int_0^{y/2} y\,dy\,dx$.

SOLUTION. We have

$$\int_1^2 \int_0^{y/2} y\,dy\,dx = \int_1^2 y(x)_0^{y/2} dy$$

$$= \int_1^2 y\left(\frac{1}{2}y\right)dy$$

$$= \frac{1}{2}\int_1^2 y^2 dy = \frac{1}{2}\left[\frac{1}{3}y^3\right]_1^2$$

$$= \frac{1}{6}(2^3 - 1^3) = 7/6.$$

2. *Evaluate* $\int_1^2 \int_0^x \frac{1}{x^2+y^2} dx\,dy$.

SOLUTION. We have

$$\int_1^2 \int_0^x \frac{dx\,dy}{x^2+y^2} = \int_1^2\left[\int_0^x \frac{dy}{x^2+y^2}\right]dx$$

$$= \int_1^2\left[\frac{1}{x}\tan^{-1}\frac{y}{x}\right]_{y=0}^{x} dx$$

$$= \int_1^2\left[\frac{1}{x}(\tan^{-1}1 - \tan^{-1}0)\right]dx$$

$$= \frac{\pi}{4}\int_1^2 \frac{dx}{x} = \frac{\pi}{4}[\log x]_1^2$$

$$= \frac{\pi}{4}.[\log 2 - \log 1] = \frac{1}{4}\pi \log 2.$$

3. *Show that*

$$\int_1^2 \int_0^{y/2} y\,dy\,dx = \int_1^2 \int_0^{x/2} x\,dx\,dy.$$

SOLUTION. We have

$$\int_1^2 \int_0^{y/2} y\,dy\,dx = \int_1^2 [y]\left[\int_0^{y/2} dx\right]dy$$

$$= \int_1^2 y[x]_0^{y/2} dy = \int_1^2 y[y/2 - 0]dy$$

$$= \frac{1}{2}\int_1^2 y^2 dy = \frac{1}{2}\left[\frac{y^3}{3}\right]_1^2 = \frac{7}{6}.$$

Again

$$\int_1^2 \int_0^{x/2} x\,dx\,dy = \int_1^2 x\left[\int_0^{x/2} dy\right]dx$$

$$= \int_1^2 x[y]_0^{x/2} dx$$

$$= \int_1^2 x\left[\frac{x}{2} - 0\right]dx = \frac{1}{2}\int_1^2 x^2 dx$$

$$= \frac{1}{2}\left[\frac{x^3}{3}\right]_1^2 = \frac{1}{6}(8-1) = \frac{7}{6}$$

Hence, $\int_1^2 \int_0^{y/2} y\,dy\,dx = \int_1^2 \int_0^{x/2} x\,dx\,dy$

4. *Evaluate the double integral of x^2y^3 over the rectangle bounded by $x = 2$, $x = 3$, $y = 2$, $y = 4$.*

SOLUTION. The required integral

$$= \int_2^3 \int_2^4 x^2 y^3 dx\,dy = \int_2^3 \left[\frac{1}{4}y^4\right]_2^4 x^2 dx$$

$$= \frac{1}{4}(4^4 - 2^4)\int_2^3 x^2 dx$$

$$= 60\left[\frac{1}{3}x^3\right]_2^3 = 20[27-8] = 380.$$

5. *Evaluate* $\int_0^3 \int_1^2 xy(1+x+y)\,dx\,dy$

SOLUTION. We have $\int_0^3 \int_1^2 xy(1+x+y)\,dx\,dy$

$$= \int_0^3 \left[x\frac{y^2}{2} + x^2\frac{y^2}{2} + x\frac{y^3}{3}\right]_{y=1}^2 dx$$

$$= \int_0^3 \left[\frac{x}{2}(4-1) + \frac{x^2}{2}(4-1) + \frac{x}{3}(8-1)\right]dx$$

$$= \int_0^3 \left[\left(\frac{3}{2} + \frac{7}{3}\right)x + \frac{3}{2}x^2\right]dx$$

$$= \left[\frac{23}{6}.\frac{x^2}{2} + \frac{3}{2}.\frac{x^2}{3}\right]_0^3$$

$$= \frac{23}{6}.\frac{9}{2} + \frac{27}{2} = \frac{123}{4}.$$

6. *Evaluate* $\iint_A (x^2+y^2)\,dx\,dy$, *where A is the region bounded by x=0, y=0, x+y=1.*

SOLUTION. Let R be the region of integration $x+y=1$ and the limit of itegration can be expressed as $0 \le x \le 1, 0 < y < 1 - x$.

From the equation $x + y = 1$, we have $x = 1$ for $y = 0$ and for the positive quadrant x varies from 0 to 1 and for y which varies from $y = 0$ to $y = 1 - x$. First integrate with respect to y, treated x as constant and then integrate with respect to 'x'.

Hence, the integral

$$= \int_0^1 \int_0^{1-x} (x^2 + y^2) dx\, dy$$

$$= \int_0^1 \left(x^2 y + \frac{1}{3} y^3 \right)_0^{1-x} dx$$

$$= \int_0^1 \left[x^2(1-x) + \frac{1}{3}(1-x)^3 \right] dx$$

$$= \int_0^1 (1-x) \left\{ x^2 + \frac{1}{3}(1-x)^2 \right\} dx$$

$$= \int_0^1 \frac{1}{3}[1 - 3x + 6x^2 - 4x^3] dx$$

$$= \frac{1}{3}\left[x - \frac{3}{2}x^2 + 2x^3 - x^4 \right]_0^1$$

$$= \frac{1}{3}\left[1 - \frac{3}{2} + 2 - 1 \right] = \frac{1}{6}$$

7. *Find the area of the region bounded by circle $x^2+y^2=a^2$.*

SOLUTION. The area of a small element at any point (x, y) is $dx\, dy$. Now to find the area bounded by the circle $x^2 + y^2 = a^2$, the region of integration R can be expressed as

$$-a \le y \le a, -\sqrt{a^2-y^2} \le x \le \sqrt{(a^2-y^2)}.$$

Now, first integration is to be performed w.r. to x regarding y as constant.

$\therefore$ The required area

$$= \iint_R dx\, dy = \int_{y=-a}^{a} \int_{x=-\sqrt{(a^2-y^2)}}^{\sqrt{(a^2-y^2)}} 1.dy\, dx$$

$$= \int_{-a}^{a} \left[2\int_0^{\sqrt{(a^2-y^2)}} 1.dx \right] dy,$$

by property of definite integral

$$= 2\int_{-a}^{a} [x]_0^{\sqrt{(a^2-y^2)}} dy = 2\int_{-a}^{a} \sqrt{(a^2-y^2)} dy$$

$$= 2.2\int_0^a \sqrt{(a^2-y^2)} dy$$

$$= 4\left[\frac{y\sqrt{(a^2-y^2)}}{2} + \frac{a^2}{2}\sin^{-1}\frac{y}{a} \right]_0^a$$

$$= 4\left[0 + \frac{a^2}{2}\sin^{-1} 1 \right] = \pi a^2.$$

8. *Evaluate $\iint (x+y)^2 dx\, dy$ over the region bounded by ellipse $\frac{x^2}{a^2} + \frac{y^2}{b^2} = 1.$ Hence find the mass of an elliptic plate whose density per unit area is given by $\rho = k(x+y)^2$.* (UKTU–2011)

SOLUTION. Since the region is bounded by ellipse $\frac{x^2}{a^2} + \frac{y^2}{b^2} = 1.$, we expressed it as:

$x = -a$ and $x = a$

$y = -b\sqrt{(1 - x^2/a^2)},$

$y = b\sqrt{(1 - x^2/a^2)}.$

$$\therefore \iint (x+y)^2 dx\, dy$$

$$= \int_{-a}^{a} \int_{-b\sqrt{(1-x^2/a^2)}}^{b\sqrt{(1-x^2/a^2)}} (x^2 + y^2 + 2xy) dx\, dy$$

$$= \int_{-a}^{a} 2\int_0^{b\sqrt{(1-x^2/a^2)}} (x^2 + y^2) dx\, dy$$

[$\because$ $2xy$ being an odd function of f, its integration under the given limits of y is 0]

$$= 2\int_{-a}^{a} \left[x^2 y + \frac{y^3}{3} \right]_0^{b\sqrt{1-x^2/a^2}} dx$$

$$= 2\int_{-a}^{a} \left\{ x^2 b\sqrt{\left(1 - \frac{x^2}{a^2}\right)} + \frac{b^3}{3}\left(1 - \frac{x^2}{a^2}\right)^{3/2} \right\} dx$$

$$= 2 \times 2\int_0^a \left\{ x^2 b\sqrt{\left(1 - \frac{x^2}{a^2}\right)} + \frac{b^3}{3}\left(1 - \frac{x^2}{a^2}\right)^{3/2} \right\} dx$$

$$= 4b\int_0^{\pi/2} \left\{ \begin{matrix} a^2 \sin^2\theta \cos\theta \\ + \frac{b^2}{3}\cos^3\theta \end{matrix} \right\} a\cos\theta\, d\theta$$

(By putting $x = a\sin\theta$ so that $dx = a\cos\theta\, d\theta$)

$$= 4ab\int_0^{\pi/2} \left[\begin{matrix} a^2 \sin^2\theta \cos^2\theta \\ + \frac{b^2}{3}\cos^4\theta \end{matrix} \right] d\theta$$

$$= 4ab \left[\begin{matrix} a^2 \int_0^{\pi/2} \sin^2\theta \cos^2\theta\, d\theta \\ + \frac{b^2}{3}\int_0^{\pi/2} \cos^4\theta\, d\theta \end{matrix} \right]$$

$$= 4ab\left[\frac{1}{16}\pi a^2 + \frac{1}{16}\pi b^2 \right]$$

$$= \frac{1}{4}\pi ab(a^2 + b^2)$$

The mass of elliptic plate whose density is given by $\rho = k(x+y)^2$

$$= \iint_A k(x+y)^2 dx\, dy$$

(where integration is to be performed over the area A of ellipse.)

$$= k.\frac{1}{4}\pi ab(a^2 + b^2)$$

9. *Evaluate* $\iint xy(x+y)\,dx\,dy$ *over the region between* $y = x^2$ *and* $y = x$.

SOLUTION. When we draw the given curve, the parabola $y = x^2$ and line $y = x$ intersect at the point (0, 0) and (1, 1) ,

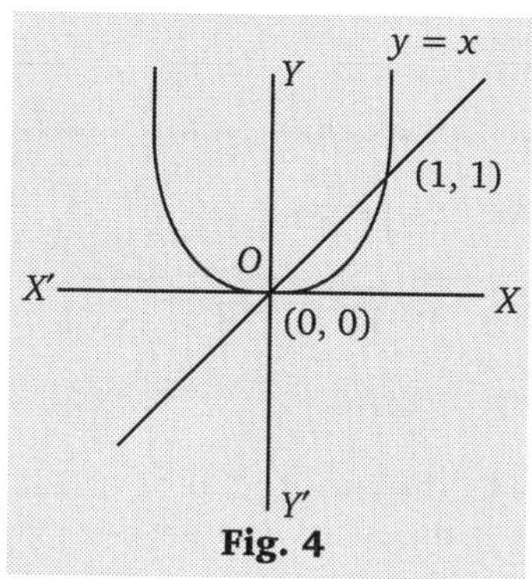

Fig. 4

Here $x^2 = x$ or $x(x-1) = 0$ *i.e.*, $x=0$ or 1, when $x=0, y = 0$, and $x=1, y=1$]. So the area of integration for x is from $x=0$ to $x = 1$ and for y from x^2 to x.

$\therefore$ Given integral

$$= \int_0^1 \int_{x^2}^x xy(x+y)\,dx\,dy$$

$$= \int_0^1 \int_{x^2}^x x(yx+y^2)\,dx\,dy$$

$$= \int_0^1 x\left[x.\frac{y^2}{2}+\frac{1}{3}y^3\right]_{x^2}^x dx$$

$$= \int_0^1 x.\left[\left(x.\frac{x^2}{2}+\frac{1}{3}x^3\right)-\left(x.\frac{x^4}{2}+\frac{1}{3}x^6\right)\right]$$

$$= \int_0^1 x\left[\frac{5x^3}{6}-\frac{1}{2}x^5-\frac{1}{3}x^6\right]dx$$

$$= \int_0^1\left[\frac{5}{6}x^4-\frac{1}{2}x^6-\frac{1}{3}x^7\right]dx$$

$$= \left[\frac{1}{6}x^5-\frac{1}{14}x^7-\frac{1}{24}x^8\right]_0^1$$

$$= \frac{1}{6}-\frac{1}{14}-\frac{1}{24}=\frac{3}{56}$$

Exercise-17.1

1. Evaluate $\int_2^3 dx \int_0^1 (x^2+3y^2)dy$.
2. Evaluate $\int_0^2 \int_0^{\sqrt{4+x^2}} \frac{dx\,dy}{(4+x^2+y^2)}$.
3. Evaluate $\int_0^{\pi/2} \int_{\pi/2}^{\pi} \cos(x+y)dx\,dy$.
4. Evaluate $\int_0^2 \int_0^{\sqrt{2x-x^2}} x\,dx\,dy$. (SRM-2010)
5. Evaluate $\int_0^1 \int_0^{x^2} e^{y/x}\,dx\,dy$.
6. Evaluate $\int_0^1 \int_0^1 \frac{dx\,dy}{\sqrt{(1-x^2)(1-y^2)}}$ (UPTU (AG)-2006)
7. Evaluate $\iint e^{2x+3y}dx\,dy$ over the triangle bounded by $x = 0, y = 0$ and $x + y = 1$.
8. Evaluate $\iint_p x\sin(x+y)dx\,dy$, where p is a rectangle $[0 \le x \le \pi, 0 \le y \le \pi/2]$.
9. Show that

   $$\int_1^2 \int_3^4 (xy+e^y)dx\,dy = \int_3^4 \int_1^2 (xy+e^y)dy\,dx.$$
10. Evaluate $\iint x^2y^2 dx\,dy$ over the region bounded by $x = 0$, $y = 0$, where A is the region bounded by $x^2+y^2=1$.
11. Find the area of the ellipse $\frac{x^2}{a^2}+\frac{y^2}{b^2}=1$ by double integration.
12. Show by double integration that the area between the parabolas $y^2 = 4ax$ and $x^2 = 4by$ is $(16/3)\,ab$.
13. Find by double integration the region included between the parabola $x^2 = 4ay$ and the curve $y = 8a^3/(x^2+4a^2)$.
14. Evaluate $\iint y\,dx\,dy$ over the region between the parabolas $y^2 = 4x$ and $x^2 = 4y$.
15. Find the double integration the region lying between the parabola $y = 4x - x^2$, and the line $y = x$.
16. Find by double integration the area of the region lying between the parabola $y^2=4ax$, and line $y=mx$.
17. Find by double integration the area of the region lying between the semi-cubical parbola $y^2 = x^3$, and line $y=mx$.
18. Find by double integration the area of the region lying between the circle $x^2+y^2=a^2$, and line $x+y=a$ (in first quadrant)
19. Find by double integration the area of the region lying between the curves $(x^2+4a^2)y = 8a^3$, $2y = x$ and $x = 0$.

20. Evaluate

(i) $\int_0^1\int_0^{\sqrt{1+x^2}} \frac{dx\,dy}{1+x^2+y^2}$

(ii) $\int_0^a\int_0^{\sqrt{a^2+y^2}} (a^2-x^2-y^2)dx\,dy$

21. (i) Evaluate $\iint_R\left(1-\frac{x^2}{a^2}+\frac{y^2}{b^2}\right)dx\,dy$ over the first quadrant of the ellipse $\frac{x^2}{a^2}+\frac{y^2}{b^2}=1$.

(ii) Evaluate $\iint xy\,dx\,dy$ where A is the domain bounded by x-axis, ordinate $x = 2a$ and the curve $x^2=4ay$.

Hints to the Selected Problems

5. $I=\int_0^1\int_0^{x^2} e^{y/x}dx\,dy=\int_0^1 x[e^{y/x}]_{y=0}^{x^2}dx$

$=\int_0^1 x(e^x-1)dx=\int_0^1 xe^x dx-\int_0^1 x\,dx$

$=\left(xe^x\right)_0^1-\left[e^x\right]_0^1-\left(\frac{x^2}{2}\right)_0^1$

$=(e-0)-(e-1)-\frac{1}{2}=\frac{1}{2}$

10. $I=\iint_A x^2y^2dx\,dy=\int_0^1\int_0^{\sqrt{1-x^2}} x^2y^2dx\,dy$

$=\int_0^1 x^2\left[\frac{y^3}{3}\right]_0^{\sqrt{1-x^2}} dx=\frac{1}{3}\int_0^1 x^2(1-x^2)^{3/2}dx$

Now put $x^2 = t$.

11. $I=\iint_A dx\,dy=\int_{-a}^{a}\int_{-b/a\sqrt{a^2-x^2}}^{b/a\sqrt{a^2-x^2}} dx\,dy$

12. $A=\int_0^{4a^{1/3}b^{2/3}}\int_{x^2/4b}^{\sqrt{4ax}} dx\,dy$.

13. $A=\int_{-2a}^{2a}\int_{x^2/4a}^{8a^3/x^2+4a^2} dx\,dy$.

14. The curves $y^2 = 4a$ and $x^2 = 4y$ intersect at the points where $x = 0$ and $x = 4$. Also, when

$$0<x<4, \sqrt{4x}>\frac{x^2}{4}.$$

$\therefore \quad I=\int_0^4\int_{x^2/4}^{\sqrt{4x}} y\,dx\,dy.$

16. Since, the two corners cut at the point where $x = 0$ and $x=\frac{4a}{m^2}$

$\therefore\ I=\int_0^{4a/m^2}\int_{mx}^{\sqrt{4ax}} dx\,dy$

ANSWERS

1. $\frac{22}{3}$ **2.** $\frac{\pi}{4}\log(1+\sqrt{2})$ **3.** -2 **4.** $\frac{\pi}{2}$ **5.** $\frac{1}{2}$ **6.** $\frac{\pi^2}{4}$

7. $\frac{1}{6}(e-1)^2(2e+1)$ **8.** $\pi+2$ **9.** $\frac{21}{4}+e^4-e^3$ **10.** $\pi/96$ **11.** πab **13.** $\left(2\pi-\frac{4}{3}\right)a^2$

14. 48/5 **15.** 9/2 **16.** $8a^2/3m^2$ **17.** $1/10\,m^5$ **18.** $\frac{1}{4}(\pi-2)a^2$

19. $(\pi-1)a^2$ **20.**(i) $\frac{\pi}{4}\log(1+\sqrt{2})$ (ii) $\frac{\pi a^4}{8}$ **21.** (i) $\frac{\pi ab}{4}$ (ii) $\frac{a^4}{3}$.

17.4 DOUBLE INTEGRAL IN POLAR CO-ORDINATES

Let us consider a function $f(r, \theta)$ of polar co-ordinates (r, θ) over a certain area A with whose boundary is also given in terms of polar co-ordinates. We divide the area into n parts of elementary areas $\delta A_1, \delta A_2, \delta A_3, \ldots \delta A_n$ and let

$$s_n=\sum_{r=1}^{n} f(r,\theta)\delta A$$

where (r_1, θ_1) is a point inside the elementary area δA_1, the dobule integral of $f(r, \theta)$ is then defined as

$$\iint_A f(r,\theta)dA=\lim_{\substack{n\to\infty\\ \delta A_i\to 0}}\sum_{i=1}^{n} f(r_i,\theta_i)\delta A_i,$$

provided limit toward right hand side exists.

- In case of cartesian co-ordinates when the double integral $\iint_A f(x,y)dA$ is expressed in the form of repeated integral, dA represents the area of the rectangle with sides dx and dy and hence $dA = dx\, dy$.

If the radius vector of OS and OP are r and $r + \delta r$ respectively and

$$\angle POQ = d\theta \Rightarrow RS = rd\theta$$

as RS and PQ are arcs of circles. Then

$$dA = RS \times SP = r\,d\theta.\,dr = r\,dr\,d\theta$$

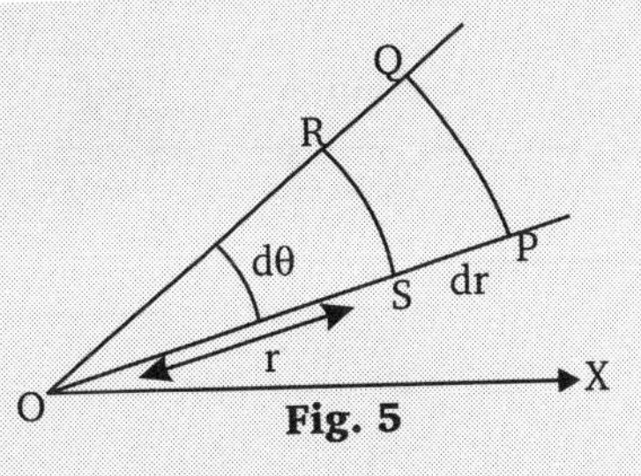

Fig. 5

Solved Examples

1. *Evaluate the double integral*
$$\int_0^{\pi/2}\int_0^{2a\cos\theta} r^2 \sin\theta.\cos\theta.d\theta\,dr.$$

SOLUTION. We have

$$\int_0^{\pi/2}\int_0^{2a\cos\theta} r^2 \sin\theta.\cos\theta.d\theta\,dr$$
$$= \int_0^{\pi/2}\int_0^{2a\cos\theta} (r^2 \sin\theta.\cos\theta)\,dr\,d\theta$$
$$= \int_0^{\pi/2}\left[\frac{r^3}{3}.\sin\theta.\cos\theta\right]_0^{2a\cos\theta} d\theta$$
$$= \frac{1}{3}\int_0^{\pi/2}(2a\cos\theta)^3.\sin\theta.\cos\theta\,d\theta$$
$$= \frac{8a^3}{3}\int_0^{\pi/2}\sin\theta.\cos^4\theta\,d\theta$$
$$= -\frac{8a^3}{3}\int_0^{\pi/2}\cos^4\theta\,d(\cos\theta)$$
$$= -\frac{8a^3}{3}\left[\frac{\cos^5\theta}{5}\right]_0^{\pi/2}$$
$$= -\frac{8a^3}{3}\left[0-\frac{1}{5}\right] = \frac{8a^3}{15}.$$

2. *Evaluate* $\iint \frac{r\,d\theta\,dr}{\sqrt{a^2+r^2}}$ *over one loop of the lemniscate* $r^2 = a^2\cos 2\theta$.

SOLUTION. In lemniscate, there are two loops. We see that when $-\pi/4 < \theta < \pi/4$ or $3\pi/4 < \theta < 5\pi/4$, where r is real. We want to evaluate the given integral over the right loop of the leminscate. [Fig. (6)]

Therefore, $\iint \frac{r\,d\theta\,dr}{\sqrt{a^2+r^2}}$
$$= \int_{-\pi/4}^{\pi/4}\int_{-a\sqrt{\cos 2\theta}}^{a\sqrt{\cos 2\theta}} \frac{r}{\sqrt{r^2+a^2}}\,dr\,d\theta$$

as $r^2 = a^2\cos 2\theta$. $\therefore\ r = \pm a\sqrt{\cos 2\theta}$

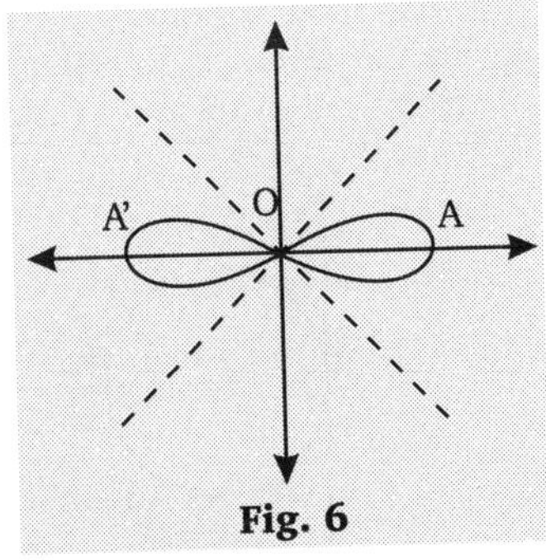

Fig. 6

Thus, r varies from
$$-a\sqrt{\cos 2\theta} \text{ to } a\sqrt{\cos 2\theta}.$$
Since, there is a symmetry about X-axis, we should evaluate the double integral over half of the right loop as follows:

$$\iint \frac{r\,d\theta\,dr}{\sqrt{a^2+r^2}}$$
$$= \int_0^{\pi/4}\int_0^{a\sqrt{\cos 2\theta}} \frac{r}{\sqrt{a^2+r^2}}\,dr\,d\theta$$
$$= \frac{1}{2}\int_0^{\pi/4}\int_0^{a\sqrt{\cos 2\theta}} \frac{2r}{\sqrt{a^2+r^2}}\,dr\,d\theta$$
$$= \frac{1}{2}\int_0^{\pi/4}\int_0^{a\sqrt{\cos 2\theta}} \frac{d(a^2+r^2)}{\sqrt{a^2+r^2}}\,d\theta$$
$$= \frac{1}{2}\int_0^{\pi/4}\left[2\sqrt{a^2+r^2}\right]_0^{a\sqrt{\cos 2\theta}} d\theta$$
$$= \int_0^{\pi/4}\left[\sqrt{a^2+a^2\cos 2\theta} - \sqrt{a^2+0}\right]d\theta$$
$$= \int_0^{\pi/4}[\sqrt{2}.a\cos\theta - a]\,d\theta$$

$$= \sqrt{2}.a\int_0^{\pi/4}\cos\theta\,d\theta - a\int_0^{\pi/4}d\theta$$

$$= \sqrt{2}.a[\sin\theta]_0^{\pi/4} - a[\theta]_0^{\pi/4}$$

$$= \sqrt{2}.a.\frac{1}{\sqrt{2}} - a.\frac{\pi}{4} = a - \frac{a}{4}\pi$$

∴ Value of double integral over the complete right loop

$$= 2a - \frac{2a\pi}{4} = 2a(1-\pi/4).$$

- If we evaluate the double integral as $\int_{-\pi/4}^{\pi/4}\int_{-a\sqrt{\cos 2\theta}}^{a\sqrt{\cos 2\theta}}\frac{r}{\sqrt{a^2+r^2}}d\theta\,dr$, then it will become zero due to oddness of function $\frac{r}{\sqrt{a^2+r^2}}$ therefore we must not calculate the double integral over the complete loop.

3. *Evaluate $\iint r^2 d\theta\,dr$ over the area of circle $r = a\cos\theta$.*

SOLUTION. In the given region of circle, θ varies from $-\pi/2$ to $\pi/2$ and r varies from 0 to a.

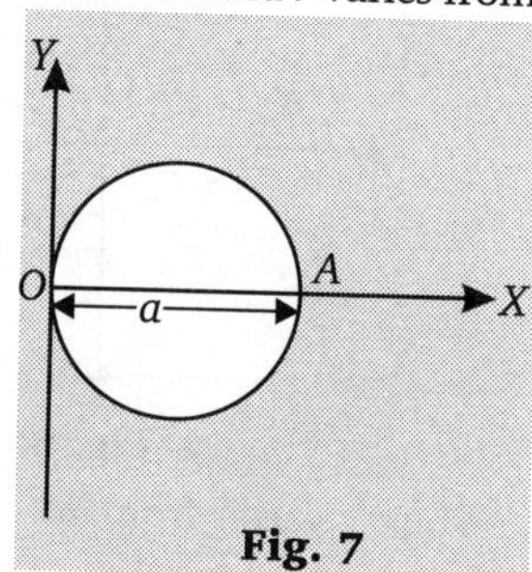

Fig. 7

$$\therefore \iint r^2 d\theta\,dr = \int_{-\pi/2}^{\pi/2}\int_0^{a\cos\theta} r^2 d\theta\,dr$$

$$= \int_{-\pi/2}^{\pi/2}\left[\frac{r^3}{3}\right]_0^{a\cos\theta} d\theta$$

$$= \frac{a^3}{3}\int_{-\pi/2}^{\pi/2}\cos^3\theta\,d\theta$$

$$= \frac{a^3}{3}\int_{-\pi/2}^{\pi/2}\left(\frac{3}{4}\cos\theta + \frac{1}{4}\cos 3\theta\right)d\theta$$

$$= \frac{a^3}{3}\times\frac{3}{4}\int_{-\pi/2}^{\pi/2}[\cos\theta\,d\theta] + \frac{a^3}{12}\int_{-\pi/2}^{\pi/2}\cos 3\theta\,d\theta$$

$$= \frac{a^3}{4}[\sin\theta]_{-\pi/2}^{\pi/2} + \frac{a^3}{12}\left[\frac{\sin 3\theta}{3}\right]_{-\pi/2}^{\pi/2}$$

$$= \frac{a^3}{4}.2 + \frac{a^3}{12}\times\frac{1}{3}\left[\sin\frac{3\pi}{2} + \sin\frac{3\pi}{2}\right]$$

$$= \frac{a^3}{2} - \frac{a^3}{18} = \frac{4}{9}a^3.$$

4. *Evaluate $\int_0^{\pi}\int_0^{a(1+\cos\theta)} r^2\cos\theta\,d\theta\,dr$.*

SOLUTION. We have $\int_0^{\pi}\int_0^{a(1+\cos\theta)} r^2\cos\theta\,d\theta\,dr$

$$= \int_0^{\pi}\cos\theta\left[\frac{r^3}{3}\right]_0^{a(1+\cos\theta)} d\theta$$

$$= \frac{1}{3}\int_0^{\pi}\cos\theta.a^3(1+\cos\theta)^3 d\theta$$

$$= \frac{a^3}{3}\int_0^{\pi}\cos\theta(1+3\cos\theta+3\cos^2\theta + \cos^3\theta)d\theta$$

$$= \frac{a^3}{3}\int_0^{\pi}[\cos\theta+3\cos^2\theta+3\cos^3\theta + \cos^4\theta)d\theta$$

$$= 2.\frac{a^3}{3}\int_0^{\pi/2}[3\cos^2\theta+\cos^4\theta]d\theta$$

$$\left[\because \int_0^{\pi}\cos^n\theta\,d\theta = 0, \text{since } n \text{ is odd}\right]$$

$$= \frac{2a^3}{3}\left[3.\frac{1}{2}.\frac{\pi}{2} + \frac{3}{4}.\frac{1}{2}.\frac{\pi}{2}\right]$$

$$= \frac{2a^3}{3}.\frac{3\pi}{4}\left[1+\frac{1}{4}\right]$$

$$= \frac{2a^3}{3}.\frac{3\pi}{4}.\frac{5}{4} = \frac{5\pi a^3}{8}$$

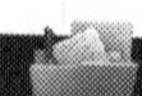

Similar Problem

(1) Evaluate $\int_0^{\pi/2}\int_0^{\sin\theta} r\,d\theta\,dr$. **Ans.** $\frac{\pi}{8}$

Exercise-17.2

1. Integrate r sinθ over the area of cardiod $r=a(1+\cos\theta)$ lying above the initial line.
2. Find by double integration that the area lying inside the cardiod $r= a(1+\cos\theta)$and outside the circle $r=a$.
3. Find by double integration the area lying inside the cardiod $r=1+\cos\theta$ and outside the parabola $r(1+\cos\theta)=1$.
4. Find by double integration the area lying inside the circle $r = a\sin\theta$ and outside the cardioid $r = a(1-\cos\theta)$.

ANSWERS

1. $\dfrac{4a^3}{3}$ 2. $\dfrac{1}{4}a^2(\pi+8)$ 3. $\dfrac{9\pi+16}{12}$ 4. $\dfrac{a^2}{4}(4-\pi)$.

17.5 APPLICATIONS OF DOUBLE INTEGRATION

Double integration is generally used to find the area of curves, volume and surface of solids of revolution.

(1) *Area of curves.* Let AD be an arc of the curve $y=f(x)$.

Let area $ABCD$ be divided into sub-area by drawing lines parallel to X and Y axis respectively such that distance between two adjoining lines drawn parallel to Y-axis be δx and those drawn parallel to X-axis be δy.

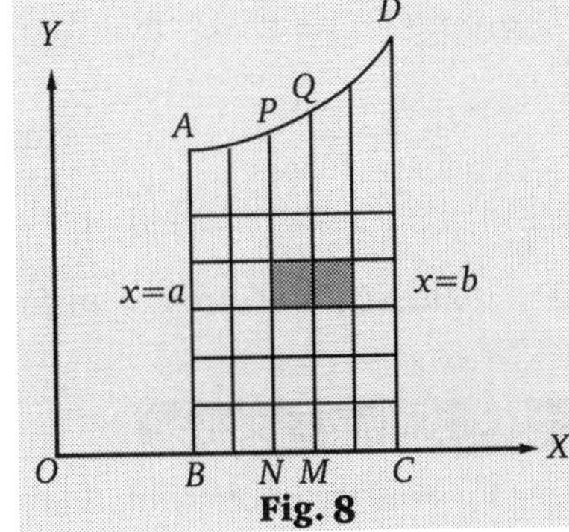

Fig. 8

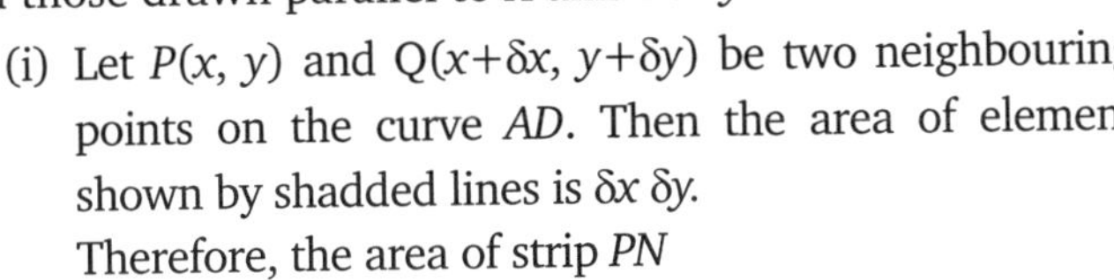

(i) Let $P(x, y)$ and $Q(x+\delta x, y+\delta y)$ be two neighbouring points on the curve AD. Then the area of element shown by shadded lines is $\delta x\,\delta y$.
Therefore, the area of strip PN

$$= \int_{y=0}^{f(x)} dx\,dy \text{ where } y = f(x).$$

The required area

$$ABCD = \int_{x=a}^{b}\int_{y=0}^{f(x)} dx\,dy\,.$$

(ii) We can find the area bounded by the two curves $y = f_1(x)$ and $y = f_2(x)$ and the ordinates $x=a$ and $x=b$

$$\int_{x=a}^{b}\int_{y=f_1(x)}^{f_2(x)} dx\,dy\,.$$

(iii) *In polar co-ordinates.* The area bounded by curve $r= f(\theta)$ where $f(\theta)$ is a single valued function of θ in the domain (α, β) and the radii vector $\theta=\alpha$ and $\theta=\beta$ is

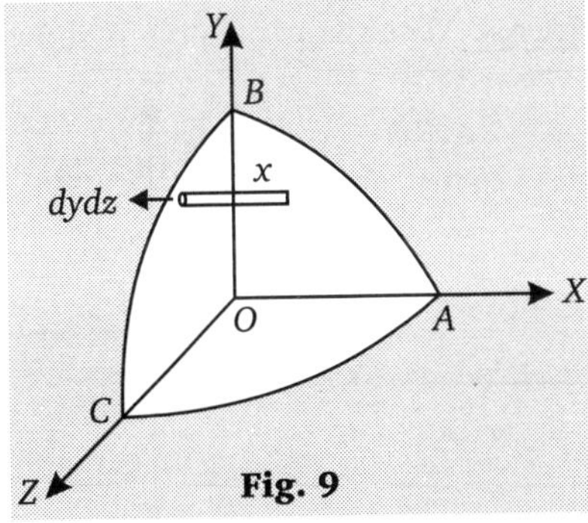

Fig. 9

$$\int_{\theta=\alpha}^{\beta}\int_{r=0}^{f(\theta)} r\,d\theta\,dr\,.$$

(2) *Volume of a solid.* Consider the area $dy\,dz$ on the plane $x=0$ through each point on the boundary of this small area. Draw the lines parallel to X-axis. This cylinder cuts the given surface, and volume of this cylinder

$$= x\,dy\,dz\,.$$

$\therefore$ Volume of solid $= \iint x\,dy\,dz\,.$

- By considering area $dx\,dy$ on plane $z=0$ the volume of solid $= \iint z\,dx\,dy$.
- By considering area $dx\,dz$ on plane $y=0$ the volume of solid $= \iint y\,dx\,dz$.

(3) *Area of surface of a solid.* Let the equation of surface be $z= f(x, y)$. Consider a point $P(x, y, z)$ on this surface surrounding this point P. Consider an element of area δs of the surface. Let $\delta x\ \delta y$ be the projection of this area δs on the plane $z = 0$, then we have

$$\delta x\ \delta y = \delta s \cos \alpha \quad \text{... (1)}$$

where α is the angle between the tangent plane to the given surface at $P(x, y, z)$ and the plane $z = 0$, then by co-ordinate geometry, we have

$$\sec\alpha = \sqrt{\left[1+\left\{\frac{\partial z}{\partial x}\right\}^2+\left\{\frac{\partial z}{\partial y}\right\}^2\right]} \quad \text{...(2)}$$

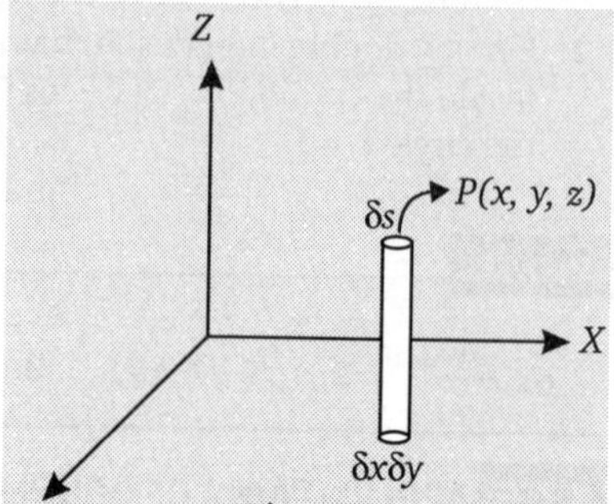

Fig. 10

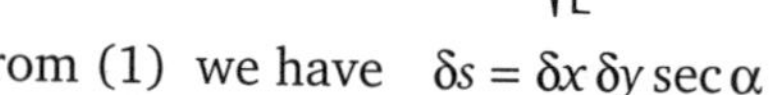

From (1) we have $\delta s = \delta x\,\delta y \sec\alpha$

$$= \delta x \delta y \sqrt{\left[1+\left\{\frac{\partial z}{\partial x}\right\}^2+\left\{\frac{\partial z}{\partial y}\right\}^2\right]} \quad \text{[From (2)]}$$

$\therefore$ The required area of surface $= \iint \sqrt{\left[1+\left\{\frac{\partial z}{\partial x}\right\}^2+\left\{\frac{\partial z}{\partial y}\right\}^2\right]}\,dx\,dy$.

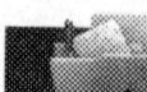

Solved Examples

1. *Find the whole area of curve*

$$a^2x^2 = y^3(2a-y).$$

SOLUTION. The shape of curve is shown in fig. 11.

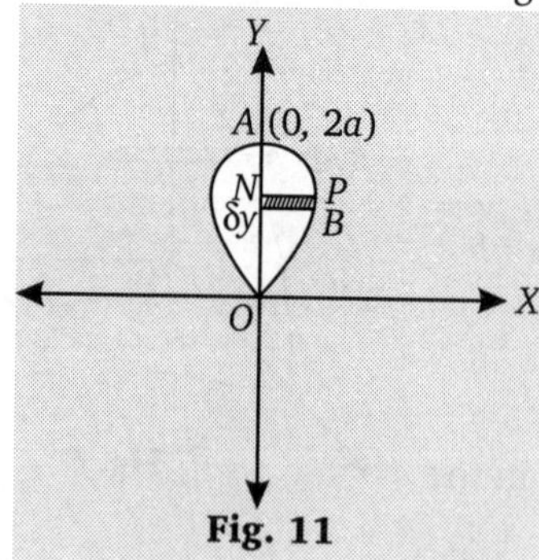

Fig. 11

The required area $= 2 \times \text{area}\, OAB$

$$= 2\int_{y=0}^{2a}\int_{x=0}^{f(y)} dy\,dx$$

where $x= f(y)$ *i.e.*, $x = y^{3/2}\dfrac{\sqrt{2a-y}}{a}$ is the equation of curve.

$\therefore$ The required area

$$= 2\int_{y=0}^{2a} [x]_0^{f(y)} dy$$

$$= 2\int_0^{2a} f(y)\,dy$$

$$= 2\int_0^{2a} \frac{y^{3/2}\sqrt{2a-y}}{a}\,dy$$

$$\left[\because f(y) = x = y^{3/2}\frac{\sqrt{2a-y}}{a}\right]$$

Put $\quad y = 2a\sin^2\theta$

$\Rightarrow \quad dy = 4a\sin\theta\cos\theta\,d\theta$

at $y = 0, \theta = 0$ and $y = 2a, \theta = \pi/2$

$\therefore$ Required area

$$= \frac{2}{a}\int_0^{\pi/2} (2a\sin^2\theta)^{3/2}\sqrt{(2a-2a\sin^2\theta)}\ 4a\sin\theta\cos\theta\,d\theta$$

$$= 32a^2\int_0^{\pi/2} \sin^4\theta\cos^2\theta\,d\theta$$

$$= \frac{32a^2\Gamma(5/2)\Gamma(3/2)}{2\Gamma 4}$$

$$= \frac{32a^2.(3/2).(1/2).\sqrt{\pi}.(1/2).\sqrt{\pi}}{2.3.2.1}$$

$$= \pi a^2.$$

2. *Find by double integration the area between* $y = \dfrac{3x}{(x^2+2)}$ *and* $4y = x^2$.

SOLUTION. We have $4y = x^2$, and $y = \dfrac{3x}{(x^2+2)}$

$$\Rightarrow \quad 4y = \frac{12x}{(x^2+2)}, \quad \text{and} \quad 4y = x^2$$

$$\Rightarrow \quad x^2 = \frac{12x}{(x^2+2)}$$

$$\Rightarrow \quad x^4 + 2x^2 - 12x = 0$$

$$\Rightarrow \quad x(x^3 + 2x - 12) = 0$$

$$x = 0, 2$$

$\therefore$ Required area

$$= \int_{x=0}^{2}\int_{y=x^2/4}^{3x/(x^2+2)} dx\,dy$$

$$= \int_0^2 [y]_{x^2/4}^{3x/(x^2+2)} dx$$

$$= \int_0^2 \left[\frac{3x}{x^2+2} - \frac{x^2}{4}\right] dx$$

$$= \frac{3}{2}\int_0^2 \frac{2x\,dx}{x^2+2} - \frac{1}{4}\int_0^2 x^2\,dx$$

$$= \frac{3}{2}\left[\log(x^2+2)\right]_0^2 - \frac{1}{4}\left(\frac{1}{3}x^3\right)_0^2$$

$$= \frac{3}{2}[\log(6) - \log(2)] - \frac{1}{12}(8-0)$$

$$= \frac{3}{2}\log 3 - \frac{2}{3}.$$

Similar Problem

(1) Find the area of curve $r = a(1 + \cos\theta)$. **Ans.** $(3/2)a^2\pi$

3. *Find the volume bounded by the cylinder* $x^2 + y^2 = 4$ *and the hyperboloid* $-x^2 - y^2 + z^2 = 1$.

SOLUTION. Here, surfaces $x^2 + y^2 = 4$ and $-x^2 - y^2 + z^2 = 1$ are symmetrical about all the three axes. Therefore, volume

$$V = \iint z\,dx\,dy$$

$$= 8\int_0^2\int_0^{\sqrt{4-x^2}} \sqrt{(x^2+y^2+1)}\,dx\,dy.$$

Change to polar co-ordinates and change the limits of integrations for the region of quadrant of circle $r = 2$ and $\theta = 0$ to $\pi/2$

$$V = 8\int_0^{\pi/2}\int_0^2 \sqrt{(r^2+1)}\,r\,d\theta\,dr$$

$$= 8\int_0^{\pi/2}\left[\frac{1}{3}(r^2+1)^{3/2}\right]_0^2 d\theta$$

$$= 8\int_0^{\pi/2}\frac{1}{3}(5\sqrt{5}-1)\,d\theta$$

$$= \frac{4\pi}{3}(5\sqrt{5}-1).$$

4. *Transform the integral*

$$\int_0^2\int_0^{\sqrt{2x-x^2}} \frac{x\,dx\,dy}{\sqrt{(x^2+y^2)}}$$

by changing into polar co-ordinates and hence evaluate it.

SOLUTION. We have the limit of integration be

$$y = 0, y = \sqrt{(2x - x^2)} \text{ and } x = 0, x = 2.$$

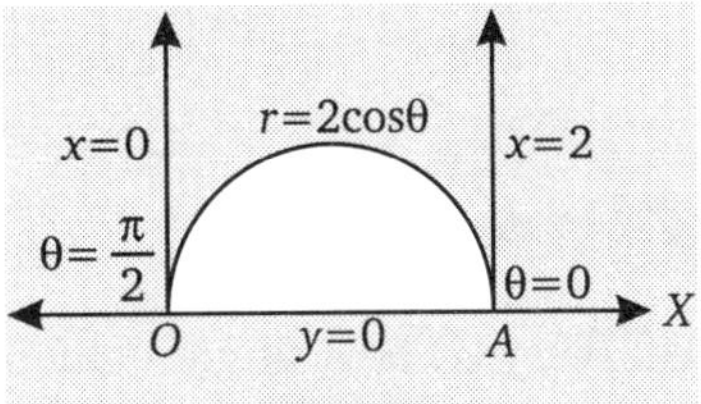

x=0
r=2cosθ
x=2
θ=π/2
θ=0
X
O
y=0
A

Fig. 12

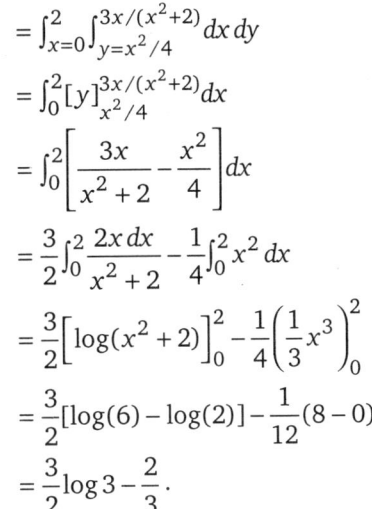

$x^2 + y^2 - 2x = 0$ which is change into

$$r^2(\cos^2\theta + \sin^2\theta) - 2r\cos\theta = 0$$

or $\quad r = 2\cos\theta$.

Now r varies from 0 to $2\cos\theta$ and θ varies from 0 to $\pi/2$.

Note that at the point A of the circle, $\theta = 0$ and at point O, $r = 0$ and so from $r = 2\cos\theta$, we get

$$\theta = \frac{\pi}{2} \text{ at } O$$

the polar equivalent of the elementary area $dx\,dy$ is $r\,d\theta\,dr$.

$$\therefore \iint_A f(x,y)\,dx\,dy$$

$$= \iint_A f(r\cos\theta, r\sin\theta)\,r\,d\theta\,dr$$

where A is the region of integration.

Therefore, transforming to polar co-ordinates, the given double integral

$$= \int_{\theta=0}^{\pi/2}\int_{r=0}^{2\cos\theta}\frac{r\cos\theta}{r}\, r\, d\theta\, dr$$

$$= \int_0^{\pi/2}\cos\theta\left[\frac{r^2}{2}\right]_0^{2\cos\theta} d\theta$$

$$= \int_0^{\pi/2}\frac{1}{2}\cos\theta . 4\cos^2\theta\, d\theta = 2\int_0^{\pi/2}\cos^3\theta d\theta$$

$$= 2.\frac{2}{3} = \frac{4}{3}.$$

5. *Find the area of the surface $z^2 = 2xy$ included between planes $x = 0$, $x = a$, $y = 0$, $y = b$.*

SOLUTION. The given surface is $z^2 = 2xy$.

$$\therefore \quad 2z\frac{\partial z}{\partial x} = 2y \text{ or } \frac{\partial z}{\partial x} = \frac{y}{z}$$

Similarly $\dfrac{\partial z}{\partial y} = \dfrac{x}{z}$

Then required area of the surface

$$= \iint \sqrt{\left[1 + \left(\frac{\partial z}{\partial x}\right)^2 + \left(\frac{\partial z}{\partial y}\right)^2\right]}\, dx\, dy$$

$$= \int_{x=0}^{a}\int_{y=0}^{b}\sqrt{\left\{1 + \left(\frac{y}{z}\right)^2 + \left(\frac{x}{z}\right)^2\right\}}\, dx\, dy$$

$$= \int_{x=0}^{a}\int_{y=0}^{b}\sqrt{\left(\frac{z^2 + y^2 + x^2}{2xy}\right)}\, dx\, dy$$

$$= \int_{x=0}^{a}\int_{y=0}^{b}\sqrt{\left(\frac{x^2 + y^2 + z^2}{2xy}\right)}\, dx\, dy$$

$$= \int_{x=0}^{a}\int_{y=0}^{b}\sqrt{\frac{x^2 + y^2 + z^2}{2xy}}\, dx\, dy$$

$$= \int_{x=0}^{a}\int_{y=0}^{b}\frac{(x+y)}{\sqrt{2}\sqrt{(xy)}}\, dx\, dy$$

$$= \frac{1}{\sqrt{2}}\int_{x=0}^{a}\int_{y=0}^{b}\left(\sqrt{x}\frac{1}{\sqrt{y}} + \sqrt{y}.\frac{1}{\sqrt{x}}\right) dx\, dy$$

$$= \frac{1}{\sqrt{2}}\int_{x=0}^{a}\sqrt{x}(2\sqrt{y})_0^b\, dx$$

$$+ \frac{1}{\sqrt{2}}\int_{x=0}^{a}\frac{1}{\sqrt{x}}\left(\frac{2}{3}y^{3/2}\right)_0^b dx$$

$$= \sqrt{(2b)}\int_0^a\sqrt{x}dx + \frac{\sqrt{2}}{3}b^{3/2}\int_0^a\frac{1}{\sqrt{x}}dx$$

$$= \sqrt{2b}\left[\frac{2}{3}x^{3/2}\right]_0^a + \frac{1}{3}\sqrt{2b^3}(2x^{1/2})_0^a$$

$$= \frac{2}{3}\sqrt{2}\sqrt{(ab)}(a+b).$$

17.6 TRIPLE INTEGRAL

Let $f(x, y, z)$ be a single-valued function of the independent variables x, y, z in finite region V. Divide the region V into n subregions $\delta V_1, \delta V_2, \delta V_3, \ldots$ Let P be any point on the boundary or inside.

Take a point in each part and form the sum

$$s_n = f(x_1, y_1, z_1)\delta V_1 + f(x_2, y_2, z_2)\delta V_2 + \ldots + f(x_n, y_n, z_n)\delta V_n$$

$$= \sum_{r=1}^{n} f(x_r, y_r, z_r)\delta V_r \qquad \ldots(1)$$

when n tends to infinity, the limit of sum (1) tends to zero is called the triple integral of function $f(x, y, z)$ over the region V and is denoted by

$$\iiint_V f(x,y,z)dv.$$

The triple integral can be utilised in evaluating a number of physical quantities like, volume, suface etc.

We find volume, $V = \iiint_V dV$ and putting $f(x, y, z) = \rho$

We get, $\quad mass = \iiint_V \rho dV$.

17.6.1 EVALUATION OF TRIPLE INTEGRALS

The region V divide into elementary cuboids by drawing parallel co-ordinate planes. The volume V can then be considered as the sum of number of columns parallel to z-axis extending from the lower surface of V say $z = z_1(x, y)$ to the upper surface of V say $z = z_2(x, y)$ the bases of these as column (only one column has been shown in fig. 13) are the elementary area δs_r, which cover a certain area S in x- y plane *i.e.* plane $z=0$.

$\therefore$ Summing up over the elementary cuboids in the same column first and then taking the sum of all such columns we can write

$$\sum_{r=1}^{n} f(x_r, y_r, z_r) \text{ as } \sum_{r=1}^{n} [f(x_r, y_r, z_r)\delta z]\delta s_r$$

where (x_r, y_r, z_r) is a point in the mth cuboid.

When δS_r and δz tend to zero this becomes equal to

$$\iint_S \left\{\int_{z=z_1(x,y)}^{z_2(x,y)} f(x,y,z)dz\right\} ds$$

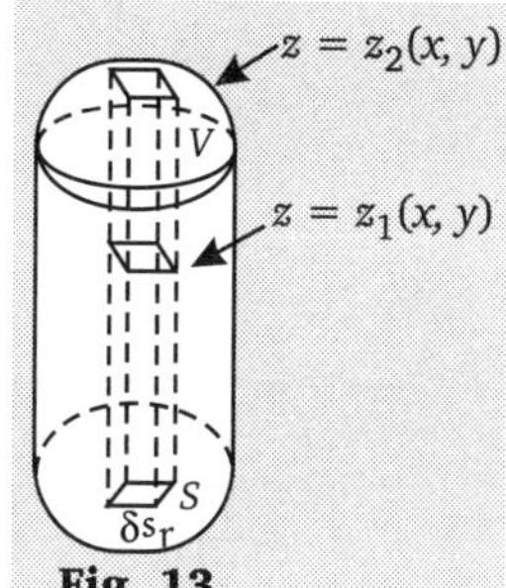

Fig. 13

(a) If the region V be specified by inequalities $a \le x \le b$, $c \le y \le d$, $e \le z \le f$ then triple integral

$$\iiint_V f(x,y,z)\,dx\,dy\,dz = \int_a^b \int_c^d \int_e^f f(x,y,z)\,dx\,dy\,dz$$
$$= \int_a^b dx \int_c^d dy \int_e^f f(x,y,z)\,dz.$$

Here, we integrate first with respect to z keeping x and y constant and then the remaining integration is done as in the case of double integrals.

The integration with respect to z is performed first regarding x and y as constant then integration w.r to y regarding x as a constant and then integrate w.r to x.

(b) If the limits of z are function of x and y and y as function of x and x takes the constant values as from $x = a$ to $x = b$.

$$\iiint_V f(x,y,z)\,dx\,dy\,dz = \int_a^b dx \int_{y_1(x)}^{y_2(x)} dy \int_{z_1(x,y)}^{z_2(x,y)} f(x,y,z)dz$$

The integration with respect to z perform first regarding x and y as constant, then integral w.r.t. y regarding x as a constant and then integrate w.r.t. x.

Solved Examples

1. *Evaluate* $\int_0^1 \int_{y^2}^1 \int_0^{1-x} x\,dy\,dx\,dz$.

SOLUTION. We have

$$I = \int_0^1 \int_{y^2}^1 (z)_0^{1-x}\, x\,dy\,dx$$
$$= \int_0^1 \int_{y^2}^1 x(1-x)\,dy\,dx$$
$$= \int_0^1 \int_{y^2}^1 (x - x^2)dy\,dx$$
$$= \int_0^1 \left[\frac{1}{2}x^2 - \frac{1}{3}x^3\right]_{y^2}^1 dy$$
$$= \int_0^1 \left[\left\{\frac{1}{2}(1)^2 - \frac{1}{3}(1)^3\right\} - \left\{\frac{1}{2}(y^2)^2 - \frac{1}{3}(y^2)^3\right\}\right] dy$$
$$= \int_0^1 \left[\left(\frac{1}{2} - \frac{1}{3}\right) - \left(\frac{1}{2}y^4 - \frac{1}{3}y^6\right)\right] dy$$
$$= \int_0^1 \left(\frac{1}{6} - \frac{1}{2}y^4 + \frac{1}{3}y^6\right) dy$$
$$= \left(\frac{1}{6}y - \frac{1}{10}y^5 + \frac{1}{21}y^7\right)_0^1$$
$$= \frac{1}{6} - \frac{1}{10} + \frac{1}{21} = \frac{4}{35}.$$

2. *Evaluate*

$$\int_{x=0}^1 \int_{y=0}^{\sqrt{1-x^2}} \int_{z=0}^{\sqrt{1-x^2-y^2}} xyz\,dx\,dy\,dz$$

SOLUTION. The given integral

$$I = \int_{x=0}^1 \int_0^{\sqrt{1-x^2}} xy\left(\frac{1}{2}z^2\right)_0^{\sqrt{1-x^2-y^2}} dx\,dy$$
$$= \frac{1}{2}\int_{x=0}^1 \int_{y=0}^{\sqrt{1-x^2}} xy(1-x^2-y^2)dx\,dy$$
$$= \frac{1}{2}\int_{x=0}^1 \int_{y=0}^{\sqrt{1-x^2}} x[y(1-x^2) - y^3)]dx\,dy$$
$$= \frac{1}{2}\int_{x=0}^1 x\left[\frac{1}{2}(1-x^2)y^2 - \frac{1}{4}y^4\right]_0^{\sqrt{1-x^2}} dx$$

$$= \frac{1}{2}\int_0^1 x \left[\begin{array}{c} \frac{1}{2}(1-x^2)(1-x^2) \\ -\frac{1}{4}(1-x^2)^2 \end{array} \right] dx$$

$$= \frac{1}{2}\int_0^1 x\left(\frac{1}{2}-\frac{1}{4}\right)(1-x^2)^2 dx$$

$$= \frac{1}{8}\int_0^1 (x - 2x^3 + x^5)\,dx$$

$$= \frac{1}{8}\left[\frac{1}{2}x^2 - \frac{1}{2}x^4 + \frac{1}{6}x^6\right]_0^1$$

$$= \frac{1}{8}\left(\frac{1}{2}-\frac{1}{2}+\frac{1}{6}\right) = \frac{1}{48}.$$

3. *Evaluate* $\int_0^4 \int_0^{2\sqrt{z}} \int_0^{\sqrt{4z-x^2}} dz\,dx\,dy$.

SOLUTION. The given triple integral

$$I = \int_0^4 \int_0^{2\sqrt{z}} \left[\int_0^{\sqrt{4z-x^2}} dy\right] dz\,dx$$

$$= \int_0^4 \int_0^{2\sqrt{z}} [y]_0^{\sqrt{4z-x^2}} dz\,dx$$

$$= \int_0^4 \left[\int_0^{2\sqrt{z}} \sqrt{4z-x^2}\,dx\right] dz$$

$$= \int_0^4 \left[\begin{array}{c} \frac{x}{2}\sqrt{4z-x^2} \\ +\frac{4z}{2}\sin^{-1}\frac{x}{2\sqrt{z}} \end{array} \right]_0^{2\sqrt{z}} dz$$

$$= \int_0^4 \left[0 + \frac{4z}{2}\sin^{-1}\frac{2\sqrt{z}}{2\sqrt{z}}\right] dz$$

$$= \int_0^4 2z.\frac{\pi}{2}dz = \int_0^4 \pi z\,dz$$

$$= \pi\left[\frac{z^2}{2}\right]_0^4 = \frac{\pi}{2}[16] = 8\pi$$

4. *Evaluate* $\int_0^{\log a} \int_0^x \int_0^{x+y} e^{x+y+z}\,dx\,dy\,dz.$

SOLUTION. Let

$$I = \int_0^{\log a} \int_0^x \int_0^{x+y} e^{x+y} e^z\,dx\,dy\,dz$$

$$= \int_0^{\log a} \int_0^x e^{x+y} (e^z)_0^{x+y} dx\,dy$$

$$= \int_0^{\log a} \int_0^x e^{x+y} [e^{x+y} - 1] dx\,dy$$

$$= \int_0^{\log a} \int_0^x e^{2(x+y)} dx\,dy - \int_0^{\log a} \int_0^x e^{x+y}\,dx\,dy$$

$$= \int_0^{\log a} \int_0^x e^{2x}.e^{2y}\,dx\,dy - \int_0^{\log a} \int_0^x e^{x+y}\,dx\,dy$$

$$= \int_0^{\log a} e^{2x}\left(\frac{1}{2}e^{2y}\right)_0^x dx - \int_0^{\log a} e^x (e^y)_0^x dx$$

$$= \frac{1}{2}\int_0^{\log a} e^{2x}(e^{2x} - e^0)dx - \int_0^{\log a} e^x (e^x - e^0)dx$$

$$= \frac{1}{2}\int_0^{\log a} (e^{4x} - e^{2x})dx - \int_0^{\log a} (e^{2x} - e^x)dx$$

$$= \frac{1}{2}\int_0^{\log a} (e^{4x} - 3e^{2x} + 2e^x)dx$$

$$= \frac{1}{2}\left[\frac{1}{4}e^{4x} - \frac{3}{2}e^{2x} + 2e^x\right]_0^{\log a}$$

$$= \frac{1}{8}(e^{4\log a} - e^0) - \frac{3}{4}(e^{2\log a} - e^0) + (e^{\log a} - e^0)$$

$$= \frac{1}{8}(a^4 - 1) - \frac{3}{4}(a^2 - 1) + (a - 1)$$

$$= \frac{1}{8}a^4 - \frac{3}{4}a^2 + a - \frac{3}{8}$$

$$= \frac{1}{8}[a^4 - 6a^2 + 8a - 3].$$

5. *Evaluate* $\iiint_V (x^2 + y^2 + z^2)\,dx\,dy\,dz$, *where V is the volume of cube bounded by the co-ordinates planes and the planes* $x = y = z = a$.

SOLUTION. Here, the limits of x, y and z are varies from 0 to a.

Therefore, the given integral

$$I = \int_0^a \int_0^a \int_0^a (x^2 + y^2 + z^2)\,dx\,dy\,dz$$

$$= \int_0^a \int_0^a \left[x^2 z + y^2 z + \frac{1}{3}z^3\right]_0^a dx\,dy$$

$$= \int_0^a \int_0^a \left(x^2 a + y^2 a + \frac{1}{3}a^3\right) dx\,dy$$

$$= \int_0^a \left[x^2 ay + \frac{1}{3}y^3 a + \frac{1}{3}ya^3\right]_0^a dx$$

$$= \int_0^a \left(x^2a^2 + \frac{1}{3}a^4 + \frac{1}{3}a^4 \right) dx$$

$$= \left[\frac{1}{3}x^3a^2 + \frac{1}{3}a^4x + \frac{1}{3}a^4x \right]_0^a = a^5.$$

6. *Evaluate the volume of tetrahedron bounded by the co-ordinate planes and the planes $x + y + z = 1$.*

SOLUTION. The volume of tetrahedron can be expressed as

$0 \le x \le 1, 0 \le y \le 1-x, 0 \le z \le 1-x-y.$

$\therefore$ The integral

$$I = \iiint dx\,dy\,dz$$

$$= \int_0^1 \int_0^{1-x} \int_0^{1-x-y} dx\,dy\,dz$$

$$= \int_0^1 \int_0^{1-x} [z]_0^{1-x-y} dx\,dy$$

$$= \int_0^1 \int_0^{1-x} (1-x-y) dx\,dy$$

$$= \int_0^1 \left[(1-x)y - \frac{y^2}{2} \right]_0^{1-x} dx$$

$$= \int_0^1 \left[(1-x)^2 - \frac{(1-x)^2}{2} \right] dx$$

$$= \int_0^1 \frac{1}{2}(1-x)^2 dx$$

$$= \frac{1}{2}\left[\frac{(1-x)^3}{3.(-1)} \right]_0^1 = -\frac{1}{6}(0-1) = \frac{1}{6}.$$

7. *Evaluate $\iiint_V zy^2 dx\,dy\,dz$, where V is the region bounded between the xy plane and the sphere, $x^2 + y^2 + z^2 = 1$.*

SOLUTION. Here the column parallel to z-axis is bounded by the plane $z=0$ and the surface of sphere $x^2 + y^2 + z^2 = 1$

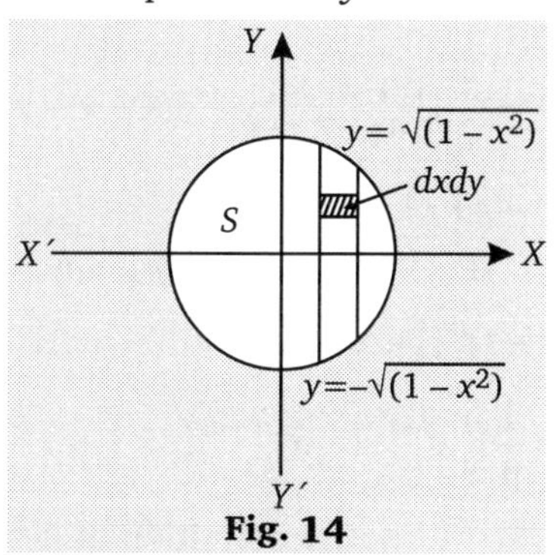

Fig. 14

i.e., $z = \sqrt{1 - x^2 - y^2}$.

The region S above which the volume V stands, is the area of circle of intersection of sphere $x^2 + y^2 + z^2 = 1$ by the xy plane.

Hence, the region S is the circle

$$x^2 + y^2 = 1.$$

It is clear from the figure that limits of integration for y are $-\sqrt{1-x^2}$ to $\sqrt{1-x^2}$ and for x are -1 to 1.

Hence, the given integral.

$$I = \int_{x=-1}^{1} \int_{y=-\sqrt{1-x^2}}^{\sqrt{1-x^2}} \int_{z=0}^{\sqrt{1-x^2-y^2}} zy^2\,dx\,dy\,dz$$

$$= \int_{x=-1}^{1} \int_{y=-\sqrt{1-x^2}}^{\sqrt{1-x^2}} y^2 \left(\frac{1}{2}z^2 \right)_0^{\sqrt{1-x^2-y^2}} dx\,dy$$

$$= \frac{1}{2}\int_{x=-1}^{1} \int_{y=-\sqrt{1-x^2}}^{\sqrt{1-x^2}} y^2(1-x^2-y^2)\,dx\,dy$$

$$= \frac{1}{2}\int_{x=-1}^{1} \int_{y=-\sqrt{1-x^2}}^{\sqrt{1-x^2}} (y^2 - x^2y^2 - y^4)\,dx\,dy$$

$$= \frac{1}{2}\int_{x=-1}^{1} \left(\frac{1}{3}y^3 - \frac{1}{3}x^2y^3 - \frac{1}{5}y^5 \right)_{-\sqrt{1-x^2}}^{\sqrt{1-x^2}} dx$$

$$= \frac{1}{2}\int_{x=-1}^{1} \left[\begin{matrix} \left(\frac{2}{3}\right)(1-x^2)^{3/2} \\ -\frac{2}{3}x^2(1-x^2)^{3/2} - \frac{2}{5}(1-x^2)^{5/2} \end{matrix} \right] dx$$

$$= \int_{x=-1}^{1} \left[\frac{1}{3}(1-x^2)^{5/2} - \frac{1}{5}(1-x^2)^{5/2} \right] dx$$

$[\because (1-x^2)^{3/2} - x^2(1-x^2)^{3/2} = (1-x^2)^{5/2}]$

$$= \frac{2}{15}\int_{x=-1}^{1} (1-x^2)^{5/2} dx = \frac{4}{15}\int_0^1 (1-x^2)^{5/2} dx$$

$$= \frac{4}{15}\int_0^{\pi/2} (1-\sin^2\phi)^{5/2} \cos\phi\,d\phi$$

(putting $x = \sin\phi$)

$$= \frac{4}{15}\int_0^{\pi/2} \cos^6\phi\,d\phi = \frac{4}{15}.\frac{5}{6}.\frac{3}{4}.\frac{1}{2}.\frac{\pi}{2} = \frac{\pi}{24}.$$

Exercise-17.3

1. Evaluate $\int_{x=0}^{1}\int_{y=0}^{2}\int_{z=1}^{2} x^2\, yz\, dx\, dy\, dz$.

2. Evaluate $\int_{-a}^{a}\int_{-b}^{b}\int_{-c}^{c}(x^2+y^2+z^2)\, dx\, dy\, dz$.

3. Evaluate $\int_{-1}^{1}\int_{0}^{z}\int_{x-z}^{x+z}(x+y+z)\, dy\, dx\, dz$. (GBTU-2010)

4. Evaluate $\int_0^1\int_0^{1-x}\int_0^{1-x-y}\dfrac{dy\, dx\, dz}{(1+x+y+z)^3}$.

5. Evaluate $\int_0^{\pi/2} d\theta \int_0^{a\sin\theta} dr \int_0^{(a^2-r^2)/a} r\, dz$.

6. Evaluate $\int_0^a\int_0^{a-x}\int_0^{a-x-y} x^2\, dx\, dy\, dz$.

7. Evaluate $\int_0^2\int_0^x\int_0^{x+y} e^x(y+2z)\, dx\, dy\, dz$.

8. Evaluate $\int_0^{\log 2}\int_0^x\int_0^{x+\log y} e^{x+y+z}\, dx\, dy\, dz$.

9. Evaluate the integral $\iiint xyz\, dx\, dy\, dz$ over the the volume enclosed by three co-ordinates plane and the plane $x+y+z=1$

10. Evaluate $\iiint \dfrac{dx\, dy\, dz}{(x+y+z+1)^2}$ over the region $x \ge 0, y \ge 0, z \ge 0, x+y+z \le 1$.

11. Evaluate $\iiint (z^5+z)\, dx\, dy\, dz$ over the sphere $x^2+y^2+z^2=1$.

12. Evaluate $\iiint_R u^2v^2w\, du\, dv\, dw$, where R is the region $u^2+v^2 \le 1$, $0 \le w \le 1$. (VTU-2011; SRM-2009)

13. Find the volume of the tetrahedron bounded by the plane $\dfrac{x}{a}+\dfrac{y}{b}+\dfrac{z}{c}=1$ and $(x+z = a)$ and coordinate plane.

14. Evaluate $\int_0^2\int_0^x\int_0^{x+y} e^x(y+2z)dx\, dy\, dz$.

15. Evaluate $\iiint_R (x-2y+z)$ where R is the region determined by $0 \le x \le 1$, $0 < y \le x^2$, $0 \le z \le x+y$.

ANSWERS

1. 1 **2.** $\frac{2}{3}abc(a^2+b^2+c^2)$ **3.** 0 **4.** $\frac{1}{2}\left(\log 2-\frac{5}{8}\right)$ **5.** $\frac{5a^3\pi}{64}$ **6.** $\frac{a^5}{60}$ **7.** $19[(1/3)e^2+1]$ **8.** $\frac{8}{3}\log 2-\frac{19}{9}$ **9.** 0 **10.** $\frac{1}{2}\left(\log 2-\frac{5}{8}\right)$ **11.** 0 **12.** $\pi/48$ **13.** $abc/5$ **14.** $\frac{19}{3}(e^2+3)$ **15.** 8/35

17.7 DIRICHLET'S THEOREM FOR THREE VARIABLES

Statements. *Let V be the region given by* $x \ge 0, y \ge 0, z \ge 0, x+y+z \le 1, l, m, n$ *are positive. Then*

$$\int_V x^{l-1}y^{m-1}z^{n-1}dx\, dy\, dz = \frac{\Gamma(l)\Gamma(m)\Gamma(n)}{\Gamma(l+m+n+1)}.$$

Proof. We evaluate the given integral over the volume enclosed by the three co-ordinates planes and the plane $x+y+z=1$, $x=0$, $y=0$, $z=0$. The limits of integration for this region can be expressed as $0 \le x \le 1$, $0 \le y \le 1-x$, $0 < z \le 1-x-y$.

Hence we may write the given triple integral as

$$\int_0^1\int_0^{1-x}\int_0^{1-x-y} x^{l-1}y^{m-1}z^{n-1}dx\, dy\, dz$$

$$= \int_0^1\int_0^{1-x} x^{l-1}y^{m-1}[z^n/n]_0^{1-x-y}\, dx\, dy = \frac{1}{n}\int_0^1\int_0^{1-x} x^{l-1}y^{m-1}(1-x-y)^n\, dx\, dy$$

$$= \frac{1}{n}\int_0^1\int_0^1 x^{l-1}\{(1-x)t\}^{m-1}[1-x-(1-x)t]^n(1-x)dx\, dt$$

(Putting $y=(1-x)t, \Rightarrow dy=(1-x)dt$))

$$= \frac{1}{n}\int_0^1\int_0^1 x^{l-1}(1-x)^{m-1}t^{m-1}(1-x)^n(1-t)^n(1-x)dx\, dt$$

$$= \frac{1}{n}\int_0^1\int_0^1 x^{l-1}(1-x)^{m+n}t^{m-1}(1-t)^n\, dx\, dt = \frac{1}{n}\int_0^1 x^{l-1}(1-x)^{m+n}dx \times \int_0^1 (t)^{m-1}(1-t)^n\, dt$$

$$= \frac{1}{n}B(l, m+n+1)B(m, n+1)$$ (By definition of Beta function)

$$= \frac{1}{n} \cdot \frac{\Gamma(l)\Gamma(m+n+1)}{\Gamma(l+m+n+1)} \cdot \frac{\Gamma(m)\Gamma(n+1)}{\Gamma(m+n+1)} \qquad \left[\because B(m,n) = \frac{\Gamma(m)\Gamma(n)}{\Gamma(m+n)}\right]$$

$$= \frac{\Gamma(l)\Gamma(m)}{\Gamma(l+m+n+1)} \cdot \frac{n\Gamma(n)}{n} \qquad [\because \Gamma(n+1) = n\,\Gamma(n)]$$

$$= \frac{\Gamma(l)\Gamma(m)\Gamma(n)}{\Gamma(l+m+n+1)}.$$

- Dirichlet's theorem holds good even if the conditions is taken as $x+y+z<1$ in place of $x+y+z \le 1$.
- The triple integral $\iiint x^{l-1} y^{m-1} z^{n-1} dx\,dy\,dz = h^{l+m+n} \frac{\Gamma(l)\Gamma(m)\Gamma(n)}{\Gamma(l+m+n+1)}$

  where the integral is extended to all positive values of the variables x, y and z, when $x+y+z \le h$.

17.8 DIRICHLET'S THEOREM FOR *n* VARIABLES

If the integral is extended to all positive values of the variables $x_1, x_2, .., x_n$ subject to the condition $x_1 + x_2 + ... + x_n \le 1$. Then

$$\iint ... \int x_1^{l_1-1} x_2^{l_2-1} ... x_n^{l_n-1} dx_1 dx_2 ... dx_n = \frac{\Gamma(l_1)\Gamma(l_2)...\Gamma(l_n)}{\Gamma(1+l_1+l_2+...+l_n)}$$

Solved Examples

1. *Evaluate* $\iiint x^{l-1} y^{m-1} z^{n-1} dx\,dy\,dz$ *in which* $x \ge 0, y \ge 0, z = 0$ *and* $(x/a)^{1/2} + (y/b)^{1/2} + (z/c)^{1/2} \le 1$.

SOLUTION. Let $(x/a)^{1/2} = u, (y/b)^{1/2} = v$ and $(z/c)^{1/2} = w$

Then $x = au^2, y = bv^2, z = cw^2$

$dx = 2au\,du; dy = 2bv\,dv; dz = 2cw\,dw,$

$u \ge 0, v \ge 0, w \ge 0$ and $u + v + w \le 1$

Hence,

$$\iiint (au^2)^{l-1} (bv^2)^{m-1} (cw^2)^{n-1} .2au.2bv.2cw\,du\,dv\,dw$$

$$= 8a^l b^m c^n \iiint u^{2l-1} v^{2m-1} w^{2n-1} du\,dv\,dw$$

$$= 8a^l b^m c^n \frac{\Gamma(2l)\Gamma(2m)\Gamma(2n)}{\Gamma(2l+2m+2n+1)}$$

2. *Evaluate* $\iint dx\,dy$ *over the region in the positive quadrant for which* $x+y \le 1$.

SOLUTION. We have $x + y \le 1$ and $x \ge 0, y \ge 0$ and so by Dirichlet's theorem, we get

$$I = \iint x^{2-1} y^{2-1} dx\,dy = \frac{\Gamma(2)\Gamma(2)}{\Gamma(2+2+1)}$$

$$= \frac{1}{4} \cdot \frac{1}{\Gamma(3)}$$

$$= \frac{1}{4.3.2\Gamma(1)} = \frac{1}{24 \times 1} = \frac{1}{24}.$$

3. *Show that the integral* $\iiint x^{l-1} y^{m-1} z^{n-1}\,dx\,dy\,dz$ *integrand over the region in the first octant below the surface* $(x/a)^p + (y/b)^q + (z/c)^r = 1$ *is*

$$\frac{a^l b^m c^n}{pqr} \cdot \frac{\Gamma(l/p)\Gamma(m/q)\Gamma(n/r)}{\Gamma[(l/p)+(m/q)+(n/r)+1]}.$$

SOLUTION. Putting $\left(\frac{x}{a}\right)^p = u$ or $x = au^{1/p}$

$\Rightarrow dx = a(1/p)u^{(1/p)-1}.du.$

Similarly putting $(y/b)^q = v$ and $(z/c)^r = w$, we get

$$dy = b(1/q)v^{(1/q)-1} dv$$

and $dz = c(1/r)w^{(1/r)-1} dw$.

$\therefore x^{l-1} dx = a^{l-1} u^{(l-1)/p} a(1/p) u^{(1-p)/p} du$

$$= a^l (1/p) u^{(l/p)-1} du$$

Similarly,

$$y^{m-1} dy = b^m (1/q) v^{(m/q)-1} dv \;;$$

$$z^{n-1} dz = c^n (1/r) w^{(n/r)-1} dw$$

Hence, subject to the condition $u+v+w \leq 1$, the given integral

$$= \frac{a^l b^m c^n}{pqr} \iiint u^{(l/p)-1} v^{(m/q)-1} w^{(n/r)-1} du\, dv\, dw$$

$$= \frac{a^l b^m c^n}{pqr} \cdot \frac{\Gamma(l/p)\Gamma(m/q)\Gamma(n/r)}{\Gamma[(l/p)+(m/q)+(n/r)+1]}$$

4. *Evaluate* $\iiint dx\, dy\, dz$ *where* $\frac{x^2}{a^2}+\frac{y^2}{b^2}+\frac{z^2}{c^2} \leq 1$ *or find the volume of* $(x^2/a^2)+(y^2/b^2)+(z^2/c^2)=1$.

SOLUTION. Let $\frac{x^2}{a^2} = u, x = au^{1/2}$ so that

$$dx = \frac{1}{2} a u^{-1/2} du\,.$$

Similarly, putting $\frac{y^2}{b^2} = v$ and $\frac{z^2}{c^2} = w$, we get

$$dy = \frac{1}{2} b v^{-1/2} dv \text{ and } dz = \frac{1}{2} c w^{-1/2} dw\,.$$

$$\therefore \iiint dx\, dy\, dz$$

$$= \iiint \frac{1}{2} a u^{-1/2} du . \frac{1}{2} b v^{-1/2} . dv . \frac{1}{2} c w^{-1/2} dw$$

$$= \frac{1}{8} abc \iiint u^{1/2-1} v^{1/2-1} w^{1/2-1} du\, dv\, dw$$

$$= \frac{1}{8} abc \frac{\Gamma(1/2)\Gamma(1/2)\Gamma(1/2)}{\Gamma(1/2+1/2+1/2+1)}$$

$$= \frac{1}{8} abc \frac{\sqrt{\pi}\sqrt{\pi}\sqrt{\pi}}{\Gamma(5/2)} = \frac{\pi\sqrt{\pi}\, bca}{8 \cdot 3/2 \cdot 1/2\sqrt{\pi}}$$

$$= \frac{1}{6} \pi abc$$

5. *Find the volume enclosed by the surface* $(x/a)^{2n}+(y/b)^{2n}+(z/c)^{2n}=1$.

SOLUTION. The given surface is symmetrical in all the eight octants. Now we want to find the volume V in the positive octant.

Clearly $V = \iiint dx\, dy\, dz$

where the integral is extended to all positive values of the variables x, y, z subject to the condition

$$(x/a)^{2n}+(y/b)^{2n}+(z/c)^{2n} \leq 1\,.$$

Now put

$$(x/a)^{2n} = u, (y/b)^{2n} = v, (z/c)^{2n} = w$$

$$\Rightarrow x = au^{1/2n}, y = bv^{1/2n}, z = cw^{1/2n}$$

So that $\quad dx = \frac{a}{2n} u^{(1/2n)-1} du$

$$\therefore \; V = \frac{abc}{8n^3} \iiint u^{(1/2n)-1} v^{(1/2n)-1} w^{(1/2n)-1} du\, dv\, dw$$

$$= \frac{abc}{8n^3} \frac{[\Gamma(1/2n)]^3}{\Gamma\{(3/2n)+1\}}$$

$$= \frac{abc}{8n^3} \frac{[\Gamma(1/2n)]^3}{(3/2n).\Gamma(3/2n)}$$

$$= \frac{abc}{12n^2} \frac{[\Gamma(1/2n)]^3}{\Gamma(3/2n)}\,.$$

Hence, the total volume enclosed by given surface

$$= 8V = \frac{2}{3} . \frac{abc}{n^2} \frac{[\Gamma(1/2n)]^3}{\Gamma(3/2n)}\,.$$

6. *Find the volume of the tetrahedron bounded by the plane* $\frac{x}{a}+\frac{y}{b}+\frac{z}{c}=1$ *and the co-ordinate planes.*

(GBTU-2012, MTU-2012)

SOLUTION. The volume of a small element at a point $(x, y, z) = dx\, dy\, dz$

$\therefore$ the volume of the given tetrahedron $= \iiint dx\, dy\, dz$ where the integral is extended to all positive values of variables x, y, z.

Put $\quad x/a = u, y/b = v, z/c = w$

subject to the condition so that

$$\frac{x}{a}+\frac{y}{b}+\frac{z}{c} \leq 1$$

$$dx = a.du, dy = b.dv \text{ and } dz = c.dw$$

then the required volume

$$= \iiint abc\, du\, dv\, dw \quad \text{where } u+v+w \leq 1$$

$$= abc\iiint u^{1-1}v^{1-1}w^{1-1}\,du\,dv\,dw$$

[By Dirichlet's theorem]

$$= abc\frac{[\Gamma(1)]^3}{\Gamma(1+1+1+1)} = abc\frac{1}{\Gamma(4)} = \frac{abc}{3.2.1} = \frac{abc}{6}$$

17.9 LIOUVILLE'S EXTENSION OF DIRICHLET'S THEOREM

Statement. *If x, y, z are all positive and such that* $h_1 < x+y+z \le h_2$ *then*

$$\iiint f(x+y+z)x^{l-1}y^{m-1}z^{n-1}dx\,dy\,dz = \frac{\Gamma(l)\Gamma(m)\Gamma(n)}{\Gamma(l+m+n)}\int_{h_1}^{h_2} f(u)u^{l+m+n-1}du.$$

Proof. From Dirichlet's theorem, we have

$$I = \iiint x^{l-1}y^{m-1}z^{n-1}dx\,dy\,dz = \frac{\Gamma(l)\Gamma(m)\Gamma(n)}{\Gamma(l+m+n+1)}u^{(l+m+n)} \quad ...(1)$$

subject to the condition that $x, y, z \ge 0$ and $x+y+z \le u$.

Now if $x, y, z \ge 0$ and $x+y+z \le u+\delta u$, then we have

$$I = \iiint x^{l-1}y^{m-1}z^{n-1}dx\,dy\,dz = \frac{\Gamma(l)\Gamma(m)\Gamma(n)}{\Gamma(l+m+n+1)}(u+\delta u)^{(l+m+n)} \quad ...(2)$$

So the value of integral given above extended to all such positive value of *x, y, z* such that $x+y+z$ lies between u and $u+\delta u$, is given by

$$I = \iiint x^{l-1}y^{m-1}z^{n-1}dx\,dy\,dz$$

$$= \frac{\Gamma(l)\Gamma(m)\Gamma(n)}{\Gamma(l+m+n+1)}[(u+\delta u)^{l+m+n} - u^{l+m+n}]$$

$$= \frac{\Gamma(l)\Gamma(m)\Gamma(n)}{\Gamma(l+m+n+1)}u^{l+m+n}\left[\left(1+\frac{\delta u}{u}\right)^{l+m+n} - 1\right]$$

$$= \frac{\Gamma(l)\Gamma(m)\Gamma(n)}{\Gamma(l+m+n+1)}u^{l+m+n}\left[1+(l+m+n)\frac{\delta u}{u}+\ldots-1\right]$$

[On expanding by Taylor's series]

$$= \frac{\Gamma(l)\Gamma(m)\Gamma(n)}{\Gamma(l+m+n+1)}(l+m+n)u^{(l+m+n-1)}\delta u$$

[Neglecting the second and higher degree terms of δu]

$$= \frac{\Gamma(l)\Gamma(m)\Gamma(n)}{\Gamma(l+m+n)}u^{(l+m+n-1)}\delta u \quad [\because \Gamma(l+m+n+1) = (l+m+n)\Gamma(l+m+n)]$$

Now, consider the intergral $\iiint f(x+y+z)x^{l-1}y^{m-1}z^{n-1}dx\,dy\,dz$.

Since $u \le x+y+z \le \delta u$, so the function *f(x+y+z)* will differ by a small quantity of same order of solution. Hence, the integral

$$\iiint f(x+y+z)x^{l-1}y^{m-1}z^{n-1}dx\,dy\,dz = \frac{\Gamma(l)\Gamma(m)\Gamma(n)}{\Gamma(l+m+n)}f(u)\cdot u^{(l+m+n-l)}\delta u$$

subject to the condition that $x, y, z \ge 0$ and $u \le x+y+z \le u+\delta u$, to the first approximation.

So finally for the given condition that for positive *x, y, z* such that $h_1 < x+y+z \le h_2$,

we get $\iiint f(x+y+z)x^{l-1}y^{m-1}z^{n-1}dx\,dy\,dz = \dfrac{\Gamma(l)\Gamma(m)\Gamma(n)}{\Gamma(l+m+n)}\displaystyle\int_{h_1}^{h_2} f(u)\cdot u^{(l+m+n-1)}du$

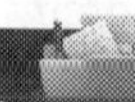

Solved Examples

1. *Evaluate* $\iiint e^{x+y+z} dx\,dy\,dz$ *taken over the positive octant such that* $x+y+z \le 1$.

(UPTU-2008)

SOLUTION. In the positive octant x, y, z are all positive and therefore $0<(x+y+z)\le 1$. Therefore, we have

$$\iiint e^{x+y+z} dx\,dy\,dz$$

$$= \frac{\Gamma(1)\Gamma(1)\Gamma(1)}{\Gamma(1+1+1)}\int_0^1 e^h h^{1+1+1-1} dh$$

[By Liouville's theorem]

$$= \frac{1}{\Gamma(3)}\int_0^1 h^2 e^h dh$$

$$= \frac{1}{2!}\left[(h^2 e^h)_0^1 - \int_0^1 2he^h dh\right]$$

$$= \frac{1}{2}\left[e - 2\left\{(he^h)_0^1 - \int_0^1 e^h dh\right\}\right]$$

$$= \frac{1}{2}\left[e - 2\left\{e - (e^h)_0^1\right\}\right]$$

$$= \frac{1}{2}[e - 2\{e - e + 1\}] = \frac{1}{2}(e-2).$$

2. *Evaluate* $\iiint \log(x+y+z)\,dx\,dy\,dz$ *taken over all positive values of x, y, z subject to the condition* $x+y+z \le 1$.

SOLUTION. Since x, y, z are to be taken positive value only, we have $0 <(x+y+z) \le 1$. Therefore, we have

$$\iiint \log(x+y+z)\,dx\,dy\,dz$$

$$= \iiint \log(x+y+z)x^{1-1}y^{1-1}z^{1-1}\,dx\,dy\,dz$$

$$= \frac{\Gamma(1)\Gamma(1)\Gamma(1)}{\Gamma(1+1+1)}\int_0^1 (\log h)h^{1+1+1-1}dh,$$

[By Liouville's theorem]

$$= \frac{1}{\Gamma(3)}\int_0^1 h^2(\log h)dh$$

$$= \frac{1}{2!}\left[\left\{(\log h)\frac{1}{3}h^3\right\}_0^1 - \int_0^1 \frac{1}{h}\cdot\frac{1}{3}h^3 dh\right]$$

$$= \frac{1}{6}\left[h^3 \log h - \frac{h^3}{3}\right]_0^1 = -\frac{1}{18}$$

3. *Evaluate* $\iiint (x+y+z)dx\,dy\,dz$ *over the tetrahedron* $x=0, y=0, z=0$ *and* $x+y+z \le 1$.

SOLUTION. We are given that: $0\le x+y+z\le 1$ therefoe, by Liouville's extension of Dirichlets theorem $\iiint (x+y+z)dx\,dy\,dz$

$$= (x+y+z)x^{1-1}y^{1-1}z^{1-1}dx\,dy\,dz$$

$$= \frac{\Gamma(1)\Gamma(1)\Gamma(1)}{\Gamma(1+1+1)}\int_0^1 u.u^{1+1+1-1}du$$

$$= \frac{1}{\Gamma(3)}\int_0^1 u^3 du = \frac{1}{2!}\left[\frac{u^4}{4}\right]_0^1 = \frac{1}{2}\left[\frac{1}{4}\right] = \frac{1}{8}.$$

4. *Prove that*

$$\iiint \frac{dx\,dy\,dz}{\sqrt{(1-x^2-y^2-z^2)}} = \frac{\pi^2}{8};$$ *the integral being extended to a positive values of variables for which the expression is real.*

SOLUTION. Since x, y, z are to be taken positive values only, we have $0<x^2+y^2+z^2<1$. Put $x^2 = u$ or $x = u^{1/2}$ so that $dx = 1/2u^{-1/2}\,du$.

Similarly putting $y^2 = v$ and $z^2 = w$, we get $dy = 1/2\,v^{-1/2}\,dv$, $dz=\frac{1}{2}w^{-1/2}dw$.

Now, given integral

$$= \iiint \frac{(1/2)u^{-1/2}(1/2)v^{-1/2}(1/2)w^{-1/2}}{\sqrt{1-(u+v+w)}}\,du\,dv\,dw$$

where $0<u+v+w<1$

$$= \frac{1}{8}\iiint \frac{u^{1/2-1}v^{1/2-1}w^{1/2-1}}{\sqrt{1-(u+v+w)}}du\,dv\,dw$$

$$= \frac{1}{8}\frac{\Gamma(1/2)\Gamma(1/2)\Gamma(1/2)}{\Gamma(1/2+1/2+1/2)}$$

$$\int_0^1 \frac{1}{\sqrt{1-h}}h^{1/2+1/2+1/2-1}dh$$

$$= \frac{1}{8}\frac{\sqrt{\pi}\sqrt{\pi}\sqrt{\pi}}{\Gamma(3/2)}\int_0^1 \sqrt{\left(\frac{h}{1-h}\right)}dh$$

$$= \frac{1}{4}\pi\int_0^{\pi/2}\sqrt{\left(\frac{\sin^2\theta}{\cos^2\theta}\right)}2\sin\theta\cos\theta d\theta$$

Putting $h = \sin^2\theta$

$$= \frac{1}{4}\pi\int_0^{\pi/2} 2\sin^2\theta d\theta$$

$$= \frac{1}{4}\pi\int_0^{\pi/2}(1-\cos 2\theta)d\theta$$

$$= \frac{1}{4}\pi\left[\theta - \frac{1}{2}\sin 2\theta\right]_0^{\pi/2} \qquad = \frac{1}{4}\pi(\pi/2) = \frac{1}{8}\pi^2.$$

Similar Problems

(1) Evaluate $\iiint x^{\alpha} y^{\beta} z^{\gamma} (1-x-y-z)^{\lambda}\, dx\, dy\, dz$ over the interior of tetrahedron formed by the co-ordinate plane and the plane $x+y+z=1$. **Ans.** $\dfrac{\Gamma(\alpha+1)\Gamma(\beta+1)\Gamma(\gamma+1)\Gamma(\lambda+1)}{\Gamma(\alpha+\beta+\gamma+\lambda+4)}$

(2) Evaluate $\iiint \sqrt{(a^2b^2c^2 - b^2c^2x^2 - c^2a^2y^2 - a^2b^2z^2)}\,dx\,dy\,dz$ taken throughout the ellipsoid $\dfrac{x^2}{a^2}+\dfrac{y^2}{b^2}+\dfrac{z^2}{c^2}=1$. **Ans.** $\dfrac{\pi^2a^2b^2c^2}{4}$

(3) Evaluate $\iiint_R (x+y+z+1)^2\,dx\,dy\,dz$ where R defined by $x\geq 0, y\geq 0, z\geq 0, x+y+z\leq 1$. **Ans.** $\dfrac{31}{60}$

5. *Show that*

$$\iint\left(\frac{1-x^2-y^2}{1+x^2+y^2}\right)^{1/2} dx\,dy = \frac{\pi}{8}(\pi-2)$$

over the positive quadrant of circle $x^2+y^2=1$.

SOLUTION. The given integral is to be extended to all positive values of x and y such that

$$0 \leq x^2+y^2 \leq 1 \qquad ...(1)$$

Put $x^2=u, y^2=v \Rightarrow x=u^{1/2}, y=v^{1/2}$ so that

$$dx = \frac{1}{2}u^{-1/2}\,du,\ dy = \frac{1}{2}v^{-1/2}dv$$

With these substitution, the condition (1) become $0 \leq u+v \leq 1$.

Therefore the integral

$$= \iint\left[\frac{1-(u+v)}{1+(u+v)}\right]^{1/2}\frac{1}{4}u^{-1/2}v^{-1/2}du\,dv$$

$$= \frac{1}{4}\iint\left[\frac{1-(u+v)}{1+(u+v)}\right]^{1/2} u^{(1/2)-1} v^{(1/2)-1}du\,dv$$

where $0 \leq u+v \leq 1$

$$= \frac{1}{4}\frac{\Gamma(1/2)\Gamma(1/2)}{\Gamma(1/2+1/2)}\int_0^1\left[\frac{1-h}{1+h}\right]^{1/2} .h^{(1/2)+(1/2)-1}dh$$

[By Liouville's extension of Dirichlet's theorem]

$$= \frac{1}{4}\frac{\sqrt{\pi}\sqrt{\pi}}{\Gamma(1)}\int_0^1\frac{1-h}{\sqrt{(1-h^2)}}dh$$

$$= \frac{\pi}{4}\int_0^1\frac{(1-\sin\theta)}{\cos\theta}\cos\theta\,d\theta$$

Putting $h=\sin\theta$, so that $dh = \cos\theta\, d\theta$

$$= \frac{\pi}{4}[\theta+\cos\theta]_0^{\frac{\pi}{2}} = \frac{\pi}{4}\left[\frac{\pi}{2}-1\right] = \frac{\pi}{8}(\pi-2).$$

Exercise-17.4

1. Show that if l, m, n are all positive, then

$$\iiint x^{l-1}y^{m-1}z^{n-1}dx\,dy\,dz = \frac{a^lb^mc^n}{8}.\frac{\Gamma(l/2)\Gamma(m/2)\Gamma(n/2)}{\Gamma(l/2+m/2+n/2+1)}$$

where the triple integral is taken throughout the part of the ellipsoid $\dfrac{x^2}{a^2}+\dfrac{y^2}{b^2}+\dfrac{z^2}{c^2}=1$ which lies in the positive octant.

2. Evaluate $\iint x^{2l-1}y^{2m-1}dx\,dy$ such that $x^2+y^2 \leq c^2$ for all positive values of x and y.

3. Find the volume of solid surrounded by the surface $\left(\dfrac{x}{a}\right)^{2/3}+\left(\dfrac{y}{b}\right)^{2/3}+\left(\dfrac{z}{c}\right)^{2/3}=1$.

4. Evaluate the double integral
$$\iint_P x^{1/2}y^{1/2}(1-x-y)^{2/3}dx\,dy$$
over the domain D bounded by lines $x = 0$, $y = 0, x + y = 1$.

5. Evaluate $\iint_T x^{1/2}y^{1/2}(1-x-y)^{3/2}dx\,dy$, where T is the region bounded by $x \geq 0, y\geq 0$, $x+y \leq 1$.

6. Evaluate $\iiint \sqrt{\left(\dfrac{1-x^2-y^2-z^2}{1+x^2+y^2+z^2}\right)}dx\,dy\,dz$, integral being taken over all positive values of x, y, z such that $x^2+y^2+z^2 \leq 1$.

7. Evaluate $\iint \sqrt{\left\{\dfrac{1-(x^2/a^2-y^2/b^2)}{1+(x^2/a^2+y^2/b^2)}\right\}}dx\,dy$ where $\dfrac{x^2}{a^2}+\dfrac{y^2}{b^2} \leq 1$.

8. Evaluate $\iint_R \sqrt{(x^2+y^2)}dx\,dy$, where R is the region in the xy plane bounded by $x^2+y^2 = 4$ and $x^2+y^2 = 9$.

9. Prove that $\iiint \dfrac{dx\,dy\,dz}{(x+y+z+1)^2} = \dfrac{1}{2}\left[\log 2 - \dfrac{5}{8}\right]$ throughout the volume bounded by the co-ordinates planes and plane $x + y + z = 1$.

10. Evaluate the integral
$$\iiint_R (ax^2+by^2+cz^2)dx\,dy\,dz$$
where R is the region given by $x^2+y^2+z^2 \leq d^2$

11. Find the value of $\iiint xyz \sin(x+y+z)\,dx\,dy\,dz$, the integral being extended to all positive values of variables subject to the condition $x+y+z \leq \pi/2$.

12. Evaluate $\iiint_R x^2y^2z^2\,dx.dy.dz$ where R is the region given by $x^2+y^2 < 1, 0 \leq z \leq 1$.

13. Find the value of $\iint x^{l-1}y^{-1}e^{x+y}\,dx, dy, 0 < l < 1$ to all positive values subject to $x+y < h$.

14. A triangular prism is formed by planes whose equations are $ay=bx$, $y= 0$ and $x = a$. Show that the volume of the prism between the planes $z = 0$ and surface $z= c+xy$ is $\dfrac{ab}{8}(4c+ab)$.

15. Show that the volume of the paraboloid of revolution $x^2+y^2=4z$ cut off by the plane $z=4$ is $32\,\pi$.

16. Show that the volume common to the cylinder $x^2+y^2 = a^2$ and $x^2+z^2=a^2$ is $\dfrac{16a^3}{3}$.

17. Show that the volume of the solid which is 4bounded by the surface $2z = x^2+y^2$ and $z=x$ is $\pi/4$. (MTU–2012)

18. Show that the volume enclosed between the two surfaces $z = 8-x^2-y^2$ and $z = x^2+3y^2$ is $8\pi\sqrt{2}$. (GBTU–2011)

19. Show that the volume bounded by the elliptic paraboloids $z = x^2 + 9y^2$ and $z = 18-x^2-9y^2$ is $27\,\pi$.

20. Apply Dirichlet's integral to find the mass of an octant of the ellipsoid $\dfrac{x^2}{a^2}+\dfrac{y^2}{b^2}+\dfrac{z^2}{c^2}=1$, the density at any point being $\rho = kxyz$.

Hint to Selected Problems

1. Put $\dfrac{x^2}{a^2} = u$ i.e., $x = au^{1/2}$, $\dfrac{y^2}{b^2} = v$ i.e., $y = bv^{1/2}$ and $z = cw^{1/2}$

   Then apply Dirichlet's theorem.

2. Put $x^2 = c^2u, y^2 = c^2v$

3. Put $\left(\dfrac{x}{a}\right)^{2/3} = u, \left(\dfrac{y}{b}\right)^{2/3} = v, \left(\dfrac{z}{c}\right)^{2/3} = w$.

4. The given integral can be written as
$$I = \iint x^{(3/2)-1}y^{(3/2)-1}[1-(x+y)]^{2/3}dx\,dy.$$

   Then apply Liouville's extension of Dirichlet's theorem.

6. Put $x^2 = u, y^2 = v, z^2 < w$ and apply Liouville's extension of Dirichlet's theorem.

7. Put $\dfrac{x^2}{a^2} = u$ and $\dfrac{y^2}{b^2} = v$ and apply Liouville's extension of Dirichlet's theorem.

18. Put $x^2 = u, y^2 = v$ and Liouville's extension of Dirichlet's theorem.

10. Put $x^2 = d^2u, y^2 = d^2v, z^2 = d^2w$.

ANSWERS

2. $\dfrac{c^{2l+2m}}{4}\dfrac{\Gamma(l)\Gamma(m)}{\Gamma(l+m+1)}$ 3. $\dfrac{4}{35}\pi abc$ 4. $\dfrac{27\pi}{1760}$ 5. $\dfrac{2\pi}{315}$ 6. $\dfrac{abc}{6}$

7. $\frac{\pi}{8}\left[B\left(\frac{3}{4},\frac{1}{2}\right)-B\left(\frac{5}{4},\frac{1}{2}\right)\right]$ 8. $\pi ab\left[\frac{\pi}{2}-1\right]$ 9. $\frac{38\pi}{3}$ 10. $\frac{4}{15}\pi(a+b+c)d^5$

11. $\frac{1}{384}[\pi^4-48\pi^2+384]$ 12. $\frac{\pi}{48}$ 13. $\frac{\pi}{\sin l\pi}(e^n-1)$ 14. $\frac{ka^2b^2c^2}{48}$.

17.10 CHANGE OF VARIABLES

Some times, we change the variables from one system to another system for more convenient way to find the double integrals. The variables x, y in $\iint_R f(x,y)dx\,dy$ are changed to u, v by means of the relations $x = f_1(u,v)$, $y = f_2(u,v)$ then the double integral is transformed into

$$\iint f\{f_1(u,v), f_2(u,v)\}\,|J|\,du\,dv$$

where $J = \begin{vmatrix} \frac{\partial x}{\partial u} & \frac{\partial x}{\partial v} \\ \frac{\partial y}{\partial u} & \frac{\partial y}{\partial v} \end{vmatrix}$ and R' is the region in the u-v plane corresponding to region R in the x-y plane.

WORKING PROCEDURE

- Replace x, y by their equivalent in terms of u and v, the element of area $dx\,dy$ by $(J)\,du\,dv$ and the region R of integration in xy plane by the region R', in the uv plane.

17.10.1 CHANGE TO POLAR CO-ORDINATES

To change the variable from cartesian to polar form we put $x = r\cos\theta$, $y = r\sin\theta$.

Then $J = \begin{vmatrix} \frac{\partial x}{\partial r} & \frac{\partial x}{\partial \theta} \\ \frac{\partial y}{\partial r} & \frac{\partial y}{\partial \theta} \end{vmatrix} = \begin{vmatrix} \cos\theta & -r\sin\theta \\ \sin\theta & r\cos\theta \end{vmatrix} = r$

$$\iint_R f(x,y)dx\,dy = \iint_{R'} f(r\cos\theta, r\sin\theta)\,|J|\,dr\,d\theta = \iint_{R'} f(r\cos\theta, r\sin\theta)\,|\,r\,dr\,d\theta$$

Solved Examples

1. *Transform $\iint f(x,y)dx\,dy$, by the substitution $x+y = u$, $y = vu$.*

SOLUTION. We have $x+y = u$ and $y = uv$ therefore,

$x = u - y = u - uv$ and $y = uv$.

$\therefore \quad \frac{\partial x}{\partial u} = 1 - v, \frac{\partial x}{\partial v} = -u, \frac{\partial y}{\partial u} = v$

and $\frac{\partial y}{\partial v} = u$ ...(1)

$$\therefore \quad J = \frac{\partial(x,y)}{\partial(u,v)} = \begin{vmatrix} \frac{\partial x}{\partial u} & \frac{\partial x}{\partial v} \\ \frac{\partial y}{\partial u} & \frac{\partial y}{\partial v} \end{vmatrix}$$

$$= \begin{vmatrix} 1-v & -u \\ v & u \end{vmatrix} = u$$

$\therefore$ *$dx\,dy = J\,du\,dv = u\,du\,dv$.*

Hence, the given integral transforms to

$$\iint F(u,v)u\,du\,dv$$

2. *Transform to polar co-ordinate and integrate $\iint\sqrt{\left(\frac{1-x^2-y^2}{1+x^2+y^2}\right)}dx\,dy$ the integral being extended over all positive values of x and y subject to $x^2+y^2 \le 1$.*

SOLUTION. Here, x varies from 0 to 1 and y varies from 0 to $\sqrt{1-x^2}$ in the first quadrant where x and y are both positive.

$\therefore$ Given integral

$$I = \int_0^1\int_0^{\sqrt{1-x^2}}\sqrt{\frac{(1-x^2-y^2)}{1+x^2+y^2}}\,dx\,dy$$

Now change it into polar form by putting $x = r\cos\theta$, $y = r\sin\theta$

then the circle $x^2+y^2 = 1$ transform into $r^2 = 1$ to $r = 1$ and its first quadrant

θ varies from 0 to $\pi/2$ and r varies from 0 to 1, then integral

$$I = \int_{\theta=0}^{\pi/2}\int_{r=0}^{1}\sqrt{\left(\frac{1-r^2}{1+r^2}\right)}\, r\, d\theta\, dr$$

$$= \int_0^{\pi/2} d\theta \int_0^1 \sqrt{\left(\frac{1-r^2}{1+r^2}\right)}\, r\, dr$$

$$= [\theta]_0^{\pi/2}\left[\frac{1}{2}\left(\frac{\pi}{2}-1\right)\right]$$

$$= \frac{1}{2}\pi.\frac{1}{2}\left(\frac{1}{2}\pi-1\right) = \frac{1}{4}\pi\left(\frac{1}{2}\pi-1\right).$$

3. *Evaluate* $\iint\sqrt{(a^2-x^2-y^2)}\,dx\,dy$, *over the semi-circle* $x^2+y^2 = ax$ *in the positive quadrant.*

SOLUTION. The region of integration is a semi-circle, we change it into the polar co-ordinate by putting $x = r\cos\theta$, and $y = r\sin\theta$ in $x^2+y^2 = ax$, then we have

$$r^2\cos^2\theta + r^2\sin^2\theta = ar\cos\theta$$

$$r^2(\sin^2\theta+\cos^2\theta) = ar\cos\theta$$

$$r = a\cos\theta.$$

The equation $r = a\cos\theta$ represent a circle which passing through the pole for the given region where r varies from 0 to $a\cos\theta$ and θ varies from 0 to $\pi/2$.

$$\therefore \iint\sqrt{(a^2-x^2-y^2)}\,dx\,dy$$

$$= \int_0^{\pi/2}\int_0^{a\cos\theta}\sqrt{a^2-r^2}\,.r\,d\theta\,dr$$

$$[\because x^2+y^2 = r^2 \text{ and } dx\,dy = r\,d\theta\,dr]$$

$$= \int_0^{\pi/2}\left[\int_0^{a\cos\theta}\left\{-\frac{1}{2}(a^2-r^2)^{1/2}(-2r)\right\}dr\right]d\theta$$

$$= \int_0^{\pi/2}\left[-\frac{1}{2}.\frac{2}{3}(a^2-r^2)^{3/2}\right]_0^{a\cos\theta} d\theta$$

$$= \frac{-1}{3}\int_0^{\pi/2}(a^3\sin^3\theta - a^3)\,d\theta$$

$$= \frac{-a^3}{3}\left[\frac{2}{3.1}-\frac{\pi}{2}\right] = \frac{1}{3}a^3\left(\frac{\pi}{2}-\frac{2}{3}\right).$$

4. *By using the transformation* $x+y = u$, $y = vu$, *show that*

$$\int_0^1\int_0^{1-x} e^{y/(x+y)}\,dx\,dy = \frac{1}{2}(e-1)$$

SOLUTION. We have $dx\,dy = u\,du\,dv$

The region of integration is bounded by the lines $y = 0$, $y = 1-x$, $x=0$ and $x=1$ Changing these equations into new variables u and v by using the relation

$$x = u-y = u-uv = u(1-v)$$

and $y = uv$, we have $uv = 0$, $uv = 1-u(1-v)$, $u(1-v)=0$ and $u(1-v)=1$

giving $v=0$ to $v=1$, $u = 0$ to $u=1$. Therefore for the given region v varies from 0 to 1 and u varies from 0 to 1.

and $e^{y/(x+y)} = e^{uv/u} = e^v$.

Changing the variables to u, v the given integral becomes

$$I = \int_0^1\int_0^1 e^v u\,du\,dv = \int_0^1 [e^v]_0^1 u\,du$$

$$= \int_0^1 (e^1-e^0)u\,du$$

$$= (e-1)\int_0^1 u\,du = (e-1)\left[\frac{u^2}{2}\right]_0^1$$

$$= \frac{1}{2}(e-1).$$

5. *Evaluate the integral* $\int_0^a\int_0^{\sqrt{a^2-y^2}}(x^2+y^2)\,dy\,dx$ by changing into polar co-ordinates. (UPTU–2009)

SOLUTION. Putting $x = r\cos\theta$, $y = r\sin\theta$, we have

$$J = \begin{vmatrix}\frac{\partial x}{\partial r} & \frac{\partial x}{\partial\theta}\\ \frac{\partial y}{\partial r} & \frac{\partial y}{\partial\theta}\end{vmatrix} = \begin{vmatrix}\cos\theta & -r\sin\theta\\ \sin\theta & r\cos\theta\end{vmatrix} = r$$

$\therefore$ $dx\,dy$ is to be replaced by $J\,dr\,d\theta$.

$$x^2+y^2 = r^2\cos^2\theta + r^2\sin^2\theta = r^2.$$

Again we find that in the upper limit $x = \sqrt{a^2-y^2}$, y varies from 0 to a and x varies from 0 to any point on the circle $x^2+y^2 = a^2$.

In the polar form of the circle $r^2 = a^2$ *i.e.*, $r = a$ we find that r varies from 0 to a and θ varies from 0 to $\pi/2$.

$$\therefore \int_0^a\int_0^{\sqrt{a^2-y^2}}(x^2+y^2)\,dy\,dx$$

$$= \int_{\theta=0}^{\pi/2}\int_{r=0}^{a} r^2.r\,d\theta\,dr$$

$$= \int_{\theta=0}^{\pi/2}\left[\frac{r^4}{4}\right]_0^a d\theta$$

$$= \frac{1}{4}a^4(\theta)_0^{\pi/2} = \left(\frac{1}{8}\right)\pi a^4.$$

Exercise-17.5

1. Transform $\int_0^a \int_0^{a-x} f(x,y)dx\,dy$, by the substitution $x+y = u$, $y=uv$.
2. By using the transformation $x+y = u$, $y = uv$ show that $\iint \{xy(1-x-y)\}^{1/2} dx\,dy$ taken over the area of the triangle bounded by lines $x=0, y=0, x+y=1$ is $\frac{2\pi}{105}$.
3. Transform the integral
$$\int_0^a \int_0^{\sqrt{a^2-x^2}} y\sqrt{x^2+y^2}\,dx\,dy$$
by changing to polar co-ordinates and hence solve it.
4. Evaluate $\iint (x^2+y^2)^{7/2} dx\,dy$, over the circle $x^2+y^2=1$.
5. Evaluate $\iint xy(x^2+y^2)^{3/2} dx\,dy$, over the positive axes of circle $x^2+y^2=1$.
6. Transform the integral $\int_0^{\pi/2} \int_0^{\pi/2} \sqrt{\frac{\sin\phi}{\sin\theta}}\, d\phi\, d\theta$ by the substitutions $x = \sin\phi\cos\theta$, $y = \sin\phi\sin\theta$ and show that its value is π.

Hint to Selected Problems

1. $x+y = u$ and $y = uv \Rightarrow x = u-uv$ and $y = uv$

Now, $J = \frac{\partial(x,y)}{\partial(x,v)} = \begin{vmatrix} \frac{\partial x}{\partial u} & \frac{\partial x}{\partial v} \\ \frac{\partial y}{\partial u} & \frac{\partial y}{\partial v} \end{vmatrix} = \begin{vmatrix} 1-v & -u \\ v & u \end{vmatrix} = u$

$\Rightarrow \quad dx\,dy = u\,du\,dv.$

2. Proceed same as (1), we have $dx\,dy = u\,du\,dv$

$\therefore \{xy(1-x-y)\}^{1/2} = [u(1-v)uv(1-u)]^{1/2}$

$= u(1-u)^{1/2} v^{1/2} (1-v)^{1/2}.$

3. $x = r\cos\theta$, $y = r\sin\theta$, $J = r$

$\Rightarrow \quad dx\,dy = r\,d\theta\,dr$

$\therefore \int_0^a \int_0^{\sqrt{(a^2-x^2)}} y\sqrt{(x^2+y^2)}\,dx\,dy$

$= \int_{\theta=0}^{\pi/2} \int_{r=0}^{a} r\sin\theta . r d\theta\, dr.$

ANSWERS

1. $\int_0^a \int_0^1 F(u,v)u\,du\,dv$ 3. $\frac{a^4}{4}$ 4. $\frac{2\pi}{9}$ 5. $\frac{1}{14}$ 6. $\int_0^1 \int_0^{\sqrt{1-y^2}} \frac{dx\,dy}{\sqrt{y-y(x^2+y^2)}}$

17.11 CHANGE OF ORDER OF INTEGRATIONS

If the limits of integration are constants in the double integration then the value of integration can be obtained by integrating with respect to any independent variable.

When the limits are not constant but are the function of x and y then firstly we integrate with respect to first independent variable and then with respect to second.

In this case the limits of integration are determined in the given region by drawing the strips parallel to Y-axis or X-axis.

In this case limits of y are function of x then we find the new limits of x as function of y and new constant.

WORKING PROCEDURE

STEP 1. If we perform the integration first with respect to y, we take the elementary strip parallel to y-axis and determine the limits of y and add up the vertical strip from extreme left to the extreme right of the region.

STEP 2. If the order of integration is performed first with respect to x, we take the elementary strip parallel to x-axis and proceed.

Solved Examples

1. *Evaluate the following integral by changing the order of integration*

$$\int_0^{2a} \int_0^{\sqrt{2ax-x^2}} a - \sqrt{(a^2-y^2)}\,dx\,dy.$$

SOLUTION. Here, we have the following figure.

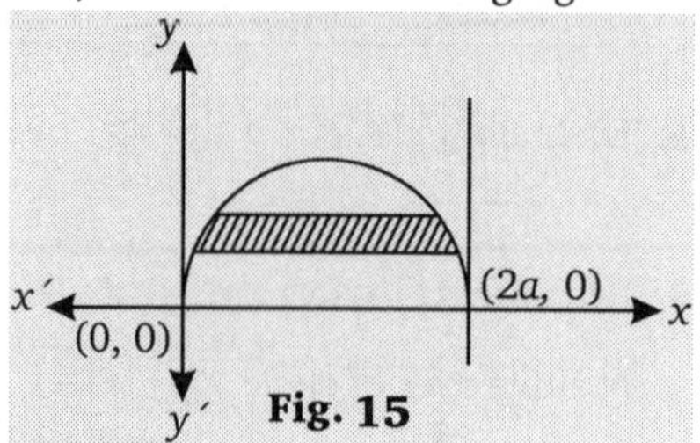

Fig. 15

The limits of y are from $y = 0$ to $y = \sqrt{2ax - x^2}$ or between x-axis and semicircle

$$x^2 + y^2 - 2ax = 0$$

or $$(x-a)^2 + y^2 = a^2$$

In the figure, the region x varies from one end of the circle to other end

i.e., $$(x-a)^2 = a^2 - y^2$$

$\Rightarrow$ $$x = a \pm \sqrt{a^2 - y^2}.$$

The strips are taken parallel to x-axis and y varies from 0 to a. So the order of integration is changed as

$$I = \int_0^{2a}\int_0^{\sqrt{2ax-x^2}} (a - \sqrt{a^2 - y^2})\,dx\,dy$$

$$= \int_0^{a}\int_{a-\sqrt{a^2-y^2}}^{a+\sqrt{a^2-y^2}} (a - \sqrt{a^2 - y^2})\,dx\,dy.$$

2. *Change the order of integration in the integral* $\int_0^a \int_0^x f(x,y)dx\,dy$.

SOLUTION. The given limits shows that the region of integration is bounded by the curve $y = 0, y = x, x = 0, x = a$.

Hence $y = 0$ represent X-axis and $y=x$ represent a straight line through the origin. Also $x = 0$ and $x = a$, represent straight lines parallel to y-axis therefore the region of the integration is the triangle OAB in the figure 16 and B is (a, a).

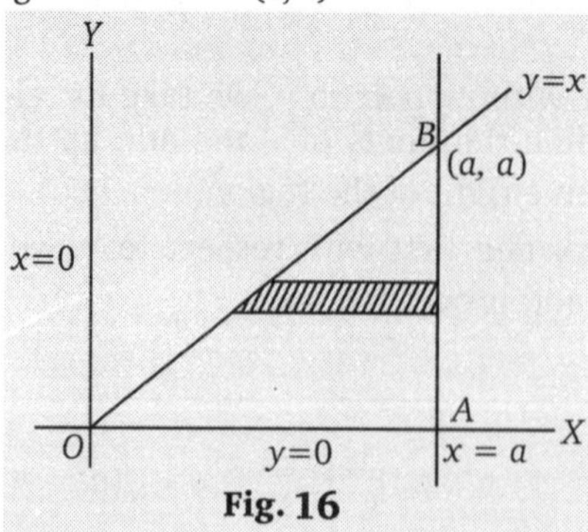

Fig. 16

In the given integral, the limits of integration of y being variable, we are required to integrate first w.r. to y regarding x as constant and then w.r. to x. To change the order of integration drawn parallel strip along x-axis, straight from the line OB and terminating on the line AB.

Thus in region OBA, x varies from y to a and y varies from 0 to a.

Hence, by changing the order of integration we have

$$\int_0^a \int_0^x f(x,y)\,dx\,dy = \int_0^a \int_y^a f(x,y)\,dy\,dx.$$

3. *Change the order of integration and evaluate* $\int_0^1 \int_{e^x}^{e} \frac{dx\,dy}{\log y}$.

SOLUTION. The region of integration is bounded by $e^x = y, y = e, x = 0$ and $x = 1$.

Here $y = e^x$ represents a curve. Putting $x = 0$ and $x = 1$ in $y = e^x$, then we get $y = 1$ and $y = e$. So $A(0, 1)$ and $B(1, e)$ are the points on this curve.

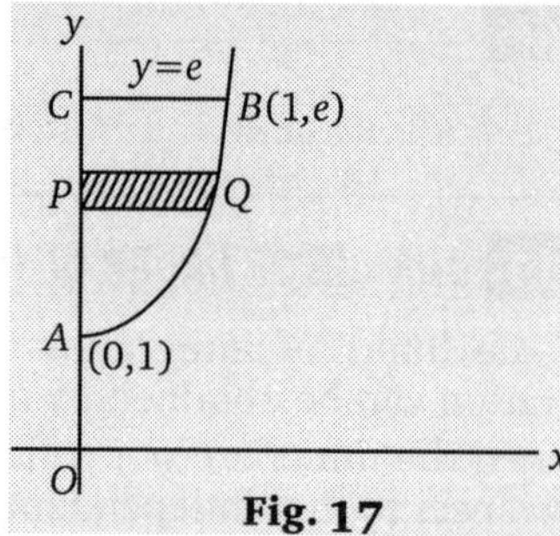

Fig. 17

When we integrate with respect to x, first drawn a strip parallel to x-axis.

The strip starts from $x = 0$ and extends upto the curve $y = e^x$ *i.e.,* $x = \log y$. Also for the given region y varies from $y = 1$ to $y = e$. On changing the order of integration, the given integral

$$I = \int_1^e \int_0^{\log y} \frac{dy\,dx}{(\log y)} = \int_1^e \frac{1}{\log y}(x)_0^{\log y}\,dy$$

$$= \int_1^e \frac{1}{\log y}(\log y - 0)dy$$

$$= \int_1^e dy = (y)_1^e = e - 1.$$

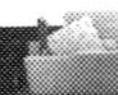

Similar Problem

(1) Change the order of integration in $\int_0^a \int_{\sqrt{a^2+x^2}}^{x+2a} f(x,y)\,dx dy$.

5. *Change the order of integration in*

$$\int_0^a \int_x^{a^2/x} \phi(x,y)\,dx\,dy.$$

SOLUTION. We observe that the region is bounded by $y = x$ and $y = a^2/x$ and $x = 0$ to $x=a$. Clearly the region is OAC.

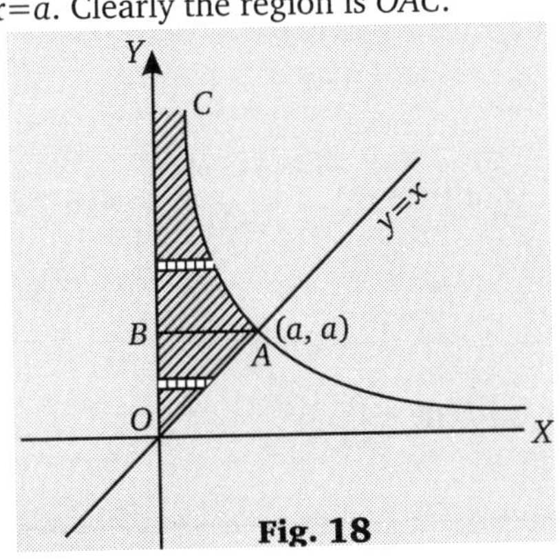

Fig. 18

Now draw a line AB parallel to x-axis, which divides the given region into two parts, OAB and BAC, Therefore, we draw a strip parallel to x-axis in OAB, where the left end of the strip is at y-axis and the right end is at $y = x$ and y takes the values from 0 to a. Also in region BAC, the left end of this strip is at y-axis whereas the right end is at the curve $y = a^2/x$, and y takes the values from $y = a$ to $y = \infty$. Hence ,the given integral becomes

$$\int_0^a \int_x^{a^2/x} \phi(x,y)\,dx\,dy$$
$$= \int_0^a \int_0^y \phi(x,y)\,dx\,dy + \int_a^\infty \int_0^{a^2/y} \phi(x,y)\,dx\,dy.$$

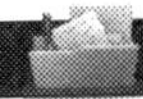

Exercise-17.6

Change the order of integration in the following integral (Ques. 1-9)

1. $\int_0^{a/2} \int_{x^2/2}^{x-x^2/a} dy\,dx$.

2. $\int_0^a \int_x^{a^3/x} f(x,y)\,dx\,dy$.

3. $\int_0^1 \int_x^{x(2-x)} f(x,y)\,dx\,dy$.

4. $\int_0^{a\cos\alpha} \int_{x\tan\alpha}^{\sqrt{a^2-x^2}} f(x,y)\,dx\,dy$.

5. $\int_0^a \int_{-mx}^{lx} f(x,y)\,dx\,dy$.

6. $\int_0^a \int_{(b/a)\sqrt{a^2-x^2}}^b f(x,y)\,dx\,dy$, where $c < a$.

7. $\int_0^{2a} \int_{\sqrt{2a-x^2}}^{\sqrt{2ax}} f(x,y)\,dx\,dy$.

8. $\int_0^{\pi/2} \int_0^{2a\cos\theta} f(r,\theta)\,r d\theta\,dr$.

9. $\int_0^a \int_0^{b/(b+x)} f(x,y)\,dx\,dy$.

10. Change the order of integration in $\int_0^\infty \int_0^\infty \frac{e^{-y}}{y}\,dx\,dy$ and hence find its value.

11. Change the order of integration in $\int_0^\infty \int_x^\infty f(x,y)\,dx\,dy$.

12. Change the order of integration in $\int_0^{2a} \int_{x(2a-x)/2a}^{\sqrt{2a-x^2}} f(x,y)\,dxdy$.

13. Change the order of integration and evaluate $\int_0^\infty \int_0^x xe^{-x^2/y}\,dx\,dy$.

14. Change the order of integration in $\int_0^a \int_{\sqrt{ax-x^2}}^{\sqrt{ax}} f(x,y)\,dx\,dy$.

15. Change the order of integration to evaluate $\int_0^1 \int_{2y}^2 e^{x^2}\,dx\,dy$. (GBTU-2010)

ANSWERS

1. $\int_0^{a/4} \int_{1/2\left[a-\sqrt{a^2-4ay}\right]}^{\sqrt{ay}} f(x,y)\,dy\,dx$.

2. $\int_0^a \int_0^y f(x,y)\,dy\,dx + \int_a^\infty \int_0^{a^2/y} f(x,y)\,dy\,dx$

3. $\int_0^1 \int_{1-\sqrt{1-y}}^y f(x,y)\,dy\,dx$.

4. $\int_0^{a\sin\alpha} \int_0^{y\cot\alpha} f(x,y)\,dy\,dx + \int_{a\sin\alpha}^a \int_0^{\sqrt{a^2-y^2}} f(x,y)\,dy\,dx$

5. $\int_0^{am} \int_{y/l}^{y/m} f(x,y)\,dy\,dx + \int_{am}^{al} \int_{y/l}^a f(x,y)\,dy\,dx$

6. $\int_0^{b\sqrt{1-(c^2/a^2)}} \int_{a\sqrt{1-y^2/b^2}}^{a} f(x,y)\,dy\,dx + \int_{b\sqrt{1-c^2/a^2}}^{b} \int_c^a f(x,y)\,dy\,dx$

7. $\int_0^a \int_{y^2/2a}^{a-\sqrt{a^2-y^2}} f(x,y)\,dy\,dx + \int_0^a \int_{a+\sqrt{a^2-y^2}}^{2a} f(x,y)\,dy\,dx + \int_a^{2a} \int_{y^2/2a}^{2a} f(x,y)\,dy\,dx$

8. $\int_0^{2a} \int_0^{\cos^{-1}(r/2a)} f(r,\theta)\,dr\,d\theta$

9. $\int_0^{b/(a+b)} \int_0^a f(x,y)\,dy\,dx + \int_{b/(a+b)}^{1} \int_0^{b(1-y)/y} f(x,y)\,dy\,dx$

10. 1

11. $\int_0^\infty \int_0^y f(x,y)\,dy\,dx$

12. $\int_0^{a/2} \int_{a-\sqrt{a^2-y^2}}^{a-\sqrt{a^2-2ay}} f(x,y)\,dx\,dy + \int_{a/2}^{a} \int_{a-\sqrt{a^2-y^2}}^{a+\sqrt{a^2-y^2}} f(x,y)\,dx\,dy + \int_a^{a/2} \int_{a+\sqrt{a^2-2ay}}^{a+\sqrt{a^2-y^2}} f(x,y)\,dx\,dy$

13. $\int_0^\infty \int_0^y xe^{-x^2/y}\,dx\,dy$

14. $\int_0^{a/2} \int_{y^2/a}^{a/2-\sqrt{(a^2/4)-y^2}} f(x,y)\,dx\,dy + \int_{a/2}^{a} \int_{y^2/a}^{a} f(x,y)\,dx\,dy + \int_0^{a/2} \int_{a/2+\sqrt{a^2/4-y^2}}^{a} f(x,y)\,dx\,dy$

15. e^2-3

❑❑❑❑❑❑

Chapter

18

Rectification of Curves

18.1 INTRODUCTION

Rectification is a process for finding the length of an arc of a plane curve between two given points on a curve.

18.2 FORMULAE FOR FINDING THE LENGTH OF THE CURVES

(a) Let the equation of a curve be $y = f(x)$ and let A and B be two points on this curve. Between A and B, the length of curve is to be required. Let s be the length of an arc from a fixed point on the curve to any point on it.

Therefore, we have

$$\frac{ds}{dx} = \pm\sqrt{\left[1+\left(\frac{dy}{dx}\right)^2\right]} \qquad \text{or} \qquad ds = \pm\sqrt{\left[1+\left(\frac{dy}{dx}\right)^2\right]}dx$$

where positive and negative sign will have to take according as x increases and decreases

as s increases. Thus, the length of an arc between the points A and B where at A, $x = a$ and at B, $x = b$ is given by

$$s = \int_a^b \sqrt{\left[1+\left(\frac{dy}{dx}\right)^2\right]}dx \qquad (a < b)$$

(b) If the equation of the curve is $x = f(y)$, then the length of an arc between c and d is given by

$$s = \int_c^d \sqrt{\left[1+\left(\frac{dx}{dy}\right)^2\right]}dy \qquad (c < d)$$

(c) If the equation of the curve is in parametric form, *i.e.*, $x = f(t)$, $y = g(t)$, then we have

$$\frac{ds}{dt} = \sqrt{\left[\left(\frac{dx}{dt}\right)^2+\left(\frac{dy}{dt}\right)^2\right]} \qquad \text{or} \qquad ds = \sqrt{\left(\frac{dx}{dt}\right)^2+\left(\frac{dy}{dt}\right)^2}\,dt$$

Thus the length of an arc between A and B where at point A, $t = t1$ and at point B, $t = t2$ is given by

$$s = \int_{t_1}^{t_2} \sqrt{\left[\left(\frac{dx}{dt}\right)^2+\left(\frac{dy}{dt}\right)^2\right]}dt$$

(d) If the equation of the curve is $r = f(\theta)$ (in polar form), then

$$\frac{ds}{d\theta} = \sqrt{\left[r^2 + \left(\frac{dr}{d\theta}\right)^2\right]} \quad \text{or} \quad ds = \sqrt{r^2 + \left(\frac{dr}{d\theta}\right)^2}\, d\theta$$

and s is measured in the direction of θ increasing. Let at point A, $\theta = \theta_1$ and at B, $\theta = \theta_2$. Therefore, the length of an arc between A and B is given by

$$s = \int_{\theta_1}^{\theta_2} \sqrt{\left[r^2 + \left(\frac{dr}{d\theta}\right)^2\right]} d\theta$$

(e) If the equation of the curve is $\theta = f(r)$, then the length of an arc between A and B is given by

$$s = \int_{r_1}^{r_2} \sqrt{\left[1 + \left(r\frac{d\theta}{dr}\right)^2\right]} dr$$

(f) If the equaton of the curve is in pedal form *i.e.*, $p = f(r)$. Since we know that

$$\frac{ds}{dr} = \frac{r}{\sqrt{(r^2 - p^2)}}$$

Then the length of an arc between $A(r = r_1)$ and $B(r = r_2)$ is given by

$$s = \int_{r_1}^{r_2} \frac{r\,dr}{\sqrt{(r^2 - p^2)}}$$

- If the curve is symmetrical about some line, then in order to find the length of an arc, we first find the length of one of the symmetrical part and multiply this length by the number of symmetrical parts.

Solved Examples

1. *Find the length of the arc of the parabola $y^2 = 4ax$ cut off by its latus rectum.*

(VTU–2008, MUMBAI–2006)

SOLUTION. **Latus rectum.** A line which passes through the focus of the given parabola and perpendicular to the axis of that parabola.

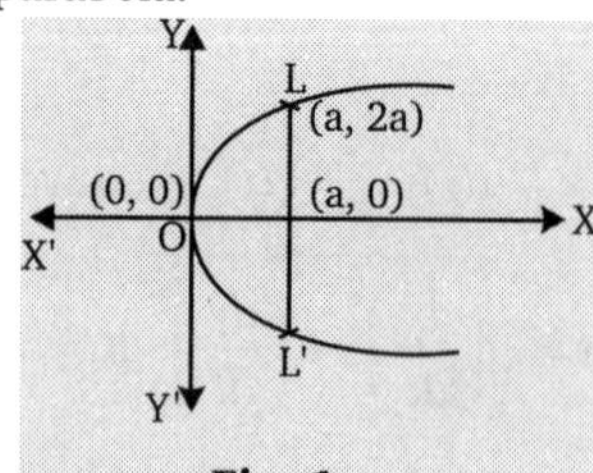

Fig. 1

Here the equation of the parabola is $y^2=4ax$ whose trace is shown above in the figure, LL' is the latus rectum, the co-ordinates of L and L' are respectively $(a, 2a)$ and $(a, -2a)$. Since $y^2=4ax$ is symmetrical about the line OX. Therefore the required arc length

$$= 2\times \text{ arc length } OL.$$

Since $\quad y^2 = 4ax.$

$\therefore \quad y = 2\sqrt{a}\sqrt{x}$

$\therefore \quad \frac{dy}{dx} = \frac{\sqrt{a}}{\sqrt{x}}.$

Now arc length

$$OL = \int_0^a \sqrt{\left[1 + \left(\frac{dy}{dx}\right)^2\right]} dx$$

($\because$ At point O, $x = 0$ and at point L, $x = a$)

$$= \int_0^a \sqrt{\left(1 + \frac{a}{x}\right)} dx = \int_0^a \frac{\sqrt{x+a}}{\sqrt{x}} dx$$

$$= \int_0^a \frac{x+a}{\sqrt{x^2+ax}} dx = \frac{1}{2}\int_0^a \frac{2x+2a}{\sqrt{(x^2+ax)}} dx$$

$$= \frac{1}{2}\int_0^a \frac{(2x+a)dx}{\sqrt{x^2+ax}} + \frac{a}{2}\int_0^a \frac{dx}{\sqrt{(x^2+ax)}}$$

$$= \frac{1}{2}\int_0^a \frac{(2x+a)dx}{\sqrt{x^2+ax}} + \frac{a}{2}\int_0^a \frac{dx}{\sqrt{\left[\left(x+\frac{a}{2}\right)^2 - \left(\frac{a}{2}\right)^2\right]}}$$

$$= \frac{1}{2}\left(2\sqrt{x^2+ax}\right)_0^a + \frac{a}{2}\left[\log\left\{\left(x+\frac{a}{2}\right)+\sqrt{x^2+ax}\right\}\right]_0^a$$

$$= a\sqrt{2} + \frac{a}{2}\log(3+2\sqrt{2})$$

$$= a\sqrt{2} + \frac{a}{2}\log(1+\sqrt{2})^2$$

Arc length $OL = a\sqrt{2} + a\log(1+\sqrt{2})$.

Hence the required arc length

$$= 2 \times \text{arc length } OL$$

$$= 2\sqrt{2}a + 2a\log(1+\sqrt{2}).$$

2. *Find the length of the curve $y = \log \sec x$ between the points $x = 0$ and $x = \pi/3$.*

(VTU–2010, PTU–2007)

SOLUTION. Since the equation of the curve is

$$y = \log \sec x$$

$$\therefore \quad \frac{dy}{dx} = \frac{1}{\sec x}.\sec x \tan x = \tan x.$$

Now $\sqrt{\left[1+\left(\frac{dy}{dx}\right)^2\right]} = \sqrt{(1+\tan^2 x)}$

$$= \sqrt{\sec^2 x} = \sec x.$$

Therefore the length of the given curve between $x = 0$ and $x = \pi/3$ is

$$s = \int_0^{\pi/3} \sqrt{\left[1+\left(\frac{dy}{dx}\right)^2\right]}dx$$

$$= \int_0^{\pi/3} \sec x dx$$

$$= \left[\log\left\{\tan\left(\frac{\pi}{4}+\frac{x}{2}\right)\right\}\right]_0^{\pi/3}$$

$$s = \log\left[\tan\left(\frac{\pi}{4}+\frac{\pi}{6}\right)\right] - \log\left[\tan\left(\frac{\pi}{4}\right)\right]$$

$$= \log\left[\frac{\tan\frac{\pi}{4}+\tan\frac{\pi}{6}}{1-\tan\frac{\pi}{4}\tan\frac{\pi}{6}}\right] - \log 1$$

$$\left[\because \tan\left(\frac{\pi}{4}+\theta\right) = \frac{1+\tan\theta}{1-\tan\theta}\right]$$

$$= \log\left[\frac{1+1/\sqrt{3}}{1-1/\sqrt{3}}\right] - 0 \qquad (\because \log 1 = 0)$$

$$= \log\left(\frac{\sqrt{3}+1}{\sqrt{3}-1}\right)$$

$$s = \log(2+\sqrt{3})$$

3. *Find the whole length of the astroid*

$$x^{2/3} + y^{2/3} = a^{2/3}.$$

or $\quad x = a\cos^3\theta, y = a\sin^3\theta$

(VTU–2010, RAJASTHAN–2006, MARATHWADA–2008)

SOLUTION. The equation of the curve is

$$x^{2/3} + y^{2/3} = a^{2/3} \qquad \ldots(1)$$

Since the curve is symmetrical about both the axis, *i.e.*, curve lies in all the four quadrants as shown in fig. 2.

Therefore the whole length of the given curve = 4 × arc length of the curve in first quadrant.

Since the co-ordinates of A and B are $(a, 0)$ and $(0, a)$ respectively. Thus in the first quadrant x varies from 0 to a.

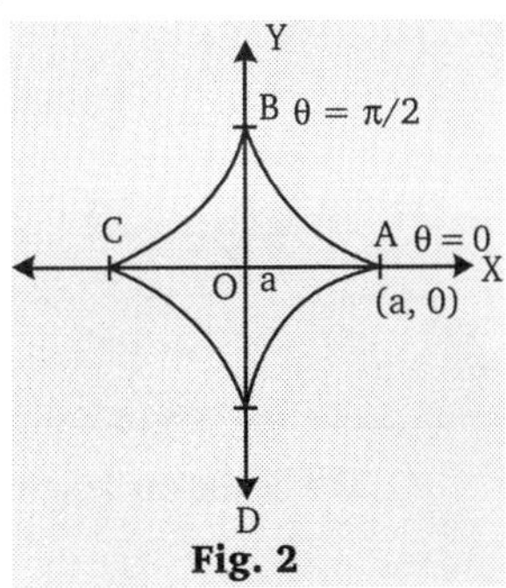

Fig. 2

Now differentiating (1) *w.r.t.* x, we get

$$\frac{2}{3}x^{-1/3} + \frac{2}{3}y^{-1/3}\frac{dy}{dx} = 0$$

or $$\frac{dy}{dx} = -\left(\frac{y}{x}\right)^{1/3}$$

Therefore, the length of the curve in the first quadrant

$$= \int_0^a \sqrt{\left[1+\left(\frac{dy}{dx}\right)^2\right]}dx = \int_0^a \sqrt{\left(1+\frac{y^{2/3}}{x^{2/3}}\right)}dx$$

$$= \int_0^a \sqrt{\left(\frac{x^{2/3}+y^{2/3}}{x^{2/3}}\right)}dx$$

$$= \int_0^a \sqrt{\left(\frac{a^{2/3}}{x^{2/3}}\right)}dx \qquad \text{[Using (1)]}$$

$$= a^{1/3}\int_0^a x^{-1/3}dx = a^{1/3}\left[\frac{3}{2}x^{2/3}\right]_0^a$$

$$= a^{1/3}\left[\frac{3}{2}a^{2/3}\right] = \frac{3}{2}a$$

Hence, the whole length of the astroid

$$= 4 \times \frac{3a}{2} = 6a$$

4. *Find the entire length of the cardioid*

$$r = a(1 + \cos\theta).$$

(PTU–2010, KURUKSHETRA–2005, BHOPAL–2008, BHILLAI–2005)

SOLUTION. From the equation of the cardioid $r = a(1 + \cos\theta)$ it is obvious, that the curve is symmetrical about the initial line (x-axis) and r will become zero, when $\theta = \pi$ and maximum, *i.e.*, $r = 2a$, when $\theta = 0$. Thus r varies from 0 to $2a$. As θ varies from π to 0. Therefore curve is shown in the fig.3.

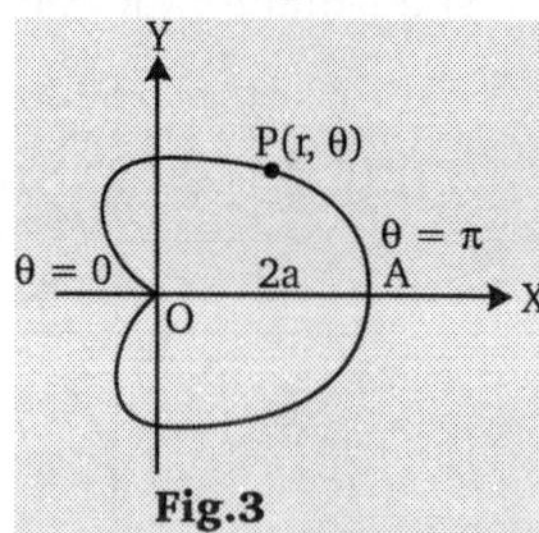

Fig.3

Let s be the arc length from O to any point $P(r, \theta)$.

∴ Entire length of the cardioid

= 2 × Arc length of the upper half of the cardioid.

Now the arc length of the upper half

$$= \int_\pi^0 \sqrt{\left[r^2+\left(\frac{dr}{d\theta}\right)^2\right]}d\theta \qquad \ldots(1)$$

Since we have

$$r = a\,(1 + \cos\theta).$$

$$\therefore \quad \frac{dr}{d\theta} = -a\sin\theta$$

and
$$\frac{ds}{d\theta} = \sqrt{\left[r^2+\left(\frac{dr}{d\theta}\right)^2\right]}$$

$$= \sqrt{a^2(1+\cos\theta)^2 + a^2\sin^2\theta}$$

$$= \sqrt{[2a^2(1+\cos\theta)]}$$

$$= \sqrt{\left[2a^2\left(2\cos^2\frac{\theta}{2}\right)\right]}$$

$$\frac{ds}{d\theta} = 2a\cos\theta/2.$$

Here we have to measure the arc length 's' from the cusp O where $\theta = \pi$ to any point $P(r, \theta)$ in the direction of θ decreasing, then the arc length 's' increases as θ decreases. Therefore, we will take $\frac{ds}{d\theta}$ to be negative. Thus from (1), we obtain

$$s = \int_\pi^0 \left(-2a\cos\frac{\theta}{2}\right)d\theta$$

$$= -2a\int_\pi^0 \cos\theta/2\,d\theta$$

$$= -2a\left[2\sin\frac{\theta}{2}\right]_\pi^0$$

$$= -4a\left[0-\sin\frac{\pi}{2}\right] = 4a.$$

Hence, the entire length of the given cardioid $= 2s = 8a$.

5. *Find the length of an arc of the curve*

$$x = a\,(t + \sin t),\ y = a(1 - \cos t)$$

(PTU–2009, VTU–2004)

SOLUTION. The given equation of the curve is

$$x = a\,(t + \sin t),\ y = a(1 - \cos t).$$

$$\therefore \quad \frac{dx}{dt} = a(1+\cos t), \frac{dy}{dt} = a\sin t.$$

Since,

$$\left(\frac{ds}{dt}\right)^2 = \left(\frac{dx}{dt}\right)^2 + \left(\frac{dy}{dt}\right)^2$$

$$= a^2(1+\cos t)^2 + a^2\sin^2 t$$

$$= 2a^2(1+\cos t)$$

$$\therefore \quad \left(\frac{ds}{dt}\right)^2 = 4a^2\cos^2 t/2$$

From the equation of the curve it is obvious when cos $t = 1$, $y = 0$ *i.e.*, when $t=0$, $y=0$. This implies when $t = 0$, $x = 0$ and $y = 0$. Therefore the curve will passes through the point (0, 0) and at the point (0, 0) tangent is the x-axis. Also y will always positive. Thus the tracing of the given curve is shown in fig. 4.

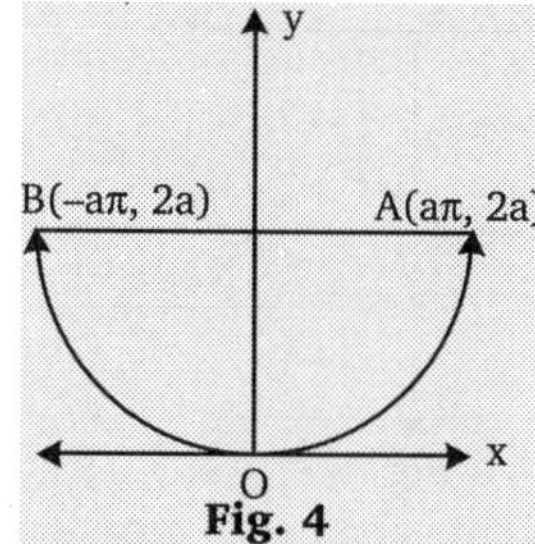

Fig. 4

From the fig. 4 it is obvious that the curve is symmetrical about the y-axis. Therefore, the entire length of the arc of the given curve will be twice of the arc OA. At O, $t = 0$ and at A, $t = \pi$.

Let s be the arc length measured from O to any point P on the curve towards the point A, then s increases as t increases so that $\frac{ds}{dt}$ will be taken positive.

$\therefore$ Arc length OA

$$= \int_0^{\pi}\frac{ds}{dt}.dt = \int_0^{\pi} 2a\cos t/2\,dt \text{ [Using(1)]}$$

$$= 2a\left[2\sin t/2\right]_0^{\pi} = 4a.$$

Hence, the entire length of the given curve $= 2 \times$ arc $OA = 2 \times 4a = 8a$.

6. *Find the length of the curve* $x\sin\theta + y\cos\theta = f'(\theta)$ *and* $x\cos\theta - y\sin\theta = f''(\theta)$.

SOLUTION. We have

$$x\sin\theta + y\cos\theta = f'(\theta) \qquad \ldots(1)$$

$$x\cos\theta - y\sin\theta = f''(\theta) \qquad \ldots(2)$$

Solving (1) and (2), we have

$$x = \sin\theta f'(\theta) + \cos\theta f''(\theta)$$

and $y = \cos\theta f'(\theta) - \sin\theta f''(\theta)$

$$\therefore \quad \frac{dx}{d\theta} = \cos\theta f'(\theta) + \sin\theta f''(\theta) - \sin\theta f''(\theta) + \cos\theta f'''(\theta)$$

$$= \cos\theta f'(\theta) + \cos\theta f'''(\theta)$$

and
$$\frac{dy}{d\theta} = \cos\theta f''(\theta) - \sin\theta f'(\theta) - \cos\theta f''(\theta) - \sin\theta f'''(\theta)$$

$$= -\sin\theta f'(\theta) - \sin\theta f'''(\theta)$$

If s is the arc length of the curve in the direction of θ increasing, then

$$\left(\frac{ds}{d\theta}\right)^2 = \left(\frac{dx}{d\theta}\right)^2 + \left(\frac{dy}{d\theta}\right)^2$$

$$= \{\cos\theta[f'(\theta) + f''(\theta)]\}^2 + \{-\sin\theta[f'(\theta) + f'''(\theta)]\}^2$$

$$= [f'(\theta) + f'''(\theta)]^2(\cos^2\theta + \sin^2\theta)$$

$$= [f'(\theta) + f'''(\theta)]^2$$

$$\therefore \quad \frac{ds}{d\theta} = f'(\theta) + f'''(\theta)$$

Now integrating both sides *w.r.t.* θ, we get

$$s = \int[f'(\theta) + f'''(\theta)]d\theta + c$$

$$= f(\theta) + f''(\theta) + c,$$

where c is a constant of integration.

7. *Find the length of the curve* $y = \log\frac{e^x - 1}{e^x + 1}$ *from* $x = 1$ *to* $x = 2$.

SOLUTION. We have $y = \log\frac{e^x - 1}{e^x + 1}$

$$= \log(e^x - 1) - \log(e^x + 1).$$

Differentiating w.r.t. x, we get

$$\frac{dy}{dx} = \frac{e^x}{e^x - 1} - \frac{e^x}{e^x + 1} = \frac{2e^x}{e^{2x} - 1}.$$

If s is the arc length of the curve in the direction of x increasing, then

$$\left(\frac{ds}{dx}\right)^2 = 1 + \left(\frac{dy}{dx}\right)^2 = 1 + \left(\frac{2e^x}{e^{2x} - 1}\right)^2$$

$$= 1 + \frac{4e^{2x}}{(e^{2x} - 1)^2}$$

$$= \frac{(e^{2x} - 1)^2 + 4e^{2x}}{(e^{2x} - 1)^2} = \left(\frac{e^{2x} + 1}{e^{2x} - 1}\right)^2.$$

$$\therefore \quad \frac{ds}{dx} = \frac{e^{2x} + 1}{e^{2x} - 1}.$$

Integrating *w.r.t.* x from $x = 1$ to $x = 2$, we get

$$s = \int_1^2 \frac{e^{2x}+1}{e^{2x}-1}dx = \int_1^2 \frac{e^x + e^{-x}}{e^x - e^{-x}}dx$$
$$= \left[\log(e^x - e^{-x})\right]_1^2$$
$$= \log(e^2 - e^{-2}) - \log(e^1 - e^{-1})$$
$$= \log\left[\frac{e^2 - e^{-2}}{e^1 - e^{-1}}\right]$$
$$= \log\frac{(e^1 - e^{-1})(e^1 + e^{-1})}{(e^1 - e^{-1})}$$
$$[\because a^2 - b^2 = (a-b)(a+b)]$$

$\therefore\ s = \log(e^1 + e^{-1})$.

8. *Find the length of the arc of the equiangular spiral $r = ae^{\theta \cot \alpha}$ between the points for which radii vectors are r_1 and r_2.*

SOLUTION. Since we have

$$r = ae^{\theta \cot \alpha} \qquad \ldots(1)$$

Now differentiating (1) *w.r.t.* θ, we get

$$\frac{dr}{d\theta} = a\cot\alpha e^{\theta\cot\alpha} = r\cot\alpha.$$

If s is the arc length of the spiral in the direction of r increasing, then

$$\frac{ds}{dr} = \sqrt{\left[1 + \left(r\frac{d\theta}{dr}\right)^2\right]}$$
$$= \sqrt{(1+\tan^2\alpha)}$$
$$\left(\because r\frac{d\theta}{dr} = \tan\alpha\right)$$
$$= \sqrt{(\sec^2\alpha)}$$
$$\frac{ds}{dr} = \sec\alpha \Rightarrow ds = \sec\alpha\, dr$$

Now integrating *w.r.t.* r from $r = r_1$ to $r = r_2$, we get

$$s = \int_{r_1}^{r_2} \sec\alpha\, dr = \sec\alpha \int_{r_1}^{r_2} dr$$
$$= \sec\alpha\left[r\right]_{r_1}^{r_2} = (r_2 - r_1)\sec\alpha$$

9. *Find the length of the loop of the curve*

$$3ay^2 = x(x-a)^2.$$

SOLUTION. The equation of the curve is

$$3ay^2 = x(x-a)^2. \qquad \ldots(1)$$

This curve is symmetrical about the x-axis and passes through the origin. The tangent at (0, 0) is the y-axis. The curve cuts the x-axis only at the point $(a, 0)$.

Now differentiating (1) *w.r.t. x, we get*

$$\frac{dy}{dx} = \frac{3x - a}{2\sqrt{3ax}}. \qquad \ldots(2)$$

$\therefore$ At $(a, 0)$ $\frac{dy}{dx} = \pm\frac{1}{\sqrt{3}}$. Thus at $(a, 0)$, tangents make the angles $\pi/6$ and $-\pi/6$ with positive x-axis.

Therefore, we have

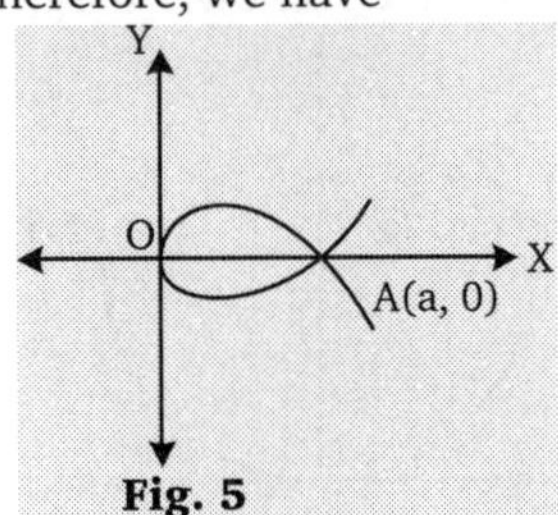

Fig. 5

If s is the arc length measured from 0 to any point on the curve in the direction of x-increasing. Then we will take $\frac{ds}{dx}$ positive.

$$\therefore\ \frac{ds}{dx} = \sqrt{\left[1 + \left(\frac{dy}{dx}\right)^2\right]}$$
$$= \sqrt{\left[1 + \frac{(3x-a)^2}{12ax}\right]}$$
$$= \sqrt{\left(\frac{12ax + 9x^2 + a^2 - 6xa}{12ax}\right)}$$
$$\Rightarrow \quad \frac{ds}{dx} = \frac{3x+a}{2\sqrt{3ax}}.$$

If s_1 denotes the length of the loop of the curve between the points $x = 0$ to $x = a$. Therefore, we have

$$s_1 = 2\int_0^a \left(\frac{ds}{dx}\right).dx$$

or
$$s_1 = 2\int_0^a \frac{3x+a}{2\sqrt{3ax}}dx$$
$$= \frac{1}{\sqrt{3a}}\int_0^a \frac{3x+a}{\sqrt{x}}dx$$
$$= \frac{1}{\sqrt{3a}}\int_0^a (3x^{1/2} + ax^{-1/2})dx$$
$$= \frac{1}{\sqrt{3a}}\left[2x^{3/2} + 2ax^{1/2}\right]_0^a$$

$$= \frac{1}{\sqrt{3a}}[2a\sqrt{a} + 2a\sqrt{a}]$$

$$= \frac{4a\sqrt{a}}{\sqrt{3}\sqrt{a}}$$

Hence, $s_1 = \dfrac{4a}{\sqrt{3}}$

10. *Find the length of the cardioid $r = a(1 - \cos\theta)$ lying outside the circle $r = a \cos\theta$.*

SOLUTION. Both curves intersect. Therefore, we have $a(1 - \cos\theta) = a\cos\theta$

or $\quad 2\cos\theta = 1$ or $\cos\theta = \dfrac{1}{2}$

or $\quad \theta = \pm\dfrac{\pi}{3}$

$\therefore$ The intersection points are $\left(\dfrac{a}{2}, \dfrac{\pi}{3}\right)$ and $\left(\dfrac{a}{2}, -\dfrac{\pi}{3}\right)$:

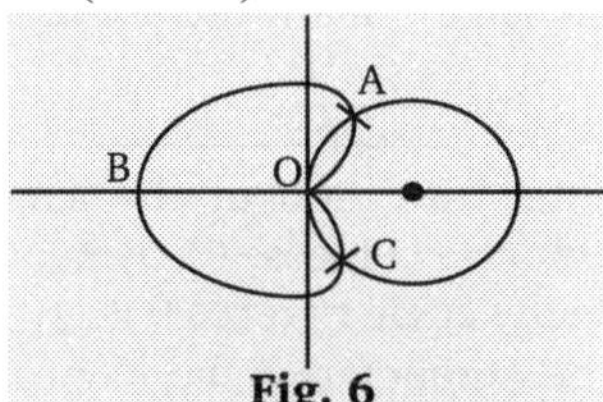

Fig. 6

The equation of the cardioid is

$$r = a(1 - \cos\theta)$$

$$\therefore \quad \frac{dr}{d\theta} = a\sin\theta$$

$$\Rightarrow \quad \frac{ds}{d\theta} = \sqrt{\left[r^2 + \left(\frac{dr}{d\theta}\right)^2\right]}$$

$$= \sqrt{[a^2(1-\cos\theta)^2 + a^2\sin^2\theta]}$$

or $\quad \dfrac{ds}{d\theta} = 2a\sin\theta/2.$

Since s is the arc length of the cardioid to any point $P(r, \theta)$ in the direction of θ increasing so we will take $\dfrac{ds}{d\theta}$ positive. But we have to find the length of the cardioid lying outside the circle. Therefore if s_1 is the required length, then

$s_1 = 2\times$ upper portion of the cardioid from A to B.

At the point A, $\theta = \pi/3$ and at B, $\theta = \pi$.

$$\therefore \quad s_1 = 2\int_{\pi/3}^{\pi}\left(\frac{ds}{d\theta}\right).d\theta$$

$$= 2\int_{\pi/3}^{\pi} 2a\sin\theta/2\,d\theta$$

$$= 4a\left[-2\cos\theta/2\right]_{\pi/3}^{\pi}$$

$$= 4a\left[-2\cos\frac{\pi}{2} + 2\cos\frac{\pi}{6}\right]$$

$$= 4a\left[2.\frac{\sqrt{3}}{2}\right]$$

Hence, $\quad s_1 = 4a\sqrt{3}.$

Similar Problems

(1) Prove that the line $4r\cos\theta = 3a$ divides the cardioid $r = a(1 + \cos\theta)$ into two equal lengths of the arc.

(2) If s be the length of the curve $r = a\tanh\dfrac{\theta}{2}$ between the origin and $\theta = 2\pi$, and Δ be the area under the curve between the same two points, prove that $\Delta = a(s - a\pi)$.

Exercise-18.1

1. Find the whole length of the curve $x^2 + y^2 = b^2$.
2. Find the length of the arc of the curve $x^2 = 8y$ from the vertex to an extremity of the latusrectum.
3. Find the arc length of the curve $y = \dfrac{1}{2}x^2 - \dfrac{1}{4}\log x$ from $x = 1$ to $x = 2$.
4. Find the length of the arc from $\theta = 0$ to $\theta = 2\pi$ of the curve $x = a(\cos\theta + \theta\sin\theta), y = a(\sin\theta - \theta\cos\theta)$.
5. Find the length of the arc of the curve $ay^2 = x^3$ between the points $(0, 0)$ and (a, a).
6. Show that the length of the curve $$x = e^{\theta}\left(\sin\frac{\theta}{2} + 2\cos\frac{\theta}{2}\right), y = e^{\theta}\left(\cos\frac{\theta}{2} - 2\sin\frac{\theta}{2}\right)$$ between $\theta = 0$ to $\theta = \pi$ is $\dfrac{5}{2}(e^{\pi} - 1)$.
7. Show that the length of the arc of the curve $y^2 = 4ax$ which is intercepted between the points of intersection of the curve and the line $3y = 8x$ is $a(\log 2 + 15/16)$.

8. Find the length of the loop of the curve $9ay^2 = (x-2a)(x-5a)^2$.

9. Find the length of an arc of the curve
$$x = a\left(\sin t + \frac{1}{3}\sin 3t\right), y = a\left(\cos t - \frac{1}{3}\cos 3t\right)$$
between $t = 0$ and $t = \pi/4$.

10. Find the whole length of the hypo-cycloid $x = a \cos^3 t, y = b \sin^3 t$.

11. Find the length of the loop of the curve $x = t^2, y = t - \frac{1}{3}t^3$.

12. Show that the whole length of the curve $x^2(a^2 - x^2) = 8a^2y^2$ is $\pi a^2\sqrt{2}$.

13. Find the length of an arc of the cycloid
$$x = a(\theta - \sin\theta), y = a(1 - \cos\theta).$$
(VTU–2004, PTU–2009)

14. Find the length of the arc of the curve $x = e^\theta \sin\theta$, $y = e^\theta \cos\theta$ between $\theta = 0$ to $\theta = \pi/2$.

15. Find the entire length of the cardioid $r = a(1 - \cos\theta)$.

16. Show that the arc of the upper half of the curve $r = a(1 - \cos\theta)$ is bisected by $\theta = 2\pi/3$.

17. In the ellipse $x = a\cos\theta$, $y = b\sin\theta$, show that $ds = a\sqrt{(1 - e^2\cos^2\theta)}d\theta$, and hence show that the whole length of the ellipse is
$$2\pi a\left[1 - \left(\frac{1}{2}\right)^2 \cdot \frac{e^2}{1} - \left(\frac{1.3}{2.4}\right)^2 \cdot \frac{e^4}{3} - \left(\frac{1.3.5}{2.4.6}\right)^2 \cdot \frac{e^6}{5} - \ldots\right].$$

18. Find the perimeter of curve $r = a(1 + \cos\theta)$ and show that the arc of the upper half is bisected by $\theta = \pi/3$. (JNTU–2003)

19. Prove that the perimeter of the limacon $r = a + b\cos\theta$, $a > b$ is approximately $2\pi a(1 + b^2/4a^2)$.

20. Find the length of the arc of the curve $r = ae^{\theta \cot \alpha}$ taking $s = 0$ when $\theta = 0$.

21. Show that $\theta = \pi/3$ divides the length of the cycloid $x = a(\theta - \sin\theta)$, $y = a(1 - \cos\theta)$ in the ratio 1:3.

22. Find the length of the arc of the curve
$$x = a(3\sin\theta - \sin^3\theta), y = a\cos^3\theta$$
between $\theta = 0$ and $\theta = \pi/2$.

23. Find the length of the arc of the curve $x = a\sin 2\theta(1 + \cos 2\theta)$, $y = a\cos 2\theta(1 - \cos 2\theta)$ between $\theta = 0$ and $\theta = \pi/2$.

24. Show that $\theta = \pi/6$ divides the arc in the first quadrant of the curve $x = a\cos^3\theta$, $y = a\sin^3\theta$ in the ratio 1:3.

25. Find the length of any arc of the cissoid
$$r = \frac{a\sin^2\theta}{\cos\theta}.$$

26. Show that the ratio of the lengths of the cardioid $r = a(1 - \cos\theta)$ lying inside and outside the circle $r = a\cos\theta$ is $(2 - \sqrt{3}) : \sqrt{3}$.

27. Find the perimeter of the loop of the curve $3ay^2 = x^2(a - x)$.

28. Show that the length of the arc of the curve $x\cos\theta - y\sin\theta = f''(\theta)$, $x\sin\theta + y\cos\theta = f(\theta)$ is given by $S = f(\theta) = \text{constant}$.

Hints to the Selected Problems

1. The given equation of the curve $x^2 + y^2 = b^2$, which is a circle.

$\therefore$ Therefore, $s = 4\int_0^b \frac{ds}{dx}dx$.

Here $\frac{dy}{dx} = -\left(\frac{x}{y}\right)$ which implies
$$\frac{ds}{dx} = \sqrt{1 + \left(\frac{dy}{dx}\right)^2} = \frac{b}{\sqrt{b^2 - x^2}}.$$

2. Let s be the length from the vertex (0, 0) to $L(4,2)$. Then, we have

$s = \int_0^4 \frac{ds}{dx}dx$ and using
$$\int\sqrt{16 + x^2}dx = \frac{x}{2}\sqrt{16 + x^2}$$
$$= 8\log\left(x + \sqrt{16x^2}\right)$$
Then proceed as in (1).

4. $\frac{dx}{d\theta} = a\theta\cos\theta, \frac{dy}{d\theta} = a\theta\sin\theta$

$\Rightarrow \frac{dy}{dx} = \tan\theta$. Therefore,
$$\frac{ds}{dx} = \sqrt{1 + \left(\frac{dy}{dx}\right)^2} = \sqrt{1 + \tan^2\theta} = \sec\theta.$$
Then obtained the arc using the following formula $s = \int_0^{2\pi} \frac{ds}{dx}.dx$.

5. $\frac{dy}{dx} = \frac{3x^2}{2ay}$
$$\therefore \frac{ds}{dx} = \sqrt{1 + \left(\frac{dy}{dx}\right)^2} = \sqrt{1 + \frac{9x}{4a}}$$
Now using the following formula $s = \int_0^a \frac{ds}{dx}.dx$.

6. $\frac{dx}{d\theta} = \frac{5}{2}e^\theta\cos\frac{\theta}{2}, \quad \frac{dy}{d\theta} = -\frac{5}{2}e^\theta\sin\frac{\theta}{2}$
$$\Rightarrow \frac{dy}{dx} = \frac{dy/d\theta}{dx/d\theta} = -\tan\frac{\theta}{2}$$

$\therefore \quad \frac{ds}{dx} = \sqrt{1+\tan^2\theta/2} = \sec\frac{\theta}{2}.$

Now $\frac{ds}{d\theta} = \frac{ds}{dx}\cdot\frac{dx}{d\theta} = \frac{5}{2}e^{\theta}$. Now using the formula $s = \int_0^{\pi}\frac{ds}{d\theta}d\theta.$

7. The points of intersection of the given curves are (0, 0) and $\left(\frac{9a}{16}, \frac{3a}{2}\right)$.

Also $\frac{dy}{dx} = \frac{2a}{y}$. Now find $\frac{ds}{dx}$ and then use the formula, $s = \int_0^{9a/16}\frac{ds}{dx}.dx$.

10. $\frac{dx}{dt} = -3a\cos^2 t\sin^2 t, \frac{dy}{dt} = 3b\sin^2 t\cos t$

$\therefore \frac{ds}{dt} = \sqrt{\left(\frac{dx}{dt}\right)^2+\left(\frac{dy}{dt}\right)^2} \quad \therefore s = 4\int_0^{\pi/2}\frac{ds}{dt}.dt$

11. Eliminate t between the given curve, we get $9y^2 = x(3-x)^2$.

Now $\quad \frac{dx}{dt} = 2t, \frac{dy}{dt} = (1-t^2).$

Then use $\frac{ds}{dt} = \sqrt{\left(\frac{dx}{dt}\right)^2+\left(\frac{dy}{dt}\right)^2}$

and $s = 2\int_0^{\sqrt{3}}\frac{ds}{dt}.dt$

15. $\frac{dr}{d\theta} = a\sin\theta.$

Since the given curve is symmetrical about the initial line, therefore, the entire length is twice the arc measure from 0 to π.

Here, $\frac{ds}{d\theta} = \sqrt{r^2+\left(\frac{dr}{d\theta}\right)^2} = 2a\sin\frac{\theta}{2}$. Then using the formula, we get $s = 2\int_0^{\pi}\frac{ds}{d\theta}.d\theta.$

26. The points of the intersection of the given curve are $\theta = \pm\frac{\pi}{3}$.

Let s_1 be the arc length of the cardioid inside the circle and s_2 be the arc length of the cardioid outside of the circle.

Therefore, $s_1 = 2\int_0^{\pi/3}\frac{ds}{d\theta}.d\theta$

and $s_2 = 2\int_{\pi/3}^{\pi}\frac{ds}{d\theta}.d\theta$

27. Do same as ex. 9 by taking $a = 1$.

28. Do same as ex. 6.

ANSWERS

1. $2\pi b$ **2.** $2[\sqrt{2}+\log(1+\sqrt{2})]$ **3.** $\frac{3}{2}+\frac{1}{4}\log 2$ **4.** $2a\pi^2$ **5.** $\frac{1}{27}a[13\sqrt{13}-8]$

8. $4a\sqrt{3}$ **9.** a **10.** $4(a^2+ab+b^2)/(a+b)$ **11.** $4\sqrt{3}$ **13.** $8a$

14. $\sqrt{2}[e^{\pi/2}-1]$ **15.** $8a$ **18.** $8a$ **20.** $a\sec\alpha\,(e^{\theta\cot\alpha}-1)$ **22.** $3a\pi/4$

23. $4a/3$ **25.** $s_1(\theta_2)-s_1(\theta_1)$ where $s_1(\theta) = a\sqrt{(\sec^2\theta+3)} - a\sqrt{3}[\log\{\cos\theta+\sqrt{(\cos^2\theta+\frac{1}{3})}\}]$

27. $\frac{4a}{\sqrt{3}}$

18.3 INTRINSIC EQUATION OF CURVES

The relation between s and ψ is called an intrinsic equation of any curve, where s is the length of an arc of the curve measured from a fixed point on the curve to any point P on it and ψ is the angle which the tangent to the curve at P makes with the positive x-axis. Thus the co-ordinates (s, ψ) is known as Intrinsic co-ordinates.

18.4 DERIVATION OF INTRINSIC EQUATION OF THE CURVES

(a) If the equation of a curve is in cartesian form. Let the equation of the curve be $y = f(x)$ as shown in fig. 7.

Let us consider a point A as fixed on this curve and let $P(x, y)$ be any point on this curve such that $AP = s$. Suppose the tangent at P makes the angle ψ with the fixed straight line (*i.e.*, x-axis). Since, we have

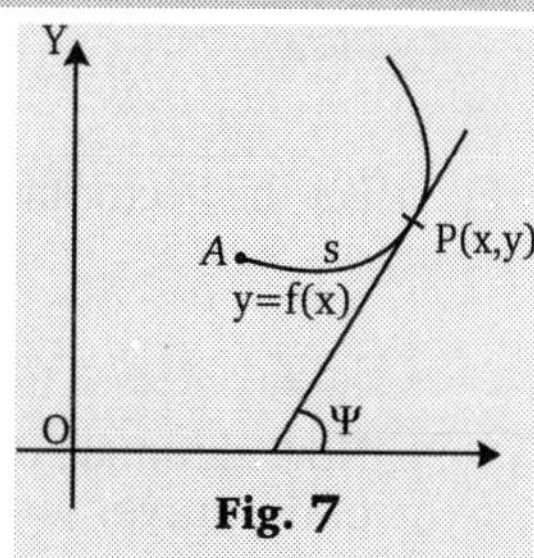

Fig. 7

$$\frac{dy}{dx} = \tan\psi\,\cdot$$

$$\therefore \qquad \tan\psi = \frac{d}{dx} f(x) = f'(x). \qquad \ldots(1)$$

Further since we know that $\dfrac{ds}{dx} = \sqrt{\left[1 + \left(\dfrac{dy}{dx}\right)^2\right]}$. ...(2)

Let x_1 be the x-co-ordinate of the fixed point A. Therefore, we have

$$s = \int_a^{x_1} \left(\frac{ds}{dx}\right) dx \quad \text{or} \quad s = \int_a^{x_1} \sqrt{\left[1 + \left(\frac{dy}{dx}\right)^2\right]} dx \qquad \text{[Using (2)]}$$

or $$s = \int_a^{x_1} \sqrt{1 + [f'(x)]^2}\, dx \qquad \text{[Using (1)]} \qquad \ldots(3)$$

Now eliminate x and $f'(x)$ between (1) and (3), we obtain the relation between s and ψ and thus obtain the intrinsic equations.

- If $x = f(t), y = g(t)$, then $\dfrac{dy}{dx} = \dfrac{dy}{dt} \Big/ \dfrac{dx}{dt}$.

(b) Equations of a curve in polar form. Let the equations of a curve be $r = f(\theta)$ and consider a point A as fixed on this curve. Let $P(r, \theta)$ be any point on this curve such that arc $AP = s$ and the tangent at P makes an angle ψ with the positive x-axis as shown in fig. 8.

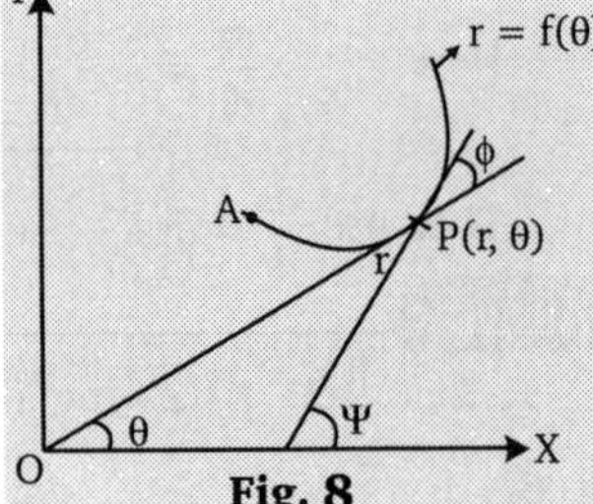

Fig. 8

Let ϕ be the angle between the radius vector and the tangent at P. Thus, we have

$$\psi = \theta + \phi \qquad \ldots(1)$$

Since we know that

$$\tan\phi = r\frac{d\theta}{dr}. \qquad \ldots(2)$$

But, the equation of a curve is

$$\left.\begin{aligned} r &= f(\theta) \\ \therefore \quad \frac{dr}{d\theta} &= f'(\theta) \end{aligned}\right\} \qquad \ldots(3)$$

Now using (2) and (3), we get

$$\tan\phi = \frac{f(\theta)}{f'(\theta)}. \qquad \ldots(4)$$

Now $$\frac{ds}{d\theta} = \sqrt{\left[r^2 + \left(\frac{dr}{d\theta}\right)^2\right]}. \Rightarrow \quad \frac{ds}{d\theta} = \sqrt{[[f(\theta)]^2 + [f'(\theta)]^2]}. \qquad \ldots(5)$$

Let the vectorial angle of the point A be α. Then, we have

$$s = \int_\alpha^\theta \left(\frac{ds}{d\theta}\right) d\theta \quad \Rightarrow \quad s = \int_\alpha^\theta \sqrt{[\{f(\theta)\}^2 + \{f'(\theta)\}^2]}\, d\theta \qquad \ldots(6)$$

[Using (5)]

Now eliminate θ and ϕ between (1), (4) and (6), we obtain the required intrinsic equation of the curve.

(c) Equation of curve in Pedal form. Let the equation of a curve in pedal form be $p=f(r)$ and let A be the fixed point on the curve such that at A, $r = a$ (say), then, we have

$$s = \int_a^r \frac{rdr}{\sqrt{(r^2 - p^2)}} \Rightarrow s = \int_a^r \frac{rdr}{\sqrt{[r^2 - \{f(r)\}^2]}} \quad ...(1)$$

where s is an arc measured from A to any point $P(p, r)$. Let ρ be the radius of curvature of the given curve at P, then we have $\rho = \frac{ds}{d\psi} = r\frac{dr}{dp} = r / f'(r)$. ...(2)

Now eliminating r between (1) and (2), we obtain the required intrinsic equation.

Solved Examples

1. *Show that the intrinsic equation of the curve $x = a(t + \sin t)$, $y = a(1 - \cos t)$ is $s = 4a \sin \psi$.*

SOLUTION. Since, we have

$$x = a(t + \sin t),\ y = a(1 - \cos t)$$

$$\therefore \frac{dx}{dt} = a(1 + \cos t), \frac{dy}{dt} = a \sin t$$

$$\therefore \frac{dy}{dx} = \frac{dy}{dt}\Big/\frac{dx}{dt} = \frac{\sin t}{1 + \cos t}$$

$$= \frac{2 \sin t/2 \cos t/2}{2\cos^2 t/2} = \tan t/2$$

Since, we know that $\frac{dy}{dx} = \tan\psi$.

$$\tan\psi = \tan t/2$$

or $\psi = t/2$ or $t = 2\psi$.

If s is the length of the arc of the curve measured from the vertex $A(0, 0)$ to any point $P(x, y)$ in the direction of t increasing, then

$$s = \int_0^t \left(\frac{ds}{dt}\right).dt$$

or $s = \int_0^t \sqrt{\left[\left(\frac{dx}{dt}\right)^2 + \left(\frac{dy}{dt}\right)^2\right]}.dt$

where $\left(\frac{ds}{dt}\right)^2 = \left(\frac{dx}{dt}\right)^2 + \left(\frac{dy}{dt}\right)^2$

$$\therefore s = \int_0^t \sqrt{[a^2(1 + \cos t)^2 + a^2 \sin^2 t]}.dt$$

$$= \int_0^t 2a \cos t/2\, dt$$

$$s = 2a[2 \sin t/2]_0^t = 4a \sin t/2$$

But $t = 2\psi$.

$$\therefore \quad s = 4a \sin\psi.$$

2. *Show that the intrinsic equation $3ay^2 = 2x^3$ taking its cusp as the fixed point is $9s = 4a(\sec^3\psi - 1)$.*

SOLUTION. The equation of the curve is

$$3ay^2 = 2x^3 \text{ or } y = \frac{\sqrt{2}x^{3/2}}{\sqrt{3a}}$$

$$\therefore \frac{dy}{dx} = \sqrt{\frac{2}{3a}}.\frac{3}{2}x^{1/2} = \sqrt{\frac{3x}{2a}}.$$

Further since, we have

$$\frac{dy}{dx} = \tan\psi$$

$$\therefore \tan\psi = \sqrt{\frac{3x}{2a}} \text{ or } x = \frac{2a}{3}\tan^2\psi \quad ...(1)$$

But $\frac{ds}{dx} = \sqrt{\left[1 + \left(\frac{dy}{dx}\right)^2\right]} = \sqrt{\left[1 + \frac{3x}{2a}\right]}$.

If s is the arc length of the given curve measure from the cusp at which $x = 0$ to any point $P(x, y)$ in the direction of x decreasing. Then

$$\frac{ds}{dx} = \sqrt{\left(1 + \frac{3x}{2a}\right)} \quad ...(2)$$

$$\therefore \quad s = \int_0^x \left(\frac{ds}{dx}\right)dx$$

or $s = \int_0^x \sqrt{\left(1 + \frac{3x}{2a}\right)}dx$ [Using (2)]

$$= \left[\frac{\frac{2}{3}\left(1+\frac{3x}{2a}\right)^{3/2}}{3/2a} \right]_0^x$$

$$\Rightarrow \quad s = \frac{4a}{9}\left[\left(1+\frac{3x}{2a}\right)^{3/2} - 1\right] \quad ...(3)$$

Now eliminating x between (1) and (3), we get

$$s = \frac{4a}{9}\left[(1+\tan^2\psi)^{3/2} - 1\right]$$

$$s = \frac{4a}{9}[\sec^3\psi - 1]$$

or $9s = 4a[\sec^3\psi - 1]$.

3. *Find the intrinsic equation of the cardioid $r = a(1 - \cos\theta)$.*

SOLUTION. The equation of the curve is

$$r = a(1 - \cos\theta). \quad ...(1)$$

$$\therefore \quad \frac{dr}{d\theta} = a\sin\theta.$$

$$\text{Now, } \frac{ds}{d\theta} = \sqrt{\left[r^2 + \left(\frac{dr}{d\theta}\right)^2\right]}$$

$$= \sqrt{[a^2(1-\cos\theta)^2 + a^2\sin^2\theta]}$$

$$= \sqrt{2a^2(1-\cos\theta)} = \pm 2a\sin\theta/2.$$

If s is the length of the arc of the curve measured from pole (0, 0) to any point $P(r, \theta)$ in the direction of θ increasing, then we will take the sign of $\frac{ds}{d\theta}$ positive.

$$s = \int_0^\theta \left(\frac{ds}{d\theta}\right) d\theta = \int_0^\theta 2a\sin(\theta/2)d\theta$$

$$= 2a\left[-2\cos(\theta/2)\right]_0^\theta$$

$$s = 4a(1-\cos(\theta/2)) \quad ...(2)$$

Further since, we know that

$$\tan\phi = r\frac{d\theta}{dr} = a(1-\cos\theta).\frac{1}{a\sin\theta}$$

$$= \frac{1-\cos\theta}{\sin\theta} = \frac{2\sin^2(\theta/2)}{2\sin(\theta/2)\cos(\theta/2)}$$

$$\therefore \quad \tan\phi = \tan\theta/2$$

$$\therefore \quad \phi = \theta/2 \quad \text{or} \quad \theta = 2\phi.$$

But we have

$$\psi = \theta + \phi = \theta + \theta/2 \quad (\because \phi = \theta/2)$$

$$\psi = \frac{3}{2}\theta \text{ or } \theta = \frac{2}{3}\psi.$$

Substitute the value of θ in (2), we get

$$s = 4a\left(1 - \cos\frac{2}{6}\psi\right)$$

$$= 4a\left(2\sin^2\frac{1}{6}\psi\right)$$

Hence, $s = 8a\sin^2\left(\frac{\psi}{6}\right)$.

4. *Find the intrinsic equation of the curve $p = r\sin\alpha$.*

SOLUTION. Since the equation of the curve is in pedal form

i.e., $p = r\sin\alpha$

$$\therefore \quad \frac{dp}{dr} = \sin\alpha$$

$$\text{Now, } \rho = \frac{ds}{d\psi} = r\frac{dr}{dp}$$

$$\therefore \quad \frac{ds}{d\psi} = r.\frac{1}{\sin\alpha} = r\,\mathrm{cosec}\,\alpha \quad ...(1)$$

If s is the length of arc measured from the point $r = 0$ to any point P in the direction of r increasing. Then, we have $s = \int_0^r \frac{rdr}{\sqrt{r^2 - p^2}}$

$$= \int_0^r \frac{rdr}{\sqrt{r^2 - r^2\sin^2\alpha}}$$

$$(\because p = r\sin\alpha)$$

$$= \int_0^r \sec\alpha dr = \sec\alpha[r]_0^r$$

$$s = r\sec\alpha \quad ...(2)$$

Now eliminate r between (1) and (2), we get

$$\frac{ds}{d\psi} = s\cot\alpha \quad \text{or} \quad \frac{ds}{s} = \cot\alpha\, d\psi.$$

Integrating, we get

$$\log s = \psi \cot \alpha + \log c$$

or $$s = ce^{\psi \cot \alpha}$$

where c is the constant of integration. This is the required intrinsic equation of the curve.

Exercise-18.2

1. Show that the intrinsic equation of the curve $y^2 = 4ax$ is
$s = a \cot \psi \operatorname{cosec} \psi + a \log (\cot \psi + \operatorname{cosec} \psi)$.
2. Find the intrinsic equation of the curve $y = c \cosh (x/c)$.
3. Find the intrinsic equation of the curve $x^2 = 4ay$.
4. Find the intrinsic equation of the curve $x = a(1 + \sin t), y = a(1 + \cos t)$.
5. Find the intrinsic equation of the curve $x^{2/3} + y^{2/3} = a^{2/3}$.
   (i) If s is measured from the vertex.
   (ii) If s is measured from the cusp on x-axis.
6. Find the intrinsic equation of the cardioid $r = a(1 + \cos \theta), \theta = 0$ being the fixed point.
7. Find the intrinsic equation of the curve $r = ae^{\theta \cot \alpha}$, where s is measured from the point $(a, 0)$.
8. Find the intrinsic equation of the curve $r = a\theta$, s being measured from $(0, 0)$.
9. Find the intrinsic equation of the curve $p = \sqrt{(r^2 - a^2)}$.
10. Prove that the intrinsic equation of the curve $x^2 = 4ay$ is
$$s = a \tan \psi \sec \psi + a \log(\tan \psi + \sec \psi).$$
11. Find the intrinsic equation of the curve $x = e^t \sin t$, $y = e^t \cos t$, where $t = \pi/4$ being the fixed point.
12. Find the intrinsic equation of the curve $y = a \log \sec \dfrac{x}{a}$.

Hint to Selected Problems

1. Since $y^2 = 4\,ax$. Therefore, $\dfrac{dy}{dx} = \dfrac{2a}{y}$.
$$\left[\because \frac{dy}{dx} = \tan \psi\right]$$
$\therefore \quad y = 2a \cot \psi$

Now using $\dfrac{ds}{dy} = \sqrt{1 + \left(\dfrac{dx}{dy}\right)^2} = \dfrac{1}{2a}\sqrt{4a^2 + y^2}$

Then integrating after separating the variables.

2. $\dfrac{dy}{dx} = \sinh\left(\dfrac{x}{c}\right) \therefore \dfrac{ds}{dx} = \cosh \dfrac{x}{c}$.

Now using the formula given below
$$\int_0^s ds = \int_0^x \cosh\left(\frac{x}{c}\right) dx.$$

3. Do same as (1)

4. $\dfrac{dx}{dt} = a \cos t, \dfrac{dy}{dt} = -a \sin t$
$$\therefore \quad \frac{dy}{dx} = -\tan t = \tan \psi \Rightarrow t = -\psi.$$
Now $\dfrac{ds}{dt} = \sqrt{\left(\dfrac{dx}{dt}\right)^2 + \left(\dfrac{dy}{dt}\right)^2} = a.$

Then use $\int_0^s ds = a\int_0^t dt$.

6. $\dfrac{dr}{d\theta} = -a \sin \theta.$

Also, $\tan \phi = r\dfrac{d\theta}{dr} = -\cot \dfrac{\theta}{2} = \tan\left(\dfrac{\pi}{2} + \dfrac{\theta}{2}\right)$.

Now using $\psi = \theta + \phi = \dfrac{3\theta}{2} + \dfrac{\pi}{2}$
$$\Rightarrow \theta = \frac{2}{3}\left(\psi - \frac{\pi}{2}\right)$$
$$\frac{ds}{d\theta} = \sqrt{r^2 + \left(\frac{dr}{d\theta}\right)^2} = 2a \cos \frac{\theta}{2}.$$
$$\therefore \quad \int_0^s ds = \int_0^\theta 2a \cos \frac{\theta}{2} d\theta.$$

7. $\dfrac{dr}{d\theta} = r \cot \alpha.$ Also, we have
$$\tan \phi = r\frac{d\theta}{dr} = r.\frac{1}{r \cot \alpha} = \tan \alpha$$
$\Rightarrow \tan \phi = \tan \alpha \Rightarrow \phi = \alpha$.

Now $\psi = \theta + \phi \Rightarrow \phi = \psi - \alpha$
$$\therefore \quad \frac{ds}{d\theta} = \sqrt{r^2 + \left(\frac{dr}{d\theta}\right)^2}$$
$$\Rightarrow \quad ds = a \operatorname{cosec} \alpha e^{\theta \cot \alpha} d\theta$$

then integrating *w.r.t.* θ.

8. Do same as (7).

11. $\frac{dx}{dt} = e^t \sin t + e^t \cos t, \frac{dy}{dt} = e^t \cos t - e^t \sin t.$

$\therefore \frac{dy}{dx} = \frac{1-\tan t}{1+\tan t} = \tan\left(\frac{\pi}{4} - t\right) \Rightarrow \psi = \frac{\pi}{4} - t$ *i.e.*,

$t = \frac{\pi}{4} - \psi.$

Now proceed as above.

12. $y = a \log \sec (x/a) \quad \Rightarrow \quad \frac{dy}{dx} = \tan(x/a)$

$\Rightarrow \tan \psi = \tan (x/a) \Rightarrow \quad x = a\psi$

$\Rightarrow \frac{ds}{dx} = \sqrt{1 + \left(\frac{dy}{dx}\right)^2} = \sqrt{1 + \tan^2 \frac{x}{a}}$

$\Rightarrow \frac{ds}{dx} = \sec \frac{x}{a}$

$\Rightarrow \quad s = \int_0^x \frac{ds}{dx} . dx .$

ANSWERS

2. $s = c \tan \psi$ **3.** $s = a \tan \psi \sec \psi + a \log (\tan \psi + \sec \psi)$ **4.** $s + a\psi = 0$

5. (i) $4s = 3a \cos 2\psi$ (ii) $2s = 3a \sin^2 \psi$ **6.** $s = 4a \sin\left(\frac{\psi}{3} - \frac{\pi}{6}\right)$ **7.** $s = a \sec \alpha \, [e^{(\psi - \alpha)\cot \alpha} - 1]$

8. $s = \frac{1}{2} a[\theta\sqrt{(1+\theta)^2} + \log\{\theta + \sqrt{(1+\theta)^2}\}]$ **9.** $s = \frac{1}{2} a(\psi^2 + 1)$ **11.** $s = \sqrt{2} e^{\pi/4} [e^{-\psi} - 1]$

12. $s = a \log [\tan \psi + \sec \psi]$

❑❑❑❑❑❑

Chapter

19 Area of Bounded Curves

19.1 AREA OF CURVE IN CARTESIAN FORM

Let $y = f(x)$ be a continuous curve in cartesian form and let A be the area of the region bounded by the curve $y = f(x)$, the axis of x and the two ordinates $x = a$ and $y = b$. Then

$$A = \int_a^b y\,dx = \int_a^b f(x)\,dx$$

Proof. Let BC be the arc of the curve $y = f(x)$ cut by the lines $x = a$ and $y = b$ as shown in fig. 1.

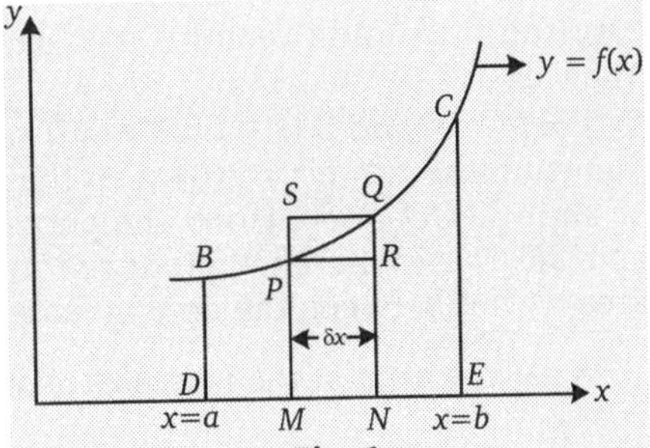

Let $P(x, y)$ and $Q(x + \delta x, y + \delta y)$ be two neighbouring points on the cuve between B and C. Now draw the perpendicular PM and QN on the axis of x such that $PM = y$ and $QN = y+dy$ and $MN = \delta x$. Since we observe that the area of $DMPB$ increases as P moves along arc BC from B to C. Draw the perpendicular PR on QN and QS to MP produced to S. Let δA be the area of $MNQP$, this area lies between the area $MNRP$ and the area $MNQS$.

Fig. 1

Since $MNRP$ and $MNQS$ both are rectangles and the area of $MNRP$ is $y\,\delta x$ and the area of $MNQS$ is $(y+\delta y)\,\delta x$.

$\therefore$ Area of $MNRP < \delta A <$ area of $MNQS$

or $$y\,\delta x < \delta A < (y + \delta y)\,\delta x \text{ or } y < \frac{\delta A}{\partial x} < y + \delta y.$$

Taking the limit as $\delta x \to 0$ and $\delta y \to 0$, where $Q \to P$.

$\therefore$ $$y < \lim_{\delta x \to 0} \frac{\delta A}{\partial x} < y \text{ or } y < \frac{dA}{dx} < y$$

$\Rightarrow$ $$\frac{dA}{dx} = y \text{ or } \frac{dA}{dx} = f(x) \qquad [\because y = f(x)]$$

or $$dA = f(x)\,dx.$$

Now integrating *w.r.t.* '*x*' from $x = a$ to $x = b$, *we get*

$$\int_{x=a}^{x=b} dA = \int_a^b f(x)\,dx$$

$\Rightarrow$ $$[A]_{x=a}^{x=b} = \int_a^b f(x)\,dx$$

or $$\text{Area } DECB = \int_a^b f(x)\,dx$$

or $$A = \int_a^b f(x)\,dx = \int_a^b y\,dx.$$

Similarly, the area bounded by the curve $x = f(y)$, the axis of y and the ordinates $y = a$ and $y = b$ is given by

$$A = \int_a^b f(y)dy = \int_a^b x\,dy\,.$$

- If the given curve is symmetrical either about x-axis or about y-axis or both, then find the area of one of the symmetrical part and multiply this area by the number of symmetrical parts, we get the whole area of the bounded region.
- Area bounded by two curves = | Area bounded by one curve – Area bounded by other curve |.

19.2 AREA OF CURVE IN POLAR FORM

Let $r = f(\theta)$ be the equation of a curve in polar form where $f(\theta)$ is a continuous function of θ, then the area of the sector bounded by the curve $r = f(\theta)$ and two radii vectors $\theta = \theta_1$ and $\theta = \theta_2$ such that $\theta_2 > \theta_1$ is given by

$$A = \frac{1}{2}\int_{\theta_1}^{\theta_2} r^2\,d\theta\,\cdot$$

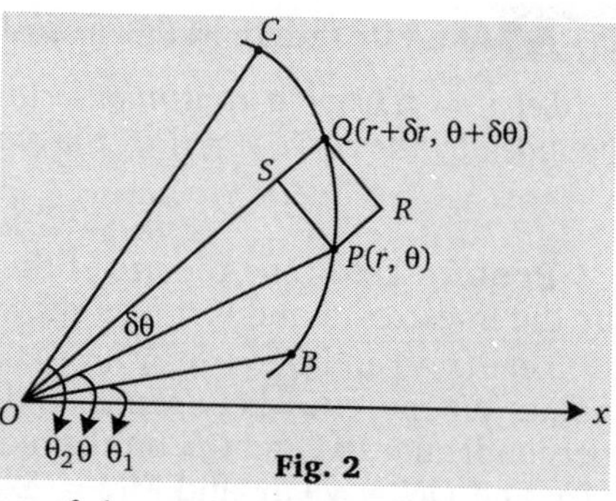

Fig. 2

Proof. Since the equation of curve in polar form is $r = f(\theta)$.

Let A be the area of the sector OBC bounded by the curve and two radii vector $\theta = \theta_1$ and $\theta = \theta_2$ as shown in fig. 2.

Let $P(r, \theta)$ and $Q\,(r + \delta r, \theta + \delta\theta)$ be two neighbouring points on the curve $r = f(\theta)$ such that $OP = r$, $OQ = r + \delta r$ and $\angle POQ = \delta\theta$. Draw the perpendicular PS to OQ and QR to OR where OP produced to R. Let δA be the area of the sector OPQ. Obviously, this area δA lies between the area of isosceles triangle OPS and the area of isosceles triangle ORQ.

Now, the area of the isosceles triangle $OPS = \frac{1}{2}OP \times OS \sin\delta\theta = \frac{1}{2}r \times r\cdot\delta\theta$ $\quad(\therefore \sin\delta\theta \approx \delta\theta)$

$$= \frac{1}{2}r^2\delta\theta \qquad (\delta\theta \text{ is very small})$$

and the area of isosceles triangle, $\quad ORQ = \frac{1}{2}OR \times OQ \sin\delta\theta$

$$= \frac{1}{2}(r + \delta r)^2\delta\theta$$

$(\because \delta\theta$ is very small so $\sin\delta\theta \approx \delta\theta)$

Since δA lies between the areas of triangle OPS and ORQ, then

$$\frac{1}{2}r^2\delta\theta < \delta A < \frac{1}{2}(r + \delta r)^2\,\delta\theta\,.$$

Divide by $\delta\theta$, we have

$$\frac{1}{2}r^2 < \frac{\delta A}{\delta\theta} < \frac{1}{2}(r + \delta r)^2.$$

As $Q \to P$, $\delta\theta > 0$ and $\delta r \to 0$ so taking the limit as $\delta\theta \to 0$, we get

$$\frac{1}{2}r^2 < \lim_{\delta\theta\to 0}\frac{\delta A}{\delta\theta} < \frac{1}{2}r^2$$

or

$$\frac{1}{2}r^2 < \frac{dA}{d\theta} < \frac{1}{2}r^2$$

or

$$\frac{dA}{d\theta} = \frac{1}{2}r^2 \text{ or } dA = \frac{1}{2}r^2 d\theta.$$

Integrating *w.r.t.* θ from $\theta = \theta_1$ to $\theta = \theta_2$, we get

$$\int_{\theta=\theta_1}^{\theta=\theta_2} dA = \int_{\theta_1}^{\theta_2} \frac{1}{2} r^2 \, d\theta$$

Hence, $$A = \frac{1}{2}\int_{\theta_1}^{\theta_2} r^2 d\theta \qquad \left(\because \int_{\theta_1}^{\theta_2} dA = \int_B^C dA = A\right)$$

- In case of $r = a \cos n\theta$ or $r = a \sin n\theta$, the number of loops are n and $2n$ according as n is odd and n is even.
- Area by double integration bounded by $r = f(\theta)$ and $\theta = \theta_1$ and $\theta = \theta_2$ is given by $\int_{\theta_1}^{\theta_2} \int_{r=0}^{r=f(\theta)} r \, d\theta \, dr$.

Solved Examples

1. *Find the area of the region bounded by the line $x = 2$ and the parabola $y^2 = 8x$.*

SOLUTION. The equation of the parabola is $y^2 = 8x$ which is symmetrical about x-axis and the line $x=2$ intersects the parabola $y^2 = 8x$ in two points (2,4) and (2, –4) as shown in fig. 3.

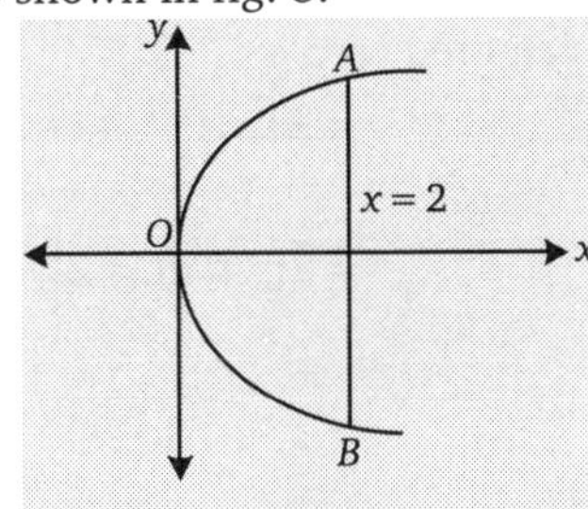

Fig. 3

∴ The required area

$$= 2\int_0^2 y \, dx = 2\int_0^2 \sqrt{8x} \, dx$$

$$= 4\sqrt{2}\left[\frac{2}{3}x^{3/2}\right]_0^2 = \frac{32}{3} \text{ sq. units.}$$

2. *Find the area bounded by the parabola $y^2 = 4ax$ and its latus rectum.*

SOLUTION. We know that a line through the focus of the parabola and perpendicular to its axis is called latus-rectum. Since the equation of the parabola is $y^2 = 4\,ax$.

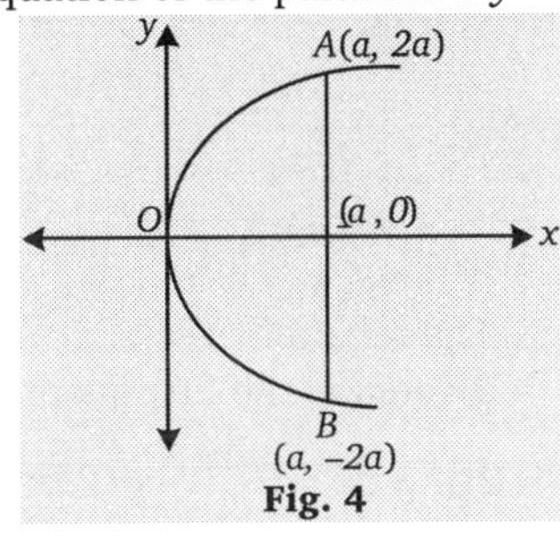

Fig. 4

∴ Extremities of latus rectum are $(a, 2a)$ and $(a, -2a)$ which is shown in fig. 4.

∴ The required area

$$= 2\int_0^a y \, dx = 2\int_0^a \sqrt{4ax} \, dx$$

$$= 4\sqrt{a}\left[\frac{2}{3}x^{3/2}\right]_0^a = 4\sqrt{a}\left[\frac{2}{3}a\sqrt{a}\right]$$

$$= \frac{8}{3}a^2 \text{ sq. units.}$$

3. *Find the whole area of the ellipse*

$$\frac{x^2}{a^2} + \frac{y^2}{b^2} = 1.$$

SOLUTION. The ellipse $\frac{x^2}{a^2} + \frac{y^2}{b^2} = 1$ is symmetrical about both axes and whose trace is shown in fig. 5.

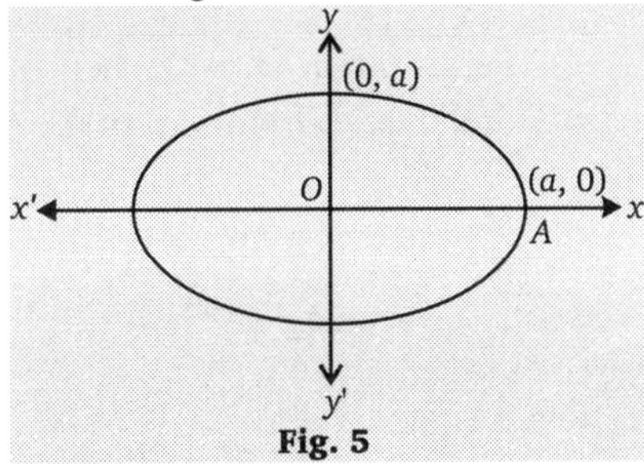

Fig. 5

∴ Required area

$$= 4\int_0^a y \, dx = 4\int_0^a b\sqrt{\left(1 - \frac{x^2}{a^2}\right)} dx$$

$$= 4b\int_0^a \sqrt{\left(1 - \frac{x^2}{a^2}\right)} dx.$$

Let us put $x = a \sin \theta$.

∴ $dx = a \cos\theta \, d\theta$ and θ varies from 0 to $\pi/2$.

$\therefore \quad A. = 4b\int_0^{\pi/2} \cos\theta . a\cos\theta \, d\theta$

$$= 4ab\int_0^{\pi/2} \cos^2\theta \, d\theta$$

$$= 4ab\left[\frac{(2-1)}{2}.\frac{\pi}{2}\right]$$

(By Walli's formula)

$$= \pi \, ab \text{ sq. units.}$$

4. *Find the area of the loop of the curve* $ay^2 = x^2(a-x)$.

(SVTU–2009, OSMANIA–2000)

SOLUTION. Since the curve is symmetrical about x-axis and $y = 0$ when $x = 0$ and $x = a$ so the loop exists between $x = 0$ and $x = a$ as shown in fig. 6.

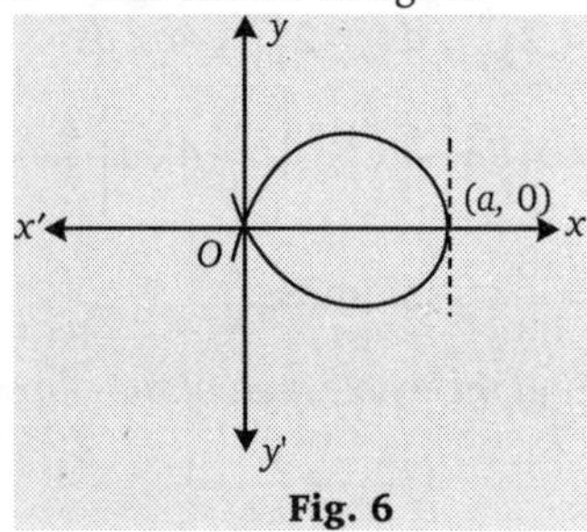

Fig. 6

$\therefore$ Required area

$$= 2\int_0^a y\,dx$$

$$= 2\int_0^a x\sqrt{\frac{a-x}{a}}\,dx.$$

Let us put $a - x = t^2$, then $-dx = 2t\,dt$ and t varies from $\sqrt{a}$ to 0.

$$\therefore \quad = \frac{2}{\sqrt{a}}\int_{\sqrt{a}}^0 (a-t^2)t(-2t\,dt)$$

$$= \frac{2}{\sqrt{a}}.2\int_0^{\sqrt{a}} (at^2 - t^4)\,dt$$

$$= \frac{4}{\sqrt{a}}\left[\frac{at^3}{3} - \frac{t^5}{5}\right]_0^{\sqrt{a}}$$

$$= \frac{4}{\sqrt{a}}\left[\frac{a^2\sqrt{a}}{3} - \frac{a^2\sqrt{a}}{5}\right]$$

$$= \frac{8}{15}a^2 \text{ sq. units.}$$

5. *Find the area of the one loop of the curve* $y^2 = x^2(a^2 - x^2)$.

SOLUTION. Clearly, the given curve is symmetrical about both axes and $y = 0$ when $x = 0, x = \pm a$. Thus the curve has two loops one of them lies between $x = 0$ and $x = a$ and other lies between $x = -a$ and $x=0$ as shown in fig. 7.

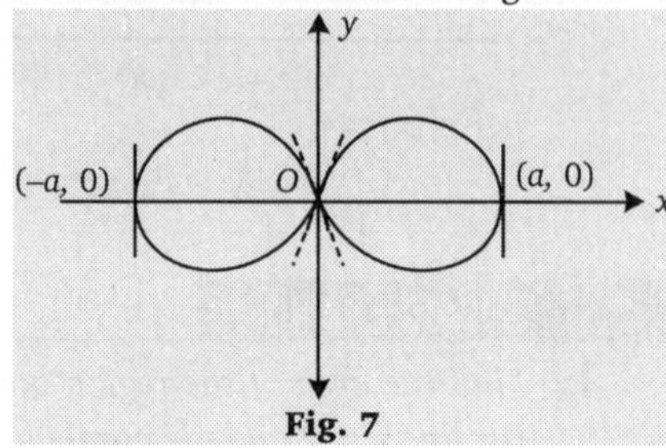

Fig. 7

$\therefore$ The required area

$$= 2\int_0^a y\,dx = 2\int_0^a x\sqrt{(a^2 - x^2)}\,dx.$$

Let us put $a^2 - x^2 = t^2$, then $x\,dx = -t dt$ and t lies between a and 0. Thus the required area is

$$= 2\int_a^0 t(-t\,dt) = -2\int_a^0 t^2 dt$$

$$= 2\int_0^a t^2 dt = 2\left[\frac{t^3}{3}\right]_0^a$$

$$= \frac{2}{3}a^3 \text{ sq. units.}$$

6. *Find the whole area of the curve* $a^2y^2 = x^3(2a - x)$.

SOLUTION. Clearly, the curve is symmetrical about x-axis and $y=0$ when $x = 0$ and $x = 2a$ so the curve has a loop between $x=0$ and $x=2a$ and curve does not exist in the regions $x < 0$ and $x > 2a$. The tracing of the curve is shown in fig. 8.

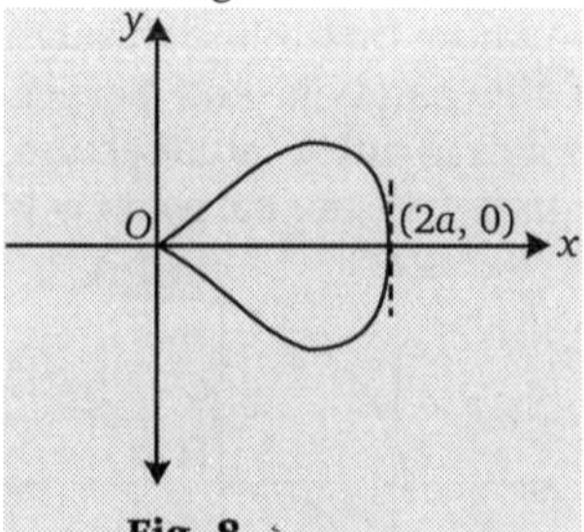

Fig. 8

$\therefore$ The required area

$= 2\times$area in the first quadrant

$$= 2\int_0^{2a} y\,dx = 2\int_0^{2a} \frac{x}{a}\sqrt{(2ax - x^2)}\,dx$$

$= \frac{2}{a}\int_0^{2a} x\sqrt{(2ax - x^2)}\, dx.$

Let us put $x=2a\sin^2\theta$, then $dx=4a\sin\theta\cos\theta d\theta$ and θ varies from $\theta=0$ to $\theta=\pi/2$.

Thus, we have

$$= \frac{2}{a}\int_0^{\pi/2} 2a\sin^2\theta . 2a\sin\theta\cos\theta . 4a\sin\theta\cos\theta\, d\theta$$

$$= 32a^2\int_0^{\pi/2}\sin^4\theta\cos^2\theta\, d\theta$$

$$= 32a^2\left[\frac{(4-1)(4-3)}{6.4.(6-4)}.(2-1).\frac{\pi}{2}\right]$$

[By Walli's formula]

$= \pi a^2$ sq. units.

7. *Find the common area between the curves $y^2=4ax$ and $x^2 = 4ay$.*

(SVTU-2008, KURUKSHETRA-2005)

SOLUTION. The curve $y^2 = 4ax$ is symmetrical about x-axis and the curve $x^2 = 4ay$ is symmetrical about y-axis. Both curves intersects at two points (0,0) and $(4a, 4a)$ which are obtained by solving both equations of curves. The tracing of the curves is shown in fig. 9.

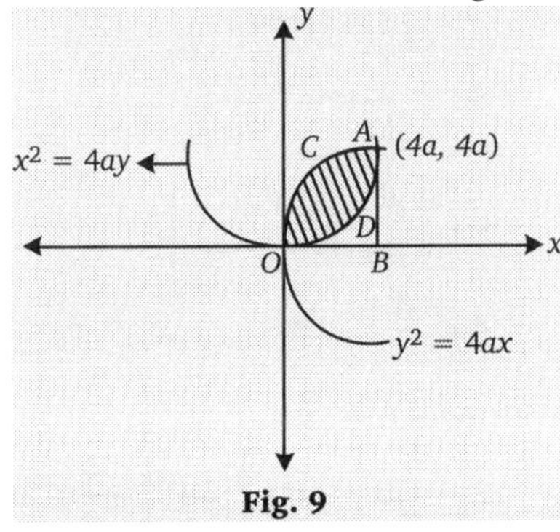

Fig. 9

The required area

= area of *OBACO* – area of *OBADO* ...(1)

Now area of *OBACO*

$= \int_0^{4a} y\,dx$, where $y^2 = 4ax$

$$= \int_0^{4a}\sqrt{4ax}\,dx = 2\sqrt{a}\left[\frac{2}{3}x^{3/2}\right]_0^{4a}$$

$$= \frac{32}{3}a^2$$

and area of *OBADO* $= \int_0^{4a} y\,dx$,

where $y = \frac{x^2}{4a} = \int_0^{4a}\frac{x^2}{4a}dx$

$$= \frac{1}{4a}\left[\frac{x^3}{3}\right]_0^{4a} = \frac{16a^2}{3}.$$

From (1), we get

Required area

$$= \frac{32}{3}a^2 - \frac{16}{3}a^2 = \frac{16}{3}a^2 \text{ sq. units.}$$

8. *Find the area common of the curves $y^2 = ax$, $x^2 + y^2 = 4ax$.*

SOLUTION. Both the curves are symmetrical about x-axis and intersect, then we have

$$x^2+y^2 = 4ax,\ y^2 = ax.$$

$\therefore \quad x^2+ax = 4ax$

or $\quad x^2 - 3ax = 0$

or $\quad x = 0, x = 3a$

$\therefore$ If $x = 0, y = 0$ and $x = 3a, y = \pm a\sqrt{3}$

Thus both curves intersect at three points (0,0) and $(3a, \pm a\sqrt{3})$. The tracing of the curves are shown in fig. 10.

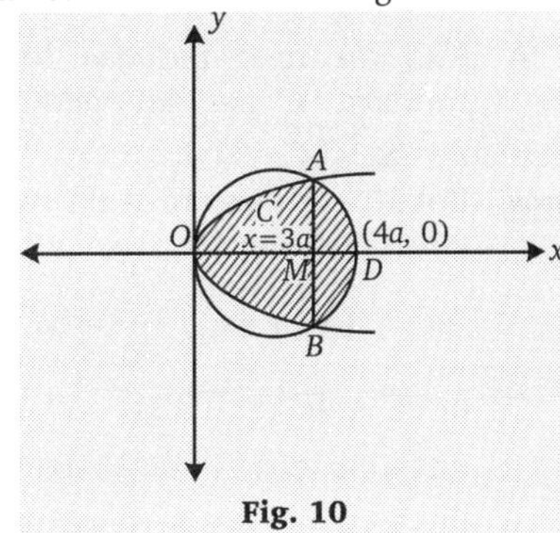

Fig. 10

The required area

= 2[area *OMACO*+area *MDAM*] ...(1)

Now area *OMACO*

$= \int_0^{3a} y\,dx$, *where* $y^2 = ax$

$$= \int_0^{3a}\sqrt{ax}\,dx$$

$$= \sqrt{a}\left[\frac{2}{3}x^{3/2}\right]_0^{3a} = 2\sqrt{3}\,a^2$$

and area *MDAM* $= \int_{3a}^{4a} y\,dx$

(where $y = \sqrt{4ax - x^2}$ and at M, $x=3a$, at D, $x = 4a$.)

$$= \int_{3a}^{4a}\sqrt{4ax - x^2}\,dx$$

$$= \int_{3a}^{4a} \sqrt{[(2a)^2 - (x-2a)^2]}\, dx$$

$$= \left[\frac{x-2a}{2}\sqrt{[(2a)^2 - (x-2a)^2]} + \frac{(2a)^2}{2}\sin^{-1}\frac{x-2a}{2a}\right]_{3a}^{4a}$$

$$= 2a^2 \sin^{-1} 1 - \frac{a}{2}.a\sqrt{3} - 2a^2 \sin^{-1}\frac{1}{2}$$

$$= \left(a^2\pi - \frac{\sqrt{3}}{2}a^2 - \frac{a^2\pi}{3}\right)$$

$$= \frac{2\pi a^2}{3} - \frac{\sqrt{3}}{2}a^2.$$

From (1), we get Required area

$$= 2\left[2\sqrt{3}a^2 + \frac{2\pi}{3}a^2 - \frac{\sqrt{3}}{2}a^2\right]$$

$$= 2\left(\frac{2\pi}{3}a^2 + \frac{3\sqrt{3}}{2}a^2\right)$$

$$= a^2\left(\frac{4\pi}{3} + 3\sqrt{3}\right) \text{ sq. units.}$$

9. *Find the area included between the parabola $x^2 = 4ay$ and the curve $y = 8a^3/(x^2+4a^2)$.*

SOLUTION. Both the curves are symmetrical about y-axis and intersect, then we have

$$(x^2 + 4a^2).\frac{x^2}{4a} = 8a^3$$

or $x^4 + 4a^2x^2 - 32a^4 = 0$

$$(x^2 + 8a^2)(x^2 - 4a^2) = 0$$

or $x^2 + 8a^2 = 0, x^2 - 4a^2 = 0$

$$x = \pm 2\sqrt{2}ai \text{ or } x = \pm 2a.$$

$x = \pm 2\sqrt{2}\,ai$ are not possible point, therefore both curves intersect at two points $(2a, a)$ and $(-2a, a)$. The tracing of the curves are shown Fig. 11.

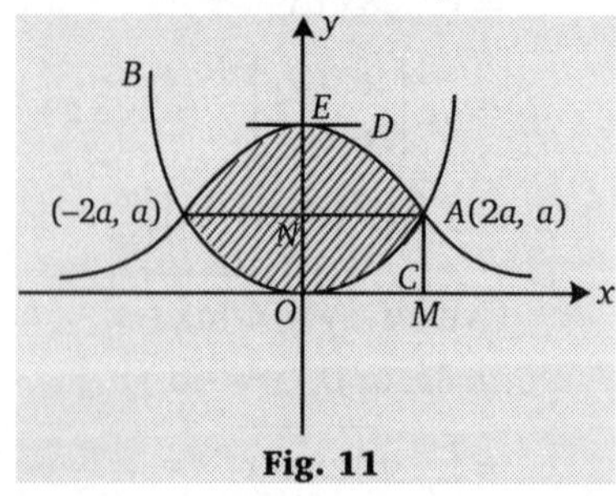

Fig. 11

The required area

$= 2[\text{area } OCANO + \text{area } NADEN] \ldots(1)$

Now area $OCANO$ + area $NADEN$

$= -$ area $OMACO$ + aera $OMADEO$

$\therefore$ From (1), we get

Required area

$= 2[-\text{area } OMACO + \text{area } OMADEO] \ldots(2)$

Now, area $OMACO$

$$= \int_0^{2a} y\, dx, \text{ where } y = \frac{x^2}{4a}$$

$$= \int_0^{2a} \frac{x^2}{4a} dx = \frac{1}{4a}\left[\frac{x^3}{3}\right]_0^{2a}$$

$$= \frac{1}{4a}\left[\frac{8a^3}{3}\right] = \frac{2}{3}a^2$$

and area $OMADEO$

$$= \int_0^{2a} y\, dx,\ y = \frac{8a^3}{(x^2 + 4a^2)}$$

$$= \int_0^{2a} \frac{8a^3}{x^2 + 4a^2} dx$$

$$= 8a^3 \int_0^{2a} \frac{dx}{x^2 + 4a^2}$$

$$= 8a^3\left[\frac{1}{2a}\tan^{-1}\frac{x}{2a}\right]_0^{2a}$$

$$= 8a^3\left[\frac{1}{2a}\tan^{-1} 1 - 0\right]$$

$$= 4a^2.\frac{\pi}{4} = a^2\pi.$$

From (2), we get, Required area

$$= 2\left[-\frac{2}{3}a^2 + a^2\pi\right] = a^2\left(-\frac{4}{3} + 2\pi\right)$$

$$= a^2\left(2\pi - \frac{4}{3}\right) \text{ sq. units.}$$

10. *Find the area included between the curve $x = a(t+\sin t)$, $y = a(1-\cos t)$ and its base.* (VTU–2000)

SOLUTION. Since the equation of the curve is

$$x = a(t + \sin t)$$
$$y = a(1 - \cos t).$$

Obviously, $y = 0$ when $\cos t = 1$ *i.e.,* $t = 0$ and $x = 0$. Thus the curve passes through the point (0,0). Also

$$\frac{dy}{dx} = \tan t/2, \text{ at } t = 0,\ \frac{dy}{dx} = 0.$$

Therefore, the tangent at (0,0) is the x-axis. The tracing of the curve is shown in fig 12.

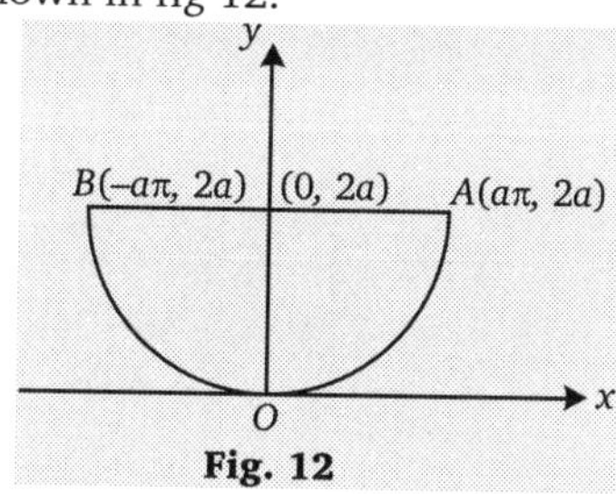

Fig. 12

Obviously, curve is symmetrical about y-axis so the required area is given by $A = 2\times$area bounded by the axis of y and $y=2a$

$$A = 2\int_{y=0}^{y=2a} x\,dy.$$

Since $x = a(t+\sin t), y = a(1-\cos t)$

$\therefore\ dy = a\sin t\,dt.$

$$\therefore\ A = 2\int_0^{\pi} a(t+\sin t).a\sin t\,dt$$

$$= 2a^2\int_0^{\pi}(t\sin t+\sin^2 t)dt$$

$$= 2a^2\left[\int_0^{\pi} t\sin t\,dt+\int_0^{\pi}\sin^2 t\,dt\right]$$

$$= 2a^2\left[(-t\cos t+\sin t)_0^{\pi} + \frac{1}{2}\left(t-\frac{\sin 2t}{2}\right)_0^{\pi}\right]$$

$$= 2a^2\left[\pi+\frac{\pi}{2}\right] = 3\pi a^2 \text{ sq. units.}$$

11. *Find the area bounded by the curve $y^2(a+x)=x^2(a-x)$ and its asymptotes.*

SOLUTION. Clearly, the given curve is symmetrical about x-axis and cuts the x-axis only at two points (0,0) and $(a, 0)$ and $x = -a$ is the asymptote of this curve. This curve has a loop lying between $x = 0$ and $x = a$. Therefore, the tracing of this curve is shown in fig. 13.

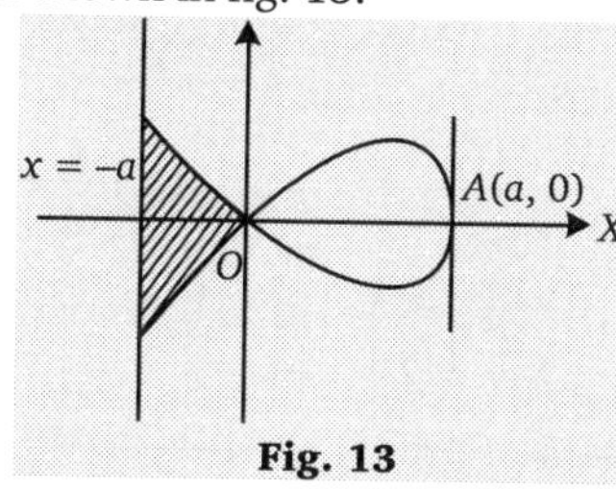

Fig. 13

The required area $= 2\int_{-a}^{0} y\,dx$

$$A = 2\int_{-a}^{0} x\sqrt{\frac{a-x}{a+x}}dx.$$

Let us put $x = a\cos 2\theta$ so $dx = -2a\sin 2\theta d\theta$ and θ will take the value from $\pi/2$ to $\pi/4$. Therefore, we have

$$A = 2\int_{\pi/2}^{\pi/4} a\cos 2\theta.\sqrt{\frac{1-\cos 2\theta}{1+\cos 2\theta}}.(-2a\sin 2\theta)d\theta$$

$$= -4a^2\int_{\pi/4}^{\pi/2}\frac{\sin\theta}{\cos\theta}.\cos 2\theta.\sin 2\theta\,d\theta$$

$$= 4a^2\int_{\pi/4}^{\pi/2}\frac{\sin\theta}{\cos\theta}.\cos 2\theta.2\sin\theta\cos\theta\,d\theta$$

$$= 8a^2\int_{\pi/4}^{\pi/2}\sin^2\theta\cos 2\theta\,d\theta$$

$$= 8a^2\int_{\pi/4}^{\pi/2}\sin^2\theta(1-2\sin^2\theta)d\theta$$

$$= 8a^2\int_{\pi/4}^{\pi/2}(\sin^2\theta-2\sin^4\theta)d\theta$$

$$= 8a^2\left[\int_{\pi/4}^{0}(\sin^2\theta-2\sin^4\theta)d\theta + \int_0^{\pi/2}(\sin^2\theta-2\sin^4\theta)d\theta\right]$$

$$= 8a^2\left[\int_{\pi/4}^{0}\sin^2\theta(1-2\sin^2\theta)d\theta + \int_0^{\pi/2}\sin^2\theta\,d\theta - 2\int_0^{\pi/2}\sin^4\theta\,d\theta\right]$$

$$= 8a^2\left[\int_{\pi/4}^{0}\frac{(1-\cos 2\theta)}{2}.\cos 2\theta\,d\theta + \frac{(2-1)}{2}.\frac{\pi}{2} - 2.\frac{(4-1)(4-3)}{4.2}\frac{\pi}{2}\right]$$

(Walli's formula)

$$= 8a^2\left[\frac{1}{2}\int_{\pi/4}^{0}(\cos 2\theta-\cos^2 2\theta)d\theta + \frac{\pi}{4}-\frac{3\pi}{8}\right]$$

Now let us put $2\theta = \phi$ so $d\theta = \frac{1}{2}d\phi$ and ϕ takes the value from $\pi/2$ to 0. Then

$$= 8a^2\left[\frac{1}{2}\int_{\pi/2}^{0}(\cos\phi-\cos^2\phi)\frac{1}{2}d\phi-\frac{\pi}{8}\right]$$

$$= 8a^2\left[\frac{1}{4}\int_{\pi/2}^{0}\cos\phi\,d\phi-\frac{1}{4}\int_{\pi/2}^{0}\cos^2\phi\,d\phi - \frac{\pi}{8}\right]$$

$$= 8a^2\left[\frac{1}{4}(\sin\phi)_{\pi/2}^{0}+\frac{1}{4}\left(\frac{2-1}{2}.\frac{\pi}{2}\right)-\frac{\pi}{8}\right]$$

$$= 8a^2\left[-\frac{1}{4}+\frac{\pi}{16}-\frac{\pi}{8}\right] = 8a^2\left[-\frac{1}{4}-\frac{\pi}{16}\right]$$

$$= -a^2\left(2+\frac{\pi}{2}\right).$$

Hence, $A = a^2\left(2+\frac{\pi}{2}\right)$.

(Taking magnitude value)

12. *Find the whole area between the curve $x^2y^2 = a^2(y^2 - x^2)$ and its asymptotes.*

(VTU–2007)

SOLUTION. The given curve is symmetrical about both axes and curve passes through only (0,0). The tangents at (0, 0) are given by

$$y^2 - x^2 = 0$$

or $$y = \pm x.$$

Thus we obtained two distinct tangents at (0, 0) so (0, 0) is a node and its two real asymptotes are $x = \pm a$. The tracing of the curve is shown in fig. 14.

The required area = 4 × area between curve and asymptote in the first quadrant.

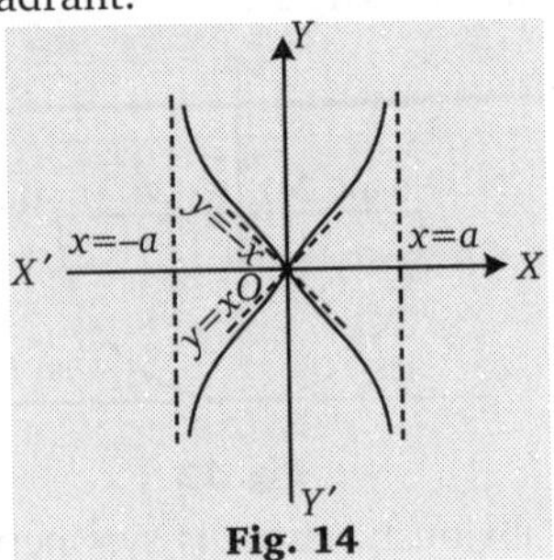

Fig. 14

$\therefore \quad A = 4\int_0^a y\,dx$

or $\quad A = 4\int_0^a \frac{ax\,dx}{\sqrt{(a^2 - x^2)}}$

Let us put $a^2 - x^2 = t^2$, so $x\,dx = -t\,dt$ and t takes the values from a to 0. Then

$$A = 4a\int_a^0 \frac{-t\,dt}{t} = 4a\int_0^a dt$$

$$= 4a[t]_0^a = 4a^2 \text{ sq. units.}$$

Similar Problem

(1) Show that the area bounded by the cissoid $x = a\sin^2 t$, $y = \frac{a\sin^3 t}{\cos t}$ and its asymptote is $3\pi a^2/4$.

13. *Find by double integration the area of the region closed by the curves $x^2 + y^2 = a^2$, $x + y = a$ (in the first quadrant).*

SOLUTION. The given equations of the circle

$$x^2 + y^2 = a^2.$$

The straight line $x + y = a$ shown in fig. 15.

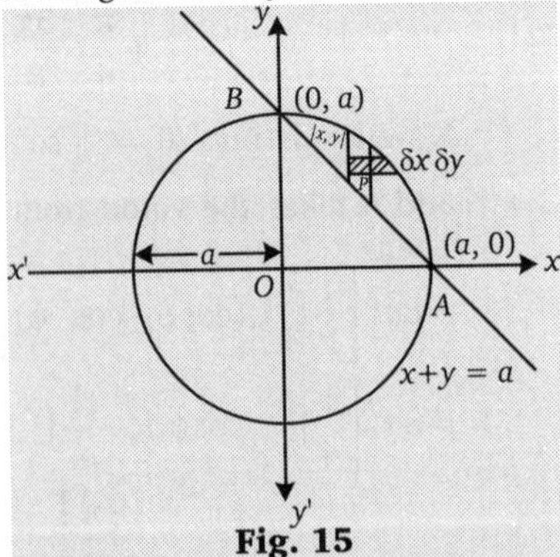

Fig. 15

To find the required area of the arc AB and the line AB by double integration take any point $P(x, y)$ and consider an area $\delta x\,\delta y$ at P. The arc of the circle $x^2 + y^2 = a^2$ and then moving x from 0 to a.

$\therefore$ The required area

$$= \int_{x=0}^{a}\int_{y=(a-x)}^{\sqrt{a^2-x^2}} dx\,dy.$$

$$= \int_0^a [y]_{a-x}^{\sqrt{a^2-x^2}}\,dx$$

$$= \int_0^a \left[\sqrt{a^2 - x^2} - (a - x)\right]dx$$

$$= \left[\left\{\frac{1}{2}x\sqrt{(a^2 - x^2)} + \frac{1}{2}a^2\sin^{-1}\left(\frac{x}{a}\right)\right\} - ax + \frac{1}{2}x^2\right]_0^a$$

$$= \frac{1}{2}a^2.\left(\frac{\pi}{2}\right) - a^2 + \frac{1}{2}a^2$$

$$= \frac{1}{2}a^2\left(\frac{\pi}{2} - 1\right) = \frac{1}{4}a^2(\pi - 2) \text{ sq. units.}$$

Exercise-19.1

1. Find the area of the region bounded by the following curves, and the axis of x and the given ordinates:
   (i) $y = \log x; x = a, x = b$
   (b) $y = c \cosh (x/c); x = 0, x = a$
   (c) $y = \sin^2 x; x = 0, x = \pi/2$
2. Find the area of the region bounded by the parabola $y^2 = 4x$ and the line $y = 2x$.
3. Find the area of a quadrant of the ellipse $x^2/a^2 + y^2/b^2 = 1$. (VTU–2003, KERALA–2005)
4. Find the area of a loop of the curve $xy^2 + (x+a)^2(x+2a) = 0$.
5. Find the area of the loop of the curve $3ay^2 = x(x-a)^2$. (RAJASTHAN–2005)
6. Find the whole area of the curve $a^2x^2 = y^3(2a-y)$. (NAGPUR-2009)
7. Prove that the area of a loop of the curve $a^4y^2 = x^4(a^2 - x^2)$ is $\pi a^2/8$.
8. Find the area bounded by the curve $xy^2 = a^2(a-x)$ and y-axis.
9. Find the area of the loop of the curve $y^2 = x(x-1)^2$.
10. Find the whole area of the curve $y^2 = x^2(a^2 - x^2)$.
11. Find the area between the curve $y^2(a-x) = x^2$ and its asymptote.
12. Find the area between the curve $y^2(2a-x) = x^3$ and its asymptote. (VTU 2003)
13. Find the area between the curve $xy^2 = 4a^2(2a - x)$ and its asymptote.
14. Find the area between the $y^2(a-x) = x^3$ and its asymptote. Also find the ratio in which the ordinate $x = a/2$ divides this area.
15. Find the area of the region bounded by the parabola $y^2 = 4ax$ and $x^2 = 4by$.
16. Find the area bounded by the curves $x^2+y^2 \le 2ax$ and $y^2 \ge ax$, $a > 0, x > 0, y > 0$.
17. Find the area bounded by the curves $y \ge x^2$ and $y \le |x|$.
18. Find the area of the segment cut off from the parabola $y^2 = 4x$ by the line $y = 8x - 1$.
19. Find the area bounded by the parabola $4y = 3x^2$ and the line $3x - 2y + 12 = 0$.
20. Find the area enclosed by the curves $y^2 \le 3x$ and $3x^2 + 3y^2 \ge 16$.
21. Find the area included between the cycloid $x = a(\theta - \sin\theta), y = a(1 - \cos\theta)$ and its base. (GORAKHPUR-1999)
22. Find the area enclosed between the curve $y = x^3$ and the line $y = x$.
23. Find whole area of the curve $x^{2/3} + y^{2/3} = a^{2/3}$. (VTU–2005)
24. Find the area of the loop of the curve $x^3 + y^3 = 3axy$.
25. Find the area enclosed between the parabola $y^2 = 4a(x+a)$ and $y^2 = -4a(x-a)$.
26. Find the area of the smaller portion enclosed by the curves $x^2 + y^2 = 9$ and $y^2 = 8x$.
27. Find the area between the parabola $y = 4x - x^2$ and the line $y = x$. (VTU–2010, SVTU–2008, UPTU–2008)

Hints to the Selected Problems

1. Required area $A = \int_a^b y\,dx$.
2. Required area $A = \int_0^1 (\sqrt{4x})\,dx - \int_0^1 (2x)\,dx$.
3. Required area $A = \int_0^a y\,dx$. (Do same example 3.)
4. $A = 2\int_{-2a}^{a} y\,dx = \pm 2\int_{-2a}^{a} \frac{\sqrt{(x+a)^2(x+2a)}}{-x}\,dx$.
   Put $-x = t$. Then integrate.
5. $3ay^2 = x(x-a)^2 \Rightarrow y = (x-a)\sqrt{\frac{x}{3a}}$.
   Then $A = 2\int_0^a y\,dx$.
6. Here $x = 0, 0$ be two real tangents. Therefore
   $$A = 2\int_0^{2a} x\,dy.$$
8. $A = 2\int_0^\infty x\,dy$.
9. $A = 2\int_0^1 y\,dx$.
12. $x = 2a$ is the asymptote of the given curve, therefore, the required area $A = 2\int_0^{2a} y\,dx$.
13. $x = 0$ is the asympotote. Therefore,
   $$A = 2\int_0^{2a} y\,dx.$$
14. $A = 2\int_0^a y\,dx \Rightarrow A = 2\int_0^a x\sqrt{\frac{x}{a-x}}\,dx$
   $$A_1 = 2\int_0^{a/2} y\,dx \Rightarrow A_1 = 2\int_0^{a/2} x\sqrt{\frac{x}{a-x}}\,dx$$
   Put $x = a\sin^2\theta$ and integrate.
16. $A = \int_0^a (\sqrt{2ax - x^2})\,dx - \int_0^a (\sqrt{ax})\,dx$.
17. $A = 2\int_0^1 x\,dx - \int_0^1 x^2\,dx$.
21. Do same as example 10.

24. Put $x = r\cos\theta$, $y = r\sin\theta$, in the equation of the given curve, we get $r = \dfrac{3a\sin\theta\cos\theta}{(\cos^3\theta + \sin^3\theta)}$.

Required area $= \int_0^{\pi/2} \dfrac{r^2}{2} d\theta$.

ANSWERS

1. (i) $b \log (b/e) - a \log (a/e)$ (ii) $c^2 \sinh (a/c)$ (iii) $\pi/4$ **2.** 1/3 **3.** $\frac{1}{4}\pi ab$ **4.** $2a^2(1-\pi/4)$
5. $8a^2/(15\sqrt{3})$ **6.** πa^2 **8.** πa^2 **9.** 8/15 **10.** $4a^3/3$ **11.** $(8/3)a^3$ **12.** $3\pi a^2$ **13.** $4\pi a^2$
14. $3\pi a^2/4$; $(3\pi-8) : (3\pi+8)$ **15.** $(16/3)ab$ **16.** $(a^2/12)(3\pi-8)$ **17.** 1/3 **18.** 9/64 **19.** 27
20. $\frac{4}{3}a^{3/2} + \frac{8\pi}{3} - \frac{a}{2}\sqrt{\left(\frac{16}{3}\right) - a^2} - \frac{8}{3}\sin^{-1}\left(\frac{a}{4\sqrt{3}}\right)$, where $a = (-a + \sqrt{273})/6$
21. $3\pi a^2$ **22.** 1/2 **23.** $\frac{3}{8}\pi a^2$ **24.** $3a^2/2$ **25.** $(16/3)a^2$ **26.** $2\left[\frac{\sqrt{2}}{3} + \frac{9\pi}{4} - \frac{9}{2}\sin^{-1}\left(\frac{1}{3}\right)\right]$
27. 9/2

19.3 PROBLEM BASED ON POLAR FORM

1. *Find the area of the cardioid $r = a(1+\cos\theta)$.* (VTU-2008)

SOLUTION. The equation of the cardioid $r = a(1+\cos\theta)$ is symmetrical about the initial line and $r = 0$ when $\cos\theta = -1$ *i.e.*, $\theta = \pi$ and r is maximum when $\cos\theta = 1$ *i.e.*, $\theta = 0$. Thus the tracing of the curve is shown in fig. 17.

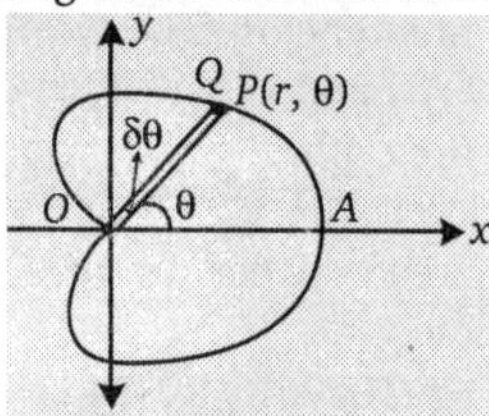

Fig. 16

Let A be the area of the cardiod $r = a(1+\cos\theta)$. This area A is the twice the area of the upper half of the curve between $\theta = 0$ and $\theta = \pi$.

Now the required area

$$A = 2\int_0^{\pi} \frac{1}{2} r^2 \, d\theta = \int_0^{\pi} a^2(1+\cos\theta)^2 d\theta$$

$$= a^2 \int_0^{\pi} (2)^2 \cos^4 \frac{\theta}{2} d\theta.$$

$$= 4a^2 \int_0^{\pi} \cos^4 \theta/2 \, d\theta.$$

Let us put $\theta/2 = \phi$ so $d\theta = 2\,d\phi$ and ϕ runs from 0 to $\pi/2$.

$$\therefore \quad A = 8a^2 \int_0^{\pi/2} \cos^4 \phi \, d\phi$$

$$= 8a^2 \left[\frac{(4-1)(4-3)}{4.2} \cdot \frac{\pi}{2}\right]$$

[By Walli's formula]

$$= \frac{3}{2}\pi a^2.$$

2. *Find the area of a loop of the curve $r^2 = a^2 \cos 2\theta$.* (VTU–2006)

SOLUTION. The curve is symmetrical about pole and initial line both and $r=0$ when $\cos 2\theta = 0$ *i.e.*, $\theta = \pm\,\pi/4$. Thus a loop of the curve lies betwen $\theta = -\pi/4$ and $\theta = \pi/4$.

Let A be the area of this loop. Then

$$A = \int_{-\pi/4}^{\pi/4} \frac{1}{2} r^2 d\theta = \frac{1}{2}\int_{-\pi/4}^{\pi/4} a^2 \cos 2\theta \, d\theta$$

$$= \frac{a^2}{2}\int_{-\pi/4}^{\pi/4} \cos 2\theta \, d\theta$$

$$= \frac{a^2}{2}\left[\frac{1}{2}\sin 2\theta\right]_{-\pi/4}^{\pi/4}$$

$$= \frac{a^2}{2}\left[\frac{1}{2} + \frac{1}{2}\right] = \frac{a^2}{2}.$$

3. *Find the whole area of the curve $r = a \sin 3\theta$.*

SOLUTION. The given curve is not symmetrical and $r = 0$ when $\sin 3\theta = 0$ *i.e.*, $\theta = 0$, $\theta = \pm\,\pi/3$ and r is maximum when $\sin 3\theta = 1$ *i.e.*, $\theta = \pi/6$. Also this curve has three loops so the whole area of the curve is thrice the area of one loop. Let whole area be A. Then

$$A = 3\int_{\theta=0}^{\theta=\pi/3} \frac{1}{2} r^2 d\theta$$

$$= \frac{3}{2}\int_0^{\pi/3} a^2 \sin^2 3\theta \, d\theta$$

$(\because r = a \sin 3\theta)$

$$= \frac{3}{2}a^2\int_0^{\pi/3}\left(\frac{1-\cos 6\theta}{2}\right)d\theta$$

$$= \frac{3}{4}a^2\left[\theta - \frac{1}{6}\sin 6\theta\right]_0^{\pi/3} = \frac{3}{4}a^2\left[\frac{\pi}{3}\right]$$

$$A = \frac{1}{4}\pi a^2.$$

4. *Find the area common to the circle $r = a$ and the cardioid $r = a(1+\cos\theta)$.*

SOLUTION. The points of intersection of the given curves $r = a$ and $r = a(1+\cos\theta)$ are given by $\theta = \pm\pi/2$.

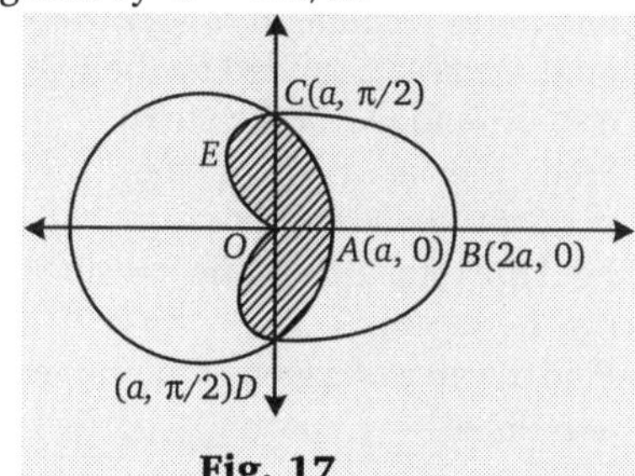

Fig. 17

Required area = 2 [area ACO + area $CEOC$]

Now area $ACO = \int_0^{\pi/2}\frac{1}{2}r^2 d\theta$ for $r = a$

$$= \frac{1}{2}a^2\int_0^{\pi/2}d\theta = \frac{\pi a^2}{4}$$

Area $CEOC = \int_{\pi/2}^{\pi}\frac{1}{2}r^2 d\theta$ for $r = a(1+\cos\theta)$

$$= \frac{a^2}{2}\int_{\pi/2}^{\pi}(1+\cos\theta)^2 d\theta$$

$$= \frac{a^2}{2}\int_{\pi/2}^{\pi}(1+\cos^2\theta + 2\cos\theta)d\theta$$

$$= \frac{a^2}{2}\left[\theta + \frac{1}{2}\left\{\theta + \frac{\sin 2\theta}{2}\right\} + 2\sin\theta\right]_{\pi/2}^{\pi}$$

$$= \frac{a^2}{2}\left[\frac{\pi}{2} + \frac{1}{2}\left(\frac{\pi}{2}\right) - 2\right] = \frac{3\pi a^2}{8} - a^2.$$

Hence, required area

$$= 2\left(\frac{\pi a^2}{4} + \frac{3\pi a^2}{8} - a^2\right)$$

$$= a^2\left(\frac{5\pi}{4} - 2\right).$$

5. *Find the area of common to the cardioids $r = a(1+\cos\theta)$ and $r = a(1-\cos\theta)$.*

(VTU-2006, KURUKSHETRA-2006)

SOLUTION. Clearly both the cardioids are symmetrical about the initial line OX and intersect at B and B' as shown in the adjoining figure.

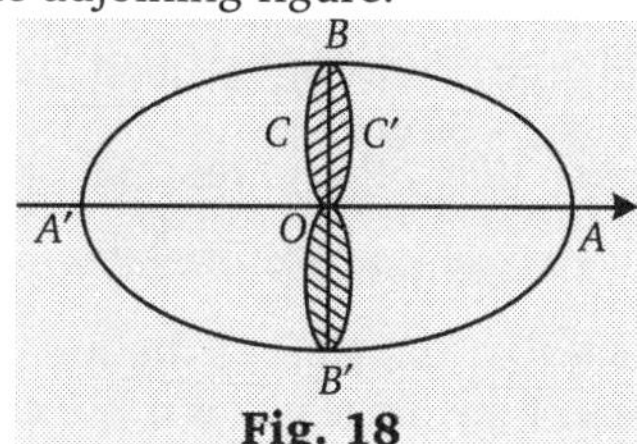

Fig. 18

Required area = 2 . Area $OC'BCO$

= 2[area $OC'BO$ + area $OBCO$]

$$= 2\left\{\left[\int_0^{\pi/2}\frac{1}{2}r^2 d\theta\right]_{r=a(1-\cos\theta)} + \left[\int_{\pi/2}^{\pi}\frac{1}{2}r^2 d\theta\right]_{r=a(1+\cos\theta)}\right\}$$

$$= a^2\int_0^{\pi/2}(1-\cos\theta)^2 d\theta + a^2\int_{\pi/2}^{\pi}(1+\cos\theta)^2 d\theta$$

$$= a^2\left\{\int_0^{\pi/2}(1-2\cos\theta+\cos^2\theta)d\theta + \int_{\pi/2}^{\pi}(1+2\cos\theta+\cos^2\theta)d\theta\right\}$$

$$= a^2\left\{\int_0^{\pi}(1+\cos^2\theta)d\theta - 2\int_0^{\pi/2}\cos\theta\, d\theta + 2\int_{\pi/2}^{\pi}\cos\theta\, d\theta\right\}$$

$$= a^2\left\{\int_0^{\pi}\left(1+\frac{1+\cos 2\theta}{2}\right)d\theta - 2|\sin\theta|_0^{\pi/2} + 2|\sin\theta|_{\pi/2}^{\pi}\right\}$$

$$= a^2\left\{\left|\frac{3}{2}\theta + \frac{\sin 2\theta}{4}\right|_0^{\pi} - 2(1-0) + 2(0-1)\right\}$$

$$= \left(\frac{3\pi}{2} - 4\right)a^2.$$

Exercise-19.2

1. Find the area of the parabola $r(1 + \cos\theta) = l$ between $\theta = 0, \theta = \alpha$.
2. Find the area of one loop of the curve $r = a\cos 4\theta$.
3. Find the whole area of the curve $r^2 = a^2\cos^2\theta + b^2\sin^2\theta$.
4. Find the area of a loop of the curve $x^3 + y^3 = 3axy$.
5. Show that the area of the limacon $r = a + b\cos\theta$, $(a > b)$ is $\pi\left(a^2 + \frac{1}{2}b^2\right)$.
6. Prove that the sum of the areas of the two loops of the limacon $r = a + b\cos\theta$ $(a<b)$ is $\pi(2a^2 + b^2)/2$.
7. Find the ratio of the two parts into which the parabola $2a = r(1 + \cos\theta)$ divides the area of the cardioid $r = 2a(1 + \cos\theta)$.
8. Find the area outside the circle $r = 2a\cos\theta$ and inside the cardioid $r = a(1 + \cos\theta)$. (KURUKSHETRA-2006)
9. Find the area between the curve $r = a(\sec\theta + \cos\theta)$ and its asymptote.
10. Find the area of a loop of the curve $x^4 + y^4 = 4a^2xy$.
11. Prove that the area of a loop of the curve $x^6 + y^6 = a^2x^2y^2$ is $\pi a^2/12$.
12. Find the area lying between the cardioid $r = (1 - \cos\theta)$ and its double tangent. (VTU–2004)
13. Find the area common to the circles $r = a\sqrt{2}$ and $r = 2a\cos\theta$.
14. If O is the pole of the lemniscate $r^2 = a^2\cos 2\theta$ and PQ is a common tanget to its two loops. Find the area bounded by the line PQ and the arcs OP and OQ of the curve.
15. Find the area of a loop of the curve $x^4 + 3x^2y^2 + 2y^4 = a^2xy$.
16. Find the total area inside $r = \sin\theta$ and outside $r = 1 - \cos\theta$. (ANNA-2009)
17. Find the area of a loop of the curve $r = a\cos 3\theta + b\sin 3\theta$.

Hint to Selected Problems

1. $A = \frac{1}{2}\int_0^{\alpha} r^2\, d\theta.$

2. $A = \frac{1}{2}\int_{-\pi/8}^{\pi/8} r^2\, d\theta.$

3. The curve is symmetrical about the initial line and line $\theta = \pi/2$. Also it is symmetric about the pole. $A = 4 \times$ Area lying in the first quadrant $= 4 \times \frac{1}{2}\int_0^{\pi/2} r^2\, d\theta.$

4. In polar form the given equation becomes $r = \dfrac{3a\cos\theta\sin\theta}{\cos^3\theta + \sin^3\theta}$. Then $A = \int_0^{\pi/2} \frac{1}{2}r^2\, d\theta.$

5. $A = 2\int_0^{\pi} \frac{1}{2}r^2\, d\theta.$

6. $A = 2\left[\int_0^{\cos^{-1}\left(-\frac{a}{b}\right)} \frac{1}{2}r^2 d\theta + \int_{\cos^{-1}\left(-\frac{a}{b}\right)}^{\pi} \frac{1}{2}r^2 d\theta\right].$

7. Smaller area
$$A_1 = \frac{1}{2}\int_0^{\pi/2} \frac{4a^2}{(1+\cos\theta)^2} d\theta + \frac{1}{2}\int_{\pi/2}^{\pi} 4a^2(1+\cos\theta)^2\, d\theta.$$
Larger area $A_2 =$ whole area $- A_1$. Then find $\dfrac{A_1}{A_2}$.

13. The points of intersection are given by $\theta = \pm\frac{\pi}{4}$. Required area $= 2(A_1 + A_2)$ where $A_1 = \int_{\pi/4}^{\pi/2} \frac{1}{2}r^2\, d\theta$ for $r = 2a\cos\theta$ and $A_2 = \int_0^{\pi/4} \frac{1}{2}r^2\, d\theta$ for $r = a\sqrt{2}$.

16. The both curve intersect at (0, 0) and $(1, \pi/2)$. Therefore, the required area $= A_1 - A_2$ where $A_1 = \frac{1}{2}\int_0^{\pi/2} r^2\, d\theta$ or $r = \sin\theta$ and $A_2 = \frac{1}{2}\int_0^{\pi/2} r^2\, d\theta$ for $r = 1 - \cos\theta$.

ANSWERS

1. $\frac{1}{4}l^2\left[\tan\frac{\alpha}{2} + \frac{1}{3}\tan^3\frac{\alpha}{2}\right]$ 2. $\frac{1}{16}\pi a^2$ 3. $\frac{1}{2}\pi(a^2 + b^2)$ 4. $\frac{3a^2}{2}$ 7. $(9\pi + 16) : (9\pi - 16)$

8. $\frac{1}{2}\pi a^2$ 9. $\frac{5}{4}\pi a^2$ 10. $\frac{1}{2}\pi a^2$ 12. $\frac{1}{16}(15\sqrt{3} - 8\pi)a^2$ 13. $a^2(\pi - 1)$

14. $\frac{1}{8}a^2(3\sqrt{3} - 4)$ 15. $\frac{1}{4}a^2\log 2$ 16. $\left(1 - \frac{\pi}{4}\right)$ 17. $(a^2 + b^2)\frac{\pi}{12}$.

□□□□□□

Chapter

20 Surface and Volume of Solid of Revolutions

20.1 INTRODUCTION

When a plane curve is revolved about a certain fixed line lying in its own plane, a surface is generated. This surface is called a surface of revolution. Also the fixed line is called the axis of revolution.

20.2 REVOLUTION ABOUT X-AXIS

Let S be the surface area (curved surface) of a solid which is generated by the revolution of the curve $y = f(x)$ about x-axis between the ordinates $x = a$ and $x = b$ and let s be the arc length measured from the point $(a, f(a))$ to any point $P(x, y)$. Then

$$S = \int_a^b 2\pi y\, ds = \int_a^b 2\pi y \frac{ds}{dx}.dx.$$

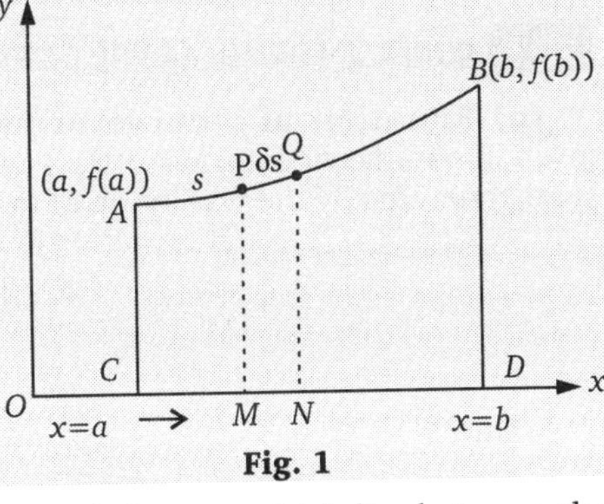

Fig. 1

Proof. Let $A\ (a, f(a))$ and $B\ (b, f(b))$ be the points on the curve $y = f(x)$and assuming that the curve $y = f(x)$ is continuous in (a, b) and does not intersect the axis of x. Let $P(x, y)$ be any point on the curve and s be the arc length of the curve measured from A as shown in fig. 1.

Let $Q(x + \delta x, y + \delta y)$ be any other point very near to $P(x, y)$. Then $PQ = \delta s$, because $AP = s$ and $AQ = s + \delta s$. Draw the perpendiculars PM and QN to the axis of x from P and Q respectively. As the curve revolves about x-axis, the arc length $PQ = \delta s$ also revolves and form a right circular cydinder of thickness δs of radii y and $y + \delta y$. Let δS be the surface area of this cylinderical element which lies between the surface areas $2\pi y \delta s$ and $2\pi\ (y + \delta y)\delta s$. That is,

$$2\pi y\ \delta s < \delta S < 2\pi(y + \delta y)\ \delta s.$$

Divide by δs, we get
$$2\pi y < \frac{\delta S}{\delta s} < 2\pi(y + \delta y).$$

As $Q \to P$, $\delta s \to 0$ and $\delta y \to 0$, then taking the limit as $\delta s \to 0$, we obtain

$$2\pi y < \lim_{\delta s \to 0} \frac{\delta S}{\delta s} < 2\pi y.$$

$$\therefore \qquad \lim_{\delta s \to 0} \frac{\delta S}{\delta s} = 2\pi y \text{ or } \frac{dS}{ds} = 2\pi y \text{ or } dS = 2\pi y\, ds.$$

Now integrating, we get $\int_{x=a}^{x=b} dS = \int_{x=a}^{x=b} 2\pi y\, ds$

or
$$S = \int_a^b 2\pi y\, ds = \int_a^b 2\pi y \frac{ds}{dx}.dx$$

where $\frac{ds}{dx} = \sqrt{\left[1+\left(\frac{dy}{dx}\right)^2\right]}$ and S is the surface area of the solid of revolution of the curve $y = f(x)$ about x-axis between $x = a$ and $x = b$.

20.3 REVOLUTION ABOUT Y-AXIS

Let S be the surface area of a solid generated by the revolution of the curve $x = f(y)$ about y-axis between $y = a$ and $y=b$. Then

$$S = \int_a^b 2\pi\, x\, ds = \int_a^b 2\pi x \frac{ds}{dy}.dy$$

where $\frac{ds}{dy} = \sqrt{\left[1+\left(\frac{dx}{dy}\right)^2\right]}$ and s the arc length being measured from the point $(f(a), a)$.

Proof. Similar as before given in § 20.2.

20.4 REVOLUTION ABOUT ANY LINE

Let S be the surface area of a solid generated by the curve about any line between certain points. Let s be the arc length of the curve measured from one of the two given points to any point P on the curve and let Q be any point very near to P such that $PQ = \delta s$. Now draw a perpendicular PM from the point P to the line of axis of the revolution. Then

$$S = \int 2\pi (PM)\, ds$$

Here the limits of integration are taken the given points between them.

20.5 SURFACE FORMULAE FOR DIFFERENT FORM OF EQUATIONS

(a) Equation of a curve in parametric form. Suppose the equation of a curve is given in parametric form $x = f(t)$, $y=g(t)$ where t is the parameter, then the surface area of a solid generated by the revolution of the given curve about x-axis between the suitable limits is

$$S = \int 2\pi y \left(\frac{ds}{dt}\right) dt$$

where
$$\frac{ds}{dt} = \sqrt{\left[\left(\frac{dx}{dt}\right)^2 + \left(\frac{dy}{dt}\right)^2\right]}.$$

Similarly for y-axis as the axis of revolution we may find the surface area.

(b) Equation of a curve in polar form. Suppose the equation of a curve is given in polar form $r = f(\theta)$. Then the formula for finding the surface area between the proper limits is given by

$$S = \int 2\pi (r \sin\theta) \frac{ds}{d\theta}.d\theta \qquad ...(1)$$

where
$$\frac{ds}{d\theta} = \sqrt{\left[r^2 + \left(\frac{dr}{d\theta}\right)^2\right]}.$$

The formula given in (1) can also be taken as

$$S = \int 2\pi (r \sin\theta) \frac{ds}{dr}.dr \qquad ...(2)$$

where $$\frac{ds}{dr} = \sqrt{\left[1+\left(r\frac{d\theta}{dr}\right)^2\right]}.$$

WORKING PROCEDURE

To find the surface area of a solid generated by the revolution of the curve about any line, use the following steps :

STEP 1. Take any point P on the curve between the given points.

STEP 2. Draw the perpendicular from P to the line of axis which meets the axis at the point M (say).

STEP 3. Find the perpendicular PM.

STEP 4. And use the formula given in § 20.4.

Solved Examples

1. *Find the surface of a sphere of radius a.*

SOLUTION. The sphere is generated, if a semi-circle is revolved about its diameter. Let the equation of a circle of radius a is

$$x^2 + y^2 = a^2. \quad \quad ...(1)$$

$$\therefore \quad 2x + 2y\frac{dy}{dx} = 0 \text{ or } \frac{dy}{dx} = -\frac{x}{y}.$$

$$\Rightarrow \quad \frac{ds}{dx} = \sqrt{\left[1+\left(\frac{dy}{dx}\right)^2\right]} = \sqrt{\left(1+\frac{x^2}{y^2}\right)}$$

$$= \sqrt{\left(\frac{x^2+y^2}{y^2}\right)} = \frac{a}{y} \text{ [Using (1)]}$$

Let $A(-a,\ 0)$ and $B(a,\ 0)$ be the bounding points of the semi-circle as shown in fig. 2.

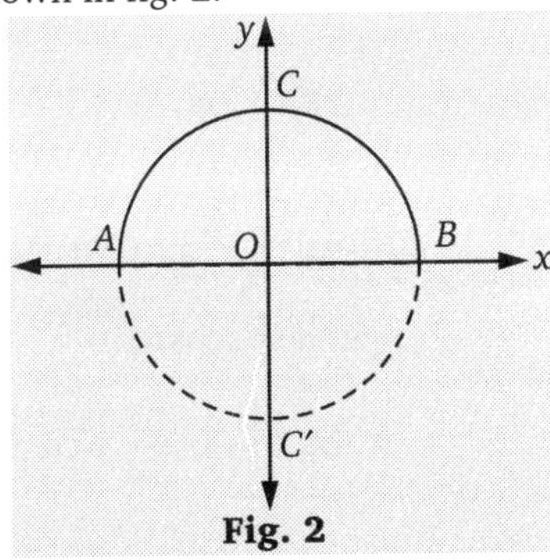

Fig. 2

Here the diameter is taken as x-axis. Let S be the surface area of the sphere, then

$$S = \int_{-a}^{a} 2\pi y.\frac{ds}{dx}.dx$$

$$= \int_{-a}^{a} 2\pi y.\frac{a}{y}.dx \quad \left(\because \frac{ds}{dx} = \frac{a}{y}\right)$$

$$= 2\pi a\int_{-a}^{a} dx = 2\pi a\left[x\right]_{-a}^{a}$$

$$\therefore \quad S = 4\,\pi a^2.$$

2. *Find the surface of the solid generated by the revolution of the ellipse $x^2 + 4y^2 = 16$ about its major axis.*

SOLUTION. The equation of the curve is

$$x^2 + 4\,y^2 = 16 \quad \quad ...(1)$$

or $$\frac{x^2}{16} + \frac{y^2}{4} = 1.$$

The end points of major axis are $A(-4,0)$ and $B(4,\ 0)$ which are on the x-axis so the major axis is the axis of x. Thus the curve is revolved about the x-axis.

Now differentiating (1) *w.r.t.* 'x', we get

$$2x + 8y\frac{dy}{dx} = 0 \text{ or } \frac{dy}{dx} = -\frac{x}{4y}.$$

$$\therefore \quad \frac{ds}{dx} = \sqrt{\left[1+\left(\frac{dy}{dx}\right)^2\right]}$$

$$= \sqrt{\left(1+\frac{x^2}{16y^2}\right)} = \frac{\sqrt{(16y^2+x^2)}}{4y}$$

$$= \frac{\sqrt{4(16-x^2)+x^2]}}{4\,y} \text{ [Using (1)]}$$

$$\therefore \quad \frac{ds}{dx} = \frac{\sqrt{(64-3x^2)}}{4y}.$$

Let S be the surface area of the solid so formed by the revolution of the ellipse given in (1) about its major axis (x-axis is)

$$S = \int_{-4}^{4} 2\pi y \frac{ds}{dx}.dx$$

$$= \int_{-4}^{4} 2\pi y.\frac{\sqrt{(64-3x^2)}}{4y}dx$$

$$= \frac{\pi}{2}\int_{-4}^{4}\sqrt{(64-3x^2)}\,dx$$

$$= \pi\int_{0}^{4}\sqrt{(64-3x^2)}\,dx$$

$$= \sqrt{3}\pi\int_{0}^{4}\sqrt{\left[\left(\frac{8}{\sqrt{3}}\right)^2 - x^2\right]}dx$$

$$= \sqrt{3}\pi\left[\frac{x}{2}\sqrt{\left[\left(\frac{8}{\sqrt{3}}\right)^2 - x^2\right]} + \frac{32}{3}\sin^{-1}\frac{\sqrt{3}x}{8}\right]_0^4$$

$$= \sqrt{3}\pi\left[2\sqrt{\left(\frac{64}{3}-16\right)} + \frac{32}{3}\sin^{-1}\left(\frac{\sqrt{3}}{2}\right)\right]$$

$$= \sqrt{3}\pi\left[2.\frac{4}{\sqrt{3}} + \frac{32}{(\sqrt{3})^2}.\frac{\pi}{3}\right]$$

$$= \pi\left[8 + \frac{32}{3\sqrt{3}}\pi\right]$$

$$\therefore\ S = 8\pi\left[1 + \frac{4\pi}{3\sqrt{3}}\right].$$

3. *Find the surface of the solid generated by the revolution of the lemniscate $r^2=a^2\cos 2\theta$ about the initial line.*

SOLUTION. The equation of the curve is

$$r^2 = a^2\cos 2\theta. \qquad ...(1)$$

From (1) $r = 0$, when $\cos 2\theta = 0$ *i.e.*, $2\theta = \pm\pi/2$ or $\theta = \pm\pi/4$ and maximum value of r is a, when $\cos 2\theta = 1$ *i.e.*, $\theta = 0$. Thus the tracing of this curve is as fig. 3.

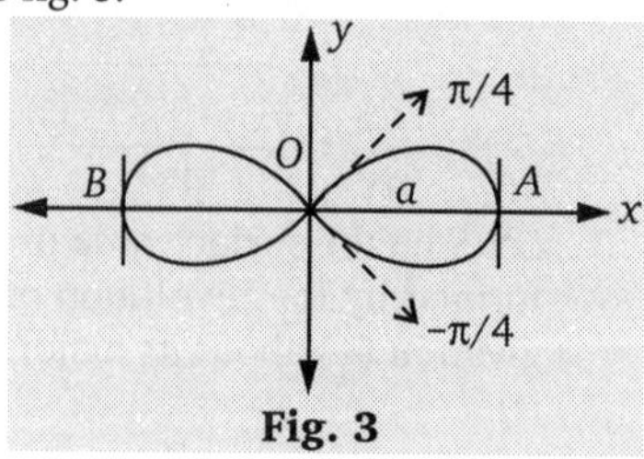

Fig. 3

Now differentiating (1) w.r.t. θ, we get

$$2r\frac{dr}{d\theta} = -2a^2\sin 2\theta$$

or
$$\frac{dr}{d\theta} = -\frac{a^2\sin 2\theta}{r}. \qquad ...(2)$$

$$\therefore\quad \frac{ds}{d\theta} = \sqrt{\left[r^2 + \left(\frac{dr}{d\theta}\right)^2\right]}$$

$$= \sqrt{\left[a^2\cos 2\theta + \frac{a^4\sin^2 2\theta}{r^2}\right]}$$

[Using (1) and (2)]

$$= \frac{\sqrt{(r^2a^2\cos 2\theta + a^4\sin^2 2\theta)}}{r}$$

$$= \frac{\sqrt{(a^4\cos^2 2\theta + a^4\sin^2 2\theta)}}{r}$$

[Using (1)]

$$= \frac{a^2}{r}.$$

Since there are two loops in the curve and one loop of the curve lies between $\theta = -\pi/4$ and $\theta = \pi/4$. Also the curve is symmetrical about the pole as well as about the initial line. Let S be the surface of the solid generated by the revolution of the given curve. Then

$$S = 2\int_0^{\pi/4} 2\pi y\frac{ds}{d\theta}.d\theta,$$

where $y = r\sin\theta$

$$= 2\int_0^{\pi/4} 2\pi(r\sin\theta).\frac{a^2}{r}.d\theta$$

[Using (2)]

$$= 4\pi a^2\int_0^{\pi/4}\sin\theta\,d\theta$$

$$= 4\pi a^2\left[-\cos\theta\right]_0^{\pi/4}$$

$$= 4\pi a^2\left[-\cos\frac{\pi}{4} + \cos 0\right]$$

$$= 4\pi a^2\left(-\frac{1}{\sqrt{2}} + 1\right)$$

$$\therefore\quad S = 4\pi a^2\left(1 - \frac{1}{\sqrt{2}}\right).$$

Similar Problem

(1) A quadrant of a circle of radius a revolves about its chord. Show that the surface of the spindle generated is $2\pi a^2\left(1-\frac{\pi}{4}\right)\sqrt{2}$.

4. *The lemniscate $r^2 = a^2\cos 2\theta$ revolves about a tangent at the pole. Find the surface of the solid thus generated.*

SOLUTION. We have $r^2 = a^2 \cos 2\theta$. ...(1)

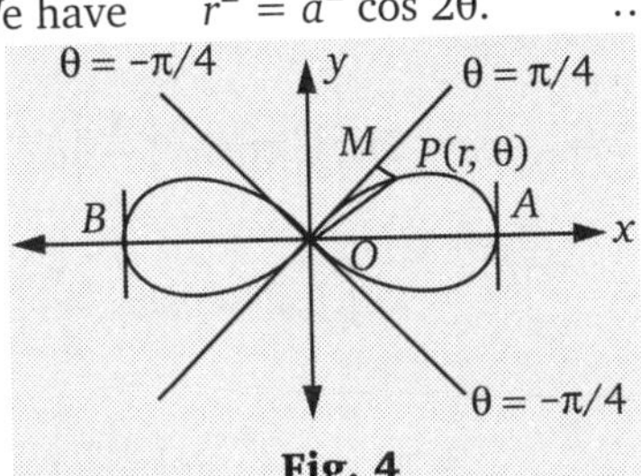

Fig. 4

Clearly, $\theta = \pi/4$ is one of the tangent at the pole.

Let $P(r, \theta)$ be any point on the curve. Draw PM as perpendicular from P to the line $\theta = \pi/4$. Then

$$\angle POM = \frac{\pi}{4} - \theta.$$

So in $\Delta\, PMO$, $\dfrac{PM}{PO} = \sin\left(\dfrac{\pi}{4} - \theta\right)$

$\therefore\ PM = r\sin\left(\dfrac{\pi}{4} - \theta\right)$.

Now differentiating (1) w.r.t. θ, we get

$$2r\frac{dr}{d\theta} = -2a^2 \sin 2\theta$$

or $$\frac{dr}{d\theta} = -\frac{a^2 \sin 2\theta}{r}$$

$\therefore$ $$\frac{ds}{d\theta} = \sqrt{r^2 + \left(\frac{dr}{d\theta}\right)^2}$$

$$= \sqrt{a^2 \cos 2\theta + \frac{a^4 \sin^2 2\theta}{r^2}}$$

$$= \frac{1}{r}\sqrt{a^4 \cos^2 2\theta + a^4 \sin^2 2\theta}$$

$$= \frac{a^2}{r}$$

There are two loops in the curve and loop lies between $\theta = -\pi/4$ and $\theta = \pi/4$. Also the curve is symmetrical about the pole as well as about the initial line.

Let S be the surface of the solid generated by the revolution of the given curve about the line $\theta = \pi/4$. Then

$$S = 2\int_{-\pi/4}^{\pi/4} 2\pi(PM)\frac{ds}{d\theta}d\theta$$

$$= 4\pi\int_{-\pi/4}^{\pi/4} r\sin\left(\frac{\pi}{4}-\theta\right)\frac{a^2}{r}d\theta$$

$$= 4\pi a^2 \int_{-\pi/4}^{\pi/4} \sin\left(\frac{\pi}{4}-\theta\right)d\theta$$

$$= 4\pi a^2\left[\cos\left(\frac{\pi}{4}-\theta\right)\right]_{-\pi/4}^{\pi/4}$$

$$= 4\pi a^2\left[1-\cos\frac{\pi}{2}\right] = 4\pi a^2(1-0)$$

$$= 4\pi a^2.$$

5. *Find the surface of the solid generated by the revolution of the curve $x = a\cos^3 t$ and $y = a\sin^3 t$ about the x-axis.*

SOLUTION. We have $x = a \cos^3 t$ and $y = a \sin^3 t$. This curve is symmetrical about both the axes.

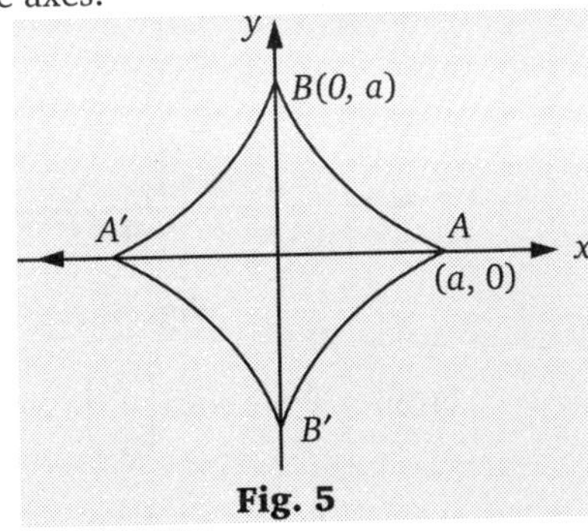

Fig. 5

At $A(a, 0)$, $t = 0$ and at $B(0, a)$, $t = \pi/2$.

Now $$\frac{dx}{dt} = -3a\cos^2 t\sin t$$

$$\frac{dy}{dt} = 3a\sin^2 t\cos t$$

$$\therefore \quad \frac{ds}{dt} = \sqrt{\left(\frac{dx}{dt}\right)^2 + \left(\frac{dy}{dt}\right)^2}$$

$$= 3a\sqrt{\cos^4 t \sin^2 t + \sin^4 t \cos^2 t}$$

$$= 3a \sin t \cos t = \frac{3a}{2}\sin 2t.$$

Let S be the surface of a solid of revolution of the given curve about x-axis. Then

$$S = 2\int_0^{\pi/2} 2\pi y \frac{ds}{dt} dt$$

$$= 4\pi\int_0^{\pi/2} a\sin^3 t . \frac{3a}{2}\sin 2t\, dt$$

$$= 12\pi a^2 \int_0^{\pi/2} \sin^4 t \cos t\, dt$$

$$= 12\pi a^2 \left[\frac{\sin^5 t}{5}\right]_0^{\pi/2} = \frac{12\pi a^2}{5}.$$

6. *Find the surface generated by the revolution of an arc of the catenary* $y = c\cosh\left(\frac{x}{c}\right)$ *about the x-axis.*

SOLUTION. Let S be the surface generated by the revolution of an arc DP of $y = c\cosh\left(\frac{x}{c}\right)$ about x-axis.

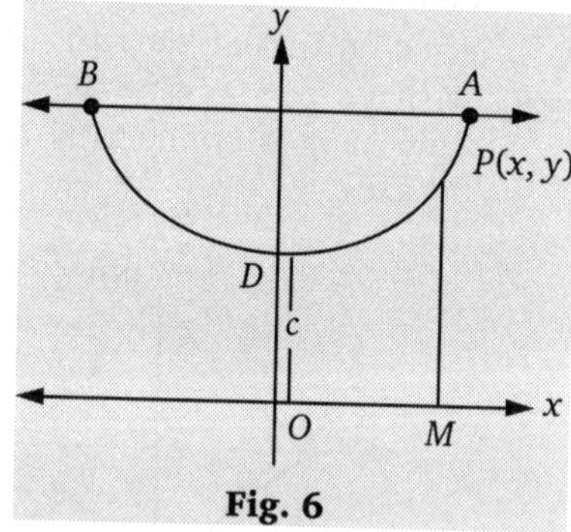

Fig. 6

From $\quad y = c\cosh\left(\frac{x}{c}\right)$, we have

$$\frac{dy}{dx} = \sinh\left(\frac{x}{c}\right)$$

Then $\dfrac{ds}{dx} = \sqrt{1 + \left(\dfrac{dy}{dx}\right)^2}$

$$= \sqrt{1 + \sinh^2\left(\frac{x}{c}\right)}$$

$$= \cosh\left(\frac{x}{c}\right)$$

Now, $\quad S = 2\pi\int_0^x y\frac{ds}{dx}dx$

$$= 2\pi\int_0^x c\cosh\left(\frac{x}{c}\right)\cosh\left(\frac{x}{c}\right)dx$$

$$= 2\pi c\int_0^x \cosh^2\left(\frac{x}{c}\right)dx$$

$$= \pi c\int_0^x \left[1 + \cosh\left(\frac{2x}{c}\right)\right]dx$$

$$= \pi c\left[x + \frac{c}{2}\sinh\frac{2x}{c}\right]_0^x$$

$$= \pi c\left[x + \frac{c}{2}\sinh\frac{2x}{c}\right].$$

7. *Find the surface of the solid generated by revolving the arc of the parabola* $y^2 = 4ax$ *bounded by its latusrectum about x-axis.* (ROHTAK–2003)

SOLUTION. Let S be the surface of solid of revolution of arc LOL' of the parabola $y^2 = 4ax$ about x-axis. Then

$$S = \int_0^a 2\pi y\, ds$$

or $\quad S = \int_0^a 2\pi y\, dx . \dfrac{ds}{dx} \qquad$ ...(1)

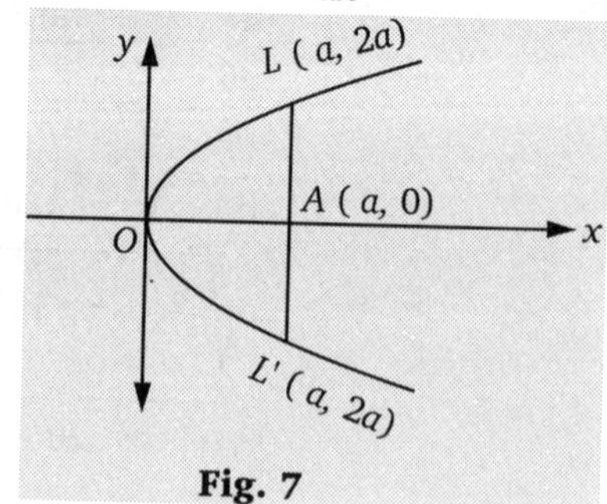

Fig. 7

We have $y^2 = 4ax$

$\Rightarrow \qquad y = 2\sqrt{ax} \quad \Rightarrow \dfrac{dy}{dx} = \dfrac{\sqrt{a}}{\sqrt{x}}$

$$\therefore \quad \frac{ds}{dx} = \sqrt{1+\left(\frac{dy}{dx}\right)^2} = \sqrt{1+\frac{a}{x}}$$
$$= \sqrt{\frac{x+a}{x}}$$

Therefore,

$$S = 2\pi\int_0^a 2\sqrt{ax}\left[\sqrt{\frac{x+a}{x}}\right]dx$$

$$= 4\pi\sqrt{a}\int_0^a \sqrt{x+a}\,dx$$
$$= 4\pi\sqrt{a}\left[\frac{2}{3}(x+a)^{3/2}\right]_0^a$$
$$= \frac{8\pi\sqrt{a}}{3}[(2a)^{3/2} - a^{3/2}]$$
$$= \frac{8\pi}{3}(2^{3/2}-1)a^2 = \frac{8\pi}{3}(2\sqrt{2}-1)a^2$$

Exercise-20.1

1. Find the curved surface of a hemi-sphere of radius a.
2. For a catenary $y = a \cosh (x/a)$, prove that
$$aS = \pi a\,(ax + sy).$$
where s is the length of the arc measured from the vertex, S is the area of curved surface of the solid generated by the revolution of the arc about x-axis.
3. Find the surface of the solid generated by the revolution of the astroid $x^{2/3} + y^{2/3} = a^{2/3}$ aboul x-axis.
4. Find the surface of the solid formed by the revolution, about the axis of y, of the part of the curve $ay^2 = x^3$ from $x = 0$ to $x = 4a$ which is above the x-axis.
5. Prove that the surface of the prolate spheroid formed by the revolution of the ellipse of essentricity e about its major axis is equal to $2\pi ab\left[\sqrt{(1-e^2)} + \frac{1}{e}\sin^{-1} e\right]$.
6. Prove that the surface of the oblate spheroid formed by the revolution of the ellipse of essentricity e about its minor axis is $2\pi a^2\left[1+\frac{1-e^2}{2e}\log\left(\frac{1+e}{1-e}\right)\right]$.
7. Find the surface area of the solid generated by revolution of the cycloid $x = a\,(\theta - \sin\theta)$, $y = a(1 - \cos\theta)$about x-axis. (VTU-2003)
8. The portion between two consecutive cusps of the cycloid, $x = a\,(\theta + \sin\theta)$, $y = a\,(1+ \cos\theta)$ is revolved about x-axis. Prove that the area of the surface so formed is to the area of the cycloid as 64 : 9.
9. Prove that the surface area of the solid generated by the revolution of the loop of the curve $x = t^2,\ y = t - \frac{1}{3}t^3$ about x-axis is 3π.
10. Find the surface of the solid formed by the revolution of the cardioid $r = a\,(1 + \cos\theta)$ about the initial line. (VTU-2009, JNTU-2003, RAJASTHAN-2006)
11. Find the area of the surface of revolution formed by revolving the curve $r = 2a\cos\theta$ about the initial line. (VTU–2009)
12. A circular arc revolves aboul its chord. Find the area of the surface generated, when 2α is the angle subtended by the arc at the centre.

Hint to the Selected Problems

1. $S = 2\pi\int_0^a 2\pi\, x\, ds = 2\pi\int_0^a \sqrt{a^2 - y^2}\cdot\frac{ds}{dy}\cdot dy.$

2. $y = a\cosh\frac{x}{a} \Rightarrow \frac{dy}{dx} = \sinh\left(\frac{x}{a}\right)$
$$\Rightarrow \frac{ds}{dx} = \cosh\frac{x}{a} \Rightarrow s = a\sinh\frac{x}{a}.$$
Now $S = 2\pi\int_0^x y\frac{ds}{dx}.dx$
$$= 2\pi\int_0^x a\cosh\frac{x}{a}.\ \cosh\frac{x}{a}.dx.$$

3. From the given curve, we obtained
$$\frac{dy}{dx} = -\left(\frac{y}{x}\right)^{1/3}$$
$$\therefore \quad \frac{ds}{dx} = \sqrt{1+\left(\frac{dy}{dx}\right)^2} = \frac{a^{1/3}}{x^{1/3}}.$$
Now use $S = 4\pi\int_0^a y.\frac{ds}{dx}.dx$
$$= 4\pi\int_0^a (a^{2/3} - x^{2/3})^{3/2}\frac{a^{1/3}}{x^{1/3}}dx.$$
Then put $x^{2/3} = a^{2/3}\sin^2\theta$.

4. $S = \int_0^{8a} 2\pi x . \frac{ds}{dy} . dy.$ ...(1)

Also $\frac{ds}{dy} = \sqrt{1 + \left(\frac{dx}{dy}\right)^2} = \frac{\sqrt{9x^4 + 4a^2y^2}}{3x^2}.$

Put in (1) and then solve.

5. Given that $\frac{x^2}{a^2} + \frac{y^2}{b^2} = 1$ ...(1)

and $b^2 = a^2 (1 - e^2)$

Then $S = 2\int_0^a 2\pi y \, ds.$

From (1), $\frac{ds}{dx} = -\left(\frac{b^2 x}{a^2 y}\right).$

Then find $\frac{ds}{dx}$ and put in $S = 2\int_0^a 2\pi y \, ds.$

9. $x = t^2,\ y = t - \frac{t^3}{3} \Rightarrow \frac{dx}{dt} = 2t, \frac{dy}{dt} = 1 - t^2.$

$\therefore \quad \frac{dy}{dx} = \frac{1 - t^2}{2t}.$

Now by using the formula

$$\left(\frac{ds}{dt}\right)^2 = \left(\frac{dx}{dt}\right)^2 + \left(\frac{dy}{dt}\right)^2.$$

We obtained $\frac{ds}{dt} = 1 + t^2.$

Then $S = \int_0^{\sqrt{3}} 2\pi y . \frac{ds}{dt} . dt.$

10. $r = a(1 + \cos\theta) \Rightarrow \frac{dr}{d\theta} = -a\sin\theta$

$\Rightarrow \frac{ds}{d\theta} = \sqrt{r^2 + \left(\frac{dr}{d\theta}\right)^2} = 2a\cos\frac{\theta}{2}$

Then use $S = \int_0^{\pi} 2\pi(r\sin\theta) . \frac{ds}{d\theta} d\theta.$

11. Here, we have $\frac{dr}{d\theta} = -2a\sin\theta.$

$\therefore \quad \frac{ds}{d\theta} = \sqrt{r^2 + \left(\frac{dr}{d\theta}\right)^2} = 2a.$

Then we use $S = \int_0^{\pi/2} 2\pi y \frac{ds}{d\theta} d\theta.$

ANSWERS

1. $2\pi a^2$ **3.** $\frac{12\pi a^2}{5}$ **4.** $\frac{128}{1215}\pi a^2[125\sqrt{10} + 1]$ **7.** $\frac{64}{3}\pi a^2$ **10.** $\frac{32}{5}\pi a^2$

11. $4\pi a^2$ **12.** $4\pi a^2 (\sin\alpha - \alpha\cos\alpha).$

20.6 VOLUME OF SOLID OF REVOLUTIONS

When a plane area is revolved about any fixed line lying in the same plane, a solid (body) is generated. This solid (body) is called a solid of revolution. Also about the x-axis, two right circular cylinders are formed of volumes $\pi y^2 \delta x$ and $\pi(y+\delta y)^2 \delta x$ respectively. Since the plane area $PMNQ$ lies between $PMNP'$ and $Q'MNQ$. Therefore δV_1 lies between $\pi y^2 \delta x$ and $\pi(y + \delta y)^2 \delta x$. Then

$$\pi y^2 \delta x < \delta V_1 < \pi (y + \delta y)^2 \delta x.$$

Divide by δx, we get

$$\pi y^2 < \frac{\delta V_1}{\delta x} < \pi(y + \delta y)^2.$$

As $Q \to P$, $\delta x \to 0$ and $\delta y \to 0$ so taking the limit as $\delta x \to 0$, we get

$$\pi y^2 < \lim_{\delta x \to 0} \frac{\delta V_1}{\delta x} < \pi y^2 \quad \text{or} \quad \lim_{\delta x \to 0} \frac{\delta V_1}{\delta x} = \pi y^2$$

or $\quad \frac{dV_1}{dx} = \pi y^2 \quad$ or $\quad dV_1 = \pi y^2 \, dx.$

Now integrating w.r.t. x between the limits $x = a$ to $x = b$, we get $\int_a^b dV_1 = \int_a^b \pi y^2 \, dx$.

$\therefore$ Volume generated by the plane area $ABDC = \int_a^b \pi y^2 dx$

or $$V_1 = \int_a^b \pi y^2 \, dx$$

Where V_1 is the required volume of a solid formed by the plane area bounded by the curve $y = f(x)$, the ordinates $x = a$ and $x = b$ and x-axis about x-axis fixed line is called axis of revolution.

20.6.1 Revolution about x-axis

Let V be the volume of a solid which is generated by the revolution of a plane area bounded by the curve y = f(x), the ordinates x = a, x = b and x-axis about the x-axis. Then

$$V = \int_a^b \pi y^2 \, dx$$

where $y = f(x)$ is a continuous and single valued function defined on $[a, b]$.

Proof. Let us assume that the curve $y = f(x)$does not cut the x-axis and let AB be the arc of $y = f(x)$ between the ordinates $x = a$ and $x = b$ as shown in fig. 8.

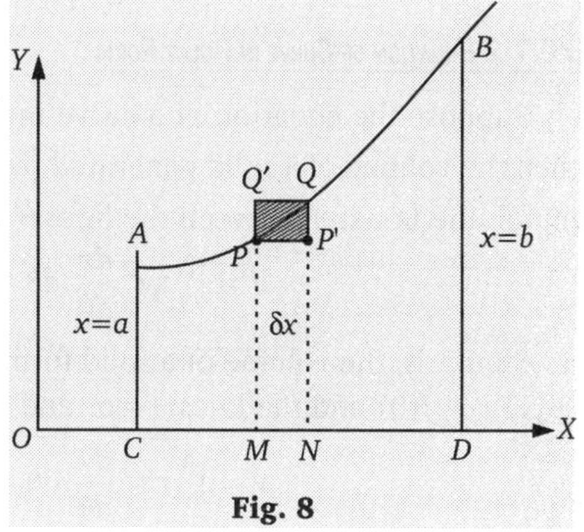

Fig. 8

Let P(x, y) and Q $(x + \delta x, y + \delta y)$ be two neighbouring points on the curve $y = f(x)$. Draw the perpendiculars PM and QN to the x-axis about which the plane area $ACDB$ is revolved. Also PP' is the perpendicular to QN and QQ' is the perpendicular to PM, where (Q' is a point on MP when P produced to Q'. Let V_1 be the volume of the solid formed by the revolution of plane area $ACMP$ about x-axis and $(V_1 + \delta V_1)$ be the volume of the solid formed by the revolution of the plane area $ACNQ$. Then δV_1 is the volume of a solid formed by the revolution of the plane area $PMNQ$ about x-axis.

20.6.2 Revolution About y-axis

The volume of a solid formed by the revolution of a plane area bounded by the curve $x = f(y)$and the lines $y = a$ and $y = b$ and y-axis about y-axis is

$$V = \int_a^b \pi x^2 \, dy.$$

20.6.3 Revolution About Any Line

The volume of a solid formed by the revolution of a plane area bounded by the arc AB and the lines AC and BD and the axis CD about any line CD (different from x-axis and y-axis) is

$$V = \int_{OC}^{OD} \pi (PM)^2 \, d(OM)$$

where PM is the length of perpendicular from any point P on the arc AB to the axis CD and O be any fixed point on the axis CD.

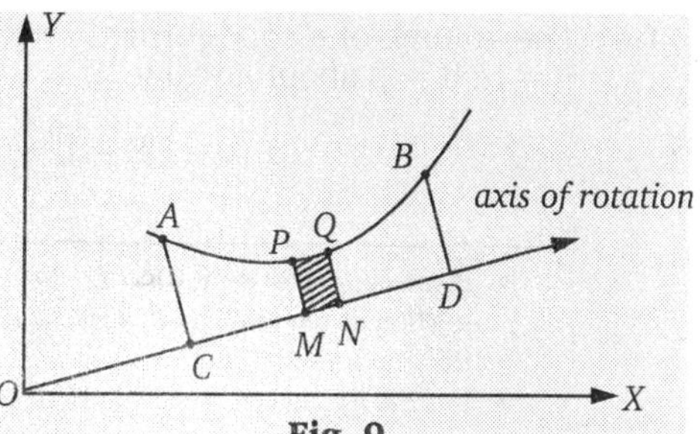

Fig. 9

20.7 VOLUME OF A SOLID OF REVOLUTION WHEN THE EQUATION OF THE CURVE ARE IN DIFFERENT FORMS

20.7.1 EQUATION OF CURVE IN PARAMETRIC FORM

Suppose the equation of a generating curve are in parametric form $x = f(t)$ and $y = g(t)$, then the volume of the solid generated by the revolution of the plane area bounded by the given curve, axis of x and the ordinates at the points where $t = a$ and $t = b$, about x-axis is

$$V = \int_a^b \pi y^2 \left(\frac{dx}{dt}\right).dt = \int_a^b \pi[g(t)]^2 \frac{dx}{dt}.dt \text{ where } \frac{dx}{dt} = \frac{d}{dt}[f(t)].$$

Similarly, the volume of a solid formed by the revolution of a plane area bounded by $x = f(t),\ y = g(t)$ axis of y and the two absciassae where $t = a$ and $t = b$ about y-axis is

$$V = \int_a^b \pi x^2 \left(\frac{dy}{dt}\right).dt = \int_a^b \pi[f(t)]^2 \frac{dy}{dt}.dt \text{ where } \frac{dy}{dt} = \frac{d}{dt}[g(t)].$$

20.7.2 EQUATION OF CURVE IN POLAR FORM

Suppose the equation of a curve in polar form is $r = f(\theta)$ where $x = r\cos\theta, y = r\sin\theta$, then the volume of a solid generated by the revolution of the plane area of the curve about the initial line (x-axis) between the lines $\theta = \alpha$ and $\theta = \beta$ is given by

$$V = \int_\alpha^\beta \pi y^2 \frac{dx}{d\theta}.d\theta = \int_\alpha^\beta \pi(r\sin\theta)^2 \frac{d}{d\theta}(r\cos\theta)d\theta \qquad \text{where} \quad r = f(\theta).$$

Similarly, the volume of a solid formed by the revolution of the plane area bounded by the curve $r = f(\theta)$ and the lines $\theta = \alpha$ and $\theta = \beta$ about the line $\theta = \pi/2$ (y-axis) is given by

$$V = \int_\alpha^\beta \pi x^2 \frac{dy}{d\theta}.d\theta = \int_\alpha^\beta \pi(r\cos\theta)^2 \frac{d}{d\theta}(r\sin\theta)d\theta \qquad \text{where} \quad r = f(\theta).$$

20.7.3 FORMULAE FOR FINDING THE VOLUME IN CASE OF POLAR FORM

(i) The volume of a solid formed by the revolution of the plane area bounded by the curve $r = f(\theta)$ and the radii vectors $\theta = \alpha$ and $\theta = \beta$ about the initial line *i.e.*, $\theta = 0$ (x-axis) is

$$V = \int_\alpha^\beta \frac{2}{3}\pi r^3 \sin\theta\, d\theta.$$

(ii) The volume of a solid formed by the revolution of a plane area bounded by $r = f(\theta)$ and $\theta = \alpha, \theta = \beta$ about the line $\theta = \pi/2$ (y-axis) is given by

$$V = \int_\alpha^\beta \frac{2}{3}\pi r^3 \cos\theta\, d\theta.$$

(iii) The volume of a solid formed by the revolution of a plane area bounded by $r = f(\theta)$ and $\theta = \alpha, \theta = \beta$ about any line $\theta = \gamma$ is given by

$$V = \int_\alpha^\beta \frac{2}{3}\pi r^3 \sin(\theta - \gamma)\, d\theta.$$

- If the curve is symmetrical about x-axis. then the portion of the curve above x-axis overlaps the other portion of the curve below x-axis during the revolution. So that the volume shall not double between the bounding points.
- If the curve is symmetrical about x-axis and the volume of a solid generated by the revolution of the plane area about y-axis is required, then the required volume will be double the volume which is obtained by the revolution of half of the symmetrical curve.

Solved Examples

1. *Find the volume of a spherical cap of height h cut off from a sphere of radius a.*

SOLUTION. The spherical cap is generated by the revolution of a plane area bounded by the curve $x^2 + y^2 = a^2$, the axis of y and the line $y = a - h$ and $y = a$ in the first quadrant about y-axis as shown in fig. 10.

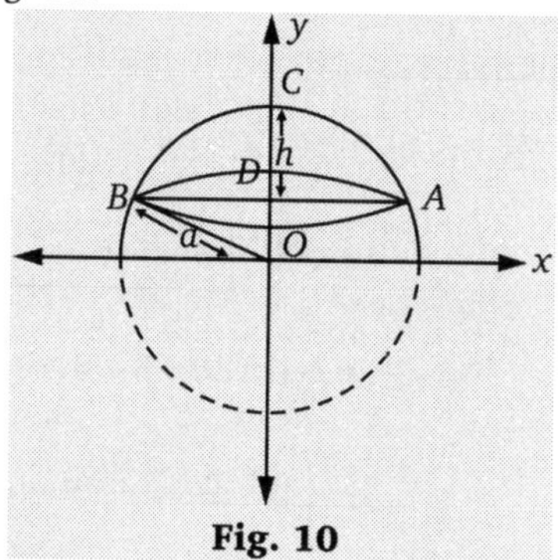

Fig. 10

Let V be the volume of this spherical cap, then

$$V = \int_{a-h}^{a} \pi x^2 \, dy$$

$$= \pi \int_{a-h}^{a} (a^2 - y^2) dy \quad (\therefore x^2 + y^2 = a^2)$$

$$= \pi \left[a^2 y - \frac{y^3}{3} \right]_{a-h}^{a}$$

$$= \pi \left[\left(a^3 - \frac{a^3}{3} \right) - (a-h) \left\{ a^2 - \frac{(a-h)^2}{3} \right\} \right]$$

$$= \pi \left[\frac{2a^3}{3} - \frac{a-h}{3} \{3a^2 - (a-h)^2\} \right]$$

$$= \frac{\pi}{3} [2a^3 - (a-h)\{2a^2 - h^2 + 2ah\}]$$

$$= \frac{\pi}{3} [2a^3 - 2a^2(a-h) + (a-h)h^2 - 2ah(a-h)]$$

$$= \frac{\pi}{3} (3ah^2 - h^3)$$

Hence, $V = \pi h^2 \left(a - \frac{h}{3} \right)$ cubic units.

2. *Find the volume of the solid generated by the revolution of the curve $y = a^3/(a^2+x^2)$ about its asymptote.*

SOLUTION. Clearly the curve cuts only y-axis at the point $(0, a)$ and $y = 0$ *i.e.*, x-axis is *its asymptote*. Therefore the solid is generated by the revolution of the curve about x-axis. The tracing of the curve is shown in fig. 11.

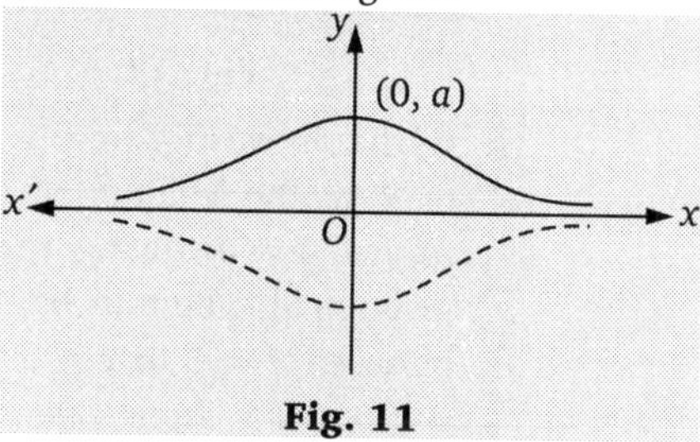

Fig. 11

Let V be the volume of the solid generated by the revolution of the curve about x-axis from $x = -\infty$ to $x = \infty$, then

$$V = \int_{-\infty}^{\infty} \pi y^2 \, dx$$

$$= \pi \int_{-\infty}^{\infty} \frac{a^6}{(a^2 + x^2)^2} dx \qquad \left[\because y = \frac{a^3}{(a^2 + x^2)} \right]$$

$$= 2\pi \int_{0}^{\infty} \frac{a^6}{(a^2 + x^2)^2} dx.$$

Let us put $x = a \tan \theta$, then $dx = a \sec^2\theta \, d\theta$ and θ varies from $\theta = 0$ to $\theta = \pi/2$.

$$\therefore V = 2\pi a^6 \int_{0}^{\pi/2} \frac{a \sec^2 \theta \, d\theta}{a^4 \sec^4 \theta}$$

$$= 2\pi a^3 \int_{0}^{\pi/2} \cos^2 \theta \, d\theta$$

$$= 2\pi a^3 \left[\frac{(2-1)}{2} \cdot \frac{\pi}{2} \right]$$

(By walli's formula)

Hence, $V = \frac{1}{2} \pi^2 a^3$ cubic units

3. *Find the volume of the solid formed by revolving the cycloid*

$x = a(\theta - \sin \theta)$, $y = (1 - \cos \theta)$

(i) about its base

(ii) about y-axis.

(VTU–2003, 05; KURUKSHETRA–2006)

SOLUTION. Since the equation of the cycloid is

$x = a(\theta - \sin\theta),\ y = a(1 - \cos\theta)$ ...(1)

The tracing of this curve is given below:

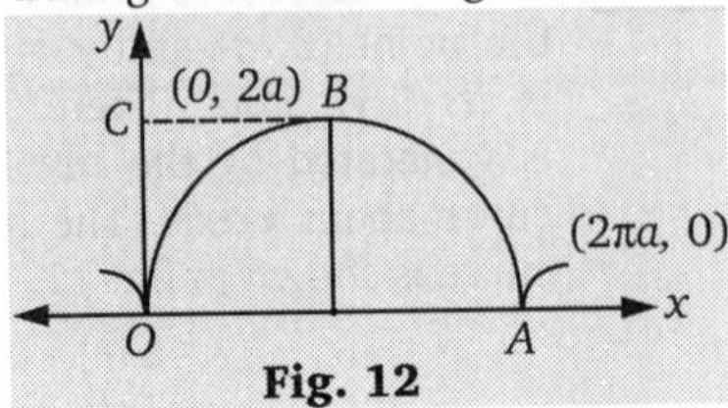

Fig. 12

(i) In the above fig. base is the axis of x so the volume of the solid formed by revolving the cycloid given in (1) about its base (x-axis) between $x = 0$ to $x = 2\pi a$ where $\theta = 0$ to $\theta = 2\pi$, is given by

$$\Rightarrow V = \int_0^{2\pi a} \pi y^2 dx = \pi\int_0^{2\pi} y^2\left(\frac{dx}{d\theta}\right).d\theta$$

$$= \pi\int_0^{2\pi} a^2(1-\cos\theta)^2.a(1-\cos\theta)d\theta$$

[Using (1)]

$$= \pi a^3\int_0^{2\pi}(1-\cos\theta)^3 d\theta$$

$$\Rightarrow V = \pi a^3\int_0^{2\pi} 8\sin^6(\theta/2)d\theta. \quad ...(2)$$

Let us put $\theta/2 = \phi$ so $d\theta = 2d\phi$ and ϕ varies from 0 to π, then (2) becomes

$$V = 8\pi a^3\int_0^{\pi}\sin^6\phi(2d\phi)$$

$$= 16\pi a^3\int_0^{\pi}\sin^6\phi\, d\phi$$

$$= 16\pi a^3.2\int_0^{\pi/2}\sin^6\phi\, d\phi$$

$$= 32\pi a^3\int_0^{\pi/2}\sin^6\phi\, d\phi$$

$$= 32\pi a^3\left[\frac{(6-1)(6-3)(6-5)}{6.4.2}.\frac{\pi}{2}\right]$$

(By Walli's formula)

$V = 5\pi^2a^3$ cubic units.

(ii) Let V be the volume of the solid formed by revolving of the cycloid about y-axis. This volume is the difference of the volume generated by the revolution of the area $OABCO$ and the volume generated by the revolution of the area $OBCO$. Since we have that at A, $\theta = 2\pi$, at O, $\theta = 0$ and at B, $\theta = \pi$. Therefore, the volume generated by the revolution of the area $OABCO$ about y-axis is given by V_1 (say)

$$V_1 = \int_{2\pi}^{\pi}\pi x^2\frac{dy}{d\theta}.d\theta$$

$$= \pi\int_{2\pi}^{\pi} a^2(\theta-\sin\theta)^2.a\sin\theta\, d\theta$$

$$= \pi a^3\int_{2\pi}^{\pi}(\theta^2+\sin^2\theta-2\theta\sin\theta)\sin\theta\, d\theta$$

$$= \pi a^3\int_{2\pi}^{\pi}(\theta^2\sin\theta+\sin^3\theta-2\theta\sin^2\theta)\, d\theta$$

$$= \pi a^3\int_{2\pi}^{\pi}\left(\theta^2\sin\theta+\frac{3}{4}\sin\theta - \frac{1}{4}\sin 3\theta-\theta+\theta\cos 2\theta\right)d\theta$$

$$= \pi a^3\Big[-\theta^2\cos\theta+2\theta\sin\theta+2\cos\theta - \frac{3}{4}\cos\theta+\frac{1}{12}\cos 3\theta-\frac{\theta^2}{2}+\frac{1}{2}\theta\sin 2\theta + \frac{1}{4}\cos 2\theta\Big]_{2\pi}^{\pi}$$

(where $\int\theta^2\sin\theta\, d\theta$ and $\int\theta\cos 2\theta\, d\theta$ are solved by integration by parts.)

$$= \pi a^3\left[\left(\pi^2-2+\frac{3}{4}-\frac{1}{12}-\frac{\pi^2}{2}+\frac{1}{4}\right) - \left(-4\pi^2+2-\frac{3}{4}+\frac{1}{12}-2\pi^2+\frac{1}{4}\right)\right]$$

$$= \pi a^3\left(\frac{13}{2}\pi^2-\frac{8}{3}\right)$$

and let V_2 be the volume generated by the revolution of the area $OBCO$ about y-axis, then

$$V_2 = \int_0^{\pi}\pi x^2\frac{dy}{d\theta}d\theta$$

$$= \pi\int_0^{\pi} a^2(\theta-\sin\theta)^2 a\sin\theta\, d\theta$$

$$= \pi a^3\int_0^{\pi}(\theta^2\sin\theta+\sin^3\theta-2\theta\sin^2\theta)\, d\theta$$

$$= \pi a^3\Big[-\theta^2\cos\theta+2\theta\sin\theta+2\cos\theta$$

$$-\frac{3}{4}\cos\theta+\frac{1}{12}\cos 3\theta-\frac{\theta^2}{2}$$

$$\left.+\frac{1}{2}\theta\sin 2\theta+\frac{1}{4}\cos 2\theta\right]_0^{\pi}$$

$$=\pi a^3\left[\left(\pi^2-2+\frac{3}{4}-\frac{1}{12}-\frac{\pi^2}{2}+\frac{1}{4}\right)\right.$$

$$\left.-\left(2-\frac{3}{4}+\frac{1}{12}+\frac{1}{4}\right)\right]$$

$$V_2=\pi a^3\left(\frac{1}{2}\pi^2-\frac{8}{3}\right).$$

$$\therefore \quad V=V_1-V_2$$

$$=\pi a^3\left(\frac{13}{2}\pi^2-\frac{8}{3}\right)-\pi a^3\left(\frac{1}{2}\pi^2-\frac{8}{3}\right)$$

$$=\pi a^3(6\pi^2)$$

$$V=6\pi^3a^3 \text{ cubic units}$$

4. *Find the volume of a solid formed by the revolution of the loop of the curve $y^2(a+x)=x^2(a-x)$ about x-axis.*

SOLUTION. Clearly, the given curve is symmetrical about x-axis and the curve cuts the x-axis only at the points (0, 0) and $(a, 0)$ so the loop exists between these points. The tracing of this curve is shown in fig. 13.

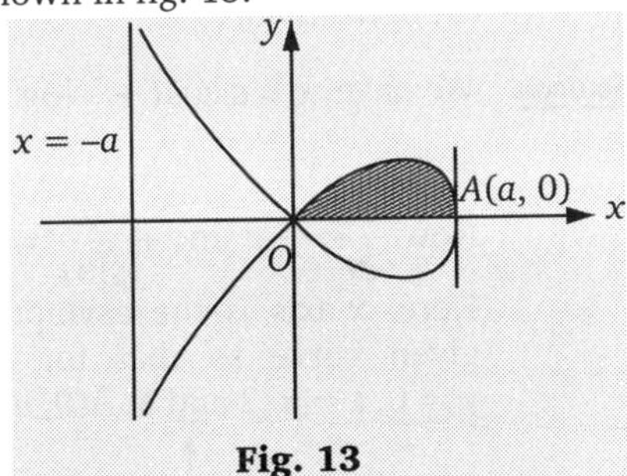

Fig. 13

Therefore, the required volume is the volume of a solid formed by the revolution of upper half of the loop of the curve about x-axis where x varies from 0 to a. Then

$$V=\int_0^a \pi y^2\,dx$$

$$=\pi\int_0^a \frac{x^2(a-x)}{a+x}dx \qquad [\because y^2(a+x)=x^2(a-x)]$$

$$=\pi\int_0^a \frac{x^2(2a-a-x)}{a+x}dx$$

$$=\pi\int_0^a \frac{2ax^2}{a+x}dx-\pi\int_0^a x^2\,dx$$

$$=2a\pi\int_0^a \frac{(x^2-a^2+a^2)}{a+x}dx-\pi\int_0^a x^2dx$$

$$=2a\pi\left[\int_0^a (x-a)\,dx+a^2\int_0^a\frac{dx}{a+x}\right]-\pi\int_0^a x^2dx$$

$$=2a\pi\left[\frac{x^2}{2}-ax+a^2\log(a+x)\right]_0^a-\pi\left[\frac{x^3}{3}\right]_0^a$$

$$=2a\pi\left[\frac{a^2}{2}-a^2+a^2\log 2a-a^2\log a\right]-\frac{\pi a^3}{3}$$

$$=2a\pi\left[-\frac{a^2}{2}+a^2\log\frac{2a}{a}\right]-\frac{\pi a^3}{3}$$

$$=-\pi a^3+2a^3\pi\log 2-\frac{\pi a^3}{3}$$

$$=2a^3\pi\log 2-\frac{4\pi}{3}a^3$$

$$\Rightarrow V=2\pi a^3\left[\log 2-\frac{2}{3}\right] \text{cubic units}$$

5. *Find the volume of the solid generated by the revolution of the cardioid $r=a(1+\cos\theta)$ about the initial line.*

(VTU–2010; KURUKSHETRA–2009)

SOLUTION. Obviously, the curve is symmetrical about the initial line and $r=0$ when $\cos\theta=-1$, *i.e.*, $\theta=\pi$ and the maximum value of $r=2a$ when $\cos\theta=1$, *i.e.*, $\theta=0$. Thus the tracing of the curve is as under:

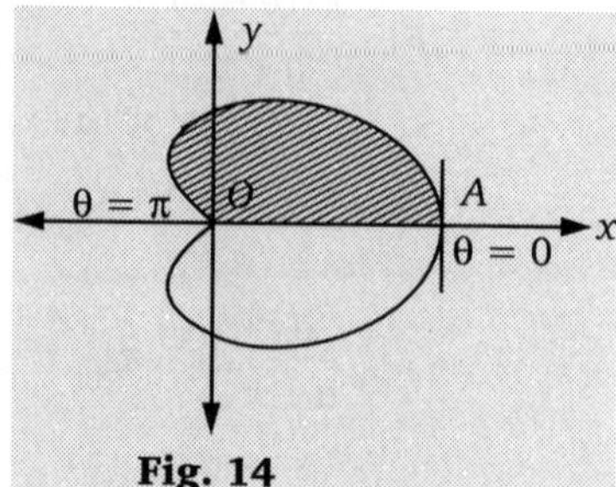

Fig. 14

Therefore, the required volume is the volume of solid generated by the revolution of the upper half of the curve between θ = 0 and θ = π about initial line (x-axis). Let this volume be V. Then $V = \int_{\theta=0}^{\theta=\pi} \pi y^2 \frac{dy}{d\theta}.d\theta$

(as θ increases x decreases so $\frac{dx}{d\theta}$ will have to take negative.)

$$= -\pi\int_0^\pi (r\sin\theta)^2.\frac{d}{d\theta}(r\cos\theta)\,d\theta$$

$(\because x = r\cos\theta, y = r\sin\theta)$

$$= -\pi\int_0^\pi a^2(1+\cos\theta)^2\sin^2\theta\frac{d}{d\theta}[a(1+\cos\theta)\cos\theta]d\theta$$

$[\because r = a(1+\cos\theta)]$

$$= -\pi a^3\int_0^\pi (1+\cos\theta)^2\sin^2\theta.(-\sin\theta - 2\cos\theta\sin\theta)d\theta$$

$$= +\pi a^3\int_0^\pi (1+\cos^2\theta+2\cos\theta)(1+2\cos\theta).\sin^3\theta d\theta$$

$$= +\pi a^3\int_0^\pi (\sin^3\theta + 4\cos\theta\sin^3\theta + 5\cos^2\theta\sin^3\theta + 2\cos^3\theta\sin^3\theta)d\theta$$

$$= +\pi a^3\left[\int_0^\pi \sin^3\theta d\theta + 4\int_0^\pi \cos\theta\sin^3\theta d\theta + 5\int_0^\pi \cos^2\theta\sin^3\theta d\theta + 2\int_0^\pi \cos^3\theta\sin^3\theta d\theta\right]$$

$$= \pi a^3\left[\int_0^\pi \sin^3\theta d\theta + 5\int_0^\pi \cos^2\theta\sin^3\theta d\theta\right]$$

(The second and fourth integral vanish by the property of definite integral.)

$$= \pi a^3\left[2\int_0^{\pi/2}\sin^3\theta d\theta + 10\int_0^{\pi/2}\cos^2\theta\sin^3\theta d\theta\right]$$

(By the property of definite integral)

$$= \pi a^3\left[2.\frac{(3-1)}{3.1}.1 + 10.\frac{(2-1)(3-1)}{5.3.1}.1\right]$$

(By Walli's formula)

$$= \pi a^3\left[\frac{4}{3}+\frac{4}{3}\right] = \frac{8}{3}\pi a^3.$$

$\therefore \quad V = \frac{8}{3}\pi a^3$ cubic units

Aliter. The required volume is also taken as

$$V = \int_0^\pi \frac{2}{3}\pi r^3\sin\theta d\theta$$

$$= \frac{2}{3}\pi\int_0^\pi a^3(1+\cos\theta)^3\sin\theta d\theta$$

$$= \frac{2}{3}\pi a^3\int_0^\pi (1+\cos\theta)^3\sin\theta d\theta$$

$$= \frac{2}{3}\pi a^3\left[-\frac{(1+\cos\theta)^4}{4}\right]_0^\pi = \frac{2}{3}\pi a^3\left[\frac{16}{4}\right].$$

$\therefore \quad V = \frac{8}{3}\pi a^3$ cubic units

6. *Find the volume of the solid generated by the revolution of the tractrix*

$$x = a\cos t + \frac{a}{2}\log\tan^2\left(\frac{t}{2}\right),\ y = a\sin t$$

about its asymptote.

SOLUTION. We have $x = a\cos t + \frac{a}{2}\log\tan^2\left(\frac{t}{2}\right)$

and $\quad y = a\sin t.$

Now $\frac{dx}{dt} = -a\sin t + \frac{a}{\sin t} = \frac{a\cos^2 t}{\sin t}.$

Here, x-axis is the asymptote of the given curve so that for x-axis *i.e.*, y = 0, t = π/2 and at A(0, a), t = 0.

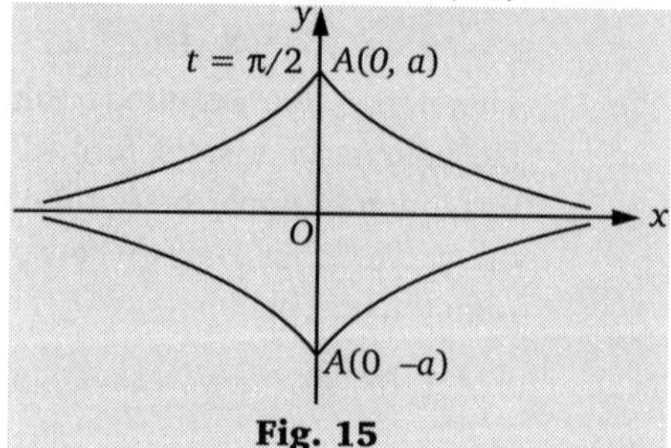

Fig. 15

Let V be the volume of the solid generated by the revolution of the tractrix. Then

$$V = 2\int_{\pi/2}^{0} \pi y^2 \frac{dx}{dt} dt$$

$$= 2\pi \int_{\pi/2}^{0} a^2 \sin^2 t \frac{a\cos^2 t}{\sin t} dt$$

$$= 2\pi a^3 \int_{\pi/2}^{0} \cos^2 t \sin t \, dt$$

$$= 2\pi a^3 \left[\frac{\cos^3 t}{3}\right]_{\pi/2}^{0}$$

$$= 2\pi a^3 \left[\frac{1}{3} - 0\right] = \frac{2}{3}\pi a^3.$$

7. *Find the volume of the solid generated by revolution of one loop of the lemniscate $r^2 = a^2 \cos 2\theta$ about the line $\theta = \pi/2$.*

SOLUTION. We have $r^2 = a^2 \cos 2\theta$. ...(1)

Clearly one loop of the curve lies between

$\theta = -\pi/4$ and $\theta = \pi/4$.

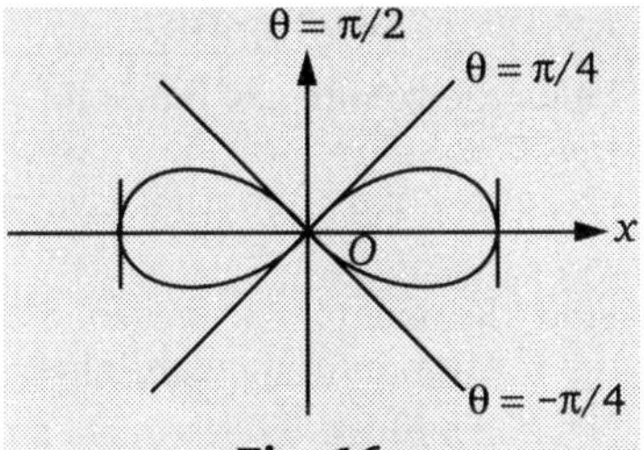

Fig. 16

Let V be the volume of the solid generated by revolving one loop of the curve (1) about the line $\theta = \pi/2$. Then

$$V = \int_{-\pi/4}^{\pi/4} \frac{2}{3}\pi r^3 \cos\theta \, d\theta$$

$$= \frac{2}{3}\pi \int_{-\pi/4}^{\pi/4} a^3 (\cos 2\theta)^{3/2} \cos\theta \, d\theta$$

$$= \frac{2\pi a^3}{3} \int_{-\pi/4}^{\pi/4} (1 - 2\sin^2\theta)^{3/2} \cos\theta \, d\theta$$

$$= \frac{4\pi a^3}{3} \int_{0}^{\pi/4} (1 - 2\sin^2\theta)^{3/2} \cos\theta \, d\theta$$

$$= \frac{4\pi a^3}{3} \int_{0}^{\pi/4} (1 - \sin^2\phi)^{3/2} \frac{1}{\sqrt{2}} \cos\phi \, d\phi$$

Put $\sqrt{2}\sin\theta = \sin\phi$

$$= \frac{4\pi a^3}{3\sqrt{2}} \int_{0}^{\pi/2} \cos^4\phi \, d\phi$$

$$= \frac{4\pi a^3}{3\sqrt{2}} \left[\frac{(4-1)(4-3)}{4.(4-2)} \cdot \frac{\pi}{2}\right] = \frac{\pi^2 a^3}{4\sqrt{2}}.$$

8. *Find the volume of the solid generated by the revolution of the cissoid $y^2(2a-x) = x^3$ about its asymptotes.* (VTU–2000)

SOLUTION. Let $P(x, y)$ be any point on the curve and let V be the volume of the solid generated by revolution of $y^2 (2a-x) = x^3$ about its asymptote $x = 2a$ then $V = \int_{-\infty}^{\infty} \pi (PM)^2 dy$

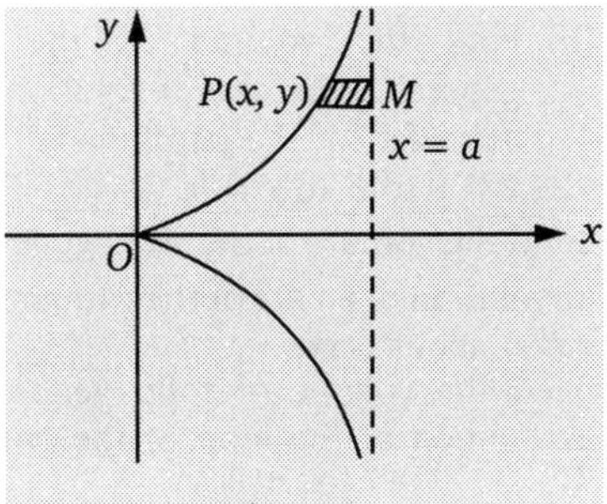

Fig. 17

$$= 2\int_{0}^{\infty} \pi (PM)^2 dy$$

$$V = 2\pi \int_{0}^{\infty} (2a - x)^2 dy \qquad ...(1)$$

Now, $y^2(2a - x) = x^3$

$$\Rightarrow y = \frac{x^{3/2}}{\sqrt{2a - x}} \Rightarrow \frac{dy}{dx} = \frac{\sqrt{x}.(3a - x)}{(2a - x)^{3/2}}$$

Then

$$V = 2\pi \int_{0}^{2a} \frac{(2a - x)^2 (3a - x)\sqrt{x}}{(2a - x)^{3/2}} dx$$

[as $y \to 0$ to ∞, $x \to 0$ to $2a$]

$$= 2\pi \int_{0}^{2a} \sqrt{2ax - x^2} (3a - x) dx$$

$$= \pi \left[\int_{0}^{2a} 2(a - x)\sqrt{2ax - x^2} \, dx + 4a\int_{0}^{2a} \sqrt{a^2 - (x - a)^2} dx\right]$$

$$= \pi\left[\frac{2}{3}(2ax - x^2) + 4a\left\{\frac{(x-a)}{2}\sqrt{a^2-(x-a)^2} + \frac{a^2}{2}\sin^{-1}\frac{(x-a)}{a}\right\}\right]_0^{2a}$$

$$= \pi\left\{0 + 4a\left\{\frac{a^2\pi}{2}\right\}\right\} = 2\pi^2 a^3.$$

Exercise-20.2

1. Show that the volume of sphere of radius a is $\frac{4}{3}\pi a^3$.
2. Find the volume of a hemi-sphere.
3. (i) The part of a parabola $y^2 = 4ax$ cut off by the latus rectum revolves about the tangent at the vertex. Find the volume of a solid thus generated.
   (ii) Find the volume of the paraboloid generated by the revolution about the axis of x, of the parabola $y^2 = 4ax$ from $x = 0$ to x to $x = h$.
4. Find the volume of the solid generated by the revolution of an arc of the catenary $y = c \cosh (x/c)$ about x-axis.
5. Find the volume of solid generated by the revolution of the loop of the curve $y^2 = x^2 (a - x)$ about the axis of x.
6. Prove that the volume of this solid generated by the revolution of an ellipse around its minor axis is a mean proportional between those generated by the revolution of the ellipse and of the auxiliary circle about the major axis.
7. Find the volume of a solid generated by the loop of the curve $y^2(a+ x)= x^2(3a - x)$ about x-axis. (MARATHWADA–2008)
8. The area of the curves $x^{2/3} + y^{2/3} = a^{2/3}$ lying in the first quadrant revolves about x-axis. Find the volume of the solid generated. (UPTU-2010, SVTU-2008)
9. Show that the volume of the solid generated by the revolution of the upper half of the loop of the curve $y^2 = x^2(2-x)$ about x-axis is $\frac{4}{3}\pi$.
10. Find the volume of the solid generated by revolving the loop of the curve $a^2y^2 = x^2(2a-x)(x-a)$ about x-axis.
11. Show that the volume of the solid generated by the revolution of the curve $(a-x)y^2 = a^2x$, about its asymptote is $\frac{1}{2}\pi^2a^3$.
12. The area cut off from the parabola $y^2 = 4ax$ by the chord joining the vertex to an end of the latusrectum is rotated through four right angles about the chord. Find the volume of the solid thus generated.
13. Prove that the volume of the reel formed by the revolution of the cycloid $x = a\ (t + \sin t)$, $y = a\ (1 - \cos t)$ about the tangent at the vertex is $\pi^2 a^3$.
14. Find the volume of the solid generated by the revolution of the cycloid $x = a(t + \sin t)$, $y = a(t - \cos t)$, $0 \le t \le n$.
    (i) about the x-axis (ii) about its base.
15. Find the voiume of the solid generated by the revolution of the loop of the curves $x = t^2$, $y = t - \frac{1}{2}t^3$ about x-axis.
16. Find the volume of ihe solid generated by the revolution of the cissoid $x=2a\sin^2 t$, $y=2a\sin^3 t/\cos t$ about its asymptote. (PTU–2001)
17. Find the volume of the solid generated by the revolution of the cardioid $r= a(1- \cos \theta)$ about the initial line. (PTU–2006)
18. (i) Find the volume of the solid formed by revolving one loop of the curve $r^2 = a^2 \cos 2\theta$ about the initial line.
    (ii) The lemniscate $r^2 = a^2 \cos 2\theta$ revolves about a tangent at the pole. Show that the volume generated is $\frac{\pi^2 a^3}{4}$.
19. Show that the volume of the solid formed by the revolution of the curve $r = a + b \cos \theta (a > b)$ about the initial line is $\frac{4}{3}\pi a(a^2+b^2)$.
20. Show that if the area lying within the cardioid $r=2a(1+\cos \theta)$ and without the parabola $r(1 + \cos \theta)= 2a$ revolves about the initial line, the volume of a solid thus generated is $18\pi a^3$.
21. Find the volume of the solid generated by the revolution of the curve $r =2a \cos \theta$ about the initial line.

Hint to Selected Problems

1. We know that, when a circle $x^2 + y^2 = a^2$ is revolved about its diameter a sphere is formed, therefore $V = \int_{-a}^{a} \pi y^2 dx = \pi \int_{-a}^{a} (a^2 - x^2)\, dx.$

2. When a quadrant of a circle $x^2 + y^2 = a^2$ is revolved about its one of bounding radius, a hemi-sphere is generated.

$\therefore \quad V = \int_0^a \pi x^2 dy = \pi \int_0^a (a^2 - y^2)\, dy.$

4. Use the formula $V = \int_0^x \pi y^2\, dx.$

6. The equation of the ellipse is given by $\frac{x^2}{a^2} + \frac{y^2}{b^2} = 1$. Therefore,

$$V = \int_{-b}^{b} \pi x^2 dy = \frac{4\pi a^2 b}{3}.$$

Let V_1 be the volume generated by an ellipse about major axis between $x = -a$ to $x = a$.

Therefore $= \sqrt{\frac{4\pi}{3} b^2 a}.$

Now let V_2 be the volume, when the circle revolves about major axis.

$$\therefore \quad V_2 = \int_{-a}^{a} \pi y^2\, dx = \frac{4\pi}{3a^2}.$$

7. Let V be the volume of a solid generated by the revolution of the loop about x-axis between $x = 0$ and $x = 3a$. Then, we have

$$V = \int_0^{3a} \pi y^2\, dx = \pi \int_0^{3a} \frac{x^2(3a - x)}{a + x} dx.$$

8. Here $V = \int_0^a \pi y^2\, dx.$ Change the given equation into polar form by assuming

$$x = a \cos^3\theta \text{ and } y = a \sin^3\theta.$$

13. $\frac{dx}{dt} = a(1 + \cos t), \frac{dy}{dt} = a(1 - \cos t)$

$$\Rightarrow \frac{dy}{dx} = \tan\frac{t}{2}.$$

Then, the required volume $V = \int_{-a\pi}^{a\pi} \pi y^2\, dx.$

17. The required volume is given by

$$V = \int_0^{\pi} \frac{2}{3}\pi r^3 \sin\theta\, d\theta.$$

18. The required volume is given by

$$V = 2\int_0^{\pi/4} \frac{2}{3}\pi r^3 \sin\theta\, d\theta.$$

21. The required volume is given by

$$V = \int_0^{\pi/2} \frac{2}{3}\pi r^3 \sin\theta\, d\theta.$$

ANSWERS

2. $\frac{2}{3}\pi a^3$ **3. (i)** $\frac{4}{5}\pi a^3$ **(ii)** $2ah^2$ **4.** $\frac{\pi c^2}{2}\left[x + \frac{c}{2}\sinh\left(\frac{2x}{c}\right)\right]$ **5.** $\frac{1}{12}\pi a^4$ **7.** $\pi a^3[8\log 2 - 3]$

8. $\frac{16}{105}\pi a^3$ **10.** $\frac{23}{60}\pi a^3$ **12.** $\frac{2}{75}\sqrt{5}\,\pi a^3$ **14.(i)** $\frac{1}{2}\pi^2 a^3$ **(ii)** $\frac{5}{2}\pi^2 a^3$ **15.** $\frac{4}{3}\pi$ **16.** $2\pi^2 a^3$

17. $\frac{8}{3}\pi a^3$ **18.** $\frac{\pi a^3}{24}\sqrt{2}[3\log(\sqrt{2} + 1) - \sqrt{2}]$ **21.** $\frac{4}{3}\pi a^3$

20.8 PAPPUS AND GULDIN'S THEOREMS

20.8.1 For the Volume of a Solid of Revolution

Statement. *When a closed plane curve revolves about any straight line lying in the same plane but not intersecting the closed curve, then the volume of a ring shape solid thus generated, is equal to the product of the area of a closed curve and the perimeter of a circle described by the centroid of the closed curve.*

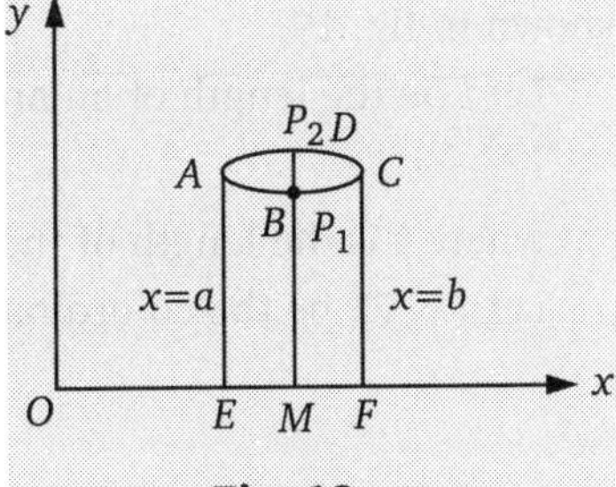

Fig. 18

Proof. Let $ABCDA$ be a closed curve which revolves about x-axis. Let the lines $x = a$ and $x = b$ touch the closed plane curve at the points A and C as shown in fig. 18.

Now draw a line through the centroid of the closed curve and parallel to the line $x = a$ and $x = b$. This line intersects the given curve at two points P_1 and P_2 such that $MP_1 = y_1$ and $MP_2 = y_2$ provided y_1 and y_2 both are the functions of x only. Therefore the required volume of a solid of revolution of the closed plane curve about x-axis is equal to the difference of the volume generated by the plane area $AEFCDA$ and the volume generated by the plane area $AEFCBA$ about x-axis.

Now the volume generated by $AEFCDA$ $= \int_a^b \pi y_2^2 \, dx$

and the volume generated by $AEFCBA$ $= \int_a^b \pi y_1^2 \, dx.$

$\therefore$ Required volume, $V = \int_a^b \pi y_2^2 \, dx - \int_a^b \pi y_1^2 \, dx = \pi \int_a^b (y_2^2 - y_1^2) dx.$ ...(1)

Let $(\bar{x}, \bar{y})$ be the co-ordinates of the centroid of the closed plane curve $ABCDA$. Then by the method of finding the centre of gravity, we have

$$\bar{y} = \frac{\int_a^b \frac{1}{2}(y_2 + y_1)(y_2 - y_1) dx}{A}$$ where A is the area of the closed plane curve.

$$\therefore \quad \bar{y}A = \frac{1}{2}\int_a^b (y_2^2 - y_1^2) dx \qquad ...(2)$$

Now from (1) and (2), we get

Required volume $= 2\pi \, \bar{y} A = A \times 2\pi \, \bar{y}$

$=$ (area of the closed curve) $\times$ (perimeter of the circle whose radius is $\bar{y}$)

$V =$ (area of the closed curve) $\times$ (perimeter of the circle described by the centroid of the closed curve)

20.8.2 For the Surface of a Solid of Revolution

Statement. *When an arc of a plane curve revolves about any straight line lying in the plane of curve but not intersecting it, then the surface area of a solid of revolution thus generated is equal to the product of the length of the arc and the perimeter of a circle described by the centroid of that arc.*

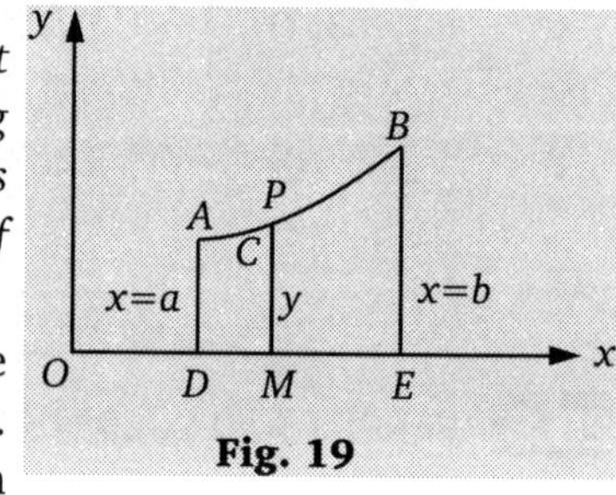

Fig. 19

Proof. Let ACB be an arc of a plane curve cut off by the lines $x = a$ and $x = b (a<b)$. Let $P(x, y)$ be any point on the arc. Now draw a line parallel to the lines $x = a$ and $x = b$ through P which meets the x-axis at M such that $PM = y$. Suppose the arc revolves about the x-axis as shown in fig. 19.

Let l be the length of an arc ACB. Therefore the surface area is given by

$$S = \int_a^b 2\pi y \, ds \qquad ...(1)$$

where s is the length of the arc measured from A to any point P.

Let $(\bar{x}, \bar{y})$ be the co-ordinates of the centroid of the arc ACB, then we know that

$$\bar{y} = \frac{\int_a^b y \, ds}{\int_a^b ds} = \frac{\int_a^b y \, ds}{l}$$

or $$l\bar{y} = \int_a^b y \, ds. \qquad ...(2)$$

From (1) and (2), we get

$$S = 2\pi \bar{y}\, l = l \times 2\pi \bar{y} = \text{length of the arc } ACB \times \text{perimeter of the circle of radius } y$$

$\therefore$ $S =$ (length of an arc ACB) $\times$ (perimeter of the circle described by the centroid of that arc)

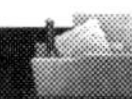

- These theorems are only applicable when the closed curve or arc donot intersect the line of revolution.
- These theorems are also used to find the centroid of the closed curve or an arc only when volume and surface area of revolution are known.

Solved Examples

1. *The volume generated by the revolution of an ellipse having semi-axes a and b about a tangent at vertex.*

SOLUTION. Let the equation of an ellipse be

$$\frac{x^2}{a^2} + \frac{y^2}{b^2} = 1$$

The centroid of this ellipse is (0, 0)and the area is πab. There are four vertices $(\pm\, a, 0)$and $(0, \pm\, b)$. Now first we revolve the ellipse about tangent at $(a, 0)$, then the distance of the centroid (0, 0)from this tangent is a.

Thus the generated volume

= (area of ellipse)

$\times$ (perimeter of the circle of radius a)

$= \pi ab \times 2\pi a = 2\pi^2 a^2 b.$

Similarly, if we revolve the ellipse about the tangent at $(0, b)$, then the distance of the centroid (0, 0) from this tangent is b.

Thus the required volume is

= (area of an ellipse)

$\times$ (perimeter of the circle of radius b)

$= \pi ab \times 2\pi b = 2\pi^2 ab^2$.

2. *Find the position of the centroid of a semi-circular area.*

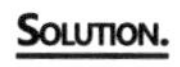

SOLUTION. Let the equation of a circle whose radius is a and centre is (0,0) be

$$x^2 + y^2 = a^2$$

Let the semi-circular area be obtained by the circle $x^2 + y^2 = a^2$ and the x-axis as shown in fig. 20.

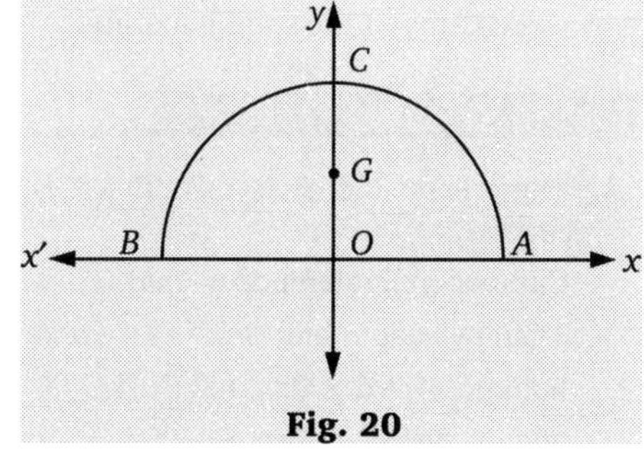

Fig. 20

Let V be the volume of a solid generated by the semi-circular area about the x-axis, between $x = -\,a$ to $x = a$. Then

$$V = \int_{-a}^{a} \pi y^2\, dx$$

$$= \pi \int_{-a}^{a} (a^2 - x^2)\, dx$$

$$= \pi \left[a^2 x - \frac{x^3}{3} \right]_{-a}^{a} = \frac{4}{3}\pi a^3$$

and let A be the area of this semi-circle.

Then $A = \dfrac{1}{2}(\pi a^2) = \dfrac{\pi a^2}{2}$.

Let G be the centroid of this semi-circular area whose position be $\bar{y}$ from x-axis (axis of revolution).

Then by Pappus theorem, we have

$$V = (\text{area of the semi-circle}) \times 2\pi \bar{y}$$

$$\Rightarrow \frac{4}{3}\pi a^3 = \frac{\pi a^2}{2} \times 2\pi \bar{y}$$

$$\therefore \quad \bar{y} = \frac{4a}{3\pi}.$$

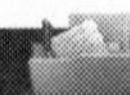

Exercise-20.3

1. Find the volume and surface area of the anchor-ring generated by the revolution of a circle of radius a about an axis in its own plane distance b from its centre ($b < a$).
2. The volume of the ring generated by the revolution of an ellipse of eccentricity $1/\sqrt{2}$ about a straight line parallel to the minor axis and situated at a distance from the centre equal to three times the major axis.
3. The loop of the curve $2ay^2 = x(x - a)^2$ revolves about the straight line $y = a$. Find the volume of the solid generated.
4. The volume of a ring generated by the revolution of the cardioid $r = a(1 + \cos\theta)$ about the line $r\cos\theta + a = 0$, given that the centroid of the cardioid is at a distance $5a/6$ from the pole.
5. Using Pappus theorem, determine the position of the centre of gravity of the quadrant of a uniform circular lamina of radius a, where the volume of the solid generated by the revolution of the quadrant of circular lamina about the tangent at either of its extremities is $\dfrac{\pi(3\pi - 4)}{6}a^3$.

Hint to Selected Problems

1. The area of the circle of radius A is given by $A = \pi a^2$.

   Circular circumference $= 2\pi b$.

   Then by Pappus and Guldin's theorem,

   Volume, $V = A \times 2\pi b = 2\pi^2 a^2 b$

   and surface $= 2\pi a \times 2\pi b = 4\pi^2 ab$.

2. Here $A = \pi a\left(\dfrac{a}{\sqrt{2}}\right) = \dfrac{1}{\sqrt{2}}\pi a^2$.

   Let l be the distance of straight line parallel to the minor axis from C.G. of the ellipse.

   Then $l = 3$ (Major axis) $= 6a$

   length of the circular path $= 12\pi a$

   $\therefore$ Required volume $V = \dfrac{1}{\sqrt{2}}\pi a^2 \times 12\pi a$.

4. $A = 2\int_0^{\pi}\frac{1}{2}r^2 d\theta = \dfrac{11\pi a}{3}$.

   The volume $V = A \times \dfrac{11\pi a}{3}$.

Answers

1. Volume $= 2\pi^2 a^2 b$, surface $= 4\pi^2 ab$ **2.** $6\sqrt{2}\pi^2 a^3$, a being the semi-major axis. **3.** $\dfrac{8}{15}\sqrt{2}\pi a^3$
4. $\dfrac{11}{2}\pi^2 a^3$ **5.** $d = \dfrac{(3\pi - 4)a}{3\pi}$, d being the distance of centroid from the tangent.

❑❑❑❑❑❑

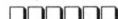

Chapter

21 Sequences

21.1 INTRODUCTION

George Cantor (1845-1918) is known as the creater of the set theory. He made a considerable contribution to the development of the theory of real sequence, and found a firm base for most of the fundamental concepts of real analysis in the sequence of rational numbers. Though his lay-outs are not convenient in the initial stages, they are quite advantageous while making advanced investigations. The study of many important and advanced concepts becomes easy if the notion of the sequence is employed.

21.2 SEQUENCES

Let **N** be the set of all natural numbers and S be any set of real numbers. A function whose domain is the set of natural numbers and range is a subset of S, is called a sequence in S.

Symbolically, if we define a function $f : \mathbf{N} \to S$, then f is a sequence. As in the case of function, we shall denote a sequence in a number of ways.

(i) Usually a sequence is denoted by its images. For a sequence f, the image corresponding to $n \in \mathbf{N}$ is denoted by f_n or $f\langle n \rangle$ and is called the nth term of the sequence f.
For example: $\langle 1, 4, 9, ... \rangle$ is the sequence whose n^{th} terms is n^2.

(ii) Using in order, the first few elements of a sequence, till the rule for writing down different elements becomes clear.
For example: $\langle 1, 2, 3, ... \rangle$ is the sequence whose n^{th} term is n.

(iii) Defining a sequence by a recurrence formula *i.e.* , by a rule which expresses the nth term by the $(n-1)th$ term.
For example : Let $a_1 = 1, a_{n+1} = 2a_n$, for all $n \geq 1$.

Above relations define a sequence whose n^{th} term is 2^{n-1}.

- A sequence is represented as $\langle s_n \rangle$ or $\{s_n\}$, where s_n is the nth term of the sequence.
- The set of all distinct terms of a sequence is called the range set of that sequence.
- A sequence whose range, is a subset of **R** is called a real sequence or a sequence of real numbers.
- Here, we shall study only real numbers. Therefore, the term sequence will be used to denote a real sequence.

ILLUSTRATIONS

(1) $\left\langle \frac{1}{n} \right\rangle$ is the sequence $\left\langle 1, \frac{1}{2}, \frac{1}{3}, \frac{1}{4}, ..., \frac{1}{n}, ... \right\rangle$

(2) $\left\langle \frac{1}{n^3} \right\rangle$ is the sequence $\left\langle 1, \frac{1}{8}, \frac{1}{27}, ..., \frac{1}{n^3}, ... \right\rangle$

(3) $\langle -2n \rangle$ is the sequence $\langle -2, -4, -6, ..., -2n, ... \rangle$

(4) $\left\langle \frac{n}{n+1} \right\rangle$ is the sequence $\left\langle \frac{1}{2}, \frac{2}{3}, \frac{3}{4}, ..., \frac{n}{n+1}, ... \right\rangle$.

21.2.1 RANGE OF A SEQUENCE

The set of all distinct terms of a sequence is known as its range.

21.2.2 CONSTANT SEQUENCE

A sequence $\langle s_n \rangle$ defined by $s_n = a$ for all $n \in \mathbf{N}$, is called a constant sequence.

21.2.3 EQUALITY OF TWO SEQUENCES

Two sequences $\langle s_n \rangle$ and $\langle t_n \rangle$ are said to be equal, if $s_n = t_n$; $\forall\, n \in \mathbf{N}$.

21.2.4 OPERATION ON SEQUENCES

Since the sequences are real valued functions, therefore, the sum, difference, product etc. of two sequences are defined as follows:

(1) If $\langle s_n \rangle$ and $\langle t_n \rangle$ be any two sequences, then the sequences whose n^{th} terms are $s_n + t_n$, $s_n - t_n$ and $s_n \cdot t_n$ are respectively known as the sum, difference and product of the sequences $\langle s_n \rangle$ and $\langle t_n \rangle$ and are denoted by $\langle s_n + t_n \rangle$, $\langle s_n - t_n \rangle$ and $\langle s_n \cdot t_n \rangle$ respectively.

(2) If $s_n \neq 0$, $\forall\, n \in \mathbf{N}$, then the sequence whose n^{th} term is $\frac{1}{s_n}$ is called the reciprocal of the sequence $\langle s_n \rangle$ and is denoted by $\left\langle \frac{1}{s_n} \right\rangle$.

(3) The sequence whose n^{th} term is s_n / t_n ($t_n \neq 0$, $\forall\, n \in \mathbf{N}$) is known as the quotient of the sequence $\langle s_n \rangle$ by the sequence $\langle t_n \rangle$ and is denoted by $< \frac{s_n}{t_n} >$.

(4) The sequence whose n^{th} term is ks_n, where $k \in \mathbf{R}$ is known as the scalar multiple of the sequence $\langle s_n \rangle$ by k and is denoted by $\langle ks_n \rangle$

21.3 BOUNDED SEQUENCES

21.3.1 BOUNDED BELOW SEQUENCE

A sequence $\langle s_n \rangle$ is said to be bounded below if there exists a real number l such that $s_n \geq l$, $\forall\, n \in \mathbf{N}$. The number l is known as the lower bound of the sequence $\langle s_n \rangle$.

21.3.2 BOUNDED ABOVE SEQUENCE

A sequence $\langle s_n \rangle$ is said to be bounded above if there exists a real number u such that $sn \leq u$; $\forall\, n \in \mathbf{N}$. The number u is said to be upper bound of the sequence $<s_n>$.

21.3.3 BOUNDED SEQUENCE

A sequence $\langle s_n \rangle$ is said to be bounded if it is bounded above as well as bounded below.

or A sequence $\langle s_n \rangle$ is bounded if there exist two real numbers l and $u (l \leq u)$ such that $l \leq s_n \leq u$, $\forall\, n \in \mathbf{N}$. Equivalently, a sequence is bounded iff there exists a real number $k > 0$ such that $| s_n | \leq k$, $\forall\, n \in \mathbf{N}$.

21.3.4 UNBOUNDED SEQUENCE

A sequence $\langle s_n \rangle$ is said to be unbounded if it is not bounded.

- In sequences, terms with equal values can occur. Therefore, a sequence may have more than one term with the smallest value. In such a case any of those is taken for the smallest value. In fact while talking about the smallest value we are interested in the value of the term rather than the position of the term in the sequence. Similar explanation holds for the greatest value. Note that, like sets of real numbers, a sequence bounded below or above may or may not have a smallest or a greatest member accordingly. Clearly, an unbounded sequence cannot have a smallest or a greatest member.

21.3.5 Least Upper Bound

If a sequence $\langle s_n \rangle$ is bounded above, then there exists a number u_1 such that

$$s_n \le u_1, \forall n \in \mathbf{N}. \quad \text{... (1)}$$

This number u_1 is called an upper bound of the sequence $\langle s_n \rangle$. If $u_1 < u_2$, then from (1) we find that $s_n \le u_2, \forall n \in \mathbf{N}$. Which implies, u_2 is also an upper bound of the sequence $\langle s_n \rangle$. Hence, we can say any number greater than u_1 is an upper bound of $\langle s_n \rangle$.

Hence, a sequence has an infinite number of upper bounds if it is bounded above. Let u be the least of all the upper bounds of the sequence $\langle s_n \rangle$. Then u is defined as the least upper bound (l.u.b.) or supremum of the sequence $\langle s_n \rangle$.

21.3.6 Greatest Lower Bound

If a sequence $\langle s_n \rangle$ is bounded below then there exists a number $l_1 \in \mathbf{R}$ such that

$$l_1 \le s_n ; \forall n \in \mathbf{N} \quad \text{...(1)}$$

This number l_1 is known as the lower bound of $\langle s_n \rangle$. If $l_2 < l_1$, then from (1) we have

$$l_2 \le s_n ; \forall n \in \mathbf{N} \quad \text{...(2)}$$

which implies, l_2 is also a lower bound of the sequence $\langle s_n \rangle$. Hence, we can say any number less than l_1 is a lower bound of $\langle s_n \rangle$.

Hence, a sequence has infinite number of lower bounds, if it is bounded below. Let l is the greatest of all the lower bounds of the sequence $\langle s_n \rangle$. Then l is known as greatest lower bound (g.l.b.) or infimum of the sequence $\langle s_n \rangle$.

ILLUSTRATIONS

(1) The sequence $\langle n^2 \rangle$ is bounded below by 1 but not bounded above.

(2) The sequence $\left\langle \frac{n}{n+1} \right\rangle$ is bounded as $\frac{1}{2} \le \frac{n}{n+1} < 1; \forall n \in \mathbf{N}$

(3) The sequence $\langle -n^2 \rangle$ is bounded above by -1 but not bounded below.

(4) The sequence $\left\langle \frac{1}{n} \right\rangle$ is bounded since $\left| \frac{1}{n} \right| \le 1; \forall n \in \mathbf{N}$.

(5) The sequence $\langle (-1)^n \rangle$ is bounded since $|(-1)^n| \le 1; \forall n \in \mathbf{N}$. $[\because |(-1)^n| = 1; \forall n \in \mathbf{N}]$

(6) The sequence $\langle s_n \rangle$ defined by $s_n = 1 + (-1)^n$ for all $n \in \mathbf{N}$ is bounded since the range set of the sequence is $\{0, 2\}$, which is a finite set.

(7) The sequence $\langle (-1)^n / n \rangle$ is bounded since $|(-1)^n / n| \le 1$ for all $n \in \mathbf{N}$.

(8) The sequence $\langle 2^n \rangle$ is bounded below and has smallest term as 2. Every member of $]-\infty, 2]$ is a lower bound of the sequence and the sequence is unbounded above.

21.4 LIMIT POINT OF A SEQUENCE

A real number l is called a limit point of a sequence $\langle s_n \rangle$ if every nbd of l contains infinite number of terms of the sequence. Thus $l \in \mathbf{R}$ is a limit point of the sequence $\langle s_n \rangle$ if for given $\varepsilon > 0$, $s_n \in]l - \varepsilon, l + \varepsilon[$, for infinitely many points.

- Limit point of a sequence need not be a member of the sequence.
- A limit point of a sequence may or may not be a limit point of the range of the sequence but the limit point of the range of a sequence is always a limit point of the sequence.
- In the case of set of real numbers, limit points of a sequence may also be called accumulation, cluster or condensation points.

21.4.1 CLASSIFICATON OF LIMIT POINTS

The limit points of a sequence may be classified in two types :
(i) those for which $l = s_n$ for infinitely many values of $n \in \mathbf{N}$.
(ii) those for which $l = s_n$ for only a finite number of values of $n \in \mathbf{N}$.

But this distinction is not very much needed. As such we do not distinguish the above mentioned two types of limit points of sequences by different titles.

☛ ILLUSTRATIONS

(1) The sequence $\left\langle \frac{1}{n} \right\rangle$ has one limit point namely 0.

(2) The sequence $\left\langle (-1)^n \right\rangle$ has two limit points 1 and –1.

(3) The sequence $\langle n \rangle$ has no limit point.

(4) The sequence $\left\langle 1 + \frac{(-1)^n}{n} \right\rangle$ has one limit point *i.e.*, 1.

(5) The sequence $\left\langle 1, \frac{1}{2}, 1, \frac{1}{3}, 1, \frac{1}{4} \ldots \right\rangle$ has one limit point *i.e.*, 1.

(6). The sequence $\langle n + 1 \rangle$ has no limit point.

21.4.2 SUFFICIENT CONDITION FOR NUMBER l TO BE OR NOT TO BE A LIMIT POINT OF THE SEQUENCE $< s_n >$

(1) If for every $\varepsilon > 0$, $\exists\, m \in \mathrm{N}$ such that $s_n \in]l - \varepsilon, l + \varepsilon[\; \forall\, n \geq m$ or equivalently $|s_n - l| < \varepsilon$ $\forall\, n \geq m$, then l is the limit point of the sequence $\langle s_n \rangle$.

(2) If for any $\varepsilon > 0$. $s_n \in]\, l - \varepsilon, l + \varepsilon$ [for only a finite number of values of n, then l is not a limit point of the sequence $\langle s_n \rangle$. Such a condition is also necessary for a number l not to be a limit point of the sequence $\langle s_n \rangle$.

- Whenever we simply write $\varepsilon > 0$, it is implied that ε may be however small positive number.
- A positive number δ is said to be arbitrary small if given $\varepsilon > 0$, δ may be chosen such that $0 < \delta < \varepsilon$.
- If δ be an arbitrarily small positive number and given any $k > 0$, then $k\delta$ is also an arbitrarily small positive numbers.
- If ε_1, ε_2, are any two arbitrarily small positive numbers then it follows that l is the limit point of the sequence s_n iff $s_n \in]\, l - \varepsilon_1, l + \varepsilon_2$ [for infinitely many values of n.

THEOREM 1. **(Bolzano-Weirstrass Theorem for sequence).** *Every bounded sequence has at least one limit point.*

PROOF. Let $S = \{s_n : n \in \mathbf{N}\}$ be the range set of the bounded sequence $\langle s_n \rangle$. Then S is bounded set. Now there may be two cases :

Case I. Let S be a finite set. Then $s_n = p$ for infinitely many indices n. Here $p \in \mathbf{R}$. Obviously p is a limit point of $\langle s_n \rangle$.

Case II. Let S be an infinite set. Since S is bounded, then by Bolzano-Weierstrass theorem for sets of real numbers, S has a limit point, say p. Therefore every nbd of p contains infinitely many distinct point of S *i.e.*, infinitely many terms of $\langle s_n \rangle$ and hence p is a limit point of the sequence $\langle s_n \rangle$.

21.5 LIMIT SUPERIOR AND LIMIT INFERIOR

The greatest limit point of a bounded sequence is called the upper limit or limit superior and is denoted by $\overline{\lim}\ s_n$ and the smallest limit point of a bounded sequence is called the lower limit or limit inferior and is denoted by $\underline{\lim}\ s_n$.

By definition, it is obvious that $\underline{\lim}\ s_n \leq \overline{\lim}\ s_n$

A bounded sequence $\langle s_n \rangle$ for which the upper limit and lower limit coincide with real number l is said to converge to l.

21.5.1 LIMIT OF SEQUENCE

A sequence $\langle s_n \rangle$ is said to have a limit l if for a given $\varepsilon > 0$ there exists a positive integer m such that

$$|s_n - l| < \varepsilon, \forall\ n \geq m.$$

21.6 CONVERGENT SEQUENCES

Definition 1. *A sequence $\langle s_n \rangle$ is said to converge to a number l, if for a given $\varepsilon > 0$ there exists a positive integer m such that*

$$|s_n - l| < \varepsilon\ \forall\ n \geq m.$$

The number l is called the limit of the sequence $\langle s_n \rangle$ and can be written as

$$s_n \to l \text{ as } n \to \infty \text{ or } \lim_{n\to\infty} s_n = l \text{ or } \lim s_n = l.$$

Definition 2. *A sequence $\langle s_n \rangle$ is said to be convergent iff it is bounded and has one and only one limit point.*

In such a case the sequence is said to converge to this limit point l.

21.7 SUBSEQUENCES

Let $\langle s_n \rangle$ be any sequence. If $\langle n_1, n_2, \ldots, n_k \rangle$ be a strictly increasing sequence of positive integers *i.e.*, $i > j \Rightarrow n_i > n_j$, then the sequence

$$\left\langle s_{n_1}, s_{n_2}, \ldots, s_{n_k} \right\rangle \text{ is called a subsequence of } \langle s_n \rangle.$$

THEOREM 1. *If $\langle s_n \rangle$ is a sequence of non-negative numbers such that $\lim s_n = l$, then $l \geq 0$.*

PROOF. Let if possible $l < 0$ then $-l > 0$. Now $\lim s_n = l$, therefore, for $\varepsilon = -\frac{l}{2} > 0$, there exists a positive integer m such that

$$|s_n - l| < -\frac{l}{2}\ \forall\ n \geq m.$$

In particular $\quad |s_m - l| < -\frac{l}{2} \Rightarrow l + \frac{l}{2} < s_m < l - \frac{l}{2} \Rightarrow s_m < \frac{l}{2} < 0$

which is a contradiction, because $s_m \geq 0$. Therefore our assumption is wrong. Hence, we must have $l \geq 0$.

THEOREM 2. *A sequence cannot converge to more than one limit.*

PROOF. Let if possible, a sequence $\langle s_n \rangle$ converges to two distinct numbers l_1 and l_2.

Now $\quad l_1 \neq l_2 \quad \Rightarrow l_1 - l_2 \neq 0 \quad \Rightarrow |l_1 - l_2| > 0$

Let $\varepsilon = \frac{1}{2}|l_1 - l_2|$; then $\varepsilon > 0$.

Since $\langle s_n \rangle$ converges to l_1, there must exists a positive integer m_1 such that

$$|s_n - l_1| < \varepsilon, \forall\ n \geq m_1 \qquad \ldots(1)$$

Similarly $\langle s_n \rangle$ converges to l_2, there must exists a positive integer m_2 such that

$$|s_n - l_2| < \varepsilon, \forall\ n \geq m_2 \qquad \ldots(2)$$

Now, let $m = \max\{m_1, m_2\}$

Then result (1) and (2) hold for all $n \geq m$. So for all $n \geq m$, we have

$$|l_1 - l_2| = |(s_n - l_1) - (s_n - l_2)|$$
$$\leq |(s_n - l_1)| + |(s_n - l_2)|$$

$$< \varepsilon + \varepsilon \qquad \text{[Using (1) and (2)]}$$
$$= 2\varepsilon = |l_1 - l_2|$$
$$\Rightarrow \quad |l_1 - l_2| < |l_1 - l_2|$$

which is absurd, hence we must have $l_1 = l_2$ *i.e.*, the limit of the sequence is unique.

THEOREM 3. *Every convergent sequence is bounded.*

PROOF. Let $\langle s_n \rangle$ be a sequence which converges to l. Take $\varepsilon = 1$. Then there exists a positive integer m such that

$$|s_n - l| < 1, \forall\, n \geq m$$

i.e., $(l-1) < s_n < (l+1), \forall\, n \geq m.$

Let $k_1 = \min\{s_1, s_2, \ldots, s_{m-1}, l-1\}$

and $k_2 = \max\{s_1, s_2, \ldots, s_{m-1}, l+1\}$

therefore $k_1 \leq s_n \leq k_2, \forall n \in \mathbf{N}$

Hence, the sequence $\langle s_n \rangle$ is bounded.

- The converse of the above theorem is *not* necessarily true *i.e.*, a bounded sequence need not be convergent. For example $\langle (-1)^n \rangle$ is bounded but not convergent.

THEOREM 4. *If $\langle s_n \rangle$ converges to l, then any subsequence of $\langle s_n \rangle$ also converges to l.*

PROOF. Let $\langle s_{n_k} \rangle$ be any subsequence of $\langle s_n \rangle$. Then by definition of subsequence $n_1, n_2, \ldots, n_k$, are positive integers such that

$$n_1 < n_2 < \ldots < n_k < \ldots$$

Now $n_1 \geq 1 \Rightarrow n_k \geq k$ [By induction]

Since $\langle s_n \rangle$ converges to l, so given $\varepsilon > 0$, there exists a positive integer m such that

$$|s_k - l| < \varepsilon \;\forall\, k \geq m$$

for $k \geq m$, we have $n_k \geq k \geq m$

therefore $|s_{n_k} - l| < \varepsilon$, for all $n_k \geq m$

Hence, $\langle s_{n_k} \rangle$ converges to l.

- All subsequences of a convergent sequence, converges to the same limit.
- To show that, a given sequence is not convergent, it is enough to show that two of its subsequences converges to different limits.
  (**Ex.** The sequence $\langle s_n \rangle = \langle (-1)^n \rangle$ is not convergent. Since the two subsequences $\langle 1, 1, \ldots \rangle$ and $\langle -1, -1, -1, \ldots \rangle$ of the given sequence converges to 1 and –1 respectively, which are not same.)
- If the subsequences $\langle s_{2n-1} \rangle$ or $\langle s_{2n+1} \rangle$ and $\langle s_{2n} \rangle$ of the sequences $\langle s_n \rangle$ converges to the same lmit l, then the sequence $\langle s_n \rangle$ converge to l.

THEOREM 5. *The limit of the sum of two convergent sequences is the sum of their limits.*

PROOF. Let $\langle s_n \rangle$ and $\langle t_n \rangle$ be the two given sequences such that

$$\lim s_n = l_1 \qquad \ldots(1)$$

and

$$\lim t_n = l_2 \qquad \ldots(2)$$

Since, $\lim s_n = l_1$, therefore for a given $\varepsilon > 0$, there exists a positive integer m_1 such that

$$|s_n - l_1| < \varepsilon/2, \;\forall\, n \geq m_1.$$

Similarly, $\lim t_n = l_2$, therefore, for a given $\varepsilon > 0$, there must exists a positive integer m_1 such that

$$|t_n - l_2| < \varepsilon/2, \;\forall\, n \geq m_2.$$

Let $m = \max\{m_2, m_2\}$.

Therefore $|s_n - l_1| < \varepsilon/2, \;\forall\, n \geq m.$

and $|t_n - l_2| < \varepsilon/2, \;\forall\, n \geq m.$

Now, consider $|(s_n + t_n) - (l_1 + l_2)| = |(s_n - l_1) + (t_n - l_2)|, \forall\, n \geq m$

$$\leq |s_n - l_1| + |t_n - l_2|, \forall\ n \geq m$$
$$< \varepsilon/2 + \varepsilon/2 = \varepsilon, \forall\ n \geq m$$

Therefore, the sequence $\langle s_n + t_n \rangle$ is convergent and

$$\lim (s_n + t_n) = l_1 + l_2 = \lim s_n + \lim t_n.$$

- The converse of the theorem need not be true. For example, the sequence $\langle s_n \rangle = \langle (-1)^n \rangle$ and $\langle t_n \rangle = \langle (-1)^{n+1} \rangle$ are not convergent, but the sequence $\langle s_n + t_n \rangle = \langle (-1)^n + (-1)^{n+1} \rangle$ converges to 0.
- The limit of the differences of two convergent sequence is the difference of their limits. (Proof is similar as Theorem 5).
- If $\langle s_n \rangle$ and $\langle t_n \rangle$ are convergent sequences such that $s_n \leq t_n$, $\forall n$ and $\lim s_n = a$, $\lim t_n = b$, then $a \leq b$.

SIMILAR RESULTS

(1) If $\lim s_n = l_1$ and $\lim t_n = l_2$, then $\lim (s_n t_n) = l_1 . l_2$.

(2) If $\lim s_n = l_1$, $l_1 \neq 0$ and $s_n \neq 0$, $\forall\ n \in \mathbf{N}$ then $\lim \left(\dfrac{1}{s_n}\right) = \dfrac{1}{l_1}$

(3) If $\lim s_n = l_1$ and $\lim t_n = l_2$ $(l_2 \neq 0)$, $t_n \neq 0$, $\forall n \in \mathrm{N}$ then $\lim \dfrac{s_n}{t_n} = \dfrac{l_1}{l_2}$

21.8 DIVERGENT SEQUENCES

Definition 1. *A sequence $\langle s_n \rangle$ is said to diverge to $+\infty$, if for every real number $k > 0$, there exists a positive integer m such that, $s_n > k$, $\forall\ n \geq m$*

Definition 2. *A sequence $\langle s_n \rangle$ is said to diverge to $-\infty$, if for every real number $k > 0$, there exists a positive integer m such that, $s_n < k$, $\forall\ n \geq m$*

Definition 3. *A sequence is said to be divergent sequence if it diverges to either $+\infty$ or $-\infty$.*

Definition 4. *A sequence which is not convergent, is known as divergent sequence.*

ILLUSTRATIONS

(1) $\langle 3, 3^2, 3^3, \ldots \rangle$ diverges to $+\infty$.

(2) $\langle -2, -2^2, -2^3, \ldots \rangle$ diverges to $-\infty$.

(3) $\langle 2, 4, 6, \ldots, 2n, \ldots \rangle$ diverges to $+\infty$.

(4) $\langle -2, -4, -6, \ldots, -2n, \ldots \rangle$ diverges to $-\infty$.

21.9 OSCILLATORY SEQUENCES

A sequence $\langle s_n \rangle$ is said to be oscillatory if it is neither convergent nor divergent.

An oscillatory sequence is said to oscillate finitely or infinitely according as it is bounded or unbounded.

In other words, we can say

(i) A bounded sequence, which is not convergent is said to oscillate finitely.

(ii) An unbounded sequence which does not diverge, is said to oscillate infinitely.

(iii) A bounded sequence which does not converge and has at least two limit points, is said to be oscillate finitely.

ILLUSTRATIONS

(1) $\langle 1 + (-1)^n \rangle$ oscillate finitely.

(2) $\langle (-1)^n \rangle$ oscillate finitely.

(3) $\left\langle (-1)^n \left(1 + \dfrac{1}{n}\right) \right\rangle$ oscillate finitely.

(4) $\langle n(-1)^n \rangle$ oscillate infinitely.

SOME RESULTS

(1) If a sequence $\langle s_n \rangle$ diverges to infinity, then any subsequence of $\langle s_n \rangle$ also diverges to infinity.
(2) If the sequence $\langle s_n \rangle$ diverges to infinity and the sequence $\langle t_n \rangle$ is bounded, then $\langle s_n + t_n \rangle$ diverges to infinity.
(3) If the sequences $\langle s_n \rangle$ and $\langle t_n \rangle$ both diverges to infinity, then the sequences $\langle s_n + t_n \rangle$ and $\langle s_n . t_n \rangle$ diverges to infinity.

Solved Examples

1. *Show that the sequence* $\left\langle \frac{1}{n} \right\rangle$ *converges to 0.*

SOLUTION. Let $\langle s_n \rangle = \left\langle \frac{1}{n} \right\rangle$

Now $\lim_{n\to\infty} s_{2n} = \lim_{n\to\infty} \frac{1}{2n} = 0$

and $\lim_{n\to\infty} s_{2n+1} = \lim_{n\to\infty} \frac{1}{2n+1} = 0$

Therefore $\lim_{n\to\infty} s_{2n} = \lim_{n\to\infty} s_{2n+1} = 0$

$\Rightarrow \lim_{n\to\infty} s_n = 0, \forall n \in \mathbf{N}$.

Since 0 is a finite quantity. Hence, the sequence $\langle s_n \rangle$ is convergent and converges to 0.

2. *Discuss the convergence of the sequence* $\left\langle \frac{1}{3^n} \right\rangle$.

SOLUTION. Let $\langle s_n \rangle = \left\langle \frac{1}{3^n} \right\rangle$

Then $\lim_{n\to\infty} s_{2n} = \lim_{n\to\infty} \frac{1}{3^{2n}} = 0$

and $\lim_{n\to\infty} s_{2n+1} = \lim_{n\to\infty} \frac{1}{3^{2n+1}} = 0$

which implies $\lim_{n\to\infty} s_{2n} = \lim_{n\to\infty} s_{2n+1} = 0$

Therefore, $\lim_{n\to\infty} s_n = 0, \forall n \in \mathbf{N}$.

Since 0 is a finite quantity, hence, the given sequence $\langle s_n \rangle$ is a convergent sequences.

3. *Show that the sequence $\langle s_n \rangle$ defined by $s_n = \left\langle \left(\sqrt{n+1} - \sqrt{n}\right) \right\rangle, \forall n \in \mathbf{N}$ is convergent.*

SOLUTION. We have $s_n = \sqrt{n+1} - \sqrt{n}$

For any $\varepsilon > 0$,

$$| s_n - 0 | = \sqrt{n+1} - \sqrt{n} < \varepsilon$$

$$\Rightarrow \quad \sqrt{n+1} < (\varepsilon + \sqrt{n})$$

$$\Rightarrow \quad n+1 < \varepsilon^2 + 2\varepsilon\sqrt{n} + n$$

$$\Rightarrow \quad 1 < \varepsilon^2 + 2\varepsilon\sqrt{n}$$

i.e., if $\frac{1}{4\varepsilon^2} < n$

Then, for any given $\varepsilon > 0, \exists m \left(> \frac{1}{4\varepsilon^2} \right) \in \mathbf{N}$ such that

$$| s_n - 0 | < \varepsilon, \forall n \geq m$$

Therefore, $\lim s_n = 0$.

Since, 0 is a finite quantity. Hence, the given sequence $\langle s_n \rangle$ is convergent.

4. *Show that the sequence $\langle s_n \rangle$ defined by $s_n = r^n$ converges to 0 if $|r| < 1$.*

SOLUTION. If $|r| < 1$. Then

$$| r | = \frac{1}{1+h}, \text{ where } h > 0$$

Since,

$$(1+h)^n = 1 + nh + \frac{n(n-1)}{2!} h^2 + ... + h^n$$

$$\geq 1 + nh \, \forall n.$$

$$\text{Now} | s_n - 0 | = | r^n |$$

$$= | r |^n = \frac{1}{(1+h)^n} \leq \frac{1}{1+nh} \forall n.$$

Let $\varepsilon > 0$. Then

$$| s_n - 0 | < \varepsilon \text{ if } \frac{1}{1+nh} < \varepsilon$$

$$\text{or} \quad n > \left(\frac{1}{\varepsilon} - 1 \right) / h.$$

Now, if we take a positive integer m such that $m > \left(\frac{1}{\varepsilon} - 1 \right) / h$, then, for all $n \geq m$.

$$|s_n - 0| < \varepsilon.$$

Hence, the sequence $\langle s_n \rangle$ converges to 0.

5. *Show that the sequence $\langle s_n \rangle = \frac{3n}{n + 5n^{1/2}}$ has the limit 3.*

SOLUTION. Let ε be any positive number.

Consider, $\left|\dfrac{3n}{n+5n^{1/2}}-3\right| = \dfrac{15n^{1/2}}{n+5n^{1/2}} < \dfrac{15}{n^{1/2}}$

Therefore,

$$\left|\frac{3n}{n+5n^{1/2}}-3\right| < \varepsilon \text{ if } \frac{15}{n^{1/2}} < \varepsilon \text{ or } n > \frac{225}{\varepsilon^2}$$

If we choose a positive integer $m > \dfrac{225}{\varepsilon^2}$ then, we get

$$|s_n - 3| < \varepsilon, \ \forall\ n \geq m$$

Hence $\lim\limits_{n\to\infty} s_n = 3$

6. *Show that* $\lim\limits_{n\to\infty} \sqrt[n]{n} = 1$

SOLUTION. Let $\sqrt[n]{n} = 1+h$, where $h \geq 0$

$$\Rightarrow n = (1+h)^n$$
$$= 1 + nh + \frac{n(n-1)}{2!}h^2 + \ldots + h^n$$

$$\Rightarrow n > \frac{n(n-1)}{2}h^2, \forall n \qquad [h \geq 0]$$

$$\Rightarrow h^2 < \frac{2}{n-1}, \qquad \text{for } n \geq 2$$

$$\Rightarrow |h| < \sqrt{\left(\frac{2}{n-1}\right)}, \qquad \text{for } n \geq 2$$

Let ε > 0 (any positive number, however small) then

$$|h| < \sqrt{\left(\frac{2}{n-1}\right)} < \varepsilon \text{ provided,}$$

$$\frac{2}{n-1} < \varepsilon^2 \text{ or } n > \frac{2}{\varepsilon^2}+1$$

If we take $m \in \mathbf{N}$ such that $m > \dfrac{2}{\varepsilon^2}+1$

then $|h| < \varepsilon\ \forall n \geq m$

or $|\sqrt[n]{n} - 1| < \varepsilon\ \forall n \geq m \Rightarrow \lim\limits_{n\to\infty} \sqrt[n]{n} = 1$

Similar Problems

(1) Prove that $\lim\left(\dfrac{1}{n^p}\right) = 0, p > 0$.

(2) Prove that the sequence $\langle n^p \rangle$, where $p > 0$, diverges to infinity.

(3) If $\langle s_n \rangle$ is a sequence such that $s_n \neq 0$ for any $n \in \mathbf{N}$, and $\dfrac{s_{n+1}}{s_n} \to l$. Then prove that if $|l| < 1$, then $s_n \to 0$.

7. Show that the sequence $\left\langle \log\dfrac{1}{n} \right\rangle$ diverges to $-\infty$.

SOLUTION. Let $s_n = \log\dfrac{1}{n}$

Take any $h < 0$. Then $s_n < h$ if $\log\dfrac{1}{n} < h$

$$\Rightarrow \text{if } (-\log n) < h$$
$$\Rightarrow \text{if } \log n > -h$$
$$\Rightarrow \text{if } n > e^{-h}$$

If we take $m \in$ N such that $m > e^{-h}$, then $s_n < h$ for all $n \geq m$.

Hence, $s_n \to -\infty$ as $n \to \infty$

21.10 CAUCHY SEQUENCE

A sequence $\langle s_n \rangle$ is said to be Cauchy sequence if, for given ε > 0 there exists $m \in \mathbf{N}$ such that

$$|s_n - s_m| < \varepsilon, \ \forall\ n \geq m$$

or

$$|s_p - s_q| < \varepsilon, \ \forall\ p, q \geq m$$

or

$$|s_{n+p} - s_n| < \varepsilon, \ \forall\ n \geq m \text{ and } p \geq 0.$$

- Cauchy sequence is also known as fundamental sequence.
- A sequence cannot converge if even one ε > 0 can be found such that for every positive integer m,

$$|s_{n+p} - s_n| > \varepsilon, \ \forall\ n \geq m \text{ and } p > 0$$

- Here, $|s_p - s_q| < \varepsilon, \ \forall\ p, q \geq m$ means that s_p and s_q are arbitrarily close together for large values of p and q.
- The inequality $n \geq m$ in the definition may be replaced by $n > m$.
- If $\langle s_n \rangle$ and $\langle t_n \rangle$ are two Cauchy sequences, then $\langle s_n + t_n \rangle$, $\langle s_n t_n \rangle$ and $\langle s_n / t_n \rangle$ ($t_n \neq 0$ for any n) are also Cauchy sequences.

☛ ILLUSTRATIONS

(1) The sequence $\left\langle \frac{1}{2^n} \right\rangle$ is a Cauchy sequence.

(2) The sequence $\left\langle \frac{1}{n} \right\rangle$ is a Cauchy sequence.

(3) The sequence $\left\langle \frac{1}{n^2} \right\rangle$ is not a Cauchy sequence.

(4) The sequence $\left\langle (-1)^n \right\rangle$ is not a Cauchy sequence.

THEOREM 1. *Every Cauchy sequence is bounded.*

PROOF. Let $\langle s_n \rangle$ be a Cauchy sequence.

Taking $\varepsilon = 1$, there exists a positive integer m such that

$$|s_n - s_m| < 1, \forall n \geq m$$

$\Rightarrow$ $(s_m - 1) < s_n < (s_m + 1), \ \forall\, n \geq m$

Let $k = \min\{s_m - 1, s_1, s_2, ..., s_{m-1}\}$

and $K = \max\{s_m + 1, s_1, s_2, ..., s_{m-1}\}$

Then $k \leq s_n \leq K, \forall n.$

Hence, the sequence $\langle s_n \rangle$ is bounded.

- Converse of the above theorem is not necessarily true, *i.e.*, a bounded sequence need not be a Cauchy sequence, for example, the sequence $\left\langle (-1)^n \right\rangle$ is bounded, but not a Cauchy sequence.

THEOREM 2. **(Cauchy's General Principle of Convergence).** *A sequence is convergent if and only if it is a Cauchy sequence.*

PROOF. Let us first suppose $\langle s_n \rangle$ be a convergent sequence. Let, this sequence be converge to l.

$\therefore$ for a given $\varepsilon > 0$ these exists a positive integer m such that

$$|s_n - l| < \varepsilon / 2, \forall\, n \geq m. \quad ...(1)$$

In particular, for $n = m$

$$|s_m - l| < \varepsilon / 2. \quad ...(2)$$

Now, consider $|s_n - s_m| = |s_n - l + l - s_m| \leq |s_n - l| + |s_m - l|$

$< \varepsilon/2 + \varepsilon/2, \ \forall\, n \geq m$ (Using (1) and (2))

$= \varepsilon, \ \forall\, n \geq m$

i.e., $|s_n - s_m| < \varepsilon, \ \forall\, n \geq m$

$\Rightarrow$ $\langle s_n \rangle$ is a cauchy sequence.

Conversely, let $\langle s_n \rangle$ be a Cauchy sequence.

$\Rightarrow$ $\langle s_n \rangle$ is a bounded sequence. [By Theorem 1]

$\Rightarrow$ By Bolzano-Weirstress theorem $\langle s_n \rangle$ has at least one limit point, say l. We shall show that sequence $\langle s_n \rangle$ converges to l.

Let $\varepsilon > 0$ be given. Since, $\langle s_n \rangle$ is a Cauchy sequence

$\therefore$ $\exists$ a positive integer m such that

$$|s_n - s_m| < \varepsilon/3, \ \forall\, n \geq m. \quad ...(3)$$

Since, l is the limit point of $\langle s_n \rangle$.

$\therefore$ For above choice of ε and m, $\exists$ a positive integer $k > m$ such that

$$|s_k - l| < \varepsilon/3. \quad ...(4)$$

Since, $k > m$, therefore from (3)

$$|s_k - s_m| < \varepsilon/3. \quad \ldots(5)$$

Now, consider $|s_n - l| = |s_n - s_m + s_m - s_k + s_k - l|$

$\leq |s_n - s_m| + |s_m - s_k| + |s_k - l|$ [By Triangle inequality]

$< \varepsilon/3 + \varepsilon/3 + \varepsilon/3 = \varepsilon$

i.e., $|s_n - l| < \varepsilon, \forall\, n \geq m.$

Hence, $\langle s_n \rangle$ is convergent.

- Cauchy's general principle of convergence, also termed as "Necessary and sufficient condition for the convergence".

Solved Examples

1. *If $\langle s_n \rangle$ is a sequence in* **R**, *where*

$$s_n = 1 + \frac{1}{2} + \frac{1}{3} + \ldots + \frac{1}{n}$$

Evaluate, $\lim_{n\to\infty} |a_{n+1} - a_n|$. *Verify, is this sequence satisfy the Cauchy criterion?*

SOLUTION. Here $s_n = 1 + \frac{1}{2} + \frac{1}{3} + \ldots + \frac{1}{n}$

$\Rightarrow s_{n+1} = 1 + \frac{1}{2} + \frac{1}{3} + \ldots + \frac{1}{n} + \frac{1}{n+1}$

$\therefore s_{n+1} - s_n = \frac{1}{n+1}$

$\Rightarrow \lim_{n\to\infty} |s_{n+1} - s_n| = 0$.

Also, we have

$$s_{2n} - s_n = \left(1 + \frac{1}{2} + \frac{1}{3} + \ldots + \frac{1}{n} + \frac{1}{n+1} + \frac{1}{n+2} + \ldots + \frac{1}{2n}\right) - \left(1 + \frac{1}{2} + \frac{1}{3} + \ldots + \frac{1}{n}\right)$$

$$= \frac{1}{n+1} + \frac{1}{n+2} + \ldots + \frac{1}{2n} \geq n\left(\frac{1}{2n}\right).$$

$$\left(\frac{1}{n+1} > \frac{1}{2n} \text{ etc.}\right)$$

$\Rightarrow |s_{2n} - s_n| > \frac{1}{2} \forall n \in \mathbf{N}$

$\Rightarrow$ There exists a positive integer k such that $|s_n - s_k| \geq \frac{1}{2}$ whenever $n \geq k$

$\Rightarrow$ Cauchy criterion is not satisfied.

2. *Show by applying Cauchy's convergence criterion that the sequence $\langle s_n \rangle$ given by*

$s_n = 1 + \frac{1}{3} + \frac{1}{5} + \ldots + \frac{1}{2n-1}$ *diverges.*

SOLUTION. Here, we have

$$s_{n+1} = 1 + \frac{1}{3} + \frac{1}{5} + \ldots + \frac{1}{2n-1} + \frac{1}{2(n+1)-1}$$

$$= 1 + \frac{1}{3} + \frac{1}{5} + \;\; + \frac{1}{2n-1} + \frac{1}{2n+1}$$

$$\therefore s_{n+1} - s_n = \left[1 + \frac{1}{3} + \frac{1}{5} + + \frac{1}{2n-1} + \frac{1}{2n+1}\right] - \left[1 + \frac{1}{3} + \frac{1}{5} + \ldots + \frac{1}{2n-1}\right]$$

$$= \frac{1}{2n+1} > 0, \forall n \in \mathbf{N}$$

Thus, $s_{n+1} > s_n, \forall n \in \mathbf{N}$

$\Rightarrow$ The sequence $\langle s_n \rangle$ is increasing sequence.

Also, we have

$$s_{2n} = 1 + \frac{1}{3} + \frac{1}{5} + \ldots + \frac{1}{2n-1} + \frac{1}{2n+1} + \ldots + \frac{1}{4n-1}$$

$$\therefore \quad s_{2n} - s_n = \left[1 + \frac{1}{3} + \frac{1}{5} + \ldots + \frac{1}{2n-1} + \frac{1}{2n+1} + \ldots + \frac{1}{4n-1}\right] - \left[1 + \frac{1}{3} + \frac{1}{5} + \ldots + \frac{1}{2n-1}\right]$$

$$= \frac{1}{2n+1} + \frac{1}{2n+3} + \ldots + \frac{1}{4n-1}$$

$$\Rightarrow \quad s_{2n} - s_n > n\left(\frac{1}{4n}\right)$$

$$\left(\frac{1}{2n+1} > \frac{1}{4n} \text{ etc. and there are } n \text{ terms}\right)$$

$$\Rightarrow \quad |s_{2n} - s_n| > \frac{1}{4}, \forall n \in \mathbf{N}$$

$\Rightarrow$ There exists a positive integer k such that $|s_{2n} - s_k| > \frac{1}{4}$ whenever $n \geq k$.

$\Rightarrow$ Cauchy criterion is not satisfied.
$\Rightarrow$ The sequence $\langle s_n \rangle$ cannot converge.
$\Rightarrow$ The sequence $\langle s_n \rangle$ diverges to $+\infty$.

THEOREM 1. **(Squeeze Principle).** If $\langle s_n \rangle$, $\langle t_n \rangle$ and $\langle u_n \rangle$ are three sequences such that

(i) $s_n \leq t_n \leq u_n$; $\forall$ n

and (ii) $\langle s_n \rangle$ *converges to* l *and* $\langle u_n \rangle$ *also converges to* l, *then* $\langle t_n \rangle$ *also converges to* l.

PROOF. Let $\varepsilon > 0$ be given. Since the sequences $\langle s_n \rangle$ and $\langle u_n \rangle$ converges to l, there must exist positive integers m_1 and m_2 such that

$$|s_n - l| < \varepsilon \ \forall\, n \geq m_1 \qquad ...(1)$$

$$|u_n - l| < \varepsilon \ \forall\, n \geq m_2 \qquad ...(2)$$

Let $m = \max\{m_1, m_2\}$. Then for $n \geq m$, we have

$$l - \varepsilon < s_n \leq t_n \leq u_n < l + \varepsilon$$

or $$l - \varepsilon < t_n < l + \varepsilon$$

or $$|t_n - l| < \varepsilon,\ \forall\, n \geq m$$

$\Rightarrow$ $$\lim t_n = l$$

Hence, $\langle t_n \rangle$ converges to l.

- If $\langle s_n \rangle$ and $\langle t_n \rangle$ are two sequences such that $|s_n| \leq |t_n|\ \forall\, n \geq m$ where m is a positive integer and $\lim t_n = 0$, then $\lim s_n = 0$.
- The above theorem is also called Sandwitch theorem.

THEOREM 2. **(Cauchy's first theorem on limits).** *If* $\lim_{n\to\infty} s_n = l$, *then*

$$\lim_{n\to\infty} \frac{s_1 + s_2 + ... + s_n}{n} = l.$$

PROOF. Let us define a sequence $\langle t_n \rangle$ in such a way that $t_n = s_n - l$

then $$\lim t_n = \lim(s_n - l) = \lim s_n - l = l - l = 0$$

and $$\frac{s_1 + s_2 + ... + s_n}{n} = l + \frac{t_1 + t_2 + ... + t_n}{n}$$

In order to prove this theorem, we have to show that

$$\lim \frac{t_1 + t_2 + ... + t_n}{n} = 0$$

Now, sequence $\langle t_n \rangle$ is convergent ($\because$ $\langle s_n \rangle$ is convergent.), therefore it is bounded and hence there must exists a positive number k such that

$$|t_n| < k,\ \forall\, n \in \mathrm{N}$$

Also, $\langle t_n \rangle$ converges to zero. Therefore, for a given $\varepsilon > 0$ there must exists *a* positive integer m such that

$$|t_n| < \varepsilon/2,\ \forall\, n \in \mathrm{N}$$

Now, consider $$\left|\frac{t_1 + t_2 + ... + t_n}{n}\right| = \left|\frac{t_1 + t_2 + ... + t_m}{n} + \frac{t_{m+1} + ... + t_n}{n}\right|$$

$$\leq \frac{|t_1| + |t_2| + ... + |t_n|}{n} + \frac{|t_{m+1}| + ... + |t_n|}{n}$$

$$< \frac{mk}{n} + \frac{\varepsilon}{2}, \forall n \geq m$$

Keeping m fixed, we have $\frac{mk}{n} < \varepsilon / 2$ if $n > \frac{2mk}{\varepsilon}$

Let μ be any positive integer $> \frac{2mk}{\varepsilon}$, so that $n \geq \mu$, we have

$$\frac{mk}{n} \leq \frac{\varepsilon}{2}$$

Let $\lambda = \max\{m, \mu\}$.

Therefore, for each $n \geq \lambda$, we have

$$\left|\frac{t_1 + t_2 + \ldots + t_n}{n}\right| < \frac{\varepsilon}{2} + \frac{\varepsilon}{2} = \varepsilon.$$

This gives $\lim\limits_{n\to\infty} \dfrac{t_1 + t_2 + \ldots + t_n}{n} = 0$

Hence, we have $\lim\limits_{n\to\infty} \dfrac{s_1 + s_2 + \quad + s_n}{n} = l$

- Here, we can state that the limit of the nth term of the given sequence is equal to limit of the arithmetic mean of first n terms of the sequence.
- The converse of the above theorem need not be true. For example :

  Let $s_n = (-1)^n$

  $$s_n = (-1)^n \Rightarrow \frac{s_1 + s_2 + \ldots + s_n}{n} = 0 \text{, if } n \text{ is even}$$

  $$= -\frac{1}{n}, \text{ if } n \text{ is odd}$$

  Therefore, $\lim\limits_{n\to\infty} \dfrac{s_1 + s_2 + \quad + s_n}{n} = 0$

  But the sequence $\langle s_n \rangle = \langle (-1)^n \rangle$ is not convergent.

THEOREM 3. **(Cauchy's second theorem on limits).** *If $\langle s_n \rangle$ is a sequence of positive terms and $\lim\limits_{n\to\infty} s_n = l$, then $\lim (s_1 \cdot s_2 \cdot \ldots \cdot s_n)^{1/n} = l$.*

PROOF. Let $\langle t_n \rangle$ be a sequence, such that $t_n = \log s_n, \forall\, n \in \mathrm{N}$

Now $\lim s_n = l \Rightarrow \lim t_n = \lim \log s_n = \log l$

$(\because \lim s_n = l \Leftrightarrow \lim \log s_n = \log l$ provided $s_n > 0, \forall\, n$ and $l > 0)$

Then, by Cauchy first theorem on limits, we have

$$\lim_{n\to\infty} \frac{t_1 + t_2 + \ldots + t_n}{n} = \lim t_n = \log l$$

$$\Rightarrow \quad \lim_{n\to\infty} \frac{\log s_1 + \log s_2 + \ldots + \log s_n}{n} = \log l$$

$$\Rightarrow \quad \lim_{n\to\infty} \frac{1}{n} \log(s_1 \cdot s_2 \cdot \ldots \cdot s_n) = \log l$$

$$\Rightarrow \quad \lim \log(s_1 \cdot s_2 \cdot \ldots \cdot s_n)^{1/n} = \log l$$

$$\Rightarrow \quad \lim(s_1, s_2, \ldots, s_n)^{1/n} = l$$

- Here, we can state that the limit of the nth term of a sequence of positive terms is equal to limit of the geometric mean of first n terms of the given sequence.
- Cauchy's second theorem on limits can also be stated as follows:

  If $\langle s_n \rangle$ be a sequence of positive terms then

  $$\lim s_n^{1/n} = \lim_{n\to\infty} \frac{s_{n+1}}{s_n}$$

  provided, the limit of right hand sides exists.

THEOREM 4. If $\langle s_n \rangle$ is a sequence such that

$$\lim_{n\to\infty} \frac{s_{n+1}}{s_n} = l \, where \, |l| < 1 \, then \, \lim_{n\to\infty} s_n = 0.$$

PROOF. Since $|l| < 1$, let us choose a positive small number ε such that $|l| + \varepsilon < 1$.

Now, $\lim \frac{s_{n+1}}{s_n} = l$, therefore for $\varepsilon > 0$, there must exists a positive integer m such that, for all $n \geq m$

$$\left| \frac{s_{n+1}}{s_n} - l \right| < \varepsilon$$

$$\Rightarrow \quad \left| \frac{s_{n+1}}{s_n} \right| - |l| \leq \left| \frac{s_{n+1}}{s_n} - l \right| < \varepsilon$$

$$\Rightarrow \quad \left| \frac{s_{n+1}}{s_n} \right| < |l| + \varepsilon = k \, (\text{say}).$$

Now, putting $n = m, m+1, ..., n-1$ in the above inequality and multiplying them, we get

$$\left| \frac{s_n}{s_m} \right| < k^{n-m}$$

or

$$|s_n| < \frac{|s_m|}{k^m} . k^n$$

But $k < 1 \Rightarrow k^n \to 0$ as $n \to \infty$, which gives $\lim s_n = 0$.

- The general result obtained here, gives the following important results on limit :

  (i) $\lim \frac{n^s}{n!} = 0$ (ii) $\lim \frac{n^r}{s^n} = 0, |s| > 1$ (iii) $\lim \frac{m(m-1) \ (m-m+1)s^n}{n!} = 0 \ |s| < 1$

THEOREM 5. *If $\langle s_n \rangle$ is a sequence such that $s_n > 0$ and $\lim \frac{s_{n+1}}{s_n} = l$, then $\lim \sqrt[n]{s_n} = l$*

PROOF. Let us define a sequence $\langle t_n \rangle$ such that

$$t_1 = s_1, t_2 = \frac{s_2}{s_1}, \ldots, t_n = \frac{s_n}{s_{n-1}}, \ldots$$

Then $\quad t_1 . t_2 \ldots t_n = s_n.$

Also $\quad \lim \frac{s_{n+1}}{s_n} = l \Rightarrow \lim \frac{s_n}{s_{n-1}} = l \Rightarrow \lim t_n = l$

Now $\quad s_n > 0 \Rightarrow t_n > 0, \forall \, n \in \mathbf{N}$

Hence, the sequence $\langle t_n \rangle$ is of positive terms and $\lim t_n = l$.

Now, by Cauchy's second theorem on limits we have

$$\lim (t_1 . t_2 \ldots t_n)^{1/n} = l$$

or

$$\lim (s_n)^{1/n} = l$$

THEOREM 6. **(Cesaro's Theorem).** *If* $\lim s_n = l_1$ *and* $\lim t_n = l_2$. *Then*

$$\lim \frac{s_1 t_n + s_1 t_{n-1} + \ldots + s_n t_1}{n} = l_1 l_2.$$

PROOF. Let us define $s_n = l_1 + u_n$ and $|u_n| = U_n$.

Then $\quad \lim u_n = 0$ and therefore $\lim Un = 0$.

Now, by Cauchy's first theorem on limits, we have

$$\lim \frac{1}{n}[U_1 + U_2 + ... + U_n] = 0 \quad ...(1)$$

Consider, $\frac{1}{n}[s_1 t_n + s_2 t_{n-1} + ... + s_n t_1]$

$$= \frac{l_1}{n}[t_1 + t_2 + ... + t_n] + \frac{1}{n}[u_1 t_n + u_2 t_{n-1} + ... + u_n t_1] \quad ...(2)$$

Since, the sequence $\langle t_n \rangle$ is convergent. Therefore, it is bounded. Hence, there must exists a positive real number k such that $|t_n| < k$, $\forall n \in \mathbf{N}$.

Therefore, $$\left|\frac{1}{n}(u_1 t_n + u_2 t_{n-1} + ... + u_n t_1\right| \geq 0$$

$$\Rightarrow \quad \frac{1}{n}[|u_1||t_n| + |u_2||t_{n-1}| + ... + |u_n||t_1|] \geq 0$$

$$\Rightarrow \quad \frac{k}{n}[|u_1| + |u_2| + ... + |u_n|] > 0$$

$$\Rightarrow \quad \frac{k}{n}[U_1 + U_2 + ... + U_n] > 0$$

$$\Rightarrow \quad \frac{k}{n}[U_1 + U_2 + ... + U_n] \to 0 \text{ as } n \to \infty \quad \text{[By using (1)]}$$

Thus $\lim \frac{1}{n}[u_1 t_n + u_2 t_{n-1} + ... + u_n t_1] = 0$

Since, $\lim t_n = l_2$, therefore

$$\lim \frac{t_1 + t_2 + \quad + t_n}{n} = l_2$$

Hence, from (2), we have

$$\lim \frac{1}{n}\ (s_1 t_n + s_2 t_{n-1} + ... + s_n t_1) = l_1 l_2$$

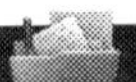

Solved Examples

1. *Prove that* $\lim_{n\to\infty} s_n = 1$, *where* $s_n = n^{1/n}$.

SOLUTION. For $n = 1$, $s_n = 1$

For $n \geq 2$, $s_n > 1$

Let $s_n = 1 + t_n$,

$n = s_n^n = (1 + t_n)^n$,

$t_n > 0, n \geq 2$

$$= 1 + nt_n + \frac{n(n-1)}{2!}t_n^2 + ... + t_n^n$$

(By Binomial Theorem)

$$\geq \frac{n(n-1)}{2!}t_n^2$$

$$\Rightarrow 0 \leq t_n^2 \leq \frac{2}{n-1}$$

$$\Rightarrow 0 < t_n \leq \sqrt{\frac{2}{n-1}}$$

Since $\sqrt{\frac{2}{n-1}} \to 0$ as $n \to \infty$

$\Rightarrow \quad t_n \to 0$ as $n \to \infty$.

Hence $s_n \to 1$ as $n \to \infty$.

2. *If* $s_n = \left[\left(\frac{2}{1}\right)^1\left(\frac{3}{2}\right)^2\left(\frac{4}{3}\right)^3 ... \left(\frac{n+1}{n}\right)^n\right]^{1/n}$ *then show that* $<s_n> \to e$. *Show also that*

$$\lim_{n\to\infty}\left[\frac{n^n}{n!}\right]^{1/n} = e.$$

SOLUTION. Let $t_n = \left(\frac{2}{1}\right)^1\left(\frac{3}{2}\right)^2\left(\frac{4}{3}\right)^3 ... \left(\frac{n+1}{n}\right)^n$

so that $s_n = t_n^{1/n}$

Also, $\frac{t_n + 1}{t_n} = \left(\frac{n+2}{n+1}\right)^{n+1} = \left(1 + \frac{1}{n+1}\right)^{n+1}$

$$\Rightarrow \quad \lim_{n\to\infty} \frac{t_n+1}{t_n} = e$$

Hence, by Cauchy's second theorem on limits, we have

$$\lim_{n\to\infty} s_n = \lim_{n\to\infty} t_n^{1/n} = e$$

$$\text{Also } s_n = \left[2.\left(\frac{3}{2}\right)^2.\left(\frac{4}{3}\right)^3 \ldots \left(\frac{n+1}{n}\right)^n\right]^{1/n}$$

$$= \left[\frac{(n+1)^n}{n!}\right]^{1/n} = \left[\frac{(n+1)^n}{n^n}.\frac{n^n}{n!}\right]^{1/n}$$

$$= \frac{n+1}{n}\left(\frac{n^n}{n!}\right)^{1/n}$$

$$\therefore \lim_{n\to\infty} s_n = \lim_{n\to\infty}\left[\left(\frac{n+1}{n}\right)\left(\frac{n^n}{n!}\right)^{1/n}\right]$$

$$= \lim_{n\to\infty}\frac{n+1}{n}\lim_{n\to\infty}\left[\frac{n^n}{n!}\right]^{1/n}$$

$$= 1\cdot \lim_{n\to\infty}\left(\frac{n^n}{n!}\right)^{1/n}$$

$$\text{Hence, } \lim_{n\to\infty}\left(\frac{n^n}{n!}\right)^{1/n} = e.$$

3. *Show that the sequence $\langle s_n\rangle$ when $s_n = 1+\frac{1}{2}+\frac{1}{3}+\ldots+\frac{1}{n}$ cannot converge.*

SOLUTION. Let us take $\varepsilon = \frac{1}{2}$ and $n = k = m$ and apply them in Cauchy's general principle of convergence, we have

$$|s_{n+k} - s_n| = |s_{2m} - s_m|$$

$$= \frac{1}{m+1}+\frac{1}{m+2}+\ldots+\frac{1}{2m}$$

$$> \frac{1}{2m}+\frac{1}{2m}+\ldots+\frac{1}{2m} = \frac{m}{2m} = \frac{1}{2},$$

which is a contradiction.

Hence, the given sequence is not convergent.

Similar Problems

(1) Show that the sequence $\langle s_n\rangle$ where $s_n = \left\{\frac{1}{\sqrt{n^2+1}}+\frac{1}{\sqrt{n^2+2}}+\ldots+\frac{1}{\sqrt{n^2+n}}\right\}$ converges to 1.

(2) Prove that $\lim_{n\to\infty}\left[\frac{(n+1)(n+2)(n+3)\ldots(n+n)}{n^n}\right]^{1/n} = \frac{4}{e}$.

4. *If $r > 0$, show that $\lim r^{1/n} = 1$.*

SOLUTION. There are following three cases :

Case I. When $r > 1$.

Let $s_n = r^{1/n} - 1$, then $s_n > 0\ \forall\ n \in N$, therefore

$$r^{1/n} = 1 + s_n$$

$$\Rightarrow \quad r = [1+s_n]^n = 1 + ns_n + \ldots + s_n{}^n$$

$$\geq 1 + ns_n + \ \forall\ n \in N$$

$$\Rightarrow \quad \frac{r-1}{n} \geq s_n, \forall n \in \mathbf{N}$$

$$\text{Hence} \quad 0 \leq s_n \leq \frac{r-1}{n}, \forall n \in \mathbf{N}$$

Then, by Sandwitch theorem, we have $\lim s_n = 0$

Hence, $\lim r^{1/n} = 1$

Case II. When $r = 1$

Here, $r^{1/n} = 1,\ \forall\ n \in N$

$$\Rightarrow \quad \lim r^{1/n} = 1$$

Case III. When $0 < r < 1$, then $\frac{1}{r} > 1$

$$\therefore \lim\left(\frac{1}{r}\right)^{1/n} = 1 \Rightarrow \lim \frac{1}{r^{1/n}} = 1$$

$$\Rightarrow \quad \lim r^{1/n} = 1.$$

5. *Prove that*

$$\lim \frac{1}{n}[1 + 2^{1/2} + 3^{1/3} + \ldots + n^{1/n}] = 1.$$

SOLUTION. Let $s_n = n^{1/n}$

$$\Rightarrow \lim s_n = \lim n^{1/n} = 1$$

Then, by Cauchy's first theorem on limits, we have

$$\lim \frac{1}{n}(s_1 + s_1 + \quad + s_n) = 1$$

$$\Rightarrow \lim \frac{1}{n}[1+2^{1/2}+3^{1/3}+ \quad +n^{1/n}]=1$$

21.11 MONOTONIC SEQUENCES

(1) A sequence $\langle s_n \rangle$ is said to be monotonically increasing (or non-decreasing).

if $\quad s_n \le s_{n+1}, \forall n$

or $\quad s_n \le s_m, \forall n < m$

(2) A sequence $\langle s_n \rangle$ is said to be strictly increasing if $s_n < s_{n+1}, \forall n \in \mathrm{N}$

(3) A sequence $\langle s_n \rangle$ is said be monotonically decreasing (or non- increasing)

if $\quad s_n \ge s_{n+1}, \forall n$

or $\quad s_n \ge s_m, \forall n < m$

(4) A sequence $\langle s_n \rangle$ is said to be strictly decreasing if $s_n > s_{n+1}, \forall n \in \mathrm{N}$.

(5) A sequence $\langle s_n \rangle$ is said to be monotonic if it is either monotonically increasing or monotonically decreasing.

☛ ILLUSTRATIONS

(1) $\langle 2, 2, 4, 4, 6, \ldots \rangle$ is monotonically increasing.

(2) $\langle 1, 2, 3, \ldots n \ldots \rangle$ is strictly increasing.

(3) $\left\langle 1, 1, \frac{1}{3}, \frac{1}{5}, \frac{1}{5} \quad \right\rangle$ is monotonically decreasing.

(4) $\langle -2, -4, -6, -8, \ldots \rangle$ is strictly decreasing.

(5) $\langle 0, 1, 0, 1, \ldots \rangle$ is not monotonic.

- Strictly monotonic sequences are special case of monotonic sequences.
- A strictly monotonic sequence may be monotonic after a certain number of terms.

THEOREM 1. (Monotone Convergence Theorem). *Every bounded monotonically increasing sequence converges.*

PROOF. Let $\langle s_n \rangle$ be a bounded monotonically increasing sequence.

Let $\quad S = \{s_n : n \in \mathbf{N}\}$ be its range.

Then, obviously S is a non-empty set, which is bounded above. Therefore there exists a number l, which is the supremum of S. We shall show that the sequence $\langle s_n \rangle$ converges to l.

Let $\varepsilon > 0$ be a given number. Since $l - \varepsilon < l$, therefore $l - \varepsilon$ is not an upper bound of S. Hence, there exists a positive integer m such that $s_n > l - \varepsilon$.

Now, since $\langle s_n \rangle$ is monotonically increasing sequence. Therefore

$$s_n \ge s_m > l - \varepsilon \ \forall\ n \ge m. \quad \ldots(1)$$

$$\text{Sup. } S = l \ \Rightarrow \ s_n \le l < l + \varepsilon, \forall\ n. \quad \ldots(2)$$

From (1) and (2), we have

$$l - \varepsilon < s_n < l + \varepsilon \ \forall n \ge m$$

$$\Rightarrow \quad | s_n - l | < \varepsilon, \forall\ n \ge m$$

Hence, $\langle s_n \rangle$ converges to l.

THEOREM 2. *Every bounded monotonically decreasing sequence converges.*

PROOF. Let $\langle s_n \rangle$ be a bounded monotonically decreasing sequence. Consider a sequence $\langle t_n \rangle$ such that $t_n = -s_n, \forall n \in \mathbf{N}$. Then, $\langle t_n \rangle$ is bounded monotonically increasing sequence and therefore it converges. [By Theorem 1]

If $\lim t_n = l$, then $\lim s_n = \lim (-t_n) = -l$.

THEOREM 3. *A non-decreasing sequence (increasing), which is not bounded above diverges to ∞.*

PROOF. Let $\langle s_n \rangle$ be a monotonic non-decreasing sequence, which is not bounded above. Let c be any positive number. Since, the sequence $\langle s_n \rangle$ is unbounded and monotonically increasing, therefore, there must exists a positive integer m such that

$$s_n \geq s_m > c, \forall n > m$$

$$\Rightarrow \quad s_n > c, \quad \forall n > m$$

Hence, the sequence $\langle s_n \rangle$ diverges to ∞.

THEOREM 4. *A non-increasing (decreasing) sequence, which is not bounded below diverges to –∞.*

PROOF. Proof is exactly on same lines and left as an exercise for the students.

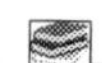

- Every monotonically increasing sequence which is bounded above converges to the least upper bound.
- Every monotonically decreasing sequence which is bounded below converges to the greatest-lower bound.

21.12 NESTED SEQUENCE

A sequence of closed intervals $\langle I_n \rangle$ is said to be nested if either

$$I_1 \subset I_2 \subset I_3 \subset \ldots \quad \text{or} \quad I_1 \supset I_2 \supset I_3 \supset \ldots$$

THEOREM 1. **(Nested Interval Theorem (Cantor's Intersection Theorem).** *If a sequence $\langle I_n = [a_n, b_n] \rangle$ of closed intervals is such that each member $[a_{n+1}, b_{n+1}]$ is contained in preceding one $[a_n, b_n]$ and*

$$\lim_{n \to \infty} [b_n - a_n] = \lim_{n \to \infty} (\textit{length of } I_n) = 0.$$

Then $\bigcap_{n=1}^{\infty} I_n$ contains precisely one point.

PROOF. Since $I_{n+1} \subset I_n, \forall n \in \mathbf{N}$, it follows $a_n \leq a_{n+1} \leq b_{n+1} \leq b_n, \forall n \in \mathbf{N}$, which implies that $\langle a_n \rangle$ is a monotonic increasing sequence bounded above by b_1 and $\langle b_n \rangle$ is a monotonic decreasing sequence bounded below by a_1.

$\Rightarrow$ Both sequence $\langle a_n \rangle$ and $\langle b_n \rangle$ converges.

Also $\lim (b_n - a_n) = 0 \Rightarrow \lim b_n - \lim a_n = 0$

$$\Rightarrow \quad \lim b_n = \lim a_n = l \text{ (say)}.$$

Obviously, l is the upper bound of sequence $\langle a_n \rangle$ and the lower bound of the sequence $\langle b_n \rangle$. So

$$a_n \leq l \leq b_n, \forall n \in \mathbf{N}$$

$$\Rightarrow \quad l \in I_n, \forall n \in \mathbf{N}$$

Therefore $$l \in \bigcap_{n=1}^{\infty} I_n$$

Now we shall show that l is the only point such that $l \in \bigcap_{n=1}^{\infty} I_n$.

Let if possible $\quad l \neq l_1 \in \bigcap_{n=1}^{\infty} I_n$

Then $\quad 0 \leq |l_1 - l| \leq |b_n - a_n|, \forall n \cdot$

$\Rightarrow \quad |l_1 - l| = 0 \qquad (\because \lim |b_n - a_n| = 0)$

$\Rightarrow \quad l = l_1$

$\Rightarrow \quad \bigcap_{n=1}^{\infty} I_n$ consist of exactly one point.

- The word "closed" in the statement of Cantor's intersection theorem cannot be dropped *i.e*, the intersection of a decreasing sequence of open intervals may be empty.

For Example: let $I_n = \left]0, \frac{1}{n}\right[\; n \in \boldsymbol{N}$, then $\bigcap_{n=1}^{\infty} I_n = \phi$.

For, if $x \leq 0$, then $x \notin I_n$ for any n and if $x > 0$, then by Archimedean property of real numbers, there exists a positive integer m such that $m > \frac{1}{x}$

$\Rightarrow \quad \frac{1}{m} < x \quad \Rightarrow x \notin I_m \quad \Rightarrow x \notin \bigcap_{n=1}^{\infty} I_n$

Solved Examples

1. *Show that the sequence $\langle s_n \rangle$ defined by*

$$s_n = \frac{1}{n+1} + \frac{1}{n+2} + \ldots + \frac{1}{n+n}$$

converges.

SOLUTION. The sequence $\langle s_n \rangle$ is defined by

$$s_n = \frac{1}{n+1} + \frac{1}{n+2} + \ldots + \frac{1}{n+n}$$

Now $s_{n+1} - s_n$

$$= \left(\frac{1}{n+2} + \frac{1}{n+3} + \ldots + \frac{1}{2n+2}\right) - \left(\frac{1}{n+1} + \frac{1}{n+2} + \ldots + \frac{1}{2n}\right)$$

$$= \frac{1}{2n+1} + \frac{1}{2n+2} - \frac{1}{n+1}$$

$$= \frac{1}{2n+1} - \frac{1}{2n+2} > 0, \ \forall n.$$

Hence, the sequence $\langle s_n \rangle$ is monotonically increasing.

$$\text{Now } |s_n| = \left|\frac{1}{n+1} + \frac{1}{n+2} + \ldots + \frac{1}{n+n}\right|$$

$$< \frac{1}{n} + \frac{1}{n} + \ldots + \frac{1}{n} = n.\frac{1}{n} = 1$$

i.e,. $|s_n| < 1, \forall n$

$\Rightarrow$ sequence $\langle s_n \rangle$ is bounded.

Then, by monotonic convergence criterion, the sequence $\langle s_n \rangle$ converges.

2. *Show that the sequences $\langle s_n \rangle$ where $s_n = \sqrt{n^2 + m} - n$ is convergent. Also find its limit.*

SOLUTION. Obviously, $\quad s_n > 0, \forall n \in \mathbf{N}$

Further,

$$s_n = \frac{(\sqrt{n^2 + m} - n)(\sqrt{n^2 + m} + n)}{(\sqrt{n^2 + m} + n)}$$

$$= \frac{m}{\sqrt{n^2 + m} + n}$$

Also $\quad s_{n+1} = \dfrac{m}{\sqrt{(n+1)^2 + m} + (n+1)}$

But $\sqrt{(n+1)^2 + m} + (n+1) > \sqrt{n^2 + m} + n$

$$\Rightarrow \frac{m}{\sqrt{(n+1)^2 + m} + (n+1)} < \frac{m}{\sqrt{n^2 + m} + n}$$

$\Rightarrow s_{n+1} < s_n, \ \forall n \in \mathbf{N}$

$\Rightarrow \ \langle s_n \rangle$ is monotonic decreasing sequence and bounded below by 0.

Hence, $\langle s_n \rangle$ is convergent.

Further $\lim_{n\to\infty} u_n = \lim_{n\to\infty} \frac{m}{\sqrt{n^2+m+n}} = 0$.

3. *If* $s_n = \sqrt{n}(\sqrt{n+1}-\sqrt{n})$, *does* $\langle s_n \rangle$ *converge?*

SOLUTION. We have, $s_n = \frac{\sqrt{n}(\sqrt{n+1}-\sqrt{n})(\sqrt{n+1}+\sqrt{n})}{(\sqrt{n+1}+\sqrt{n})}$

$$= \frac{\sqrt{n}(n+1-n)}{(\sqrt{n+1}+\sqrt{n})} = \frac{\sqrt{n}}{(\sqrt{n+1}+\sqrt{n})}$$

Also $s_{n+1} = \frac{\sqrt{n+1}}{\sqrt{n+2}+\sqrt{n+1}}$

$$\therefore \quad s_{n+1} - s_n = \frac{\sqrt{n+1}}{(\sqrt{n+2}+\sqrt{n+1})} - \frac{\sqrt{n}}{(\sqrt{n+1}+\sqrt{n})}$$

$$= \frac{n+1+\sqrt{n}\sqrt{n+1} - \sqrt{n}\sqrt{n+2} - \sqrt{n}\sqrt{n+1}}{(\sqrt{n+2}+\sqrt{n+1})(\sqrt{n+1}+\sqrt{n})}$$

$$= \frac{n+1-\sqrt{n(n+2)}}{(\sqrt{n+2}+\sqrt{n+1})(\sqrt{n+1}+\sqrt{n})}$$

$$= \frac{\sqrt{(n+1)^2} - \sqrt{(n^2+2n)}}{(\sqrt{n+2}+\sqrt{n+1})(\sqrt{n+1}+\sqrt{n})}$$

$$= \frac{\sqrt{(n^2+2n+1)} - \sqrt{(n^2+2n)}}{(\sqrt{n+2}+\sqrt{n+1})(\sqrt{n+1}+\sqrt{n})} > 0, \forall n,$$

as $n^2 + 2n + 1 > n^2 + 2n$

$\Rightarrow s_{n+1} > s_n \Rightarrow \langle s_n \rangle$ is monotonically increasing sequence.

Also $1 - s_n = 1 - \frac{\sqrt{n}}{\sqrt{n+1}+\sqrt{n}}$

$$= \frac{\sqrt{n+1}}{(\sqrt{n+1}+\sqrt{n})} > 0$$

$\Rightarrow \quad s_n < 1, \forall n \in \mathbf{N}$

$\Rightarrow \langle s_n \rangle$ is monotonically increasing and bounded (above) sequence.

Hence $\langle s_n \rangle$ is convergent.

Further $\lim_{n\to\infty} s_n = \lim_{n\to\infty} \frac{\sqrt{n}}{\sqrt{n+1}+\sqrt{n}}$

$$= \lim_{n\to\infty} \frac{\sqrt{n}}{\sqrt{n}\left(\sqrt{1+\frac{1}{n}}+1\right)}$$

$$= \lim_{n\to\infty} \frac{1}{\left(\sqrt{1+\frac{1}{n}}+1\right)} = \frac{1}{2}.$$

Hence $\langle s_n \rangle$ converges to 1/2.

Similar Problems

(1) Show that the sequence $\langle n/n+1 \rangle$ is a bounded monotonically increasing sequence and convergent too.

(2) Prove that the sequence $\left\langle \frac{2^n}{n!} \right\rangle$ is a monotonic decreasing. Also prove that it is bounded.

(3) Show that the sequence $\langle x_n \rangle$ where $x_1 = 1$ and $x_n = (2 + x_{n-1})^{1/2}$ is convergent and converge to 2.

4. *Show that* $\lim_{n\to\infty}\left(1+\frac{1}{n}\right)^n$ *exists and lies between 2 and 3.*

SOLUTION. Let $s_n = \left(1+\frac{1}{n}\right)^n$

$\therefore \quad s_1 = 2$

Now, $s_n = 1 + n\frac{1}{n} + \frac{n(n-1)}{2!}\frac{1}{n^2} + \ldots + \frac{1}{n^n}$

[By binomial theorem for positive integral index]

$$= 1 + 1 + \frac{1}{2!}\left(1-\frac{1}{n}\right) + \ldots + \frac{1}{n!}\left(1-\frac{1}{n}\right)\left(1-\frac{2}{n}\right)\ldots\left(1-\frac{n-1}{n}\right) \quad \ldots (1)$$

Similarly $s_{n+1} = 1+1+\frac{1}{2!}\left(1-\frac{1}{n+1}\right)+\ldots$

$$+\frac{1}{(n+1)!}\left(1-\frac{1}{n+1}\right)$$

$$\left(1-\frac{2}{n+1}\right)\ldots\left(1-\frac{n}{n+1}\right) \quad \ldots(2)$$

Comparing (1) and (2), we see that $s_{n+1} \geq s_n \ \forall n$.

$\Rightarrow$ The sequence $\langle s_n \rangle$ is monotonically increasing.

Now from (1), we have

$$2 < s_n < 1+1+\frac{1}{2!}+\frac{1}{3!}+\ldots+\frac{1}{n!}$$

$$\leq 1+1+\frac{1}{2}+\frac{1}{2^2}+\ldots+\frac{1}{2^{n-1}},$$

which is a G.P.

$$= 1+\frac{1-\frac{1}{2^n}}{1-\frac{1}{2}} = 3-\frac{1}{2^{n-1}} < 3, \forall n.$$

$\Rightarrow$ The sequence $\langle s_n \rangle$ is bounded.

Thus, the sequence $\langle s_n \rangle$, being a monotonically increasing sequence bounded above by 3, is convergent.

Since $2 < s_n < 3 \forall n \Rightarrow 2 \leq \lim_{n\to\infty} s_n \leq 3, \forall n.$

$\Rightarrow$ limit of the sequence $\langle s_n \rangle$ lies between 2 and 3.

5. *Show that the sequence* $\langle s_n \rangle$ *defined by* $s_1 = \sqrt{2}, s_{n+1} = \sqrt{(2s_n)}$ *converges to 2.*

SOLUTION. We have $s_{n+1} = \sqrt{(2s_n)}$

For $n = 1 \Rightarrow s_2 = \sqrt{(2s_1)}$

$\Rightarrow \quad s_2 = \sqrt{(2\sqrt{2})}$

Since $\Rightarrow 1 < \sqrt{2} \quad \Rightarrow 2 < 2\sqrt{2}$

$\Rightarrow \quad \sqrt{2} < \sqrt{(2\sqrt{2})} \quad \Rightarrow s_1 < s_2$

Now, let us suppose that $s_m < s_{m+1}$ then $\sqrt{(2s_m)} < \sqrt{(2s_{m+1})}$

$\Rightarrow \quad s_{m+1} < s_{m+2}.$

Now, by the principle of mathematical induction, we have $s_n < s_{n+1}, \forall n \in \mathrm{N}$

i.e., $\langle s_n \rangle$ is monotonically increasing sequence.

Now we shall show that $<s_n>$ is bounded.

Since $\quad s_1 = \sqrt{2} < 2.$

Let us suppose that $s_m < 2$. Then $\sqrt{(2s_m)} < \sqrt{2.2} = 2$

$\Rightarrow \quad s_{m+1} < 2.$

By the principle of mathematical induction, we have $s_n < 2, \forall n \in \mathbf{N}$

$\Rightarrow \langle s_n \rangle$ is bounded above by 2.

$\Rightarrow \langle s_n \rangle$ is monotonically increasing sequence which is bounded above.

Then, by monotone convergence ctiterion, $\langle s_n \rangle$ is convergent.

Now, let $\lim_{n\to\infty} s_n = l \Rightarrow \lim_{n\to\infty} s_{n+1} = l$

Given that $s_{n+1} = \sqrt{(2s_n)}$

$\Rightarrow \qquad \lim s_{n+1} = \lim \sqrt{2s_n}$

$\Rightarrow \qquad l = \sqrt{2l}$

$\Rightarrow l(l-2) = 0$ which gives $l = 2, l = 0$.

But, since $\langle s_n \rangle$ is positive terms sequence with first term $= \sqrt{2}$. Therefore, l cannot be equal to 0. Hence, $l=2$.

6. *Show that the sequence* $\langle s_n \rangle$ *defined by formula* $s_1 = 1, \quad s_{n+1} = \sqrt{(3s_n)}$ *converges to 3.*

SOLUTION. Solution is exactly same as Example 5 and left as an exercise for the students.

7. *Show that the sequence* $\langle s_n \rangle$ *defined by*

$$s_1 = 1, s_{n+1} = \frac{4+3s_n}{3+2s_n}, \forall n \in \mathbf{N}$$

is convergent and find its limit.

SOLUTION. Since $s_1 = 1, s_2 = \frac{4+3s_1}{3+2s_1} = \frac{7}{5}$

$\therefore \qquad s_2 > s_1.$

Now, let us assume that for some positive integer n, $s_{n+1} > s_n$.

We shall show that $s_{n+2} > s_{n+1}$

Consider, $s_{n+2} - s_{n+1} = \frac{4+3s_{n+1}}{3+2s_{n+1}} - \frac{4+3s_n}{3+2s_n}$

$$= \frac{(4+3s_{n+1})(3+2s_n) - (4+3s_n)(3+2s_{n+1})}{(3+2s_{n+1})(3+2s_n)}$$

$$= \frac{s_{n+1} - s_n}{(3+2s_{n+1})(3+2s_n)} > 0$$

$(\because \ s_{n+1} > s_n)$

$\Rightarrow \qquad s_{n+2} > s_{n+1}.$

Then, by the principle of mathematical induction $s_{n+1} > s_n, \forall n \in \mathbf{N}$

$\Rightarrow$ The sequence $\langle s_n \rangle$ is monotonically increasing.

Now we have

$$s_{n+1} = \frac{3s_n + 4}{2s_n + 3} = \frac{\frac{3}{2}(2s_n + 3) - \frac{1}{2}}{2s_n + 3}$$

$$= \frac{3}{2} - \frac{1}{2(2s_n + 3)}$$

$$\Rightarrow \quad s_{n+1} < \frac{3}{2}, \forall n \in \mathbf{N}$$

$\Rightarrow$ The sequence $\langle s_n \rangle$ is bounded above by $\frac{3}{2}$ $\quad \left(\because s_1 = 1 < \frac{3}{2} \Rightarrow s_n < \frac{3}{2}\right)$

$\Rightarrow$ The sequence $\langle s_n \rangle$ is bounded, monotonically increasing sequence.

Then, by monotone convergence theorem, $\langle s_n \rangle$ is convergent.

Now, let $\lim s_n = l \Rightarrow \lim s_{n+1} = l$

Consider $s_{n+1} = \dfrac{4 + 3s_n}{3 + 2s_n}$

$$\Rightarrow \quad \lim s_{n+1} = \frac{4 + 3\lim s_n}{3 + 2\lim s_n}$$

$$\Rightarrow l = \frac{4 + 3l}{3 + 2l} \Rightarrow l^2 = 2 \text{ i.e., } l = \pm\sqrt{2}.$$

Since $\langle s_n \rangle$ is a positive terms sequence, hence l cannot be negative therefore, $l = \sqrt{2}$

8. *If $a > 1$, $s_1 = 1$, $s_{n+1} = \sqrt{a + s_n}$, then show that the sequence is bounded and monotonic and converges to the positive root of the equation $x^2 - x - a = 0$.*

SOLUTION. Since $1 \le s_1 = 1 < a + 1$

$$1 \le s_2 = \sqrt{a+1} < (a+1).$$

Let us suppose $1 \le s_m < a+1$, then

$$1 \le s_{m+1} = \sqrt{a + s_m}$$

$$< \sqrt{a + a + 1} = \sqrt{2a} + 1 < a + 1.$$

Then, by the method of mathematical induction, we have $1 \le s_n < a + 1$

$\Rightarrow \langle s_n \rangle$ is bounded.

Now, we shall show that $\langle s_n \rangle$ is monotonically increasing sequence.

Consider $s_{n+1}^2 - s_n^2 = (a + s_n) - (a + s_{n-1})$

$$= s_n - s_{n-1}$$

$$\Rightarrow s_{n+1}^{2(n-1)} - s_n^{2(n-1)} = s_2 - s_1 > 0$$

$$\Rightarrow a + 1 > s_{n+1} > s_n > 1, \forall n \in \mathbf{N}.$$

$\Rightarrow$ The sequence is monotonically increasing.

Then, by monotone convergence theorem, $\langle s_n \rangle$ is convergent.

Now, let $\lim_{n\to\infty} s_n = l$. Then

$$\lim_{n\to\infty} s_{n+1} = \lim_{n\to\infty} \sqrt{a + s_n}$$

$$\Rightarrow \quad l = \sqrt{a + l} \Rightarrow l^2 = a + l$$

$$\Rightarrow \quad l^2 - l - a = 0$$

By the theory of equation we can say this equation has only one positive root.

$\Rightarrow$ The given sequences $\langle s_n \rangle$ converges to the positive root of $x^2 - x - a = 0$.

9. *Prove that the sequence $\langle a_n \rangle$ is convergent where $a_n = 1 + \frac{1}{1!} + \frac{1}{2!} + \frac{1}{3!} + \ldots + \frac{1}{n!}$.*

SOLUTION. Since $a_n = 1 + \dfrac{1}{1!} + \dfrac{1}{2!} + \dfrac{1}{3!} + \ldots + \dfrac{1}{n!}$

and $a_{n+1} = 1 + \dfrac{1}{1!} + \dfrac{1}{2!} + \dfrac{1}{3!} + \ldots + \dfrac{1}{n!} + \dfrac{1}{(n+1)!}$

then $a_{n+1} - a_n = \dfrac{1}{(n+1)!} > 0, \forall n \in \mathbf{N}$

Thus, $\langle a_n \rangle$ is monotonically increasing.

Further, $a_n = 1 + \dfrac{1}{1!} + \dfrac{1}{2!} + \dfrac{1}{3!} + \ldots + \dfrac{1}{n!}$

$$\Rightarrow 2 < a_n < 1 + 1 + \frac{1}{2^2} + \frac{1}{2^3} + \ldots + \frac{1}{2^{n-1}}$$

$$\Rightarrow 2 < a_n \le 1 + \frac{1 - \frac{1}{2^n}}{1 - \frac{1}{2}} = 3 - \frac{1}{2^{n-1}} < 3, \forall n$$

$\Rightarrow \quad \langle a_n \rangle$ is bounded.

Hence, $\langle a_n \rangle$ is convergent.

10. *Show that $\lim_{n\to\infty} \dfrac{n}{(n!)^{1/n}} = e$.*

SOLUTION. Let $s_n = \dfrac{n^n}{n!}$, then $s_{n+1} = \dfrac{(n+1)^{n+1}}{(n+1)!}$

$$\therefore \quad \frac{s_{n+1}}{s_n} = \frac{(n+1)^{n+1}}{(n+1)} \cdot \frac{1}{n^n} = \left(\frac{n+1}{n}\right)^n$$

$$\Rightarrow \lim_{n\to\infty} \frac{s_{n+1}}{s_n} = \lim_{n\to\infty} (1 + 1/n)^n$$

$$= e > 0, \forall n \in \mathbf{N}.$$

So, by Cauchy second theorem

$$\lim_{n\to\infty} s_n^{1/n} = \lim_{n\to\infty} \frac{s_{n+1}}{s_n} = e$$

Hence $\lim_{n\to\infty} \frac{n}{(n!)^{1/n}} = e$.

Similar Problem

(1) Prove that the sequence $\left\langle \frac{2n-7}{3n+2} \right\rangle$ is monotonically increasing, bounded above and bounded below.

Exercise-21.1

1. Discuss the boundedness of the following sequences $\langle s_n \rangle$, where s_n is given by

(i) $s_n = 6$ (ii) $s_n = (-1)^n.4$

(iii) $s_n = \frac{2n+3}{3n+4}$ (iv) $s_n = \left(1+\frac{1}{n}\right)^n$

(v) $s_n = \frac{1}{n^2} + \frac{1}{(n+1)^2} + \quad + \frac{1}{(2n)^2}$

(vi) $s_n = n^3$ (vii) $s_n = 1+(-1)^n$.

2. Discuss the convergence and divergence of sequences in Ques. 1.

3. Give examples of sequence $\langle s_n \rangle$ for which

$\lim_{n\to\infty} \frac{s_{n+1}}{s_n} = 1$ and

(i) $s_n \to \infty$ (ii) $s_n \to 2$

(iii) $s_n \to 0$.

4. Verify the following:

(i) $\lim_{n\to\infty} \frac{3n-5}{4-2n} = -\frac{3}{2}$

(ii) $\lim_{n\to\infty} [(n^2+1)^{1/8} - (n+1)^{1/4}] = 0$

(iii) $\lim_{n\to\infty} \left[\frac{1}{n^2} + \frac{1}{(n+1)^2} + \ldots + \frac{1}{(2n)^2}\right] = 0$

(iv) $\lim_{n\to\infty} \left(1-\frac{1}{n}\right)^{-n} = e$

5. If $\langle s_n \rangle$ diverges to $+\infty$ and $\langle t_n \rangle$ diverges to $-\infty$, then show by example that $\langle s_n + t_n \rangle$ may :

(i) converge (ii) diverge to ∞

(ii) diverge to $-\infty$ (iv) oscillate

6. Prove by definition that the following sequences whose n^{th} term are given below, are Cauchy sequence:

(i) $\frac{1}{n}$ (ii) $\frac{1}{n^2}$

(iii) $(-1)^n.\frac{1}{n}$ (iv) $\frac{n}{n+1}$

7. Show that the sequences whose n^{th} terms are given below are not Cauchy sequences.

(i) $(-1)^n$ (ii) n (iii) $(-1)^n.n$.

8. If $\langle s_n \rangle$ and $\langle t_n \rangle$ are two Cauchy sequences, then show that

(i) $\langle s_n + t_n \rangle$ (ii) $\langle s_n - t_n \rangle$

(iii) $\langle s_n t_n \rangle$ and (iv) $\left\langle \frac{s_n}{t_n} \right\rangle (t_n \neq 0)$

are Cauchy sequences.

9. Show that the sequences $\langle s_n \rangle$ defined by $s_1 = \frac{1}{2}, s_{n+1} = \frac{2s_n+1}{3}, \forall n \in \mathbf{N}$ is convergent. Also find its limit.

10. Show that the sequence $\left\langle \frac{n^2+3n+5}{2n^2+5n+7} \right\rangle$ converges to $\frac{1}{2}$.

11. Show that the sequence $\langle s_n \rangle$ defined by $s_1 = \sqrt{7}, s_{n+1} = \sqrt{7+s_n}$ converges to the positive root of $x^2 - x - 7 = 0$.

12. Show that the sequence where $s_n = \frac{1}{(\log n)^{\log n}}$ is convergent.

13. Show that the sequence $\langle s_n \rangle$ where $s_n = \frac{2n^2 \cdot\cdot 1}{2n^2 - 1}$ converges to 1.

Hints to the Selected Problems

1. (iii) $s_n = \frac{2n+3}{3n+4} \Rightarrow \langle s_n \rangle = \left\langle \frac{5}{7}, \frac{7}{10}, \frac{9}{13}, \right\rangle$

$\Rightarrow |s_n| \leq \frac{5}{7} \Rightarrow \langle s_n \rangle$ is bounded.

4. (i) Let $\varepsilon > 0$ be given. Therefore

$$\left|\frac{3n-5}{4-2n} - \frac{3}{2}\right| = \left|\frac{1}{4-2n}\right| = \frac{1}{-4+2n}$$

$< \varepsilon$ if $\frac{1}{-4+2n} < \varepsilon$ or $n > \frac{4+\varepsilon}{2}$

6. (i) $s_n = \frac{1}{n}$. Take $\varepsilon > 0$. If $n \geq m$ then

$$|s_n - s_m| = \left|\frac{1}{n} - \frac{1}{m}\right| = \left|\frac{m-n}{mn}\right|$$

$$= \frac{n-m}{mn} = \frac{n-m}{n} \cdot \frac{1}{m} < \frac{1}{m}$$

If we take m as positive integer, such that $m > \frac{1}{\varepsilon}$ *i.e.*, $\frac{1}{m} < \varepsilon$. Then $|s_n - s_m| < \varepsilon$

$\Rightarrow \langle s_n \rangle = \left\langle \frac{1}{n} \right\rangle$ is a Cauchy sequence.

9. $s_{n+1} = \frac{2s_{n+1}}{3}$

If $\lim s_n = l$. Then $\lim s_{n+1} = l \Rightarrow \frac{2l+1}{3} \Rightarrow l = 1$

10. $s_n = \frac{n^2 + 3n + 5}{2n^2 + 5n + 7}$

$$\Rightarrow \lim_{n\to\infty} s_n = \lim_{n\to\infty} \left[\frac{1 + \frac{3}{n} + \frac{5}{n^2}}{2 + \frac{5}{n} + \frac{7}{n^2}}\right] = \frac{1}{2}.$$

12. $s_n = \frac{1}{(\log n)^{\log n}}$

Since we know that $\log(n+1) > \log n, \forall n \in \mathbf{N}$

$\Rightarrow [\log (n+1)]^{\log(n+1)} > (\log n)^{\log(n+1)}, \forall n \in \mathbf{N}$

$> (\log n)^{\log n}, \forall n \in \mathbf{N}$

$$\Rightarrow \frac{1}{(\log n)^{\log n}} > \frac{1}{[\log(n+1)]^{\log(n+1)}}, \forall n \in \mathbf{N}$$

$\Rightarrow s_n > s_{n+1} \Rightarrow \langle s_n \rangle$ is monotonically decreasing sequence. Similarly we can show that $\langle s_n \rangle$ is bounded.

ANSWERS

1. (i), (ii), (iii), (iv), (v), (vii) bounded (vi) unbounded.

2. (i), (iii), (iv), (v) converges (ii), (vii) oscillate (vi) diverges to ∞

3. (i) $s_n = n$ (ii) $s_n = \frac{2n+1}{n}$ (iii) $s_n = \frac{1}{n}$

5. (i) $s_n = n, t_n = -n$ (ii) $s_n = n^2, t_n = -n$ (iii) $s_n = n, t_n = -n^2$ **9.** $l = 1$

□□□□□□

Chapter

22

Infinite Series

22.1 INTRODUCTION

Infinite series are essential in the calculation of values of many functions, and can frequently be used for the evaluation of definite integrals. They can also serve to define new and useful functions that are fundamental in many investigations in advanced mathematics and its applications.

Problems connected with the concept of series attracted the Indian mathematician as early as the third century A.D. Their work on series continued till late fourteenth century, but they never took up a critical study of series. In Europe, it was during the sixth century A.D., that the wider significance of finite and infinite series was realized.

The English mathematicians, Brook Taylor (1685-1731) and James Sterling (1692-1770), and the Scotch mathematician Colin Maclaurin (1698-1746), made important contributions to the study of infinite series. The question of convergent of infinite series was first subjected to rigorous investigation by the German Mathematician Carl Friedrich Gauss (1777-1855).

In this chapter, we are going to discuss the convergence behaviour of infinite series of real numbers and shall obtain a few tests for ascertaining the convergence of the infinite series. Some writer use the word Progression instead of word series. But here the word Series, which is due to the writers of the 17th century and is most commonly used in preferred.

22.2 INFINITE SERIES

Let $<u_n>$ be a sequence of real numbers, then an expression of the form

$$u_1+u_2+\ldots+u_n+\ldots \qquad \ldots(1)$$

is called an infinite series. In symbols, it is generally written as

$$\sum_{n=1}^{\infty} u_n \text{ or } \sum u_n$$

If all the terms of $<u_n>$ after a certain number are zero then the expression

$$u_1+u_2+\ldots+u_m, \text{ written as } \sum_{n=1}^{m} u_n \text{ is called a finite series.}$$

The term u_n is called the nth term or general term of the series (1). The sum of first n terms of the series is denoted by s_n. Thus, $s_n = u_1+u_2+\ldots+u_n = \sum_{r=1}^{n} u_r$

22.3 SEQUENCE OF PARTIAL SUM OF AN INFINITE SERIES

An expression of the form $u_1 + u_2 + \ldots + u_n \ldots$ which involves addition of infinitely many terms has in itself no meaning. In order to give a meaning to the value of such as infinite sum, we form a sequence of partial sums. It is the limit of such a sequence which gives meaning to the infinite series.

Let us associate to the infinite series $u_1 + u_2 + ... + u_n ....$; a sequence $<s_n>$ defined by $s_n = u_1 + u_2 + ... + u_n$.

Then the sequence $<s_n>$ is called the sequence of partial sums of the given series $u_1 + u_2 + ... + u_n ...$

22.4 CONVERGENCE, DIVERGENCE OR OSCILLATION OF AN INFINITE SERIES

An infinite series $\sum_{n=1}^{\infty} u_n$ is said to be

(i) convergent if the sequence $<s_n>$ of its partial sums converges to a real number l and in that case l is called the sum of the series $\sum_{n=1}^{\infty} u_n$ and we write $\sum_{n=1}^{m} u_n = l$. In this case, we also say that the series is convergent to l.

(ii) converges absolutely if $\sum_{n=1}^{\infty} |u_n|$ converges.

(iii) converges conditionally if $\sum_{n=1}^{\infty} u_n$ converges but $\sum_{n=1}^{\infty} |u_n|$ does not converge.

(iv) diverges to ∞ (or $-\infty$) if the sequence $<s_n>$ diverges to ∞ (or $-\infty$) and in that case $\sum_{n=1}^{\infty} u_n = \infty \left(\text{or } \sum_{n=1}^{\infty} u_n = -\infty \right)$

(v) oscillate finitely if the sequence $<s_n>$ oscillates finitely.

(vi) oscillate infinitely if the sequence $<s_n>$ oscillates infinitely.

(vii) oscillatory if s_n, the sum of its first n terms, neither tends to a definite finite limit nor to $+\infty$ or $-\infty$ as $n \to \infty$.

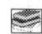

- Divergent and oscillatory series are often called non-convergent series.
- The value of s_n of oscillate finitely series fluctuate within a finite range as $n \to \infty$.
- The value of s_n of oscillate infinitely series, tends to infinity as $n \to \infty$ and its sign is alternatively positive and negative.

☛ ILLUSTRATIONS

(1) The series $1 + \frac{2}{3} + \left(\frac{2}{3}\right)^2 + ... + \left(\frac{2}{3}\right)^{n-1} + ...$ is convergent.

(2) The series $\frac{1}{2} + \frac{1}{2^2} + \frac{1}{2^3} + ...$ is convergent.

(3) The series $1 + 2 + 3 + ... + n + ...$ is divergent.

(4) The series $3 - 3 + 3 - 3 + ...$ is oscillatory.

THEORM 1. **(Necessary condition for convergence).** *For a series Σu_n to be convergent, it is necessary that $\lim u_n = 0$.* (PTU–2009)

PROOF. Let us suppose, the series Σu_n be convergent. Let s_n denote the sum of n terms of the series

Therefore $\left.\begin{aligned} s_n &= u_1 + u_2 + ... + u_n \\ \Rightarrow \quad s_{n-1} &= u_1 + u_2 + ... + u_{n-1} \end{aligned}\right] \Rightarrow u_n = s_n - s_{n-1}$ ...(1)

The series Σu_n is convergent, therefore s_n and s_{n-1} both will tend to the same finite limit, say l as $n \to \infty$.

Now, from (1) $\lim u_n = \lim s_n - \lim s_{n-1} = l - l = 0$.

Hence, for a convergent series, it is necessary that $\lim u_n = 0$.

- The converse of the above theorem is not necessarily true :

  For example, in the series $\Sigma u_n = 1 + \frac{1}{2} + \frac{1}{3} + \ldots ; u_n = \frac{1}{n} \to 0$ as $n \to \infty$ but the series is not convergent.
- If a series Σu_n be such that u_n does not tend to zero as $n \to \infty$ then the series does not converge.

THEOREM 2. (Cauchy's General principle of convergence of series). *A necessary and sufficient condition for a series Σu_n to be convergent is that to each $\varepsilon > 0$, there exists a positive integer m such that $|u_{n+1} + u_{n+2} + \ldots + u_{n+p}| < \varepsilon \ \forall \ n > m, \ p \geq 1$.*

PROOF. Let $<s_n>$ be the sequence of partial sums of the series Σu_n. The series Σu_n will converge if and only if the sequence $<s_n>$ of its partial sums converges. But by Cauchy's general principle of convergence for sequences, we know that a necessary and sufficient condition for the convergence of $<s_n>$ is that for each $\varepsilon > 0$, there exists $m \in N$ such that

$$|s_n - s_m| < \varepsilon, \ \forall \ n > m$$

$$\Rightarrow \quad |u_{n+1} + u_{n+2} + \ldots + u_{n+p}| < \varepsilon, \ \forall \ n > m \text{ and } p \geq 1.$$

- The nature of a series remains unaltered if :
  (a) the sign of all terms are changed.
  (b) a finite number of terms are added or omitted.
  (c) each term of the series is multiplied or divided by the same fixed number k $(k \neq 0)$.
- If Σu_n converges to l and $k \in \mathbf{R}$, then $\Sigma k u_n$ converges to lk.
- If Σu_n converges to l_1 and Σv_n converges to l_2 then $\Sigma(u_n + v_n)$ converges to $(l_1 + l_2)$.
- If Σu_n diverges and $k \in \mathbf{R}$, $k \neq 0$, then $\Sigma k u_n$ diverges.
- If Σu_n and Σv_n are two divergent series having all terms positive, then $\Sigma(u_n + v_n)$ also diverges.

THEOREM 3. *A series of positive terms is convergent if s_n, the sum of n terms is less than a fixed number for all values of n.*

PROOF. Let $u_1 + u_2 + \ldots u_n + \ldots$ be the series of positive terms.

Then $s_n = u_1 + u_2 + \ldots u_n$.

Obviously if n increases, then s_n increases and may tend to a finite limit or to $+\infty$. The series cannot oscillate. If s_n remains less than a fixed number for all values of n it cannot tend to infinity and so it must tend to a finite limit. Hence, the series is convergent.

22.5 FUNDAMENTAL RESULTS FOR THE CONVERGENCE OF POSITIVE TERM SERIES

THEOREM 1. *A series Σu_n of positive term is convergent if and only if the sequence $<s_n>$ (where $s_n = u_1 + u_2 + \ldots + u_n$) of its partial sum is bounded above.*

PROOF. Since $u_n > 0 \ \forall \ n$, the sequence $<s_n>$ of partial sums of the series is monotonically increasing. Now the series Σu_n is convergent iff the sequence $<s_n>$ is convergent, *i.e.*, iff the sequence $<s_n>$ is bounded above.

($\because$ a monotonically increasing sequence is convergent iff it is bounded above.)

- To show that a series of positive term is convergent it is enough to show the sequence of its partial sum is bounded above and to show that the series of positive term is divergent, we have to show that the sequence of its partial sum is unbounded above.
- A series Σu_n where the terms are not necessarily positive, may fail to the convergent even if the sequence of its partial sums is bounded above.

  For example, consider the series $\sum_{n=1}^{\infty} u_n$ where $u_n = (-1)^n$. Then $s_n = \begin{cases} -1 & \text{if } n \text{ is odd} \\ 0 & \text{if } n \text{ is even.} \end{cases}$

  The sequence $<s_n>$ is bounded above but not convergent and as such, the series is not convergent. Hence, boundedness of the sequence of partial sums of a series Σu_n is only a necessary condition and not a sufficient one. However, it is a sufficient condition for a positive term series.

THEOREM 2. **(Pringsheim theorem).** *If a series Σu_n of positive monotonic decreasing terms converges then not only u_n tends to zero but also nu_n tends to zero as n tends to infinity.*

PROOF. By Cauchy's general principle of convergence, we have for a convergent series, that for given $\varepsilon > 0$ there exists a positive integer k such that $|u_{m+1} + u_{m+2} + \ldots + u_{m+p}| < \varepsilon/2$ $\forall\ m \geq k; p \geq 1$

Choose $m+p = n > 2k$ and $m = \left[\frac{n}{2}\right]$ where $\left[\frac{n}{2}\right]$ denote the greatest integer not greater than $\left(\frac{n}{2}\right)$.

Then $$|u_{m+1} + u_{m+2} + \ldots + u_n| < \frac{\varepsilon}{2}$$

But Σu_n is monotonic decreasing sequence of positive terms. Therefore,

$$(n-m)u_n < |u_{m+1} + u_{m+2} + \ldots + u_n| < \frac{\varepsilon}{2}$$

$$\Rightarrow \quad \frac{1}{2}nu_n < \frac{\varepsilon}{2} \quad \Rightarrow nu_n < \varepsilon, \forall n \in \mathrm{N} \quad \Rightarrow \quad \lim_{n\to\infty} nu_n = 0.$$

THEOREM 3. *If each term of a series Σu_n of positive terms does not exceed the corresponding terms of a convergent series Σv_n of positive terms, then Σu_n is convergent. On the other hand, if each term of Σu_n exceed (or equals) the corresponding terms of a divergent series of positive terms, then Σu_n is divergent.*

PROOF. Let us suppose $u_n < v_n \ \forall\ n \in \mathbf{N}$. Now let $s_n = u_1 + u_2 + \ldots + u_n$ and $s'_n = v_1 + v_2 + \ldots + v_n$

Since $u_n \leq v_n\ \forall\ n$, therefore $s_n \leq s'_n$.

Now Σv_n is convergent, therefore $\lim s_n \leq \lim s'_n = s'$ (a finite quantity).

Thus s_n tends to a finite limit as $n \to \infty$. Hence, the series Σu_n is convergent.

Now, if $u_n > v_n$, $\forall\ n$ then $s_n > s'_n$.

But Σv_n is divergent, therefore $s'_n \to \infty$ as $n \to \infty$ and hence $s_n \to \infty$ as $n \to \infty$ which gives that Σu_n is divergent.

THEOREM 4 **(Convergence of geometric series).** *The geometric series $1+r+r^2+\ldots+r^{n-1}+\ldots$*

(i) converges to $\frac{1}{1-r}$ if $|r| < 1$ *(ii) diverges to $+\infty$ if $r \geq 1$*

(iii) oscillate finitely if $r = -1$. *(iv) oscillate infinitely if $r < -1$.*

PROOF. Here $$s_n = 1 + r + r^2 + \ldots + r^{n-1} = \begin{cases} \dfrac{1-r^n}{1-r} & \text{if } r \neq 1 \\ n & \text{if } r = 1 \end{cases}$$

Now, there are following cases :

Case (I). If $|r| < 1$.

Then $\lim_{n\to\infty} r^n = 0$ so that $\lim_{n\to\infty} s_n = \frac{1}{1-r}$ $\Rightarrow$ the series is convergent to $\frac{1}{1-r}$.

Case (II). If $r > 1$.

Then $\lim_{n\to\infty} r^n = \infty$ so that $s_n = \frac{1-r^n}{1-r} = \frac{1}{1-r} + \frac{r^n}{r-1} \to \infty$ as $n \to \infty$.

Hence, the series diverges to ∞.

if $r=1$, then $s_n = 1 + 1 + \ldots + 1 + \ldots$ to n times

$= n$

Thus, the sequence $< s_n >$ diverges and hence the series diverges.

Case (III). If $r = -1$.

Then, $s_n = \begin{cases} 0 \text{ if } n \text{ is even} \\ 1 \text{ if } n \text{ is odd} \end{cases}$

Therefore the sequence $<s_n>$ oscillate between 0 and 1. $\Rightarrow$ The series oscillates finitely between 0 and 1.

Case (IV). If $r < -1$

Let $r = -a$ where $a > 1$ Then $s_n = \frac{1}{1+a} - \frac{(-1)^n \cdot a^n}{1+a}$ so that $s_{2n} \to \infty$ and $s_{2n+1} \to \infty$

Therefore, the sequence $<s_n>$ oscillate infinitely between $-\infty$ and $+\infty$.

Hence, the series oscillate infinitely.

THEOREM 5. *A positive terms series Σu_n either converges to a finite limit or diverges to ∞.*

PROOF. Let $s_n = u_1 + u_2 + \ldots + u_n$

$\Rightarrow$ $s_{n+1} = u_1 + u_2 + \ldots u_{n+1}$

Therefore, $s_{n+1} - s_n = u_{n+1} > 0 \Rightarrow s_{n+1} > s_n, \forall n$

$\Rightarrow$ $<s_n>$ is monotonically increasing sequence.

Since, a monotonically increasing sequence is either convergent to a finite limit or divergent to ∞, the sequence $< s_n>$ of partial sums of the series Σu_n is either convergent a finite limit or divergent to ∞.

Hence, the series Σu_n is either converges or diverges to ∞.

- In view of the above theorem, a positive term series has only two possible behaviours, *i.e.* convergence or divergence while a general term has got five behaviour (*i.e.*, convergent, divergent to ∞, divergent to $-\infty$, oscillate finitely and oscillate infinitely).
- If, in a positive terms series Σu_n, u_n does not tend to 0 as $n \to \infty$, the series is divergent.
- Similarly, it can be proved that a negative term series either converges to a finite limit or diverges to $-\infty$.

THEOREM 6. $\left(\textbf{The Auxillary series } \Sigma \frac{1}{n^p}\right)$. *The infinite series* $\Sigma\left(\frac{1}{n^p}\right) = \frac{1}{1^p} + \frac{1}{2^p} + \ldots + \frac{1}{n^p} + \ldots$ *is convergent if $p > 1$ and divergent if $p \le 1$.* (PTU–2009, VTU–2006, ROHTAK–2003)

PROOF. **Case (I).** *When $p > 1$.*

Since each term of the given series is positive so that the given series can be written as :

$$\Sigma\left(\frac{1}{n^p}\right) = \frac{1}{1^p} + \left(\frac{1}{2^p} + \frac{1}{3^p}\right) + \left(\frac{1}{4^p} + \frac{1}{5^p} + \frac{1}{6^p} + \frac{1}{7^p}\right) + \left(\frac{1}{8^p} + \frac{1}{9^p} + \frac{1}{10^p} + \frac{1}{11^p} + \frac{1}{12^p} + \frac{1}{13^p} + \frac{1}{14^p} + \frac{1}{15^p}\right) + \ldots \quad \ldots(1)$$

Since $p > 1$, then

$$3^p > 2^p \Rightarrow \frac{1}{3^p} < \frac{1}{2^p} \quad \Rightarrow \quad \frac{1}{2^p} + \frac{1}{3^p} < \frac{1}{2^p} + \frac{1}{2^p} = \frac{2}{2^p} = \frac{1}{2^{p-1}}$$

Also, $5^p > 4^p, 6^p > 4^p, 7^p > 4^p \quad \Rightarrow \quad \frac{1}{5^p} < \frac{1}{4^p}, \frac{1}{6^p} < \frac{1}{4^p}, \frac{1}{7^p} < \frac{1}{4^p}$

$$\Rightarrow \quad \frac{1}{4^p} + \frac{1}{5^p} + \frac{1}{6^p} + \frac{1}{7^p} < \frac{1}{4^p} + \frac{1}{4^p} + \frac{1}{4^p} + \frac{1}{4^p} = \left(\frac{1}{2^{p-1}}\right)^2$$

Similarly $\frac{1}{8^p} + \frac{1}{9^p} + \frac{1}{10^p} + \ldots + \frac{1}{15^p} < \frac{8}{8^p} = \left(\frac{1}{2^{p-1}}\right)^3$ ... and so on.

Now using above inequalities, equation (1) becomes

$$\Sigma\left(\frac{1}{n^p}\right) < 1 + \frac{1}{2^{p-1}} + \left(\frac{1}{2^{p-1}}\right)^2 + \left(\frac{1}{2^{p-1}}\right)^3 + \ldots \quad \ldots(2)$$

The R.H.S. of (2) is a geometric series with common ratio less than 1 as $p > 1$, which is therefore convergent thus the series on L.H.S of (2) is convergent, hence, $\Sigma\left(\frac{1}{n^p}\right)$ is convergent, when $p > 1$.

Case (II). *When* $p = 1$. Then the given series becomes

$$\Sigma\frac{1}{n^p} = 1 + \frac{1}{2} + \frac{1}{3} + \ldots$$

Now, this series may be written as follows

$$\Sigma\frac{1}{n^p} = 1 + \frac{1}{2} + \left(\frac{1}{3} + \frac{1}{4}\right) + \ldots > 1 + \frac{1}{2} + \left(\frac{1}{4} + \frac{1}{4}\right) + \ldots$$

$$= 1 + \frac{1}{2} + \frac{2}{4} + \ldots. = 1 + \frac{1}{2} + \frac{1}{2} \ldots.$$

Now since $\lim u_n = \frac{1}{2} \neq 0$, the series is divergent.

Case (III). *When* $p < 1$. Then

$$2^p < 2,\ 3^p < 3,\ 4^p < 4 \text{ and so on.}$$

Hence, the given series reduces to $\sum\frac{1}{n^p} > 1 + \frac{1}{2} + \frac{1}{3} + \frac{1}{4} + \ldots$

Clearly, the series on the right hand side is divergent. [By case (II)]
Hence, the given series is divergent when $p < 1$.

22.6 COMPARISON TESTS

The most important technique for deciding whether a series is convergent or not is to compare it with another suitable chosen series which is already known to be convergent or divergent.

(i) First form. Let Σu_n and Σv_n be two series of positive terms such that $u_n < kv_n$, $\forall\, n$ Then,

(i) Σv_n converges $\Rightarrow \Sigma u_n$ converges (ii) Σu_n diverges $\Rightarrow \Sigma v_n$ diverges.

(ii) Second form. Let Σu_n and Σv_n be two series of positive terms and let k_1 and k_2 be positive real numbers such that $k_1 v_n < u_n < k_2 v_n$, $\forall\, n$ then series Σu_n and Σv_n converge or diverge together.

(iii) Third form. If Σu_n and Σv_n be two given positive terms series such that $u_n < kv_n$, $\forall\, n > m$, $k>0$ and $m \in \mathbf{N}$

Then

(i) Σv_n *is* convergent $\Rightarrow \Sigma u_n$ is convergent (ii) Σu_n is divergent $\Rightarrow \Sigma v_n$ is also divergent.

(iv) Fourth form. Let Σu_n and Σv_n be two series of positive terms and let k_1, k_2 be positive real numbers such that $k_1 v_n < u_n < k_2 v_n$ $\forall\, n > m$, m being a fixed positive integer. Then the series Σu_n and Σv_n converge or diverge together.

(v) Fifth form. Let Σu_n and Σv_n be two sereis of positive terms such that

$$\lim_{n\to\infty}\frac{u_n}{v_n} = l \text{ (finite and non-zero)}$$

then both the series converge or diverge together.

- In the above form of the comparison test, the condition $\lim_{n\to\infty} \frac{u_n}{v_n}$ be finite and non-zero cannot be dropped. For example, if $u_n = \frac{1}{n}$ and $v_n = \frac{1}{n^2}$ then $\lim \frac{u_n}{v_n} = +\infty$, Σu_n is divergent and Σv_n is convergent.
In this case, neither the hypothesis nor the conclusion of the comparison test happens to be true.
- The comparison test is usually applied when the nth term u_n of the given series Σu_n contains the powers of n only which may be positive or negative, integral or fractional.
- v_n can be choosen such that $v_n = \frac{1}{n^{p-q}}$ where p and q are respectively the highest indices of n in the denominator and numerator of u_n when it is in the form of fraction, if u_n can be expanded in ascending powers of $\frac{1}{n}$ then to get v_n we should retain only the lowest power of $\frac{1}{n}$ the numerical factor being disregarded.
- We always denote the given series by Σu_n and the series which is used for comparison is Σv_n
- The series Σv_n is known as auxiliary series. We select the auxiliary series in such a way that $\lim_{n\to\infty}\left(\frac{u_n}{v_n}\right)$ exists finitely and non-zero.

(vi) Sixth form. Let Σu_n and Σv_n be two series of positive terms and let $\exists$ a positive integer m such that $\frac{u_n}{u_{n+1}} > \frac{v_n}{v_{n+1}}, \forall n \geq m$ then Σu_n and Σv_n both converge or diverge together.

Solved Examples

1. *If $u_n \geq 0$ for all n and Σu_n converges then show that $\sum \frac{\sqrt{u_n}}{n}$ also converges.*

SOLUTION. Since $u_n \geq 0$, then for all $n \in \boldsymbol{N}$

or $$\frac{u_n}{n^2} < u_n^2 + \frac{2u_n}{n^2} + \frac{1}{n^4}$$

or $$0 \leq \frac{u_n}{n^2} < \left(u_n + \frac{1}{n^2}\right)^2$$

or $$0 \leq \frac{\sqrt{u_n}}{n} < u_n + \frac{1}{n^2}$$

Since Σu_n and $\sum \frac{1}{n^2}$ are convergent, therefore $\sum\left(u_n + \frac{1}{n^2}\right)$ is convergent.

Hence, by comparison test $\sum \frac{\sqrt{u_n}}{n}$ is convergent.

2. *If Σu_n is a sereis of positive terms and Σu_n is convergent then show that $\sum \frac{u_n}{1+u_n}$ is convergent.*

SOLUTION. Since $u_n > 0$, then for all $n \in \boldsymbol{N}$, $1 + u_n > 1$

$$\Rightarrow \quad \frac{1}{1+u_n} < 1 \forall n \in N$$

$$\therefore \quad 0 < \frac{u_n}{1+u_n} < u_n \ \forall n \in N$$

$$\Rightarrow \quad 0 < \frac{u_n}{1+u_n} < \Sigma u_n$$

Since Σu_n is convergent, hence by comparison test $\sum \frac{u_n}{1+u_n}$ is convergent.

3. *If Σu_n is a convergent series of positive terms, prove that $\sum u_n^2$ is also convergent. Is the converse true?*

SOLUTION. Since Σu_n is convergent, then $\lim_{n\to\infty} u_n = 0$

$\therefore$ For given $\in > 0$ there exists a positive integer m such that

$$|u_n| < \varepsilon \quad \forall n \geq m$$

$$\Rightarrow \quad -\varepsilon < u_n < \varepsilon \ \forall n \geq m$$

Since $u_n > 0 \ \forall n$, choose $\varepsilon < 1$, then

$$0 < u_n < 1 \ \forall n$$

$$\Rightarrow \quad 0 < u_n^2 < u_n \ \forall n$$

$$[\because u_n < 1 \Rightarrow u_n^2 < u_n]$$

$$\Rightarrow \quad 0 < \Sigma u_n^2 < \Sigma u_n \ \forall n$$

Since Σu_n is convergent, hence by comparison test $\sum u_n^2$ is convergent.

Converse is not always true :

For example if $u_n = \frac{1}{n}$, then $u_n^2 = \frac{1}{n^2}$.

Clearly if $\sum u_n^2 = \sum \frac{1}{n^2}$ convergent but $\sum u_n = \sum \frac{1}{n}$ is divergent.

4. *If $\sum u_n^2$ and $\sum v_n^2$ are both convergent series, prove that the series $\Sigma u_n v_n$ also convergent.*

SOLUTION. Since $\sum u_n^2$ and $\sum v_n^2$ both are convergent, therefore $\Sigma(u_n^2 + v_n^2)$ is also convergent

$\Rightarrow \sum \frac{1}{2}(u_n^2 + v_n^2)$ is also convergent.

We know that G. M. < A. M.

$$\Rightarrow \sqrt{u_n^2 v_n^2} < \frac{1}{2}(u_n^2 + v_n^2)$$

$$\Rightarrow u_n v_n < \frac{1}{2}(u_n^2 + v_n^2)$$

Hence, by comparison test $\Sigma u_n v_n$ is convergent.

5. *Examine the following series for convergence :*

(i) $\sum \frac{1}{(\log n)^{\log n}}$

(ii) $\sum \frac{1}{(\log\log n)^{\log n}}$

SOLUTION. (i) Since we have $\lim_{n\to\infty} \log(\log n) = \infty$

$\Rightarrow$ There exists a large positive integer n such that $\log(\log n) > 2$

$$\Rightarrow [\log(\log n)] \log n > 2 \log n$$

$$\Rightarrow (\log n)[\log(\log n)] > \log n^2$$

$$\Rightarrow \log[(\log n)^{\log n}] > \log n^2$$

$$\Rightarrow (\log n)^{\log n} > n^2$$

$$\Rightarrow \frac{1}{(\log n)^{\log n}} < \frac{1}{n^2}$$

since $\sum \frac{1}{n^2}$ is convergent hence by comparison test $\Sigma \frac{1}{(\log n)^{\log n}}$ is also convergent.

(ii) Similarly, $\lim_{n\to\infty} \log(\log\log n) = \infty$

$\Rightarrow$there exists a positive integer n is so large such that $\log(\log\log n) > 2$

$$\Rightarrow \log n\,[\log(\log\log n)] > 2 \log n$$

$$\Rightarrow \log[\{\log(\log n)\}^{\log n}] > \log n^2$$

$$\Rightarrow [\log(\log n)]^{\log n} > n^2$$

$$\Rightarrow \frac{1}{[\log(\log n)]^{\log n}} < \frac{1}{n^2}$$

Since $\sum \frac{1}{n^2}$ is convergent, hence by comparison test $\sum \frac{1}{[\log(\log n)]^{\log n}}$ is convergent.

6. *Test the convergence of the series*

$$\frac{2}{1} + \frac{3}{4} + \frac{4}{9} + \ldots + \frac{n+1}{n^2} + \ldots$$

SOLUTION. Here $u_n = \frac{n+1}{n^2}$.

Take $v_n = \frac{n}{n^2} = \frac{1}{n}$

Then $\frac{u_n}{v_n} = \frac{\frac{n+1}{n^2}}{\frac{1}{n}} = \frac{n+1}{n^2} \cdot \frac{n}{1} = \frac{n+1}{n}$

Therefore

$$\lim_{n\to\infty} \frac{u_n}{v_n} = \lim_{n\to\infty} \frac{n+1}{n} = \lim_{n\to\infty}\left(1 + \frac{1}{n}\right)$$

= 1, which is finite and non-zero.

Thus, by the comparison test two series are either both convergent or both divergent. But the auxiliary series $\sum v_n = \frac{1}{n}$ is divergent, Hence, the given series Σu_n is also divergent.

7. *Test the convergence of the series*

$$\frac{1}{1\cdot 2} + \frac{1}{2\cdot 3} + \ldots + \frac{1}{n(n+1)} + \ldots$$

(VTU–2006)

SOLUTION. Here $u_n = \frac{1}{n(n+1)} = \frac{1}{n} - \frac{1}{n+1}$

If s_n is the partial sum of n terms of the series Σu_n, then

$$s_n = u_1 + u_2 + \ldots + \ldots + u_n$$

$$= \left(1 - \frac{1}{2}\right) + \left(\frac{1}{2} - \frac{1}{3}\right) + \ldots + \left(\frac{1}{n} - \frac{1}{n+1}\right)$$

$$= 1 - \frac{1}{n+1}$$

Now, $\lim_{n\to\infty} s_n = \lim_{n\to\infty}\left[1 - \frac{1}{n+1}\right] = 1,$

which is finite and non-zero.
Hence, the given series is convegent.

- This type of series is calld "Telescoping series".

8. *Show that the series* $1 + \frac{1}{2!} + \frac{1}{3!} + \ldots$ *is convergent.*

SOLUTION. Since,

$$\frac{1}{2!} = \frac{1}{2}$$
$$\frac{1}{3!} < \frac{1}{2^2}$$
$$\ldots \quad \ldots \quad \ldots$$
$$\ldots \quad \ldots \quad \ldots$$
$$\frac{1}{n!} < \frac{1}{2^{n-1}}$$

Therefore,

$$1 + \frac{1}{2!} + \frac{1}{3!} + \ldots + \frac{1}{n!} + \ldots < 1 + \frac{1}{2} + \frac{1}{2^2} + \ldots$$

The series on the right hand side is a geometric series with common ratio $\frac{1}{2}$ and hence convergent. So the series on the left hand side will also be convergent.

9. *Test the convergence or divergence of*

$$\frac{1}{1\cdot2\cdot3} + \frac{3}{2\cdot3\cdot4} + \frac{5}{3\cdot4\cdot5} + \ldots + \frac{2n-1}{n(n+1)(n+2)} + \ldots$$

(PTU–2009)

SOLUTION. Here, $u_n = \frac{2n-1}{n(n+1)(n+1)}$

Take $v_n = \frac{n}{n(n)(n)} = \frac{1}{n^2}$

Then,

$$\frac{u_n}{v_n} = \frac{2n-1}{n(n+1)(n+2)} \cdot \frac{n^2}{1} = \frac{\left(2 - \frac{1}{n}\right)}{\left(1 + \frac{1}{n}\right)\cdot\left(1 + \frac{2}{n}\right)}$$

$$\Rightarrow \lim_{n\to\infty} \frac{u_n}{v_n} = \lim_{n\to\infty} \frac{\left(2 - \frac{1}{n}\right)}{\left(1 + \frac{1}{n}\right)\left(1 + \frac{2}{n}\right)} = 2,$$

which is finite.

Now, the auxiliary series $\sum v_n = \sum \frac{1}{n^2}$ is convergent ($\because$ $p = 2 > 1$). Hence the given series is convergent.

10. *Test the convergence or divergence of the series* $1 + \frac{1}{2^2} + \frac{2^2}{3^3} + \frac{3^3}{4^4} + \ldots$

SOLUTION. Leaving the first term, we get

$$u_n = \frac{n^n}{(n+1)^{n+1}} = \frac{1}{n\left(1 + \frac{1}{n}\right)^{n+1}}$$

$$= \frac{1}{n}\left[1 + \frac{1}{n}\right]^{-[n+1]}$$

$$= \frac{1}{n}\left[1 - \frac{(n+1)}{n} + \ldots\right] = \frac{1}{n} - \left(1 + \frac{1}{n}\right)\frac{1}{n} + \ldots$$

Let $\sum v_n = \sum \frac{1}{n}$, where $v_n = \frac{1}{n}$ be the auxiliary series.

$$\text{Then } \lim_{n\to\infty} \frac{u_n}{v_n} = \lim_{n\to\infty} \frac{\frac{1}{n}\left[\frac{1}{(1+1/n)^{n+1}}\right]}{\frac{1}{n}}$$

$$= \lim_{n\to\infty}\left[\frac{\frac{1}{(1+1/n)^n}}{\left(1 + \frac{1}{n}\right)}\right]$$

$= \frac{1}{e}$, which is finite and non-zero.

Now, since $\sum v_n = \sum \frac{1}{n}$ is divergent, therefore by comparsion test the given series is also divergent.

11. *Test the convergence of the series whose general term is* $[n^3 + 1]^{1/3} - n]$.

(PTU–2007, ROHTAK–2003)

SOLUTION. Here, we have

$$u_n = (n^3 + 1)^{1/3} - n$$

$$= n\left[\left(1 + \frac{1}{n^3}\right)^{1/3} - 1\right]$$

$$= n\left[\left(1+\frac{1}{3n^3}+\frac{\frac{1}{3}\left(\frac{1}{3}-1\right)}{2!}\cdot\frac{1}{n^6}+\ldots\right)-1\right]$$

$$= \frac{1}{n^2}\left[\frac{1}{3}-\frac{1}{9n^3}+\ldots\right]$$

Let $v_n = \frac{1}{n^2}$, then the auxiliary series

$$\sum v_n = \sum \frac{1}{n^2}$$

Now, $\lim \frac{u_n}{v_n} = \frac{1}{3}-\frac{1}{9n^3}+\ldots = \frac{1}{3}$

which is finite and non-zero.

Since the series $\sum v_n = \sum \frac{1}{n^2}$ is convergent ($\because p = 2 > 1$), therefore, the given series is also convergent.

12. *Test the convergence of the series whose n^{th} term is $[\sqrt{(n^4+1)}-\sqrt{(n^4-1)}]$.*

SOLUTION. Here, we have,

$$u_n = \sqrt{(n^4+1)}-\sqrt{(n^4-1)}$$

$$= n^2\left[\left(1+\frac{1}{n^4}\right)^{1/2}-\left(1-\frac{1}{n^4}\right)^{1/2}\right]$$

$$= n^2\left[\left(1+\frac{1}{2n^4}+\frac{\frac{1}{2}\left(\frac{1}{2}-1\right)}{2!}\cdot\frac{1}{n^8}+\frac{\frac{1}{2}\left(\frac{1}{2}-1\right)\left(\frac{1}{2}-2\right)}{3!}\cdot\frac{1}{n^{12}}+\ldots\right)-\left(1-\frac{1}{2n^4}+\frac{\frac{1}{2}\left(\frac{1}{2}-1\right)}{2!}\cdot\frac{1}{n^8}-\frac{\frac{1}{2}\left(\frac{1}{2}-1\right)\left(\frac{1}{2}-2\right)}{3!}\cdot\frac{1}{n^{12}}+\ldots\right)\right]$$

$$= n^2\left[\frac{1}{n^4}+\frac{1}{8n^{12}}+\ldots\right]$$

$$= \frac{1}{n^2}+\frac{1}{8n^{10}}+\ldots$$

Let $v_n = \frac{1}{n^2}$, then the auxillary series is $\sum v_n = \sum \frac{1}{n^2}$, which is convergent.

Now $\lim_{n\to\infty}\frac{u_n}{v_n} = \lim_{n\to\infty}\left[\frac{1}{n^2}+\frac{1}{8n^{10}}+\ldots\right]\Big/\frac{1}{n^2}$

$$= \lim_{n\to\infty}\left[1+\frac{1}{8n^8}+\ldots\right]$$

= 1, which is finite and non-zero.

Therefore, by comparsion test the given series is also convergent.

13. *Test the convergence of the series $\sum \sin\frac{1}{n}$.*

SOLUTION. Here, we have $u_n = \sin\frac{1}{n}$

Let $v_n = \frac{1}{n}$, therefore, the auxiliary series $\sum v_n = \sum \frac{1}{n}$ is divergent.

Now $\lim_{n\to\infty}\frac{u_n}{v_n} = \lim_{n\to\infty}\frac{\sin 1/n}{1/n} = 1$,

which is finite and non-zero.

Therefore, by comparison test the given series is also divergent.

Similar Problems

(1) Test the convergence of the series $\frac{1}{a\cdot 1^2+b}+\frac{2}{a\cdot 2^2+b}+\frac{3}{a\cdot 3^2+b}+\ldots$ **Ans.** Divergent

(2) Test the convergence or divergence of the series $\sum_{n=1}^{\infty}\frac{1}{x^n+x^{-n}}, x > 0$.

Ans. $x > 1$ Convergent, $x < 1$ Convergent, $x = 1$ Divergent

14. *Test the convergence of the series whose n^{th} term is $\sqrt{n^3+1}-\sqrt{n^3}$.*

SOLUTION. Here, we have

$$u_n = \sqrt{n^3+1}-\sqrt{n^3}$$

$$= n^{3/2}\left[1+\frac{1}{n^3}\right]^{1/2} - n^{3/2}$$

$$= n^{3/2}\left[1+\frac{1}{2n^3}+\frac{1}{8n^6}+\ldots\right]-n^{3/2}$$

$$= \frac{1}{2n^{3/2}}-\frac{1}{8n^{9/2}}+\ldots$$

Let us take $v_n = \frac{1}{n^{3/2}}$ ($\because$ when u_n is in the form of the series in powers of $1/n$, v_n is taken as the term of lowest power of $1/n$, by ignoring the numerical factor).

Then we have

$$\lim_{n\to\infty}\frac{u_n}{v_n} = \lim_{n\to\infty}\left[\frac{1}{2n^{3/2}}-\frac{1}{8n^{9/2}}+\ldots\right]\times\frac{n^{3/2}}{1}$$

$$= \lim_{n\to\infty}\left[\frac{1}{2}-\frac{1}{8n^3}+\ldots\right]$$

$$= \frac{1}{2}, \text{ which is finite and non-zero.}$$

But the auxillary series $\sum v_n = \sum \frac{1}{n^{3/2}}$ is convergent ($p = 3/2 > 1$). Hence, the given series is also convergent.

Exercise-22.1

Check the convergence of the following series:

1. $\sum u_n = 1+\frac{1}{3}+\frac{1}{5}+\frac{1}{7}+\ldots$
2. $\sum u_n = 1+\frac{1}{\sqrt{2}}+\frac{1}{\sqrt{3}}+\frac{1}{\sqrt{4}}+\ldots$
3. $\sum u_n = 1+\frac{4}{5}+\frac{6}{10}+\frac{8}{17}+\ldots+\frac{2n}{n^2+1}\ldots$
4. $\sum u_n = \sqrt{\frac{1}{2^3}}+\sqrt{\frac{2}{3^3}}+\sqrt{\frac{3}{4^3}}+\ldots$
5. $\sum u_n = \frac{1}{2}+\frac{\sqrt{2}}{5}+\frac{\sqrt{3}}{10}+\ldots\frac{\sqrt{n}}{n^2+1}+\ldots$
6. $\sum u_n = \frac{\sqrt{1}}{1+\sqrt{1}}+\frac{\sqrt{2}}{2+\sqrt{2}}+\frac{\sqrt{3}}{3+\sqrt{3}}+\ldots.$
7. $\sum u_n = \frac{1}{a+b}+\frac{1}{a+2b}+\frac{1}{a+3b}+\ldots+\frac{1}{a+nb}+\ldots$
8. $\sum u_n = \frac{1}{a(a+b)}+\frac{1}{(a+2b)(a+3b)}+\frac{1}{(a+4b)(a+5b)}+\ldots$
9. $\sum u_n = \sum\frac{n}{n^2+\sqrt{n}}$
10. $\sum u_n = \sum\frac{n}{(a+nb)^2}$
11. $\sum u_n = \sum\frac{\sqrt{n+1}+\sqrt{n-1}}{n}$
12. $\sum u_n = \sum\frac{1}{n}\sin\frac{1}{n}$
13. $\sum u_n = \sum\tan^{-1}\frac{1}{n}$
14. $\sum u_n = \sum\frac{n^p}{(n+1)^q}$
15. $\sum u_n = \sum\frac{n^2-1}{n^2+1}$
16. $\sum u_n = \sum\frac{1}{n}\sqrt{n^2+n+1}-\sqrt{n^2-n+1}$
17. $\frac{1}{4.7.10}+\frac{4}{7.10.13}+\frac{9}{10.13.16}+\ldots+\infty$
18. $\sum_{n=1}^{\infty}\frac{1}{\sqrt{n}+\sqrt{(n+1)}}$
19. $\sum_{n=1}^{\infty}\sqrt{\frac{3^n-1}{2^n+1}}$
20. $1-\frac{1}{3}+\frac{1}{3^2}-\frac{1}{3^3}+\frac{1}{3^4}-\ldots\infty$
21. $\frac{1}{1.2}+\frac{2}{3.4}+\frac{3}{5.6}+\ldots\infty$ (COCHIN–2001)
22. $\frac{1}{1.3}+\frac{2}{3.5}+\frac{3}{5.7}+\ldots\infty$ (PTU–2009)
23. $\sum_{n=1}^{\infty}[\sqrt{(n^2+1)}-n]$
24. $\frac{1}{1.3.5}+\frac{2}{3.5.7}+\frac{3}{5.7.9}+\ldots\infty$
25. $\sum\frac{\sqrt{n}}{n^2+1}$ (OSMANIA–2000S)
26. $\sum\frac{(n+1)(n+2)}{n^2\sqrt{n}}$
27. $\sum_{n=1}^{\infty}\frac{\sqrt{(n+1)}-1}{(n+2)^3-1}$

Hints to the Selected Problems

1. $\Sigma u_n = \sum_{n=1}^{\infty}\left(\frac{1}{2n-1}\right) \Rightarrow \lim_{n\to\infty} u_n = \lim_{n\to\infty}\left(\frac{1}{2n-1}\right) = 0$

Now apply comparison test .

4. $u_n = \frac{\sqrt{n}}{(n+1)\sqrt{n+1}}$

Then $\lim_{n\to\infty}\frac{u_n}{v_n} = \lim_{n\to\infty}\sqrt{\frac{1}{1+\frac{1}{n}}}\cdot\frac{1}{\left(1+\frac{1}{n}\right)} = n \neq 0$

7. $u_n = \frac{1}{a+nb}$ Let $v_n = \frac{1}{n}$.

Then $\lim_{n\to\infty}\frac{u_n}{v_n} = \lim_{n\to\infty}\frac{n}{a+nb} = \frac{1}{b} \neq 0.$

8. Here, we have $u_n = \frac{1}{[a+(2n-2)b][a+(2n-1)b]}$

Let $v_n = \frac{1}{n^2}$

Then $\lim_{n\to\infty}\frac{u_n}{v_n} = \frac{1}{4b^2} \neq 0$

12. $u_n = \frac{1}{n}\sin\frac{1}{n} = \frac{1}{n}\left[\frac{1}{n} - \frac{1}{6n^3} + \frac{1}{120n^5} - ....\right]$

Let $v_n = \frac{1}{n^2}$. Then $\lim_{n\to\infty}\frac{u_n}{v_n} = 1 \neq 0$

14. Here we have $u_n = \frac{n^p}{(n+1)^q}$

Let $v_n = \frac{1}{n^{q-p}}$

Then $\lim_{n\to\infty}\frac{v_n}{u_n} = \lim_{n\to\infty} n^{q-p}\left[\frac{n^p}{(n+1)^q}\right]$

$= \lim_{n\to\infty}\frac{1}{\left(1+\frac{1}{n}\right)^q} = 1 \neq 0$

15. $\lim_{n\to\infty} u_n = \lim_{n\to\infty}\frac{\left(1-\frac{1}{n^2}\right)}{\left(1+\frac{1}{n^2}\right)} = 1 \neq 0$

ANSWERS

1. Divergent **2.** Divergent **3.** Divergent **4.** Divergent
5. Convergent **6.** Divergent **7.** Divergent **8.** Convergent
9. Divergent **10.** Divergent **11.** Divergent **12.** Convergent
13. Divergent **14.** Convergent if $p - q + 1 < 0$ and divergent if $p - q + 1 \geq 0$
15. Divergent **16.** Divergent **17.** Divergent **18.** Divergent
19. Divergent **20.** Convergent **21.** Divergent **22.** Divergent
23. Divergent **24.** Convergent **25.** Convergent **26.** Divergent
27. Convergent

22.7 CAUCHY'S ROOT TEST

Let Σu_n be a series of positive terms and let $\lim_{n\to\infty} u_n^{1/n} = l.$
If,

(i) $l < 1$, *then* Σu_n *converges;* (ii) $l > 1$, *then* Σu_n *diverges;*

(iii) $l = 1$, *then the test fails and the series may either converge or diverge.*

Proof. Case (I). Let $u_n^{1/n} = l < 1$.

Since $l < 1$, we can choose an $\varepsilon > 0$ such that $l + \varepsilon < 1$.

Let $l + \varepsilon = r$ such that $0 < r < 1$.

Since $\lim_{n\to\infty} u_n^{1/n} = l$, therefore there exists a positive integer m_1 such that.

$$|u_n^{1/n} - l| < \varepsilon, \forall\, n > m_1 \quad \Rightarrow \quad l - \varepsilon < u_n^{1/n} < l + \varepsilon \;\forall\, n > m_1$$

$$\Rightarrow \quad (l-\varepsilon)^n < u_n < (l+\varepsilon)^n \;\forall\, n > m_1$$

Since $u_n < r^n\; \forall\, n > m_1$ and since Σr^n converges (being a geometric series with common ratio less than one). Then by comparison test Σu_n converges.

Case (II). Let $u_n^{1/n} = l > 1$.

Since $l > 1$, we can choose an $\varepsilon > 0$ such that $l - \varepsilon > 1$.

Let $\quad l - \varepsilon = R \quad$ then $\quad R > 1$.

Since $R^n < u_n \; \forall \; n > m_2$ and since ΣR^n diverges (being a G.P. with common ratio greater than one). Then by comparison test Σu_n diverges.

Case (III). Let $\quad u_n = \dfrac{1}{n} \quad$ then $\quad \lim\limits_{n\to\infty} u_n^{1/n} = 1.$

Since $\sum\left(\dfrac{1}{n}\right)$ diverges, therefore we find that if $\lim\limits_{n\to\infty} u_n^{1/n} = 1$, then the series Σu_n may diverge.

Again, let $u_n = \dfrac{1}{n^2}$. In this case also $\lim\limits_{n\to\infty} u_n^{1/n} = 1$ but the series Σu_n converges. Thus we find that if $\lim\limits_{n\to\infty} u_n^{1/n} = 1$, then the series Σu_n may converge. The above two examples show that if

$$\lim_{n\to\infty} (u_n)^{1/n} = 1$$

Then the test fail.

- Cauchy's root test can be applied with advantage to series in which the nth term happens to be an exponential fraction of n.
- In this test, it is understood that $u_n^{1/n}$ stands for the positive n^{th} root of u_n.
- The Cauchy's root test can also be stated as follows :
- "A series Σu_n of positive terms is convergent if for every value of $n \geq m$, m being finite, $(u_n)^{1/n}$ less than a fixed number, which is less than unity, and the series is divergent if $(u_n)^{1/n} \geq 1$ for every value of $n \geq m$."

22.8 D'ALEMBERT RATIO TEST

Let Σu_n be a series of positive terms and let

(a) $\lim\limits_{n\to\infty} \dfrac{u_n}{u_{n+1}} = l$

Then if,

(i) $l > 1$, *the series converges,* (ii) $l < 1$, *the series diverges*

(iii) $l = 1$, *the series may converge or diverge and therefore the test fails.*

(b) $\dfrac{u_n}{u_{n+1}} = \infty$ *as $n \to \infty$. Then Σu_n converges.*

Proof. (a) Case(I). When $l > 1$, Let $\varepsilon > 0$ be a positive number such that $l - \varepsilon > 1$.

Now since $\lim\limits_{n\to\infty} \dfrac{u_n}{u_{n+1}} = l$, therefore $\exists$ a positive integer m such that $l - \varepsilon < \dfrac{u_n}{u_{n+1}} < l + \varepsilon$, whenever $n > m$

Now, putting $n = m + 1, m + 2, \ldots p - 1$, in succession in the above inequality, we get

$$l - \varepsilon < \frac{u_{m+1}}{u_{m+2}} < l + \varepsilon$$

$$l - \varepsilon < \frac{u_{m+2}}{u_{m+3}} < l + \varepsilon$$

$$\ldots \quad \ldots. \quad \ldots \quad \ldots.$$

$$l - \varepsilon < \frac{u_{p-1}}{u_p} < l + \varepsilon$$

Multiplying the corresponding sides of the first part of the above inequalities, we get

$$(l-\varepsilon)^{p-1-m} < \frac{u_{m+1}}{u_{m+2}} \cdot \frac{u_{m+2}}{u_{m+3}} \cdots \frac{u_{p-1}}{u_p}$$

$$\Rightarrow \quad (l-\varepsilon)^{p-1-m} < \frac{u_{m+1}}{u_p}$$

$$\Rightarrow \quad u_p < u_{m+1}(l-\varepsilon)^{m+1} \cdot (l-\varepsilon)^{-p}$$

$$\Rightarrow \quad u_p < k(l-\varepsilon)^{-p}, \forall p \geq m+2 \text{ and } k = u_{m+1}(l-\varepsilon)^{m+1}$$

Since, the series $\Sigma(l-\varepsilon)^{-P}$ converges (being a geometric series with common ratio $(l-\varepsilon)^{-1}$, which is certainly less than unity), then by comparison test it follows that Σu_n converges,

Case (II). When $l < 1$, let $\varepsilon > 0$ be a positive number such that $l + \varepsilon < 1$.

Now since $\lim_{n\to\infty} \frac{u_n}{u_{n+1}} = l$, therefore, $\exists$ a positive intger m such that $l - \varepsilon < \frac{u_n}{u_{n+1}} < l + \varepsilon, \forall n > m$

Putting $n = m+1, m+2, \ldots, p-1$ in succession in the second part of the above inequality, we get

$$\frac{u_{m+1}}{u_{m+2}} < l+\varepsilon, \frac{u_{m+2}}{u_{m+3}} < l+\varepsilon, \ldots \ldots \ldots \frac{u_{p-1}}{u_p} < l+\varepsilon.$$

Multiplying the corresponding sides of the above inequalities, we have

$$\frac{u_{m+1}}{u_p} < (l+\varepsilon)^{p-1-m} \quad \Rightarrow \quad u_p > u_{m+1}(l+\varepsilon)^{m+1}(l+\varepsilon)^{-p}$$

$$\Rightarrow \quad u_p > A(l+\in)^{-p} \; \forall p \geq m+2 \text{ and } A = u_{m+1}(l+\varepsilon)^{m+1}$$

Since, $\Sigma(l+\varepsilon)^{-p}$ is a divergent series (being a geometric series with common ratio $(l+\varepsilon)^{-1}$, which is certainly greater than unity), then by comparison test, it follows that Σu_n diverges.

Case (III). Let $l = 1$.

Now, first consider the harmonic series $1 + \frac{1}{2} + \frac{1}{3} + \frac{1}{5} + \ldots + \frac{1}{n} + \ldots$

Then $$\frac{u_n}{u_{n+1}} = \frac{n+1}{n} = 1 + \frac{1}{n} \Rightarrow \lim_{n\to\infty} \frac{u_n}{u_{n+1}} = 1$$

Since, the harmonic series is divergent, we find that if $l = 1$, a series may diverge.

Now, consider the series $\frac{1}{1^2} + \frac{1}{2^2} + \ldots + \frac{1}{n^2} + \ldots$

Then $$\frac{u_n}{u_{n+1}} = \frac{(n+1)^2}{n^2} = \left(1 + \frac{1}{n}\right)^2 \Rightarrow \lim_{n\to\infty} \frac{u_n}{u_{n+1}} = 1$$

since, the series $\sum \frac{1}{n^2}$ converges, we find that if $l = 1$, a series may converge.

(b) Let us suppose $\lim_{n\to\infty} \frac{u_n}{u_{n+1}} = +\infty$ then there exists positive integers m and p such

$$\frac{u_n}{u_{n+1}} > p \; \forall n \geq m, p > 1$$

Replacing n by $m, m+1, m+2, \ldots, n-1$, we have

$$\frac{u_m}{u_{m+1}} > p, \frac{u_{m+1}}{u_{m+2}} > p \; \ldots \; \ldots \ldots \; \frac{u_{n-1}}{u_n} > p.$$

Multiplying the corresponding sides of the above inequalities, we have

$$\frac{u_m}{u_n} > p^{n-m} \quad \Rightarrow \quad u_n < p^{m-n} \cdot u_m,$$

$$\Rightarrow \quad u_n < A.p^{-n} \forall n \geq m \quad \text{and} \quad A = p^m u_m.$$

Since Σp^{-n} is convergent, then by comparison test, the series Σu_n is convergent.

- The ratio test is generally applied when the nth term of the series involves factorials, products of several factors, or combination of powers and factorials.
- The ratio test can also be stated as follows:
  "An inifinite series of positive terms is convergent if from and after some terms the ratio of each term to the preceding term is less than a fixed number which is less than unity and series is divergent if the ratio, defined above is greater than or equal to unity."
- The ratio test is easier to apply than the root test. However, the root test is stronger than the ratio test.
- The ratio test does not tell us anything about the convergence of the series Σu_n if we only have
  $$\frac{u_n}{u_{n+1}} > 1 \forall n.$$

Solved Examples

1. *Test the series for convergence of the series* $1+\frac{1}{2^2}+\frac{1}{3^3}+\frac{1}{4^4}+\ldots$

SOLUTION. Here, we have $u_n = \frac{1}{n^n}$

$$\Rightarrow \lim_{n\to\infty} (u_n)^{1/n} = \lim_{n\to\infty} \frac{1}{n} = 0 < 1$$

Hence by Cauchy's root test the given series is convergent.

2. *Test the convergence of the series*

$$\Sigma\left(1+\frac{1}{n}\right)^{-n^2}.$$

SOLUTION. Here we have

$$u_n = \left(1+\frac{1}{n}\right)^{-n^2} \Rightarrow (u_n)^{1/n} = \left(1+\frac{1}{n}\right)^{-n}$$

$$\Rightarrow \lim_{n\to\infty} (u_n)^{1/n} = \lim_{n\to\infty}\left(1+\frac{1}{n}\right)^{-n} = \frac{1}{e} < 1.$$

Hence, by Cauchy's root test the given series Σu_n is convergent.

3. *Examine the convergene of the following series :*

(i) $\Sigma\left(1+\frac{1}{\sqrt{n}}\right)^{-n^{3/2}}$ (PTU–2009, KURUKSHETRA–2005)

(ii) $\Sigma \frac{(n-\log n)^n}{2^n . n^n}$

(iii) $\sum_{n=2}^{\infty} \frac{1}{(\log n)^n}$ (PTU–2005)

SOLUTION. (i) We have $u_n = \left(1+\frac{1}{\sqrt{n}}\right)^{-n^{3/2}}$

$$\therefore \lim_{n\to\infty} u_n^{1/n} = \lim_{n\to\infty}\left(1+\frac{1}{\sqrt{n}}\right)^{-\sqrt{n}}$$

$$= \lim_{n\to\infty}\left[\left(1+\frac{1}{\sqrt{n}}\right)^{\sqrt{n}}\right]^{-1}$$

$$= e^{-1} = \frac{1}{e} < 1$$

Hence, the given series is convergent.

(ii) We have $u_n = \frac{(n-\log n)^n}{2^n . n^n}$

$$\therefore u_n^{1/n} = \frac{n-\log n}{2n} = \frac{1}{2}\left(1-\frac{\log n}{n}\right)$$

$$\therefore \lim_{n\to\infty} u_n^{1/n} = \lim_{n\to\infty}\frac{1}{2}\left(1-\frac{\log n}{n}\right)$$

$$= \frac{1}{2}(1-0) = \frac{1}{2} < 1$$

$$\left[\because \lim_{n\to\infty}\frac{\log n}{n} = 0\right]$$

Hence, by Cauchy's root test the given series is convergent.

(iii) We have $u_n = \dfrac{1}{(\log n)^n}$

$\therefore \quad u_n^{1/n} = \dfrac{1}{(\log n)}$

$\therefore \lim_{n\to\infty} u_n^{1/n} = \lim_{n\to\infty} \dfrac{1}{(\log n)} = 0 < 1$

Hence, by Cauchy's root test the given series is convergent.

4. *Test the convergence of the series*

$$\left(\frac{2^2}{1^2}-\frac{2}{1}\right)^{-1}+\left(\frac{3^3}{2^3}-\frac{3}{2}\right)^{-2}+\left(\frac{4^4}{3^4}-\frac{4}{3}\right)^{-3}+\ldots$$

(VTU–2006)

SOLUTION. Here we have $u_n = \left[\dfrac{(n+1)^{n+1}}{n^{n+1}} - \dfrac{(n+1)}{n}\right]^{-n}$

Therefore
$$\lim_{n\to\infty} u_n^{1/n} = \lim_{n\to\infty}\left[\frac{(n+1)^{n+1}}{n^{n+1}}-\frac{n+1}{n}\right]^{-1}$$

$$= \lim_{n\to\infty}\left[\left(1+\frac{1}{n}\right)^{n+1}-\left(1+\frac{1}{n}\right)\right]^{-1}$$

$$= \lim_{n\to\infty}\left(1+\frac{1}{n}\right)^{-1}\left[\left(1+\frac{1}{n}\right)^{n}-1\right]^{-1}$$

$$= (1+0)^{-1}[e-1)^{-1} = \frac{1}{e-1} < 1.$$

Hence, by Cauchy's root test the given series is convergent.

5. *Test the convergence of the series* $x + 2x^2 + 3x^3 + 4x^4 + \ldots$

SOLUTION. Here, we have $u_n = nx^n$

$\Rightarrow \quad (u_n)^{1/n} = n^{1/n} . x$

$\Rightarrow \lim_{n\to\infty} (u_n)^{1/n} = \lim_{n\to\infty} (x.n^{1/n}) = x.1 = x$

$\left[\because \lim_{n\to\infty} n^{1/n} = 1\right]$

Then, by Cauchy's root test, Σu_n is convergent if $x < 1$ and is divergent if $x > 1$. For $x = 1$, the Cauchy's root test fails.

In this case, the given series becomes

$1 + 2 + 3 + \ldots$

s_n = sum of n terms of the series = $\frac{1}{2} n(n+1)$, which is finite.

Thus the given series is convergent if $x < 1$ and is divergent if $x \geq 1$.

6. *Test the convergence of the series*

$$\frac{1}{2}+\left(\frac{2}{3}\right)x+\left(\frac{3}{4}\right)^2 x^2+\left(\frac{4}{5}\right)^3 x^3+\ldots\infty, x>0$$

(JNTU–2006)

SOLUTION. Omitting the first term of the series (because it will not effect the convergence or divergence of the series),

we have $u_n = \left(\dfrac{n+1}{n+2}\right)^n \cdot x^n$

Therefore
$$\lim_{n\to\infty} u_n^{1/n} = \lim_{n\to\infty}\left[\frac{\left(1+\frac{1}{n}\right)x}{1+\left(\frac{2}{n}\right)}\right].$$

$$= x$$

Therefore by Cauchy's root test, the given series Σu_n converges if $x < 1$, divegent if $x > 1$.

For $x = 1$, test fails

$$\therefore \lim_{n\to\infty} u_n = \lim_{n\to\infty}\frac{\left(1+\frac{1}{n}\right)^n}{\left(1+\frac{2}{n}\right)^n} = \frac{e}{e^2} = \frac{1}{e} > 0.$$

$\therefore$ The series Σu_n diverges if $x = 1$.

Hence, the given series is convergent if $x < 1$ and divergent if $x \geq 1$.

7. *Test the convergence of the series*

$$\Sigma\left[\frac{\log n}{\log(n+1)}\right]^{n^2 \log n}.$$

SOLUTION. Here we have

$$u_n = \left[\frac{\log n}{\log(n+1)}\right]^{n^2 \log n}$$

$$\Rightarrow u_n^{1/n} = \left[\frac{\log n}{\log(n+1)}\right]^{n \log n}$$

$$= \left[\frac{\log n\left(1+\frac{1}{n}\right)}{\log n}\right]^{-n\log n}$$

$$= \left[\frac{\log n + \log\left(1+\frac{1}{n}\right)}{\log n}\right]^{-n\log n}$$

$$= \left[\frac{\log n + \frac{1}{n} - \frac{1}{2n^2} + \ldots}{\log n}\right]^{-n\log n}$$

$$= \left[1 + \frac{1}{n\log n} - \frac{1}{2n^2\log n} + \ldots\right]^{-n\log n} = k \text{ (say)}$$

Then

$$\log k = \log\left[1 + \frac{1}{n\log n} - \frac{1}{2n^2\log n} + \ldots\right]^{-n\log n}$$

$$= (-n\log n)\log\left[\left(1 + \frac{1}{n\log n} - \frac{1}{2n^2\log n} + \ldots\right)\ldots\right]$$

$$= -n\log n\left[\left(\frac{1}{n\log n} - \frac{1}{2n^2\log n} + \ldots\right)\ldots\right]$$

$$= -1 + \frac{1}{2n} - \ldots$$

$$\Rightarrow \lim_{n\to\infty} \log k = -1$$

$$\Rightarrow \lim_{n\to\infty} k = e^{-1}$$

$$\Rightarrow \lim_{n\to\infty} u_n^{1/n} = \frac{1}{e} < 1. \quad [\because 2 < e < 3]$$

Then, by Cauchy's root test the given series is convergent.

8. *Test the convergence of* $\sum\left(\frac{n+1}{n+2}\right)^n x^n, (x > 0)$.

SOLUTION. The nth term of the given series is

$$u_n = \left(\frac{n+1}{n+2}\right)^n x^n$$

Then we have

$$u_n^{1/n} = \left(\frac{n+1}{n+2}\right)x = \left(\frac{1+1/n}{1+2/n}\right)x$$

$$\therefore \lim_{n\to\infty} u_n^{1/n} = \lim_{n\to\infty}\left(\frac{1+\frac{1}{n}}{1+\frac{2}{n}}\right)x = x$$

Now we have the followings cases.

Case I : If $x < 1$ then by Cauhy's root test Σu_n is convergent.

Case II : If $x > 1$ then by Cauchy's root test Σu_n is divergent.

Case III : If $x = 1$, the test fails.

Now, when $x = 1$, we have

$$u_n = \left(\frac{n+1}{n+2}\right)^n = \left(\frac{1+\frac{1}{n}}{1+\frac{2}{n}}\right)^n$$

$$\Rightarrow \lim_{n\to\infty} u_n = \lim_{n\to\infty}\frac{(1+1/n)^n}{(1+2/n)^n} = \frac{e}{e^2} = \frac{1}{e} \neq 0$$

$\Rightarrow \Sigma u_n$ is divergent.

Hence, the given series is convergent if $x < 1$ and divergent if $x \geq 1$.

9. *Test for convergence the series*

$$1 + \frac{2^p}{2!} + \frac{3^p}{3!} + \frac{4^p}{4!} + \ldots$$

(KURUKSHETRA–2005)

SOLUTION. Here, we have

$$u_n = \frac{n^p}{n!} \Rightarrow u_{n+1} = \frac{(n+1)^p}{(n+1)!}$$

$$\text{Now } \lim_{n\to\infty}\frac{u_{n+1}}{u_n} = \lim_{n\to\infty}\frac{(n+1)^p}{(n+1)!}\frac{n!}{n^p}$$

$$= \lim_{n\to\infty}\left[1+\frac{1}{n}\right]^p \cdot \frac{1}{(n+1)}$$

$$= 0 < 1$$

Hence, by ratio test, the given series is convergent.

10. *Test the series* $x + \frac{x^3}{3!} + \frac{x^5}{5!} + \frac{x^7}{7!} + \ldots$ *for convergence, for all positive value of x.*

SOLUTION. Since x is positive. Hence the given series is of positive term series.

$$\text{Here } u_n = \frac{x^{2n-1}}{(2n-1)!}, u_{n+1} = \frac{x^{2n+1}}{(2n+1)!}$$

$$\Rightarrow \lim_{n\to\infty}\frac{u_n}{u_{n+1}} = \lim_{n\to\infty}\frac{x^{2n-1}}{(2n-1)!}\frac{(2n+1)!}{x^{2n+1}}$$

$$= \lim_{n\to\infty}\frac{2n(2n+1)}{x^2}$$

$$= +\infty, \forall \text{ positive value of } x.$$

Then, by ratio test the given series converges for all positive value of x.

11. *Test for convergence the series*

$$1 + \frac{x}{2^2} + \frac{x^2}{3^2} + \frac{x^3}{4^2} + \ldots$$

SOLUTION. Here we have

$$u_n = \frac{x^{n-1}}{n^2}$$

$$\Rightarrow \quad u_{n+1} = \frac{x^n}{(n+1)^2}$$

Now $\frac{u_n}{u_{n+1}} = \frac{x^{n-1}(n+1)^2}{n^2.x^n} = \frac{1}{x}\cdot\left(1+\frac{1}{n}\right)^2$

$$\Rightarrow \lim_{n\to\infty}\frac{u_n}{u_{n+1}} = \lim_{n\to\infty}\frac{1}{x}\left(1+\frac{1}{n}\right)^2 = \frac{1}{x}.$$

Hence, by ratio test the series converges if $\frac{1}{x} > 1$ *i.e.*, $x < 1$, diverges if $x > 1$ and the test fails if $x = 1$.

For $x = 1$, $u_n = \frac{1}{n^2}$. Therefore in this case the series $\Sigma u_n = \Sigma\frac{1}{n^2}$ is convergent.

12. *Test for convergence of the series*

$$\frac{1}{2\sqrt{1}} + \frac{x^2}{3\sqrt{2}} + \frac{x^4}{4\sqrt{3}} + \ldots$$

SOLUTION. $u_n = \frac{x^{2n-2}}{(n+1)\sqrt{n}}, u_{n+1} = \frac{x^{2n}}{(n+2)\sqrt{(n+1)}}$

$$\Rightarrow \frac{u_n}{u_{n+1}} = \frac{x^{2n-2}}{(n+1)\sqrt{n}}\cdot\frac{(n+2)\sqrt{(n+1)}}{x^{2n}}$$

$$= \frac{(1+2/n)}{(1+1/n)}\sqrt{\left(1+\frac{1}{n}\right)}\cdot\frac{1}{x^2}$$

$$\Rightarrow \lim_{n\to\infty}\frac{u_n}{u_{n+1}} = \frac{1}{1}.\sqrt{1}.\frac{1}{x^2} = \frac{1}{x^2}$$

Therefore, by ratio test the given series Σu_n is

(i) convergent if $\frac{1}{x^2} > 1$ *i.e.*, if $x^2 < 1$.

(ii) divergent if $\frac{1}{x^2} < 1$ *i.e.*, if $x^2 > 1$.

and (iii) The test fails if $x^2 = 1$

When $x^2 = 1$, we have $u_n = \frac{1}{(n+1)\sqrt{n}}$

Take $v_n = \frac{1}{n\sqrt{n}}$. Then $\lim_{n\to\infty}\frac{u_n}{v_n} = 1.$ which is finite and non-zero. Hence, by comparison test Σu_n and Σv_n are either both convergent or both divergent.

Since $\Sigma v_n = \Sigma\frac{1}{n^{3/2}}$ is convergent as $p = 3/2 > 1$.

Hence, the given series Σu_n is also convergent if $x^2 = 1$.

Similar Problems

(1) Test for convergence the series $x + \frac{3}{5}x^2 + \frac{8}{10}x^3 + \frac{15}{17}x^4 + \ldots + \frac{n^2-1}{n^2+1}x^n + \ldots.$

Ans. convergent if $x < 1$ and divergent if $x \geq 1$.

(2) Test the convergence of the series $\sum_{n=1}^{\infty}\frac{1\cdot3\cdot5\ldots.\cdot(2n-1)}{2\cdot4\cdot6\ldots.\cdot(2n)}(1-x^2)^n,\quad 0 \leq x^2 < 1$

Ans. Convergent.

13. *Test the following series for convergence*

$$\frac{x^2}{2\sqrt{1}} + \frac{x^3}{3\sqrt{2}} + \frac{x^4}{4\sqrt{3}} + \ldots.$$

SOLUTION. The nth term of the given series is

$$u_n = \frac{x^{n+1}}{(n+1)\sqrt{n}}$$

$$\Rightarrow \quad u_{n+1} = \frac{x^{n+2}}{(n+2)\sqrt{n+1}}$$

$$\therefore \quad \frac{u_n}{u_{n+1}} = \frac{n+2}{n+1}.\sqrt{\frac{n+1}{n}}.\frac{1}{x}$$

$$= \left(\frac{1+\frac{2}{n}}{1+\frac{1}{n}}\right).\sqrt{1+\frac{1}{n}}.\frac{1}{x}$$

$$\therefore \lim_{n\to\infty}\frac{u_n}{u_{n+1}} = \lim_{n\to\infty}\left(\frac{1+\frac{2}{n}}{1+\frac{1}{n}}\right).\sqrt{1+\frac{1}{n}}.\frac{1}{x}$$

$$= \frac{1}{x}$$

Therefore, by D'Alembert ratio test the given series is convergent if $x < 1$ and is divergent if $x > 1$.

When $x = 1$, we have

$$u_n = \frac{1}{(n+1)\sqrt{n}}$$

Then $v_n = \frac{1}{n\sqrt{n}}$

$$\therefore \lim_{n\to\infty} \frac{u_n}{v_n} = \lim_{n\to\infty} \frac{n\sqrt{n}}{(n+1)\sqrt{n}} = \lim_{n\to\infty} \frac{1}{\left(1+\frac{1}{n}\right)} = \frac{1}{1+0} = 1 \neq 0$$

$\Rightarrow$ By comparison test, $\Sigma v_n = \Sigma \frac{1}{n^{3/2}}$ is convergent, then Σu_n is convergent. Hence, the given series is convergent if $x \le 1$ and is divergent if $x > 1$.

Exercise-22.2

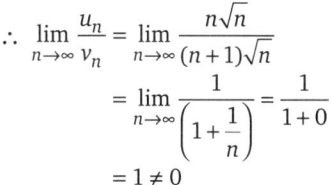

Based on Cauchy's Root Test :

1. Test the convergence of the following series :

(i) $\sum_{n=1}^{\infty}\left(1+\frac{2}{n}\right)^{-n^2}$ (ii) $\sum_{n=1}^{\infty}\frac{n^{n^2}}{(n+1)^{n^2}}$

(iii) $\sum_{n=1}^{\infty} 2^{-n-(-1)^n}$ (iv) $\sum_{n=1}^{\infty} 5^{-n-(-1)^n}$

(v) $\sum_{n=1}^{\infty}(n^{1/n}+x)$ for all positive values of x

(vi) $\sum_{n=1}^{\infty}\frac{n^3}{3^n}$ (vii) $\sum_{n=1}^{\infty}\frac{x^n}{n^n},\ x>0$

2. Test the convergence of the following series :

(i) $\sum\left(\frac{n}{n+1}\right)^{n^2}$ (ii) $\sum n^n x^n,\ x>0$

(iii) $\sum\left(\frac{n+1}{3n}\right)^n$ (iv) $\sum\left(\frac{nx}{n+1}\right)^n$

(v) $\sum\frac{(1+nx)^n}{n^n}$ (vi) $\sum(n^{1/n}-1)^n$

3. Test the convergence of the following series :

(i) $\frac{1^3}{3}+\frac{2^3}{3^2}+\frac{3^3}{3^3}+\frac{4^3}{3^4}+\ldots.$

(ii) $\frac{2}{1^2}x+\frac{3^2}{2^3}x^2+\frac{4^3}{3^4}x^3+\ldots+\frac{(n+1)^n x^n}{n^{n+1}}+\ldots.$ if $x>0$

(iii) $\sum q^{n^2} r^2,\ q, r>0$ (iv) $\sum_{n=2}^{\infty}\frac{1}{[\log(\log n)]^n}$

Based on D'Alembert's Ratio test

4. Test the convergence of the following series :

(i) $\sum_{n=1}^{\infty}\frac{2^{n-1}}{3^n+1}$ (ii) $\sum_{n=1}^{\infty}\frac{n!}{n^n}$

(iii) $\sum_{n=1}^{\infty}\frac{x^n}{n!}, x>0$ (iv) $\sum_{n=1}^{\infty}\frac{x^n}{n^n}, x>0$

(v) $\sum_{n=1}^{\infty}\frac{2^n n!}{n^n}$ (vi) $\sum_{n=1}^{\infty}\frac{n^n x^n}{n!}$

(vii) $\sum_{n=1}^{\infty}\frac{5^n}{n^2+5}$ (viii) $\sum_{n=1}^{\infty}\frac{n^3+a}{2^n+a}$

(ix) $\sum_{n=1}^{\infty}\frac{\sqrt{n}}{\sqrt{n^2+1}}x^n,\ x>0$ (PTU–2006)

(x) $\sum_{n=1}^{\infty}\sqrt{\frac{n-1}{n^3+1}}\,x^n,\ x>0$

5. Test the convergence of the series with n^{th} term :

(i) $\frac{1}{x^n+x^{-n}}$ (ii) $\left[\sqrt{n^2+1}-n\right]x^{2n}$

(iii) $\frac{1}{2^n+x},\ x\ge 0$ (iv) $\frac{x^n}{n^2+1}$

(v) $\frac{a^n}{x^n+a^n}$ (vi) $\sqrt{\frac{2^n-1}{3^n-1}}$

6. Test the convergence of the following series :

(i) $\frac{2!}{3}+\frac{3!}{3^2}+\frac{4!}{3^3}+\ldots+\frac{(n+1)!}{3^n}+\ldots.$

(ii) $\frac{1^2.2^2}{1!}+\frac{2^2.3^2}{2!}+\frac{3^2.4^2}{3!}+\ldots$

(iii) $\frac{1}{1+2}+\frac{2}{1+2^2}+\frac{3}{1+2^3}+\ldots$

(iv) $1+3x+5x^2+7x^3+\ldots$

(v) $1+\frac{x}{2^2}+\frac{x^2}{3^2}+\frac{x^3}{4^2}+\ldots$

(vi) $2x+\frac{3x^2}{8}+\frac{4x^3}{27}+\ldots+\frac{(n+1)x^n}{n^3}+\ldots$

(vii) $\frac{1}{\sqrt{1}+\sqrt{2}}+\frac{1}{\sqrt{2}+\sqrt{3}}+\frac{1}{\sqrt{3}+\sqrt{4}}+\ldots$

(viii) $\frac{\sqrt{2}-1}{3^3-1}+\frac{\sqrt{3}-1}{4^3-1}+\frac{\sqrt{4}-1}{5^3-1}+\ldots$

(ix) $\frac{1}{2}+\frac{2!}{8}+\frac{3!}{32}+\frac{4!}{128}+\ldots$

(x) $1+\frac{1}{2\cdot 2^{1/100}}+\frac{1}{3\cdot 3^{1/100}}+\frac{1}{4\cdot 4^{1/100}}+\ldots$

7. Test for convergence the following series :

(i) $\frac{1}{2\cdot 3}+\frac{1}{3\cdot 4}+\frac{1}{4\cdot 5}+\frac{1}{5\cdot 6}+\ldots$

(ii) $\frac{1}{1\cdot 2\cdot 3}+\frac{3}{2\cdot 3\cdot 4}+\frac{5}{3\cdot 4\cdot 5}+\ldots$

(iii) $\frac{1\cdot 2}{3^2.4^2}+\frac{3\cdot 4}{5^2.6^2}+\frac{5\cdot 6}{7^2.8^2}+\ldots$

(iv) $\frac{1}{3}+\frac{1\cdot 2}{3\cdot 5}+\frac{1\cdot 2\cdot 3}{3\cdot 5\cdot 7}+\frac{1\cdot 2\cdot 3\cdot 4}{3\cdot 5\cdot 7\cdot 9}+\ldots$

8. Test the series : $1+\frac{x^2}{2}+\frac{x^4}{4}+\frac{x^6}{6}+\ldots$

for convergence for all positive values of x.

9. Test for convergence the series :

$$\frac{x}{1\cdot 2}+\frac{x^2}{2\cdot 3}+\frac{x^3}{3\cdot 4}+\frac{x^4}{4\cdot 5}+\ldots, x>0$$

10. Show that the series ($\alpha > 0, \beta > 0$)

$$1+\frac{\alpha+1}{\beta+1}+\frac{(\alpha+1)(2\alpha+1)}{(\beta+1)(2\beta+1)}+\frac{(\alpha+1)(2\alpha+1)(3\alpha+1)}{(\beta+1)(2\beta+1)(3\beta+1)}+\ldots$$

converges if $\beta > \alpha > 0$ and diverges if $\alpha \geq \beta > 0$

11. Test for convergence the series :

$$\frac{x}{1\cdot 3}+\frac{x^2}{2\cdot 4}+\frac{x^3}{3\cdot 5}+\frac{x^4}{4\cdot 6}+\ldots$$

12. Test for convergence the following series :

(i) $1+\frac{x}{2}+\frac{x^2}{3^2}+\frac{x^3}{4^3}+\ldots, x>0$

(ii) $x+2x^2+3x^3+4x^4+\ldots$

(iii) $2+\frac{3}{2}x+\frac{4}{3}x^2+\frac{5}{4}x^3+\ldots, x>0$

(iv) $\frac{(1+a)(1+b)}{1\cdot 2\cdot 3}+\frac{(2+a)(2+b)}{2\cdot 3\cdot 4}+\frac{(3+a)(3+b)}{3\cdot 4\cdot 5}+\ldots$

(v) $x\log x+x^2\log 2x+x^3\log 3x+\ldots+x^n\log nx+\ldots$

(vi) $\sum_{n=1}^{\infty}\frac{n!}{(n^n)^2}$

(vii) $1+\frac{2!}{2^2}+\frac{3!}{3^3}+\frac{4!}{4^4}+\ldots\infty$

(viii) $\sum_{n=1}^{\infty}\frac{n!3^n}{n^n}$ (KERALA–2005)

(ix) $\frac{2}{3.4}+\frac{2.4}{3.5.6}+\frac{2.4.6}{3.5.7.8}+\ldots$

(x) $\sum_{n=2}^{\infty}\frac{x^n}{n(n-1)(n-2)}$

(xi) $\sum_{n=1}^{\infty}\left(\frac{n^2}{2^n}+\frac{1}{n^2}\right)$ (ROHTAK–2005)

(xii) $\sum_{1}^{\infty}\frac{n^3-n+1}{n!}$ (MADRAS–2000)

(xiii) $1+\frac{1^2.2^2}{1.3.5}+\frac{1^2.2^2.3^3}{1.3.5.7.9}+\ldots\infty$ (DELHI–2002)

(xiv) $\frac{4}{18}+\frac{4.12}{18.27}+\frac{4.12.20}{18.27.36}+\ldots\infty$

(MADRAS–2000, 12)

(xv) $\frac{1}{1^P}+\frac{x}{3^P}+\frac{x^2}{5^P}+\ldots\frac{x^{n-1}}{(2n-1)^P}+\ldots\infty$

(xvi) $\sum_{n=1}^{\infty}\frac{3.6.9\ldots 3n}{4.7.10\ldots(3n+1)}\cdot\frac{5^n}{3n+2}$

(xvii) $\frac{3}{4}x+\left(\frac{4}{5}\right)^2x^2+\left(\frac{5}{6}\right)^3x^3+\ldots+\infty\ (x>0)$

13. Test for convergence the series with n^{th} term :

(i) $\frac{n^3-1}{n^3+1}x^n, x>0$ (ii) $\frac{x^n}{a+\sqrt{n}}$

(iii) $\frac{x^n}{x+n}$ (iv) $\frac{3n+1}{4n+3}x^n, x>0$

(v) $\frac{x^n}{(2n+1)^P}$

(vi) $\frac{3^n-2}{3^n+1}x^{n-1}, x>0$

ANSWERS

1. (i) Convergent (ii) Convergent (iii) Convergent (iv) Convergent (v) Divergent (vi) Convergent (vii) Convergent

2. (i) Convergent (ii) Divergent (iii) Convergent (iv) Convergent if $x<1$, divergent if $x \geq 1$ (v) Convergent if $x < 1$, divergent if $x \geq 1$ (vi) Convergent

3. (i) Convergent (ii) Convergent if $x < 1$ and divergent if $x \geq 1$

(iii) Convergent if $0 < q < 1$ and divergent if $q > 1$, Convergent if $0 < r < 1$, when $q = 1$, divergent if $q > 1$ or $q = 1, r \geq 1$ (iv) Convergent

4. (i) Convergent (ii) Convergent (iii) Convergent (iv) Convergent (v) Convergent (vi) Convergent if $x < 1$, divergent if $x \geq 1$ (vii) Divergent (viii) Convergent (ix) Convergent if $x < 1$, divergent if $x \geq 1$ (x) Convergent if $x < 1$, divergent if $x \geq 1$

5. (i) Convergent if $x > 1$ or $x < 1$, and divergent if $x = 1$ (ii) Convergent if $x < 1$, divergent if $x \geq 1$ (iii) Convergent (iv) Convergent if $x \leq 1$, divergent if $x > 1$ (v) Convergent if $x > a$, divergent if $x \leq a$, (vi) Convergent.

6. (i) Divergent (ii) Convergent (iii) Convergent (iv) Convergent if $x < 1$, divergent if $x \geq 1$ (v) Convergent if $x \leq 1$, divergent if $x > 1$ (vi) Convergent if $x \leq 1$, divergent if $x > 1$ (vii) Divergent (viii) Convergent (ix) Divergent (x) Convergent

7. (i) Convergent (ii) Convergent (iii) Convergent (iv) Convergent

8. Convergent if $x < 1$, divergent if $x \geq 1$ **9.** Convergent if $x \leq 1$, divergent if $x > 1$

11. Convergent if $x \leq 1$, divergent $x > 1$

12. (i) Convergent (ii) Convergent if $x < 1$, divergent if $x \geq 1$ (iii) Convergent if $x < 1$, divergent if $x \geq 1$ (iv) Divergent (v) Convergent if $x < 1$, divergent if $x \geq 1$ (vi) Convergent (vii) Convergent (viii) Convergent (ix) Convergent (x) Convergent for $x \geq 1$, divergent for $x < 1$ (xi) Convergent (xii) Convergent (xiii) Divergent (xiv) Convergent (xv) Convergent $x < 1$, divergent for $x > 1$; Covergent for $P > 1$ and divergent for $P \leq 1$ (xvi) Divergent (xvii) Convergent

13. (i) Convergent if $x < 1$, divergent if $x \geq 1$ (ii) Convergent if $x < 1$, divergent if $x \geq 1$ (iii) Convergent if $x < 1$, divergent if $x \geq 1$ (iv) Convergent if $x < 1$, divergent if $x \geq 1$ (v) Convergent if $x < 1$, divergent if $x > 1$, when $x = 1$, then convergent if $p > 1$ and divergent if $p \leq 1$ (vi) Convergent if $x < 1$, divergent if $x \geq 1$

22.9 RAABE'S TEST

If $\Sigma\, u_n$ be a series of positive terms such that $\lim\limits_{n\to\infty}\left\{n\left(\dfrac{u_n}{u_{n+1}}-1\right)\right\}=l.$

Then, if

(i) $l > 1$, *the series converges,* (ii) $l < 1$, *the series diverges,*

(iii) $l = 1$, *the series may either converge or diverge and therefore the test fails.*

Proof. Case (I) When $l > 1$. We can write $l = 1 + r$, where $r > 0$. Choosing $\varepsilon = r/2$, we can find a positive integer m such that

$$l-\varepsilon < n\left(\frac{u_n}{u_{n+1}}-1\right) < l+\varepsilon \;\forall\; n \geq m$$

Now, from the first part of the above inequality, we have

$$(1+r)-\frac{1}{2}r < n\left(\frac{u_n}{u_{n+1}}-1\right) \;\forall\; n \geq m$$

$$\Rightarrow \quad \frac{1}{2}ru_{n+1} < nu_n-(n+1)u_{n+1} \;\forall\, n \geq m \qquad ...(1)$$

Putting $n = m+1, m+2, ..., p-1$ in succession in (1), we have

$$\frac{1}{2}ru_{m+2} < (m+1)u_{m+1}-(m+2)u_{m+2}$$

... ...

$$\frac{1}{2}ru_p < (p-1)u_{p-1} - pu_p.$$

Now, adding the corresponding sides of the above inqualities, we have

$$\frac{1}{2}r[u_{m+2} + u_{m+3} + ... + u_p] < (m+1)u_{m+1} - pu_p,$$

$$\Rightarrow \qquad \frac{1}{2}r[u_{m+2} + ... + u_p] < (m+1)u_{m+1},$$

or $$u_1 + u_2 + ... + u_p < \frac{2(m+1)}{r}u_{m+1} < u_1 + u_2 + ... + u_{m+1}, \forall p \geq m+2.$$

The above inequality shows that the sequence $\langle s_n \rangle$ of the partial sums of the series Σu_n is bounded and therefore Σu_n converges.

Case (II) When $l < 1$. Let us choose $\varepsilon = 1 - l$, then we can find a positive integer m such that

$$l - \varepsilon < n\left(\frac{u_n}{u_{n+1}} - 1\right) < 1 (= l + \varepsilon) \forall n \geq m \qquad \text{or } nu_n < (n+1)u_{n+1} \forall n \geq m$$

Putting $n = m+1, m+2, ..., p-1$ ($p \geq m+2$), in succession, we get

$$(m+1)u_{m+1} < (m+2)u_{m+2},$$
$$(m+2)u_{m+2} < (m+3)u_{m+3},$$
... .
$$(p-1)u_{p-1} < pu_p.$$

From the above inequality, we have by transitivity

$$(m+1)u_{m+1} < pu_p \ \forall p \geq m+2 \qquad \text{or} \qquad u_p > k(1/p) \ \forall p \geq m+2 \text{ and } k = (m+1)u_{m+1}.$$

Now, since the series $\Sigma\left(\frac{1}{p}\right)$ diverges, then by comparison test the given series diverges.

Case (III) When $l = 1$. In this case the test fails to give any definite information. For example, consider the series $\Sigma\frac{1}{n}$ and $\Sigma\frac{1}{n(\log n)^2}$ then, we have

$$\lim_{n\to\infty} n\left[\frac{u_n}{u_{n+1}} - 1\right] = 1.$$

But the former series is divergent, while the latter is convergent.

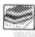

- Raabe's test is to be applied when D'Alembert's ratio test fails.
- Raabe's test is stronger than D'Alembert ratio test.
- It can be shown as in the proof of case (I) above that if $\lim_{n\to\infty}\left\{n\left[\frac{u_n}{u_{n+1}} - 1\right]\right\} = +\infty$. Then, Σu_n converges.
- The case in which $\lim_{n\to\infty}\left\{n\left[\frac{u_n}{u_{n+1}} - 1\right]\right\} = -\infty$. The given series Σu_n diverges.

22.10 LOGARITHMIC TEST

If Σu_n be a series of positive terms such that $\lim_{n\to\infty}\left(n\log\frac{u_n}{u_{n+1}}\right) = l.$

then Σu_n converges if $l > 1$ and diverges when $l < 1$.

Proof. Case (I) When $l > 1$. In this case, we can choose $\varepsilon > 0$ such that $l - \varepsilon > 1$. Let $l - \varepsilon = p$ (say).

Since $\lim_{n\to\infty}\left(n\log\frac{u_n}{u_{n+1}}\right) = l.$ Therefore, we can find a positive integer m such that

$$l-\varepsilon < n\log\frac{u_n}{u_{n+1}} < l+\varepsilon \ \forall\ n \geq m.$$

Consider the first part of the above inequality, we have

$$n\log\frac{u_n}{u_{n+1}} > p \ \ \forall\ n \geq m. \qquad \Rightarrow \qquad \frac{u_n}{u_{n+1}} > e^{p/n} \ \ \forall\ n \geq m. \qquad ...(1)$$

Since, $a_n = \left(1+\frac{1}{n}\right)^n$ defines a monotonically increasing sequence converging to e, therefore,

$$e \geq \left(1+\frac{1}{n}\right)^n \ \forall\ n. \qquad ...(2)$$

From (1) and (2), we have

$$\frac{u_n}{u_{n+1}} > \left(1+\frac{1}{n}\right)^p \ \forall\ n \geq m. \quad \Rightarrow \quad \frac{u_n}{u_{n+1}} > \frac{v_n}{v_{n+1}} \ \forall\ n \geq m. \qquad ...(3)$$

where $v_n = \frac{1}{n^p}$.

Now since $p > 1$, therefore Σv_n converges and from (3) it then follows by comparison test that Σu_n converges.

Case (II) When l < 1. Let the comparison series $\Sigma v_n = \Sigma \frac{1}{n^p}$ be divergent, *i.e.*, $p < 1$.

$\therefore$ Σu_n will be divergent if $\frac{v_n}{v_{n+1}} > \frac{u_n}{u_{n+1}}$

$$\Rightarrow \quad \frac{u_n}{u_{n+1}} < \left(1+\frac{1}{n}\right)^p \Rightarrow \log\left(\frac{u_n}{u_{n+1}}\right) < p\log\left(1+\frac{1}{n}\right) = p\left[\frac{1}{n}-\frac{1}{2n^2}+\frac{1}{3n^3}+...\right]$$

$$\therefore \quad n\log\left(\frac{u_n}{u_{n+1}}\right) = p\left[1-\frac{1}{2n}+\frac{1}{3n^2}+...\right]$$

$$\therefore \quad \lim_{n\to\infty}\left[n\log\frac{u_n}{u_{n+1}}\right] = p < 1$$

$\therefore$ Σu_n will be divergent if $l < 1$.

- Logarithmic test is to be applied only when :
  (a) ratio test fails (b) the ratio test involves the exponent 'e'
- This test is an alternative to Raabe's test.

22.11 SOME MODIFIED FORMS

Various test of convergence, involving limits can be modified in terms of the upper and lower limits. For example, a few modification are given below :

(i) Cauchy's Root test.

The series of non-negative term Σu_n converges or diverges according as

$$\underline{\lim}\, u_n^{1/n} < 1 \qquad \text{or} \qquad \overline{\lim}\, u_n^{1/n} > 1.$$

(ii) D' Alembert's Ratio test.

The series Σu_n of positive terms converges or diverges according as

$$\underline{\lim}\frac{u_n}{u_{n+1}} > 1 \qquad \text{or} \qquad \overline{\lim}\frac{u_n}{u_{n+1}} < 1.$$

(iii) Raabe's test.

The series Σu_n of positive terms converges or diverges according as

$$\underline{\lim}\left\{n\left(\frac{u_n}{u_{n+1}}-1\right)\right\}>1 \qquad \text{or} \qquad \overline{\lim}\left\{n\log\frac{u_n}{u_{n+1}}\right\}<1.$$

(iv) Logarithmic test.

The series Σu_n of positive terms converges or diverges according as

$$\underline{\lim}\left\{n\log\frac{u_n}{u_{n+1}}\right\}>1 \text{ or } \overline{\lim}\left\{n\log\frac{u_n}{u_{n+1}}\right\}<1.$$

Some Important Limits

- $\lim_{n\to\infty}\left(1+\frac{x}{n}\right)^n=e^x$
- $\lim_{n\to\infty} n^{1/n}=1$
- $\lim_{n\to\infty}\frac{\log n}{n}=0$
- $\lim_{n\to\infty}\left(1+\frac{x}{n}\right)^p=1$, if p is finite.
- $\lim_{n\to\infty}\left(1+\frac{x}{n}\right)^{n+p}=e^x$, if p is finite.

22.11.1 Some Other Important Tests

(1) De Morgan's and Bertrand's test : The series Σu_n of positive terms is convergent or divergent according as

$$\lim\left[n\left(\frac{u_n}{u_{n+1}}-1\right)-1\right]\log n>1 \quad \text{or} \quad <1.$$

(2) Alternative to Bertrand's test : The series Σu_n of positive terms is convergent or divergent according as

$$\lim\left[\left(n\log\frac{u_n}{u_{n+1}}-1\right)\log n\right]>1 \quad \text{or} \quad <1.$$

Solved Examples

1. *Test the convergence of the series*

$$1+\frac{3}{7}x+\frac{3\cdot6}{7\cdot10}x^2+\frac{3\cdot6\cdot9}{7\cdot10\cdot13}x^3+\ldots$$

SOLUTION. After leaving the first term we have

$$u_n=\frac{3\cdot6\cdot9\cdot\ldots\cdot3n}{7\cdot10\cdot13\cdot\ldots\cdot(3n+4)}x^n$$

$$\Rightarrow u_{n+1}=\frac{3\cdot6\cdot9\cdot\ldots\cdot3n(3n+3)}{7\cdot10\cdot13\cdot\ldots\cdot(3n+4)(3n+7)}x^{n+1}$$

Now $\lim_{n\to\infty}\frac{u_{n+1}}{u_n}=\lim_{n\to\infty}\left(\frac{3n+3}{3n+7}\right)x$

$$=\lim_{n\to\infty}\left(\frac{3+3/n}{3+7/n}\right)x=x$$

Then, by D'Alembert ratio test the series is convergent if $x<1$, divergent if $x>1$ and the test fails if $x=1$.

For $x=1$, we have

$$\frac{u_n}{u_{n+1}}=\frac{3n+7}{3n+3}$$

$$\text{or } n\left(\frac{u_n}{u_{n+1}}-1\right)=n\left(\frac{3n+7}{3n+3}-1\right)=\frac{4n}{3n+3}$$

$$\Rightarrow \lim_{n\to\infty} n\left[\left(\frac{u_n}{u_{n+1}}-1\right)\right]=\lim_{n\to\infty}\frac{4n}{3n+3}$$

$$=\lim_{n\to\infty}\frac{4}{3+3/n}$$

$$=\frac{4}{3}>1$$

Therefore, by Raabe's test the series is convergent when $x=1$.

Hence, the given series is convergent when $x\le1$ and divergent when $x>1$.

2. *Test the convergence of the following series*

$$\sum_{n=1}^{\infty}\frac{1.3.5\ldots.(2n-1)}{2.4.6\ldots.(2n)}\cdot\frac{x^{2n}}{2n},\ (x>0).$$

SOLUTION. Here, we have

$$u_n=\frac{1.3.5\ldots.(2n-1)}{2.4.6\ldots.(2n)}\cdot\frac{x^{2n}}{2n}$$

and

$$u_{n+1}=\frac{1.3.5\ldots(2n-1)(2n+1)}{2.4.6\ldots(2n)(2n+2)}\cdot\frac{x^{2n+2}}{(2n+2)}$$

$$\Rightarrow \lim_{n\to\infty}\frac{u_n}{u_{n+1}}=\lim_{n\to\infty}\left(\frac{2n+2}{2n+1}\cdot\frac{2n+2}{2n}\cdot\frac{1}{x^2}\right)$$

$$=\frac{1}{x^2}.$$

$\therefore$ By D'Alembert's ratio test, the series is convergent if $x^2 < 1$ and divergent if $x^2 > 1$.

Now since $x > 0$ this gives that the series is convergent if $x < 1$ and divergent if $x > 1$.

If $x = 1$. Then D'Alembert's ratio test fails.

Now consider

$$\lim_{n\to\infty} n\left[\frac{u_n}{u_{n+1}}-1\right]=\lim_{n\to\infty} n\left(\frac{2n+2}{2n+1}\cdot\frac{2n+2}{2n}-1\right)$$

$$=\lim_{n\to\infty}\frac{n(6n+4)}{2n(2n+1)}=\frac{3}{2}>1.$$

Then by Raabe's test, the series is convergent for $x = 1$.

Hence, the series is convergent if $x \le 1$ and divergent if $x > 1$.

3. *Test the convergence of the series*

$$\frac{a}{b}+\frac{(1+a)}{(1+b)}+\frac{(1+a)(2+a)}{(1+b)(2+b)}+\ldots$$

SOLUTION. Here, we have

$$u_n=\frac{(1+a)(2+a)\ldots(n-1+a)}{(1+b)(2+b)\ldots(n-1+b)}$$

$$\Rightarrow\ u_{n+1}=\frac{(1+a)(2+a)\ldots(n+a)}{(1+b)(2+b)\ldots(n+b)}$$

$$\therefore\ \lim_{n\to\infty}\frac{u_n}{u_{n+1}}=\lim_{n\to\infty}\left[\frac{n+b}{n+a}\right]$$

$$=\lim_{n\to\infty}\left[\frac{1+\frac{b}{n}}{1+\frac{a}{n}}\right]=1.$$

Hence, the D'Alembert's ratio test fails.

Now, consider

$$\lim_{n\to\infty} n\left[\frac{u_n}{u_{n+1}}-1\right]$$

$$=\lim_{n\to\infty} n\left[\frac{n+b}{n+a}-1\right]=\lim_{n\to\infty} n\left[\frac{b-a}{n+b}\right]$$

$$=\lim_{n\to\infty}\left[\frac{b-a}{1+b/n}\right]=(b-a).$$

Then by Raabe's test the given series is convergent if $b - a > 1$, *i.e.*, $b > a + 1$ and divergent if $b < a + 1$.

The test fails for $b = a + 1$.

Now, for $b = a + 1$, the given series becomes $\frac{a}{a+1}+\frac{1+a}{2+a}+\ldots=\Sigma\frac{1+a}{n+a}$.

Taking $v_n=\frac{1}{n}$, by comparison test, we can easily shown that the series is divergent.

Hence, the given series is convergent if $b > a + 1$ and divergent if $b \le a + 1$.

4. *Test the convergence of the series*

$$1+a+\frac{a(a+1)}{1\cdot 2}+\frac{a(a+1)(a+2)}{1\cdot 2\cdot 3}+\ldots$$

SOLUTION. On leaving the first term we have

$$u_n=\frac{a(a+1)(a+2)\ldots(a+n-1)}{1.2.\ldots.n}$$

$$\Rightarrow\ u_{n+1}=\frac{a(a+1)\ldots(a+n)}{1.2.\ldots.n(n+1)}$$

$$\therefore\ \lim_{n\to\infty}\frac{u_n}{u_{n+1}}=\lim_{n\to\infty}\frac{(n+1)}{(a+n)}=\lim_{n\to\infty}\frac{1+\frac{1}{n}}{1+\frac{a}{n}}=1.$$

$\Rightarrow$ The D' Alembert's ratio test fails.

Now $\lim_{n\to\infty} n\left[\frac{u_n}{u_{n+1}}-1\right]=\lim_{n\to\infty} n\left[\frac{n+1}{a+n}-1\right]$

$$=\lim_{n\to\infty} n\left[\frac{1-a}{a+n}\right]=\lim_{n\to\infty}\frac{(1-a)}{(1+a/n)}=(1-a).$$

Hence, by Raabe's test the given series is convergent if $1 - a > 1$, *i.e.*, $a < 0$ and divergent if $a > 0$ and test fails if $a = 0$.

In case $a = 0$, the given series becomes $1 + 0 + 0 + \ldots$

The sum of n terms is always 1. Therefore, the series is convergent if $a = 0$. Thus the given series Σu_n is convergent if $a \le 0$ and divergent if $a > 0$.

5. *Test the convergence of the series*

$$\Sigma\frac{n!x^n}{3.5.7\ldots(2n+1)}.$$

SOLUTION. Here, we have

$$u_n=\frac{n!x^n}{3.5.7\ldots(2n+1)}$$

$$\Rightarrow\ u_{n+1}=\frac{(n+1)!x^{n+1}}{3.5.7\ldots(2n+1)(2n+3)}$$

Now $\lim_{n\to\infty}\frac{u_n}{u_{n+1}}=\lim_{n\to\infty}\left(\frac{2n+3}{n+1}\right)\cdot\frac{1}{x}$

$$=\lim_{n\to\infty}\left(\frac{2+\frac{3}{n}}{1+\frac{1}{n}}\right)\cdot\frac{1}{x}=\frac{2}{x}.$$

Hence, by D'Alembert's ratio test the series is convergent if $2/x > 1$, *i.e.*, if

$x < 2$ and diverges if $2/x < 1$, *i.e.*, if $x > 2$ and test fails when $2/x = 1$, *i.e.*, when $x = 2$.

In case $x = 2$, apply Raabe's test. When $x = 2$, $\dfrac{u_n}{u_{n+1}} = \dfrac{(2n+3)}{2(n+1)}$

$$\therefore n\left(\frac{u_n}{u_{n+1}} - 1\right) = n\left(\frac{2n+3}{2n+2} - 1\right) = \frac{n}{2(n+1)} = \frac{1}{2(1+1/n)}$$

$$\therefore \lim_{n\to\infty} n\left(\frac{u_n}{u_{n+1}} - 1\right) = \lim_{n\to\infty} \frac{1}{2(1+1/n)} = \frac{1}{2} < 1.$$

Hence, by Raabe's test Σu_n is divergent if $x = 2$.

Thus, the given series Σu_n is convergent if $x < 2$ and divergent if $x \geq 2$.

6. *Test the convergence of the series*

$$1 + \frac{1}{2}x + \frac{2!}{3^2}x^2 + \frac{3!}{4^3}x^3 + \ldots$$

SOLUTION. Here, we have

$$u_n = \frac{(n-1)!}{n^{n-1}}x^{n-1} \Rightarrow u_{n+1} = \frac{n!}{(n+1)^n}x^n$$

$$\therefore \lim_{n\to\infty} \frac{u_n}{u_{n+1}} = \lim_{n\to\infty} \frac{(n+1)^n (n-1)!\, x^{n-1}}{n!\, x^n . n^{n-1}}$$

$$= \lim_{n\to\infty}\left[1 + \frac{1}{n}\right]^n . \frac{1}{x} = \frac{e}{x}.$$

Hence, the given series is convergent if $\dfrac{e}{x} > 1$, *i.e.*, if $x < e$ and divergent if $x > e$ and the test fails if $x = e$. In this case

$$\lim_{n\to\infty}\left[n \log \frac{u_n}{u_{n+1}}\right] = \lim_{n\to\infty}\left[n \log \frac{\left(1+\frac{1}{n}\right)^n}{e}\right]$$

$$= \lim_{n\to\infty}\left[n^2\left(\frac{1}{n} - \frac{1}{2n^2} + \frac{1}{3n^3} + \ldots\right) - n\right]$$

$$= \lim_{n\to\infty}\left[-\frac{1}{2} + \frac{1}{3n} - \ldots\right] = -\frac{1}{2} < 1.$$

Hence, by log test the series Σu_n is divergent if $x = e$.

Thus the given series Σu_n is convergent if $x < e$ and divergent if $x \geq e$.

7. *Test the convergence of the series*

$$x + \frac{2^2 x^2}{2!} + \frac{3^3 x^3}{3!} + \frac{4^4 x^4}{4!} + \ldots$$

(PTU–2008, COCHIN–2005, ROHTAK–2003)

SOLUTION. Here, we have $u_n = \dfrac{n^n x^n}{n!}$

$$\Rightarrow \quad u_{n+1} = \frac{(n+1)^{n+1} . x^{n+1}}{(n+1)!}$$

Therefore,

$$\lim_{n\to\infty} \frac{u_n}{u_{n+1}} = \lim_{n\to\infty} \frac{(n+1)!\, n^n x^n}{(n+1)^{n+1} x^{n+1} . n!}$$

$$= \lim_{n\to\infty} \frac{1}{\left(1+\frac{1}{n}\right)^n x} = \frac{1}{ex}.$$

Thus, by D'Alembert's ratio test the series is convergent if $ex < 1$ *i.e.*, $x < \dfrac{1}{e}$, divergent if $x > \dfrac{1}{e}$ and the test fails if $\dfrac{1}{ex} = 1$, *i.e.*, $x = \dfrac{1}{e}$.

In this case

$$\lim_{n\to\infty} n\left[\log \frac{u_n}{u_{n+1}}\right] = \lim_{n\to\infty} n \log\left[\frac{e}{\left(1+\frac{1}{n}\right)^n}\right]$$

$$= \lim_{n\to\infty} n\left[\log e - n\log\left(1 + \frac{1}{n}\right)\right]$$

$$= \lim_{n\to\infty} n\left[1 - n\left(\frac{1}{n} - \frac{1}{2n^2} + \frac{1}{3n^2} - \ldots\right)\right]$$

$$= \lim_{n\to\infty}\left[\frac{1}{2} - \frac{1}{3n} + \ldots\right] = \frac{1}{2} < 1.$$

Hence, by Logarithmic test, the series is divergent if $x = \dfrac{1}{e}$.

Thus the given series Σu_n is convergent if $x < \dfrac{1}{e}$ and divergent if $x \geq \dfrac{1}{e}$.

8. *Test the convergence of the series*

$$1 + \frac{2x}{2!} + \frac{3^2 x^2}{3!} + \frac{4^3 x^3}{4!} + \ldots$$

SOLUTION. Here, we have

$$u_n = \frac{n^{n-1} x^{n-1}}{n!} \Rightarrow u_{n+1} = \frac{(n+1)^n x^n}{(n+1)!}$$

$$\text{Now } \frac{u_n}{u_{n+1}} = \frac{(n+1)!\, n^{n-1} x^{n-1}}{(n+1)^n x^n \cdot n!} = \frac{\left(1+\frac{1}{n}\right)}{\left(1+\frac{1}{n}\right)^n} . \frac{1}{x}$$

$$\therefore \lim_{n\to\infty} \frac{u_n}{u_{n+1}} = \frac{1}{ex}.$$

Hence, by D'Alembert's ratio test the series is convergent if $\frac{1}{ex} > 1$, *i.e.*, $x < \frac{1}{e}$, divergent if $x > \frac{1}{e}$ and the test fails if $x = \frac{1}{e}$.

In this case

$$\lim_{n\to\infty}\left[n\log\frac{u_n}{u_{n+1}}\right] = \lim_{n\to\infty} n\left[\log\frac{\left(1+\frac{1}{n}\right)e}{\left(1+\frac{1}{n}\right)^n}\right]$$

$$= \lim_{n\to\infty} n\left[\log\left(1+\frac{1}{n}\right)+\log e - n\log\left(1+\frac{1}{n}\right)\right]$$

$$= \lim_{n\to\infty} n\left[\left(\frac{1}{n}-\frac{1}{2n^2}+\frac{1}{3n^3}-\ldots\right)+1 - n\left(\frac{1}{n}-\frac{1}{2n^2}+\frac{1}{3n^3}-\ldots\right)\right]$$

$$= \lim_{n\to\infty}\left[\frac{3}{2}-\frac{5}{6n}+\ldots\right] = \frac{3}{2} > 1.$$

Thus, by Logarithmic test, the series is convergent if $x = \frac{1}{e}$.

Thus the given series Σu_n is convergent if $x \le \frac{1}{e}$ and divergent if $x > \frac{1}{e}$.

Similar Problems

(1) Test the convergence of the series $\frac{(a+x)}{1!}+\frac{(a+2x)^2}{2!}+\frac{(a+3x)^3}{3!}+\ldots.$

Ans. convergent if $x < \frac{1}{e}$ and divergent if $x \ge \frac{1}{e}$.

(2) Test the convergence of the series $1^p + \left(\frac{1}{2}\right)^p + \left(\frac{1\cdot3}{2\cdot4}\right)^p + \left(\frac{1\cdot3\cdot5}{2\cdot4\cdot6}\right)^p + \ldots.$

Ans. convergent if $p/2 > 1$, *i.e.*, if $p > 2$, and divergent if $p \le 2$.

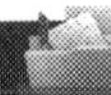

Exercise-22.3

Test the convergence of the following series

1. $1+\frac{2}{3}\left(\frac{1}{4}\right)+\frac{2.4}{3.5}\left(\frac{1}{6}\right)+\frac{2.4.6}{3.5.7}\left(\frac{1}{8}\right)+\ldots$

2. $\frac{1^2}{4^2}+\frac{1^2.5^2}{4^2.8^2}+\frac{1^2.5^2.9^2}{4^2.8^2.12^2}+\frac{1^2.5^2.9^2.13^2}{4^2.8^2.12^2.16^2}+\ldots$

3. $1+\frac{1}{2}x+\frac{1.3}{2.4}x^2+\frac{1.3.5}{2.4.6}x^3,\ldots,(x>0)$ (RAIPUR–2005)

4. $x^2+\frac{2^2}{3.4}x^4+\frac{2^2.4^2}{3.4.5.6}x^6+\ldots.$

5. $1+\frac{1}{2}\frac{x^2}{4}+\frac{1.3.5}{2.4.6}.\frac{x^4}{8}+\frac{1.3.5.7.9}{2.4.6.8.10}.\frac{x^6}{12}+\ldots$

6. $\sum_{n=1}^{\infty}\frac{n!}{(n+1)^n}x^n, x>0$

7. $\sum_{n=1}^{\infty}\left[\frac{1}{1+\log n}\right]$

8. $1+\frac{2}{3.5}+\frac{2.4}{3.5.7}+\frac{2.4.6}{3.5.7.9}+\ldots$

9. Test the convergence of the series

$x + x^{1+\frac{1}{2}} + x^{1+\frac{1}{2}+\frac{1}{3}} + x^{1+\frac{1}{2}+\frac{1}{3}+\frac{1}{4}} + \ldots$

10. Test the convergence of the following series:

(i) $\frac{1^2}{2^2}+\frac{1^2.3^2}{2^2.4^2}x+\frac{1^2.3^2.5^2}{2^2.4^2.6^2}x^2+\ldots$

(ii) $1+\frac{2^2}{3^2}+\frac{2^2.4^2}{3^2.5^2}+\frac{2^2.4^2.6^2}{3^2.5^2.7^2}+\ldots$

11. Test for convergence, the following series :

(i) $1+\frac{x}{1}+\frac{1}{2}.\frac{x^3}{3}+\frac{1.3}{2.4}.\frac{x^5}{5}+\frac{1.3.5}{2.4.6}.\frac{x^7}{7}+\ldots.$

(ii) $\frac{x}{1}+\frac{1}{2}.\frac{x^2}{3}+\frac{1.3}{2.4}.\frac{x^3}{5}+\frac{1.3.5}{2.4.6}.\frac{x^4}{7}+\ldots$ $(x>0)$

(iii) $\sum_{n=1}^{\infty}\frac{1.3.5\ldots.(4n-5)(4n-3)}{2.4.6\ldots.(4n-4)(4n-2)}\frac{x^{2n}}{4n}, x>0$

(iv) $\sum_{n=1}^{\infty}\frac{2.4.6\ldots.2n}{1.3.5\ldots(2n+1)}$

12. Test for convergence, the following series :

(i) $1+\frac{x}{1!}+\frac{2^2x^2}{2!}+\frac{3^3x^3}{3!}+...\text{for } x>0$

(ii) $\frac{1}{2}x+\frac{1.3}{2.4}x^2+\frac{1.3.5}{2.4.6}x^3+..., x>0$

(iii) $1+\frac{2!}{2^2}x+\frac{3!}{3^3}x^2+..., x>0$

13. Test for convergence, the following series :

(i) $1+\frac{a(1-a)}{1^2}+\frac{(1+a)a(1-a)(2-a)}{1^2.2^2}+\frac{(2+a)(1+a)a(1-a)(2-a)(3-a)}{1^2.2^2.3^2}+...$

(ii) $\frac{(1+a)(1+b)}{1.2.3}+\frac{(2+a)(2+b)}{2.3.4}+\frac{(3+a)(3+b)}{3.4.5.}+...$

14. Test for convergence the following series :

(i) $1+\frac{\alpha}{1.\beta}x+\frac{\alpha(\alpha+1)^2}{1.2\beta(\beta+1)^2}x^2+\frac{\alpha(\alpha+1)^2(\alpha+2)^2}{1.2.3\beta(\beta+1)(\beta+2)}x^3+...$

(ii) $1+\frac{\alpha.\beta}{1.\gamma}x+\frac{\alpha(\alpha+1)\beta(\beta+1)}{1.2.\gamma(\gamma+1)}x^2+\frac{\alpha(\alpha+1)(\alpha+2)\beta(\beta+1)(\beta+2)}{1.2.3.\gamma(\gamma+1)(\gamma+2)}x^3+...$

(KURUKSHETRA–2005)

15. Test for convergence the following series :

$\frac{a}{a+3}+\frac{a(a+2)}{(a+3)(a+5)}x+\frac{a(a+2)(a+4)}{(a+3)(a+5)(a+7)}x^2+...$

16. Test for convergence the following series :

$\left(\frac{1}{2.4}\right)^{2/3}+\left(\frac{1.3}{2.4.6}\right)^{2/3}+\left(\frac{1.3.5}{2.4.6.8}\right)^{2/3}+....$

17. Test for convergence the following series :

(i) $\sum_{n=1}^{\infty}\frac{1\cdot3\cdot5....(2n-1)}{2\cdot4\cdot6....2n}\cdot\frac{1}{n}$

(ii) $\sum_{n=1}^{\infty}\frac{4\cdot7\cdot10....(3n+1)}{1\cdot2\cdot3....n}x^n$

(iii) $\sum_{n=1}^{\infty}\frac{3\cdot6\cdot9....(3n)}{7\cdot10\cdot13....(3n+4)}x^n, x>0$

(iv) $\sum_{n=1}^{\infty}\frac{(2n)!}{(n!)^2}x^n, x>0$

18. Test for convergence the following series :

$\frac{1^2}{2^2}+\frac{1^2.3^2}{2^2.4^2}+\frac{1^2.3^2.5^2}{2^2.4^2.6^2}+...$

19. Test for convergence the following series :

(i) $\frac{1}{(\log 2)^p}+\frac{1}{(\log 3)^p}+...+\frac{1}{(\log n)^p}+...$

(ii) $x^2(\log 2)^p+x^3(\log 3)^p+x^4(\log 4)^p+...$

20. Test for convergence the following series :

(i) $\frac{x}{1.2}+\frac{x^2}{3.4}+\frac{x^3}{5.6}+\frac{x^4}{7.8}+...\infty\ (x>0)$

(MUMBAI–2009)

(ii) $\frac{x}{1.2}+\frac{x^2}{2.3}+\frac{x^3}{3.4}+\frac{x^4}{4.5}+...\infty$

(iii) $1+\frac{2}{3}x+\frac{2.3}{3.5}x^2+\frac{2.3.4}{3.5.7}x^3+...\infty$

(iv) $\frac{x}{1}+\frac{1}{2}\frac{x^3}{3}+\frac{1.3}{2.4}\frac{x^5}{5}+\frac{1.3.5}{2.4.6}\frac{x^7}{7}+...\infty$ $(x>0)$

(RAIPUR–2005)

(v) $1+\frac{1}{2}\frac{x^2}{4}+\frac{1.3.5}{2.4.6}\frac{x^4}{8}+\frac{1.3.5.7.9}{2.4.6.8.10}\frac{x^6}{12}+...\infty$

(ROHTAK–2006S, ROORKEE–2000)

(vi) $\frac{1}{1^2}+\frac{1+2}{1^2+2^2}+\frac{1+2+3}{1^2+2^2+3^3}+...$

ANSWERS

1. Convergent **2.** Convergent **3.** $\begin{cases}\text{Convergent if } x<1,\\ \text{Divergent if } x\ge 1\end{cases}$

4. Convergent if $x^2\le 1$, divergnet if $x^2>1$ **5.** Convergent if $x\le 1$, divergent if $x>1$

6. Convergent if $x<e$, divergent if $x\ge e$ **7.** Convergent **8.** Convergent

9. Convergent if $x<\frac{1}{e}$, divergent if $x\ge\frac{1}{e}$ **10.** (i)Convergent if $x<1$, divergent if $x\ge 1$ (ii)Divergent

11. (i) Convergent if $x^2\le 1$, divergent if $x^2>1$(ii)Convergent if $0<x\le 1$, divergent if $x>1$ (iii)Convergent if $x\le 1$, divergent if $x>1$ (iv) Divergent

12. (i) Convergent if $x<\frac{1}{e}$, divergent if $x\ge\frac{1}{e}$ (ii) Convergent if $x<1$, divergent if $x\ge 1$, (iii)Convergent if $x<e$, divergent if $x\ge e$ **13.** (i) Divergent (ii) Divergent

14. (i) Convergent if $x<1$, divergent if $x>1$, When $x=1$, then convergent if $\beta>2\alpha$, divergent if $\beta\le 2\alpha$ (ii)Convergent if $x<1$, divergent if $x>1$, When $x=1$, then convergent if $\gamma>\alpha+\beta$, divergent if $\gamma\le\alpha+\beta$.

15. Convergent if $x \le 1$, divergent if $x > 1$ **16.** Divergent

17. (i) Convergent (ii) Convergent if $x < \frac{1}{3}$, divergent if $x \ge \frac{1}{3}$

(iii) Convergent if $x \le 1$, divergentif $x > 1$ (iv) Convergent if $x < \frac{1}{4}$, divergent if $x \ge \frac{1}{4}$.

18. Divergent **19.**(i) Divergent for all values of p, (ii) Convergent if $x < 1$, divergent if $x \ge 1$

20. (i) Convergent for $x \le 1$; divergent for $x > 1$ (ii)Convergent for $x \le 1$; divergent for $x > 1$

(iii) Convergent for $x < 2$; divergent for $x \ge 2$(iv)Convergent for $x \le 1$; divergent for $x > 1$

(v) Convergent for $x^2 \le 1$; divergent for $x^2 > 1$(vi) Diverges

22.12 GAUSS'S TEST

If Σu_n be a series of positive terms such that

$$\frac{u_n}{u_{n+1}} = \alpha + \frac{\beta}{n} + \frac{\gamma_n}{n^p},$$

where $\alpha > 0$, $p > 1$ and $<\gamma_n>$ is a bounded sequence. Then

(i) *Σu_n converges for $\alpha > 1$, diverges for $\alpha < 1$, whatever β may be.*

(ii) *If $\alpha = 1$, Σu_n converges whenever $\beta > 1$, and diverges whenever $\beta \le 1$.*

Proof. We have

$$\lim_{n\to\infty} \frac{u_n}{u_{n+1}} = \alpha.$$

Then by D'Alembert's ratio test Σu_n is convergent if $\alpha > 1$ and divergent if $\alpha < 1$.
For $\alpha = 1$, we have

$$n\left[\frac{u_n}{u_{n+1}} - 1\right] = \beta + \frac{\gamma_n}{n^{p-1}},$$

where $p > 1$ and $< \gamma_n >$ is a bounded sequence.

$$\therefore \quad \lim_{n\to\infty} n\left[\frac{u_n}{u_{n+1}} - 1\right] = \beta.$$

Then, by Raabe's test Σu_n is convergent if $\beta > 1$ and divergent if $\beta < 1$.
Now for $\alpha = \beta = 1$, we compare the series with the divergent series Σv_n where $v_n = \frac{1}{n\log n}$.
Now, consider

$$\frac{u_n}{u_{n+1}} - \frac{v_n}{v_{n+1}} = 1 + \frac{1}{n} + \frac{\gamma_n}{n^p} - \frac{(n+1)\log(n+1)}{n\log n} = \frac{\gamma_n}{n^p} - \frac{(n+1)}{n}\left[\frac{\log(n+1)}{\log n} - 1\right]$$

$$= \frac{1}{n^p}\left[\gamma_n - (n+1)\log\left(1+\frac{1}{n}\right).\frac{n^{p-1}}{\log n}\right].$$

But $\lim_{n\to\infty} (n+1)\log\left(1+\frac{1}{n}\right) = \lim_{n\to\infty}\left[\log\left(1+\frac{1}{n}\right)^n + \log\left(1+\frac{1}{n}\right)\right]$

Also, $\lim_{n\to\infty} \frac{n^{p-1}}{\log n} = \infty, p > 1$ and $< \gamma_n >$ is bounded.

Therefore, for large value of n, $\gamma_n - (n+1)\log\left(1+\frac{1}{n}\right)\frac{n^{p-1}}{\log n}$ remains negative.

$$\therefore \quad \frac{u_n}{u_{n+1}} - \frac{v_n}{v_{n+1}} < 0 \quad \text{or} \quad \frac{u_n}{u_{n+1}} < \frac{v_n}{v_{n+1}}.$$

Now, since Σv_n is divergent, by comparison test Σu_n is divergent.

Hence, the series Σu_n is convergent if $\alpha > 1$ or $\alpha = 1$ and $\beta > 1$ and divergent if $\alpha < 1$ or $\alpha = 1$ and $\beta \le 1$.

22.13 CAUCHY'S INTEGRAL TEST

Let $f(x)$ be non-negative monotonically decreasing integrable function on $[1, \infty[$ then the series $\sum_{n=1}^{\infty} f(n)$ and the improper integral $\int_1^{\infty} f(x)\,dx$ converge or diverge together.

22.14 CAUCHY'S CONDENSATION TEST

If $f(n)$ is a monotonically decreasing function of n for all $n \in N$ such that each $f(n)$ is positive, then two infinite series $\sum_{n=1}^{\infty} f(n)$ and $\sum_{n=1}^{\infty} a^n f(a^n)$ converge or diverge together, where a is a positive integer greater than unity.

22.15 REARRANGEMENT OF TERMS

A series Σv_n is said to be rearrangement of a series Σu_n if there exists one-one correspondence between the terms of the two series and if v_n corresponds to u_n then $v_n = u_n$.

In other words, we can say that a series Σu_n is said to be rearrangement of a series Σv_n if every term of Σu_n is a term of Σv_n and *vice-versa*.

22.16 ALTERNATING SERIES

A series, whose terms are alternatively positive and negative is called an alternating series.

Thus, a series of the form $u_1 - u_2 + u_3 - u_4 + ... + (-1)^{n-1} u_n + ...$ where $u_n > 0\ \forall\ n$, is an alternating series.

22.16.1 ABSOLUTE CONVERGENCE

A series Σu_n is said to be absolutely convergent if the series $\Sigma |u_n|$ is convergent.

22.16.2 UNCONDITIONALLY CONVERGENT SERIES

A series Σu_n is said to be unconditionally convergent if every rearrangement converge to the same sum Σu_n, *i.e*, Σu_n is conditionally convergent iff it is absolutely convergent.

22.16.3 CONDITIONAL CONVERGENCE

A series Σu_n is said to be conditionally convergent if Σu_n is convergent but $\Sigma |u_n|$ is divergent.

- The conditional convergence of a series is also known as semi-convergent or non-absolutely convergent.

☛ ILLUSTRATIONS

(1) The series $\Sigma u_n = 1 - \frac{1}{2} + \frac{1}{2^2} - \frac{1}{2^3} + ...$ is absolutely convergent.

(2) The series $\frac{1}{1^2} - \frac{1}{2^2} + \frac{1}{3^2} - \frac{1}{4^2} + ...$ is absolutely convergent.

THEOREM 1. *An absolutely convergent series is convergent.*

PROOF. Let us suppose, the series Σu_n is absolutely convergent. Then by definition $\Sigma |u_n|$ is convergent.

Now
$$u_n + |u_n| = \begin{cases} 2u_n, & \text{if } u_n \text{ is positive} \\ 0, & \text{if } u_n \text{ is negative.} \end{cases}$$

Therefore, every term of the series $\Sigma(u_n + |u_n|)$ is ≥ 0 and less than equal to the corresponding term of the convergent series $\Sigma 2|u_n|$.

Hence, $\Sigma(u_n + |u_n|)$ is convergent. Hence Σu_n is convergent.

- The converse of the above theorem is not necessarily true :
  For example : The series $\Sigma u_n = 1 - \frac{1}{2} + \frac{1}{3} - ....$ is convergent, but the series $\Sigma |u_n| = 1 + \frac{1}{2} + \frac{1}{3} + ...$ is divergent. Hence a convergent series need not be absolutely convergent.
- The usefulness of absolute convergence is partly due to the fact that it is often easier to establish absolute convergence than convergence :
  For example : Consider the series $\Sigma \frac{a^n}{2^n}$, where $a_n = 1$ if n is prime number and $a_n = -1$ otherwise. Here, $\Sigma |a_n| = \Sigma \frac{1}{2^n}$ is convergent. Accordingly $\Sigma a^n/2^n$ is absolutely convergent, and hence convergent.

THEOREM 2. *If the terms of a convergent series of positive terms are rearranged, the series remains convergent and its sum is unaltered.*

PROOF. Let us suppose Σu_n be a convergent series, and let the terms be rearranged in any manner. Denote the new series by Σv_n, so that every u is a v and every v is a u.

Let $s_n = u_1 + u_2 + ... + u_n$ and $t_n = v_1 + v_2 + ... + v_n$.

Then, for any definite value of n, s_n contains n terms each of which occurs, sooner or later, in the v series and so we can find a corresponding m such that t_m contains all the terms of s_n (and possibly other not contained in s_n).

Now, since each term is positive, therefore $s_n \le t_m$.

Also, suppose that the first m terms of Σv_n are among the first $(n+p)$ terms of Σu_n.

Therefore, $$s_n \le t_m \le s_{n+p}.$$

and m tends to infinity with n.

Let Σu_n converges to s, so that $\lim s_n = \lim s_{n+p} = s$

$$\therefore \qquad \lim t_m = s.$$

Hence, Σv_n is convergent and has the same sum as Σu_n.

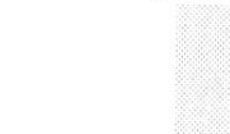

- The arrangement fails for a dearrangement such as $u_1 + u_3 + u_5 + ... + u_2 + u_4 + u_6 + ...$ where Σu_n is broken up into two (or any finite no. of) infinite series.
  Here, we cannot find an m so that the first n terms of Σu_n occur among the first m terms of Σv_n.
  For instance, u_2 does not occur even if infinitely many of the terms $u_1, u_3, u_5, ...$ have been placed.

THEOREM 3. **(Dirichlet's Theorem).** *If the terms of an absolutely convergent series are rearranged, the series remains convergent and its sum is unaltered.*

PROOF. Let Σu_n be an absolutely convergent series, and let its terms be rearranged in a different order. Let, the new series be denoted by Σv_n so that every v occurs somewhere in the u series and every u occurs somewhere in the v series.

Now, we have $u_n + |u_n| = 2u_n$ or 0 according as u_n is positive or negative. Now $\Sigma |u_n|$ is a convergent series of positive terms, so also in the series $\Sigma(u_n + |u_n|)$, because its terms are less than equal to be corresponding terms of the series $\Sigma 2|u_n|$.

Let $\Sigma |u_n| = s$ and $\Sigma(u_n + |u_n|) = s'$ so that $\Sigma u_n = s' - s$.

Also, since $\Sigma |u_n|$ and $\Sigma(u_n + |u_n|)$ are convergent series of positive terms, their sum remains unchanged by any rearrangement of term (By theorem 2).

Accordingly, $\Sigma |v_n| = s$ and $\Sigma(v_n + |v_n|) = s'$.

Hence, $\Sigma v_n = s' - s = \Sigma u_n$.

- If we rearrange the order of terms of a semi-convergent series, we may or may not changed the sum of the series.
- The sum will be changed if we interfere too much with the balance between positive and negative terms.
- By a suitable rearrangement of the terms a semi-convergent series may be made to diverge. The reason is that in a semi-convergent series the positive and negative terms taken separately from two divergent series.

THEOREM 4. **(Riemann's Rearrangement theorem).** *By a suitable rearrangement of terms of a conditionally convergent series can be made to converge to any number λ or to diverge to ∞ or $-\infty$ even to oscillate.*

In other words, this theorem can be stated as follows:

To a given conditionally convergent series and to any given number there corresponds a rearrangement of the given series which is convergent and whose sum is the given number.

THEOREM 5. **(Pringsheim theorem).** *Let f(x) be a sequence of positive terms which monotonically converges to zero and let the series $\sum_{n=1}^{\infty}(-1)^{n-1}f(x)$ be rearranged so that in the first p+n terms there are p-positive terms and n negative terms, i.e., $\lim_{n\to\infty} n\,f(x)=\lambda$ and $\lim_{n\to\infty}\frac{p}{n}=k$ then the sum of the series is increased by $\frac{1}{2}\lambda\log k$.*

22.17 LEIBNITZ'S TEST

If the alternative series $u_1 - u_2 + u_3 - \ldots (u_n > 0, \forall\, n \in \mathbf{N})$ is such that

(i) $u_{n+1} \le u_n, \forall\, n \in \mathbf{N}$ (ii) $\lim_{n\to\infty} u_n = 0$

Then the series converges.

Proof. Let $s_n = u_1 - u_2 + u_3 - \ldots + (-1)^{n-1}u_n$ so that $<s_n>$ is a sequence of partial sums of the given series.

Now for all n

$$s_{2n+2} - s_{2n} = u_{2n+1} - u_{2n+2} \ge 0 \qquad \text{[By (i)]}$$

which gives that $<s_{2n}>$ is a monotonically increasing sequence.

Further,
$$s_{2n} = u_1 - u_2 + u_3 - \ldots u_{2n-1} - u_{2n} = u_1 - (u_2 - u_3) - (u_4 - u_5) - \ldots - u_{2n}$$
$$= u_1 - [(u_2 - u_3) + \ldots + u_{2n}] = u_1 - \text{some positive number} \le u_1.$$

Therefore, the monotonically increasing sequence $<s_{2n}>$ is bounded above and consequently it is convergent.

Let $\lim_{n\to\infty} s_{2n} = s.$

Now
$$s_{2n+1} = s_{2n} + u_{2n+1} \Rightarrow \lim_{n\to\infty} s_{2n+1} = \lim_{n\to\infty} s_{2n} + \lim_{n\to\infty} u_{2n+1}$$
$$\left[\because \lim_{n\to\infty} u_n = 0\right]$$
$$= s + 0 = s$$

Thus, the subsequences $<s_{2n}>$ and $<s_{2n+1}>$ both converge to the same limit. Now we shall show that the sequence $<s_n>$ also converges to s.

Let $\varepsilon > 0$ be given. Since, the sequences $<s_{2n}>$ *and* $<s_{2n+1}>$ both converges to s, there exists positive integers m_1, m_2 such that

$$|s_{2n} - s| < \varepsilon\ \forall\, n \ge m_1,$$

and $|s_{2n+1} - s| < \varepsilon\ \forall\, n \ge m_2.$

Let $m = \max\{m_1, m_2\}.$

Then $|s_n - s| < \varepsilon\ \forall\, n \ge m$

which gives that the sequence $<s_n>$ converges to s.

Hence, the given series $\Sigma(-1)^{n-1}u_n$ converges.

- This test gives us a set of sufficient conditions for the convergence of an alternating series.
- If the test does not show a series to be convergent, we may not immediately say that the series is divergent.

Solved Examples

1. *Show that* $\lim_{n\to\infty}\left[1+\frac{1}{2}+\ldots+\frac{1}{n}-\log n\right]$ *exists.*

SOLUTION. Let $f(x)=\frac{1}{x}$, $x\in[1,\infty[$.

Then $f(x)>0$ and monotonically decreasing on $[1,\infty[$.

Let $S_n = f(1)+f(2)+\ldots+f(n)$

$$=1+\frac{1}{2}+\frac{1}{3}+\ldots+\frac{1}{n}$$

and $I_n=\int_1^n f(x)dx=\int_1^n \frac{1}{x}dx$

$$=[\log x]_1^n=\log n.$$

It can be easily shown that

$$f(n)\le S_n-I_n\le f(1)\ \forall\ n\in \mathrm{N}$$

or $0<\frac{1}{n}\le S_n-I_n\le 1\ \forall\ n\in\mathrm{N}$

which gives that the sequence $<u_n>$, where $u_n=S_n-I_n$, is bounded below. Now, it can also be shown easily that the sequence $<u_n>$ is a monotonically decreasing. Therefore it converges.

Hence, $\lim_{n\to\infty}\left(1+\frac{1}{2}+\ldots+\frac{1}{n}-\log n\right)$ exist.

- The limit of the above sequence is called Euler's constant and is denoted by γ.

2. *Show by integral test that* $\Sigma\frac{1}{n^p}$ *converges if* $p>1$ *and diverges if* $p\le 1$.

SOLUTION. Let $f(x)=\frac{1}{x^p}$, $p>0$. Then $f(x)$ is positive valued and monotonically decreasing.

Therefore by Cauchy's integral test $\Sigma\frac{1}{n^p}$ and $\int_1^\infty f(x)dx$ converges and diverges together.

Let $I_n=\int_1^n\frac{1}{x^p}dx=\int_1^n x^{-p}dx$

$$=\begin{cases}\left(\frac{n^{1-p}}{1-p}-\frac{1}{1-p}\right), & \text{if } p\ne 1\\ \log n, & \text{if } p=1.\end{cases}$$

If $n\to\infty$, $n^{1-p}=\frac{1}{n^{p-1}}\to 0$ if $p>1$

and tends to ∞ if $p<1$ and $\log n\to\infty$

$$\therefore \lim_{n\to\infty} I_n=-\frac{1}{1-p}=\frac{1}{p-1},\ \text{if } p>1$$

and $\lim_{n\to\infty} I_n=\infty$, if $p\le 1$.

Hence, $\int_1^\infty f(x)dx$ converges if $p>1$and diverges if $p\le 1$. Then by Cauchy's integral test the series $\Sigma\frac{1}{n^p}$ is convergent if $p>1$ and divergent if $p\le 1$.

3. *Show by Cauchy's integral test that the series* $\sum_{n=2}^{\infty}\frac{1}{n(\log n)^p}$ *converges if* $p>1$ *and diverges if* $0<p\le 1$. (PTU–2010)

SOLUTION. Let us suppose

$$f(x)=\frac{1}{x(\log x)^p},\ p>0$$

and $x\in[2,\infty[$; then obviously $f(x)$ is monotonically decreasing in $[2,\infty[$ and positive valued.

Let $I_n=\int_2^n\frac{dx}{x(\log x)^p}$

Then $I_n=\left[\frac{(\log x)^{1-p}}{1-p}\right]_2^n$, $p\ne 1$

$$=\frac{1}{(1-p)}[(\log n)^{1-p}-(\log 2)^{1-p}],\ p\ne 1$$

and $I_n=[\log\log x]_2^n$, $p=1$

$$=[\log\log n-\log\log 2],\ p=1.$$

Therefore, we have

$$\lim_{n\to\infty} I_n=\lim_{n\to\infty}\int_2^n f(x)dx=\infty,\ \text{if } p<1$$

and $\lim_{n\to\infty} I_n=-\frac{1}{(1-p)}(\log 2)^{1-p}$, if $p>1$.

Thus the integral $\int_2^\infty f(x)dx$ converges if $p>1$ and diverges if $0<p\le 1$.

Hence, by Cauchy's integral test, the series $\sum_{n=2}^{\infty}f(x)=\sum_{n=2}^{\infty}\frac{1}{n(\log n)^p}$ converges if $p>1$ and diverges if $0<p\le 1$.

4. *Apply the Cauchy's condensation test to discuss the convergence of the series*

$$\sum_{n=2}^{\infty} \frac{1}{(n\log n)(\log\log n)^p}.$$

SOLUTION. Here, we have

$$f(n) = \frac{1}{(n\log n)(\log\log n)^p}$$

$$\therefore a^n f(a^n) = \frac{a^n}{(a^n \log a^n)(\log\log a^n)^p}$$

$$= \frac{1}{(n\log a)[\log(n\log a)]^p}$$

Since, a is a positive integer greater than 1 and can be chosen that $\log a > 1$ so that $n \log a > n$.

Then $a^n f(a^n) < \dfrac{1}{(n\log a)(\log n)^p}$

Since, the series $\dfrac{1}{\log a}\Sigma\dfrac{1}{n(\log n)^p}$ is convergent when $p > 1$, therefore $\Sigma a^n f(a^n)$ is also convergent and consequently the given series is convergent when $p > 1$.

Now let $p \le 1$. If we take $a = 2$, then $\log a < 1$ so that $n \log a < n$

$$\therefore\ a^n f(a^n) > \frac{1}{(n\log a)(\log n)^p}$$

But the series $\dfrac{1}{\log a}\Sigma\dfrac{1}{n(\log n)^p}$ is divergent when $p \le 1$ and therefore $\Sigma a^n f(a^n)$ is also divergent. Then by Cauchy condensation test, the given series is divergent when $p \le 1$.

5. *Test the convergence of the series*

$$\frac{1^2}{2^2} + \frac{1^2.3^2}{2^2.4^2} + \frac{1^2.3^2.5^2}{2^2.4^2.6^2} + ...$$

SOLUTION. Here, we have

$$u_n = \frac{1^2.3^2.5^2...(2n-1)^2}{2^2.4^2.6^2...(2n)^2}$$

$$\therefore\ u_{n+1} = \frac{1^2.3^2...(2n-1)^2(2n+1)^2}{2^2.4^2...(2n)^2(2n+2)^2}$$

$$\therefore\ \frac{u_n}{u_{n+1}} = \frac{(2n+2)^2}{(2n+1)^2}$$

$$\Rightarrow \lim_{n\to\infty}\frac{u_n}{u_{n+1}} = \lim_{n\to\infty}\frac{\left(2+\frac{2}{n}\right)^2}{\left(2+\frac{1}{n}\right)^2} = 1$$

which gives that, the ratio test is fail. Now, we can easily see that

$$\lim_{n\to\infty} n\left[\frac{u_n}{u_{n+1}} - 1\right] = 1.$$

$\Rightarrow$ Raabe's test also fails.

Now applying Gauss test, Consider

$$\frac{u_n}{u_{n+1}} = \frac{(2n+2)^2}{(2n+1)^2} = \left(1+\frac{1}{n}\right)^2\left(1+\frac{1}{2n}\right)^{-2}$$

$$= \left(1+\frac{2}{n}+\frac{1}{n^2}\right)\left(1-2.\frac{1}{2n}+3.\frac{1}{4n^2}....\right)$$

$$= 1 + \frac{1}{n} - \frac{1}{4n^2} + ...$$

$$= \alpha + \frac{\beta}{n} + \frac{\gamma_n}{n^2}, \text{where } \gamma_n \to -\frac{1}{4} \text{ as } n \to \infty.$$

Here, $\alpha = 1$, $\beta = 1$. Therefore by Gauss test the series Σu_n is divergent.

6. *Test the convergence of the series*

$$1 + \left(\frac{2}{3}\right)^p + \left(\frac{2.4}{3.5}\right)^p + \left(\frac{2.4.6}{3.5.7}\right)^p + ...$$

SOLUTION. Neglecting first term, we have

$$u_n = \left[\frac{2.4.6...(2n)}{3.5.7...(2n+1)}\right]^p$$

$$\Rightarrow u_{n+1} = \left[\frac{2.4.6...(2n)(2n+2)}{3.5.7...(2n+1)(n+3)}\right]^p$$

$$\Rightarrow \frac{u_n}{u_{n+1}} = \left(\frac{2n+3}{2n+2}\right)^p = \frac{\left(1+\frac{3}{2n}\right)^p}{\left(1+\frac{2}{2n}\right)^p}$$

$$= \left(1+\frac{3}{2n}\right)^p\left(1+\frac{1}{n}\right)^{-p}$$

$$= \left[1 + p.\frac{3}{2n} + O\left(\frac{1}{n^2}\right)\right]\left[1 - \frac{p}{n} + O\left(\frac{1}{n^2}\right)\right]$$

$$= \left[1 + \left(\frac{3}{2} - 1\right)\frac{p}{n} + O\left(\frac{1}{n^2}\right)\right]$$

$$= 1 + \frac{\frac{1}{2}p}{n} + O\left(\frac{1}{n^2}\right).$$

Then by Gauss test, the series is convergent if $p/2 > 1$, *i.e.*, $p > 2$ and divergent if $p/2 \le 1$, *i.e*, $p \le 2$.

7. *If x, α, β, γ are all positive, discuss the convergence of hypergeometric series*

$$1+\frac{\alpha.\beta}{1.\gamma}+\frac{\alpha(\alpha+\beta)\beta(\beta+1)}{1.2.\gamma(\gamma+1)}x^2+\frac{\alpha(\alpha+1)(\alpha+2)\beta(\beta+1)(\beta+2)}{1.2.3.\gamma.(\gamma+1).(\gamma+2)}$$

SOLUTION. Since, x, α, β, γ are all positive, the given series is a series of positive terms. Neglecting first term we have,

$$u_n=\frac{\alpha(\alpha+1)...(\alpha+n-1)\beta(\beta+1)...(\beta+n-1)}{1.2...n.\gamma.(\gamma+1)...(\gamma+n-1)}.x^n$$

$$\Rightarrow u_{n+1}=\frac{\alpha(\alpha+1)...(\alpha+n-1)(\alpha+n)\beta(\beta+1)...(\beta+n-1)(\beta+n)}{1.2...n(n+1).\gamma.(\gamma+1)...(\gamma+n-1)(\gamma+n)}\cdot x^{n+1}$$

$$\therefore \frac{u_n}{u_{n+1}}=\frac{(n+1)(\gamma+n)}{(\alpha+n)(\beta+n)}.\frac{1}{x}$$

$$\Rightarrow \lim_{n\to\infty}\frac{u_n}{u_{n+1}}=\frac{(n+1)(\gamma+n)}{(\alpha+n)(\beta+n)}.\frac{1}{x}=\frac{1}{x}$$

$\therefore$ By ratio test, the series is convergent if $\frac{1}{x} > 1$, *i.e.*, $x < 1$ and divergent if $x>1$.

When $x = 1$, the ratio test is fails.

In this case, consider

$$\therefore \frac{u_n}{u_{n+1}}=\left(\frac{(n+1)(n+\gamma)}{(\alpha+n)(\beta+n)}\right)=\frac{\left(1+\frac{1}{n}\right)\left(\frac{\gamma}{n}+1\right)}{\left(1+\frac{\alpha}{n}\right)\left(1+\frac{\beta}{n}\right)}$$

$$=\left[\left(1+\frac{1}{n}\right)\left(1+\frac{\gamma}{n}\right)\right]\left(1+\frac{\alpha}{n}\right)^{-1}\left(1+\frac{\beta}{n}\right)^{-1}$$

$$=\left[1+(1+\gamma)\frac{1}{n}+O\left(\frac{1}{n^2}\right)\right]\left[1-\frac{\alpha}{n}+O\left(\frac{1}{n^2}\right)\right]\left[1-\frac{\beta}{n}+O\left(\frac{1}{n^2}\right)\right]$$

$$=1+\frac{1+\gamma-\alpha-\beta}{n}+O\left(\frac{1}{n^2}\right)$$

Then by Gauss test, the series is convergent if $1+\gamma-\alpha-\beta > 1$ and divergent if $1+\gamma-\alpha-\beta \le 1$, *i.e.*, the series is convergent if $\gamma > \alpha+\beta$ and divergent if $\gamma \le \alpha+\beta$.

Similar Problems

(1) Test the convergence of the series $1-\frac{1}{2^p}+\frac{1}{3^p}-\frac{1}{4^p}+...(p>0)$. **Ans.** Convergent.

(2) Test the convergence of the series $\frac{1}{x}-\frac{1}{x+a}+\frac{1}{x+2a}+..., x>0, a>0$. **Ans.** Convergent.

8. *Test the convergence of the series*

$$\frac{\log 2}{2^2}-\frac{\log 3}{3^2}+\frac{\log 4}{4^2}-...$$

SOLUTION. The given series is an alternating series Here, the nth term

$$t_n=(-1)^n u_n, \text{ where } u_n=\frac{\log(n+1)}{(n+1)^2}>0$$

$$\lim_{n\to\infty}u_n=\lim_{n\to\infty}\frac{\log(n+1)}{(n+1)^2}$$

$$=\lim_{n\to\infty}\frac{\log(n+1)}{(n+1)}.\frac{1}{(n+1)}=0.$$

Now, we shall show that $u_{n+1} \le u_n \ \forall\ n$.

Let $f(x)=\frac{\log x}{x^2}, x>0$

Then $f'(x)=\frac{x^2.\frac{1}{x}-2x\log x}{x^4}$

$$=\frac{1-2\log x}{x^3}<0 \text{ when } x>e^{1/2}.$$

Therefore, the function $f(x)$ is monotonically decreasing for all $x>e^{1/2}$. We know that

$$2<e<3 \Rightarrow 2^{1/2}<e^{1/2}<3^{1/2}$$

so $f(n+2) \le f(n+1)$ for all n.

i.e, $u_{n+1} \le u_n \ \forall\ n$.

Hence, by Leibnitz test the given series is convergent.

9. *Test the absolute convergence of the series* $1-\frac{1}{2\sqrt{2}}+\frac{1}{3\sqrt{3}}-...$

SOLUTION. Here, $\Sigma u_n = 1 - \frac{1}{2\sqrt{2}} + \frac{1}{3\sqrt{3}} - \ldots$

Then series Σu_n is absolutely convergent if $\Sigma|u_n|$ is convergent.

Now $\Sigma|u_n| = 1 + \frac{1}{2\sqrt{2}} + \frac{1}{3\sqrt{3}} + \ldots$

$= 1 + \frac{1}{2^{3/2}} + \frac{1}{3^{3/2}}$

$= \Sigma \frac{1}{n^{3/2}}.$

Hence, the series is convergent ($\because p = 3/2 > 1$).

$\Rightarrow$ The given series is absolutely convergent.

10. *Show that the series* $\frac{1}{\sqrt{1}} - \frac{1}{\sqrt{2}} + \frac{1}{\sqrt{3}} - \ldots$ *is conditionally convergent.*

SOLUTION. The given series is an alternating series.

$\therefore$ The nth term

$t_n = (-1)^{n-1} u_n$ where $u_n = \frac{1}{\sqrt{n}} > 0.$

Now $u_{n+1} - u_n = \frac{1}{\sqrt{n+1}} - \frac{1}{\sqrt{n}}$

$= \frac{\sqrt{n} - \sqrt{n+1}}{\sqrt{n}\sqrt{n+1}} < 0.$

$\therefore \quad u_{n+1} < u_n$

$\Rightarrow \lim_{n\to\infty} u_n = \lim_{n\to\infty} \frac{1}{\sqrt{n}} = 0.$

$\therefore$ By Leibnitz test, the given series is convergent.

But the series $\Sigma \left|\frac{(-1)^{n-1}}{\sqrt{n}}\right| = \Sigma \frac{1}{\sqrt{n}}$ is divergent. $\left(\because p = \frac{1}{2} < 1\right)$

Hence, the given series is conditionally convergent.

11. *Discuss the convergence of the series* $1 + \frac{x}{1!} + \frac{x^2}{2!} + \ldots$ *for all values of x.*

SOLUTION. Here, we have

$$u_n = \frac{x^{n-1}}{(n-1)!} \quad \Rightarrow \quad u_{n+1} = \frac{x^n}{n!}$$

So,

$$\frac{|u_n|}{|u_{n+1}|} = \frac{|x|^{n-1}}{(n-1)!} \cdot \frac{n!}{|x|^n} = \frac{n}{|x|}, \text{ for } x \neq 0$$

$$\therefore \lim_{n\to\infty} \frac{|u_n|}{|u_{n+1}|} = \lim_{n\to\infty} \frac{n}{|x|} = \infty, \text{ for } x \neq 0.$$

$\therefore$ By the ratio test, the series $\sum_{n=1}^{\infty} |u_n|$ is convergent when $x \neq 0$.

Thus $\sum_{n=1}^{\infty} u_n$ is absolutely convergent.

If $x=0$, then the series becomes $1+0+0+\ldots$ and so is convergent.

Thus the given series is absolutely convergent.

- Since for a convergent series $\sum_{n=1}^{\infty} u_n$, $\lim_{n\to\infty} u_n = 0$. Therefore, $\lim_{n\to\infty} \frac{x^n}{n!} = 0$ is a useful result.

22.17.1 MORE ABOUT CONDITIONAL AND ABSOLUTE CONVERGENCE

(i) If Σu_n is an absolute convergent series, then the series of its positive and the series of its negative terms are both convergent.

(ii) The divergence of $\Sigma|u_n|$ does not imply the divergence of Σu_n. For example, if $u_n = \frac{(-1)^{n-1}}{n}$ then $\Sigma|u_n|$ is divergent, whereas Σu_n is convergent.

(iii) Since, the series $\Sigma|u_n|$ is of positive terms, therefore, all the tests established for testing the convergence of series of positive terms, will also be the tests for determining the absolute convergence of the series Σu_n.

(iv) If Σu_n is conditionally convergent, then the series of its positive terms and the series of its negative terms are both divergent.

(v) A series with mixed signs cannot converge, if the series of its positive terms is convergent (divergent) and the series of its negative terms is divergent (convergent).

22.17.2 SUMMARY OF THE TESTS

For the guidance of the students we given below a working procedure for determining the convergence of a series.

(i) If in a series of positive terms, n^{th} term does not tend to zero, the series is divergent.

(ii) If n^{th} terms tends to zero, then a comparison test may be applied when its nth term neither involves any power of n nor involve factorials.

(iii) If the nth term is the nth power of some expression, then Cauchy's root test may be applied.

(iv) When the series involves increasing power of x or involves factorials, one should start with the ratio test.

(v) If the $\lim\limits_{n\to\infty} \frac{u_n}{u_{n+1}}$ turns out to be 1, then the ratio test fails and Raabe's test or Gauss's test is applied provided $\frac{u_n}{u_{n+1}}$ does not involves e, otherwise logarithmic test is applied.

(vi) For an arbitrary terms series, try with the ratio test for absolute convergence. If the limit turns out to be 1, then try some other tests. When the terms have alternating signs, then Leibnitz's test is suggested.

Exercise-22.4

1. Test the convergence of the following series
$$1-\frac{1}{2}+\frac{1}{3}-\frac{1}{4}+\ldots$$

2. Prove that the following series is absolute convergent.
$$\left(\frac{\sqrt{2}-1}{1}\right)-\left(\frac{\sqrt{3}-\sqrt{2}}{2}\right)+\left(\frac{\sqrt{4}-\sqrt{3}}{3}\right)-\ldots$$

3. Show that the series $\Sigma\frac{\sin n\theta}{n^2}$ is absolutely convergent.

4. Show that the series
$$\frac{1^2}{4^2}+\frac{1^2.5^2}{4^2.8^2}+\frac{1^2.5^2.9^2}{4^2.8^2.12^2}+\ldots$$ is convergent.

5. Examine the convergence of the series
$$1+a+b^2+a^3+b^4+\ldots$$

6. Test the convergence of the series
$$\frac{x}{1}+\frac{1}{2}\cdot\frac{x^2}{3}+\frac{1.3}{2.4}\cdot\frac{x^3}{5}+\ldots$$

7. Show that the series $\Sigma(-1)^{n-1}\sin\frac{1}{n}$ is conditionally convergent.

8. Test for convergence the series
$$\Sigma\left(\frac{n^{n-1}.x^{n-1}}{n!}\right).$$

9. Test the convergence of the series
$$1+\frac{a(1-a)}{1^2}+\frac{(1+a)a(1-a)(2-a)}{1^2.2^2}+\ldots$$

10. Show that the series $\frac{2}{1^2}-\frac{3}{2^2}+\frac{4}{3^2}-\frac{5}{4^2}+\ldots$ converge conditionally.

11. Show that the series $\frac{1}{x+1}-\frac{1}{x+2}+\frac{1}{x+3}-\ldots$ is convergent except when x is a negative integer.

12. Show that the series $\Sigma(-1)^n[\sqrt{n^2+1}-n]$ is conditionally convergent.

13. Show that the series $\sum\limits_{n=1}^{\infty}\frac{(-1)^{n+1}.n}{n^2+1}$ is not absolutely convergent.

14. Show that the binomial series
$$1+nx+\frac{n(n-1)}{2!}x^2+\ldots\frac{n(n-1)\ldots(n-r+1)}{r!}x^r+\ldots$$
is absolutely convergent when $|x|<1$.

15. Test the convergence of the series
$$\sum_{n=1}^{\infty}\left[\frac{1}{n}+\frac{(-1)^{n+1}}{\sqrt{n}}\right].$$

16. Show that the series
$$x+\frac{a-b}{2!}x^2+\frac{(a-b)(a-2b)}{3!}x^3+\frac{(a-b)(a-2b)(a-3b)}{4!}x^4+\ldots$$
is absolutely convergent if $|x|<\frac{1}{|b|}$.

17. Show that the series

$$1-\frac{1}{2^3}-\frac{1}{4^3}+\frac{1}{3^3}-\frac{1}{6^3}-\frac{1}{8^3}+ \ldots+\frac{1}{(2n-1)^3}-\frac{1}{(4n-2)^3}-\frac{1}{(4n)^3}+\ldots$$

is absolutely convergent.

18. Show that the series

$$2\sin\frac{x}{3}+4\sin\frac{x}{9}+8\sin\frac{x}{27}+\ldots$$

converges absolutely for all finite values of x.

19. Discuss the convergence of the series

$$x^2(\log 2)^q + x^3(\log 3)^q + x^4(\log 4)^q + \ldots$$

20. Discuss the convergence of the following series :

(i) $\frac{1}{\log 2}-\frac{1}{\log 3}+\frac{1}{\log 4}-\frac{1}{\log 5}+\ldots$

(ii) $1-\frac{1}{5}+\frac{1}{9}-\frac{1}{13}+\ldots\infty$

(iii) $\sum_{n=0}^{\infty}\frac{(-1)^n}{n!}$ (DELHI–2002)

(iv) $\frac{1}{1.2}-\frac{1}{3.4}+\frac{1}{5.6}-\frac{1}{7.8}+\ldots\infty$

(OSMANIA–2003)

(v) $1-2x+3x^2-4x^3+\ldots\infty\left(x<\frac{1}{2}\right)$

(COCHIN–2005)

(vi) $\frac{x}{1+x}-\frac{x^2}{1+x^2}+\frac{x^3}{1+x^3}-\frac{x^4}{1+x^4}+\ldots\infty$ $(0<x<1)$

(VTU–2004, DELHI–2002)

Hint to Selected Problems

1. $u_n=\frac{1}{n},\ u_{n+1}=\frac{1}{n+1}$

$u_n-u_{n+1}=\frac{1}{n+1}>0\ \forall\ n\in N\Rightarrow u_n>u_{n+1}.$

Also $\lim u_n=0.$

3. Since $\Sigma\left|\frac{\sin n\theta}{n^2}\right|\le\Sigma\frac{1}{n^2}.$

The series $\Sigma\frac{1}{n^2}$ is convergent.

7. $u_n=\sin\left(\frac{1}{n}\right)>0$

$\sin\left(\frac{1}{n+1}\right)<\frac{1}{\sin n}\Rightarrow u_{n+1}<u_n.$

Also $\lim_{n\to\infty}u_n=\lim_{n\to\infty}\sin\frac{1}{n}=0$

8. By D'Alembert's test, series is convergent for $x<\frac{1}{e}$ and divergent for $x>\frac{1}{e}$.

Then by logarithmic series, for $x=\frac{1}{e}$ the series is convergent.

18. $\sum_{n=1}^{\infty}u_n=\sum_{n=1}^{\infty}2^n\sin\left(\frac{x}{3^n}\right)$

$\therefore\quad u_n=2^n\sin\frac{x}{3^n}>0,\forall\ n\in N$

$\Rightarrow |u_n|=u_n\Rightarrow\Sigma|u_n|=\Sigma u_n$

$u_{n+1}=2^{n+1}\sin\left(\frac{x}{3^{n+1}}\right)$

$\Rightarrow\quad \lim_{n\to\infty}\left|\frac{u_n}{u_{n+1}}\right|=\frac{3}{2}>1.$

Then by D'Alembert's ratio test. The given series is absolutely convergent.

ANSWERS

1. Convergent **5.** Convergent. **6.** Convergent if $x\le 1$ and divergent if $x>1$.

20. (i) Convergent (ii) Convergent (iii) Convergent (iv) Convergent (v) Convergent

□□□□□□

Chapter

23 Differential Equations

23.1 INTRODUCTION

Sometimes in the field of Physics, Chemistry, Engineering and Biology, it is necessary to prepare a Mathematical model which represents some specific problems. In these Mathematical Models, generally we tries to find such functions who satisfies the given equation which contain the unknown function and some of its differential coefficients. These equations are called Differential equations.

23.2 DIFFERENTIAL EQUATION

An equation is said to be differential equation if it contains not only the dependent variables and independent variables but their differential coefficients also.

For example.

$$\frac{dy}{dx} = x + 9 \quad \text{...(1)}$$

$$\frac{dy}{dx} + x\cos x = 0 \quad \text{...(2)}$$

$$\frac{d^2y}{dx^2} = 0 \quad \text{...(3)}$$

$$\frac{dy}{dx} = \sin x \quad \text{...(4)}$$

$$\frac{d^2y}{dx^2} = e^x \quad \text{...(5)}$$

$$\frac{d^2y}{dx^2} + 4y^2 = x \quad \text{...(6)}$$

$$\left(\frac{d^2y}{dx^2}\right)^3 + \left(\frac{dy}{dx}\right)^3 = x^3 + 7y + 9 \quad \text{...(7)}$$

are differential equations.

23.3 KINDS OF DIFFERENTIAL EQUATIONS

(i) Ordinary Differential Equation: A differential equation is said to be ordinary differential equation if it contains only one independent variable. In article 23.2 the equations from (1) to (7) are all ordinary differential equations because in these equations only one variable x is used.

(ii) Partial Differential Equation: A differential equation is said to be partial differential equation if it contains more than one independent variable and derivatives.

For example.

$$y^2 \frac{\partial z}{\partial x} + y \frac{\partial z}{\partial y} = x$$

is a partial differential equation because it contains two independent variables x and y.

- In this chapter we shall discuss only ordinary differential equations.

23.4 ORDER OF A DIFFERENTIAL EQUATION

The order of a differential equation is the order of the derivative of the highest order appearing in it.

For example. The equation $\frac{dy}{dx} = x + 7$ is a differential equation of order 1 while the differential equation $\left(\frac{d^2y}{dx^2}\right)^2 + 5\frac{dy}{dx} = x^2 + 6y$ is a differential equation of second order.

23.4.1 DEGREE OF A DIFFERENTIAL EQUATION

The degree of a differential equation is the degree (power) of the highest order differential coefficient appearing in it. **For example.** In article 23.2,

Equation (1) is a differential equation of first order and first degree.
Equation (2) is a differential equation of first order and first degree.
Equation (3) is a differential equation of second order and first degree.
Equation (4) is a differential equation of first order and first degree.
Equation (5) is a differential equation of second order and first degree.
Equation (6) is a differential equation of second order and first degree.
Equation (7) is a differential equation of second order and third degree.

- To find the order and degree of a differential equation, it should be free from radicals and fractions.

For Example.

$$\sqrt{\left[\left(\frac{d^2y}{dx^2}\right)^2 + y\right]} = \sin x$$

$$\Rightarrow \quad \left(\frac{d^2y}{dx^2}\right)^2 + y = \sin^2 x$$

$\Rightarrow$ order = 2, degree = 2

23.5 SOLUTION OF A DIFFERENTIAL EQUATION

Any relation between the dependent and independent variable which satisfies the given differential equation is called the solution of the given differential equation.

23.5.1 GENERAL SOLUTION OF A DIFFERENTIAL EQUATION

If the solution of nth order differential equation contains n arbitrary constants, then it is called general solution or complete primitive.

23.5.2 PARTICULAR SOLUTION OF A DIFFERENTIAL EQUATION

A solution obtained from the general solution by giving particular values to the arbitrary constants in the general solution is called particular solution or particular integral.

23.6 FORMATION OF A DIFFERENTIAL EQUATION

If an equation contains n arbitrary constants, a differential equation of nth order can be obtained by eliminating these arbitrary constants from the given equations and n equations obtained by differentiate the given equations n times. Let us suppose there is an equation representing a family of curves, containing n arbitrary constants. Then in order to find its differential equation we proceed as follows.

WORKING PROCEDURE

STEP 1. Differentiate the given equation of family of curves n times to get n more equations containing n arbitrary constants and derivatives.

STEP 2. Eliminating all the n constants from the above $(n + 1)$ equations to get an equation containing a nth order derivative, which is the required differential equation of the family of curves.

23.7 METHOD OF FORMING A DIFFERENTIAL EQUATION

Making of a differential equation corresponding to a dependent variable is depend upon the given situation. Let us consider the following situations.

(a) When a geometrical fact is represented by differential calculus: Let the slope of a straight line be m. Then this fact can be represented by the differential equation as follows:

$$\frac{dy}{dx} = m$$

(b) If a scientific fact is represented by a differential equation: Let the acceleration of a moving particle be f. Then we represent it in the form of differential equation as follows:

$$\frac{d^2x}{dt^2} = f$$

(c) By eliminating arbitrary constant from the given equation:

$$y = 4\,ax \qquad \text{...(1)}$$

$$\therefore \quad \frac{dy}{dx} = 4a \qquad \text{...(2)}$$

The differential equation obtained from (1) and (2) is

$$x\frac{dy}{dx} = 4ax = y$$

$$\Rightarrow \quad x\frac{dy}{dx} = y$$

WORKING PROCEDURE

To make a differential equation from the equation of x and y use the following steps:

STEP 1. Write the given equation.

STEP 2. Differentiate the given equation w.r.t. x as many times as the number of constants.

STEP 3. Solve the equations of step (1) and step (2).

23.8 SOME SPECIAL EXAMPLES

(a) Differential equation of Simple Harmonic Motion

We know that S.H.M. is a motion in which a particle moved in straight line such that the direction of its acceleration is always towards a fixed point. Let O be the centre, known as origin. Let at A, the particle be at rest. It start to move from A to O such that $OA = a$.

Let at time t, the particle be at P such that $OP = x$.

By definition of S.H.M.

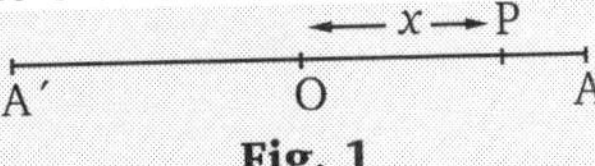

Fig. 1

$$\frac{dv}{dt} \propto x \Rightarrow \frac{dv}{dt} = \mu x$$

where μ is the constant of proportionality called intensity of force.

(b) Differential equation for the motion under gravity

Let a particle be falling from the height h to the earth. At time t, its height from the earth be x. Then by Newton's second law of motion, we have

$$m \cdot g = -\frac{\mu}{x^2}$$

where g is the gravitational force.

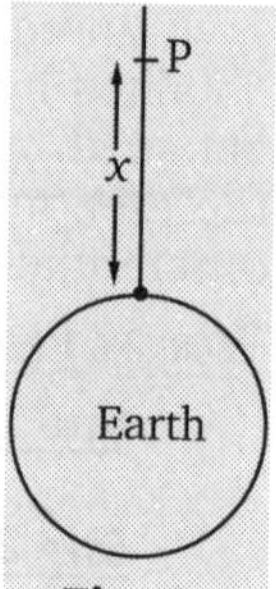

Fig. 2

23.9 GENERAL AND PARTICULAR SOLUTIONS OF A DIFFERENTIAL EQUATION

We know that if the solution of nth order differential equation contains n arbitrary constants, then it is called general solution but if we give some particular values to the arbitrary constants, then solution thus obtained is called particular solution.

For Example. Consider the differential equation

$$\frac{d^3y}{dx^3} = 0 \qquad ...(i)$$

Its primitives is $y = Ax^2 + Bx + C$, which is the general solution of the given equation. If $A = 0$, $C = 0$ and $B = 5$, then particular solution of (1) y given by $y = 5x$ and if $A = 3$, $B = 0 = C$, then particular solution of (1) y given by $y = 3x^2$

Solved Examples

1. *Find the order and degree of the following differential equation.*

(i) $\frac{dy}{dx} = 3x + 7$

(ii) $\frac{d^2y}{dx^2} + \frac{dy}{dx} + P_x = y$

(iii) $\left(\frac{dy}{dx}\right)^3 + \frac{dy}{dx} + \sin x = 0$

(iv) $\frac{dy}{dx} = xy - \sin x$

SOLUTION. (i) First order and first degree

(ii) Second order and first degree

(iii) First order and third degree

(iv) First order and first degree.

2. *The slope of a curve at every point (x, y) is two times the sum of its coordinates. Represent it by differential equation.*

SOLUTION. The coordinates of $P = (x, y)$

Sum of coordinates $= (x + y)$

Slope of the curve at $P = 2(x + y)$

Slope of the curve at $P = \frac{dy}{dx}$

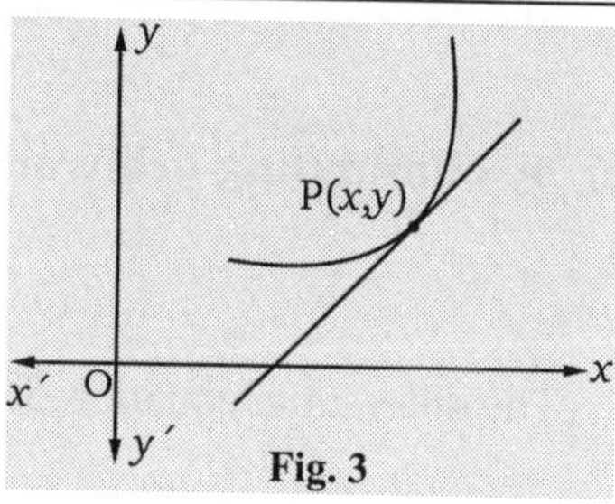

Fig. 3

As per given $\frac{dy}{dx} = 2(x + y)$

which is the required differential equation.

3. *In a city, the rate of increase of population, equal to the product of $(P - 75000)$ and P where P is the population. Express it by differential equation.*

SOLUTION. Rate of change of increase in population

$$= \frac{dP}{dt}$$

As per given $\frac{dP}{dt} = P(P - 75000)$

Which is the required differential equation.

4. *The rate of change of 100 gm sugar to dextrose is directly proportional to the original quantity. Represent the rate of change at time t in the form of differential equation.*

SOLUTION. Let in time t, m gm sugar converted into dextrose.

$\therefore$ Remains sugar = $(100 - m)$ gm

Rate of change $= \dfrac{dm}{dt}$

Now as per given

$$\frac{dm}{dt} \propto (100 - m) \qquad ...(1)$$

$$\Rightarrow \quad \frac{dm}{dt} = k(100 - m),$$

where k is a constant of proportionality. Which is the required differential equation.

Similar Problems

(1) The rate of evaporation of a spherical drop of rain water is directly proportional to its surface area. Express the rate of change of spherical drop in the form of differential equation. **Ans.** $\dfrac{dr}{dt} = k$

(2) Find the differential equation of the following equations:

(i) $xy = c^2$ (ii) $y = (c_1 + c_2x)e^x$

Ans. (i) $\dfrac{dy}{dx} = -\dfrac{y}{x}$, (ii) $\dfrac{d^2y}{dx^2} - 2\dfrac{dy}{dx} + y = 0$

5. *Represent the circles by differential equation whose centre is on x-axis and radius is r.*

SOLUTION. The equation of the circles whose centre is on x-axis and radius is r, is given by

$$(x - a)^2 + (y - 0)^2 = r^2$$

$$\Rightarrow \quad (x - a)^2 + y^2 = r^2 \qquad ...(1)$$

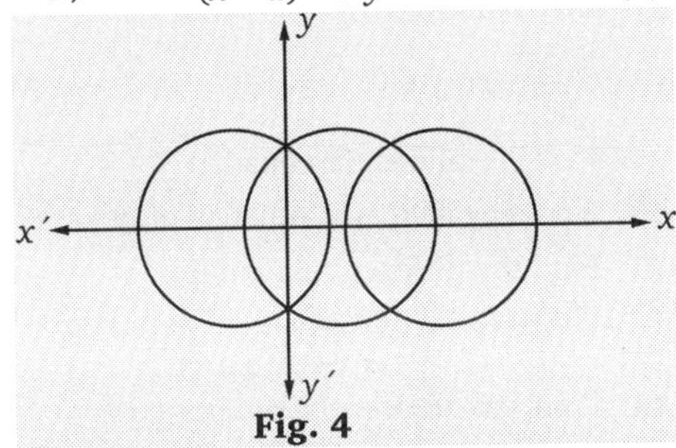

Fig. 4

Differentiating (1) w.r.t. x, we get

$$2(x - a) + 2y\frac{dy}{dx} = 0$$

$$\Rightarrow \quad (x - a) + y\frac{dy}{dx} = 0$$

Again differentiating,

$$1 - 0 + \left(\frac{dy}{dx}\right)^2 + y\left(\frac{d^2y}{dx^2}\right) = 0$$

$$\Rightarrow \quad y\frac{d^2y}{dx^2} + \left(\frac{dy}{dx}\right)^2 + 1 = 0$$

which is the required differential equation.

6. *Find the differential equation of all circles in first quadrant of xy-plane which touches with the axes.*

Fig. 5

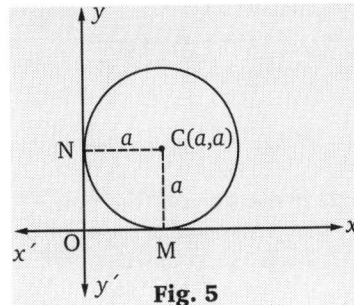

SOLUTION. Let centre of the circle be (a, a) and radius is a.

Equation of the circle

$$(x - a)^2 + (y - a)^2 = a^2 \qquad ...(1)$$

where a is arbitrary constant.

Differentiating (1) w.r.t. x, we get,

$$2(x - a) + 2(y - a)\frac{dy}{dx} = 0$$

$$\Rightarrow \quad (x - a) = -(y - a)\frac{dy}{dx} \qquad ...(2)$$

$$\Rightarrow \quad x - a + y\frac{dy}{dx} - a\frac{dy}{dx} = 0$$

$$\Rightarrow \quad x + y\frac{dy}{dx} = a\left(1 + \frac{dy}{dx}\right)$$

$$\Rightarrow \qquad a = \frac{x + y\frac{dy}{dx}}{1 + \frac{dy}{dx}}. \qquad ...(3)$$

From eq. (1) and (2), we get

$$(y-a)^2\left(\frac{dy}{dx}\right)^2 + (y-a)^2 = a^2$$

$$\Rightarrow \quad (y-a)^2\left[1+\left(\frac{dy}{dx}\right)^2\right] = a^2 \quad ...(4)$$

Putting the value of a from eq. (3) in (4), we get

$$\left[y - \frac{x + y\frac{dy}{dx}}{1+\left(\frac{dy}{dx}\right)}\right]^2 \left[1+\left(\frac{dy}{dx}\right)^2\right] = \left[\frac{x + y\frac{dy}{dx}}{1+\frac{dy}{dx}}\right]^2$$

which is the required differential equation.

Exercise-23.1

1. Find the order and degree of the following differential equation.
   (i) $dy + (3x + \cot x)dx = 0$
   (ii) $\frac{d^2y}{dx^2} + y\left(\frac{dy}{dx}\right) + 1 = 0$
   (iii) $L\frac{d^2Q}{dt^2} + R\frac{dQ}{dt} + \frac{Q}{c} = 0$
   (iv) $\frac{d^3y}{dx^3} + x\frac{d^2y}{dx^2} + 2y\left(\frac{dy}{dx}\right)^2 + xy = 0$
   (v) $\frac{d^2r}{d\theta^2} = \sqrt[4]{1+\left(\frac{dr}{d\theta}\right)^2}$
   (vi) $\left(\frac{d^2y}{dx^2}\right)^{3/2} = \left(x + \frac{dy}{dx}\right)^{1/2}$
2. If the slope of the tangent to the curve at (x, y) is equal to the three times to sum of the cubes of its abscissa and ordinate. Find the differential equation.
3. Find the differential equation for the straight lines whose distance from origin is 1 unit.
4. Find the differential equation of all circles who touches y-axis at origin.
5. Find the differential equation of all parabolas whose vertex is at origin and foci are on y-axis.
6. Find the differential equation of all ellipse $\frac{x^2}{a^2} + \frac{y^2}{b^2} = 1$, where a and b are constant.
7. Prove that $y = \frac{A}{x} + B$ is the solution of the differential equation $\frac{d^2y}{dx^2} + \frac{2}{x}\frac{dy}{dx} = 0$.
8. Prove that $y = A \cos mx + B \sin mx$ is the solution of the differential equation $\frac{d^2y}{dx^2} + m^2y = 0$.
9. Find the differential equation of $y = a + bx + cx^2$.
10. Find the differential equation of $xy = ae^x + be^{-x}$.
11. Find the differential equation of $x^2 + y^2 = a^2$.
12. Find the differential equation of $y = e^x (A \cos x + B \sin x)$.
13. Find the differential equation of $y = A \cos x^2 + B \sin x^2$.

ANSWERS

1. (i) order = 1, degree = 1 (ii) order = 2, degree = 1 (iii) order = 2 degree = 1
   (iv) order = 3, degree = 1 (v) order = 2, degree = 4 (vi) order = 2 degree = 3

2. $\frac{dy}{dx} = 3(x^3 + y^3)$ 3. $\left(x\frac{dy}{dx} - y\right)^2 = 1 + \left(\frac{dy}{dx}\right)^2$ 4. $y^2 - x^2 = 2xy\frac{dy}{dx}$ 5. $x\frac{dy}{dx} = 2y$

6. $y\frac{dy}{dx} = x\left[y\frac{d^2y}{dx^2} + \left(\frac{dy}{dx}\right)^2\right]$ 9. $\frac{d^3y}{dx^3} = 0$ 10. $x\frac{d^2y}{dx^2} + 2\frac{dy}{dx} = xy$

11. $\frac{dy}{dx} = -\frac{x}{y}$ 12. $\frac{d^2y}{dx^2} - 2\left(\frac{dy}{dx}\right) + 2y = 0$ 13. $x\frac{d^2y}{dx^2} - \frac{dy}{dx} + 4x^3y = 0$

23.10 SOLUTION OF DIFFERENTIAL EQUATIONS

(I) Type I. $\dfrac{dy}{dx} = f(x)$ ...(1)

We know that integration is the reverse process of differentiation. To solve the equation (1), integrate both sides.

WORKING PROCEDURE

STEP 1. Write the given equation of the form $dy = f(x)dx$.
STEP 2. Integrate and use the constant of integration.

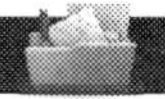

Solved Examples

1. *Solve the differential equation*

$$\frac{dy}{dx} = \cos x \cdot$$

SOLUTION. We have, $\dfrac{dy}{dx} = \cos x$

$\Rightarrow \quad dy = \cos x\, dx$

Integrating both sides, we get

$$\int dy = \int \cos x\, dx + c$$

$\Rightarrow \quad y = \sin x + c,$

where c is any constant.

2. *Solve the differential equation*

$$\frac{dy}{dx} = \sec^2 x + 3x^2.$$

SOLUTION. We have $\dfrac{dy}{dx} = \sec^2 x + 3x^2$

$\Rightarrow \quad dy = \sec^2 x\, dx + 3x^2\, dx$

Integrating both sides, we get

$$\int dy = \int \sec^2 x\, dx + 3\int x^2 dx + c$$

$\Rightarrow \quad y = \tan x + x^3 + c,$

where c is any constant.

3. *Solve the differential equation*

$$\frac{dy}{dx} = \sec x(2\sec x + \tan x).$$

SOLUTION. We have $\dfrac{dy}{dx} = \sec x(2\sec x + \tan x)$

$\Rightarrow \quad dy = 2\sec^2 x\, dx + \sec x \tan x\, dx$

Integrating both sides, we get

$$\int dy = 2\int \sec^2 x\, dx + \int \sec x \tan x dx + c$$

$\Rightarrow y = 2 \tan x + \sec x + c,$

where c is any constant.

Similar Problems

(1) Solve the differential equation $\dfrac{dy}{dx} = \sin(5x+9)$. **Ans.** $y = -\dfrac{1}{5}\cos(5x+9) + c$

(2) Solve the differential equation $\dfrac{dy}{dx} = x^3 + \sin 4x$. **Ans.** $y = \dfrac{1}{4}x^4 - \dfrac{1}{4}\cos 4x + c$

(3) Solve the differential equation $\dfrac{dy}{dx} = \dfrac{\cos x}{2 - \cos^2 x}$. **Ans.** $y = \tan^{-1}(\sin x) + c$

4. *Solve the differential equation* $\cos y\, dy + \cos x \sin y\, dx = 0$. *Given* : $x = \dfrac{\pi}{2}$, *if* $y = \dfrac{\pi}{2}$.

SOLUTION. We have $\cos y\, dy + \cos x \sin y\, dx = 0$

$\Rightarrow \quad \dfrac{\cos y}{\sin y} dy + \cos x\, dx = 0$

On integrating, we get

$$\int \frac{\cos y}{\sin y} dy + \int \cos x\, dx = c$$

$\Rightarrow \quad \log \sin y + \sin x = c$

$x = \dfrac{\pi}{2}$ if $y = \dfrac{\pi}{2}$ (given)

$\Rightarrow \quad \log \sin\dfrac{\pi}{2} + \sin\dfrac{\pi}{2} = c$

$\therefore \quad c = 1$

$\therefore \quad \log \sin y + \sin x = 1$

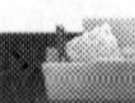

Exercise-23.2

Solve the following differential equations.

1. $\frac{dy}{dx}=e^x$
2. $\frac{dy}{dx}=\frac{1}{x}$
3. $\frac{dy}{dx}=\tan x$
4. $\frac{dy}{dx}=\cot x$
5. $\frac{dy}{dx}=\operatorname{cosec}^2 x+\sec^2 x+\cos x$
6. $\frac{dy}{dx}=\sec^2 x+4x$
7. $\frac{dy}{dx}=x^2+\sin 4x$
8. $\frac{dy}{dx}=x^3+x^2+6x+9$
9. $\frac{dy}{dx}=\sin^8 x\cos x$
10. $(1+x^2)\frac{dy}{dx}=x$
11. $\frac{dy}{dx}+\frac{1+x^2}{x}=0$
12. $\frac{dy}{dx}=\operatorname{cosec} x(3\operatorname{cosec} x+4\cot x)$
13. $\frac{dy}{dx}=\cos(ax+b)$

ANSWERS

1. $y = e^x + c$ 2. $y = \log x + c$ 3. $y = \log \sec x + c$ 4. $y = \log \sin x + c$
5. $y = -\cot x + \tan x - \sin x$ 6. $y = \tan x + 2x^2 + c$ 7. $\frac{x^3}{3}-\frac{\cos 4x}{4}+c$
8. $\frac{x^4}{4}+\frac{x^3}{3}+3x^2+9x+c$ 9. $y=\frac{\sin^9 x}{9}+c$ 10. $y=\frac{1}{2}\log(1+x^2)+c$
11. $y+\log x+\frac{1}{2}x^2=c$ 12. $y = -3\cot x - 4\operatorname{cosec} x + c$ 13. $y=-\frac{1}{a}\sin(ax+b)+c$

(II) Type II. Equation in which variables are separable

Here, the equation is of the form

$$\frac{dy}{dx}=\frac{f(x)}{\phi(y)}$$

Using transposition of terms, we get

$$f(x)\,dx = \phi(y)\,dy$$

We separate all the terms of *x* with *dx* and all the terms of *y* with *dy*.

Then adding the constant of integration after integrate.

WORKING PROCEDURE

STEP 1. Write the given equation in the form of $\frac{dy}{dx}=f(x)\cdot g(y)$

STEP 2. Write all the terms of *x* with *dx*, and all terms of *y* with *dy*, *i.e.*,

$$f(x)dx=\frac{dy}{g(y)}$$

STEP 3. Integrating both the sides.

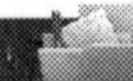

Solved Examples

1. *Solve the differential equation* $\frac{dy}{dx}=\frac{x}{y}$.

SOLUTION. We have $\frac{dy}{dx}=\frac{x}{y}$

$\Rightarrow \quad ydy = xdx$

On integrating, we get

$$\int ydy=\int xdx+c$$

$$\Rightarrow \quad \frac{y^2}{2}=\frac{x^2}{2}+c$$

$\Rightarrow y^2 = x^2 + k$, where *k* is an arbitrary constant.

2. *Solve the differential equation*

$$\frac{dy}{dx}=xy+x+y+1.$$

SOLUTION. We have $\frac{dy}{dx}=xy+x+y+1$

$$= x(y + 1) + 1(y + 1)$$

$\Rightarrow \quad \frac{dy}{dx} = (x+1)(y+1)$

$\Rightarrow \quad \frac{dy}{y+1} = (x+1)dx$

On integrating, we get

$$\int \frac{dy}{y+1} = \int (x+1)dx + c$$

$\Rightarrow \log(y+1) = \frac{x^2}{2} + x + c$, where c is an arbitrary constant.

3. *Solve the differential equation*

$$\frac{dy}{dx} + \sqrt{\left(\frac{1-y^2}{1-x^2}\right)} = 0.$$

SOLUTION. We have $\frac{dy}{dx} + \sqrt{\left(\frac{1-y^2}{1-x^2}\right)} = 0$

$\Rightarrow \quad \frac{dy}{\sqrt{1-y^2}} + \frac{dx}{\sqrt{1-x^2}} = 0$

On integrating, we get

$$\int \frac{dy}{\sqrt{1-y^2}} + \int \frac{dx}{\sqrt{1-x^2}} = c$$

$\Rightarrow \sin^{-1} y + \sin^{-1} x = c$, where c is an arbitrary constant.

4. *Solve the differential equation*

$$\frac{dy}{dx} = e^{x-y} + x^2 e^{-y}.$$

SOLUTION. We have

$$\frac{dy}{dx} = e^{x-y} + x^2 e^{-y} = \frac{e^x}{e^y} + \frac{x^2}{e^y}$$

$\Rightarrow e^y dy = e^x dx + x^2 dx$

On integrating, we get

$$\int e^y dy = \int e^x dx + \int x^2 dx + c$$

$\Rightarrow \quad e^y = e^x + \frac{1}{3}x^3 + c$, where c is an arbitrary constant.

5. *Solve the differential equation* $(1 + x^2)\sec^2 y dy + 2x \tan y dx = 0$. *Given that* $y = \frac{\pi}{4}$ *when* $x = 1$.

SOLUTION. We have $(1+x^2)\sec^2 y dy + 2x\tan y dx = 0$

$\Rightarrow \quad \frac{\sec^2 y}{\tan y}dy + \frac{2x}{1+x^2}dx = 0$

On integrating,

$$\int \frac{\sec^2 y}{\tan y}dy + \int \frac{2x}{1+x^2}dx = 0$$

$\Rightarrow \log \tan y + \log (1 + x^2) = c$

If $y = \frac{\pi}{4}$ and $x = 1$ then

$$c = \log \tan \frac{\pi}{4} + \log(1+1)$$

$\Rightarrow c = \log 2$

$\therefore \log \tan y + \log(1 + x^2) = \log 2$

$\Rightarrow \log[\tan y (1 + x^2)] = \log 2$

$\therefore \quad \tan y = \frac{2}{1+x^2}$

Similar Problems

(1) Solve the differential equation $(x - y^2x)dx - y(1 - x^2)dy = 0$. **Ans.** $(1 - x^2) = c(1 - y^2)$

(2) Solve the differential equation $\left(y - x\frac{dy}{dx}\right) = a\left(y^2 + \frac{dy}{dx}\right)$. **Ans.** $y = c(1 - ay)(a + x)$

6. *Solve the differential equation* $(3x^2y - xy)dx + (2x^3y^2 + x^3y^4)dy = 0$.

SOLUTION. We have

$(3x^2y - xy)dx + (2x^3y^2 + x^3y^4)dy = 0$

$\Rightarrow y(3x^2 - x)dx + x^3(2y^2 + y^4)dy = 0$

$\Rightarrow \left(\frac{3x^2 - x}{x^3}\right)dx + \left(\frac{2y^2 + y^4}{y}\right)dy = 0$

$\Rightarrow \left(\frac{3}{x} - \frac{1}{x^2}\right)dx + (2y + y^3)dy = 0$

On integrating, we get

$$\int \left(\frac{3}{x} - x^{-2}\right)dx + \int (2y + y^3)dy = 0$$

$\Rightarrow 3\log x + \frac{1}{x} + \frac{2y^2}{2} + \frac{y^4}{4} = c$,

where c is an arbitrary constant.

7. *Solve the differential equation* $x^2(y + 1)dx + y^2(x - 1)dy = 0$.

SOLUTION. We have $x^2(y + 1)dx + y^2(x - 1)dy = 0$

$$\Rightarrow \left(\frac{x^2}{x-1}\right)dx + \left(\frac{y^2}{y+1}\right)dy = 0$$

$$\Rightarrow \left(\frac{x^2-1+1}{x-1}\right)dx + \left(\frac{y^2-1+1}{y+1}\right)dy = 0$$

$$\Rightarrow \int\left(x+1+\frac{1}{x-1}\right)dx$$
$$+\int\left(y-1+\frac{1}{y+1}\right)dy = 0$$

On integrating, we get

$$\int\left(x+1+\frac{1}{x-1}\right)dx$$
$$+\int\left(y-1+\frac{1}{y+1}\right)dy = 0$$

$$\Rightarrow \frac{x^2}{2}+x+\log(x-1)+\frac{y^2}{2}$$
$$-y+\log(y+1) = c$$

$$\Rightarrow \frac{1}{2}(x^2+y^2)+(x-y)$$
$$+\log(x-1)(y+1) = c$$

$\Rightarrow (x^2 + y^2) + 2(x - y)$

$+ 2\log(x - 1)(y + 1) = k,$

when k is an arbitrary constant.

8. *Solve the differential equation*

$$\frac{dy}{dx} = e^{ax}\cos y, \text{ if } y(0) = 0.$$

SOLUTION. We have $\dfrac{dy}{dx} = e^{ax}\cos y$

$$\Rightarrow \quad \frac{dy}{\cos y} = e^{ax}dx$$

$$\Rightarrow \quad \sec y\,dy = e^{ax}\,dx$$

On integrating, we get

$$\int \sec y\,dy = \int e^{ax}dx + c$$

$$\Rightarrow \log(\sec y + \tan y) = \frac{1}{a}e^{ax} + c$$

$\Rightarrow a\log(\sec y + \tan y) = e^{ax} + k$ ...(1)

Now if $x = 0$, then $y = 0$

$\Rightarrow a\log(\sec 0 + \tan 0) = e^0 + k$

$\Rightarrow \quad a\log(1 + 0) = 1 + k$

$\Rightarrow \quad k = -1$

Hence, from eq. (1), we get

$$a\log(\sec y + \tan y) = e^{ax} - 1$$

Similar Problems

(1) Solve the differential equation $(1 + e^{2x})dy + (1 + y^2)e^x\,dx = 0$, where $y = 1$ if $x = 0$.

Ans. $\tan^{-1}y + \tan^{-1}(e^x) = \dfrac{\pi}{2}$

(2) Solve the differential equation $\dfrac{dy}{dx} + \dfrac{1+y^3}{xy^2(1+x^2)} = 0$. **Ans.** $(1 + y^3)^2x^6 = k(1 + x^2)^3$

Where k is an arbitrary constant.

9. *Solve the differential equation*

$\sec^2x\tan y\,dx + \sec^2y\tan x\,dy = 0.$

SOLUTION. We have

$\sec^2x\tan y\,dx + \sec^2y\tan x\,dy = 0$

$$\Rightarrow \quad \frac{\sec^2 x}{\tan x}dx + \frac{\sec^2 y}{\tan y}dy = 0$$

On integrating, we get

$$\Rightarrow \int\frac{\sec^2 x}{\tan x}dx + \int\frac{\sec^2 y}{\tan y}dy = \log k$$

$\Rightarrow \log\tan x + \log\tan y = \log k$

$\Rightarrow \quad \log\tan x\tan y = \log k$

$\Rightarrow \quad \tan x\tan y = k$

10. *Solve* $\dfrac{dy}{dx} = \tan^{-1}x$.

SOLUTION. Given $\dfrac{dy}{dx} = \tan^{-1}x$

$$\Rightarrow \int\frac{dy}{dx}dx = \int\tan^{-1}x\,dx + c$$

$$\Rightarrow \int dy = \int\tan^{-1}x\cdot 1\,dx + c$$

$$\Rightarrow y = \tan^{-1}x\cdot x - \int\left[\frac{1}{1+x^2}\cdot x\right]dx + c$$

$$\Rightarrow y = x\tan^{-1}x - \frac{1}{2}\log(1+x^2) + c$$

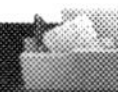

Exercise-23.3

Solve the following differential equations:

1. $\frac{dy}{dx} = -\frac{y}{x}$
2. $\frac{dy}{dx} = \frac{1}{y + \sin y}$
3. $3e^x \tan y dx + (1 - e^x)\sec^2 y dy = 0$
4. $(e^x + 1)y dy + (y + 1)dx = 0$
5. $(1 + x^2)\frac{dy}{dx} + 1 + y^2 = 0$
6. $\frac{dy}{dx} = e^{x+y} + x^2 e^y$
7. $y \sec^2 x + (y + 7)\tan x \frac{dy}{dx} = 0$
8. $\frac{dy}{dx} = \frac{1 + y^2}{1 + x^2}$
9. $\frac{dy}{dx} = \sin x \sin y$
10. $\sqrt{(a + x)}\frac{dy}{dx} + x = 0$
11. $\frac{dy}{dx} + \frac{1 + y^2}{y} = 0$
12. $(1 + x) y dx + (1 + y) x dy = 0$
13. $(1 + x^2)\frac{dy}{dx} = 2x$
14. $x\frac{dy}{dx} + y = y^2$
15. $\frac{dy}{dx} = \frac{x(2\log x + 1)}{\sin y + y \cos y}$
16. $e^{2x - 3y}dx + e^{2y - 3x}dy = 0$

ANSWERS

1. $xy = c$
2. $\frac{y^2}{2} - \cos y = x + c$
3. $\log \tan y = 3 \log(1 - e^x) + \log c$
4. $y = \log(1 + y) + \log(1 + e^{-x}) + c$
5. $\tan^{-1} x + \tan^{-1} y = c$
6. $e^x + e^{-y} + \frac{1}{3}x^3 = c_1$
7. $y^7 \tan x = e^{c - y}$
8. $\frac{y - x}{1 + xy} = c$
9. $\log(\operatorname{cosec} y - \cot y) + \cos x = c$
10. $y = \frac{2}{3}(a - x)\sqrt{a + x} + c$
11. $\frac{1}{2}\log(1 + y^2) + x = c$
12. $xy = c_1 e^{x + y}$
13. $y = \log(1 + x^2) + c$
14. $y - 1 = cxy$
15. $y \sin y = x^2 \log x + c$
16. $e^{5x} + e^{5y} = c$

(III) Type III: Solution of the differential equation of the form $\frac{d^2y}{dx^2} = f(x)$

To solve such type of differential equation, integrate the given equation two times.

Solved Examples

1. *Solve the differential equation*

$$\frac{d^2y}{dx^2} = \cos x - \sin x.$$

SOLUTION. The given differential equation is

$$\frac{d}{dx}\left(\frac{dy}{dx}\right) = \cos x - \sin x$$

Integrating both the sides w.r.t. x, we get

$$\frac{dy}{dx} = \int(\cos x - \sin x)dx + c_1$$

where c_1 is an arbitrary constant.

$$\Rightarrow \quad \frac{dy}{dx} = \sin x + \cos x + c_1$$

$$\Rightarrow \quad dy = (\sin x + \cos x + c_1)dx$$

Again, integrating both the sides w.r.t. x, we get

$$y = \int \sin x dx + \int \cos x dx + c_1 \int dx + c_2$$

where c_2 is an arbitrary constant.

$$\Rightarrow y = -\cos x + \sin x + c_1 x + c_2$$

2. *Solve the differential equation*

$$\frac{d^2y}{dx^2} = x^2 + e^x.$$

SOLUTION. The given differential equation is

$$\frac{d}{dx}\left(\frac{dy}{dx}\right) = x^2 + e^x$$

Integrating both the sides w.r.t. x, we get

$$\frac{dy}{dx} = \int(x^2 + e^x)dx + c_1,$$

where c_1 is an arbitrary constant.

$$\Rightarrow \quad \frac{dy}{dx} = \frac{x^3}{3} + e^x + c_1$$

$$\Rightarrow dy = \left(\frac{x^3}{3} + e^x + c_1\right)dx$$

$$\Rightarrow dy = \frac{x^3}{3}dx + e^x dx + c_1 dx$$

Again, integrating both the sides w.r.t. x, we get

$$y = \frac{1}{3}\int x^3 dx + \int e^x dx + c_1 \int dx + c_2\,;$$

where c_2 is an arbitrary constant.

$$\Rightarrow y = \frac{x^4}{12} + e^x + c_1 x + c_2$$

3. *Solve the differential equation*

$$\frac{d^2y}{dx^2} = xe^x.$$

SOLUTION. The given differential equation

$$\frac{d}{dx}\left(\frac{dy}{dx}\right) = xe^x$$

Integrating both the sides w.r.t. x, we get

$$\frac{dy}{dx} = \int xe^x dx$$

$$= x\int e^x dx - \int\left[\frac{d}{dx}x\int e^x dx\right]dx + c_1$$

(On integrating by parts)

$$= xe^x - \int e^x dx + c_1$$

where c_1 is an arbitrary constant.

$$\Rightarrow \frac{dy}{dx} = xe^x - e^x + c_1$$

$\Rightarrow dy = xe^x\,dx - e^x\,dx + c_1\,dx$

Again, integrating both the sides w.r.t. x, we get

$$\int dy = \int xe^x dx - \int e^x dx + c_1\int dx + c_2,$$

where c_2 is an arbitrary constant.

$$y = x\int e^x dx - \int\left[\frac{d}{dx}x\int e^x dx\right]dx - e^x + c_1 x + c_2$$

(On integrating by parts)

$$\Rightarrow \quad y = xe^x - e^x - e^x + c_1 x + c_2$$

$$= (x-2)e^x + c_1 x + c_2$$

4. *Solve the differential equation*

$$\frac{d^2y}{dx^2} = \log x.$$

Given : $y = 1, \dfrac{dy}{dx} = -1$ *when* $x = 1$

SOLUTION. The given differential equation is

$$\frac{d}{dx}\left(\frac{dy}{dx}\right) = \log x$$

Integrating both the sides w.r.t. x, we get

$$\frac{dy}{dx} = \log x\int 1dx - \int\left[\frac{d}{dx}\log x\int 1dx\right]dx + c_1$$

(On integrating by parts)

$$\Rightarrow \frac{dy}{dx} = x\log x - x + c_1$$

when $x = 1, \dfrac{dy}{dx} = -1$

$\therefore \quad -1 = 0 - 1 + c_1 \Rightarrow \quad c_1 = 0$

So, $\dfrac{dy}{dx} = x\log x - x$

Again integrating, we get

$$y = \log x\int xdx - \int\left[\frac{d}{dx}\log x\cdot\int xdx\right]dx - \int xdx + c_2$$

$$\Rightarrow y = \frac{x^2}{2}\log x - \frac{1}{2}\int xdx - \frac{x^2}{2} + c_2$$

$$y = \frac{x^2}{2}\log x - \frac{x^2}{4} - \frac{x^2}{2} + c_2$$

$$\Rightarrow y = \frac{x^2}{2}\log x - \frac{3}{4}x^2 + c_2$$

Given $x = 1 \Rightarrow y = 1$

$$\therefore \quad 1 = \frac{1}{2}\times 1^2\log 1 - \frac{(3\times 1^2)}{4} + c_2$$

$$\Rightarrow c_2 = \frac{7}{4}$$

Hence, $y = \dfrac{1}{2}x^2\log x - \dfrac{3x^2}{4} + \dfrac{7}{4}$

Exercise-23.4

Solve the following differential equations:

1. $\dfrac{d^2y}{dx^2} = 1$ **2.** $\dfrac{d^2y}{dx^2} = \sin x$ **3.** $\dfrac{d^2y}{dx^2} = x^7$ **4.** $\dfrac{d^2y}{dx^2} = e^{4x}$

5. $\frac{d^2y}{dx^2} = xe^x + \cos x$

6. $\frac{d^2y}{dx^2} = \cos x + x$

7. $\frac{d^2y}{dx^2} = x^2e^x$

8. $\frac{d^2y}{dx^2} = x\sin x + e^x$

9. $\frac{d^2y}{dx^2} = x\sin x$

10. $\frac{d^2y}{dx^2} = x\cos x$

11. $\frac{d^2y}{dx^2} = x + \sin x$, given at $y = 0$, $\frac{dy}{dx} = -1$ if $x = 0$.

12. $\frac{d^2y}{dx^2} = x^2 \sin x$, given at $x = 0$ if $y = 0$, $\frac{dy}{dx} = 1$

13. $\frac{d^2y}{dx^2} + \sin 2x = (x^2+1)e^{2x}$

14. $\frac{d^2y}{dx^2} = \cos x + e^{3x} + x^3$

15. $\frac{d^2y}{dx^2} = \frac{1}{1+x^2}$ when $x = 0, y = 0$ and $\frac{dy}{dx} = 0$

16. $x\frac{d^2y}{dx^2} + \frac{dy}{dx} + x = 0$

ANSWERS

1. $y = \frac{x^2}{2} + c_1x + c_2$
2. $y = c_1x - \sin x + c_2$
3. $y = \frac{x^9}{72} + c_1x + c_2$
4. $y = \frac{e^{4x}}{16} + c_1x + c_2$
5. $y = xe^x - 2e^x - \cos x + c_1x + c_2$
6. $y = -\cos x + \frac{x^3}{6} + c_1x + c_2$
7. $(x^2 - 4x + 6)e^x + c_1x + c_2$
8. $y = -x\sin x - 2\cos x + e^x + c_1x + c_2$
9. $y = -x\sin x - 2\cos x + c_1x + c_2$
10. $y = -x\cos x + 2\sin x + c_1x + c_2$
11. $y = \frac{x^3}{6} - \sin x$
12. $y = -x^2\sin x - 4x\cos x + 6\sin x - x$
13. $y = \frac{1}{8}(2x^2 - 4x + 5)e^{2x} + \frac{1}{4}\sin 2x + c_1x + c_2$
14. $y = -\cos x + \frac{1}{9}e^{3x} + \frac{1}{20}x^5 + c_1x + c_2$
15. $y = x\tan^{-1}x - \frac{1}{2}\log(1+x^2)$
16. $y = -\frac{x^2}{4} + c_1\log x + c_2$

23.11 HOMOGENEOUS DIFFERENTIAL EQUATIONS

We know that a function $f(x, y)$ is said to be homogenous function of degree n if each term in $f(x, y)$ is of degree n.

Definition. *A differential equation of the form* $\frac{dy}{dx} = \frac{f(x,y)}{g(x,y)}$ *is said to be homogeneous if* $f(x, y)$ *and* $g(x, y)$ *are function of same degree.*

For Example. $\frac{dy}{dx} = \frac{x^2+xy}{y^2}$

23.11.1 SOLUTION OF THE HOMOGENEOUS DIFFERENTIAL EQUATION

Let $$\frac{dy}{dx} = f(x,y) \qquad ...(1)$$

be a homogeneous equation.

To solve the above equation, put $y = vx$, *i.e.*, $\frac{dy}{dx} = v + x\frac{dv}{dx}$. Then applying the method of separation of variables, find the required solution.

Putting $y = vx \Rightarrow \frac{dy}{dx} = v + x\frac{dv}{dx}$ in eq. (1), we get

$$v + x\frac{dv}{dx} = f(v)$$

$$\Rightarrow \qquad x\frac{dv}{dx} = f(v) - v$$

$$\Rightarrow \qquad \int \frac{dv}{f(v) - v} = \int \frac{dx}{x} + c$$,where c is a constant of integration.

After integrating put $v = \dfrac{y}{x}$.

WORKING PROCEDURE

STEP 1. Write the given equation in the form of $\dfrac{dy}{dx} = f(x, y)$.

STEP 2. Check the homogeneity of the given equation, *i.e.*, $f(kx, ky) = k^n f(x, y)$.

STEP 3. Putting $y = vx$, *i.e.*, $\dfrac{dy}{dx} = v + x\dfrac{dv}{dx}$.

STEP 4. Separate the variables and then integrate.

STEP 5. Finally put $v = \dfrac{y}{x}$.

Solved Examples

1. *Solve* $x\dfrac{dy}{dx} - y = \sqrt{x^2 + y^2}$. (NCERT)

SOLUTION. We have $x\dfrac{dy}{dx} - y = \sqrt{x^2 + y^2}$

$$\Rightarrow \qquad x\frac{dy}{dx} = y + \sqrt{x^2 + y^2}$$

$$\Rightarrow \qquad \frac{dy}{dx} = \frac{y + \sqrt{x^2 + y^2}}{x},$$

which is a homogeneous equation.

Putting $y = vx \Rightarrow \dfrac{dy}{dx} = v + x\dfrac{dv}{dx}$, we get

$$v + x\frac{dv}{dx} = \frac{vx + \sqrt{x^2 + v^2x^2}}{x}$$

$$= \frac{vx + x\sqrt{1 + v^2}}{x} = v + \sqrt{1 + v^2}$$

$$\Rightarrow \quad x\frac{dv}{dx} = \sqrt{1 + v^2} \Rightarrow \frac{dv}{\sqrt{1 + v^2}} = \frac{dx}{x}$$

Integrating both the sides, we get

$$\int \frac{dv}{\sqrt{1 + v^2}} = \int \frac{dx}{x}$$

$$\Rightarrow \log|v + \sqrt{1 + v^2}| = \log|x| + \log c_1$$

$$\Rightarrow |v + (\sqrt{1 + v^2})| = c_1|x|$$

$$\Rightarrow v + \sqrt{1 + v^2} = \pm c_1 x = cx \quad (c = \pm c_1)$$

Again, putting $v = \dfrac{y}{x}$

$$\frac{y}{x} + \sqrt{1 + \frac{y^2}{x^2}} = cx$$

which is the required solution of the given differential equation.

2. *Solve* $(x^2 + xy)dy = (x^2 + y^2)dx$. (NCERT)

SOLUTION. Given $(x^2 + xy)dy = (x^2 + y^2)dx$

$$\Rightarrow \qquad \frac{dy}{dx} = \frac{x^2 + y^2}{x^2 + xy} \qquad ...(1)$$

which is a homogeneous equation.

Putting $y = vx$, *i.e.*, $\dfrac{dy}{dx} = v + x\dfrac{dv}{dx}$ in the above equation, we get

$$v + x\frac{dv}{dx} = \frac{x^2 + v^2x^2}{x^2 + x \cdot vx} = \frac{1 + v^2}{1 + v}$$

$$\Rightarrow \quad x\frac{dv}{dx} = \frac{1 + v^2}{1 + v} - v = \frac{1 - v}{1 + v}$$

$$\Rightarrow \qquad \frac{1 + v}{1 - v}dv = \frac{dx}{x}$$

Integrating both the sides, we get

$$\int \left[-1 + \frac{2}{1 - v}\right] dv = \int \frac{dx}{x} + c$$

$$\Rightarrow \quad -v - 2\log|(1-v)| = \log|x| + c$$

$$\Rightarrow \quad -\frac{y}{x} - 2\log\left|\left(1-\frac{y}{x}\right)\right| = \log|x| + c \qquad \left(\because v = \frac{y}{x}\right)$$

which is the required solution of the given differential equation.

Similar Problems

(1) Solve: $(y^2 - x^2)dy = 3xydx$. **Ans.** $y^2(4x^2 - y^2)^3 = c_1$

(2) Solve: $(x^3 + y^3)dy - x^2ydx = 0$. **Ans.** $-\dfrac{x^3}{3y^3} + \log|y| = c$

(3) Solve: $2xydx + (x^2 + 2y^2)dy = 0$. **Ans.** $3x^2y + 2y^3 = c$

(4) Solve: $x^2 \cdot \dfrac{dy}{dx} = 2xy + y^2$. **Ans.** $y = cx(x + y)$

3. *Solve* $y^2dx + (x^2 - xy + y^2)dy = 0$.

SOLUTION. Given $y^2dx + (x^2 - xy + y^2)dy = 0$

$$\Rightarrow \quad \frac{dy}{dx} = -\frac{y^2}{(x^2 - xy + y^2)} \qquad ...(1)$$

Putting $y = vx$, *i.e.*, $\dfrac{dy}{dx} = v + x\dfrac{dv}{dx}$ in eq. (1), we get

$$v + x\frac{dv}{dx} = -\frac{v^2}{(1 + v^2 - v)}$$

$$\Rightarrow \quad x\frac{dv}{dx} = -\left[\frac{v^2}{(1 - v + v^2)} + v\right]$$

$$= \frac{-(v + v^3)}{(1 - v + v^2)}$$

Separating the variables, we get

$$\frac{(1 - v + v^2)}{v(1 + v^2)}dv = -\frac{1}{x}dx$$

$$\Rightarrow \left[\frac{1 + v^2}{v(1 + v^2)} - \frac{v}{v(1 + v^2)}\right]dv = -\frac{1}{x}dx$$

Integrating both the sides, we get

$$\Rightarrow \quad \int\left(\frac{1}{v} - \frac{1}{(1 + v^2)}\right)dv = -\int\frac{1}{x}dx$$

$$\log|v| - \tan^{-1} v + \log|x| = \log c$$

$$\Rightarrow \quad \tan^{-1} v = \log\frac{|vx|}{c}$$

Again putting $v = \dfrac{y}{x}$, we get

$$\tan^{-1}\frac{y}{x} = \log\frac{(|y|)}{c}$$

$$\Rightarrow \quad \frac{|y|}{c} = e^{\tan^{-1}\frac{y}{x}}$$

$$\Rightarrow \quad y = c_1 e^{\tan^{-1}\frac{y}{x}} \qquad (c_1 = \pm c)$$

4. *Solve* $(3xy + y^2)dx + (x^2 + xy)dy = 0$.

SOLUTION. Given $(3xy + y^2)dx + (x^2 + xy)dy = 0$

$$\Rightarrow \quad \frac{dy}{dx} = -\frac{(3xy + y^2)}{(x^2 + xy)} \qquad ...(1)$$

Putting $y = vx$, *i.e.*, $\dfrac{dy}{dx} = v + x\dfrac{dv}{dx}$ in eq. (1), we get

$$v + x\frac{dv}{dx} = -\frac{(3vx^2 + v^2x^2)}{x^2 + vx^2}$$

$$\Rightarrow \quad v + x\frac{dv}{dx} = -\frac{(3v + v^2)}{(1 + v)}$$

$$\Rightarrow \quad x\frac{dv}{dx} = \left[-\frac{(3v + v^2)}{(1 + v)} - v\right]$$

$$\Rightarrow \quad x\frac{dv}{dx} = \frac{-2(2v + v^2)}{(1 + v)}$$

$$\Rightarrow \quad \frac{(1 + v)}{(2v + v^2)}dv = -\frac{2}{x}dx$$

On integrating both the sides, we get

$$\int\frac{1 + v}{(2v + v^2)}dv + \int\frac{2}{x}dx = \log c$$

$$\Rightarrow \quad \frac{1}{2}\log|2v + v^2| + 2\log|x| = \log c$$

$$\Rightarrow \log|x^2\sqrt{2v+v^2}| = \log c$$
$$\Rightarrow |x^2\sqrt{2v+v^2}| = c$$

Again putting $v = \frac{y}{x}$, we get

$$x^2\sqrt{\frac{2y}{x}+\frac{y^2}{x^2}} = c$$
$$\Rightarrow x\sqrt{(2xy+y^2)} = c$$
$$\Rightarrow x^2(2xy+y^2) = c^2$$

5. *Solve* $(y+x)\frac{dy}{dx} = (y-x)$.

SOLUTION. Given $(y+x)\frac{dy}{dx} = (y-x)$

$$\Rightarrow \frac{dy}{dx} = \frac{(y-x)}{(y+x)} \quad ...(1)$$

Putting $y = vx$, *i.e.*, $\frac{dy}{dx} = v + x\frac{dv}{dx}$ in eq. (1), we get

$$v + x\frac{dv}{dx} = \frac{(vx-x)}{(vx+x)} = \frac{(v-1)}{(v+1)}$$

$$\Rightarrow x\frac{dv}{dx} = \frac{(v-1)}{(v+1)} - v = \frac{-(1+v^2)}{(1+v)}$$

On separating the variables, we get

$$\frac{(v+1)}{(v^2+1)}\cdot dv + \frac{dx}{x} = 0$$

Integrating both the sides, we get

$$\int\frac{(v+1)}{(v^2+1)}dv + \int\frac{dx}{x} = c$$
$$\Rightarrow \int\frac{v}{(v^2+1)}dv + \int\frac{1}{(v^2+1)}dv + \int\frac{dx}{x} = c$$
$$\Rightarrow \frac{1}{2}\log(v^2+1) + \tan^{-1}v + \log|x| = c$$
$$\Rightarrow \frac{1}{2}[\log(v^2+1) + 2\log(x)] + \tan^{-1}v = c$$

Again putting $v = \frac{y}{x}$, we get

$$\frac{1}{2}\log\left(\left(\left(\frac{y}{x}\right)^2+1\right)x^2\right) + \tan^{-1}\left(\frac{y}{x}\right) = c$$
$$\Rightarrow \frac{1}{2}\log(x^2+y^2) + \tan^{-1}\left(\frac{y}{x}\right) = c$$

Similar Problem

(1) Solve $(x^3 - 3xy^2)dx = (y^3 - 3x^2y)dy$. **Ans.** $(y^2 - x^2) = c^2(y^2 + x^2)^2$

6. *Solve* $x\frac{dy}{dx} = y - x\tan\frac{y}{x}$.

SOLUTION. Given $x\frac{dy}{dx} = y - x\tan\frac{y}{x}$

$$\Rightarrow \frac{dy}{dx} = \frac{y}{x} - \tan\frac{y}{x} \quad ...(1)$$

Putting $y = vx$, *i.e.*, $\frac{dy}{dx} = v + x\frac{dv}{dx}$ in eq. (1), we get

$$v + x\frac{dv}{dx} = v - \tan v$$
$$\Rightarrow x\frac{dv}{dx} = -\tan v$$

On separating the variables, we get

$$\frac{dv}{\tan v} = -\frac{dx}{x}$$
$$\Rightarrow \cot v \cdot dv = -\frac{dx}{x}$$
$$\Rightarrow \frac{\cos v}{\sin v}\cdot dv = -\frac{dx}{x}$$

On integrating both the sides, we get

$$\int\frac{\cos v}{\sin v}\cdot dv = -\int\frac{dx}{x} + \log c$$
$$\Rightarrow \log|\sin v| + \log|x| = \log c$$
$$\Rightarrow \log|x\sin v| = \log c$$
$$\Rightarrow |x\sin v| = c$$

Again putting $v = \frac{y}{x}$, we get

$$x\sin\frac{y}{x} = c_1 \qquad (c_1 = \pm c)$$

7. *Solve*

$$\left(x\cos\frac{y}{x}+y\sin\frac{y}{x}\right)ydx = \left(y\sin\frac{y}{x}-x\cos\frac{y}{x}\right)xdy.$$

SOLUTION. Given $\left(x\cos\frac{y}{x}+y\sin\frac{y}{x}\right)ydx$

$$=\left(y\sin\frac{y}{x}-x\cos\frac{y}{x}\right)xdy$$

$$\Rightarrow \frac{dy}{dx}=\frac{\left[x\cos\left(\frac{y}{x}\right)+y\sin\left(\frac{y}{x}\right)\right]y}{\left[y\sin\left(\frac{y}{x}\right)-x\cos\left(\frac{y}{x}\right)\right]x}$$

Divide numerator and denominator by x^2

$$\frac{dy}{dx}=\frac{\left[\cos\left(\frac{y}{x}\right)+\left(\frac{y}{x}\right)\sin\left(\frac{y}{x}\right)\right]\left(\frac{y}{x}\right)}{\left[\left(\frac{y}{x}\right)\sin\left(\frac{y}{x}\right)-\cos\left(\frac{y}{x}\right)\right]} \quad ...(1)$$

Putting $y = vx$, *i.e.*, $\frac{dy}{dx}=v+x\frac{dv}{dx}$ in eq. (1), we get

$$v+x\frac{dv}{dx}=\frac{v(\cos v+v\sin v)}{(v\sin v-\cos v)}$$

$$\Rightarrow \quad x\frac{dv}{dx}=\left[\frac{v(\cos v+v\sin v)}{(v\sin v-\cos v)}-v\right]$$

$$=\frac{2v\cos v}{v\sin v-\cos v}$$

On separating the variables, we get

$$\frac{v\sin v-\cos v}{v\cos v}dv=\frac{2}{x}dx$$

Integrating both the sides, we get

$$\int\frac{v\sin v-\cos v}{v\cos v}dv=\int\frac{2}{x}dx+\log c$$

$$\Rightarrow \quad \int\tan v dv-\int\frac{dv}{v}=\int\frac{2}{x}dx+\log c$$

$$\Rightarrow \log|\cos v|+\log|v|+2\log|x|=\log c$$

$$\Rightarrow \log|x^2v\cos v|=\log c$$

$$\Rightarrow \quad x^2v\cos v=c$$

Again putting $v=\frac{y}{x}$, we get

$$x^2\cdot\frac{y}{x}\cos\frac{y}{x}=c$$

$$\Rightarrow xy\cos\left(\frac{y}{x}\right)=c,$$

8. *Solve* $2ye^{x/y}dx + (y - 2xe^{x/y})dy = 0.$

Given, $y = 1$ *then* $x = 0.$

SOLUTION. The given equation can be written as

$$\frac{dx}{dy}=\frac{2xe^{x/y}-y}{2ye^{x/y}}=\frac{2\cdot\frac{x}{y}\cdot e^{x/y}-1}{2e^{x/y}} \quad ...(1)$$

Putting $x = vy$, *i.e.*, $\frac{dx}{dy}=v+y\frac{dv}{dy}$ in eq. (1), we get

$$v+y\frac{dv}{dy}=\frac{2ve^v-1}{2e^v}$$

$$\Rightarrow \quad y\frac{dv}{dy}=\frac{2ve^v-1}{2e^v}-v=\frac{-1}{2e^v}$$

On separating the variables, we get

$$2e^v\cdot dv=-\frac{dy}{y}$$

On integrating both the sides, we get

$$\int 2e^v\cdot dv=-\int\frac{dy}{y}+c$$

$$\Rightarrow \quad 2e^v=-\log|y|+c$$

Again putting $v=\frac{x}{y}$, we get

$$2e^{x/y}+\log|y|=c \quad ...(2)$$

Given $x = 0 \Rightarrow y = 1$, therefore

$$2e^0+\log 1=c$$

$$\Rightarrow \quad 2\cdot 1+0=c$$

$$\Rightarrow \quad c=2$$

Putting the value of c in eq. (2), we get

$$2e^{x/y}+\log|y|=2$$

9. *Solve*

$$2x^2\frac{dy}{dx}-2xy+y^2=0 \textit{ when } y(e)=e.$$

SOLUTION. Given $2x^2\frac{dy}{dx}-2xy+y^2=0$

$$\Rightarrow \quad \frac{dy}{dx} = \frac{2xy - y^2}{2x^2} \qquad ...(1)$$

Which is a homogeneous equation.

Putting $y = vx$, *i.e.*, $\frac{dy}{dx} = v + x\frac{dv}{dx}$ in eq. (1), we get

$$v + x\frac{dv}{dx} = \frac{2x(vx) - (vx)^2}{2x^2}$$

$$= \frac{2v - v^2}{2} = v - \frac{1}{2}v^2$$

$$\Rightarrow x\frac{dv}{dx} = v - \frac{1}{2}v^2 - v = -\frac{1}{2}v^2$$

On separating the variables, we get

$$\Rightarrow \quad \frac{dv}{v^2} + \frac{1}{2}\frac{dx}{x} = 0$$

$$\Rightarrow \quad \int\frac{dv}{v^2} + \frac{1}{2}\int\frac{dx}{x} = 0$$

$$\Rightarrow \quad -\frac{1}{v} + \frac{1}{2}\log|x| = c$$

Again putting $v = \frac{y}{x}$,

$$-\frac{x}{y} + \frac{1}{2}\log|x| = c \qquad ...(2)$$

Given, $\qquad y(e) = e \qquad ...(3)$

Putting $x = e$ and $y = e$ in eq. (2), we get

$$-\frac{e}{e} + \frac{1}{2}\log e = c$$

$$\Rightarrow \quad -1 + \frac{1}{2}\cdot 1 = c$$

$$\Rightarrow \quad c = -\frac{1}{2}$$

Putting the value of c in eq. (2), we get

$$-\frac{x}{y} + \frac{1}{2}\log|x| = -\frac{1}{2}$$

$$\Rightarrow \quad \frac{1}{2}(\log x + 1) = \frac{x}{y}$$

$$\Rightarrow \quad \frac{1}{2}(\log x + \log e) = \frac{x}{y}$$

$$\Rightarrow \quad y \log ex = 2x$$

10. *Solve*

$$(1 + e^{x/y})dx + e^{x/y}\left(1 - \frac{x}{y}\right)dy = 0$$

SOLUTION. Given

$$(1 + e^{x/y})dx + e^{x/y}\left(1 - \frac{x}{y}\right)dy = 0$$

$$\Rightarrow \quad \frac{dx}{dy} = \frac{-e^{x/y}\left(1 - \frac{x}{y}\right)}{1 + e^{x/y}} \qquad ...(1)$$

Putting $x = vy$, *i.e.*, $\frac{dx}{dy} = v + y\frac{dv}{dy}$ in eq. (1), we get

$$v + y\frac{dv}{dy} = -\frac{e^v(1 - v)}{1 + e^v}$$

$$\Rightarrow \quad y\frac{dv}{dy} = -\frac{v + e^v}{1 + e^v}$$

Integrating after separating the variables, we get

$$\Rightarrow \int\frac{1 + e^v}{v + e^v}\cdot dv = -\int\frac{dy}{y}$$

$$\Rightarrow \log|v + e^v| = -\log|y| + c$$

$$\Rightarrow \log|y(v + e^v)| = c$$

$$\Rightarrow \quad |y(v + e^v)| = e^c = c_1 \qquad \text{(say)}$$

Again putting $v = \frac{x}{y}$, we get

$$y\left(\frac{x}{y} + e^{x/y}\right) = c_1$$

$$\Rightarrow x + ye^{x/y} = c_1$$

Exercise-23.5

Solve the following differential equations:

1. $x\frac{dy}{dx} = x + y$
2. $\frac{dy}{dx} = \frac{2xy}{x^2 - y^2}$
3. $\frac{dy}{dx} = \frac{x + y}{x - y}$
4. $x(x - y)dy + y^2\,dx = 0$
5. $(x - y)\frac{dy}{dx} = x + 2y$
6. $2xy\frac{dy}{dx} = x^2 + y^2$
7. $x^2\cdot\frac{dy}{dx} = x^2 + xy + y^2$
8. $ye^{x/y}dx = (xe^{x/y} + y)dy$

9. $x\frac{dy}{dx} = y - x\cos^2\left(\frac{y}{x}\right)$

10. $x\frac{dy}{dx} - y = 2\sqrt{y^2 - x^2}$

11. $(x^3 + 3xy^2)dx + (y^3 + 3x^2y)dy = 0$

12. $x\frac{dy}{dx} = y(\log y - \log x + 1)$

13. $(1+2e^{x/y})dx + 2e^{x/y}\left(1-\frac{x}{y}\right)dy = 0$

14. $y^2dx + (x^2 + xy + y^2)dy = 0$

15. $ydx + x\log\left(\frac{y}{x}\right)dy - 2xdy = 0$

16. $x\frac{dy}{dx} - y + x\sin\frac{y}{x} = 0$

17. $x^2dy + y(x + y)dx = 0$

18. $(x - \sqrt{xy})dy = ydx$

19. $x\frac{dy}{dx} - y = x\tan\frac{y}{x}$

20. $\left(x\sin^2\frac{y}{x} - y\right)dx + xdy = 0$, $y(1) = \frac{\pi}{4}$

21. $(x^2 - y^2)dx + 2xydy = 0, y(1) = 1$

22. Prove that the family of curve for which the slope of the tangent at the point (x, y) is $\frac{x^2+y^2}{2xy}$ is given by $x^2 - y^2 = cx$.

ANSWERS

1. $y = x\log|x| + cx$ 2. $y = c(x^2 + y^2)$ 3. $\tan^{-1}\frac{y}{x} = \frac{1}{2}\log\left(\frac{x^2+y^2}{x}\right) + c$ 4. $y = ce^{y/x}$

5. $\log|x^2+xy+y^2| = 2\sqrt{3}\tan^{-1}\left(\frac{x+2y}{\sqrt{3}\cdot x}\right) + c$ 6. $x = c(x^2 - y^2)$

7. $\tan^{-1}\frac{y}{x} = \log|x| + c$ 8. $e^{x/y} = \log cy$ 9. $\tan\frac{y}{x} = c - \log|x|$

10. $y + \sqrt{y^2 - x^2} = cx^3$ 11. $y^4 + 6x^2y^2 + x^4 = c$ 12. $y = xe^{cx}$

13. $x + 2ye^{x/y} = c{\cdot}x{\cdot}y$ 14. $\log|y| + \frac{x}{x+y} = c$ 15. $1 + \log\frac{x}{y} = cy$

16. $x\tan\left(\frac{y}{x}\right) = c$ 17. $x^2y = c(y + 2x)$ 18. $2\sqrt{\frac{x}{y}} - \log|y| = c$

19. $\left|\sin\frac{y}{x}\right| = c|x|$ 20. $\cot\left(\frac{y}{x}\right) = \log|x| + 1$ 21. $x^2 + y^2 = 2x$

23.12 LINEAR DIFFERENTIAL EQUATIONS

Definition. *A differential equation of the form*

$$\frac{dy}{dx} + Py = Q$$

where P and Q are function of x only or constant is called linear differential equation.

23.12.1 Solution of the Linear Differential Equations

Let the given equation be

$$\frac{dy}{dx} + Py = Q \quad ...(1)$$

First of all, find the value of integrating factor (I.F.) $= e^{\int Pdx}$.

Multiply both sides of eq. (1) by $e^{\int Pdx}$

$$e^{\int Pdx}\cdot\frac{dy}{dx} + Pye^{\int Pdx} = Qe^{\int Pdx}$$

$$\Rightarrow \qquad e^{\int P dx} dy + Pye^{\int P dx} dx = Qe^{\int P dx} \cdot dx$$

$$\Rightarrow \qquad d(y \cdot e^{\int P dx}) = Qe^{\int P dx} \cdot dx$$

On integrating both the sides, we get

$$ye^{\int P dx} = \int Qe^{\int P dx} dx + c,$$

which the required solution of the given equation.

WORKING PROCEDURE

STEP 1. Compare the given equation with $\frac{dy}{dx} + Py = Q$ and find the value of P and Q.

STEP 2. Find the value of $e^{\int P dx}$.

STEP 3. Putting the value of Q and $e^{\int P dx}$ in the following formula

$$y(e^{\int P dx}) = \int Qe^{\int P dx} dx + c$$

Solved Examples

1. *Solve* $\frac{dy}{dx} - \frac{y}{x} = 2x^2$.

SOLUTION. Given $\frac{dy}{dx} - \frac{y}{x} = 2x^2$ ...(1)

Clearly, it is a linear differential equation.

Comparing eq. (1) with $\frac{dy}{dx} + Py = Q$,

we get $P = -\frac{1}{x}$, $Q = 2x^2$

$\therefore$ Integrating factor (I.F.)

$$= e^{\int P dx} = e^{\int -\frac{1}{x} dx} = e^{-\log x} = e^{\log \frac{1}{x}} = \frac{1}{x}$$

Hence, solution of the given equation is $y \cdot e^{\int P dx} = \int Qe^{\int P dx} \cdot dx + c$

$$\Rightarrow y \cdot \frac{1}{x} = \int 2x^2 \cdot \frac{1}{x} dx + c = 2\int x dx + c$$

$$= x^2 + c$$

$$\Rightarrow \quad y = x^3 + cx$$

2. *Solve* $x\frac{dy}{dx} - y = x^2$.

SOLUTION. Given $x\frac{dy}{dx} - y = x^2$

$$\Rightarrow \qquad \frac{dy}{dx} - \frac{y}{x} = x \qquad ...(1)$$

which is a linear differential equation.

Comparing eq. (1) with $\frac{dy}{dx} + Py = Q$,

we get

$$P = -\frac{1}{x}, \; Q = x$$

$$\therefore \text{I.F.} = e^{\int P dx} = e^{\int -\frac{1}{x} dx} = e^{-\log x}$$

$$= e^{\log \frac{1}{x}} = \frac{1}{x}$$

Hence, solution of the given equation is

$$y \cdot e^{\int P dx} = \int Qe^{\int P dx} \cdot dx + c$$

$$\Rightarrow \qquad y \cdot \frac{1}{x} = \int x \cdot \frac{1}{x} dx + c$$

$$= \int dx + c = x + c$$

$$\Rightarrow \qquad y = x^2 + cx$$

3. *Solve* $\frac{dy}{dx} + \sec x \cdot y = \tan x ; 0 \le x < \frac{\pi}{2}$.

SOLUTION. Given $\frac{dy}{dx} + \sec x \cdot y = \tan x$ ...(1)

Comparing eq. (1) with $\frac{dy}{dx} + Py = Q$,

we get $P = \sec x$, $Q = \tan x$

Now, I.F.

$$= e^{\int P dx} = e^{\int \sec x dx} = e^{\log(\sec x + \tan x)}$$

$$= \sec x + \tan x$$

Hence, solution of the given equation is

$$y \cdot e^{\int P dx} = \int Qe^{\int P dx} \cdot dx + c$$

$\Rightarrow y\cdot(\sec x+\tan x)$
$=\int \tan x(\sec x+\tan x)dx+c$
$=\int \sec x\tan x dx+\int \tan^2 x dx+c$

$=\int \sec x\tan x dx+\int \sec^2 x dx-\int 1 dx+c$

$\Rightarrow y(\sec x + \tan x) = \sec x + \tan x - x + c$, which is the required solution.

4. *Solve* $\frac{dy}{dx}-y=x\cdot e^x$.

SOLUTION. Given $\frac{dy}{dx}-y=x\cdot e^x$ ...(1)

Comparing eq. (1) with $\frac{dy}{dx}+Py=Q$,

we get $P = -1$, $Q = xe^x$

Now, I.F. $= e^{\int Pdx}=e^{\int -1dx}=e^{-x}$

Hence, required solution is given by

$$y\cdot e^{\int Pdx}=\int Qe^{\int Pdx}\cdot dx+c$$

$$\Rightarrow y\cdot e^{-x}=\int xe^x\cdot e^{-x}\cdot dx+c$$

$$=\int xdx+c=\frac{x^2}{2}+c$$

$$\Rightarrow \quad y=\left(\frac{x^2}{2}+c\right)e^x$$

Similar Problems

(1) Solve $\frac{dy}{dx}+y\cot x=2\cos x$. **Ans.** $y=-\frac{1}{2}\cos 2x\,\text{cosec}\,x+c\,\text{cosec}\,x$

(2) Solve $\frac{dy}{dx}-y\tan x=2\sin x$. **Ans.** $y=-\frac{1}{2}\cos 2x\sec x+c\sec x$

5. *Solve* $(1+x^2)\frac{dy}{dx}+y=e^{\tan^{-1}x}$.

SOLUTION. Given $\frac{dy}{dx}+\frac{y}{1+x^2}=\frac{e^{\tan^{-1}x}}{1+x^2}$ ...(1)

Comparing eq. (1) with $\frac{dy}{dx}+Py=Q$,

we get $P=\frac{1}{1+x^2}$, $Q=\frac{e^{\tan^{-1}x}}{1+x^2}$

Now, I.F. $=e^{\int Pdx}=e^{\int \frac{1}{1+x^2}dx}=e^{\tan^{-1}x}$

Hence, required solution is given by

$$y\cdot(\text{I.F.})=\int Q\cdot(\text{I.F.})dx+c$$

$$\Rightarrow y\cdot e^{\tan^{-1}x}=\int \frac{e^{\tan^{-1}x}}{1+x^2}\cdot e^{\tan^{-1}x}\cdot dx+c$$

$$=\int \frac{e^{2\tan^{-1}x}}{1+x^2}dx+c \quad ...(2)$$

Let $\tan^{-1}x=t \Rightarrow \frac{1}{1+x^2}dx=dt$

Then from eq. (2),

$$y\cdot e^t=\int e^{2t}dt+c=\frac{1}{2}e^{2t}+c$$

$$\therefore \; y=\frac{1}{2}\frac{e^{2t}}{e^t}+\frac{c}{e^t}=\frac{1}{2}e^t+ce^{-t}$$

$$\Rightarrow y=\frac{1}{2}e^{\tan^{-1}x}+ce^{-\tan^{-1}x}$$

6. *Solve* $\sin x\frac{dy}{dx}+\cos x\cdot y=\cos x\sin^2 x$.

SOLUTION. Given

$$\sin x\frac{dy}{dx}+\cos x\cdot y=\cos x\sin^2 x$$

$$\Rightarrow \frac{dy}{dx}+\frac{\cos x}{\sin x}y=\frac{\cos x\sin^2 x}{\sin x}$$

$$\Rightarrow \frac{dy}{dx}+y\cot x=\cos x\sin x \quad ...(1)$$

Comparing eq. (1) with $\frac{dy}{dx}+Py=Q$,

we get $P = \cot x$, $Q = \cos x \sin x$

Now,

I.F. $=e^{\int Pdx}=e^{\int \cot x dx}=e^{\log \sin x}=\sin x$

$\therefore$ Solution of the given equation is

$$\Rightarrow y\cdot\sin x=\int \cos x\cdot\sin x\cdot\sin x dx+c$$

$$=\int \sin^2 x\cos x dx+c$$

$$= \frac{\sin^3 x}{3} + c$$

$$\Rightarrow y = \frac{1}{3}\sin^2 x + c \operatorname{cosec} x$$

7. *Solve* $\frac{dy}{dx} + 2\tan x \cdot y = \sin x$.

SOLUTION. Given $\frac{dy}{dx} + 2\tan x \cdot y = \sin x$ ...(1)

Comparing eq. (1) with $\frac{dy}{dx} + Py = Q$,

we get $P = 2\tan x$, $Q = \sin x$

Now,

$$\text{I.F.} = e^{\int P dx} = e^{\int 2\tan x dx} = e^{2\log \sec x}$$

$$= e^{\log \sec^2 x} = \sec^2 x$$

$\therefore$ Solution of the equation is given by

$$y \cdot (\text{I.F.}) = \int Q(\text{I.F.})dx + c$$

$$\Rightarrow y \cdot \sec^2 x = \int \sin x \cdot \sec^2 x dx + c$$

$$= \int \sec x \tan x \, dx + c$$

$$= \sec x + c$$

$$y = \frac{\sec x}{\sec^2 x} + \frac{c}{\sec^2 x} = \cos x + c\cos^2 x$$

8. *Solve* $(1+x^2)\frac{dy}{dx} + y = \tan^{-1} x$.

SOLUTION. Given $(1+x^2)\frac{dy}{dx} + y = \tan^{-1} x$

$$\Rightarrow \frac{dy}{dx} + \frac{y}{(1+x^2)} = \frac{\tan^{-1} x}{1+x^2} \qquad \text{...(1)}$$

Comparing equation (1) with $\frac{dy}{dx} + Py = Q$, we get

$$P = \frac{1}{1+x^2}, Q = \frac{\tan^{-1} x}{1+x^2}$$

Now, $\text{I.F.} = e^{\int P dx} = e^{\int \frac{1}{1+x^2} dx} = e^{\tan^{-1} x}$

$\therefore$ Solution of the given equation is

$$\Rightarrow y \cdot e^{\int P dx} = \int Q e^{\int P dx} \cdot dx + c$$

$$\Rightarrow y \cdot e^{\tan^{-1} x} = \int \frac{e^{\tan^{-1} x} \cdot \tan^{-1} x}{1+x^2} dx + c$$

Let $\tan^{-1} x = t \Rightarrow \frac{1}{1+x^2} dx = dt$

$$\therefore y \cdot e^{\tan^{-1} x} = \int t e^t dt + c$$

$$= e^t (t-1) + c$$

$$= e^{\tan^{-1} x}(\tan^{-1} x - 1) + c$$

$$\Rightarrow y = -1 + \tan^{-1} x + ce^{-\tan^{-1} x},$$

9. *Solve* $x\frac{dy}{dx} - y = \log x$.

SOLUTION. Given $x\frac{dy}{dx} - y = \log x$

$$\Rightarrow \frac{dy}{dx} - \frac{y}{x} = \frac{\log x}{x} \qquad \text{...(1)}$$

Comparing equation (1) with $\frac{dy}{dx} + Py = Q$, we get

$$P = -\frac{1}{x}, Q = \frac{\log x}{x}$$

Now, $\text{I.F.} = e^{\int P dx} = e^{\int -\frac{1}{x} dx} = e^{-\log x}$

$$= e^{\log\left(\frac{1}{x}\right)} = \frac{1}{x}$$

$\therefore$ Solution of the given equation is

$$y \cdot e^{\int P dx} = \int Q e^{\int P dx} \cdot dx + c$$

$$\Rightarrow y \cdot \frac{1}{x} = \int \frac{\log x}{x} \cdot \frac{1}{x} dx + c$$

$$= \log x\left(-\frac{1}{x}\right) - \int \frac{1}{x}\left(-\frac{1}{x}\right) dx + c$$

$$= -\frac{\log x}{x} + \int \frac{1}{x^2} dx + c$$

$$= -\frac{\log x}{x} - \frac{1}{x} + c$$

$$y = cx - (\log x + 1)$$

Similar Problems

(1) Solve $\frac{dy}{dx}+\frac{y}{x}=e^x, x>0$. **Ans.** $y_x = e^x(x-1)+c$

(2) Solve $\frac{dy}{dx}+y\cot x=x^2\cot x+2x$, when $y\left(\frac{\pi}{2}\right)=0$. **Ans.** $y=x^2-\frac{\pi^2}{4}\text{cosec}\, x$

(3) Solve $\frac{dy}{dx}+2y=xe^{4x}$. **Ans.** $y=\frac{1}{6}xe^{4x}-\frac{1}{36}e^{4x}+ce^{-2x}$

(4) Solve $\cos^2 x\frac{dy}{dx}+y=\tan x, 0\le x\le\frac{\pi}{2}$ **Ans.** $y=\tan x-1+ce^{-\tan x}$

(5) Solve $x\frac{dy}{dx}+y=x^3$, when at $x=2, y=1$. **Ans.** $y=\frac{x^3}{4}-2x^{-1}$

10. *Solve* $\frac{dy}{dx}+\frac{1}{x}\cdot y=y^3$.

SOLUTION. Given $\frac{dy}{dx}+\frac{1}{x}\cdot y=y^3$

$$\Rightarrow \frac{1}{y^3}\frac{dy}{dx}+\frac{1}{x\cdot y^2}=1 \quad ...(1)$$

Let $\frac{1}{y^2}=t\Rightarrow -\frac{2}{y^3}\frac{dy}{dx}=\frac{dt}{dx}$

$$\Rightarrow \frac{1}{y^3}\frac{dy}{dx}=-\frac{1}{2}\cdot\frac{dt}{dx}$$

$\therefore$ From eq. (1),

$$-\frac{1}{2}\frac{dt}{dx}+t\frac{1}{x}=1$$

$$\Rightarrow \frac{dt}{dx}-\frac{2}{x}t=-2 \quad ...(2)$$

which is linear equation of the form

$$\frac{dt}{dx}+Pt=Q$$

where $P=\frac{-2}{x}, Q=-2$

Now, I.F. $=e^{\int P dx}=e^{\int -\frac{2}{x}dx}=e^{-2\log x}$

$$=e^{\log\left(\frac{1}{x^2}\right)}=\frac{1}{x^2}$$

$\therefore$ Solution of the given equation

$$\Rightarrow t\cdot\frac{1}{x^2}=\int(-2)\cdot\frac{1}{x^2}dx+c=\frac{2}{x}+c$$

$$\Rightarrow \frac{1}{y^2}\cdot\frac{1}{x^2}=\frac{2}{x}+c \quad \left(\because t=\frac{1}{y^2}\right)$$

$\Rightarrow 2xy^2 + cx^2y^2 = 1$, which is the required solution.

11. *Solve* $\frac{dy}{dx}+2y\tan x=\cos 2x$.

SOLUTION. The given equation is

$$\frac{dy}{dx}+2y\tan x=\cos 2x$$

Which is a linear differential equation of the type $\frac{dy}{dx}+py=Q$

where $P = 2\tan x$, $Q = \cos 2x$

$$\text{I.F.}=e^{\int P dx}=e^{\int 2\tan x dx}=e^{-2\log\cos x}$$

$$=e^{\log(\cos x)^{-2}}=\frac{1}{\cos^2 x}$$

Hence, solution is given by

$$y\cdot(\text{I.F.})=\int Q\cdot(\text{I.F.})dx+c$$

$$\Rightarrow y\cdot\frac{1}{\cos^2 x}=\int\left(\cos 2x\cdot\frac{1}{\cos^2 x}\right)dx+c$$

$$=\int\left\{(2\cos^2 x-1)\cdot\frac{1}{\cos^2 x}\right\}dx+c$$

$$=\int 2dx-\int\sec^2 x dx+c$$

$$= 2x-\tan x+c$$

$$\Rightarrow y = 2x\cos^2 x-\cos^2 x\cdot\tan x + c\cos^2 x$$

$$= (2x+c)\cos^2 x-\cos x\sin x$$

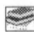

- The equation given in the above example is not a linear differential equation originally but it can be made linear by using some suitable transformation.
- The equation of the form $\frac{dy}{dx}+Py=Qy^n$ is called **Bernaulli's equation**, which can be reduce to a linear equation by dividing both sides by y^n and then by putting $t=\frac{1}{y^{n-1}}$.

Exercise-23.6

Solve the following differential equations:

1. $2x\frac{dy}{dx}+y=6x^3$
2. $(1-x^2)\frac{dy}{dx}-xy=x$
3. $\frac{dy}{dx}+y\cot x=\cos x$
4. $x\cos x\frac{dy}{dx}+y(x\sin x+\cos x)=1$
5. $4\frac{dy}{dx}+8y=5e^{-3x}$
6. $x\log x\frac{dy}{dx}+y=2\log x$
7. $x\frac{dy}{dx}+2y=x^2\log x$
8. $\frac{dy}{dx}+y=\sin x$
9. $\frac{dy}{dx}+y=e^{-2x}$
10. $(1+x^2)\frac{dy}{dx}+2xy=4x^2$
11. $(x^2-1)\frac{dy}{dx}+2xy=\frac{2}{x^2-1}$
12. $x\frac{dy}{dx}+2y=x^2, x\neq 0$
13. $\sec x\cdot\frac{dy}{dx}=y+\sin x$
14. $\frac{dy}{dx}+y=e^x$
15. $\frac{dy}{dx}+\frac{y}{x}=e^x$
16. $(1-x^2)\frac{dy}{dx}+xy=ax$
17. $\frac{dy}{dx}-y\tan x=e^x\sec x$
18. $\frac{dy}{dx}+y\cot x=x$
19. $(1+x^2)\frac{dy}{dx}+2xy=\cos x$
20. $\frac{dy}{dx}+y\tan x=2x+x^2\tan x$
21. $(x^2-1)\frac{dy}{dx}+2(x+2)y=2(x+1)$
22. $x\frac{dy}{dx}+2y=\sin x$
23. $(1+x^2)dy+2xydx=\cot x dx, x\neq 0$
24. $\left(\frac{e^{-2\sqrt{x}}}{\sqrt{x}}-\frac{y}{\sqrt{x}}\right)\frac{dx}{dy}=1, x\neq 0$
25. $\frac{dy}{dx}+y\cos x=\sin x\cos x$
26. $x\frac{dy}{dx}+y-x+xy\cot x=0, x\neq 0$
27. $x\frac{dy}{dx}-y=x+1$
28. $x\frac{dy}{dx}+2y=x\cos x$
29. $\frac{dy}{dx}+y\cot x=2x+x^2\cot x$; when $y(0)=0$
30. $\frac{dy}{dx}-2y=\cos 3x$
31. $x\frac{dy}{dx}=y(\log y-\log x-1)$
32. $(x\log x)\frac{dy}{dx}+y=\frac{2}{x}\log x$
33. $\frac{dy}{dx}+2y\cot x=3x^2\text{cosec}^2 x$
34. $\frac{dy}{dx}+2y=\sin x$
35. $x\frac{dy}{dx}-y=2x^2\sec x$
36. $\frac{dy}{dx}-3y\cot x=\sin 2x$; where at $x=\frac{\pi}{2}, y=2$
37. $y\frac{dy}{dx}\sin x=\cos x\left(\sin x-\frac{y^2}{2}\right)$; $y=1$ when at $x=\frac{\pi}{2}$
38. $\frac{dy}{dx}+y\cot x=4x\,\text{cosec}\, x$, $x=0$ and at $x=\frac{\pi}{2}$, $y=0$
39. $(1+x^2)\frac{dy}{dx}+2xy=\frac{1}{1+x^2}$ (Given: $y=0$ when $x=1$)
40. $(x+y)\frac{dy}{dx}=1$
41. $(x+2y^2)\frac{dy}{dx}=y$
42. $\frac{dy}{dx}+xy=xy^3$

43. $ydx + (x - y^2)dy = 0, y > 0$

44. $x\frac{dy}{dx} + y = y^2 \log x$

45. $\tan y \cdot \frac{dy}{dx} + \tan x = \cos y \cos^2 x$

ANSWERS

1. $y = \frac{6}{7}x^3 + cx^{-1/2}$ **2.** $y = -1 + \frac{c}{\sqrt{1-x^2}}$ **3.** $y \sin x = \frac{\sin^2 x}{2} + c$ **4.** $yx \sec x = \tan x + c$

5. $ye^{2x} = -\frac{5}{4}e^{-x} + c$ **6.** $y \log x = (\log x)^2 + c$ **7.** $y = \frac{x^2}{16}(4\log x - 1) + \frac{c}{x^2}$

8. $y = ce^{-x} + \frac{1}{2}(\sin x - \cos x)$ **9.** $ye^x = -e^{-x} + c$ **10.** $y(1+x^2) = \frac{4x^3}{3} + c$

11. $y(x^2 - 1) = 2\log\left|\frac{x-1}{x+1}\right| + c$ **12.** $y = \frac{x^2}{4} + \frac{c}{x^2}$ **13.** $y = ce^{\sin x} - (1 + \sin x)$

14. $y = \frac{e^x}{2} + ce^{-x}$ **15.** $y = e^x - \frac{e^x}{x} + \frac{c}{x}$ **16.** $y = a + c\sqrt{1-x^2}$ **17.** $y \cos x = e^x + c$

18. $(y - 1)\sin x + x \cos x = c$ **19.** $y(1 + x^2) = \sin x + c$ **20.** $y \sec x = x^2 \sec x + c$

21. $y = \frac{(x+1)}{(x-1)^3}[x^2 - 6x + 8\log(x+1)]$ **22.** $x^2y = -x \cos x + \sin x + c$

23. $y(1 + x^2) = \log \sin x + c$ **24.** $y = (2\sqrt{x} + c)e^{-2\sqrt{x}}$ **25.** $y = \sin x - 1 + ce^{-\sin x}$

26. $xy \sin x = -x \cos x + \sin x + c$ **27.** $y = x \log x - 1 + cx$

28. $y = \sin x + \frac{2}{x}\cos x - \frac{2}{x^2}\sin x + \frac{c}{x^2}$ **29.** $y = x^2$ **30.** $y = \frac{(3\sin 3x - 2\cos 3x)}{13} + ce^{2x}$

31. $y = xc^x$ **32.** $y(\log x) = \frac{-2}{x}(\log x + 1) + c$ **33.** $y(\sin^2 x) = x^3 + c$

34. $y = \frac{1}{5}(2\sin x - \cos x) + ce^{-2x}$ **35.** $y = cx + 2x \log(\sec x + \tan x)$

36. $y = -2\sin^2 x + 4\sin^3 x$ **37.** $y^2 = \sin x$ **38.** $y \sin x = 2x^2 - \frac{\pi^2}{2}$

39. $y(x^2 + 1) = \tan^{-1} x - \frac{\pi}{4}$ **40.** $x + y + 1 = ce^y$ **41.** $x = 2y^2 + cy$ **42.** $\frac{1}{y^2} = 1 + ce^{x^2}$

43. $3xy = y^3 + c$ **44.** $\frac{1}{xy} = \frac{\log x + 1}{x} + c$ **45.** $\sec x \sec y = \sin x + c$

23.13 LINEAR DIFFERENTIAL EQUATIONS WITH CONSTANT COEFFICIENTS

The equation $\frac{d^n y}{dx^n} + A_1 \frac{d^{n-1} y}{dx^{n-1}} + A_2 \frac{d^{n-2} y}{dx^{n-2}} + \ldots + A_n y = B$ ...(1)

having $A_1, \ldots, A_n$ and B either constant or function of x, is called the linear differential equation of nth order.

If $A_1, A_2, \ldots, A_n$ are all constants and B may not be constant, then equation (1) is said to be linear differential equation of nth degree with constant coefficients.

If we take $B = 0$, then the corresponding equation is called homogeneous equation.

Using the symbols $D, D^2, \ldots, D^n$ for $\frac{d}{dx}, \frac{d^2}{dx^2}, \ldots, \frac{d^n}{dx^n}$ respectively in (1), then we get

$$D^n y + A_1 D^{n-1} y + A_2 D^{n-2} y + \ldots + A_n y = B$$

$$\Rightarrow \qquad (D^n + A_1D^{n-1} + A_2D^{n-2} + ... + A_n)y = B \Rightarrow f(D)y = B \qquad ...(2)$$

where, $f(D) = D^n + A_1D^{n-1} + A_2D^{n-2} + ... + A_n$.

Now, consider the homogeneous differential equation

$$f(D)y = 0 \qquad ...(3)$$

(Obtained by putting right hand side, *i.e.*, B equal to zero).

Now, we shall show that if $y_1, y_2, ..., y_n$ are n linearly independent solutions of (3), then $(C_1y_1 + C_2y_2 + ... + C_ny_n)$ is also a solution of (3), where $C_1, C_2, ..., C_n$ are arbitrary constants.

Since, we assumed that $y_1, y_2, ..., y_n$ are solution of (3) $\Rightarrow y_1, y_2, ..., y_n$ must satisfy (3).

which gives
$$\left.\begin{array}{r} f(D)y_1 = 0 \\ f(D)y_2 = 0 \\ \dots\dots\dots\dots \\ f(D)y_n = 0 \end{array}\right] \qquad ...(4)$$

Now consider

$$f(D)(C_1y_1 + C_2y_2 + ... + C_ny_n) = f(D)(C_1y_1) + f(D)(C_2y_2) + ... + f(D)(C_ny_n)$$
$$= C_1f(D)y_1 + C_2f(D)y_2 + ... + C_nf(D)y_n$$
$$= C_1.0 + C_2.0 + ... + C_n.0 \qquad \text{(By using (4))}$$

Therefore, we have $f(D)\,[C_1y_1 + C_2y_2 + ... C_ny_n] = 0$ ...(5)

$\Rightarrow$ $(C_1y_1 + C_2y_2 + ... + C_ny_n)$ satisfies (3).

$\Rightarrow$ $(C_1y_1 + C_2y_2 + ... + C_ny_n)$ is also a solution of (3).

Hence, we can say that if $y_1, y_2, ..., y_n$ are n linearly independent solution of (3), then $(C_1y_1 + C_2y_2 + ... + C_ny_n)$ is also a solution of (3) known as complete or general solution of (3), containing n arbitrary constants $C_1, C_2, ..., C_n$.

Now, let us suppose $(C_1y_1 + C_2y_2 + ... + C_ny_n) = u$ (say).

Then, from (5), we have

$$f(D)\,u = 0 \qquad ...(6)$$

Again, let v be any particular solution of (2). Therefore, we have

$$f(D)\,v = B \qquad ...(7)$$

Now, $\quad f(D)(u + v) = f(D)u + f(D)v \quad$ (Using (6) and (7))

which shows that $(u + v)$, *i.e.*, $\{(C_1y_1 + C_2y_2 + ... + C_ny_n) + v\}$ is the general solution of (2).

WORKING PROCEDURE

STEP 1. Firstly, we find the general solution of (2), which is called the complimentary function (C.F.), contains as many arbitrary constants as is the order of the given differential equation.

STEP 2. Next, find the solution of (1), with no arbitrary constant which is called the particular integral (P.I.).

STEP 3. To find the general solution of (1), add C.F. and P.I. obtained in (1) and (2), *i.e.*, $y = u + v =$ C.F. + P.I.

- Here, the operator D stands for d / dx, D^2 for d^2 / dx^2 and so on.
- The operator D^{-1} stands for integration.
- Since, the symbol D satisfies the fundamental laws of algebra, therefore it can be regarded as an algebraic quantity.
- The general solution of (1) is $y = C.F. + P.I.$, where C.F. involves n arbitrary constants and P.I. does not involve any arbitrary constant.

- Since P.I. appears due to B in (1), therefore, if a linear differential equation with constant coefficients is given with $B = 0$, then its general solution will not involve P.I. and hence the general solution of the differential equation is given by y = C.F.
- The method (discussed above) of solving these type of equations, is given by Euler and D'Alembert.

23.13.1 AUXILIARY EQUATION

Consider the differential equation (1) with $B = 0$, *i.e.*,

$$(D^n + A_1 D^{n-1} + A_2 D^{n-2} + \ldots + A_n) y = 0 \quad \text{or} \quad f(D)y = 0. \qquad \ldots(1)$$

Substitute $y = e^{mx}$ on the trial basis, then we get $e^{mx}(m^n + A_1 m^{n-1} + A_2 m^{n-2} + \ldots + A_n) = 0$ which holds if

$$m^n + A_1 m^{n-1} + A_2 m^{n-2} + \ldots + A_n = 0 \quad \text{or} \quad f(m) = 0. \qquad \ldots(2)$$

Equation (2) is called the auxiliary equation.

From (1) and (2), we observe that the auxiliary equation $f(m) = 0$ will give the same value of m as the equation $f(D) = 0$ gives the value of D.

23.14 METHOD OF FINDING THE COMPLEMENTARY FUNCTION (C.F.)

To find the C.F., the roots of the auxiliary equation (2) are to be considered. Three different cases arise :

(i) The roots of auxiliary equation (2) are real.

(ii) The roots of auxiliary equation (2) are complex, *i.e.*, $\alpha \pm i\beta$ type.

(iii) The roots of auxiliary equation (2) are surds, *i.e.*, $\alpha \pm \sqrt{\beta}$ type.

Case (i) : (a) Suppose that the auxiliary equation (2) has n distinct roots $m_1, m_2, \ldots, m_n$, then C.F. is given by $C_1 e^{m_1 x} + C_2 e^{m_2 x} + \ldots + C_n e^{m_n x}$

where $C_1, C_2, \ldots, C_n$ are arbitrary constants.

(b) If the auxiliary equation having r roots are equal to m_1(say) and remaining roots are distinct, then the C.F. is given by

$$[C_1 + C_2 x + C_3 x^2 + \ldots + C_r x^{r-1}]\, e^{m_1 x} + C_{r+1} e^{m_{r+1} x} + \ldots + C_n e^{m_n x}.$$

Case (ii): If some of the roots of the auxiliary equation are complex, then we shall use the following procedure.

Let $\alpha \pm i\beta$ be the roots of the auxiliary equation, then the corresponding part becomes

$$= C_1 e^{(\alpha+i\beta)x} + C_2 e^{(\alpha-i\beta)x} = C_1 e^{\alpha x}.e^{i\beta x} + C_2 e^{\alpha x}.e^{-i\beta x}$$

$$= e^{\alpha x}[C_1 \cos\beta x + iC_1 \sin\beta x] + e^{\alpha x}[C_2 \cos\beta x - iC_2 \sin\beta x]$$

$$= e^{\alpha x}[(C_1 + C_2)\cos\beta x + (iC_1 - iC_2)\sin\beta x]$$

$$\text{C.F.} = e^{\alpha x}\,[B_1 \cos\beta x + B_2 \sin\beta x] \qquad \ldots(1)$$

where, B_1, B_2 are arbitrary constants.

The expression (1) can also be written as

(a) $B_1 e^{\alpha x}\cos(\beta x + B_2)$ (b) $B_1 e^{\alpha x}\sin(\beta x + B_2)$.

If, the equation has two equal pair of complex roots $\alpha + i\beta$ and $\alpha - i\beta$, say, occur twice, then the corresponding part of C.F. is written as

$$e^{\alpha x}[(B_1 + B_2 x)\cos\beta x + (B_3 + B_4 x)\sin\beta x].$$

In general, if $\alpha \pm i\beta$ occur k times, then the corresponding part of the C.F. can be written as

$$e^{\alpha x}\{(B_1 + B_2 x + \ldots + B_k x^{k-1})\cos\beta x + (B_{k+1} + B_{k+2} x + \ldots + B_{2k} x^{k-1})\}\,\sin\beta x$$

where $B_1, B_2, ..., B_k, B_{k+1}, ..., B_{2k}$ are arbitrary constants.

Case (iii) : If a pair of the roots of the auxiliary equation involves surds, say $\alpha \pm \sqrt{\beta}$, where $\beta > 0$, then the corresponding part of C.F. is one of the following three forms

(a) $e^{\alpha x}[B_1 \cosh(x\sqrt{\beta}) + B_2 \sinh(x\sqrt{\beta})]$ (b) $B_1 e^{\alpha x} \cosh(x\sqrt{\beta} + B_2)$

(c) $B_1 e^{\alpha x} \sinh(x\sqrt{\beta} + B_2)$

- The results obtained in case (iii), are exactly similar to those of case (ii) except that sin and cos replaced by sinh and cosh respectively.
- The method of finding the complimentary function (C.F.) of the following differential equation of the form

$$(D^n + A_1 D^{n-1} + A_2 D^{n-2} + ... + A_n)y = 0$$

can be concluded as follows :

S. No.	Nature of the Roots	Solution
1.	Real and distinct say $m_1, m_2, ..., m_n$	$y = B_1 e^{m_1 x} + B_2 e^{m_2 x} ... + B_n e^{m_n x}$
2.	Real and equal, say n	$y = (B_1 + B_2 x + B_3 x^2 + ... + B_n x^{n-1}) e^{nx}$
3.	Non-repeated roots : $\alpha \pm i\beta$	(a) $y = (B_1 \cos\beta x + B_2 \sin\beta x)e^{\alpha x}$ (b) $y = B_1 e^{\alpha x} \cos(\beta x + B_2)$
4.	Repeated roots : $\alpha \pm i\beta$, r times	$y = \{(B_1 + B_2 x + ... + B_r x^{r-1})\cos\beta x$ $+ (B_1' + B_2' x + ... + B_r' x^{r-1})\sin\beta x\}e^{\alpha x}$
5.	Irrational roots : $\alpha \pm \sqrt{\beta}$	(a) $y = B_1 e^{\alpha x} \cosh(x\sqrt{\beta} + B_2)$ (b) $y = B_1 e^{\alpha x} \sinh(x\sqrt{\beta} + B_2)$

Solved Examples

1. *Solve* $[D^3 + 6D^2 + 11D + 6]\, y = 0$.

[UPTU(B.PHARMA)–2001]

SOLUTION. Here, the given differential equation is

$$[D^3 + 6D^2 + 11D + 6]\, y = 0$$

To find the auxiliary equation, replace D by m, then (1) becomes,

$$m^3 + 6m^2 + 11m + 6 = 0$$

$\Rightarrow (m+1)(m^2 + 5m + 6) = 0$

$\Rightarrow (m+1)(m+2)(m+3) = 0$

$\Rightarrow m = -1, -2, -3$

i.e., Roots are real and unequal. Hence, the general solution is

$$y = C_1 e^{-x} + C_2 e^{-2x} + C_3 e^{-3x}.$$

2. *Solve* $[D^4 + 2D^3 - 3D^2 - 4D + 4]y = 0$.

SOLUTION. Here, the auxiliary equation is

$$m^4 + 2m^3 - 3m^2 - 4m + 4 = 0$$

or $(m-1)(m^3 + 3m^2 - 4) = 0$

$\Rightarrow (m-1)(m-1)(m^2 + 4m + 4) = 0$

$\Rightarrow \quad (m-1)(m-1)(m+2)^2 = 0$

$\Rightarrow m = +1, +1, -2, -2$

$\Rightarrow$ Repeated real roots exist.

Hence, general solution is

$$y_1 = (C_1 + C_2 x)e^x + (C_3 + C_4 x)e^{-2x}.$$

3. *Solve* $(D^4 + k^4)y = 0$.

SOLUTION. Here, the auxiliary equation is

$$m^4 + k^4 = 0$$

or $(m^2 + k^2)^2 - 2k^2 m^2 = 0$

$\Rightarrow (m^2 + k^2)^2 - (\sqrt{2}\,.\,km)^2 = 0$

$\Rightarrow (m^2 + k^2 - \sqrt{2}.km)(m^2 + k^2 + \sqrt{2}.km) = 0$

$\Rightarrow \quad m^2 - \sqrt{2}.km + k^2 = 0$

and $m^2 + k^2 + \sqrt{2}\,.\,km = 0$

$$\Rightarrow m = \frac{\sqrt{2}k \pm \sqrt{(2k^2 - 4k^2)}}{2}$$

$$\text{and } m = \frac{-\sqrt{2}k \pm \sqrt{(2k^2 - 4k^2)}}{2}$$

$$\Rightarrow m = \frac{k}{\sqrt{2}} \pm i\frac{k}{\sqrt{2}} \text{ and } m = -\frac{k}{\sqrt{2}} \pm i\frac{k}{\sqrt{2}}$$

Hence, the solution is

$$y = e^{kx/\sqrt{2}}\{C_1 \cos(kx/\sqrt{2}) + C_2 \sin(kx/\sqrt{2})\} + e^{-kx/\sqrt{2}}\{C_3 \cos(kx/\sqrt{2}) + C_4 \sin(kx/\sqrt{2})\}$$

4. *Solve* $[D^4 - 4D^3 + 8D^2 - 8D + 4]y = 0$.

SOLUTION. Here, the auxiliary equation is

$$m^4 - 4m^3 + 8m^2 - 8m + 4 = 0$$

$\Rightarrow \quad (m^2 - 2m + 2)^2 = 0$

$\Rightarrow \quad m = 1 \pm i,\ 1 \pm i$

$\Rightarrow$ Repeated complex roots exist.

Hence, the solution of the given equation is

$$y = e^x\{(C_1 + C_2x)\cos x + (C_3 + C_4x)\sin x\}.$$

5. *Solve* $(D^2 + 6D + 4)y = 0$.

SOLUTION. Here, the auxiliary equation is

$m^2 + 6m + 4 = 0 \quad \Rightarrow \quad m = -3 \pm \sqrt{5}$.

$\Rightarrow$ Irrational roots exist.

Hence, the solution of the given equation is

$$y = e^{-3x}(C_1 \cosh x\sqrt{5} + C_2 \sinh x\sqrt{5}).$$

Exercise-23.7

Solve the following equations :

1. $\dfrac{d^2y}{dx^2} + 3\dfrac{dy}{dx} + 2y = 0$
2. $(D^3 - 9D^2 + 23D - 15)y = 0$
3. $(D^4 - D^3 - 9D^2 - 11D - 4)y = 0$
4. $(D^2 + 1)^2 (D - 1)^2 y = 0$ [UPTU(B.PHARMA)-2002]
5. $(D^3 - D^2 - 12D)y = 0$
6. $(D^4 + 2n^2D^2 + n^4)y = 0$
7. $[D^2 - 2\lambda D + (\lambda^2 + \mu^2)]y = 0$
8. $(D^4 + D^3 + 2D^2 - D + 3)\ y = 0$
9. $(D^5 - 13D^3 + 26D^2 + 82D + 104)y = 0$
10. $\dfrac{d^4y}{dx^4} + y = 0$
11. $(D^3 - 3D^2 + 4)y = 0$
12. $(D^2 - 2D + 4)^2 y = 0$
13. $\dfrac{d^2x}{dt^2} + 5\dfrac{dx}{dt} + 6x = 0$, given $x(0) = 0$, $\dfrac{dx(0)}{dt} = 15$
14. $(D^4 - 4D + 4)y = 0$
15. $(D^2 + 1)^3 y = 0$, where $D \equiv d/dx$
16. $\dfrac{d^2x}{dt^2} - 4\dfrac{dx}{dt} + 13x = 0, x(0), \dfrac{dx(0)}{dt} = 2$
17. $\dfrac{d^3y}{dx^3} + y = 0$
18. $\dfrac{d^4y}{dx^4} + 8\dfrac{d^2y}{dx^2} + 16y = 0$
19. $(4D^4 - 8D^3 - 7D^2 + 11D + 6)y = 0$

Hint to the Selected Problems

1. $m = -1, -2$
2. $m = 1, 5, 3$
3. $m = -1, -1, -1, 4$
4. $m = \pm i, \pm i, 1, 1$
5. $m = 0, 4, 3$
6. $m = \pm ni,\ \pm ni$
7. $m = \lambda \pm \mu i$
8. $m = -1 \pm i\sqrt{2}, \dfrac{1}{2} \pm i\dfrac{\sqrt{3}}{2}$
9. $m = -1 \pm i,\ -3 \pm 2i,\ -4$
10. $m = \dfrac{-1 \pm i}{\sqrt{2}}, \dfrac{1 \pm i}{\sqrt{2}}$
11. $m = -1, 2, 2$
12. $m = 1 \pm \sqrt{3}i,\ 1 \pm \sqrt{3}i$

ANSWERS

1. $y = C_1e^{-x} + C_2e^{-2x}$
2. $y = C_1e^x + C_2e^{3x} + C_3e^{5x}$

3. $y = e^{-x}(C_1 + C_2x + C_3x^2) + C_4e^{4x}$ **4.** $y = (C_1 + C_2x)\sin x + (C_3 + C_4x)\cos x + (C_5 + C_6x)e^x$

5. $y = C_1 + C_2e^{4x} + C_3e^{-3x}$ **6.** $y = (C_1 + C_2x)\cos nx + (C_3 + C_4x)\sin nx$

7. $y = e^{\lambda x}(C_1 \cos \mu x + C_2 \sin \mu x)$

8. $y = e^{-x}\left[C_1 \cos(\sqrt{2}x) + C_2 \sin(\sqrt{2}x) + e^{x/2}\left(C_3 \cos\frac{\sqrt{3}}{2}x + C_4 \sin\frac{\sqrt{3}}{2}x\right)\right]$

9. $y = C_1e^{-x}\cos(x+\alpha) + C_2e^{-3x}\cos(2x+\beta) + C_3e^{-4x}$

10. $y = C_1e^{x/\sqrt{2}}\cos\left(\frac{x}{\sqrt{2}} + C_2\right) + C_3e^{-x/\sqrt{2}}\cos\left(\frac{x}{\sqrt{2}} + C_4\right)$

11. $y = C_1e^{-x} + (C_2 + C_3x)\,e^{2x}$ **12.** $y = e^x[(C_1 + C_2x)\cos\sqrt{3}x + (C_3 + C_4x)\sin\sqrt{3}\,x]$

13. $x = 15(e^{-2t} - e^{-3t})$ **14.** $y = ((C_1 + C_2x)e^{\sqrt{2}x} + (C_3 + C_4x)e^{-\sqrt{2}x})$

15. $y = (C_1 + C_2x + C_3x^2)\cos x + (C_4 + C_5x + C_6x^2)\sin x$ **16.** $\frac{2}{3}e^{2t}\sin 3t$

17. $y = C_1e^{-x} + e^{x/2}\left(C_2 \cos\frac{\sqrt{3}x}{2} + C_3 \sin\frac{\sqrt{3}x}{2}\right)$ **18.** $y = (C_1 + C_2x)\cos 2x + (C_3 + C_4x)\sin 2x$

19. $y = C_1e^{-x} + C_2e^{2x} + e^{x/2}\left(C_3 \cos\frac{x}{\sqrt{2}} + C_4 \sin\frac{x}{\sqrt{2}}\right)$

23.15 PARTICULAR INTEGRAL

Consider the differential equation

$$f(D)y = B \Rightarrow y = \frac{1}{f(D)}\,.\,B$$

Here, P.I. $= \frac{1}{f(D)}\,.\,B$.

23.15.1 GENERAL METHOD OF FINDING P.I.

THEOREM 1. *If B is a function of x, then* $\frac{1}{D-a}B = e^{ax}\int B\,e^{-ax}\,dx$.

PROOF. Let $y = \frac{1}{D-a}B \Rightarrow (D-a)y = B \Rightarrow \left(\frac{d}{dx} - a\right)y = B \Rightarrow \frac{dy}{dx} - ay = B$

which is the linear differential equation. I.F. $= e^{-\int a dx} = e^{-ax}$.

Hence, solution is given by $ye^{-ax} = \int B\,e^{-ax}dx$.

(Since we find the P.I., therefore we omit the constant of integration.)

$$\therefore \quad y = e^{ax}\int Be^{-ax}\,dx \quad \Rightarrow \quad \frac{1}{D-a}\,.\,B = e^{ax}\int Be^{-ax}dx$$

- P.I. never contains any arbitrary constant.
- The method discussed above can be used to evaluate P.I. in any problem. It does not depend upon the form of B.
- The method discussed above must be used when B is of the form $\sec ax$, $\operatorname{cosec} ax$, $\tan ax$, etc.

- Here, the operator $\frac{1}{f(D)}$ (known as increase operator) having the following properties :

(a) If $B = u_1 + u_2 + ... + u_n$, then $\frac{1}{f(D)}.B = \frac{1}{f(D)}.u_1 + \frac{1}{f(D)}.u_2 + ... \frac{1}{f(D)}.u_n$

(b) $\frac{1}{f(D)}(KB) = \frac{K}{f(D)}.B$ (c) $\frac{1}{f(D)}$ can be resolved into factors.

(d) $\frac{1}{f(D)}$ can be broken into partial fractions. (e) $\frac{1}{f(D)}.B$ is a particular integration.

Solved Examples

1. *Solve* $D^2 - 5D + 6 = e^{3x}$.

[UPTU(B.PHARMA)–2002, 04]

SOLUTION. The given equation can be written as

$$(D-3)(D-2)y = e^{3x}$$

$$\text{C.F.} = C_1e^{3x} + C_2e^{2x}$$

and $\text{P.I.} = \frac{1}{D-3} \cdot \frac{1}{D-2}e^{3x}$

$$= \frac{1}{D-3}e^{2x}\int e^{3x}e^{-2x}dx$$

$$= \frac{1}{D-3}e^{2x}.e^{x}$$

$$= e^{3x}\int e^{3x}.e^{-3x}dx = xe^{3x}.$$

Now, general solution = C.F. + P.I.

$$\Rightarrow \quad y = C_1e^{3x} + C_2e^{2x} + xe^{3x}.$$

2. *Solve* $(D^2+1)y = \sec^2 x$.

SOLUTION. Here, the given equation is

$$(D^2+1)y = \sec^2 x \quad ...(1)$$

The auxiliary equation of (1) is given by $m^2 + 1 = 0 \Rightarrow m = \pm i$

$\Rightarrow$ C.F. $= C_1 \cos x + C_2 \sin x$

$$\text{P.I.} = \frac{1}{D^2+1}\sec^2 x$$

$$= \frac{1}{(D+i)(D-i)}\sec^2 x$$

$$= \frac{1}{2i}\left[\frac{1}{D-i} - \frac{1}{D+i}\right]\sec^2 x$$

$$= \frac{1}{2i}\begin{bmatrix} e^{xi}\int e^{-ix}\sec^2 x\,dx \\ -e^{-ix}\int e^{ix}\sec^2 x\,dx \end{bmatrix}$$

$$= \frac{1}{2i}\begin{Bmatrix} e^{ix}\int \frac{\cos x - i\sin x}{\cos^2 x}dx \\ -e^{-ix}\int \frac{\cos x + i\sin x}{\cos^2 x}dx \end{Bmatrix}$$

$$= \frac{1}{2i}\begin{Bmatrix} e^{ix}\int(\sec x - i\sec x\tan x)dx \\ -e^{-ix}\int(\sec x + i\sec x\tan x)dx \end{Bmatrix}$$

$$= \frac{1}{2i}\begin{Bmatrix} (e^{ix} - e^{-ix})\int \sec x dx \\ -i(e^{ix} + e^{-ix})\int \tan x \sec x dx \end{Bmatrix}$$

$$= \frac{1}{2i}\{2i\sin x\log(\sec x + \tan x) - 2i\cos x\sec x\}$$

$$= \sin x\log(\sec x + \tan x) - 1.$$

Hence, the general solution is

$$y = \text{C.F.} + \text{P.I.}$$

$$\Rightarrow y = C_1\cos x + C_2\sin x + \sin x\log(\sec x + \tan x) - 1.$$

3. *Solve* $(D^2+9)y = \sec 3x$.

[UPTU(B.PHARMA)–2002]

SOLUTION. Auxiliary equation is

$$m^2 + 9 = 0 \Rightarrow m = \pm 3i$$

$$\therefore \quad \text{C.F.} = c_1\cos 3x + c_2\sin 3x$$

$$\text{P.I.} = \frac{\sec 3x}{D^2+9} = \frac{\sec 3x}{(D+3i)(D-3i)}$$

$$= \frac{1}{6i}\left[\frac{1}{D-3i} - \frac{1}{D+3i}\right]\sec 3x$$

$$= \frac{1}{6i}\begin{bmatrix} e^{3ix}\int e^{-3ix}\sec 3x dx \\ -e^{-3ix}\int e^{3ix}\sec 3x dx \end{bmatrix}$$

$$= \frac{1}{6i}\begin{bmatrix} e^{3ix}\left\{\int\left(1 - i\frac{\sin 3x}{\cos 3x}\right)dx\right\} \\ -e^{-3ix}\left\{\int\left(1 + i\frac{\sin 3x}{\cos 3x}\right)dx\right\} \end{bmatrix}$$

$$= \frac{1}{6i}\begin{bmatrix} e^{3ix}\left\{x + \frac{i}{3}\log\cos 3x\right\} \\ -e^{-3ix}\left\{x - \frac{i}{3}\log\cos 3x\right\} \end{bmatrix}$$

$$= \frac{1}{6i}\left[(\cos 3x + i\sin 3x)\left(x + \frac{i}{3}\log\cos 3x\right) - (\cos 3x - i\sin 3x)\left(x - \frac{i}{3}\log\cos 3x\right)\right]$$

$$= \frac{1}{6i}\left[\frac{2i}{3}\cos 3x \log\cos 3x + 2ix\sin 3x\right].$$

$$= \frac{1}{9}\cos 3x \log\cos 3x + \frac{x}{3}\sin 3x$$

Hence, y = C.F. + P.I.

$$= c_1\cos 3x + c_2\sin 3x + \frac{x}{3}\sin 3x + \frac{1}{9}\cos 3x\log\cos 3x.$$

Exercise-23.8

Solve the following differential equations :

1. $(D^2 + a^2)y = \sec ax$
2. $(D^2 + a^2)y = \tan ax$
3. $(D^2 + 1)y = \text{cosec } x$
4. $(D^2 + n^2)\,y = \cot nx$
5. $(D^2 + n^2)y = \tan nx$

Hint to the Selected Problems

1. $m = \pm ai \Rightarrow$ C.F. $= C_1\cos ax + C_2\sin ax$

$$\text{P.I.} = \frac{1}{D^2 + a^2}\sec ax = \frac{1}{(D+ai)(D-ai)}\sec ax$$

$$= \frac{1}{2ai}\left[\frac{1}{(D-ai)} - \frac{1}{(D+ai)}\right]\sec ax$$

$$= \frac{1}{2ai}\left\{e^{iax}\int e^{-iax}\sec ax\,dx - e^{-iax}\int e^{iax}\sec ax\,dx\right\}$$

2. $$\text{P.I.} = \frac{1}{D^2 + a^2}\tan ax$$

$$= \frac{1}{2ai}\left[\frac{1}{D - ia} - \frac{1}{D + ia}\right]\tan ax.$$

Then proceed as above.

3. $$\text{P.I.} = \frac{1}{D^2 + 1}\text{cosec } x$$

$$= \frac{1}{(D+i)(D-i)}\text{cosec } x$$

$$= \frac{1}{2i}\left[\frac{1}{D-i} + \frac{1}{D+i}\right]\text{cosec } x \cdot$$

Now proceed as above.

4. C.F. $= C_1\cos nx + C_2\sin nx$

$$\text{P.I.} = \frac{1}{D^2 + n^2}\cot nx = \frac{1}{(D - in)(D + in)}\cot nx$$

$$= \frac{1}{2in}\left[\frac{1}{D - in}\cot nx - \frac{1}{D + in}\cot nx\right]$$

ANSWERS

1. $y = C_1\cos ax + C_2\sin ax + \frac{x}{a}\sin ax + \frac{1}{a^2}\cos ax\log\cos ax$
2. $y = C_1\cos ax + C_2\sin ax - \frac{1}{a^2}\cos ax\log\tan\left(\frac{\pi}{4} + \frac{ax}{2}\right)$
3. $y = C_1\cos x + C_2\sin x + \sin x\log\sin x - x\cos x$
4. $y = C_1\cos nx + C_2\sin nx + \frac{1}{n^2}\sin nx\log(\text{cosec } nx - \cot nx)$
5. $y = C_1\cos nx + C_2\sin nx - \frac{1}{n^2}\cos nx\log(\sec nx + \tan nx)$

23.15.2 SHORT METHODS OF GETTING P.I.

The general method for getting P.I. discussed above requires lot of calculations. In certain cases, the P.I. can be obtained by methods which are shorter than the general method.

(1) To evaluate P.I., when B is of the form e^{ax} :

Here, we want to evaluate $\frac{1}{f(D)}e^{ax}$ where, $f(D) = A_0D^n + A_1D^{n-1} + ... + A_n$ with $f(a) \neq 0$.

Here, $B = e^{ax}$, we have

$$D(e^{ax}) = ae^{ax}$$
$$D^2(e^{ax}) = a^2e^{ax}$$
$$..................$$
$$..................$$
$$D^n(e^{ax}) = a^ne^{ax}$$

$\Rightarrow$ $$f(D)e^{ax} = (A_0D^n + A_1D^{n-1} + ... + A_n)e^{ax} = A_0D^ne^{ax} + A_1D^{n-1}e^{ax} + ... + A_ne^{ax}$$
$$= A_0a^ne^{ax} + A_1a^{n-1}e^{ax} + ... + A_ne^{ax} = (A_0a^n + A_1a^{n-1} + ... + A_n)\, e^{ax}$$

$\Rightarrow$ $$f(D)\, e^{ax} = f(a)\, e^{ax}.$$

Operating upon both sides with $\frac{1}{f(D)}$, we get $\frac{1}{f(D)} \cdot f(D).e^{ax} = \frac{1}{f(D)} \cdot f(a)\, e^{ax}$

$\Rightarrow$ $$e^{ax} = f(a)\frac{1}{f(D)}e^{ax}$$

$\Rightarrow$ $$\frac{1}{f(D)}e^{ax} = \frac{e^{ax}}{f(a)}, \text{ provided } f(a) \neq 0.$$

Solved Examples

1. *Solve* $(D^2 - 3D + 2)y = e^{5x}$.

SOLUTION. The given equation is

$$(D^2 - 3D + 2)y = e^{5x}$$

Auxiliary equation is $m^2 - 3m + 2 = 0$

$\Rightarrow (m-1)(m-2) = 0 \quad \Rightarrow \quad m = 1, 2$.

$\therefore \quad \text{C.F.} = C_1e^x + C_2e^{2x}$

Now,

$$\text{P.I.} = \frac{1}{D^2 - 3D + 2}.e^{5x} = \frac{1}{25 - 3\times 5 + 2}e^{5x}$$
$$= \frac{1}{12}e^{5x}$$

Hence, the general solution is

$$y = \text{C.F.} + \text{P.I.}$$

$\Rightarrow$ $$y = C_1e^x + C_2e^{2x} + \frac{1}{12} \cdot e^{5x}.$$

2. *Solve* $(D^3 + 1)y = (e^x + 1)^2$.

SOLUTION. The given equation is

$$(D^3 + 1)y = (e^x + 1)^2$$

The auxiliary equation is $m^3 + 1 = 0$

$\Rightarrow \quad (m+1)(m^2 - m + 1) = 0$

$\Rightarrow \quad m = -1, \frac{1}{2} \pm \frac{i\sqrt{3}}{2}$

Therefore,

$$\text{C.F.} = C_1e^{-x} + e^{x/2}\left[C_2\cos\left(\frac{x\sqrt{3}}{2}\right) + C_3\sin\left(\frac{x\sqrt{3}}{2}\right)\right].$$

$$\text{Now, P.I.} = \frac{1}{(D^3 + 1)}[e^x + 1]^2$$
$$= \frac{1}{(D^3 + 1)}(e^{2x} + 2e^x + 1)$$
$$= \frac{1}{D^3 + 1}(e^{2x} + 2e^x + e^{0x})$$
$$= \frac{1}{D^3 + 1}e^{2x} + 2\frac{1}{D^3 + 1}e^x + \frac{1}{D^3 + 1}e^{0x}.$$

$$=\frac{1}{2^3+1}e^{2x}+2\frac{1}{1^3+1}e^{x}+\frac{1}{0+1}e^{0x}$$

$$=\frac{1}{9}e^{2x}+e^{x}+1$$

Here, the general solution is

$$y = \text{C.F.} + \text{P.I.}$$

$$\Rightarrow y=C_1e^{-x}+e^{x/2}\left[C_2\cos\left(\frac{x\sqrt{3}}{2}\right)+C_3\sin\left(\frac{x\sqrt{3}}{2}\right)\right]+\frac{1}{9}e^{2x}+e^{x}+1$$

Exercise-23.9

Solve the following differential equations :

1. $(D^2-4D+1)y=e^{2x}-e^{-x}$

2. $(D^2+5D+6)y=e^{2x}$

3. $(4D^2+4D-3)y=e^{2x}$

4. $(D^2-2D+1)y=2e^{5x/2}$

5. $(D^2+D+1)y=e^{-x}$

6. $D^2(D+1)^2(D^2+D+1)^2y=e^{x}$

7. $[D^2+2pD+(p^2+q^2)]\,y=e^{ax}$

8. $(4D^2+12D+9)y=144e^{-3x}$

9. $(D^2-4D+3)y=e^{3x}$

10. $(D^2-a^2)y=e^{ax}-e^{-ax}$

11. $(D^2+D+1)y=(1+e^{x})^2$

12. $\frac{d^3y}{dx^3}-3\frac{d^2y}{dx^2}+3\frac{dy}{dx}-y=e^{x}+2$

Hint to the Selected Problems

1. $m=2\pm\sqrt{3}$

$$\Rightarrow \text{C.F.}=e^{2x}[C_1\cosh x\sqrt{3}+C_2\sinh x\sqrt{3}]$$

$$\text{P.I.}=\frac{1}{D^2-4D+1}[e^{2x}-e^{-x}]$$

$$=\frac{1}{D^2-4D+1}e^{2x}-\frac{1}{(D^2-4D+1)}e^{-x}$$

$$=\frac{e^{2x}}{2^2-4\times2+1}-\frac{e^{-x}}{(-1)^2-4(-1)+1}$$

$$=-\frac{e^{2x}}{3}-\frac{e^{-x}}{6}$$

4. $m=1,1\Rightarrow \text{C.F.}=(C_1+C_2x)e^{x}$

$$\text{P.I.}=\frac{1}{D^2-2D+1}(2e^{5x/2})=2.\frac{e^{5x/2}}{\frac{25}{4}-4}.$$

6. $m=0,0,-1,-1,-\frac{1}{2}\pm\frac{i\sqrt{3}}{2},\ -\frac{1}{2}\pm\frac{i\sqrt{3}}{2}.$

7. $m=-p\pm iq.$

8. $m=-\frac{3}{2},-\frac{3}{2}\Rightarrow \text{C.F.}=(C_1+C_2x)\,e^{-3x/2}$

$$\text{P.I.}=144\left(\frac{1}{4D^2+12D+9}\right)e^{-3x}=\frac{144\,e^{-3x}}{9}$$

9. $\text{P.I.}=\frac{1}{D^2-4D+3}e^{3x}=\frac{1}{2D-4}e^{3x}=\frac{x}{2}.e^{3x}$

10. $m=\pm a$

11. $m=-\frac{1}{2}\pm\frac{\sqrt{3}}{2}i$

12. $m=1,1,1$

Answers

1. $y=e^{2x}(C_1\cosh x\sqrt{3}+C_2\sinh x\sqrt{3})-\frac{1}{3}e^{2x}-\frac{1}{6}e^{-x}$

2. $y=C_1e^{-2x}+C_2e^{-3x}+\frac{1}{20}e^{2x}$

3. $y=C_1e^{x/2}+C_2e^{-3x/2}+\frac{1}{21}e^{2x}$

4. $y=(C_1+C_2x)\,e^{x}+\frac{8}{9}e^{5x/2}$

5. $y=e^{-x/2}\left[C_1\cos\left(\frac{1}{2}x\sqrt{3}\right)+C_2\sin\left(\frac{1}{2}x\sqrt{3}\right)\right]+e^{-x}$

6. $y=(C_1+C_2x)e^{0x}+(C_3+C_4x)e^{-x}+e^{-x/2}\left[(C_5+C_6x)\cos\left(\frac{1}{2}\sqrt{3}x\right)+(C_7+C_8x)\sin\left(\frac{1}{2}\sqrt{3}x\right)\right]+\frac{1}{36}e^{x}$

7. $y=e^{-px}(C_1\cos qx+C_2\sin qx)+\frac{e^{ax}}{[(p+a)^2+q^2]}$

8. $y=(C_1+C_2x)\,e^{-3x/2}+16e^{-3x}$

9. $y=C_1e^{x}+C_2e^{3x}+\frac{x}{2}e^{3x}$

10. $y=C_1e^{ax}+C_2e^{-ax}+\frac{x}{9}\cosh ax$

11. $y = e^{-x/2}\left[C_1 \cos\frac{\sqrt{3}}{2}x + C_2 \sin\frac{\sqrt{3}}{2}x\right] + 1 + \frac{1}{7}e^{2x} + \frac{2}{3}e^x$

12. $y = (C_1 + C_2 x + C_2 x^2)e^x + \frac{x^3}{6}e^x - 2$

(2) To evaluate P.I., when B is of the form $\sin ax$ or $\cos ax$:

Case (I) : ***If f(D) contains even power of D :***

Let us suppose $f(D^2) = A_0(D^2)^n + A_1(D^2)^{n-1} + \ldots + A_n$.

Here, we observe that

$$D^2 \sin ax = -a^2 \sin ax$$
$$D^4 \sin ax = (-a^2)^2 \sin ax$$
$$D^6 \sin ax = (-a^2)^3 \sin ax$$
$$\ldots\ldots\ldots\ldots\ldots\ldots\ldots\ldots$$
$$(D^2)^n \sin ax = (-a^2)^n \sin ax$$

Consider
$$f(D^2)\sin ax = [A_0(D^{2n}) + A_1(D^{2n-2}) + \ldots + A_n]\sin ax$$
$$= A_0 D^{2n} \sin ax + A_1 D^{2n-2} \sin ax + \ldots + A_n \sin ax$$
$$= A_0(-a^2)^n \sin ax + A_1(-a^2)^{n-1} \sin ax + \ldots + A_n \sin ax$$
$$= f(-a^2)\sin ax$$

Now, operating on both sides with $\frac{1}{f(D^2)}$, we get

$$\frac{1}{f(D^2)} \cdot f(D^2)\sin ax = f(-a^2)\frac{1}{f(D^2)}\sin ax$$

$$\Rightarrow \quad \sin ax = f(-a^2)\left[\frac{1}{f(D^2)}\sin ax\right] \Rightarrow \frac{1}{f(D^2)}\sin ax = \frac{1}{f(-a^2)}\sin ax.$$

Case (II) : ***If f(D) contains odd power of D :***

Let us suppose, it be put in the form $f_1(D^2) + Df_2(D^2)$, then

$$\frac{1}{f(D)}\sin ax = \frac{1}{f_1(D^2) + f_2(D^2)D}\sin ax = \frac{1}{f_1(-a^2) + f_2(-a^2)D}\sin ax$$

$$= \frac{1}{p + qD}\sin ax \text{ (say)} \qquad \text{(Where } p = f_1(-a^2), q = f_2(-a^2)]$$

$$= (p - qD)\left[\frac{1}{(p - qD)(p + qD)}\sin ax\right] = (p - qD)\left[\frac{1}{p^2 - q^2D^2}\sin ax\right]$$

$$= (p - qD)\left[\frac{1}{p^2 + q^2a^2}\sin ax\right] \qquad \text{(By putting } D^2 = -a^2)$$

$$= \frac{(p - qD)\sin ax}{(p^2 + a^2q^2)} = \frac{p\sin ax - qa\cos ax}{p^2 + a^2q^2}$$

$$\Rightarrow \quad \frac{1}{f(D)}\sin ax = \frac{f_1(-a^2)\sin ax - f_2(-a^2)a\cos ax}{\{f_1(-a^2)\}^2 + a^2\{f_2(-a^2)\}^2}$$

- To find P.I. of $\frac{1}{f(D)}\sin ax$, replace D^2 by $-a^2$ provided $f(-a^2) \neq 0$.
- If the linear factors of D contains the odd powers of D, then first multiplying the numerator and denominator by the conjugate factors $(P \pm qD)$ and then putting D^2 by$(-a^2)$.
- Similar results are true for $\frac{1}{f(D)}\cos ax$.

Solved Examples

1. *Solve* $\frac{d^2y}{dx^2} - 3\frac{dy}{dx} + 2y = \cos 3x$.

SOLUTION. The given differential equation can be written as

$$(D^2 - 3D + 2)y = \cos 3x \quad ...(1)$$

To find C.F., the auxiliary equation is

$m^2 - 3m + 2 = 0 \Rightarrow (m-1)(m-2) = 0$

which gives $m = 1$ and $m = 2$.

Therefore, C.F. $= C_1e^x + C_2e^{2x}$.

Now, P.I.

$$= \frac{1}{D^2 - 3D + 2}\cos 3x$$

$$= \frac{1}{-9 - 3D + 2}\cos 3x \quad [\because D^2 = -a^2 = -9]$$

$$= \frac{1}{-7 - 3D}\cos 3x = -\frac{(7-3D)}{(7^2 - 9D^2)}\cos 3x$$

$$= -\frac{(7-3D)}{7^2 - 9(-9)}\cos 3x$$

$$= -\frac{1}{130}[7\cos 3x - 3D\cos 3x]$$

$$= -\frac{7}{130}\cos 3x - \frac{9}{130}\sin 3x$$

$$= -\frac{1}{130}(7\cos 3x + 9\sin 3x).$$

Hence, the general solution of (1) is given by y = C.F. + P.I.

$$\Rightarrow y = C_1e^x + C_2e^{2x} - \frac{1}{130}[7\cos 3x + 9\sin 3x].$$

2. *Solve* $\frac{d^2y}{dx^2} - \frac{dy}{dx} - 2y = \sin 2x$.

SOLUTION. Here, the given equation can be written as $(D^2 - D - 2)y = \sin 2x \quad ...(1)$

To find the C.F. of (1), the auxiliary equation is $m^2 - m - 2 = 0$ which gives,

$$(m+1)(m-2) = 0 \Rightarrow m = -1, 2$$

$$\text{C.F.} = C_1e^{-x} + C_2e^{2x}.$$

Now, P.I.

$$= \frac{1}{D^2 - D - 2}\sin 2x = \frac{1}{-4 - D - 2}\sin 2x$$

$$[\because D^2 = -a^2 = -4]$$

$$= -\frac{1}{D+6}\sin 2x = -\frac{(D-6)}{(D+6)(D-6)}\sin 2x$$

$$= -\frac{(D-6)}{D^2 - 36}\sin 2x = -\frac{(D-6)}{-4-36}\sin 2x$$

$$= \frac{1}{40}[(D-6)\sin 2x]$$

$$= \frac{1}{40}[D\sin 2x - 6\sin 2x]$$

$$= \frac{1}{40}[2\cos 2x - 6\sin 2x]$$

$$= \frac{1}{20}\cos 2x - \frac{3}{20}\sin 2x$$

Hence, the complete solution is given by y = C.F. + P.I.

$$\Rightarrow y = C_1e^{-x} + C_2e^{2x} + \frac{1}{20}\cos 2x - \frac{3}{20}\sin 2x.$$

3. *Solve* $(D^2 + 4)y = \cos^2 x$.

[MTU(B.PHARMA)–2011]

SOLUTION. Here, the given differential equation is

$$(D^2 + 4)y = \cos^2 x \quad ...(1)$$

To find the C.F. of (1), the auxiliary equation is

$$m^2 + 4 = 0 \Rightarrow m = \pm 2i$$

$\therefore$ C.F. $= C_1\cos 2x + C_2\sin 2x$.

Now, P.I. $= \frac{1}{D^2 + 4}\cos^2 x$

$$= \frac{1}{2}\left[\frac{1}{D^2 + 4}(1 + \cos 2x)\right]$$

$$=\frac{1}{2}\left[\frac{1}{D^2+4}(e^{0x})+\frac{1}{D^2+4}(\cos 2x)\right]$$

$$=\frac{1}{2}\left[\frac{1}{4}+x.\frac{1}{2D}(\cos 2x)\right]$$

$$=\frac{1}{2}\left[\frac{1}{4}+\frac{x}{4}\sin 2x\right]=\frac{1}{8}(1+x\sin 2x)$$

Hence, the general solution of (1) is given by

y = C.F. + P.I.

$$=C_1\cos 2x+C_2\sin 2x+\frac{1}{8}(1+x\sin 2x)$$

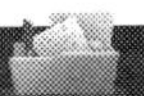

Exercise-23.10

Solve the following differential equations :

1. $(D^2+9)y=\cos 4x$ [UPTU(B.PHARMA)–2002]
2. $(D^2-2D+5)y=\sin 3x$
3. $(D^2-3D+2)y=\sin 3x$
4. $(D^4+2D^3-3D^2)y=3e^{2x}+4\sin x$
5. $(D^3-2D^2+3)y=\cos x$
6. $(D^2+16)y=\sin 2x$, given that y = 0 and $\frac{dy}{dx}=\frac{5}{6}$ when $x=0$.
7. $(D^4-2D^2+1)y=\cos x$
8. $(D^2+2D+2)y=\cos 2x$
9. $(D^2-9)y=\sin x+\cos x$
10. Solve $\frac{d^2y}{dx^2}+2\frac{dy}{dx}+10y+37\sin 3x=0$ and find the value of y when $x=\frac{\pi}{2}$ being given that y = 3, $\frac{dy}{dx}=0$ when x = 0.
11. $\frac{d^2y}{dx^2}+4y=e^x+\sin 2x$ [UPTU(B.PHARMA)–2009, 2010]
12. $(D^2+5D-6)y=\sin 3x+\cos 2x$
13. $(D^2+5D-6)y=\sin 4x\sin x$

Hint to the Selected Problems

1. $m=\pm 3i \Rightarrow$ C.F. $=C_1\cos 3x+C_2\sin 3x$

$$\text{P.I.}=\frac{1}{D^2+9}\cos 4x$$

$$=\frac{1}{-4^2+9}\cos 4x=-\frac{1}{7}\cos 4x.$$

5. $m=-1, \frac{3}{2}\pm\frac{i\sqrt{3}}{2}$

$$\Rightarrow \text{C.F.}=C_1e^{-x}+e^{3/2.x}\left[C_2\cos\left(\frac{\sqrt{3}}{2}x\right)+C_3\sin\left(\frac{\sqrt{3}}{2}x\right)\right]$$

$$\text{P.I.}=\frac{1}{(D+1)(D^2-3D+3)}\cos x.$$

9. C.F. $=C_1e^{3x}+C_2e^{-3x}$

$$\text{P.I.}=\frac{1}{D^2-9}(\sin x+\cos x)$$

$$=\frac{1}{D^2-9}\sin x+\frac{1}{D^2-9}\cos x$$

$$=\frac{1}{-1-9}\sin x+\frac{1}{-1-9}\cos x$$

$$=-\frac{1}{10}\sin x-\frac{1}{10}\cos x$$

ANSWERS

1. $y=C_1\cos 3x+C_2\sin 3x-\frac{1}{7}\cos 4x$
2. $y=e^x[C_1\cos 2x+C_2\sin 2x]+\frac{1}{26}(3\cos 3x-2\sin 3x)$
3. $y=C_1e^x+C_2e^{2x}+\frac{1}{130}(9\cos 3x-7\sin 3x)$
4. $y=(C_1+C_2x)+C_3e^x+C_4e^{-3x}+\frac{3}{20}e^{2x}+\frac{4}{5}\sin x+\frac{2}{5}\cos x$
5. $y=C_1e^{-x}+\left\{C_2\cos\left(\frac{x\sqrt{3}}{2}\right)+C_3\sin\left(\frac{x\sqrt{3}}{2}\right)\right\}e^{3x/2}+\frac{1}{26}[5\cos x-\sin x]$

6. $y = \frac{1}{6}\sin 4x + \frac{1}{12}\sin 2x$ **7.** $y = (C_1 + C_2 x)\,e^x + (C_3 + C_4 x)e^{-x} + \frac{1}{4}\cos x$

8. $y = e^{-x}[C_1 \cos x + C_2 \sin x] - \frac{1}{10}(\cos 2x - 2\sin 2x)$ **9.** $y = C_1 e^{3x} + C_2 e^{-3x} - \frac{1}{10}[\sin x + \cos x]$

10. $y = e^{-x}(C_1 \cos 3x + C_2 \sin 3x) + 6\cos 3x - \sin 3x$ and $y = 1$ at $x = \pi/2$

11. $y = C_1 \cos 2x + C_2 \sin 2x + \frac{1}{5}e^x - \frac{x}{4}\cos 2x$

12. $y = C_1 e^x + C_2 e^{-6x} - \frac{1}{30}(\cos 3x + \sin 3x) + \frac{1}{20}(\sin 2x - \cos 2x)$

13. $y = C_1 e^x + C_2 e^{-6x} + \frac{1}{2}\left[\frac{\sin 3x - \cos 3x}{30} + \frac{31\cos 5x - 25\sin 5x}{1586}\right]$

(3) To evaluate P.I., when *B* is of the form x^m, when *m* is positive integer :

i.e., to evaluate $\frac{1}{f(D)}\,x^m,\ m \in Z^+$ and $f(D) = A_0 D^n + A_1 D^{n-1} + \ldots + A_n$

Let us consider $\frac{1}{D-a}\,x^m$

$$i.e.,\ \frac{1}{(D-a)}\,x^m = e^{ax}\int e^{-ax}\,x^m\,dx$$

$$= e^{ax}\left\{-\frac{e^{-ax}x^m}{a} - \frac{mx^{m-1}e^{-ax}}{a^2} - \frac{m(m-1)x^{m-2}e^{-ax}}{a^3} - \ldots - \frac{m(m-1)\ldots 2.1e^{-ax}}{a^{m+1}}\right\} \quad \ldots(1)$$

If we expand $\frac{1}{D-a}$ in powers of *D*, we get

$$\frac{1}{(D-a)}x^m = -\frac{1}{a(1-D/a)}x^m = -\frac{1}{a}\left[1 + \frac{D}{a} + \frac{D^2}{a^2} + \ldots\right]x^m$$

$$\frac{1}{D-a}x^m = -\frac{1}{a}\left[x^m + \frac{mx^{m-1}}{a} + \frac{m(m-1)x^{m-2}}{a^2} + \ldots + \frac{m(m-1)\ldots 2.1}{a^m}\right] \quad \ldots(2)$$

Here, we observe that (1) and (2) are the same.

WORKING PROCEDURE

- Take the lowest degree term from $f(D)$ and remaining factor will be of the form $[1 + f(D)]$ or $[1 - f(D)]$. Now, this factor can be taken in the numerator with a negative index, which can be expanded by Binomial theorem. Here, it should be noted that the expansion is to be carried upto the term D^m, since we always have $D^{m+1}x^m = 0,\ D^{m+2}x^m = 0$ and all other higher differential coefficients of x^m are zero.

SOME IMPORTANT EXPANSIONS (TO BE USED DIRECTLY)

1. $[1+x]^n = 1 + nx + \frac{n(n-1)}{2!}x^2 + \frac{n(n-1)(n-2)}{3!}x^3 + \ldots$

2. $(1+x)^{-1} = 1 - x + x^2 - x^3 + x^4 - x^5 + \ldots$

3. $(1-x)^{-1} = 1 + x + x^2 + x^3 + x^4 + \ldots$ **4.** $(1-x)^{-2} = 1 + 2x + 3x^2 + 4x^3 + \ldots$

5. $(1+x)^{-2} = 1 - 2x + 3x^2 - 4x^3 + \ldots$

Solved Examples

1. *Solve* $(D^2+D-2)y = x+\sin x$.

SOLUTION. The given equation is

$$(D^2+D-2)y = x+\sin x \qquad \ldots(1)$$

To find C.F., the auxiliary equation is

$$m^2+m-2=0$$

$\Rightarrow \quad (m-1)(m+2)=0 \Rightarrow m=1,-2$

$\therefore \quad$ C.F. $= C_1e^x + C_2e^{-2x}$

Now, P.I.

$$= \frac{1}{(D^2+D-2)}(x+\sin x)$$

$$= \frac{1}{(D^2+D-2)}x + \frac{1}{(D^2+D-2)}\sin x$$

$$= \frac{1}{-2\left(1-\frac{1}{2}D-\frac{1}{2}D^2\right)}x + \frac{1}{-1+D-2}\sin x$$

$$= -\frac{1}{2}\left[1-\left(\frac{1}{2}D+\frac{1}{2}D^2\right)\right]^{-1}x + \frac{(D+3)}{(D-3)(D+3)}\sin x$$

$$= -\frac{1}{2}\left(1+\frac{1}{2}D+\ldots\right)x + \frac{(D+3)}{D^2-9}\sin x$$

$$= -\frac{1}{2}\left(x+\frac{1}{2}\right) + \frac{D+3}{-1-9}\sin x$$

$$= -\frac{1}{2}\left(x+\frac{1}{2}\right) - \left(\frac{1}{10}\right)[D(\sin x)+3\sin x]$$

$$= -\frac{1}{2}x - \frac{1}{4} - \frac{1}{10}(\cos x + 3\sin x).$$

Hence, the complete solution is given by y = C.F. + P.I.

$$\therefore \; y = C_1e^x + C_2e^{-2x} - \frac{1}{2}x - \frac{1}{4} - \frac{1}{10}(\cos x + 3\sin x)$$

2. *Solve* $(D^2-4)y = x^2$.

SOLUTION. The differential equation is

$$(D^2-4)y = x^2 \qquad \ldots(1)$$

To find the C.F. of (1), the auxiliary equation is $m^2-4=0 \Rightarrow m=\pm 2$

$\therefore \quad$ C.F. $= C_1e^{2x} + C_2e^{-2x}$

Now, P.I.

$$= \frac{1}{D^2-4}x^2 = \frac{1}{-4\left[1-\frac{1}{4}D^2\right]}x^2$$

$$= -\frac{1}{4}\left[1-\frac{1}{4}D^2\right]^{-1}x^2$$

$$= -\frac{1}{4}\left[1+\frac{1}{4}D^2+\ldots\right]x^2$$

$$= -\frac{1}{4}\left[x^2+\frac{1}{4}D^2(x^2)\right]$$

$$= -\frac{1}{4}\left[x^2+\frac{1}{2}\right]$$

Hence, the complete solution is given by y = C.F. + P.I.

$$\Rightarrow y = C_1e^{2x} + C_2e^{-2x} - \frac{1}{4}\left[x^2+\frac{1}{2}\right].$$

3. *Solve*

$$(D^2-4D+4)y = x^2+e^x+\cos 2x.$$

(UPTU(B.PHARMA)–2009)

SOLUTION. The given differential equation is

$$(D^2-4D+4)y = x^2+e^x+\cos 2x \qquad \ldots(1)$$

To find C.F., the auxiliary equation is given by

$$m^2-4m+4=0$$

$\Rightarrow (m-2)^2=0 \Rightarrow m=2,2$

$\therefore$ C.F. $= (C_1+C_2x)\,e^{2x}$

Now, P.I.

$$= \frac{1}{(D^2-4D+4)}(x^2+e^x+\cos 2x)$$

$$= \frac{1}{(D-2)^2}x^2 + \frac{1}{(D-2)^2}e^x + \frac{1}{(D^2-4D+4)}\cos 2x$$

$$= \frac{1}{4\left(1-\frac{D}{2}\right)^2}x^2 + \frac{1}{(1-2)^2}e^x + \frac{1}{(-2^2-4D+4)}\cos 2x$$

$$= \frac{1}{4}\left(1 - \frac{D}{2}\right)^{-2} x^2 + \frac{e^x}{1} - \frac{1}{4D}\cos 2x$$

$$= \frac{1}{4}\left[1 + D + \frac{3}{4}D^2 + \ldots\right]x^2 + e^x$$

$$- \frac{1}{4}\int \cos 2x\, dx$$

$$= \frac{1}{4}\left(x^2 + D(x^2) + \frac{3}{4}D^2(x^2)\right)$$

$$+ e^x - \frac{1}{4}.\frac{1}{2}\sin 2x$$

$$= \frac{1}{4}\left[x^2 + 2x + \frac{3}{2}\right] + e^x - \frac{1}{8}\sin 2x.$$

Hence, the complete solution is given by y = C.F. + P.I.

$$\Rightarrow y = (C_1 + C_2 x)e^{2x} + \frac{1}{4}\left(x^2 + 2x + \frac{3}{2}\right)$$

$$+ e^x - \frac{1}{8}\sin 2x.$$

Exercise-23.11

Solve the following differential equations :

1. $(D^3 - D^2 - 6D)y = x^2 + 1$
2. $(D^4 - a^4)y = x^4$
3. $(D^3 + 2D^2 + D)y = e^{2x} + x^2 + x$
4. $(D^3 - 3D - 2)\ y = x^3$
5. $(D^3 - 3D^2 + 2D)\ y = 4 + 60e^{5x}$
6. $(D^3 + 1)\ y = \sin 3x - \cos^2 \dfrac{x}{2}$
7. $(D^2 - 2D + 3)y = \cos x + x^2$
8. $(D^2 - 5D + 6)y = x + e^{mx}$
9. $(D^2 + 16)y = \cos 3x + e^{3x} + x^4$.
10. $(D^2 + 4)y = \sin 3x + x^2$
11. $\dfrac{d^2y}{dx^2} - \dfrac{dy}{dx} + 4y = x^2 + e^x$
12. If $\dfrac{d^2x}{dt^2} + \dfrac{g}{b}(x - a) = 0; a, b$ and g are positive numbers and $x = a', \dfrac{dx}{dt} = 0$ when t = 0, show that $x = a + (a' - a)\cos\sqrt{\dfrac{g}{b}}t$

Hint to the Selected Problems

1. $m = 0, -2, 3 \Rightarrow$ C.F. $= C_1 e^{0x} + C_2 e^{-2x} + C_3 e^{3x}$

$$\text{P.I.} = \frac{1}{D^3 - D^2 - 6D}(1 + x^2)$$

$$= -\frac{1}{6D}\left[1 + \frac{D}{6} - \frac{D^2}{6}\right]^{-1}(1 + x^2)$$

$$= -\frac{1}{6D}\left[1 - \frac{1}{6}(-D + D^2)\right]^{-1}(1 + x^2)$$

Now expand by binomial theorem and use D for differentiation and $1/D$ for integration.

7. $m = 1 \pm i\sqrt{2}$

$$\Rightarrow \text{C.F.} = e^x[C_1 \cos\sqrt{2}x + C_2 \sin\sqrt{2}x]$$

$$\text{P.I.} = \frac{1}{D^2 - 2D + 3}(\cos x + x^2)$$

$$= \frac{1}{D^2 - 2D + 3}\cos x + \frac{1}{D^2 - 2D + 3}x^2$$

$$= \frac{1}{-1 - 2D + 3}\cos x + \frac{1}{3}\left[1 - \left(\frac{2D}{3} - \frac{D^2}{3}\right)\right]^{-1} x^2.$$

10. $m = \pm 2i \Rightarrow$ C.F. $= C_1 \cos 2x + C_2 \sin 2x$

$$\text{P.I.} = \frac{1}{D^2 + 4}(\sin 3x + x^2)$$

$$= \frac{1}{D^2 + 4}\sin 3x + \frac{1}{D^2 + 4}.x^2$$

$$= \frac{1}{-9 + 4}\sin 3x + \frac{1}{4\left(1 + \frac{D^2}{4}\right)}.x^2$$

$$= -\frac{1}{5}\sin 3x + \frac{1}{4}\left(1 + \frac{D^2}{4}\right)^{-1}.x^2$$

Now expand by Binomial expansion.

ANSWERS

1. $y = C_1 + C_2 e^{3x} + C_3 e^{-2x} - \dfrac{25}{108}x - \dfrac{1}{18}x^3 + \dfrac{1}{36}x^2$

2. $y = C_1e^{ax} + C_2e^{-ax} + C_3\cos ax + C_4\sin ax - \frac{x^4}{a^4} - \frac{24}{a^8}$

3. $y = C_1 + (C_2 + C_3x)e^{-x} + \frac{1}{18}e^{2x} + \frac{1}{3}x^3 - \frac{3}{2}x^2 + 4x$

4. $y = (C_1 + C_2x)e^{-x} + C_3e^{2x} - \frac{1}{2}x^3 + \frac{9}{4}x^2 - \frac{27}{4}x + 15$ **5.** $y = C_1 + C_2e^x + C_3e^{2x} + 2x + e^{5x}$

6. $y = C_1e^{-x} + e^{x/2}\left\{C_2\cos\frac{x\sqrt{3}}{2} + C_3\sin\frac{x\sqrt{3}}{2}\right\} + \frac{1}{730}[\sin 3x + 27\cos 3x] - \frac{1}{2} - \frac{1}{4}(\cos x - \sin x)$

7. $y = e^x[C_1\cos(x\sqrt{2}) + C_2\sin(x\sqrt{2})] + \frac{1}{4}(\cos x - \sin x) + \frac{x^2}{3} + \frac{4}{9}x + \frac{2}{27}$

8. $y = C_1e^{2x} + C_2e^{3x} + \frac{1}{6}\left[x + \frac{5}{6}\right] + [e^{mx}/(m^2 - 5m + 6)]$

9. $y = C_1\cos 4x + C_2\sin 4x + \frac{1}{7}\cos 3x + \frac{1}{25}e^{3x} + \frac{1}{16}x^4 - \frac{3}{64}x^2 + \frac{3}{512}$

10. $y = C_1\cos 2x + C_2\sin 2x - \frac{1}{5}\sin 3x + \frac{1}{4}x^2 - \frac{1}{8}$

11. $y = e^{x/2}\left(C_1\cos\frac{\sqrt{15}}{2}x + C_2\sin\frac{\sqrt{15}}{2}x\right) + \frac{1}{4}\left(e^x + x^2 + \frac{x}{2} - \frac{3}{8}\right)$

(4) To evaluate $\frac{1}{f(D)}e^{ax}.X$, where X is any function of x :

Let us consider any function X_1 of x. Then, by simple differentiation, we get

$$D(e^{ax}.X_1) = e^{ax}D(X_1) + X_1ae^{ax} = e^{ax}(D+a)X_1. \quad \ldots(1)$$

Now, let us assume

$$D^n[e^{ax}.X_1] = e^{ax}(D+a)^n.X_1 \quad \ldots(2)$$

Then, consider $D^{n+1}[e^{ax}.X_1] = D[D^n(e^{ax}.X_1)] = D[e^{ax}(D+a)^n.X_1]$

$$= ae^{ax}(D+a)^n.X_1 + e^{ax}.D(D+a)^n.X_1$$
$$= e^{ax}(D+a)^{n+1}.X_1$$

Therefore, by the method of induction, we have $D^n[e^{ax}.X_1] = e^{ax}(D+a)^nX_1$, for all positive integer n

$$\therefore \quad f(D)e^{ax}.X_1 = e^{ax}f(D+a)X_1. \quad \ldots(3)$$

Now, operating on equation (3) with $\frac{1}{f(D)}$, we get

$$\frac{1}{f(D)}.f(D)e^{ax}.X_1 = \frac{1}{f(D)}e^{ax}f(D+a).X_1$$

$$\Rightarrow \quad e^{ax}.X_1 = \frac{1}{f(D)}e^{ax}f(D+a).X_1. \quad \ldots(4)$$

Let $\quad X = f(D+a).X_1 \Rightarrow X_1 = \frac{X}{f(D+a)}$.

Now, (4) becomes

$$e^{ax}.\frac{X}{f(D+a)} = \frac{1}{f(D)}e^{ax}.\frac{X}{f(D+a)}.f(D+a)$$

$$\Rightarrow \quad \frac{1}{f(D)}[e^{ax}.X] = e^{ax}\left[\frac{1}{f(D+a)}.X\right]$$

- Here, we observe that if e^{ax} is brought to the left from the right of $\frac{1}{f(D)}$, then D should be replaced by $(D + a)$.
- This method will be used if X is $\cos ax$, $\sin ax$ or x^m or a polynomial of degree m.
- This method is also capable to find $\left\{\frac{1}{f(D)}e^{ax}\right\}$, when $f(a) = 0$.

WORKING PROCEDURE

- Replace D by $(D+a)$ and brought e^{ax} before the operator $\frac{1}{f(D)}$. After that, determine $\frac{1}{f(D+a)}.X$ as usual.

Solved Examples

1. *Solve* $(D^2+4D-12)y=(x-1)e^{2x}$.

SOLUTION. The given differential equation is

$$(D^2+4D-12)y=(x-1)e^{2x} \quad ...(1)$$

To find C.F. of (1), the auxiliary equation is

$m^2+4m-12=0 \Rightarrow (m-2)(m+6)=0$

which gives $m = 2$ and $m = -6$.

$\therefore$ C.F. $= C_1e^{2x} + C_2e^{-6x}$

Now, P.I.

$$= \frac{1}{(D^2+4D-12)}e^{2x}(x-1)$$

$$= e^{2x}\frac{1}{[(D+2)^2+4(D+2)-12]}(x-1)$$

$$= e^{2x}\frac{1}{(D^2+8D)}(x-1)$$

$$= e^{2x}\frac{1}{8D\left(1+\frac{D}{8}\right)}(x-1)$$

$$= \frac{1}{8}e^{2x}\frac{1}{D}\left(1+\frac{1}{8}D\right)^{-1}(x-1)$$

$$= \frac{1}{8}e^{2x}\frac{1}{D}\left(1-\frac{1}{8}D+...\right)(x-1)$$

$$= \frac{1}{8}e^{2x}\frac{1}{D}\left(x-1-\frac{1}{8}\right) = \frac{1}{8}e^{2x}\frac{1}{D}\left(x-\frac{9}{8}\right)$$

$$= \frac{1}{8}e^{2x}\int\left(x-\frac{9}{8}\right)dx$$

$$= \frac{1}{8}e^{2x}\left(\frac{x^2}{2}-\frac{9}{8}x\right).$$

Hence, the general solution of (1), is given by y = C.F. + P.I.

$$\Rightarrow y=C_1e^{2x}+C_2e^{-6x}+\frac{1}{8}e^{2x}\left[\frac{x^2}{2}-\frac{9}{8}x\right].$$

2. *Solve* $(D^2-2D+4)y=e^x\cos x$.

SOLUTION. The differential equation is

$$(D^2-2D+4)y=e^x\cos x \quad ...(1)$$

To find the C.F. of (1), the auxiliary equation is

$m^2-2m+4=0 \Rightarrow m=1\pm i\sqrt{3}$.

Therefore, C.F.

$$= e^x(C_1\cos\sqrt{3}.x + C_2\sin\sqrt{3}.x)$$

Now, P.I.

$$= \frac{1}{(D^2-2D+4)}e^x\cos x$$

$$= e^x\frac{1}{[(D+1)^2-2(D+1)+4]}\cos x$$

$$= e^x\frac{1}{(D^2+3)}\cos x = e^x\frac{1}{-1^2+3}\cos x$$

$$= \frac{1}{2}e^x\cos x.$$

Hence, the complete solution of (1) is given by y = C.F. + P.I.

$$\Rightarrow y = e^x[C_1\cos\sqrt{3}.x + C_2\sin\sqrt{3}.x] + \frac{1}{2}e^x\cos x.$$

3. *Solve* $(D^2-5D+6)y=e^{2x}\sin 2x$.

SOLUTION. The given differential equation is

$$(D^2-5D+6)y = e^{2x}\sin 2x \quad \ldots(1)$$

To find the C.F. of (1), the auxiliary equation is given by

$$m^2-5m+6=0 \Rightarrow (m-2)(m-3)=0$$

which gives, $m = 2$ and $m = 3$.

$\therefore$ C.F. $= C_1e^{2x} + C_2e^{3x}$

Now, P.I.

$$= \frac{1}{D^2-5D+6}e^{2x}\sin 2x$$

$$= e^{2x}\frac{1}{[(D+2)^2-5(D+2)+6]}\sin x$$

$$= e^{2x}\frac{1}{D^2-D}\sin 2x = e^{2x}\frac{1}{-2^2-D}\sin 2x$$

$$= e^{2x}\frac{1}{-4-D}\sin 2x = -e^{2x}\frac{1}{(4+D)}\sin 2x$$

$$= -e^{2x}\frac{(D-4)}{(D+4)(D-4)}\sin 2x$$

$$= -e^{-2x}\left[\frac{D-4}{D^2-16}\right]\sin 2x$$

$$= -e^{2x}\left[\frac{D-4}{-4-16}\right]\sin 2x$$

$$= \frac{e^{2x}}{20}(D-4)\sin 2x$$

$$= \frac{e^{2x}}{20}[D\sin 2x - 4\sin 2x]$$

$$= \frac{e^{2x}}{20}[2\cos 2x - 4\sin 2x]$$

Hence, the complete solution of (1) is given by y = C.F. + P.I.

$$\Rightarrow y = C_1e^{2x} + C_2e^{3x} + \frac{e^{2x}}{20}[2\cos 2x - 4\sin 2x].$$

Exercise-23.12

Solve the following differential equations :

1. $(D^2-2D+1)y = e^x.x^2$ [UPTU–2004]
2. $(D^2-5D+6)y = x^3.e^{2x}$
3. $(D^2-1)y = e^x(1+x^2)$ [UPTU–2001]
4. $(D^2-4D+1)y = e^{2x}\sin x$
5. $(D^2-2D+1)y = x^2e^{3x}$
6. $(D^2-1)y = e^x\cos x$
7. $(D^2-2D+5)y = e^{2x}\sin x$
8. $(D^2-2D+6)y = e^x\cos x$
9. $(D^2-1)y = \cosh x\cos x + a^x$
10. $(D^2-4D-5)y = xe^{-x}$ given that $y=0$ and $\frac{dy}{dx}=0$ at $x=0$.
11. $(D^2-4D+4)y = e^x\cos x$ (GBTU(CO)–2010)
12. $\frac{d^2y}{dx^2}-2\frac{dy}{dx}+4y = e^{2x}\cos x$
13. $(D^2-3D+2)y = xe^x + \sin 2x$
14. $(D^2-1)y = xe^x + \cos^2 x$
15. $(D^2-1)y = x\sin x + x^2e^x$
16. $(D^2-2D+1)y = x\sin x$
17. $\frac{d^2y}{dx^2}+2\frac{dy}{dx}+y = x^2e^{-x}\cos x$

Hint to the Selected Problems

1. $m = 1,1, \therefore$ C.F. $= (C_1+C_2x)e^x$

$$\text{P.I.} = \frac{1}{D^2-2D+1}e^x.x^2 = \left[\frac{1}{(D-1)^2}e^x.x^2\right]$$

$$= e^x\left[\frac{1}{[(D+1)-1]^2}.x^2\right]$$

$$= e^x.\frac{1}{D^2}.x^2 = \frac{e^x.x^4}{12}$$

3. $m = \pm 1, \therefore$ C.F. $= C_1e^x + C_2e^{-x}$

$$\text{P.I.} = \frac{1}{D^2-1}e^x(1+x^2)$$

$$= e^x\frac{1}{(D+1)^2-1}(1+x^2)$$

$$= e^x\left[\frac{1}{D^2+2D+1-1}\right].(1+x^2)$$

$$= e^x.\frac{1}{D^2+2D}(1+x^2) = \frac{e^x}{2D}\left[1+\frac{D}{2}\right]^{-1}[1+x^2]$$

Expand by binomial expansion.

7. $m = 1 \pm 2i$, $\therefore$ C.F. $= e^x(C_1 \cos 2x + C_2 \sin 2x)$

$$\text{P.I.} = \frac{1}{D^2 - 2D + 5} e^{2x} \sin x$$

$$= e^{2x} \frac{1}{(D+2)^2 - 2(D+2) + 5} . \sin x$$

$$= e^{2x} . \frac{1}{D^2 + 2D + 5} \sin x .$$

9. C.F. $= C_1 e^x + C_2 e^{-x}$

$$\text{P.I.} = \frac{1}{D^2 - 1} \cosh x \cos x + \frac{1}{D^2 - 1} a^x$$

$$= \frac{1}{D^2 - 1}\left(\frac{e^x + e^{-x}}{2}\right)\cos x + \frac{1}{(D^2 - 1)} e^{\log a^x}$$

$$= \frac{1}{2} e^x \left\{ \frac{1}{(D+1)^2 - 1} \cos x + \frac{1}{2} e^{-x} \right.$$

$$\left. \frac{1}{(D-1)^2 - 1} \cos x + \frac{1}{(\log a)^2 - 1} e^{x \log a} \right\}.$$

ANSWERS

1. $y = (C_1 + C_2 x)e^x + \frac{1}{12} e^x . x^4$
2. $y = C_1 e^{2x} + C_2 e^{3x} - e^{2x}\left[\frac{x^4}{4} + x^3 + 3x^2 + 6x\right]$
3. $y = C_1 e^x + C_2 e^{-x} + \frac{1}{12} e^x [9x + 2x^3 - 3x^2]$
4. $y = C_1 e^{(2+\sqrt{3})x} + C_2 e^{(2-\sqrt{3})x} - \frac{1}{4} e^{2x} \sin x$
5. $y = (C_1 + C_2 x)e^x + \frac{1}{8} e^{3x}(2x^2 - 4x + 3)$
6. $y = C_1 e^x + C_2 e^{-x} - \frac{1}{5} e^x (\cos x - 2 \sin x)$
7. $y = e^x [C_1 \cos 2x + C_2 \sin 2x] - \frac{1}{10} e^{2x}(\cos x - 2 \sin x)$
8. $y = e^x [C_1 \cos \sqrt{5}.x + C_2 \sin \sqrt{5}.x] + \frac{1}{4} e^x \cos x$
9. $y = C_1 e^x + C_2 e^{-x} + \frac{1}{10} e^x [2 \sin x - \cos x] - \frac{1}{10} e^{-x}(2 \sin x + \cos x) + \frac{a^x}{(\log a)^2 - 1}$
10. $y = -\frac{1}{216} e^{-x} + \frac{1}{216} e^{5x} - \frac{1}{36} x e^{-x} - \frac{1}{12} x^2 e^{-x}$
11. $y = (C_1 + C_2 x)e^{2x} - \frac{e^x}{2} \sin x$
12. $y = e^x (C_1 \cos \sqrt{3}x + C_2 \sin \sqrt{3}x) + \frac{1}{13} e^{2x}(2 \sin x + 3 \cos x)$
13. $y = C_1 e^x + C_2 e^{2x} - e^x \left(\frac{x^2}{2} + x\right) + \frac{1}{20}(3 \cos 2x - \sin 2x)$
14. $y = C_1 e^x + C_2 e^{-x} + \frac{1}{4} e^x (x^2 - x) - \frac{1}{2} - \frac{1}{10} \cos 2x$
15. $y = C_1 e^x + C_2 e^{-x} - \frac{1}{2}(x \sin x + \cos x) + \frac{x e^x}{12}(2x^2 - 3x + 3)$
16. $y = (C_1 + C_2 x)e^x + \frac{1}{2}[(x+1)\cos x - \sin x]$
17. $y = (C_1 + C_2 x)e^{-x} + e^{-x}(-x^2 \cos x + 4x \sin x + 6 \cos x)$

(5) To evaluate $\frac{1}{f(D)} e^{ax}$, when $f(a) = 0$:

Let us suppose $f(a) = 0$. In this case $(D - a)$ is at least one factor of $f(D)$.

Let $f(D) = (D - a)^r \; g(D)$, where $g(a) \neq 0$.

$$\text{Then, } \frac{1}{f(D)} e^{ax} = \frac{1}{(D-a)^r} . \frac{1}{g(a)} e^{ax} = \frac{1}{g(a)} . \frac{1}{(D-a)^r} e^{ax}$$

$$= \frac{1}{g(a)} . \frac{1}{(D-a)^{r-1}} e^{ax} \int e^{ax} . e^{-ax} dx$$

$$= \frac{1}{g(a)} \cdot \frac{1}{(D-a)^{r-1}} xe^{ax} = \frac{1}{g(a)} \cdot \frac{1}{(D-a)^{r-2}} e^{ax} \int xe^{ax} . e^{-ax} dx$$
$$= \frac{1}{g(a)} \cdot \frac{1}{(D-a)^{r-2}} \cdot \frac{x^2}{2!} e^{ax}.$$

Proceeding in the same way, finally, we get $\frac{1}{f(D)} e^{ax} = \frac{1}{g(a)} \cdot \frac{x^r}{r!} e^{ax}$.

- Substitute $D = a$ in those factors of $f(D)$ which do not vanish for $D = a$ and then make the question as P.I. of a product of e^{ax} and 1, which is calculated by previous section and reduce to the calculation of $\frac{1}{D}.1$ or $\frac{1}{D^2}.1$ or $\frac{1}{D^3}.1$ and so on.
- Here, $\frac{1}{D^n}$ implies n times integral of 1, with respect to x.

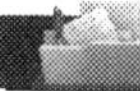

Solved Examples

1. *Solve* $(D^2 + D - 6)y = e^{2x}$. [UPTU-2002]

SOLUTION. The given equation is

$$(D^2 + D - 6)y = e^{2x} \qquad \ldots(1)$$

To find C.F. of (1), the auxiliary equation is

$$m^2 + m - 6 = 0$$

$\Rightarrow (m+3)(m-2) = 0 \Rightarrow m = 2, -3$

$\therefore$ C.F. $= C_1e^{2x} + C_2e^{-3x}$

Now, P.I.

$$= \frac{1}{D^2 + D - 6} e^{2x} = \frac{1}{(D+3)(D-2)} e^{2x}$$

$$= \frac{1}{(2+3)(D-2)} e^{2x} = \frac{1}{5(D-2)} e^{2x}.1$$

$$= \frac{1}{5} e^{2x} \frac{1}{(D+2)-2}.1 = \frac{1}{5} e^{2x} \frac{1}{D}.1 = \frac{1}{5} xe^{2x}.$$

Hence, the complete solution of (1) is given by y = C.F. + P.I.

$$\Rightarrow y = C_1e^{2x} + C_2e^{-3x} + \frac{1}{5} xe^{2x}.$$

2. *Solve* $\frac{d^2y}{dx^2} - 3\frac{dy}{dx} + 2y = e^x$.

SOLUTION. The given differential equation can be written as $(D^2 - 3D + 2)y = e^x \quad \ldots(1)$

To find the C.F. of (1), the auxiliary equation is $m^2 - 3m + 2 = 0$

$\Rightarrow (m-1)(m-2) = 0 \Rightarrow m = 1, 2$

$\therefore$ C.F. $= C_1e^x + C_2e^{2x}$

Now, P.I.

$$= \frac{1}{(D^2 - 3D + 2)} e^x = \frac{1}{(D-2)(D-1)} e^x$$

$$= \frac{1}{(1-2)(D-1)} e^x$$

(By putting 1 for D in $(D-2)$, because at $D = 1$ $(D-2) \neq 0$)

$$= -\frac{1}{D-1} e^x = -\frac{1}{D-1} e^x.1$$

$$= -e^x \frac{1}{(D+1)-1}.1 = -e^x.\frac{1}{D}.1 = -e^x.x$$

Hence, the complete solution of (1) is given by y = C.F. + P.I.

$$\Rightarrow y = C_1e^x + C_2e^{2x} - xe^x.$$

3. *Solve* $(D^3 + 3D^2 + 3D + 1)\, y = e^{-x}$.

SOLUTION. The given differential equation is

$$(D^3 + 3D^2 + 3D + 1)\, y = e^{-x} \qquad \ldots(1)$$

To find the C.F. of (1), the auxiliary equation is given by $(m+1)^3 = 0$

$\Rightarrow m = -1, -1, -1$

$\therefore$ C.F. $= (C_1 + C_2x + C_3x^2)\, e^{-x}$

Now, P.I.

$$= \frac{1}{(D+1)^3} e^{-x} = e^{-x} \frac{1}{(D-1+1)^3}.1$$

$$= e^{-x}.\frac{1}{D^3}.1 = e^{-x}.\frac{x^3}{3!}.$$

Hence, the complete solution of (1) is given by y = C.F. + P.I.

$$\Rightarrow y = (C_1 + C_2x + C_3x^2)e^{-x} + e^{-x}.\frac{x^3}{3!}.$$

Exercise-23.13

Solve the following differential equations :

1. $(D^2+4D+3)\, y = e^{-3x}$

2. $(D^2+6D+9)y = 2e^{-3x}$

3. $(D^4+D^3+D^2-D-2)y = e^x$

4. $(D^2-9D+18)y = \cosh 3x$

5. $(D-1)^2(D^2+1)^2 y = e^x$

6. $(D^2-3D+2)y = e^x$ when $y=3$, $\frac{dy}{dx}=3$ at $x=0$

7. $(D-1)^3(D+1)y = e^x + e^{-x}$

8. $(D^2-6D+9)y = 4e^{3x}$

9. $(D^2-1)y = \cosh x$

10. $(D^2-4D+4)y = 8(x^2+e^{2x}+\sin 2x)$

Hint to the Selected Problems

1. C.F. $= C_1e^{-x} + C_2e^{-3x}$

$$\text{P.I.} = \frac{1}{D^2+4D+3}e^{-3x} = \frac{1}{(D+1)(D+3)}e^{-3x}$$

$$= \frac{1}{(-3+1)(D+3)}e^{-3x} = -\frac{1}{2(D+3)}e^{-3x}.1$$

$$= -\frac{1}{2}e^{-3x}\frac{1}{[(D-3)+3]}.1$$

$$= -\frac{1}{2}e^{-3x}.\frac{1}{D}.1 = -\frac{1}{2}e^{-3x}.x$$

4. C.F. $= C_1e^{3x} + C_2e^{6x}$

$$\text{P.I.} = \frac{1}{D^2-9D+18}\cosh 3x$$

$$= \frac{1}{D^2-9D+18}\left(\frac{e^{3x}+e^{-3x}}{2}\right)$$

$$= \frac{1}{2(D-3)(D-6)}(e^{3x}+e^{-3x})$$

7. C.F. $= (C_1 + C_2x + C_3x^2)\, e^x + C_1e^{-x}$

$$\text{P.I.} = \frac{1}{(D-1)^3(D+1)}(e^x+e^{-x})$$

$$= \frac{1}{2}\frac{1}{(D-1)^3}e^x.1 - \frac{1}{8}\frac{1}{(D+1)}e^{-x}.1.$$

10. $$\text{P.I.} = \frac{1}{(D^2-4D+4)}(8x^2+8e^{2x}+8\sin 2x)$$

$$= \frac{1}{(D-2)^2}8x^2 + \frac{1}{(D-2)^2}8e^{2x} + \frac{1}{(D-2)^2}.8\sin 2x.$$

ANSWERS

1. $y = C_1e^{-x} + C_2e^{-3x} - \frac{x}{2}e^{-3x}$

2. $y = (C_1+C_2x)\, e^{-3x} + x^2e^{-3x}$

3. $y = C_1e^x + C_2e^{-x} + e^{-x/2}\left[C_3\cos\left(\frac{\sqrt{7}}{2}x\right) + C_4\sin\left(\frac{\sqrt{7}}{2}x\right)\right] + \frac{1}{8}xe^x$

4. $y = C_1e^{3x} + C_2e^{6x} - \frac{1}{6}xe^{3x} + \frac{1}{108}e^{-3x}$

5. $y = (C_1+C_2x)e^x + (C_3+C_4x)\cos x + (C_5+C_6x)\sin x + \frac{1}{8}x^2e^x$

6. $y = 2e^x + e^{2x} - xe^x$

7. $y = (C_1 + C_2x + C_3x^2)e^x + C_4e^{-x} + \frac{1}{12}x^3e^x - \frac{x}{8}e^{-x}$

8. $y = (C_1+C_2x)\, e^{3x} + 2x^2e^{3x}$

9. $y = C_1e^x + C_2e^{-x} + \frac{1}{2}x\sinh x$

10. $(C_1+C_2x)\, e^{2x} + 2x^2 + 3 + 4x + 4x^2e^{2x} + \cos 2x$

(6) To evaluate $\frac{1}{f(D^2)}\sin ax$ or $\cos ax$, when $f(-a^2)=0$:

To find the particular integral of such cases, we shall calculate P.I. for e^{iax} instead of $\sin ax$ or $\cos ax$.

Here, we have $e^{iax} = \cos ax + i\sin ax$.

Thus, P.I. for e^{iax} = P.I. for $(\cos ax + i\sin ax)$

$\Rightarrow$ P.I. for $\cos ax$ = Real part of P.I. for e^{iax} and P.I. for $\sin ax$ = imaginary part of P.I. for e^{iax}.

Therefore, $\frac{\cos ax}{D^2+a^2}$ and $\frac{\sin ax}{D^2+a^2}$ are respectively, real and imaginary part of $\frac{e^{iax}}{D^2+a^2}$

$$= \frac{e^{iax}}{(D+ai)(D-ai)} = \frac{e^{iax}}{(ai+ai)(D-ai)}$$

(By putting ai in $(D+ai)$ because at $D = ai$ it does not vanish.)

$$= \frac{e^{iax}}{2ai}\left[\frac{1}{D+ai-ai}.1\right] = \frac{e^{iax}}{2ai}\cdot\frac{1}{D}.1 = \frac{x}{2ai}(e^{aix})$$

$$= -\frac{ix(\cos ax + i\sin ax)}{2a} = -\frac{ix}{2a}\cos ax + \frac{x}{2a}\sin ax$$

$$\Rightarrow \quad \frac{1}{D^2+a^2}\sin ax = -\frac{x}{2a}\cos ax = \frac{x}{2}\int \sin ax\, dx$$

and $$\frac{1}{D^2+a^2}\cos ax = \frac{x}{2a}\sin ax = \frac{x}{2}\int \cos ax\, dx.$$

Solved Examples

1. *Solve* $(D^2+a^2)y = \sin ax$.

SOLUTION. The given equation is

$$(D^2+a^2)y = \sin ax \qquad ...(1)$$

To find the C.F. of (1), the auxiliary equation is

$$m^2+a^2 = 0 \Rightarrow m = 0 \pm ai$$

$\therefore$ C.F. $= e^{0x}[C_1\cos ax + C_2\sin ax]$
$= [C_1\cos ax + C_2\sin ax]$

Now, P.I.

$$= \frac{1}{D^2+a^2}\sin ax$$

= Imaginary part of $\left[\frac{1}{D^2+a^2}(\cos ax + i\sin ax)\right]$

= Imaginary part of $\left[\frac{1}{D^2+a^2}e^{iax}\right]$

= Imaginary part of $\left[\frac{1}{(D+ai)(D-ai)}e^{iax}\right]$

= Imaginary part of $\left[\frac{1}{(ai+ai)(D-ai)}e^{iax}\right]$

= Imaginary part of $\left[\frac{1}{2ai}\cdot\frac{1}{(D-ai)}e^{iax}\right]$

= Imaginary part of $\frac{1}{2ai}\frac{1}{(D-ai)}e^{iax}.1$

= Imaginary part of $\frac{1}{2ai}e^{iax}\frac{1}{[(D+ia)-ia]}.1$

= Imaginary part of $\frac{1}{2ai}e^{iax}\frac{1}{D}.1$

= Imaginary part of $\frac{1}{2ai}e^{iax}.x$

= Imaginary part of $\frac{1}{2ai}.x(\cos ax + i\sin ax)$

= Imaginary part of $\frac{1}{2a}x\left[\frac{1}{i}\cos ax + \sin ax\right]$

= Imaginary part of $\frac{1}{2a}x\left[\frac{i}{i^2}\cos ax + \sin ax\right]$

= Imaginary part of $\frac{1}{2a}x[-i\cos ax + \sin ax]$

$= -\frac{x}{2a}\cos ax$.

Hence, the complete solution of (1) is given by y = C.F. + P.I.

$$\Rightarrow y = C_1\cos ax + C_2\sin ax - \frac{x}{2a}\cos ax.$$

2. *Solve* $(D^2+1)y = \sin x \sin 2x$.

SOLUTION. The given equation is

$$(D^2+1)y = \sin x\sin 2x \qquad ...(1)$$

To find the C.F. of (1), the auxiliary equation is

$$(m^2+1) = 0 \Rightarrow m = \pm i$$

$\therefore$ C.F. $= C_1\cos x + C_2\sin x$

Now, P.I. $= \frac{1}{(D^2+1)}(\sin x\sin 2x)$

$$=\frac{1}{(D^2+1)}\cdot\frac{1}{2}[2\sin x\sin 2x]$$

$$=\frac{1}{2}\cdot\frac{1}{D^2+1}[\cos x-\cos 3x]$$

$$=\frac{1}{2}\left[\frac{1}{D^2+1}\cos x-\frac{1}{D^2+1}\cos 3x\right].$$

Now, $\frac{1}{D^2+1}\cos 3x=\frac{1}{-3^2+1}\cos 3x$

$$=-\frac{1}{8}\cos 3x$$

Again, $\frac{1}{D^2+1}\cos x$

$$= \text{Real part of}\left[\frac{1}{D^2+1}e^{ix}\right]$$

$$= \text{Real part of}\left[\frac{1}{(D+i)(D-i)}e^{ix}\right]$$

$$= \text{Real part of}\left[\frac{1}{(i+i)(D-i)}e^{ix}\right]$$

$$= \text{Real part of}\left[\frac{1}{2i}\cdot\frac{1}{(D-i)}e^{ix}\right]$$

$$= \text{Real part of}\left[\frac{1}{2i}\,\frac{1}{D-i}e^{ix}.1\right]$$

$$= \text{Real part of}\left[\frac{1}{2i}e^{ix}\cdot\frac{1}{(D+i-i)}.1\right]$$

$$= \text{Real part of}\left[\frac{1}{2i}\,e^{ix}\,\frac{1}{D}.1\right]$$

$$= \text{Real part of}\left[\frac{1}{2i}.e^{ix}.x\right]$$

$$= \text{Real part of}\left[\frac{x}{2i}(\cos x+i\sin x)\right]$$

$$= \text{Real part of}\left[-i.\frac{1}{2}x\cos x+\frac{1}{2}x\sin x\right]$$

$$=\frac{1}{2}x\sin x$$

Hence, the complete solution of (1) is given by y = C.F. + P.I.

$$\Rightarrow y=C_1\cos x+C_2\sin x+\frac{x}{4}\sin x-\frac{1}{16}\cos 3x\ .$$

3. *Find the solution of the equation* $\frac{d^2y}{dx^2}+4y=8\cos 2x$ *given that* $y=0$ *and* $\frac{dy}{dx}=2$ *when* $x=0$.

SOLUTION. The given differential equation can be written as $(D^2+4)y=8\cos 2x$ ...(1)

To find the C.F. of (1), the auxiliary equation is given by

$$m^2+4=0\Rightarrow m=\pm 2i$$

$\therefore$ C.F. $=C_1\cos 2x+C_2\sin 2x$

Now, P.I. $=8.\frac{1}{D^2+4}\cos 2x$

$$=8.\text{ Real part of}\left[\frac{1}{D^2+4}(\cos 2x+i\sin 2x\right]$$

$$=8.\text{ Real part of}\left[\frac{1}{D^2+4}e^{2ix}\right]$$

$$=8.\text{ Real part of}\left[\frac{1}{(D+2i)(D-2i)}e^{2ix}\right]$$

$$=8.\text{ Real part of}\left[\frac{1}{(2i+2i)(D-2i)}e^{2ix}\right]$$

$$=8.\text{ Real part of}\left[\frac{1}{4i}\,\frac{1}{(D-2i)}e^{2ix}.1\right]$$

$$=8.\text{ Real part of}\left[\frac{1}{4i}e^{2ix}\,\frac{1}{D}.1\right]$$

$$=8.\text{ Real part of}\left[\frac{1}{4i}\,e^{2ix}.x\right]$$

$$=8.\text{ Realpartof}\left[\frac{1}{4i}(\cos 2x+i\sin 2x).x\right]$$

$$=8.\text{ Real part of}\frac{1}{-4}[i\cos 2x-\sin 2x].x$$

$$=8.\frac{x}{4}\sin 2x=2x\sin 2x$$

Hence, the complete solution of (1) is given by y = C.F. + P.I.

$$\Rightarrow y=C_1\cos 2x+C_2\sin 2x+2x\sin 2x$$

$$\Rightarrow \frac{dy}{dx}=-2C_1\sin 2x+2C_2\cos 2x+2\sin 2x+4x\cos 2x.$$

Now, using the given conditions

$y=0, \frac{dy}{dx}=2$ at $x=0$ gives $C_1=0$

and $C_2=1$

$\therefore$ General solution is

$$y=\sin 2x+2x\sin 2x$$

4. *Solve the given differential equation*

$$\frac{d^2y}{dx^2}+9y=2\sin 3x+\cos 3x\cdot$$

SOLUTION. The given differential equation can be written as

$$(D^2+9)y=2\sin 3x+\cos 3x \quad \ldots(1)$$

To find the C.F. of (1), the auxiliary equation is given by

$$m^2+9=0 \Rightarrow m=\pm 3i$$

$\therefore$ C.F. $=C_1\cos 3x+C_2\sin 3x$

Now, P.I.

$$=\frac{1}{D^2+9}(2\sin 3x+\cos 3x)$$

$$=2\frac{1}{D^2+9}\sin 3x+\frac{1}{D^2+9}\cos 3x.$$

Now,

$$\frac{1}{D^2+9}\cos 3x+i.\frac{1}{D^2+9}\sin 3x$$

$$=\frac{1}{D^2+9}(\cos 3x+i\sin 3x)$$

$$=\frac{1}{D^2+9}e^{i3x}$$

$$=\frac{1}{(D+3i)(D-3i)}e^{i3x}$$

$$=\frac{1}{(3i+3i)(D-3i)}e^{3ix}.1$$

$$=\frac{e^{i3x}}{6i}.\frac{1}{[(D+3i)-3i]}.1$$

$$=\frac{1}{6i}.e^{i3x}.\frac{1}{D}.1=\frac{1}{6i}e^{i3x}.x$$

$$=\frac{x}{6i}[\cos 3x+i\sin 3x]$$

$$=\frac{x}{6}\sin 3x-i\frac{x}{6}\cos 3x.$$

Now, equating real and imaginary part of both sides, we get

$$\frac{1}{D^2+9}\cos 3x=\frac{x}{6}\sin 3x$$

and $\frac{1}{D^2+9}\sin 3x=-\frac{x}{6}\cos 3x.$

$\therefore$ Required P.I.

$$=2\left[-\frac{x}{6}\cos 3x\right]+\frac{x}{6}\sin 3x$$

$$=-\frac{x}{3}\cos 3x+\frac{x}{6}\sin 3x.$$

Hence, the complete solution of (1) is given by y = C.F. + P.I.

$$\Rightarrow y=C_1\cos 3x+C_2\sin 3x-\frac{1}{3}x\cos 3x+\frac{1}{6}x\sin 3x$$

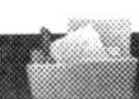

Exercise-23.14

Solve the following differential equations :

1. $(D^2+a^2)y=\cos ax$
2. $(D^2+4)y=\cos 2x$
3. $(D^2+4)y=e^x+\sin 2x$
4. $(D^3+a^2D)y=\sin ax$ [UPTU–2005]
5. $(D^3+1)y=\cos 2x$
6. $(D^4+D^2+1)y=e^{-x/2}\cos\frac{x\sqrt{3}}{2}$
7. $(D^2+2D+2)y=2e^{-x}\sin x$
8. $(D^4+2D^2+1)y=\cos x$
9. $(D^2+4)y=4+\sin 2x$

Hint to the Selected Problems

1. $m=\pm ai \Rightarrow$ C.F. $=C_1\cos ax+C_2\sin ax$

P.I. $=\frac{1}{D^2+a^2}\cos ax$

$=$ Real part of $\left[\frac{1}{D^2+a^2}e^{iax}\right].$

3. $m=\pm 2i$, C.F. $=C_1\cos 2x+C_2\sin 2x$

P.I. $=\frac{1}{(D^2+4)}(e^x+\sin 2x)$

$$=\frac{e^x}{D^2+4}+\frac{1}{D^2+4}.\sin 2x$$

$$=\frac{e^x}{1+4}+\text{ Imag. part of}\left[\frac{1}{D^2+4}.e^{2ix}\right]$$

ANSWERS

1. $y = C_1 \cos ax + C_2 \sin ax + \frac{x}{2a} \sin ax$
2. $y = C_1 \cos 2x + C_2 \sin 2x + \frac{x}{4} \sin 2x$
3. $y = C_1 \cos 2x + C_2 \sin 2x + \frac{1}{5} e^x - \frac{1}{4} x \cos 2x$
4. $y = C_1 + C_2 \cos ax + C_3 \sin ax - \frac{1}{2a^2} x \sin ax$
5. $y = C_1 e^{-x} + e^{x/2}\left[C_2 \cos \frac{\sqrt{3}}{2} x + C_3 \sin \frac{\sqrt{3}}{2} x\right] + \frac{1}{65}(\cos 2x - 8 \sin 2x)$
6. $y = e^{-x/2}\left[C_1 \cos \frac{1}{2} x\sqrt{3} + C_2 \sin \frac{1}{2} x\sqrt{3}\right] + e^{x/2}\left[C_3 \cos \frac{1}{2} x\sqrt{3} + C_4 \sin \frac{1}{2} x\sqrt{3}\right]$
$$- \frac{1}{12}\sqrt{3}\, x\, e^{-x/2} \sin \frac{\sqrt{3}x}{2} + \frac{x}{4} e^{-x/2} \cos \frac{\sqrt{3}}{2} x$$
7. $y = e^{-x}(C_1 \cos x + C_2 \sin x) - xe^{-x} \cos x$
8. $y = (C_1 + C_2 x) \cos x + (C_3 + C_4 x) \sin x - \frac{1}{8} x^2 \cos x$
9. $y = C_1 \cos 2x + C_2 \sin 2x + 1 - \frac{x}{4} \cos 2x$

(7) To evaluate $\frac{1}{f(D)} x.X$, where X is any function of x (except e^{ax}) :

Consider $D^n(x.X) = xD^n.X + {}^nC_1\ D^{n-1}.X$ (By Leibnitz's theorem)

We have $f(D)\,(xX) = x\ f(D)X + f'(D).X$

Now, taking the inverse operator, we have $\frac{1}{f(D)}(xX) = x.\frac{1}{f(D)} X + \left[\frac{d}{dD}\frac{1}{f(D)}\right] X$

But we have $\frac{d}{dD}\left[\frac{1}{f(D)}\right] = -\frac{f'(D)}{\{f(D)\}^2}$.

Therefore, $\frac{1}{f(D)}(x.X) = x.\frac{1}{f(D)} X - \frac{f'(D)}{\{f(D)\}^2} X$.

- If we want to find P.I. when B is of the form $x^m.X$, where X is any function of x, then there are two cases

(a) If $X = x^n$, then $x^m.X = x^{m+n}$.

Then B is of the form x^{m+n} (Polynomial). Here, we should apply the method of finding P.I. for polynomial discussed earlier.

(b) If $X = e^{ax}$, then $x^m.X = x^m.e^{ax}$ and we should apply the method, discussed earlier.

(c) If $X = \cos ax$, then $x^m.X = x^m \cos ax$

Then P.I. $= \frac{1}{f(D)} x^m \cos ax = \frac{1}{f(D)}$ (Real part of $x^m.e^{iax}$) = Real part of $\frac{1}{f(D)} x^m.e^{iax}$, which can be easily calculated.

Similar results hold if $X = \sin ax$, then taking imaginary part.

Solved Examples

1. *Solve* $(D^2+2D+1)y = x\cos x$.

SOLUTION. The given equation is

$$(D^2+2D+1)y = x\cos x \quad \ldots(1)$$

To find the C.F. of (1), the auxiliary equation is

$$m^2+2m+1=0 \Rightarrow m=-1,-1$$

$\therefore$ C.F. $=(C_1+C_2x)\,e^{-x}$

Now, P.I.

$$= \frac{1}{(D^2+2D+1)}.x\cos x$$

$$= x.\frac{1}{D^2+2D+1}\cos x - \frac{2D+2}{(D^2+2D+1)^2}\cos x$$

$$= x.\frac{1}{2D}\cos x - \frac{2D+2}{4D^2}\cos x$$

$$= \frac{x}{2}\sin x + \frac{(D+1)}{2}\cos x$$

$$= \frac{x}{2}\sin x + \frac{\cos x}{2} - \frac{\sin x}{2}$$

Hence, the complete solution of (1) is given by y = C.F. + P.I.

$$\Rightarrow y = (C_1+C_2x)e^{-x} + \frac{x}{2}\sin x + \frac{\cos x}{2} - \frac{\sin x}{2}.$$

2. *Solve* $(D^2-4D+4) = 8x^2e^{2x}\sin 2x$.

SOLUTION. The given equation is

$$(D^2-4D+4) = 8x^2e^{2x}\sin 2x \ \ldots(1)$$

To find the C.F. of (1), the auxiliary equation is

$$m^2-4m+4=0 \Rightarrow m=2,2$$

$\therefore$ C.F. $=(C_1+C_2x)\,e^{2x}$

Now, P.I.

$$= 8.\frac{1}{(D-2)^2}e^{2x}(x^2\sin 2x)$$

$$= 8e^{2x}.\frac{1}{(D+2-2)^2}.(x^2\sin 2x)$$

$$= 8e^{2x}.\frac{1}{D^2}(x^2\sin 2x) = 8\,e^{2x}.I_1$$

where, $I_1 = \frac{1}{D^2}(x^2\sin 2x)$

$$= \text{Imaginary part of } \frac{1}{D^2}x^2e^{2ix}$$

$$= \text{Imaginary part of } e^{2ix}\frac{1}{(D+2i)^2}x^2$$

$$= \text{Imaginary part of } \frac{e^{2ix}}{4i^2}\left(1+\frac{D}{2i}\right)^{-2}x^2$$

$$= \text{Imaginary part of } \frac{e^{2ix}}{-4}\left(1-\frac{iD}{2}\right)^{-2}x^2$$

= Imaginary part of

$$\frac{e^{2ix}}{-4}\left[1+2\left(\frac{iD}{2}\right)+3\left(\frac{iD}{2}\right)^2+\ldots\right]x^2$$

= Imaginary part of

$$\frac{e^{2ix}}{-4}\left[1+Di-\frac{3}{4}D^2+\ldots\right]x^2$$

$$= \text{Imaginary part of } \frac{e^{2ix}}{-4}\left[x^2+2ix-\frac{3}{2}\right]$$

= Imaginary part of

$$\left\{-\frac{1}{4}(\cos 2x+i\sin 2x)\left(x^2+2ix-\frac{3}{2}\right)\right\}$$

$$= -\frac{1}{4}\left[\left(x^2-\frac{3}{2}\right)\sin 2x + 2x\cos 2x\right]$$

$$= -\frac{1}{8}[(2x^2-3)\sin 2x+4x\cos 2x]$$

$\therefore$ P.I.

$$= 8e^{2x}.I_1$$

$$= 8e^{2x}\left[-\frac{1}{8}\{(2x^2-3)\sin 2x+4x\cos 2x\}\right]$$

$$= -e^{2x}[(2x^2-3)\sin 2x+4x\cos 2x].$$

Hence, the complete solution of (1) is given by y = C.F. + P.I.

$$\Rightarrow y = e^{2x}[C_1+C_2x+3\sin 2x - 2x^2\sin 2x - 4x\cos 2x].$$

3. *Solve* $(D^2-2D+1)\,y = xe^x\sin x$.

SOLUTION. The given differential equation can be written as

$$(D^2 - 2D + 1)\, y = xe^x \sin x \quad \ldots(1)$$

To find the C.F. of (1), the auxiliary equation is given by

$$m^2 - 2m + 1 = 0 \Rightarrow m = 1,1$$

$\therefore$ C.F. $= (C_1 + C_2x)\, e^x$

Now, P.I.

$$= \frac{1}{(D^2 - 2D + 1)} xe^x \sin x$$

$$= e^x \frac{1}{(D+1)^2 - 2(D+1) + 1} x \sin x$$

$$= e^x \frac{1}{D^2}(x \sin x) = e^x . \frac{1}{D}\int x \sin x\, dx$$

$$= e^x \left(\frac{1}{D}\right)(-x \cos x + \sin x)$$

$$= e^x \left[\int -x \cos x dx + \int \sin x dx\right]$$

$$= e^x\, [-x \sin x - 2\cos x].$$

Hence, the complete solution of (1) is given by y = C.F. + P.I.

$$\Rightarrow y = (C_1 + C_2x)e^x - e^x(x \sin x + 2\cos x).$$

4. *Solve* $\dfrac{d^2y}{dx^2} + 4y = x \sin x$.

SOLUTION. The given differential equation can be written as $(D^2 + 4)y = x \sin x \quad \ldots(1)$

To find the C.F. of (1), the auxiliary equation is given by

$$m^2 + 4 = 0 \Rightarrow m = \pm 2i$$

$\therefore$ C.F. $= C_1 \cos 2x + C_2 \sin 2x$

Now, P.I.

$$= \frac{1}{D^2 + 4} x \sin x$$

$$= x \frac{1}{D^2 + 4} \sin x - \frac{2D}{(D^2 + 4)^2} \sin x$$

$$= \frac{x \sin x}{-1^2 + 4} - \frac{2D}{(-1^2 + 4)^2} \sin x$$

$$= \frac{1}{3} x \sin x - \frac{2}{9} D(\sin x)$$

$$= \frac{1}{3} x \sin x - \frac{2}{9} \cos x$$

Hence, the complete solution of (1) is given by y = C.F. + P.I.

$$\Rightarrow y = C_1 \cos 2x + C_2 \sin 2x + \frac{x}{3} \sin x - \frac{2}{9} \cos x.$$

Exercise-23.15

Solve the following differential equations :

1. $(D^2 - 2D + 1)y = x \sin x$
2. $(D^2 + m^2)y = x \cos mx$
3. $(D^2 - 1) = x^2 \sin x$
4. $(D^2 + a^2)^2 y = \sin ax$
5. $(D^4 - 1)y = x \sin x$
6. $(D^4 - 1)y = e^x \cos x$
7. $(D^4 + 2D^2 + 1)y = x^2 \cos x$
8. $(D^2 + 1)y = x^2 \sin 2x$
9. $(D^2 + 1)^2 y = 24x \cos x$, given that $x = 0, y = 0, Dy = 0,\ D^2y = 0, D^3y = 0$.
10. $(D^2 + 4)y = \cos^2 x$ [UPTU–2003]

Hint to the Selected Problems

1. C.F. $= (C_1 + C_2x)\, e^x$

$$\text{P.I.} = \frac{1}{D^2 - 2D + 1} x \sin x$$

$$= x \frac{1}{D^2 - 2D + 1} \sin x - \frac{(2D - 2)}{(D^2 - 2D + 1)^2} \sin x$$

$$= x . \frac{1}{-1 - 2D + 1} \sin x - \frac{(2D - 2)}{(-1 - 2D + 1)^2} \sin x$$

$$= x . \frac{1}{-2D} \sin x - \frac{(2D - 2)}{4D^2} \sin x.$$

2. $\text{P.I.} = \dfrac{1}{D^2 + m^2} x \cos mx$

$$= \text{Real part of} \frac{1}{(D^2 + m^2)} x\, e^{imx}$$

$$= \text{Real part of}\, e^{imx} \left[\frac{1}{(D + im)^2 + m^2} . x\right]$$

8. $\text{P.I.} = \dfrac{1}{D^2 + 1} x^2 \sin 2x$

$= \text{Imaginary part of } \frac{1}{D^2+1} \cdot xe^{2ix}$

$= \text{Imag. part of } e^{2ix}\left[\frac{1}{(D+2i)^2+1}\right] \cdot x.$

10. $\text{P.I.} = \frac{1}{(D^2+1)^2} 24x\cos x = 24\frac{1}{(D^2+1)^2} x\cos x$

$= \text{Real part of } 24e^{ix} \frac{1}{[(D+i)^2+1]^2} \cdot x$

ANSWERS

1. $y = (C_1 + C_2x)\, e^x + \frac{1}{2}(x\cos x + \cos x - \sin x)$

2. $y = C_1 \cos mx + C_2 \sin mx + \frac{x^2}{4m} \sin mx + \frac{x}{4m^2} \cos mx$

3. $y = C_1e^x + C_2e^{-x} - x\cos x - \frac{1}{2}(x^2-1)\sin x$

4. $y = (C_1 + C_2x)\cos ax + (C_3 + C_4x)\sin ax - \frac{1}{8a^2}(x^2 \sin ax)$

5. $y = C_1e^x + C_2e^{-x} + C_3 \cos x + C_4 \sin x + \frac{1}{8}(x^2 \cos x - x\sin x)$

6. $y = C_1e^x + C_2e^{-x} + C_3 \cos x + C_4 \sin x - \frac{1}{5}e^x \cos x$

7. $y = (C_1 + C_2x)\cos x + (C_3 + C_4x)\sin x - \frac{1}{48}(x^4 - 9x^2)\cos x + \frac{1}{12}x^3 \sin x$

8. $y = C_1 \cos x + C_2 \sin x - \frac{1}{27}[24x\cos 2x + (9x^2 - 26)\sin 2x]$

9. $y = 3x^2 \sin x - x^3 \cos x$

10. $y = C_1e^{2x} + C_2e^{-2x} - \frac{1}{8} - \frac{1}{16}\cos 2x$

23.16 ORDINARY SIMULTANEOUS LINEAR DIFFERENTIAL EQUATIONS

In this section, we shall discuss the ordinary differential equations involving two or more dependent variables. Here, we shall discuss the case when there are as many simultaneous equations as there are dependent variables with one independent variable, by the process of elimination. After solving the derived equation, we substitute back to get the other dependent variable.

Consider the simultaneous equation as

$$\left.\begin{aligned} & f_1(D)x + f_2(D)y = f(t) \\ \text{and} \quad & g_1(D)x + g_2(D)y = g(t) \end{aligned}\right] \quad \text{with} \quad D \equiv \frac{d}{dt} \qquad \text{...(1)}$$

where, x and y are functions of t and $f_1(D), f_2(D), g_1(D)$ and $g_2(D)$ are rational integral functions with constant coefficients, $f(t)$ and $g(t)$ are the functions of the independent variable t. Now define the determinant Δ such as

$$\Delta = \begin{vmatrix} f_1(D) & f_2(D) \\ g_1(D) & g_2(D) \end{vmatrix} \qquad \text{... (2)}$$

then we can say Δ involves the operator coefficients of x and y in (1).

The equation (2) can be solved by the usual methods.

- To solve the simultaneous equations completely, we always require as many simultaneous equations as are the number of dependent variables.
- The method of solving the simultaneous differential equations with constant coefficients is similar to that of solving a set of simultaneous equations in Algebra.

- The number of arbitrary constants appearing in the general solution of the system (1) is equal to the degree in D of the determinant Δ given by (2), provided determinant is non zero.
- The determinant Δ, defined by (2), involves the operator coefficients of x and y in (1).

23.17 METHOD OF SOLVING SIMULTANEOUS LINEAR DIFFERENTIAL EQUATION WITH CONSTANT COEFFICIENTS

Let x and y be the dependent variables and t be the independent variable. Generally, there are two methods for the solution of simultaneous linear differential equations with constant coefficients.

METHOD-1: SYMBOLIC METHOD WITH USE OF D

Consider the simultaneous equation such as

$$f_1(D)x + g_1(D)y = T_1 \quad \text{... (1)}$$

and

$$f_2(D)x + g_2(D)y = T_2 \quad \text{... (2)}$$

where T_1 and T_2 are the functions of independent variable t and f_1, f_2, g_1, g_2 are polynomial functions with constant coefficients.

Operate on both sides of equation (1) by $g_2(D)$ and equation (2) by $g_1(D)$, we get

$$g_2(D)f_1(D)x + g_2(D)g_1(D)y = g_2(D)T_1 \quad \text{... (3)}$$

and

$$g_1(D)\, f_2(D)x + g_1(D)g_2(D)y = g_1(D)\, T_2 \quad \text{... (4)}$$

Now, since $g_1(D)$ and $g_2(D)$ both have the constant coefficients then

$$g_1(D)\, g_2(D)y = g_2(D)\, g_1(D)y$$

therefore, from (3) and (4)

$$[g_2(D)f_1(D) - g_1(D)f_2(D)]x = g_2(D)T_1 - g_1(D)T_2 \quad \text{... (5)}$$

Equation (5) is an ordinary differential equation with one dependent variable and can be solved by the usual methods. Thus, x can be obtained as a function of t. The value of y is then obtained by substituting the value of x in any of the given equations and integrating the resulting equation, if necessary. If however, y is obtained by an independent elimination as in the case of x, the values of x and y are to be substituted in given equation (1) and (2) and the arbitrary constants in x and y are to be so adjusted that the given equations are satisfied. Here, the number of independent arbitrary constants entering in the general solution is the index of the highest power of D.

METHOD-2: USE OF DIFFERENTIATION

If two equations containing $x, y, \frac{dx}{dt}$ and $\frac{dy}{dt}$ are given. Then we can obtain more equations containing $x, y, \frac{dx}{dt}, \frac{dy}{dt}, \frac{d^2x}{dt^2}$ and $\frac{d^2y}{dt^2}$ by differentiating the given equations with respect to t.

From these equations, we can obtain an equation containing x (or y) and its derivative, by eliminating x (or y) and its derivatives. Now, solve this new equation for x (or y) and substituting the value of x (or y) in any of the given equation and if necessary, solve the resulting equation.

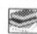

- The method of differentiation will be used when found very necessary.
- Generally t will be the independent variable and x and y will be dependent variables. In some problems any other variable, say x, will be given as the independent variable and y and z as the dependent variables.

Solved Examples

1. *Solve* $\frac{dx}{dt} - 7x + y = 0$

$\frac{dy}{dt} - 2x - 5y = 0$. [UPTU-2002]

SOLUTION. The given equation can be written as

$$(D-7)x + y = 0 \quad \text{... (1)}$$

and $(D-5)y - 2x = 0$ ... (2)

Now, eliminating y, we get

$$(D-7)(D-5)x + 2x = 0$$

$$\Rightarrow \quad \frac{d^2x}{dt^2} - 12\frac{dx}{dt} + 37x = 0 \quad \text{...(3)}$$

The auxiliary equation is

$$m^2 - 12m + 37 = 0 \Rightarrow m = 6 \pm i$$

$$\therefore \quad x = e^{6t}[C_1 \cos t + C_2 \sin t]$$

Putting this value of x in (1), we get

$$e^{6t}[-C_1 \sin t + C_2 \cos t] + 6e^{6t}[C_1 \cos t + C_2 \sin t] - 7e^{6t}(C_1 \cos t + C_2 \sin t) + y = 0$$

$$\Rightarrow y = e^{6t}(C_1 - C_2)\cos t + (C_1 + C_2)\sin t$$

Hence, the solution is

$$x = e^{6t}[C_1 \cos t + C_2 \sin t]$$

$$y = e^{6t}[(C_1 - C_2)\cos t + (C_1 + C_2)\sin t]$$

2. *Solve* $\frac{dx}{dt} = -\omega y$ ... (1)

$\frac{dy}{dt} = \omega x$ ... (2)

SOLUTION. Differentiating (1) with respect to t, we get

$$\frac{d^2x}{dt^2} + \omega\frac{dy}{dt} = 0 \Rightarrow \frac{d^2x}{dt^2} + \omega^2 x = 0$$

[By using (2)]

$$\therefore x = C_1 \cos \omega t + C_2 \sin \omega t$$

Putting this value of x in (1), we get

$$y = -C_2 \cos \omega t + C_1 \sin \omega t$$

3. *Solve* $\frac{dx}{dt} + 2\frac{dy}{dt} - 2x + 2y = 3e^t$,

$3\frac{dx}{dt} + \frac{dy}{dt} + 2x + y = 4e^{2t}$.

[UPTU(B.PHARMA)–2003, 06, 07]

SOLUTION. The given equation can be written as

$$(D-2)x + 2(D+1)y = 3e^t \quad \text{...(1)}$$

and $(3D+2)x + (D+1)y = 4e^{2t}$ ...(2)

Eliminating y between (1) and (2), we obtain

$$[2(3D+2) - (D-2)]\, x = 8e^{2t} - 3e^t$$

or $(5D+6)x = 8e^{2t} - 3e^t$

or $\frac{dx}{dt} + \frac{6}{5}x = \frac{8}{5}e^{2t} - \frac{3}{5}e^t$

which is a linear differential equation with

$$\text{I.F.} = e^{\int 6/5\, dt} = e^{6t/5}$$

Now, solution becomes

$$x.e^{6t/5} = \int e^{6t/5}\left[\frac{8}{5}e^{2t} - \frac{3}{5}e^t\right]dt + C_1$$

$$= \frac{8}{5}\int e^{16t/5} - \frac{3}{5}\int e^{11t/5}dt + C_1$$

$$= \frac{1}{2}e^{16t/5} - \frac{3}{11}e^{11t/5} + C_1$$

$$\therefore x = \frac{1}{2}e^{2t} - \frac{3}{11}e^t + C_1e^{-6t/5}$$

Now, $\frac{dx}{dt} = e^{2t} - \frac{3}{11}e^t - \frac{6}{5}C_1e^{-6t/5}$

Putting this value in (1), we get

$$2Dy + 2y + e^{2t} - \frac{3}{11}e^t - \frac{6}{5}C_1e^{-6t/5} - e^{2t} + \frac{6}{11}e^t - 2C_1e^{-6t/5} = 3e^t$$

or $2\frac{dy}{dt} + 2y = \frac{30}{11}e^t + \frac{16}{5}C_1e^{-6t/5}$

or $\frac{dy}{dt} + y = \frac{15}{11}e^t + \frac{8}{5}C_1e^{-6t/5}$

which is a linear differential equation with

$$\text{I.F.} = e^{\int dt} = e^t$$

The solution is

$$\therefore y.e^t = \frac{15}{11}\int e^{2t}dt + \frac{8}{5}C_1\int e^{-t/5}dt + C_2$$

$$= \frac{15}{22}e^{2t} - 8C_1e^{-t/5} + C_2$$

$$\therefore \quad y = C_2e^{-t} + \frac{15}{22}e^t - 8C_1e^{-6t/5}$$

Hence, the solution is given by

$$x = \frac{1}{2}e^{2t} - \frac{3}{11}e^{t} + C_1 e^{-6t/5}$$

$$y = \frac{15}{22}e^{t} - 8C_1 e^{-6t/5} + C_1 e^{-t}$$

4. *Solve* $\frac{dx}{dt} + \frac{dy}{dt} - 2y = 2\cos t - 7\sin t$

$$\frac{dx}{dt} - \frac{dy}{dt} + 2x = 4\cos t - 3\sin t$$

[UPTU–2005]

SOLUTION. The given equation can be written as

$$Dx + (D-2)y = 2\cos t - 7\sin t \quad \ldots (1)$$

and $(D+2)x - Dy = 4\cos t - 3\sin t \quad \ldots(2)$

Eliminating y between (1) and (2), we obtain $[D^2 + (D-2)(D+2)]x$

$$= D(2\cos t - 7\sin t) + (D-2)(4\cos t - 3\sin t)$$

or $(D^2 - 2)x = -9\cos t$

Auxiliary equation is

$$m^2 - 2 = 0 \Rightarrow m = \pm\sqrt{2}$$

C.F. $= C_1 e^{\sqrt{2}\cdot t} + C_2 e^{-\sqrt{2}\cdot t}$

and P.I. $= -9\frac{1}{D^2 - 2}\cos t = \frac{-9\cos t}{D^2 - 2}$

$= 3\cos t$

$$\therefore \quad x = C_1 e^{\sqrt{2}\cdot t} + C_2 e^{-\sqrt{2}\cdot t} + 3\cos t$$

$$\frac{dx}{dt} = \sqrt{2}C_1 e^{\sqrt{2}\cdot t} - C_2\sqrt{2}e^{-\sqrt{2}\cdot t} - 3\sin t$$

Now adding (1) and (2), we get

$$2Dx + 2x - 2y = 6\cos t - 10\sin t$$

or $y = \frac{dx}{dt} + x - 3\cos t + 5\sin t$

$$= \sqrt{2}C_1 e^{\sqrt{2}\cdot t} - C_2\sqrt{2}e^{-\sqrt{2}\cdot t} - 3\sin t + C_1 e^{\sqrt{2}\cdot t} + C_2 e^{-\sqrt{2}\cdot t} + 3\cos t - 3\cos t + 5\sin t$$

$$= (\sqrt{2}+1)C_1 e^{\sqrt{2}\cdot t} + (1-\sqrt{2})C_2 e^{-\sqrt{2}\cdot t} + 2\sin t$$

Hence, the solution is given as

$$x = C_1 e^{\sqrt{2}\cdot t} + C_2 e^{-\sqrt{2}\cdot t} + 3\cos t,$$

$$y = (\sqrt{2}+1)C_1 e^{\sqrt{2}\cdot t} + (1-\sqrt{2})C_2 e^{-\sqrt{2}\cdot t} + 2\sin t$$

Similar Problems

(1) Solve $\frac{dx}{dt} = ax + by,\ \frac{dy}{dt} = a'x + b'y$.

Ans. $x = C_1 e^{m_1 t} + C_2 e^{m_2 t},\ y = \frac{1}{b}[(m_1 - a)C_1 e^{m_1 t} + (m_2 - a)C_2 e^{m_2 t}]$

(2) Solve $\frac{dx}{dt} + 4x + 3y = t,\quad \frac{dy}{dt} + 2x + 5y = e^t$

Ans. $x = C_1 e^{-2t} + C_2 e^{-7t} + \frac{5}{14}t - \frac{31}{196} - \frac{1}{8}e^t,\ y = -\frac{2}{3}C_1 e^{-2t} + C_2 e^{-7t} + \frac{9}{98} - \frac{t}{7} - \frac{5e^t}{24}$

5. *Solve* $t dx = (t - 2x)dt = 0$ *and* $t\,dy = (tx + ty + 2x - t)dt$.

SOLUTION. The given equation can be written as

$$t\,dx - (t - 2x)dt = 0 \quad \ldots (1)$$

and $t\,dy - (tx + ty + 2x - t)dt = 0 \quad \ldots(2)$

From (1), we get $\frac{dx}{dt} + \frac{2}{t}x = 1$

which is a linear equation

I.F. $= e^{\int 2/t\,dt} = e^{2\log t} = t^2 \quad \ldots(3)$

$$\therefore \quad xt^2 = \int t^2.1\,dt + C_1 = \frac{1}{3}t^3 + C_1$$

$$\therefore \quad x = \frac{1}{3}t + C_1 t^{-2}$$

Now adding (1) and (2), we get

$$t(dx + dy) = t(x + y)dt$$

or $\frac{dx + dy}{x + y} = dt$

Integrating, $\log(x + y) = t + \log C_2$

$$y = C_2 e^t - C_1 t^{-2} - \frac{1}{3}t$$

Hence, solution is . $x = \frac{1}{3}t + C_1 t^{-2}$;

$$y = C_2 e^t - C_1 t^{-2} - \frac{1}{3}t$$

6. *Solve* $x\frac{dy}{dx}+z=0,\ x\frac{dz}{dx}+y=0.$

SOLUTION. Differentiating first equation w.r.t. x, we get

$$x\frac{d^2y}{dx^2}+\frac{dy}{dx}+\frac{dz}{dx}=0$$

or $$x^2\frac{d^2y}{dx^2}+x\frac{dy}{dx}+x\frac{dz}{dx}=0 \quad ...(A)$$

and from second equation,

$$x\frac{dz}{dx}=-y$$

Put this value of $x\frac{dz}{dx}$ in equation (A), we get

$$x^2\frac{d^2y}{dx^2}+x\frac{dy}{dx}-y=0 \quad ...(B)$$

This equation is a homogeneous equation.

Put $x=e^t$ so that $\frac{dy}{dx}=\frac{dy}{dt}.\frac{dt}{dx}=\frac{1}{x}\frac{dy}{dt}$

$$\therefore \quad x\frac{dy}{dx}=\frac{dy}{dt} \quad \text{or} \quad x\frac{d}{dx}\equiv\frac{d}{dt}$$

$$x\frac{d}{dx}\left[x\frac{dy}{dx}\right]=x^2\frac{d^2y}{dx^2}+x\frac{dy}{dx}$$

or $$x^2\frac{d^2y}{dx^2}=\left(x\frac{d}{dx}-1\right)x\frac{dy}{dx}=(D-1)Dy$$

$$\left[\because \frac{d}{dt}\equiv D\right]$$

$\therefore$ From (B), we get

$$\{(D-1)D+(D-1)\}y=0$$

or $$(D^2-1)y=0$$

$$\therefore \quad y=C_1e^t+C_2e^{-t}$$

or $$y=C_1x+C_2x^{-1} \quad ...(1)$$

so that $\frac{dy}{dx}=C_1-\frac{C_2}{x^2}$

$\therefore$ From first equation, we get

$$z=-x\frac{dy}{dx}$$

$$z=-C_1x+C_2x^{-1}$$

or Desired solution is

$$y=C_1x+C_2x^{-1},\ z=-C_1x+C_2x^{-1}$$

7. *Solve* $\frac{d^2x}{dt^2}+m^2y=0,\ \frac{d^2y}{dt^2}-m^2x=0.$

SOLUTION. The given equation can be written as

$$D^2x+m^2y=0 \quad ...(1)$$

$$-m^2x+D^2y=0 \quad ...(2)$$

Eliminating y between (1) and (2),

$$(D^4+m^4)x=0.$$

Auxiliary equation is $M^4+m^4=0$

or $$(M^2+m^2)^2-2M^2m^2=0$$

or $$(M^2-\sqrt{2}Mm+m^2)(M^2+\sqrt{2}Mm+m^2)=0$$

$$\therefore \quad M^2-\sqrt{2}mM+m^2=0$$

or $$M^2+\sqrt{2}\,mM+m^2=0$$

$$\therefore \quad M=\frac{\sqrt{2}m\pm\sqrt{(2m^2-4m^2)}}{2},$$

$$M=\frac{-\sqrt{2}m\pm\sqrt{(2m^2-4m^2)}}{2}$$

$$=\frac{m}{\sqrt{2}}\pm\frac{m}{\sqrt{2}}i\ ,-\frac{m}{\sqrt{2}}\pm\frac{m}{\sqrt{2}}i$$

$$\therefore \quad x=e^{mt/\sqrt{2}}\left[C_1\cos\frac{mt}{\sqrt{2}}+C_2\sin\frac{mt}{\sqrt{2}}\right]+e^{mt/\sqrt{2}}\left[C_3\cos\frac{mt}{\sqrt{2}}+C_4\sin\frac{mt}{\sqrt{2}}\right] \quad ...(3)$$

so that $$\frac{dx}{dt}=\frac{m}{\sqrt{2}}e^{mt/\sqrt{2}}\left[C_1\cos\frac{mt}{\sqrt{2}}+C_2\sin\frac{mt}{\sqrt{2}}\right]$$

$$+e^{-mt/\sqrt{2}}\frac{m}{\sqrt{2}}\left[-C_1\sin\frac{mt}{\sqrt{2}}+C_2\cos\frac{mt}{\sqrt{2}}\right]$$

$$+\left(-\frac{m}{\sqrt{2}}\right)e^{-mt/\sqrt{2}}\left[C_3\cos\frac{mt}{\sqrt{2}}+C_4\sin\frac{mt}{\sqrt{2}}\right]$$

$$+e^{-mt/\sqrt{2}}\frac{m}{\sqrt{2}}\left[-C_3\sin\frac{mt}{\sqrt{2}}+C_4\cos\frac{mt}{\sqrt{2}}\right]$$

and

$$\frac{d^2x}{dt^2} = \frac{m^2}{2}e^{mt/\sqrt{2}}\left[C_1\cos\frac{mt}{\sqrt{2}} + C_2\sin\frac{mt}{\sqrt{2}}\right]$$

$$+\frac{m^2}{2}e^{mt/\sqrt{2}}\left[-C_1\sin\frac{mt}{\sqrt{2}} + C_2\cos\frac{mt}{\sqrt{2}}\right]$$

$$-\frac{m^2}{2}e^{mt/\sqrt{2}}\left[C_1\cos\frac{mt}{\sqrt{2}} + C_2\sin\frac{mt}{\sqrt{2}}\right]$$

$$+\frac{m^2}{2}e^{-mt/\sqrt{2}}\left[C_3\cos\frac{mt}{\sqrt{2}} + C_4\sin\frac{mt}{\sqrt{2}}\right]$$

$$-\frac{m^2}{2}e^{-mt/\sqrt{2}}\left[-C_3\sin\frac{mt}{\sqrt{2}} + C_4\cos\frac{mt}{\sqrt{2}}\right]$$

$$-\frac{m^2}{2}e^{-mt/\sqrt{2}}\left[-C_3\sin\frac{mt}{\sqrt{2}} + C_4\cos\frac{mt}{\sqrt{2}}\right]$$

$$-\frac{m^2}{2}e^{-mt/\sqrt{2}}\left[C_3\cos\frac{mt}{\sqrt{2}} + C_4\sin\frac{mt}{\sqrt{2}}\right]$$

$$= m^2e^{mt/\sqrt{2}}\left[-C_1\sin\frac{mt}{\sqrt{2}} + C_2\cos\frac{mt}{\sqrt{2}}\right]$$

$$-m^2e^{-mt/\sqrt{2}}\left[-C_3\sin\frac{mt}{\sqrt{2}} + C_4\cos\frac{mt}{\sqrt{2}}\right]$$

$\therefore$ From (1) $y = -\dfrac{1}{m^2}\dfrac{d^2x}{dt^2}$

$$= e^{mt/\sqrt{2}}\left[C_1\sin\frac{mt}{\sqrt{2}} - C_2\cos\frac{mt}{\sqrt{2}}\right]$$

$$+e^{-mt/\sqrt{2}}\left[-C_3\sin\frac{mt}{\sqrt{2}} + C_4\cos\frac{mt}{\sqrt{2}}\right] \quad ...(4)$$

Hence, (3) and (4) be complete solution.

Exercise-23.16

Solve the following simultaneous differential equations :

1. $\dfrac{d^2x}{dt^2} - 3x - 4y = 0, \quad \dfrac{d^2y}{dt^2} + x + y = 0$
2. $\dfrac{dx}{dt} = 3x + 2y, \quad \dfrac{dy}{dt} = 5x + 3y$
3. $\dfrac{d^2x}{dt^2} + 4x + y = te^{3t}, \quad \dfrac{d^2y}{dt^2} + y - 2x = \cos^2 t$
4. $\dfrac{dx}{dt} + 5x + y = e^t, \quad \dfrac{dy}{dt} - x + 3y = e^{2t}$
5. $\dfrac{dx}{dt} = 3x + 2y, \quad \dfrac{dy}{dt} + 5x + 3y = 0$
6. $\dfrac{dx}{dt} + 2x - 3y = t, \quad \dfrac{dy}{dt} - 3x + 2y = e^{2t}$
7. $(D-17)y + (2D-8)z = 0, (13D-53)y - 2z = 0$
8. $2\dfrac{d^2y}{dx^2} - \dfrac{dz}{dx} - 4y = 2x, \quad 2\dfrac{dy}{dx} + 4\dfrac{dz}{dx} - 3z = 0$
9. $\dfrac{dx}{dt} + \dfrac{2}{t}(x-y) = 1, \quad \dfrac{dy}{dt} + \dfrac{1}{t}(x+5y) = t$
10. $\dfrac{dx}{dt} + 5x - 2y = t, \quad \dfrac{dy}{dt} + 2x + y = 0$
11. $\dfrac{d^2x}{dt^2} + y = \sin t, \dfrac{d^2y}{dt^2} + x = \cos t$
12. $(D^2-1)x + 8Dy = 16e^t, Dx + 3(D^2+1)y = 0$
13. $\dfrac{dx}{dt} + 7x - y = 0, \dfrac{dy}{dt} + 2x + 5y = 0)$
14. $\dfrac{dx}{dt} + x - 2y = 0, \dfrac{dy}{dt} + x + 4y = 0$; $x(0) = y(0) = 1$
15. $\dfrac{dx}{dt} = 3x + 8y, \dfrac{dy}{dt} = -x - 3y$; $x(0) = 6, y(0) = -2$
16. $\dfrac{dx}{dt} = y + 1, \dfrac{dy}{dt} = x + 1$
17. $\dfrac{dx}{dt} - y = e^t, \dfrac{dy}{dt} + x = \sin t$; $x(0) = 1, y(0) = 0$
18. $\dfrac{dx}{dt} + 5x + y = e^t, \dfrac{dy}{dt} + x + 5y = e^{5t}$
19. $\dfrac{dx}{dt} + \dfrac{dy}{dt} + 2x + y = 0, \dfrac{dy}{dt} + 5x + 3y = 0$
20. $\dfrac{dx}{dt} = -4(x+y), \dfrac{dx}{dt} + 4\dfrac{dy}{dt} = -4y$ with $x(0)=1, y(0)=0$
21. $\dfrac{dx}{dt} + y = \sin t, \dfrac{dy}{dt} + x = \cos t$ given that $x = 2$ and $y = 0$ when $t = 0$
22. $\dfrac{dx}{dt} + 2x + 3y = 0, \quad 3x + \dfrac{dy}{dt} + 2y = 2e^{2t}$
23. $\dfrac{dx}{dt} + 2y = e^t, \dfrac{dy}{dt} - 2x = e^{-t}$
24. $\dfrac{d^2x}{dt^2} - 3x - 4y = 0, \dfrac{d^2y}{dt^2} + x + y = 0$
25. $\dfrac{d^2x}{dt^2} + y = \sin t, \dfrac{d^2y}{dt^2} + x = \cos t$

Hint to the Selected Problems

1. Eliminating y , we get

$$[(D^2+1)(D^2-3)+4]x=0$$

$$\Rightarrow \qquad (D^2-1)^2 x=0$$

The auxiliary equation is $(m^2-1)^2=0$

$\Rightarrow m=\pm 1, \pm 1$

$$x=(C_1+C_2 t)e^{-t}+(C_3+C_4 t)\,e^t$$

$$\frac{dx}{dt}=-(C_1+C_2 t)e^{-t}+C_2 e^{-t}+(C_3+C_4 t)e^t+C_4 e^t$$

$$\frac{d^2x}{dt^2}=(C_1+C_2 t)e^{-t}-2C_2 e^{-t}+(C_3+C_4 t)^t+2C_4 e^t$$

Now, for given equation

$$4y=D^2x-3x$$

$$=(C_1+C_2 t)\,e^{-t}-2C_2 e^{-t}+(C_3+C_4 t)\,e^t$$
$$+2C_4 e^t-3(C_1+C_2 t)e^{-t}-3(C_2 t+C_4 t)\,e^t$$
$$=-(2C_1+2C_2+2C_2 t)e^{-t}$$
$$+(-2C_3+2C_4-2C_4 t)e^t$$
$$=-\frac{1}{2}(C_1+C_2+C_2 t)\,e^{-t}+\frac{1}{2}(C_4+C_3-C_5 t)\,e^t$$

3. The given equation can be written as

$$(D^2+4)x+y=t\,e^{3t} \qquad \ldots (1)$$

$$-2x+(D^2+1)y=\cos^2 t \qquad \ldots (2)$$

Eliminating y , we get

$$\left[(D^2+1)(D^2+4)+2\right]x=(D^2+1)t\,e^{3t}-\cos^2 t$$

$$(D^4+5D^2+6)x=10t\,e^{3t}-\cos^2 t+6e^{3t}$$

$$m^4+5m^2+6=0$$

$$(m^3+3)(m^2+2)=0$$

$$m=\pm\sqrt{3}\,i,\ \pm\sqrt{2}\,i$$

$$\text{C.F.}=(C_1\cos\sqrt{3}t+C_2\sin\sqrt{3}t)$$
$$+(C_3\cos\sqrt{2}t+C_4\sin\sqrt{2}t)$$

$$\text{P.I.}=\frac{10}{D^4+5D^2+6}t\,e^{3t}+\frac{6}{D^4+5D^2+6}e^{3t}$$
$$-\frac{1}{D^4-5D^2+6}\cos^2 t$$

$$=10\,e^{3t}.\frac{1}{(D+3)^4+5(D+3)^2+6}t$$
$$+\frac{6e^{3t}}{3^4+5.3^2+6}$$
$$-\frac{1}{(D^4+5D^2+6)}.\frac{1}{2}(1+\cos 2t)$$

$$=10e^{3t}.\frac{1}{131+138D+59D^2+\ldots}t+\frac{1}{22}e^{3t}$$
$$-\frac{1}{6+5D^2+D^4}.\frac{1}{2}-\frac{1}{D^4+5D^2+6}\left(\frac{1}{2}\cos 2t\right)$$

$$=10^{3t}\frac{1}{132}\left(1+\frac{23}{22}D+\frac{59}{132}D^2+\ldots\right)^{-1}t$$
$$+\frac{e^{3t}}{22}-\frac{1}{6}\left(1+\frac{5D^2}{6}+\frac{D^4}{6}\right)^{-1}$$
$$\frac{1}{2}-\frac{\frac{1}{2}\cos 2t}{(-2)^2+5(-2)^2+6}$$

$$=\frac{5}{66}te^{3t}-\frac{49}{1452}e^{3t}-\frac{1}{12}-\frac{1}{4}\cos 2t$$

$$x=(C_1\cos\sqrt{3}\,t+C_2\sin\sqrt{3}\,t)$$
$$+(C_3\cos\sqrt{2}\,t+C_4\sin\sqrt{2}\,t)$$
$$+\frac{5}{66}t\,e^{3t}-\frac{49}{1452}e^{3t}-\frac{1}{12}-\frac{1}{4}\cos 2t \qquad \ldots (3)$$

$$\frac{dx}{dt}=\left(-C_1\sqrt{3}\sin\sqrt{3}\,t+C_2\sqrt{3}\cos\sqrt{3}\,t\right)$$
$$+\left(-C_3\sqrt{3}\sin\sqrt{2}\,t+C_4\sqrt{2}\cos\sqrt{2}\,t\right)$$
$$+\frac{5}{66}\left(3t\,e^{3t}+e^{3t}\right)-\frac{49}{1452}3e^{3t}+\frac{1}{2}\sin 2t$$

$$\frac{d^2x}{dt^2}=-3(C_1\cos\sqrt{3}\,t+C_2\sin\sqrt{3}\,t)$$
$$-2(C_3\cos\sqrt{2}\,t+C_4\sin\sqrt{2}t)$$
$$+\frac{5}{66}(9te^{3t}+6e^{3t})-\frac{49}{1452}9e^{3t}+\cos 2t$$

Substituting in (1), we get

$$y=-\frac{d^2x}{dt^2}-4x+te^{3t}$$

$$y=-\left(C_1\cos\sqrt{3}\,t+C_2\sin\sqrt{3}\,t\right)$$
$$-2(C_3\cos\sqrt{2}\,t+C_4\sin\sqrt{2}\,t)$$
$$+\frac{1}{66}te^{2t}-\frac{23}{1452}e^{3t}+\frac{1}{3} \qquad \ldots (4)$$

6. The given equation can be written as

$$(D+2)x-3y=t \qquad \ldots (1)$$

$$-3x+(D+2)y=e^{2t} \qquad \ldots (2)$$

Eliminating y , we get

$$[(D+2)^2-9]x=(D+2)t+3e^{2t}$$

$$(D^2+4+4D-9)x=(D+2)t+3e^{2t}$$
$$=(1+2t)+3e^{2t}$$

A.E. $m^2+4m-5=0 \quad m=1,-5$

C.F. $= C_1e^{-5t}+C_2e^t$

$$\text{P.I.} = \frac{1+2t}{(D-1)(D+5)}+3\frac{e^{2t}}{(D-1)(D+5)}$$

$$= -\frac{1}{5}\left[1-\frac{4}{5}D-\frac{1}{5}D^2\right]^{-1}(1+2t)+\frac{3e^{2t}}{(2-1)(2+5)}$$

$$= -\frac{1}{5}\left[1+\frac{4}{5}D+\frac{1}{5}D^2+\ldots\right](1+2t)+\frac{3}{7}e^{2t}$$

$$= -\frac{13}{25}-\frac{2}{5}t+\frac{3}{7}e^{2t}$$

$$x = C_1e^{-5t}+C_2e^t+\frac{3}{7}e^{2t}-\frac{2}{5}t-\frac{13}{25}$$

$$\frac{dx}{dt} = -5C_1e^{-5t}+C_2e^t+\frac{6}{7}e^{2t}-\frac{2}{5}$$

From (1) :

$$3y = -5C_1e^{-5t}+C_2e^t+\frac{6}{7}e^{2t}-\frac{2}{5}+2C_1e^{-5t}$$

$$+2C_2e^t+\frac{6}{7}e^{2t}-\frac{4}{5}t-\frac{26}{25}-t$$

$$y = -C_1e^{-5t}+C_2e^t+\frac{4}{7}e^{2t}-\frac{12}{25}-\frac{3}{5}t$$

9. The given equation can be written as

$$t\frac{dx}{dt}+2(x-y)=t \qquad \ldots (1)$$

$$t\frac{dy}{dt}+x+5y=t^2 \qquad \ldots (2)$$

Differentiating (1) w.r.t. t, we have

$$t\frac{d^2x}{dt^2}+\frac{dx}{dt}+2\frac{dx}{dt}-2\frac{dy}{dt}=1$$

$$t^2\frac{d^2x}{dt^2}+t\frac{dx}{dt}+2t\frac{dx}{dt}-2t\frac{dy}{dt}=t \qquad \ldots (3)$$

Substituting the value of $t\frac{dy}{dt}$ from (2) in (1), we get

$$t^2\frac{d^2x}{dt^2}+3t\frac{dx}{dt}+2x+5\left(t\frac{dx}{dt}+2x-t\right)-2t^2=t$$

$$\Rightarrow t\frac{d^2x}{dt^2}+8t\frac{dx}{dt}+12x=2t^2+6t \qquad \ldots(4)$$

which is a homogeneous linear equation.

Put $t = e^z$

$$\frac{dx}{dt}=\frac{dx}{dz}\cdot\frac{dz}{dt}=\frac{dx}{dz}\cdot\frac{1}{t}$$

$$t\frac{d}{dt}\left(t\frac{dx}{dt}\right)=t^2\frac{d^2x}{dt^2}+t\frac{dx}{dt}$$

$$t^2D^2x=(D-1)Dx$$

Equation (4) gives

$$[(D-1)D+8D+12]x = 2e^{2z}+6e^z$$

$$(D^2+7D+12)x=2e^{2z}+6e^z$$

A.E. is $m^2+7m+12=0 \Rightarrow m=-3,-4$

C.F. $= C_1e^{-3z}+C_2e^{-4z}$

$$\text{P. I.} = \frac{2}{(D^2+7D+12)}e^{2z}+\frac{6}{(D^2+7D+12)}e^z$$

$$= \frac{2}{30}e^{2z}+\frac{6}{20}e^z=\frac{1}{15}e^z+\frac{3}{10}e^z$$

$$x = C_1e^{-3z}+C_2e^{-4z}+\frac{1}{15}e^{2z}+\frac{3}{10}e^z$$

$$x=\frac{C_1}{t^3}+\frac{C_2}{t^4}+\frac{t^2}{15}+\frac{3}{10}t$$

$$\frac{dx}{dt}=-\frac{3C_1}{t^4}-\frac{4C_2}{t^5}+\frac{2t}{15}+\frac{3}{10}$$

From (1) :

$$2y=-\frac{3C_1}{t^3}-\frac{4C_2}{t^4}+\frac{2t^2}{15}+\frac{3t}{10}$$

$$+\frac{2C_1}{t^3}+\frac{2C_2}{t^3}+\frac{2t^2}{15}+\frac{6}{10}t-t$$

$$y=-\frac{C_1}{2t^3}-\frac{C_2}{t^4}+\frac{2t^2}{15}+\frac{3}{10}$$

ANSWERS

1. $x=(C_1+C_2t)e^{-t}+(C_3+C_4t)\,e^t$, $y = -\frac{1}{2}(C_1+C_2+C_2t)e^{-t}+\frac{1}{2}(C_4-C_3-C_4t)e^t$

2. $x=C_1e^{(3+\sqrt{10})t}+C_2e^{(3-\sqrt{10})t}$, $y=\frac{1}{2}\sqrt{10}\,[C_1e^{(3+\sqrt{10})t}-C_2e^{(3-\sqrt{10})t}]$

3. $x=(C_1\cos\sqrt{3}t+C_2\sin\sqrt{3}t)+(C_3\cos\sqrt{2}t+C_4\sin\sqrt{2}t)+\frac{5}{66}t\,e^{3t}-\frac{49}{1452}e^{3t}-\frac{1}{12}-\frac{1}{4}\cos 2t$

$y=(C_1\cos\sqrt{3}t+C_2\sin\sqrt{3}t)-(C_3\cos\sqrt{2}t+C_4\sin\sqrt{2}t)+\frac{1}{60}t\,e^{3t}-\frac{23}{1452}e^{3t}+\frac{1}{3}$

4. $x=(C_1+C_2t)e^{-4t}+\frac{4}{25}e^t-\frac{1}{36}e^{2t}$, $y=-(C_1+C_2+C_3t)\,e^{-4t}+\frac{7}{36}e^{2t}+\frac{1}{25}e^t$

5. $x = C_1\cos t + C_2\sin t$, $y = \frac{1}{2}(C_2 - 3C_1)\cos t - \frac{1}{2}(C_1 + 3C_2)\sin t$

6. $x = C_1e^{-5t} + C_2e^{t} + \frac{3}{7}e^{2t} - \frac{2}{5}t - \frac{13}{25}$, $y = -C_1e^{-5t} + C_2e^{t} + \frac{4}{7}e^{2t} - \frac{3}{5}t - \frac{12}{25}$

7. $y = C_1e^{3x} + C_2e^{5x}$, $z = -7C_1e^{3x} + 6C_2e^{5x}$

8. $y = (C_1 + C_2x)\,e^{x} + C_3e^{-3x/2} - \frac{1}{2}x$, $z = -2(C_1 + C_2x - 3C_2)e^{x} - \frac{1}{3}C_3e^{-3x/2} - \frac{1}{3}$

9. $x = \frac{C_1}{t^3} + \frac{C_2}{t^4} + \frac{t^2}{15} + \frac{3}{10}t$, $y = -\frac{C_1}{2t^3} - \frac{C_2}{t^4} + \frac{2t^2}{15} - \frac{t}{20}$

10. $x = -\frac{1}{27}(1+6t)e^{-3t} + \frac{1}{27}(1+3t)$, $y = -\frac{2}{27}(2+3t)e^{-3t} + \frac{2}{27}(2-3t)$

11. $x = C_1e^{t} + C_2e^{-t} + C_3\cos t + C_4\sin t + \frac{t}{4}(\sin t - \cos t)$,

$y = -C_1e^{t} - C_2e^{-t} + C_3\cos t + C_4\sin t + \frac{1}{4}(2+t)(\sin t - \cos t)$

12. $y = C_1\cos\frac{t}{\sqrt{3}} + C_2\sin\frac{t}{\sqrt{3}} + C_3\cosh\sqrt{3}.t + C_4\sinh\sqrt{3}t + 2e^{t}$; $x = \sqrt{3}C_1\sin\frac{t}{\sqrt{3}} - \sqrt{3}C_2\cos\frac{t}{\sqrt{3}}$

$-3\sqrt{3}C_3\sinh\sqrt{3}t - 3\sqrt{3}C_4\cosh\sqrt{3}t - 6e^{t} - 3t$

13. $x = e^{-6t}(A\cos t + B\sin t), y = e^{-6t}[(A+B)\cos t - (A-B)\sin t]$

14. $x = 4e^{-2t} - 3e^{-3t}, y = -2e^{-2t} + 3e^{-3t}$

15. $x = 4e^{t} + 2e^{-t}, y = -e^{t} - e^{-t}$

16. $x = C_1e^{t} + C_2e^{-t} - 1, y = C_1e^{t} - C_2e^{-t} - 1$

17. $x = 2\sin t + \frac{3}{2}\cos t + \frac{t}{2}\cos t - \frac{1}{2}e^{t}, y = \frac{1}{2}\cos t - \frac{3}{2}\sin t + \frac{t}{2}\sin t - \frac{1}{2}e^{t}$

18. $x = C_1e^{-6t} + C_2e^{-4t} + \frac{6e^{t}}{35} - \frac{e^{5t}}{99}$, $y = C_1e^{-6t} - C_2e^{-4t} - \frac{1}{35}e^{t} + \frac{10}{99}, e^{5t}$

19. $x = \left(\frac{C_1 - 3C_2}{5}\right)\sin t - \left(\frac{C_2 + 3C_1}{5}\right)\cos t$, $y = C_1\cos t + C_2\sin t$

20. $x = (1-2t)e^{-2t}, y = te^{-2t}$

21. $x = e^{t} + e^{-t}, y = e^{-t} - e^{t} + \sin t$

22. $x = C_1e^{t} + C_2e^{-st} + \frac{6}{7}e^{2t}$; $y = C_2e^{-st} - C_1e^{t} + \frac{8}{7}e^{2t}$

23. $x = \frac{1}{5}e^{t} + \frac{2}{5}e^{-t} - C_1\sin 2t + C_2\cos 2t$, $y = \frac{2}{5}e^{t} + \frac{1}{5}e^{-t} + C_1\cos 2t + C_2\sin 2t$

24. $x = (C_1 + C_2t)e^{-t} + (C_3 + C_4t)e^{t}$, $y = -\frac{1}{2}[C_1 + C_2(1+t)]e^{-t} + \frac{1}{2}[C_4(1-t) - C_3]e^{t}$

25. $x = C_1e^{t} + C_2e^{-t} + C_3\cos t + C_4\sin t - \frac{t}{4}\cos t + \frac{t}{4}\sin t$,

$y = -C_1e^{t} - C_2e^{-t} + C_3\cos t + C_4\sin t + \frac{1}{4}(2+t)(\sin t - \cos t)$

23.18 SIMULTANEOUS EQUATIONS IN DIFFERENT FORM

Consider the equations of the type
$$P_1dx + Q_1dy + R_1dz = 0$$
$$P_2dx + Q_2dy + R_2dz = 0 \quad \ldots (1)$$
where P_1, P_2, Q_1, Q_2, R_1 and R_2 are functions of x, y, z.

Equation (1) can be written as
$$P_1\frac{dx}{dz} + Q_1\frac{dy}{dz} + R_1 = 0 \;, P_2\frac{dx}{dz} + Q_2\frac{dy}{dz} + R_2 = 0 .$$

Solving the above equations for $\frac{dx}{dz}, \frac{dy}{dz}$, we get $\frac{dx}{dz} = \frac{Q_1R_2 - Q_2R_1}{P_1Q_2 - Q_1P_2}$, $\frac{dy}{dz} = \frac{R_1P_2 - P_1R_2}{P_1Q_2 - Q_1P_2}$

Hence,
$$\frac{dx}{Q_1R_2 - Q_2R_1} = \frac{dy}{R_1P_2 - R_2P_1} = \frac{dz}{P_1Q_2 - P_2Q_1}$$

i.e., the equation can be put in the form $\frac{dx}{P} = \frac{dy}{Q} = \frac{dz}{R}$

where *P*, *Q* and *R* the functions of *x*, *y* and *z* .

WORKING PROCEDURE

Method-I

STEP 1. Take any two member of an equation (1) say $\frac{dx}{P} = \frac{dy}{Q}$ (say)

After integrating it, we may get an equation.

STEP 2. Again take two member of equation (1) say $\frac{dy}{Q} = \frac{dz}{R}$ (say)

After integrating it, we also get an equation.

STEP 3. The solution obtained from (i) and (ii) give the required general solution.

Method-II

STEP 1. The given equation is $\frac{dx}{P} = \frac{dy}{Q} = \frac{dz}{R}$

If we choose *l*, *m* and *n* such that $\frac{dx}{P} = \frac{dy}{Q} = \frac{dz}{R} = \frac{ldx + mdy + ndz}{lP + mQ + nR}$

If $lP + mQ + nR = 0$, then, $ldx + mdy + ndz = 0$

If it is an exact differential, say *du*, then $u = a$ is one equation of the complete solution.

- To find a solution of the given equation, we choose *l*, *m*, *n* such that $ldx + mdy + ndz$ is differential of $lP + mQ + nR$.
- If we have obtained one solution, then this solution can be used to simplify the other differential equations in the integrable form.
- Sometimes, we use only one set of multiples, but in some cases, we have a need of more than one set of multipliers.
- We can obtain one relation, say $u = a$ by the first method and the second relation by the second method.

23.18.1 GEOMETRICAL MEANING OF $\frac{dx}{P} = \frac{dy}{Q} = \frac{dz}{R}$

Since, we know that the direction cosines of the tangent to a curve at any point (x, y, z) are $\frac{dx}{ds}, \frac{dy}{ds}, \frac{dz}{ds}$ or proportional to dx, dy, dz. Therefore, geometrically the above situations represents a system of curves in such a way that the direction-ratios of the tangent from it at any point $A(x, y, z)$ are proportional to P, Q and R. If $u = a$ and $v = b$ are the complete solutions of $\frac{dx}{P} = \frac{dy}{Q} = \frac{dz}{R}$, then system of curves is intersection of the surfaces $u = a, v = b$.

Solved Examples

1. *Solve the simultaneous equations.*

$$\frac{a\,dx}{(b-c)\,yz} = \frac{b\,dy}{(c-a)zx} = \frac{c\,dz}{(a-b)\,xy}.$$

[UPTU–2001]

SOLUTION. Let us take the x, y, z as multipliers.

$$\text{Each fraction} = \frac{ax\,dx + by\,dy + cz\,dz}{0}$$

$$\therefore \quad axdx + bydy + cz\,dz = 0$$

Integrating $ax^2 + by^2 + cz^2 = C_1$ ...(1)

Now taking ax, by, cz as multipliers.

$$\text{Each fraction} = \frac{a^2xdx + b^2ydy + c^2zdz}{0}$$

$$\therefore \quad a^2xdx + b^2ydy + c^2zdz = 0$$

On integrating,

$$a^2x^2 + b^2y^2 + c^2z^2 = 0 \qquad \text{...(2)}$$

Hence, complete solution is

$$\phi(ax^2 + by^2 + cz^2, a^2x^2 + b^2y^2 + c^2z^2) = 0$$

2. *Solve* $\frac{xdx}{z^2 - 2yz - y^2} = \frac{dy}{y+z} = \frac{dz}{y-z}$.

SOLUTION. Let us take $1, y, z$ as multipliers, we get

$$\text{Each fraction} = \frac{xdx + ydy + zdz}{0}$$

$$xdx + ydy + zdz = 0$$

Integrating, $x^2 + y^2 + z^2 = C_1$ ...(1)

Again, last two members, we get

$$\frac{dy}{y+z} = \frac{dz}{y-z}$$

$$ydy - zdy = ydz + zdz$$

or $\quad ydy - (ydz + zdy) - zdz = 0$

Integrating $y^2 - 2yz - z^2 = C_2$ ...(2)

Complete solution is

$$x^2 + y^2 + z^2 = C_1$$

$$y^2 - 2yz - z^2 = C_2$$

Similar Problems

(1) Solve the simultaneous equation $\frac{dx}{y^2 + z^2 - x^2} = \frac{dy}{-2xy} = \frac{dz}{-2xz}$

Ans. $y = C_1 z, x^2 + y^2 + z^2 = C_2 z$

(2) Solve $\frac{dx}{x^2 + y^2 + yz} = \frac{dy}{x^2 + y^2 - xz} = \frac{dz}{z(x+y)}$. **Ans.** $z - x + y = C_1, x^2 + y^2 = z^2 C_2$

3. *Solve*

$$\frac{dx}{x(y^2 - z^2)} = \frac{dy}{-y(z^2 + x^2)} = \frac{dz}{z(x^2 + y^2)}.$$

SOLUTION. Taking $\frac{1}{x}, -\frac{1}{y}, -\frac{1}{z}$ as multipliers, we get

$$\text{Each fraction} = \frac{\frac{dx}{x} - \frac{dy}{y} - \frac{dz}{z}}{0}$$

$$\therefore \quad \frac{dx}{x} - \frac{dy}{y} - \frac{dz}{z} = 0$$

or $\quad \frac{dy}{y} + \frac{dz}{z} = \frac{dx}{x}$

Integrating,

$$\log y + \log z = \log x + \log C_1.$$

$$\therefore \quad yz = C_1 x \qquad \text{...(A)}$$

Again using x, y, z as multipliers, we get

$$\text{Each fraction} = \frac{xdx + ydy + zdz}{0}$$

$$\therefore \quad xdx + ydy + zdz = 0$$

Integrating $x^2 + y^2 + z^2 = C_2$. ...(B)

From (A) and (B), we obtain complete solution.

4. *Solve*

$$\frac{dx}{y^3x-2x^4}=\frac{dy}{2y^4-x^3y}=\frac{dz}{9z(x^3-y^3)}$$

SOLUTION. Taking first two members, we get

$$(2y^4-x^3y)dx=(y^3x-2x^4)dy \quad \ldots(1)$$

Dividing (1) by x^3y^3,

$$\left[\frac{2y}{x^3}-\frac{1}{y^2}\right]dx=\left[\frac{1}{x^2}-\frac{2x}{y^3}\right]dy$$

or $$\left[\frac{1}{x^2}dy-\frac{2y}{x^3}dx\right]+\left[\frac{1}{y^2}dx-\frac{2x}{y^3}dy\right]=0$$

Integrating $\dfrac{y}{x^2}+\dfrac{x}{y^2}=C_1 \quad \ldots(1)$

Again using $\dfrac{1}{x}\cdot\dfrac{1}{y}\cdot\dfrac{1}{3z}$ as multipliers, we get

$$=\frac{\frac{1}{x}dx+\frac{1}{y}dy+\frac{1}{3z}dz}{(y^3-2x^3)+(2y^3-x^3)+3(x^3-y^3)}$$

$$=\frac{\frac{1}{x}dx+\frac{1}{y}dy+\frac{1}{3z}dz}{0}$$

$$\therefore\ \frac{1}{x}dx+\frac{1}{y}dy+\frac{1}{3z}dz=0$$

On integrating, we get

$$\log x+\log y+\frac{1}{3}\log z=\log C_2 \quad \ldots(2)$$

or $$xyz^{1/3}=C_2$$

Hence, complete solution is given by

$$\frac{y}{x^2}+\frac{x}{y^2}=C_1, xyz^{1/3}=C_2$$

5. *Solve* $\dfrac{dx}{\cos(x+y)}=\dfrac{dy}{\sin(x+y)}=\dfrac{dz}{z}$.

SOLUTION. $\dfrac{dx}{\cos(x+y)}=\dfrac{dy}{\sin(x+y)}=\dfrac{dz}{z}$.

$$\Rightarrow \frac{dx}{\cos(x+y)}=\frac{dy}{\sin(x+y)}=\frac{dz}{z}$$
$$=\frac{dx+dy}{\cos(x+y)+\sin(x+y)}$$

Taking $\dfrac{dz}{z}=\dfrac{dx+dy}{\cos(x+y)+\sin(x+y)}$

$$\Rightarrow \frac{dz}{z}=\frac{du}{\cos u+\sin u}, u=x+y$$

$$\Rightarrow \frac{dz}{z}=\frac{du}{\sqrt{2}\sin(u+\pi/4)}$$

$$\Rightarrow \frac{dz}{z}=\frac{1}{\sqrt{2}}\operatorname{cosec}(u+\pi/4)du.$$

Integrating both sides, we get

$$\log z=\frac{1}{\sqrt{2}}\log\tan\left(\frac{u+\pi/4}{2}\right)+\frac{1}{\sqrt{2}}\log C_1$$

$$z^{\sqrt{2}}=c_1\tan\left(\frac{u}{2}+\frac{\pi}{8}\right)$$
$$=c_1\tan\left(\frac{x+y}{2}+\frac{\pi}{8}\right)$$

Also each fraction is equal to

$$\frac{dx+dy}{\cos(x+y)+\sin(x+y)}=\frac{dx-dy}{\cos(x+y)-\sin(x+y)}$$

or $$\frac{\cos(x+y)-\sin(x+y)}{\cos(x+y)+\sin(x+y)}(dx+dy)=dx-dy$$

Integrating, we get

$$\log[\cos(x+y)+\sin(x+y)]=x-y+\log c_2$$

or $\cos(x+y)+\sin(x+y)]e^{y-x}=c_2$

Hence the solution is

$$f\left\{\begin{matrix}\{\cos(x+y)+\sin(x+y)\} \\ e^{y-x}z^{\sqrt{2}}\cot\left(\dfrac{x+y}{2}+\dfrac{\pi}{8}\right)\end{matrix}\right\}=0$$

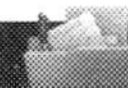

Exercise-23.17

Solve the following simultaneous differential equations :

1. $\frac{dx}{xy}=\frac{dy}{y^2}=\frac{dz}{zyx-2x^2}$

2. $\frac{dx}{x^2+y^2}=\frac{dy}{2xy}=\frac{dz}{(x+y).z}$

3. $\frac{dx}{(x^2-yz)}=\frac{dy}{y^2-zx}=\frac{dz}{z^2-xy}$

4. $\frac{dx}{yz}=\frac{dy}{zx}=\frac{dz}{xy}$

5. $\frac{dx}{y+z}=\frac{dy}{z+x}=\frac{dz}{x+y}$

6. $\frac{dx}{mz-ny}=\frac{dy}{nx-lz}=\frac{dz}{ly-mx}$

7. $\frac{dx}{z(x+y)}=\frac{dy}{z(x-y)}=\frac{dz}{x^2+y^2}$

8. $\frac{dx}{z}=\frac{dy}{-z}=\frac{dz}{z^2+(x+y)^2}$

9. $\frac{dx}{x(y-z)}=\frac{dy}{y(z-x)}=\frac{dz}{z(x-y)}$

10. $\frac{dx}{x^2+y^2}=\frac{dy}{2xy}=\frac{dz}{(x+y)^2}$

11. $\frac{dx}{y^2+yz+z^2}=\frac{dy}{z^2+zx+x^2}=\frac{dz}{x^2+xy+y^2}$

Hint to the Selected Problems

1. Taking the first two members, we get

$$\frac{dx}{xy}=\frac{dy}{y^2} \quad \text{or} \quad \frac{dx}{x}=\frac{dy}{y}$$

Integrating $\log x=\log y+\log C_1$

$$x=C_1y \qquad ...(1)$$

Again taking the last two members, we have

$$\frac{dy}{y^2}=\frac{dz}{zxy-2x^2}$$

$$\frac{dy}{y^2}=\frac{dz}{zC_1y^2-2C_1^2y^2} \qquad \text{from (1)}$$

$$dy=\frac{dz}{zC_1-2C_1^2} \quad \text{or} \quad C_1dy=\frac{dz}{z-2C_1}$$

Integrating, we get

$$C_1y=\log(z-2C_1)+C_2$$

$$x=\log\left(z-\frac{2x}{y}\right)+C_2 \qquad [\because C_1y=x]$$

$$x=\log(zy-2x)-\log y+C_3 \qquad ...(2)$$

3. Obviously, each of the given ratios

$$=\frac{dx-dy}{x^2yz-y^2+zx} \qquad ...(1)$$

$$=\frac{dy-dz}{y^2-zx-z^2+xy} \qquad ...(2)$$

$$=\frac{dz-dx}{x^2-xy-x^2+yz} \qquad ...(3)$$

From (1) and (2)

$$\frac{dx-dy}{(x-y)(x+y+z)}=\frac{dy-dz}{(y-z)(x+y+z)}$$

$$\frac{dx-dy}{x-y}=\frac{dy-dz}{y-z}$$

Integrating, we get

$$\log(x-y)=\log(y-z)+\log a$$

$$\frac{x-y}{y-z}=a \qquad ...(4)$$

From (2) and (3), similarly

$$\frac{y-z}{z-x}=b \qquad ...(5)$$

From (4) and (5), the complete solution of the equation is

$$\phi\left(\frac{x-y}{y-z},\ \frac{y-z}{z-x}\right)=0$$

7. Using $x,-y,-z$ as multipliers, we have

Each fraction

$$=\frac{xdx-ydy-zdz}{xz(x+y)-yz(x-y)-z(x^2+y^2)}$$

$$=\frac{xdx-ydy-zdz}{0}$$

$$xdx-ydy-zdz=0$$

Integrating, $x^2-y^2-z^2=C_1$ ...(1)

Similarly, using $y,x,-z$ as multipliers, we get

Each fraction

$$=\frac{ydx+xdy-zdz}{yz(x+y)+xz(x-y)-z(x^2+y^2)}$$

$$=\frac{ydx+xdy-zdz}{0}$$

$\therefore \quad ydx + xdy - zdz = 0$

Integrating, $2xy - z^2 = C_2$

9. Obviously, $\dfrac{dx}{x(y-z)} = \dfrac{dy}{y(z-x)} = \dfrac{dz}{z(x-y)}$

$$= \frac{dx + dy + dz}{xy - xz + yz - yx + zx - zy}$$

$$dx + dy + dz = 0$$

Integrating, $x + y + z = C_1$ ... (1)

Now using $\dfrac{1}{x}, \dfrac{1}{y}, \dfrac{1}{z}$ as multipliers, we have

$$\frac{\frac{1}{x}dx}{y-z} = \frac{\frac{1}{y}dy}{z-x} = \frac{\frac{1}{z}dz}{x-y}$$

$$I \qquad II \qquad III$$

$$I = II = III = \frac{\frac{1}{x}dx + \frac{1}{y}dy + \frac{1}{z}dz}{y - z + z - x + x - y}$$

$$\frac{1}{x}dx + \frac{1}{y}dy + \frac{1}{z}dz = 0$$

On integrating, we get

$$\log x + \log y + \log z = \log C_2$$

$$xyz = C_2 \qquad ...(2)$$

10. Obviously,

$$\frac{dx + dy}{x^2 + y^2 + 2xy} = \frac{dx - dy}{x^2 + y^2 - 2xy} = \frac{dz}{(x+y)^2}$$

$$\frac{dx + dy}{(x+y)^2} = \frac{dx - dy}{(x-y)^2} = \frac{dz}{(x+y)^2}$$

$$I \qquad II \qquad III$$

Taking first two members

$$\frac{dx + dy}{(x+y)^2} = \frac{dx - dy}{(x-y)^2}$$

Integrating, we get

$$-(x+y)^{-1} = -(x-y)^{-1} + C_1$$

$$\frac{1}{x-y} - \frac{1}{x+y} = C_1$$

$$\frac{2y}{x^2 - y^2} = C_1 \qquad ... (1)$$

Now, taking first and last members

$$\frac{dx + dy}{(x+y)^2} = \frac{dz}{(x+y)^2}$$

$$dx + dy - dz = 0$$

Integrating, we get $x + y - z = C_2$ ...(2)

From equation (1) and (2), the complete solution is given by

$$\phi\left(\frac{2y}{x^2 - y^2},\ x + y - z\right) = 0$$

ANSWERS

1. $\phi\left[\left(\dfrac{x}{y}\right), x - \log(zy - 2) + \log y\right] = 0$

2. $\phi\left(\dfrac{x+y}{z}, \dfrac{2y}{y^2 - x^2}\right) = 0$

3. $\phi\left(\dfrac{x-y}{y-z}, \dfrac{y-z}{z-x}\right) = 0$

4. $\phi(x^2 - y^2,\ x^2 - z^2) = 0$

5. $\phi\left[\left(\dfrac{y-x}{z-y}\right), (x-y)^2(x+y+z)\right] = 0$

6. $\phi(lx + my + nz,\ x^2 + y^2 + z^2) = 0$

7. $\phi(x^2 - y^2 - z^2,\ 2xy - z^2) = 0$

8. $\phi[x + y, \log\{z^2 + (x+y)^2\} - 2x] = 0$

9. $\phi(x + y + z,\ xyz) = 0$

10. $\phi\left(\dfrac{-2y}{x^2 - y^2},\ x + y - z\right) = 0$

11. $\phi\left(\dfrac{y-x}{z-x}, \dfrac{y-x}{z-y}\right) = 0$

□□□□□□

Chapter

24 Vector Algebra

24.1 INTRODUCTION

Physical quantities are of two types. First, which are completely known if their magnitudes are known and second, which are completely known only when their magnitude as well as their direction are known. First type of quantities which are known by their magnitude only are called scalars and second type of quantity which known by magnitude and direction both are called vectors.

Definition. (Vector quantities): *The physical quantities which are completely known only when their magnitude and direction are known are called vector. For example, force, velocity, acceleration, momentum etc.*

Vector quantities can be represented by $\vec{a}, \vec{b}, \vec{c}$.

24.2 REPRESENTATION OF THE VECTOR QUANTITY

Let $\vec{a}$ be a vector. Draw a line segment OA in the direction of $\vec{a}$. Then the line segment $\overrightarrow{OA}$ has both magnitude and direction. Hence, line segment $\overrightarrow{OA}$ represents the vector $\vec{a}$ whose initial point is O and terminal point is A.

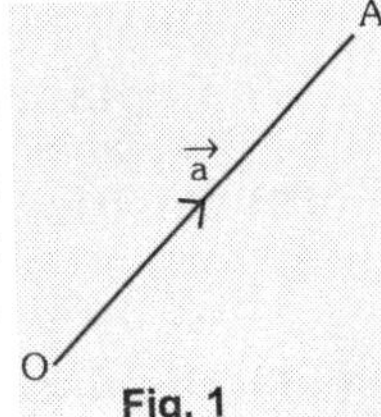

Fig. 1

24.3 MODULUS OF VECTOR QUANTITY

The magnitude of a vector is the length of the line segment OA representing it. It is always a positive quantity and is represented by $|\vec{a}|$ or $|\overrightarrow{OA}|$.

i.e., $$|\vec{a}| = a \text{ and } |\overrightarrow{OA}| = OA,$$

It is read as 'Modulus *a*'.

24.4 TYPES OF VECTORS

(1) Unit vector: A vector which has unit modulus is called unit vector. The unit vectors in the direction of *a*, *b*, *c* are respectively denoted by $\hat{a}, \hat{b}, \hat{c}$.

i.e., $$\hat{a} = \frac{\vec{a}}{|a|}, \hat{b} = \frac{\vec{b}}{|b|}, \hat{c} = \frac{\vec{c}}{|c|}$$

$\therefore$ $$|\hat{a}| = 1, |\hat{b}| = 1, |\hat{c}| = 1$$

(2) Free vector: A vector is said to be a free vector if it can be taken any where in the space. This vector is independent to its initial position.

(3) Equal vectors: Two vectors are said to be equal if their magnitude are equal and they have same direction.

(4) Like vectors: Vectors having same sense of direction are called like vectors.

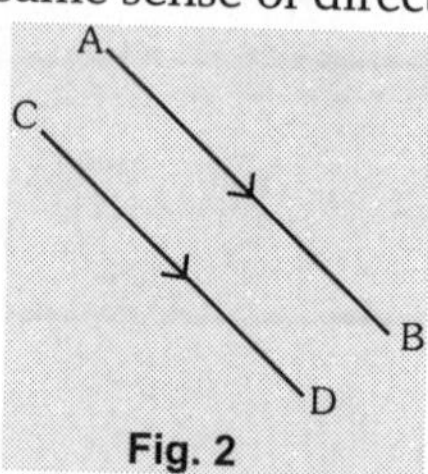

Fig. 2

(5) Unlike vectors: Vectors having the opposite sense of direction are called unlike vectors.

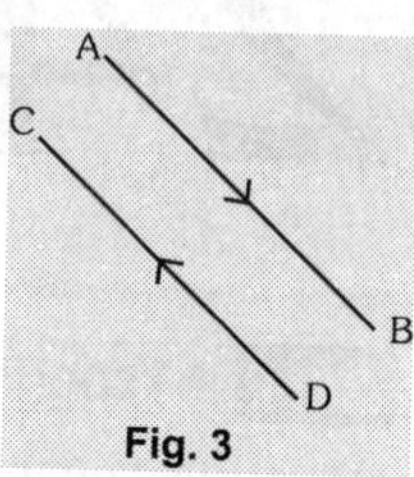

Fig. 3

(6) Negative vectors: The vector whose magnitude is same as that of $\vec{a}$ but the direction is opposite is called the negative of $\vec{a}$.

Let $\vec{a} = \overrightarrow{OA}$ be any given vector. Then its negative vector can be represented by $-\vec{a} = \overrightarrow{AO}$

Similarly, negative vector of $\overrightarrow{AB} = -\overrightarrow{BA}, \overrightarrow{DC} = -\overrightarrow{CD}$

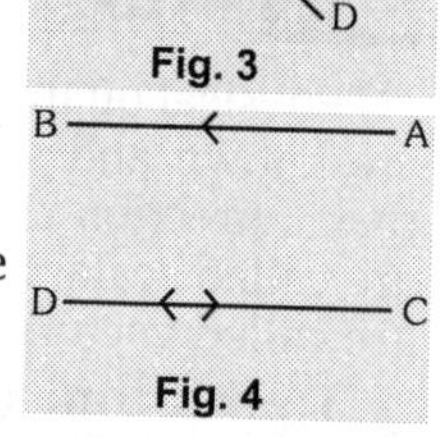

Fig. 4

(7) Zero vector: A vector whose modulus is zero and direction is indeterminate is called zero vector. The initial and terminal point of zero vector are same. It is denoted by $\vec{0}$.

(8) Collinear vectors: Vectors which are parallel to the same line are said to be collinear or parallel vectors. They need not have the same modulus and the same sense of direction.

(9) Coplanar vectors: Vectors lie in the same plane or parallel to the same plane are called coplanar vectors. A vector which is not coplanar is called non-coplanar.

(10) Position vector: Given any origin O, the position of a point P is specified uniquely by the vector $\overrightarrow{OP}$ is called the position vector of P with respect to O. Hence $\overrightarrow{OP}$ is the position vector of P relative to O.

(11) Displacement vector: If a point A is displaced from A to B then displacement AB is called the displacement vector $\overrightarrow{AB}$.

24.5 PRODUCT OF SCALAR AND VECTOR QUANTITY

Let $\vec{a}$ be any vector and m be any scalar then $m\vec{a}$ will be a vector parallel to $\vec{b}$ such that

$\therefore$ $$\vec{b} = m\vec{a}$$

and $$\vec{a} = \frac{1}{m}(\vec{b}) \Rightarrow \vec{a} = n(\vec{b})\text{ ; where } n = \frac{1}{m} \text{ is a scalar.}$$

Since scalar product of vector is distributive, therefore

$$(m+n)\vec{a} = m\vec{a} + n\vec{a} \qquad \text{and} \qquad m(\vec{a}+\vec{b}) = m\vec{a} + m\vec{b}$$

where $\vec{a}, \vec{b}$ are vectors and m, n are scalars.

24.6 ADDITION OF VECTORS

Addition of two vectors is done by using law of triangles which is known as triangle law of addition of vectors.

Let $\vec{a}$ and $\vec{b}$ be two given vectors. Draw $\vec{a} = \overrightarrow{AB}$ and $\vec{b} = \overrightarrow{BC}$ such that the terminal point of $\vec{a}$ is the initial point of $\vec{b}$. Then sum of $\vec{a}$ and $\vec{b}$ is the vector represented by the terminal point of $\vec{b}$ and initial point of $\vec{a}$, *i.e.* $\vec{R} = \overrightarrow{AC}$, then

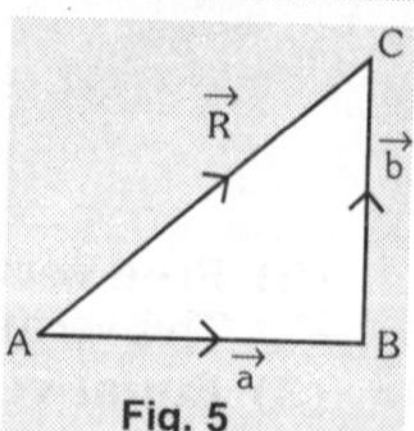

Fig. 5

$$\overrightarrow{AC} = \overrightarrow{AB} + \overrightarrow{BC} \text{ or } \vec{R} = \vec{a} + \vec{b}$$

24.7 PROPERTIES OF ADDITION OF VECTORS

(1) Commutative law: *Addition of vectors is commutative, i.e.,*

$$\vec{a}+\vec{b}=\vec{b}+\vec{a}$$

Proof. Let $\vec{a}$ and $\vec{b}$ be two vectors represented by $\overrightarrow{OA}$ and $\overrightarrow{AB}$ respectively

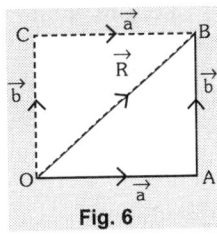

$$\overrightarrow{OB}=\overrightarrow{OA}+\overrightarrow{AB}$$

$\Rightarrow$ $$\overrightarrow{OB}=\vec{a}+\vec{b} \quad ...(1)$$

Fig. 6

Complete the parallelogram $OABC$ such that $OC = AB$, $OC \parallel AB$,

$$\overrightarrow{OC}=\overrightarrow{AB}=\vec{b}$$

and $$\overrightarrow{CB}=\overrightarrow{OA}=\vec{a}$$

similarly $$\overrightarrow{OB}=\overrightarrow{OC}+\overrightarrow{CB}=\vec{b}+\vec{a} \quad ...(2)$$

Hence from eqn. (1) and (2) we have

$$\vec{a}+\vec{b}=\vec{b}+\vec{a}$$

(2) Associative law: *Addition of vectors is associative.*

Proof. Let $\vec{a},\vec{b},\vec{c}$ be three vectors, then

$$\vec{a}+(\vec{b}+\vec{c})=(\vec{a}+\vec{b})+\vec{c}$$

Let O be the origin, then

$$\overrightarrow{OA}=\vec{a}, \overrightarrow{AB}=\vec{b}, \overrightarrow{BC}=\vec{c},$$

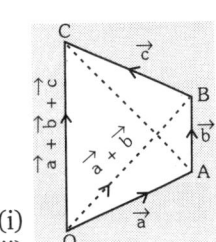

Now $$\vec{b}+\vec{c}=\overrightarrow{AB}+\overrightarrow{BC}=\overrightarrow{AC}$$

Therefore, $$\vec{a}+(\vec{b}+\vec{c})=\overrightarrow{OA}+\overrightarrow{AC}=\overrightarrow{OC} \quad ...(i)$$

Similarly, $$(\vec{a}+\vec{b})+\vec{c}=\overrightarrow{OB}+\overrightarrow{BC}=\overrightarrow{OC} \quad ...(ii)$$

Fig. 7

Hence, from eqn. (i) and (ii)

$$\vec{a}+(\vec{b}+\vec{c})=(\vec{a}+\vec{b})+\vec{c}$$

(3) Distributive law: For any scalar λ and vector $\vec{a}$ and $\vec{b}$ we have

$$\lambda(\vec{a}+\vec{b})=\lambda\vec{a}+\lambda\vec{b}$$

(4) Identity for addition: The zero vector ($\vec{0}$) is called the additive identity element.

i.e., $$\vec{a}+\vec{0}=\vec{a}=\vec{0}+\vec{a}$$

(5) Additive Inverse: Negative vector ($-\vec{a}$) will be the additive inverse of $\vec{a}$.

$\because$ $$\vec{a}+(-\vec{a})=0=(-\vec{a})+\vec{a}$$

24.8 SUBTRACTION OF VECTORS QUANTITIES

Let $\vec{a}$ and $\vec{b}$ be two vectors represented by

$$\vec{a}=\overrightarrow{AB} \text{ and } \vec{b}=\overrightarrow{BC}$$

$\therefore$ $$\vec{a}-\vec{b}=\vec{a}+(-\vec{b})$$

and $$\overrightarrow{BD}=-\overrightarrow{BC}=-\vec{b}$$

$\therefore$ $$\overrightarrow{AD}=\overrightarrow{AB}+\overrightarrow{BD}=\vec{a}+(-\vec{b})=\vec{a}-\vec{b}$$

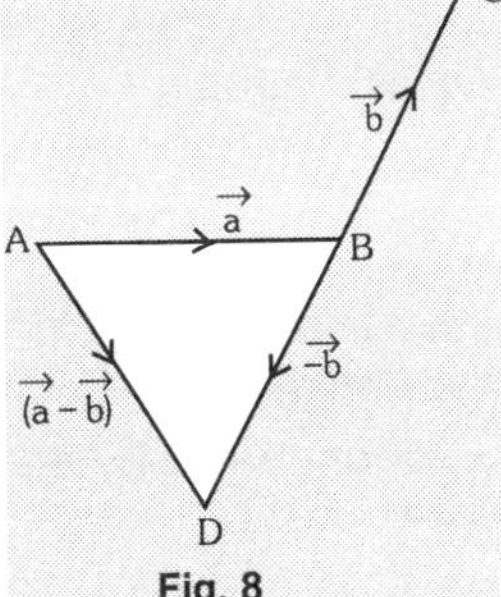

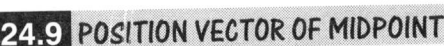

Fig. 8

24.9 POSITION VECTOR OF MIDPOINT

Let $\vec{a}$ and $\vec{b}$ be the position vectors of the point P and Q respectively.

Then position vector of the mid point PQ is $=\dfrac{\vec{a}+\vec{b}}{2}$

24.10 TO FIND THE POSITION VECTOR OF A POINT P WHICH DIVIDES THE LINE AB IN THE RATIO m : n

Let $\vec{a}$ and $\vec{b}$ be the position vectors of the point A and B respectively with respect to the origin O.

Let the point P divides the line AB in the ratio $m : n$

$$\overrightarrow{OA} = \vec{a} \text{ and } \overrightarrow{OB} = \vec{b}$$

and $$\frac{\overrightarrow{AP}}{\overrightarrow{PB}} = \frac{m}{n} \Rightarrow n \cdot \overrightarrow{AP} = m \cdot \overrightarrow{PB} \quad \text{...(i)}$$

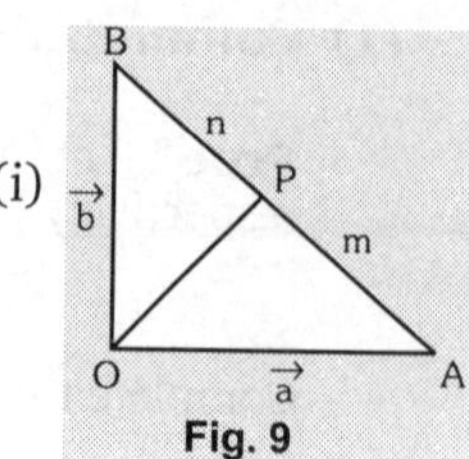

Fig. 9

but $$\overrightarrow{AP} = \overrightarrow{OP} - \overrightarrow{OA}$$

and $$\overrightarrow{PB} = \overrightarrow{OB} - \overrightarrow{OP}$$

Putting all these value in (i), we get

$$n(\overrightarrow{OP} - \overrightarrow{OA}) = m(\overrightarrow{OB} - \overrightarrow{OP})$$

$\therefore$ $$\overrightarrow{OP} = \frac{(m\overrightarrow{OB} + n\overrightarrow{OA})}{m+n} = \frac{m\vec{b} + n\vec{a}}{m+n}$$

24.11 $\lambda - \mu$ THEOREM

The resultant vectors of two vectors $\lambda\vec{a}$ and $\mu\vec{b}$ is $(\lambda + \mu)\overrightarrow{OG}$ when G, divides the line AB in the ratio of $\mu : \lambda$.

i.e., $$AG : GB = \mu : \lambda$$

Hence $$\lambda\overrightarrow{OA} + \mu\overrightarrow{OB} = (\lambda + \mu)\overrightarrow{OG}$$

24.12 RESOLUTION OF VECTOR QUANTITIES

Let $\vec{r}$ be a vector such that it can be written as the sum of vector quantities $\vec{a}, \vec{b}, \vec{c}, \vec{d}, \ldots$ then $\vec{a}, \vec{b}, \vec{c}, \vec{d}, \ldots$ are called the components of the vector $\vec{r}$.

24.13 NON-COPLANAR VECTORS

If $\vec{a}, \vec{b}, \vec{c}$ are three given non-coplanar vectors then any vector $\vec{r}$ can be expressed uniquely as $\vec{r} = x\vec{a} + y\vec{b} + z\vec{c}$ where x, y, z are scalars.

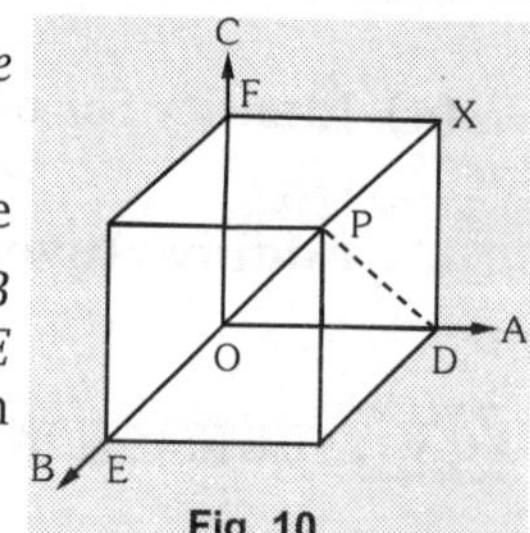

Fig. 10

Proof. Let us take any point O. Let $\overrightarrow{OA} = \vec{a}, \overrightarrow{OB} = \vec{b}, \overrightarrow{OC} = \vec{c}$. The three lines OA, OB and OC are non-coplanar and BOC, COA and AOB are different planes through P, draw parallel planes which meet at D, E and F to OA, OB and OC respectively, thus we get a parallelopiped with OP as diagonal.

$$\vec{r} = \overrightarrow{OP} = \overrightarrow{OD} + \overrightarrow{DP} = \overrightarrow{OD} + \overrightarrow{DX} + \overrightarrow{XP}$$

$$= \overrightarrow{OD} + \overrightarrow{OF} + \overrightarrow{OE} \quad \text{...(i)}$$

$\because$ $$\overrightarrow{OD} \,||\, \overrightarrow{OA}, \overrightarrow{OE} \,||\, \overrightarrow{OB} \text{ and } \overrightarrow{OF} \,||\, \overrightarrow{OC}$$

Hence $$\overrightarrow{OD} = x \cdot \overrightarrow{OA} = x\vec{a}, \overrightarrow{OE} = y \cdot \overrightarrow{OB} = y\vec{b}, \overrightarrow{OF} = z \cdot \overrightarrow{OC} = z\vec{c} \quad \text{...(ii)}$$

From eqns. (i) and (ii), we have

$$\vec{r} = x\vec{a} + y\vec{b} + z\vec{c}$$

THEOREM. *If $\vec{a}, \vec{b}, \vec{c}$ are three non-coplanar vector such that $x\vec{a} + y\vec{b} + z\vec{c} = 0$, then $x = 0, y = 0$, $z = 0$, x, y, z being scalars.*

PROOF. Let $x \neq 0$ then from $x\vec{a} + y\vec{b} + z\vec{c} = 0$

$$\vec{a} = -\frac{y}{x}\vec{b} - \frac{z}{x}\vec{c}$$

$\Rightarrow$ Vector $\vec{a}$ is coplanar to $\vec{b}$ and $\vec{c}$, which is a contradiction.

Hence, $$x = 0, y = 0, z = 0.$$

24.14 RECTANGULAR UNIT VECTOR

If OX and OY are two mutually perpendicular lines such that $OX = x$-axis and $OY = y$-axis. Then $\hat{i}$ and $\hat{j}$ are the unit vectors in the direction of x and y-axis respectively.

24.15 TWO-DIMENSIONAL UNIT VECTORS

Let $P(x, y)$ be any point. Draw perpendicular OM on OX from P.

$\because$ $\overrightarrow{OM} = x\hat{i}, \overrightarrow{MP}$ and $\hat{j}$, are parallel.

$\therefore$ $\overrightarrow{MP} = y\hat{j}$

In Δ OPM, $\vec{r} = \overrightarrow{OP} = \overrightarrow{OM} + \overrightarrow{MP}$

$= x\hat{i} + y\hat{j}$

where $OP = \sqrt{x^2 + y^2}$

unit vector in the direction of $\vec{r} = \dfrac{\vec{r}}{|r|} = \dfrac{\vec{r}}{r} = \hat{r}$

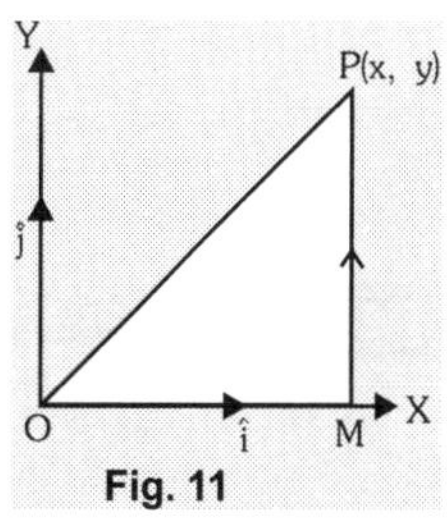

Fig. 11

24.16 THREE-DIMENSIONAL UNIT VECTORS

Let OX, OY and OZ be three mutually perpendicular lines and co-ordinate of the point $P = (x, y, z)$. Let $\hat{i}, \hat{j}, \hat{k}$ be the unit vectors along OX, OY and OZ respectively.

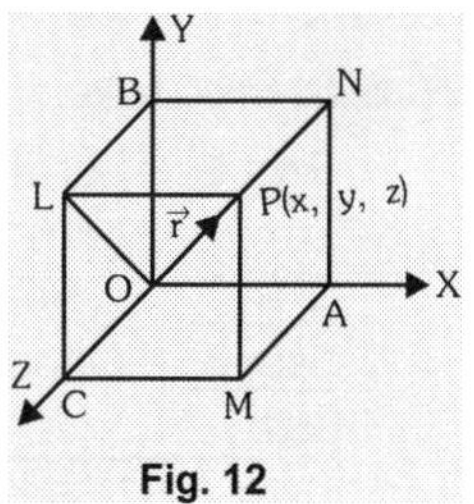

Fig. 12

$$\overrightarrow{OA} = x\hat{i}, \overrightarrow{OB} = y\hat{j} \text{ and } \overrightarrow{OC} = z\hat{k}$$

$$\vec{r} = \overrightarrow{OP} = \overrightarrow{OL} + \overrightarrow{LP} = (\overrightarrow{OB} + \overrightarrow{BL}) + \overrightarrow{LP}$$

$$= \overrightarrow{OB} + \overrightarrow{OA} + \overrightarrow{OC} \qquad (\because \overrightarrow{BL} = \overrightarrow{OC}, \overrightarrow{LP} = \overrightarrow{OA})$$

$$= \overrightarrow{OA} + \overrightarrow{OB} + \overrightarrow{OC}$$

$$\vec{r} = x\hat{i} + y\hat{j} + z\hat{k}$$

Now unit vector along $\vec{r}$ is $\vec{r} = \dfrac{\vec{r}}{|r|} = \dfrac{\vec{r}}{r} = \dfrac{x\hat{i} + y\hat{j} + z\hat{k}}{r}$

and $r = \sqrt{x^2 + y^2 + z^2}$

24.17 RELATIVE VELOCITY

It is possible to find the velocity of a particle w.r.t. the other. Here we subtract the velocity of first particle from the velocity of other.

Let $\overrightarrow{v_1}$ be the velocity of the particle A and $\overrightarrow{v_2}$ be the velocity of the particle B then relative velocity of A w.r.t. B is given by

$$\vec{V} = \overrightarrow{v_1} - \overrightarrow{v_2}$$

- Unit vector in north-east direction $= \dfrac{\hat{i} + \hat{j}}{\sqrt{2}}$
- Unit vector in north-west direction $= \dfrac{(-\hat{i} + \hat{j})}{\sqrt{2}}$
- Unit vector in south-east direction $= \dfrac{\hat{i} - \hat{j}}{\sqrt{2}}$
- Unit vector in south-west direction $= \dfrac{(-\hat{i} - \hat{j})}{\sqrt{2}}$

24.18 DIRECTION COSINES OF VECTORS

If a vector $\overrightarrow{AB}$ makes the angles α, β, γ with the positive direction of rectangle axes OX, OY

and OZ respectively. Then direction cosine of these vectors can be defined as follows:

$$\cos\alpha = \frac{a_1}{|\overrightarrow{OS}|} = \frac{a_1}{\sqrt{a_1^2 + a_2^2 + a_3^2}}$$

$$\cos\beta = \frac{a_2}{|\overrightarrow{OS}|} = \frac{a_2}{\sqrt{a_1^2 + a_2^2 + a_3^2}}$$

$$\cos\gamma = \frac{a_3}{|\overrightarrow{OS}|} = \frac{a_3}{\sqrt{a_1^2 + a_2^2 + a_3^2}}$$

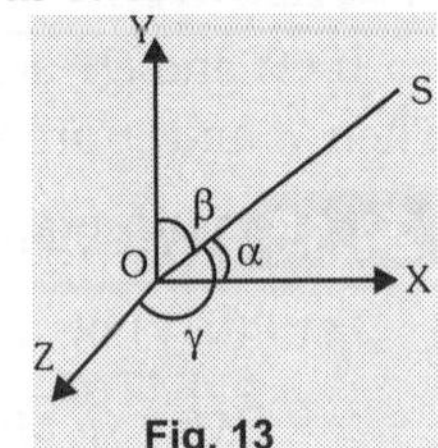

Fig. 13

and $\cos^2\alpha + \cos^2\beta + \cos^2\gamma = 1$

24.19 LINEARLY DEPENDENT AND INDEPENDENT VECTORS

A set of vectors $\vec{a_1}, \vec{a_2}, \vec{a_3}, ..., \vec{a_n}$ is said to be linearly dependent if there exist n scalars x_1, x_2, x_3, ..., x_n (not all zero) such that

$$x_1\vec{a_1} + x_2\vec{a_2} + x_3\vec{a_3} + ... + x_n\vec{a_n} = 0$$

But, if $x_1 = 0, x_2 = 0, x_3 = 0, ..., x_n = 0$ then $\vec{a_1}, \vec{a_2}, \vec{a_3}, ..., \vec{a_n}$ are called linearly independent vectors.

WORKING PROCEDURE

STEP 1. Letting as many scalar quantities as the vectors and put each of them equal to zero separately.

STEP 2. Compare the coefficients of vectors.

STEP 3. Obtained scalar quantities by solving the equations.

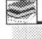

- If the values of all scalars are zero then given vectors are said to be linearly independent otherwise dependent.

24.20 EQUATION OF A LINE PASSING THROUGH A POINT AND PARALLEL TO THE GIVEN VECTOR

The required equation is $\vec{r} = \vec{a} + t\vec{b}$

where $\vec{a}$ = position vector of the given point

and $\vec{b}$ = given vector

- If the line passes through the origin then its equation is $\vec{r} = t\vec{b}$.

24.21 CONDITION FOR THREE POINTS TO BE COLLINEAR

If $\vec{a}$, $\vec{b}$ and $\vec{c}$ are the position vector of three points A, B and C respectively, then points A, B, C will be collinear if and only if there exists scalars x, y, z such that $x\vec{a} + y\vec{b} + z\vec{c} = 0, x + y + z = 0$.

Proof. Let $z \neq 0$ then $x + y = -z$

$$x\vec{a} + y\vec{b} = -z\vec{c} = (x + y)\cdot\vec{c} \qquad ...(i)$$

$$\Rightarrow \qquad \vec{c} = \frac{x\vec{a} + y\vec{b}}{x + y}$$

Hence, points are collinear and $\vec{c}$ be the position vector of the point which divide the line joining the points $\vec{a}$ and $\vec{b}$ in the ratio of $y : x$.

24.22 EQUATION OF THE LINE PASSING THROUGH TWO GIVEN POINTS

The required equation is $\vec{r} = \vec{a} + t(\vec{b} - \vec{a})$

or $\vec{r} = (1-t)\vec{a} + t\vec{b}$

where $\vec{a}$ = position vector of one point

and $\vec{b}$ = position vector of other point

24.23 VECTOR EQUATION OF A PLANE

Plane passing through a given point and parallel to two given non-parallel vectors.

Let $\vec{b}$ and $\vec{c}$ be two non-parallel vectors parallel to the vector $\vec{a}$.

Also $\vec{r}$ be position vector of P about O.

Then $\overrightarrow{AM} = t\vec{b}$ and $\overrightarrow{MP} = s\vec{c}$ where t, s are scalars.

$$\vec{r} = \overrightarrow{OP} = \overrightarrow{OA} + \overrightarrow{AP} = \overrightarrow{OA} + \overrightarrow{AM} + \overrightarrow{MP}$$

$$\boldsymbol{\vec{r} = \vec{a} + t\vec{b} + s\vec{c}}$$

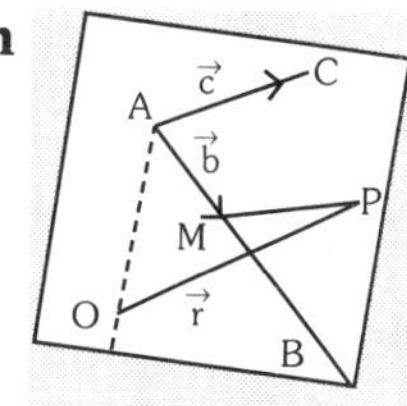

Fig. 14

24.24 EQUATION OF A PLANE PASSING THROUGH THREE POINTS

Let $\vec{a}$, $\vec{b}$ and $\vec{c}$ be the position vectors of three given points

Then $\overrightarrow{AB} = \overrightarrow{OB} - \overrightarrow{OA} = \vec{b} - \vec{a}$

and $\overrightarrow{AC} = \overrightarrow{OC} - \overrightarrow{OA} = \vec{c} - \vec{a}$

This plane is parallel to $\overrightarrow{AB}$ and $\overrightarrow{AC}$. Hence equation of the plane is

$$\vec{r} = \vec{a} + t(\vec{b} - \vec{a}) + s(\vec{c} - \vec{a})$$

$$\vec{r} = (1-s-t)\vec{a} + t\vec{b} + s\vec{c}$$

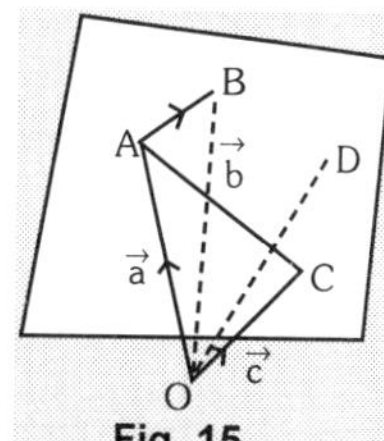

Fig. 15

24.25 CONDITION FOR FOUR POINTS TO BE COPLANAR

Let A, B, C and D be the four points in which A, B and C are not collinear. The position vectors of the points A, B, C and D are respectively given by $\vec{a}, \vec{b}, \vec{c}$ and $\vec{d}$. Then the condition for four points to be coplanar is given by:

$$\vec{a} + \lambda\vec{b} + \mu\vec{c} + \nu\vec{d} = 0$$

Where $1 + \lambda + \mu + \nu = 0$

WORKING PROCEDURE

STEP 1. Write the relation $\vec{a} + \lambda\vec{b} + \mu\vec{c} + \nu\vec{d} = 0$.

STEP 2. Equating the coefficients of $\vec{a}, \vec{b}, \vec{c}$ and $\vec{d}$ on both the sides.

STEP 3. On solving the equation, find λ, μ, ν.

STEP 4. If value of λ, μ, ν satisfies $1 + \lambda + \mu + \nu = 0$, then given four points will be coplanar.

- For proving the three points $\vec{a}, \vec{b}$ and $\vec{c}$ to be collinear, consider the equation

$$\vec{a} = \lambda\vec{b} + \mu\vec{c}$$

where λ and μ are scalars.

Solved Examples

1. *If the vectors $a\hat{i} + b\hat{j} + c\hat{k}$ and $-2\hat{i} + \hat{j} + 3\hat{k}$ are equal, find the values of a, b and c.*

SOLUTION. $a\hat{i} + b\hat{j} + c\hat{k} = -2\hat{i} + \hat{j} + 3\hat{k}$

Equating the coefficients of both the sides, we get

we get $a = -2, b = 1, c = 3$

2. *If $\hat{i}$ and $\hat{j}$ are the unit vectors corresponding to the sides a and b of a rectangle. Find the unit vector along its* *diagonals. In case of a square, what will be its value?*

SOLUTION. Let $ABCD$ be rectangle such that $AB = a$, $AD = b$ and AC be the diagonal.

Vector along $\overrightarrow{AB} = a\hat{i}$

Vector along $\overrightarrow{AD} = b\hat{j}$

$$\therefore \quad \overrightarrow{AC} = \overrightarrow{AB} + \overrightarrow{BC} = \overrightarrow{AB} + \overrightarrow{AD} = a\hat{i} + b\hat{j}$$

and magnitude $= \sqrt{a^2 + b^2}$

Hence, unit vector along

$$\overrightarrow{AC} = \frac{a\hat{i} + b\hat{j}}{\sqrt{a^2 + b^2}}$$

If BD be the another diagonal of the rectangle then

$$\overrightarrow{BD} = \overrightarrow{AD} - \overrightarrow{AB} = bj - ai$$

Unit vector along $\overrightarrow{BD} = \dfrac{b\hat{j} - a\hat{i}}{\sqrt{a^2 + b^2}}$

If rectangle is a square then $a = b$ and hence unit vectors of the diagonals are $\dfrac{\hat{i} + \hat{j}}{\sqrt{2}}, \dfrac{\hat{j} - \hat{i}}{\sqrt{2}}$.

3. *Find the sum of the vectors* $3\hat{i} + 7\hat{j} - 4\hat{k}$, $\hat{i} - 5\hat{j} - 8\hat{k}$ *and* $6\hat{i} - 2\hat{j} + 12\hat{k}$.

SOLUTION. Clearly, $(3\hat{i} + 7\hat{j} - 4\hat{k}) + (\hat{i} - 5\hat{j} - 8\hat{k}) + (6\hat{i} - 2\hat{j} + 12\hat{k})$

$$= (3\hat{i} + \hat{i} + 6\hat{i}) + (7\hat{j} - 5\hat{j} - 2\hat{j}) + (-4\hat{k} - 8\hat{k} + 12\hat{k}) = 10\hat{i}$$

4. *The position vectors of two vectors* $\overrightarrow{OA}$ *and* $\overrightarrow{OB}$ *along O are respectively given by* $3\hat{i} + 2\hat{j} - 3\hat{k}$ *and* $2\hat{i} + 5\hat{j} - \hat{k}$. *Find* $\overrightarrow{AB}$.

SOLUTION. Since $\overrightarrow{OA} = 3\hat{i} + 2\hat{j} - 3\hat{k}$

$$\overrightarrow{OB} = 2\hat{i} + 5\hat{j} - \hat{k}$$

$$\therefore \quad \overrightarrow{AB} = \overrightarrow{OB} - \overrightarrow{OA}$$
$$= (2\hat{i} + 5\hat{j} - \hat{k}) - (3\hat{i} + 2\hat{j} - 3\hat{k})$$
$$= (2\hat{i} - 3\hat{i}) + (5\hat{j} - 2\hat{j}) + (-\hat{k} + 3\hat{k})$$
$$= -\hat{i} + 3\hat{j} + 2\hat{k}$$

5. *If* $\vec{a} = 2\hat{i} + \hat{j} - 3\hat{k}, \vec{b} = 3\hat{i} - 2\hat{j} + \hat{k}$ *and* $\vec{c} = \hat{i} + \hat{j} + \hat{k}$, *find the value of* $-\vec{a} + 2\vec{b} + 3\vec{c}$.

SOLUTION. We have $-\vec{a} + 2\vec{b} + 3\vec{c}$

$$= -(2\hat{i} + \hat{j} - 3\hat{k}) + 2(3\hat{i} - 2\hat{j} + \hat{k}) + 3(\hat{i} + \hat{j} + \hat{k})$$
$$= (-2\hat{i} - \hat{j} + 3\hat{k}) + (6\hat{i} - 4\hat{j} + 2\hat{k}) + (3\hat{i} + 3\hat{j} + 3\hat{k})$$
$$= (-2\hat{i} + 6\hat{i} + 3\hat{i}) + (-\hat{j} - 4\hat{j} + 3\hat{j}) + (3\hat{k} + 2\hat{k} + 3\hat{k})$$
$$= 7\hat{i} - 2\hat{j} + 8\hat{k}$$

6. *If* $\vec{a} = 4\hat{i} - \hat{j} + \hat{k}, \vec{b} = 2\hat{i} + \hat{j} - 7\hat{k}$, $\vec{c} = -3\hat{i} - 4\hat{j} + 2\hat{k}$ *and* $\vec{d} = \hat{i} + \hat{j} + \hat{k}$, *find the value of* $3\vec{a} + 2\vec{b} - 4\vec{c} - \vec{d}$.

SOLUTION. We have $3\vec{a} + 2\vec{b} - 4\vec{c} - \vec{d}$

$$= 3(4\hat{i} - \hat{j} + \hat{k}) + 2(2\hat{i} + \hat{j} - 7\hat{k}) - 4(-3\hat{i} - 4\hat{j} + 2\hat{k}) - (\hat{i} + \hat{j} + \hat{k})$$
$$= (12\hat{i} - 3\hat{j} + 3\hat{k}) + (4\hat{i} + 2\hat{j} - 14\hat{k}) + (12\hat{i} + 16\hat{j} - 8\hat{k}) - (\hat{i} + \hat{j} + \hat{k})$$
$$= (12\hat{i} + 4\hat{i} + 12\hat{i} - \hat{i}) + (-3\hat{j} + 2\hat{j} + 16\hat{j} - \hat{j}) + (3\hat{k} - 14\hat{k} - 8\hat{k} - \hat{k})$$
$$= 27\hat{i} + 14\hat{j} - 20\hat{k}$$

7. *The position vectors of the points A, B, C and D are respectively given by* $\hat{i} + \hat{j} + \hat{k}$, $2\hat{i} + 3\hat{j}, 3\hat{i} + 5\hat{j} - 2\hat{k}$ *and* $\hat{k} - \hat{j}$. *Prove that AB and CD are parallel.*

SOLUTION. Let O be the origin. Then

$$\overrightarrow{OA} = \hat{i} + \hat{j} + \hat{k}, \overrightarrow{OB} = 2\hat{i} + 3\hat{j}$$
$$\overrightarrow{OC} = 3\hat{i} + 5\hat{j} - 2\hat{k},$$
$$\overrightarrow{OD} = \hat{k} - \hat{j} = -\hat{j} + \hat{k}$$
$$\overrightarrow{AB} = \overrightarrow{OB} - \overrightarrow{OA} = (2\hat{i} + 3\hat{j}) - (\hat{i} + \hat{j} + \hat{k})$$
$$= (2\hat{i} - \hat{i}) + (3\hat{j} - \hat{j}) + (0 - \hat{k})$$
$$= \hat{i} + 2\hat{j} - \hat{k}$$

and $\overrightarrow{CD} = \overrightarrow{OD} - \overrightarrow{OC}$

$= (-\hat{j} + \hat{k}) - (3\hat{i} + 5\hat{j} - 2\hat{k})$

$= -3\hat{i} + (-\hat{j} - 5\hat{j}) + (\hat{k} + 2\hat{k})$

$= -3\hat{i} - 6\hat{j} + 3\hat{k}$

$= -3(\hat{i} + 2\hat{j} - \hat{k}) = -3(\overrightarrow{AB})$

$\overrightarrow{CD} = m(\overrightarrow{AB})$ where $m = -3$

Hence, lines AB and CD are parallel.

8. *The position vector of the point A and B are $2\hat{i} + 3\hat{j}$ and $3\hat{j} + 8\hat{k}$ respectively. Find the position vector of C if it divides the line in the ratio of 1 : 2.*

SOLUTION. Let O be the origin. Then, we have

$\overrightarrow{OA} = 2\hat{i} + 3\hat{j}, \overrightarrow{OB} = 3\hat{j} + 8\hat{k}$

Hence $\overrightarrow{OC} = \dfrac{1\cdot(\overrightarrow{OB}) + 2\cdot(\overrightarrow{OA})}{1+2}$

$= \dfrac{(3\hat{j} + 8\hat{k}) + 2(2\hat{i} + 3\hat{j})}{3}$

$= \dfrac{4\hat{i} + 9\hat{j} + 8\hat{k}}{3}$

$= \dfrac{4}{3}\hat{i} + \dfrac{9}{3}\hat{j} + \dfrac{8}{3}\hat{k}$

$= \dfrac{4}{3}\hat{i} + 3\hat{j} + \dfrac{8}{3}\hat{k}$

9. *Write the position vectors of the point A and B of their co-ordinates are (1, 2, –1) and (2, –3, 1) respectively. Also find $\overrightarrow{AB}$.*

SOLUTION. Let O be the origin. Then

$\overrightarrow{OA} = 1(\hat{i}) + 2(\hat{j}) - 1(\hat{k}) = \hat{i} + 2\hat{j} - \hat{k}$

$\overrightarrow{OB} = 2(\hat{i}) - 3(\hat{j}) + 1(\hat{k}) = 2\hat{i} - 3\hat{j} + \hat{k}$

Hence $\overrightarrow{AB} = \overrightarrow{OB} - \overrightarrow{OA}$

$= (2\hat{i} - 3\hat{j} + \hat{k}) - (\hat{i} + 2\hat{j} - \hat{k})$

$= (2\hat{i} - \hat{i}) + (-3\hat{j} - 2\hat{j}) + (\hat{k} + \hat{k})$

$= \hat{i} - 5\hat{j} + 2\hat{k}$

10. *Find the modulus of $\hat{i} + \hat{j} + \hat{k}$.*

SOLUTION. Required modulus

$= |\hat{i} + \hat{j} + \hat{k}| = \sqrt{(1^2 + 1^2 + 1^2)} = \sqrt{3}$

11. *The position vectors of the point P and Q are $3\hat{i} + 5\hat{j} - 7\hat{k}$ and $3\hat{i} - 4\hat{j} + \hat{k}$ respectively. Find $|\overrightarrow{PQ}|$.*

SOLUTION. Let O be the origin. Then

$\overrightarrow{OP} = 3\hat{i} + 5\hat{j} - 7\hat{k}$ and $\overrightarrow{OQ} = 3\hat{i} - 4\hat{j} + \hat{k}$

$\therefore\ \overrightarrow{PQ} = \overrightarrow{OQ} - \overrightarrow{OP}$

$= (3\hat{i} - 4\hat{j} + \hat{k}) - (3\hat{i} + 5\hat{j} - 7\hat{k})$

$= 0\hat{i} - 9\hat{j} + 8\hat{k}$

and $|\overrightarrow{PQ}| = |0\hat{i} - 9\hat{j} + 8\hat{k}|$

$= \sqrt{(-9)^2 + (8)^2}$

$= \sqrt{81 + 64} = \sqrt{145}$

12. *Find the sum of the vectors $3\hat{i} - 4\hat{j} + 7\hat{k}$ and $\hat{i} - 2\hat{j} - 5\hat{k}$. Also find the resultant of the sum.*

SOLUTION. We have $(3\hat{i} - 4\hat{j} + 7\hat{k}) + (\hat{i} - 2\hat{j} - 5\hat{k})$

$= 4\hat{i} - 6\hat{j} + 2\hat{k}$

and modulus $= 4\hat{i} - 6\hat{j} + 2\hat{k}$

$= |4\hat{i} - 6\hat{j} + 2\hat{k}|$

$= \sqrt{(4)^2 + (-6)^2 + (2)^2}$

$= \sqrt{16 + 36 + 4} = \sqrt{56}$

$= 2\sqrt{14}$

13. *Find the sum of $3\hat{i} + 7\hat{j} - 4\hat{k}$ and $\hat{i} - 5\hat{j} - 8\hat{k}$. Also find the modulus of the resultant of sum.*

SOLUTION. We have $(3\hat{i} + 7\hat{j} - 4\hat{k}) + (\hat{i} - 5\hat{j} - 8\hat{k})$

$= (3\hat{i} + \hat{i}) + (7\hat{j} - 5\hat{j}) + (-4\hat{k} - 8\hat{k})$

$= 4\hat{i} + 2\hat{j} - 12\hat{k}$

and modulus

$= |4\hat{i} + 2\hat{j} - 12\hat{k}|$

$= \sqrt{(4)^2 + (2)^2 + (-12)^2}$

$= \sqrt{16 + 4 + 144} = \sqrt{164} = 2\sqrt{41}$

14. *If position vectors of A and B are respectively given by $5\hat{i} - 2\hat{j} + 4\hat{k}$ and $\hat{i} + 3\hat{j} - 7\hat{k}$. Find $|\overrightarrow{AB}|$.*

SOLUTION. Let O be the origin. Then

$\overrightarrow{OA} = 5\hat{i} - 2\hat{j} + 4\hat{k}$ and $\overrightarrow{OB} = \hat{i} + 3\hat{j} - 7\hat{k}$

and $\overrightarrow{AB} = \overrightarrow{OB} - \overrightarrow{OA}$

$= (\hat{i} + 3\hat{j} - 7\hat{k}) - (5\hat{i} - 2\hat{j} + 4\hat{k})$

$= (\hat{i} - 5\hat{i}) + (3\hat{j} + 2\hat{j}) + (-7\hat{k} - 4\hat{k})$

$= -4\hat{i} + 5\hat{j} - 11\hat{k}$

$$|\overrightarrow{AB}| = |-4\hat{i} + 5\hat{j} - 11\hat{k}|$$
$$= \sqrt{(-4)^2 + (5)^2 + (-11)^2}$$
$$= \sqrt{16 + 25 + 121}$$
$$= \sqrt{162} = 9\sqrt{2}$$

15. *Prove that the line joining the point represented by $\hat{i} + \hat{j} - \hat{k}$ and $3\hat{i} - 2\hat{j} - \hat{k}$ is parallel to xy-plane. Also find its length.*

SOLUTION. Let O be the origin, then

$\overrightarrow{OA} = \hat{i} + \hat{j} - \hat{k}$ and $\overrightarrow{OB} = 3\hat{i} - 2\hat{j} - \hat{k}$

$$\overrightarrow{AB} = \overrightarrow{OB} - \overrightarrow{OA}$$
$$= (3\hat{i} - 2\hat{j} - \hat{k}) - (\hat{i} + \hat{j} - \hat{k})$$
$$= (3\hat{i} - \hat{i}) + (-2\hat{j} - \hat{j}) + (-\hat{k} + \hat{k})$$
$$= 2\hat{i} - 3\hat{j} + 0\hat{k}$$

Coefficient of $\hat{k}$ in the vector $\overrightarrow{AB}$ is 0.

Hence, line AB is parallel to xy-plane.

$\therefore$ Length $= |\overrightarrow{AB}| = \sqrt{4+9} = \sqrt{13}$ unit

16. *Find the unit vector parallel to the vector $\vec{a} = 3\hat{i} + 4\hat{j} - 2\hat{k}$? Which vector is to be added to $\vec{a}$ to get the resultant $\hat{i}$?*

SOLUTION. We have $|\vec{a}| = \sqrt{(3)^2 + (4)^2 + (-2)^2}$

$$= \sqrt{9 + 16 + 4} = \sqrt{29}$$

Unit vector $e = \dfrac{\vec{a}}{|\vec{a}|} = \dfrac{3\hat{i} + 4\hat{j} - 2\hat{k}}{\sqrt{29}}$

Let $\vec{b}$ be the required vector such that

$$\vec{a} + \vec{b} = \hat{i}$$
$$(3\hat{i} + 4\hat{j} - 2\hat{k}) + \vec{b} = \hat{i}$$
$$\Rightarrow \quad \vec{b} = \hat{i} - (3\hat{i} + 4\hat{j} - 2\hat{k})$$
$$= -2\hat{i} - 4\hat{j} + 2\hat{k}$$

17. *Find two unit vectors parallel to the diagonals of a parallelogram whose adjacent sides are $2\hat{i} + 4\hat{j} - 5\hat{k}$ and $\hat{i} + 2\hat{j} + 3\hat{k}$.*

SOLUTION. Let $PQRS$ be a parallelogram.

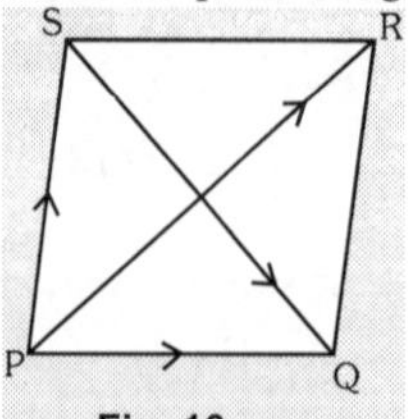

Fig. 16

Then $\overrightarrow{PQ} = 2\hat{i} + 4\hat{j} - 5\hat{k} = \overrightarrow{SR}$

$$\overrightarrow{PS} = \hat{i} + 2\hat{j} + 3\hat{k} = \overrightarrow{QR}$$

The unit vector is parallel to $\overrightarrow{PR}$.

In $\Delta\, PQR$,

$$\overrightarrow{PR} = \overrightarrow{PQ} + \overrightarrow{QR} = \overrightarrow{SR} + \overrightarrow{PS}$$
$$= (2\hat{i} + 4\hat{j} - 5\hat{k}) + (\hat{i} + 2\hat{j} + 3\hat{k})$$
$$= 3\hat{i} + 6\hat{j} - 2\hat{k}$$
$$|\overrightarrow{PR}| = |3\hat{i} + 6\hat{j} - 2\hat{k}|$$
$$= \sqrt{3^2 + 6^2 + (-2)^2}$$
$$= \sqrt{9 + 36 + 4} = \sqrt{49} = 7$$

Let e_1 be the unit vector parallel to diagonal PR.

$$\text{Then } e_1 = \frac{\overrightarrow{PR}}{|\overrightarrow{PR}|} = \frac{3\hat{i} + 6\hat{j} - 2\hat{k}}{\sqrt{3^2 + 6^2 + (-2)^2}}$$
$$= \frac{3\hat{i} + 6\hat{j} - 2\hat{k}}{7}$$

Now, in $\Delta\, QRS$,

$$\overrightarrow{SQ} = \overrightarrow{SR} + \overrightarrow{RQ} = \overrightarrow{SR} - \overrightarrow{QR} = \overrightarrow{PQ} - \overrightarrow{PS}$$
$$= (2\hat{i} + 4\hat{j} - 5\hat{k}) - (\hat{i} + 2\hat{j} + 3\hat{k})$$
$$= \hat{i} + 2\hat{j} - 8\hat{k}$$
$$|\overrightarrow{SQ}| = \sqrt{(1)^2 + (2)^2 + (-8)^2}$$
$$= \sqrt{1 + 4 + 64} = \sqrt{69}$$

Let e_2 be the unit vector parallel to diagonal SQ. Then

$$e_2 = \frac{\overrightarrow{SQ}}{|\overrightarrow{SQ}|} = \frac{\hat{i} + 2\hat{j} - 8\hat{k}}{\sqrt{69}}$$

18. *If the position vector of the vertices A, B and C are respectively given by $2\hat{i} - \hat{j} + \hat{k}$, $\hat{i} - 3\hat{j} - 5\hat{k}$ and $3\hat{i} - 4\hat{j} - 4\hat{k}$, show that triangle is right angled.*

SOLUTION. We have $\overrightarrow{AB}$

= position vector of B – position vector of A

$$= (\hat{i} - 3\hat{j} - 5\hat{k}) - (2\hat{i} - \hat{j} + \hat{k})$$
$$= (\hat{i} - 2\hat{i}) + (-3\hat{j} + \hat{j}) + (-5\hat{k} - \hat{k})$$
$$= -\hat{i} - 2\hat{j} - 6\hat{k}$$
$$|\overrightarrow{AB}| = \sqrt{(-1)^2 + (-2)^2 + (-6)^2}$$
$$= \sqrt{1 + 4 + 36} = \sqrt{41}$$

$\overrightarrow{BC}$
= position vector of C
– position vector of B
$= (3\hat{i} - 4\hat{j} - 4\hat{k}) - (\hat{i} - 3\hat{j} - 5\hat{k})$
$= (3\hat{i} - \hat{i}) + (-4\hat{j} + 3\hat{j}) + (-4\hat{k} + 5\hat{k})$
$= 2\hat{i} - \hat{j} + \hat{k}$
$|\overrightarrow{BC}| = \sqrt{(2)^2 + (-1)^2 + (1)^2}$
$= \sqrt{4 + 1 + 1} = \sqrt{6}$

$\overrightarrow{CA}$
= position vector of A
– position vector of C
$= (2\hat{i} - \hat{j} + \hat{k}) - (3\hat{i} - 4\hat{j} - 4\hat{k})$
$= (2\hat{i} - 3\hat{i}) + (-\hat{j} + 4\hat{j}) + (\hat{k} + 4\hat{k})$
$= -\hat{i} + 3\hat{i} + 5\hat{k}$
$|\overrightarrow{CA}| = \sqrt{(-1)^2 + (3)^2 + (5)^2}$
$= \sqrt{1 + 9 + 25} = \sqrt{35}$

$|\overrightarrow{AB}| = \sqrt{41} \Rightarrow |\overrightarrow{AB}|^2 = 41$

$|\overrightarrow{BC}| = \sqrt{6} \Rightarrow |\overrightarrow{BC}|^2 = 6$

$|\overrightarrow{CA}| = \sqrt{35} \Rightarrow |\overrightarrow{CA}|^2 = 35$

$|\overrightarrow{AB}|^2 = |\overrightarrow{BC}|^2 + |\overrightarrow{CA}|^2$

41 = 6 + 35 = 41

Hence, it is right angled triangle.

19. *Show that the points $A(-2\hat{i} + 3\hat{j} + 5\hat{k})$, $B(\hat{i} + 2\hat{j} + 3\hat{k})$ and $C(7\hat{i} - \hat{k})$ are collinear.*

SOLUTION. We know that $\overrightarrow{AB}$
= (position vector of B)
– (position vector of A)
$= (\hat{i} + 2\hat{j} + 3\hat{k}) - (-2\hat{i} + 3\hat{j} + 5\hat{k})$
$= (3\hat{i} - \hat{j} - 2\hat{k})$

and $\overrightarrow{BC}$
= (position vector of C)
– (position vector of B)
$= (7\hat{i} - \hat{k}) - (\hat{i} + 2\hat{j} + 3\hat{k})$
$= (6\hat{i} - 2\hat{j} - 4\hat{k})$

Since $\overrightarrow{AB} = 2\overrightarrow{BC}$, therefore $\overrightarrow{AB}$ and $\overrightarrow{AC}$ are parallel vectors. Thus A, B and C are collinear.

20. *What is the cosine of the angle which the vector $(\sqrt{2}\hat{i} + \hat{j} + \hat{k})$ makes with y-axis?*

SOLUTION. It is given that $\vec{a} = (\sqrt{2}\hat{i} + \hat{j} + \hat{k})$
and direction ratios are $\sqrt{2}, 1, 1$

$\therefore |\vec{a}| = \sqrt{(\sqrt{2})^2 + 1^2 + 1^2} = \sqrt{4} = 2$

Since direction cosines are $\frac{\sqrt{2}}{2}, \frac{1}{2}, \frac{1}{2}$.

Let us assume that $\vec{a}$ makes angle β with y-axis.

Hence, $\cos\beta = \frac{1}{2}$

21. *Find the value of p for which $p(\hat{i} + \hat{j} + \hat{k})$ is a unit vector.*

SOLUTION. It is given that $p(\hat{i} + \hat{j} + \hat{k})$ is a unit vector.

$\Rightarrow \quad |p(\hat{i} + \hat{j} + \hat{k})|^2 = 1$

$\Rightarrow \quad (p^2 + p^2 + p^2) = 1$

$\Rightarrow \quad 3p^2 = 1$

$\Rightarrow \quad p^2 = \frac{1}{3}$

$\Rightarrow \quad p = \pm\frac{1}{\sqrt{3}}$

22. *Find the position vector of the midpoint of the vector joining the points P(2, 3, 4) and Q(4, 1, –2).*

SOLUTION. Here, the position vectors of P and Q are $\vec{a} = (2\hat{i} + 3\hat{j} + 4\hat{k})$ and $\vec{b} = (4\hat{i} + \hat{j} - 2\hat{k})$ respectively.
Hence, position vector of the mid point of P and Q is,

$$\frac{(2\hat{i} + 3\hat{j} + 4\hat{k}) + (4\hat{i} + \hat{j} - 2\hat{k})}{2}$$

$$= \frac{6\hat{i} + 4\hat{j} + 2\hat{k}}{2}$$

$$= 3\hat{i} + 2\hat{j} + \hat{k}$$

23. *If $\vec{a} = 4\hat{i} - \hat{j} + \hat{k}$ and $\vec{b} = 2\hat{i} - 2\hat{j} + \hat{k}$, then find a unit vector parallel to the vector $(\vec{a} + \vec{b})$.*

SOLUTION. Given vectors are
$\vec{a} = 4\hat{i} - \hat{j} + \hat{k}, \vec{b} = 2\hat{i} - 2\hat{j} + \hat{k}$

Now, $\vec{a} + \vec{b} = (4\hat{i} - \hat{j} + \hat{k}) + (2\hat{i} - 2\hat{j} + \hat{k})$
$= 6\hat{i} - 3\hat{j} + 2\hat{k}$

$$|a+b| = \sqrt{6^2+(-3)^2+(2)^2}$$
$$= \sqrt{36+9+4} = \sqrt{49} = 7$$

∴ The unit vector parallel to the vector $(\vec{a}+\vec{b})$ is

$$\Rightarrow \frac{\vec{a}+\vec{b}}{|\vec{a}+\vec{b}|} = \frac{6\hat{i}-3\hat{j}+2\hat{k}}{7}$$

24. *Find the position vector of a point which divides the join of points with position vectors $\vec{a}-2\vec{b}$ and $2\vec{a}+\vec{b}$ externally in the ratio 2 : 1.*

SOLUTION. Let given position vectors are $\overrightarrow{OA} = \vec{a}-2\vec{b}$ and $\overrightarrow{OB} = 2\vec{a}+\vec{b}$.

Let $\overrightarrow{OC}$ be the position vector of a point C which divides the join of points, with position vectors $\overrightarrow{OA}$ and $\overrightarrow{OB}$ externally in the ratio 2 : 1.

$$\therefore \quad \overrightarrow{OC} = \frac{2\overrightarrow{OB}-1\overrightarrow{OA}}{2-1}$$
$$= \frac{2(2\vec{a}+\vec{b})-1(\vec{a}-2\vec{b})}{1}$$
$$= 4\vec{a}+2\vec{b}-\vec{a}+2\vec{b}$$
$$= 3\vec{a}+4\vec{b}$$

Exercise-24.1

1. If $\vec{a}$ and $\vec{b}$ are the position vectors of A and B respectively. Prove that the position vector of the mid point of AB is $\frac{\vec{a}+\vec{b}}{2}$.
2. Prove that the diagonals of a parallelogram bisects each other.
3. Prove that median of a triangle divides each other in the ratio of 2:1.
4. If $\vec{a} = 2\hat{i}-3\hat{j}+4\hat{k}$ and $\vec{b} = \hat{i}-2\hat{j}-\hat{k}$, prove that
   (i) $\vec{a}+\vec{b} = 3\hat{i}-\hat{j}+3\hat{k}$
   (ii) $\vec{a}-\vec{b} = \hat{i}-5\hat{j}+5\hat{k}$
5. If $\overrightarrow{OA} = 2\hat{i}+\hat{j}-3\hat{k}$ and $\overrightarrow{OB} = 5\hat{i}+3\hat{j}+\hat{k}$, prove that $\overrightarrow{AB} = 3\hat{i}+2\hat{j}+4\hat{k}$.
6. Prove that modulus of the vector $2\hat{i}-\hat{j}+5\hat{k}$ is $\sqrt{30}$.
7. If $\vec{a} = 2\hat{i}+\hat{j}-3\hat{k}, \vec{b} = -\hat{i}+\hat{j}+2\hat{k}, \vec{c} = 4\hat{i}+3\hat{k}$, prove that $\vec{a}-\vec{b} = 3\hat{i}-5\hat{k}$. Also, prove that its modulus is $\sqrt{54}$ and direction cosines are $\frac{3}{\sqrt{34}}, 0$ and $\frac{-5}{\sqrt{34}}$.
8. Prove that the line passing through the points $\hat{i}-\hat{j}+2\hat{k}$ and $2\hat{i}+\hat{k}$ is
   $$\vec{r} = (\hat{i}-\hat{j}+2\hat{k})+t(\hat{i}+\hat{j}-\hat{k})$$
9. Prove that the following vectors are coplanar.
   (i) $\vec{a}-2\vec{b}+3\vec{c}, 2\vec{a}+3\vec{b}-4\vec{c}, \vec{a}-3\vec{b}+5\vec{c}$
   (ii) $\vec{a}-2\vec{b}+3\vec{c}, -2\vec{a}+3\vec{b}-4\vec{c}, -\vec{b}+2\vec{c}$
   (iii) $\vec{a}-2\vec{b}+5\vec{c}, \vec{a}-2\vec{b}+2\vec{c}, \vec{a}-2\vec{b}+\vec{c}$
10. For what value of a, the vectors $2\hat{i}-3\hat{j}+4\hat{k}$ and $a\hat{i}+6\hat{j}-8\hat{k}$ are collinear?

Hint to the Selected Problems

5. $\overrightarrow{AB} = \overrightarrow{OB}-\overrightarrow{OA}$

7. $\vec{a}-\vec{b} = (2\hat{i}+\hat{j}-3\hat{k})-(-\hat{i}+\hat{j}+2\hat{k})$
$$= 3\hat{i}-5\hat{k}$$
$$|3\hat{i}-5\hat{k}| = \sqrt{34}$$
$$\text{d'cs} = \frac{3}{\sqrt{34}}, \frac{0}{\sqrt{34}}, \frac{-5}{\sqrt{34}}$$

10. For the given points to be collinear we have
$$1(2\hat{i}-3\hat{j}+4\hat{k})+\lambda(a\hat{i}+6\hat{j}-8\hat{k}) = 0$$
$$\Rightarrow (2+a\lambda)\hat{i}+(6\lambda-3)\hat{j}+(4-8\lambda)\hat{k} = (0\hat{i}+0\hat{j}+0\hat{k})$$
$$\Rightarrow 2+a\lambda = 0, 6\lambda-3 = 0, 4-8\lambda = 0$$
Now solve these equations.

ANSWERS

2. $a = -4$.

24.26 SCALAR PRODUCT OR DOT PRODUCT

Let $\vec{a}$ and $\vec{b}$ be two vectors represented by $\overrightarrow{OA}$ and $\overrightarrow{OB}$. Let θ be the angle between $\overrightarrow{OA}$ and $\overrightarrow{OB}$ and let $|\vec{a}| = a$ and $|\vec{b}| = b$.

Then scalar product of $\vec{a}$ and $\vec{b}$, denoted by $\vec{a}\cdot\vec{b}$ is defined by

$$\vec{a}\cdot\vec{b}=|\vec{a}|\cdot|\vec{b}|\cos\theta=ab\cos\theta,\quad 0\le\theta\le\pi$$

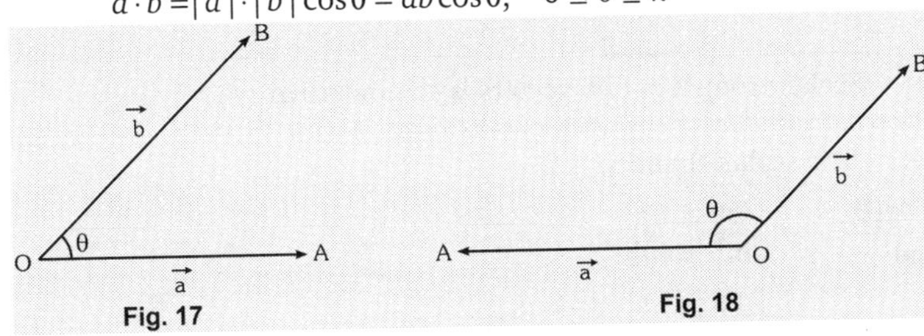

Fig. 17 Fig. 18

- Scalar product does not depend on the direction of θ because cos(− θ) = cos θ.
- Scalar product is also called dot product.
- If θ is acute then $\vec{a}\cdot\vec{b}>0$.
- If θ is obtuse then $\vec{a}\cdot\vec{b}<0$.

24.27 GEOMETRICAL MEANING OF SCALAR PRODUCT

Let $\overrightarrow{OA}=\vec{a},\overrightarrow{OB}=\vec{b}$ be two vectors. Then angle between them is θ.

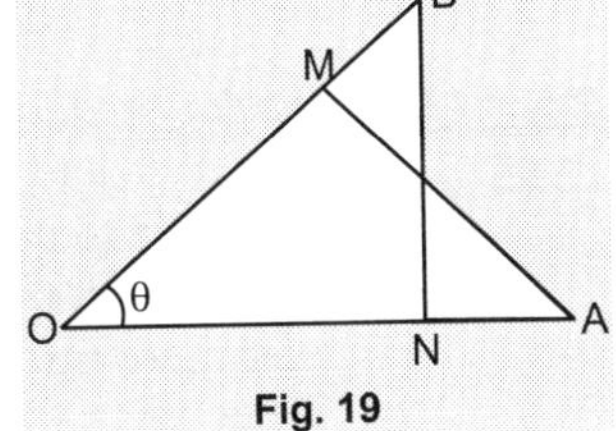

Fig. 19

Let $|\vec{a}|=OA=a$ and $|\vec{b}|=OB=b$,

Draw perpendicular AM from A to OB and BN from B to OA.

$$OM = OA\cos\theta = a\cos\theta$$
$$ON = OB\cos\theta = b\cos\theta$$

By definition, $\vec{a}\cdot\vec{b}=ab\cos\theta=a(b\cos\theta)$

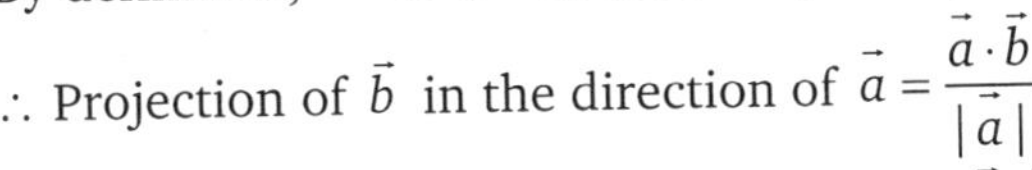

∴ Projection of $\vec{b}$ in the direction of $\vec{a}=\dfrac{\vec{a}\cdot\vec{b}}{|\vec{a}|}$

and projection of $\vec{a}$ in the direction of $\vec{b}=\dfrac{\vec{a}\cdot\vec{b}}{|\vec{b}|}$

24.28 ANGLE BETWEEN TWO VECTORS

We know that $\vec{a}\cdot\vec{b}=ab\cos\theta$

$$\Rightarrow\qquad \cos\theta=\frac{\vec{a}\cdot\vec{b}}{ab}=\frac{\vec{a}}{a}\cdot\frac{\vec{b}}{b}=\hat{a}\cdot\hat{b}$$

So $\theta=\cos^{-1}(\hat{a}\cdot\hat{b})$

24.29 SCALAR PRODUCT OF TWO PARALLEL VECTORS

If $\vec{a}$ and $\vec{b}$ are parallel, then θ = 0°

$$\therefore\qquad \vec{a}\cdot\vec{b}=ab\cos 0^\circ=ab$$

24.30 SCALAR PRODUCT OF TWO PERPENDICULAR VECTORS

If $\vec{a}$ and $\vec{b}$ are perpendicular ⇒ θ = 90°

$$\therefore\qquad \vec{a}\cdot\vec{b}=ab\cos 90^\circ=0$$

24.31 PROPERTIES OF SCALAR PRODUCT

PROPERTY 1. *Scalar product of two vectors is commutative.*

PROOF. Let $\vec{a}$ and $\vec{b}$ be two vector quantities such that $|\vec{a}|=a$ and $|\vec{b}|=b$.

Then by definition,

$$\vec{a} \cdot \vec{b} = ab\cos\theta$$
$$= ba \cos\theta \qquad (\because ab = ba)$$
$$= \vec{b} \cdot \vec{a}$$

$\Rightarrow$ Scalar product of two vectors is commutative.

PROPERTY 2. *The scalar product of two vectors is associative with respect to some scalar.*

PROOF. Let m be a scalar quantity.

Clearly $|m\vec{a}| = ma$

and $|m\vec{b}| = mb$

$\therefore$ $|m\vec{a}| = m|\vec{a}| = ma$

and $|m\vec{b}| = m|\vec{b}| = mb$

$$(m\vec{a}) \cdot \vec{b} = |m\vec{a}||\vec{b}|\cos\theta$$
$$= (ma)(b)\cos\theta$$
$$= m(ab)\cos\theta = m(\vec{a} \cdot \vec{b}) \qquad \text{...(i)}$$

Similarly $\vec{a} \cdot (m\vec{b}) = |\vec{a}||m\vec{b}|\cos\theta$

$$= (a)(mb)\cos\theta = a(bm)\cos\theta$$
$$= m(ab)\cos\theta = m(\vec{a} \cdot \vec{b}) \qquad \text{...(ii)}$$

From (i) and (ii), we have

$$(m\vec{a}) \cdot \vec{b} = \vec{a} \cdot (m\vec{b}) = m(\vec{a} \cdot \vec{b})$$

PROPERTY 3. *Scalar product is distributive over vector addition.*

PROOF. Let $\vec{a}, \vec{b}$ and $\vec{c}$ be three vector quantities.

We have to prove that

$$\vec{a} \cdot (\vec{b} + \vec{c}) = \vec{a} \cdot \vec{b} + \vec{a} \cdot \vec{c}$$

Let these three vectors $\vec{a}, \vec{b}$ and $\vec{c}$ be represented by $\overrightarrow{OP}, \overrightarrow{OQ}$ and $\overrightarrow{QR}$ respectively. Then by triangle law of addition, we have

In Δ OQR,

$$\overrightarrow{OQ} + \overrightarrow{QR} = \overrightarrow{OR}$$

$\Rightarrow$ $$\overrightarrow{OR} = \vec{b} + \vec{c}$$

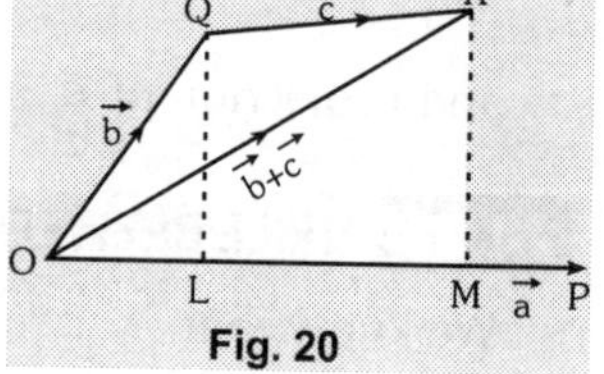

Fig. 20

Draw the perpendicular QL and RM from Q and R respectively.

Then OL, LM and OM are the projections of $\vec{b}$, $\vec{c}$ and $(\vec{b} + \vec{c})$ respectively in the direction of $\vec{a}$.

Now, $\vec{a} \cdot (\vec{b} + \vec{c})$ = projection of $(\vec{b} + \vec{c})$ in the direction of $\vec{a}$

$= a(OM) = a(OL + LM)$

$= a(OL) + a(LM)$

$= a$(projection of $\vec{b}$ in the direction of $\vec{a}$) + a(projection of $\vec{c}$ in the direction of $\vec{a}$)

$= \vec{a} \cdot \vec{b} + \vec{a} \cdot \vec{c}$

PROPERTY 4. *For any three vectors* $\vec{a}$, $\vec{b}$ *and* $\vec{c}$.

(i) $\vec{a} \cdot (-\vec{b}) = -(\vec{a} \cdot \vec{b})$ (ii) $\vec{a} \cdot (\vec{b} - \vec{c}) = \vec{a} \cdot \vec{b} - \vec{a} \cdot \vec{c}$

(iii) $(\vec{a} + \vec{b}) \cdot (\vec{c} + \vec{d}) = \vec{a} \cdot \vec{c} + \vec{a} \cdot \vec{d} + \vec{b} \cdot \vec{c} + \vec{b} \cdot \vec{d}$

(iv) $(\vec{a} + \vec{b})^2 = (\vec{a})^2 + (\vec{b})^2 + 2(\vec{a} \cdot \vec{b})$

(v) $(\vec{a} - \vec{b})^2 = (\vec{a})^2 + (\vec{b})^2 - 2(\vec{a} \cdot \vec{b})$ (vi) $(\vec{a} + \vec{b})(\vec{a} - \vec{b}) = (\vec{a})^2 - (\vec{b})^2$

PROOF. (i) Let $\overrightarrow{OA} = \vec{a}$ and $\overrightarrow{OB} = \vec{b}$ and angle between $\vec{a}$ and $\vec{b}$ is θ.

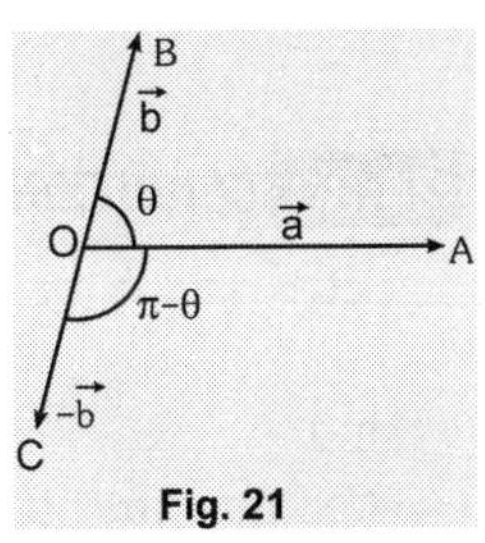

Fig. 21

$$OC = OB$$

Then $$\overrightarrow{OC} = -\overrightarrow{OB} = -\vec{b}$$

$\angle AOC$ = angle between $\vec{a}$ and $-\vec{b}$ = π – θ

$$\therefore \quad \vec{a}\cdot(-\vec{b}) = \overrightarrow{OA}\cdot\overrightarrow{OC} = |\overrightarrow{OA}|\,|\overrightarrow{OC}|\cos(\pi-\theta)$$
$$= OA\cdot OC\cdot(-\cos\theta)$$
$$= -OA\cdot OB\cos\theta = -(\vec{a}\cdot\vec{b})$$

(ii) $$\vec{a}\cdot(\vec{b}-\vec{c}) = \vec{a}\cdot[\vec{b}+(-\vec{c})]$$
$$= \vec{a}\cdot\vec{b}+\vec{a}\cdot(-\vec{c}) \quad \text{(By prop. 3)}$$
$$= \vec{a}\cdot\vec{b}+[-(\vec{a}\cdot\vec{c})] = \vec{a}\cdot\vec{b}-\vec{a}\cdot\vec{c}$$

(iii) Let $$\vec{a}+\vec{b} = \vec{p}$$

Then, $$\text{LHS} = \vec{p}\cdot(\vec{c}+\vec{d}) = \vec{p}\cdot\vec{c}+\vec{p}\cdot\vec{d} = \vec{c}\cdot\vec{p}+\vec{d}\cdot\vec{p}$$
$$= \vec{c}\cdot(\vec{a}+\vec{b})+\vec{d}\cdot(\vec{a}+\vec{b}) = \vec{c}\cdot\vec{a}+\vec{c}\cdot\vec{b}+\vec{d}\cdot\vec{a}+\vec{d}\cdot\vec{b}$$
$$= \vec{a}\cdot\vec{c}+\vec{b}\cdot\vec{c}+\vec{a}\cdot\vec{d}+\vec{b}\cdot\vec{d} = \text{RHS}$$

(iv) $$(\vec{a}+\vec{b})^2 = (\vec{a}+\vec{b})\cdot(\vec{a}+\vec{b}) = \vec{a}\cdot\vec{a}+\vec{a}\cdot\vec{b}+\vec{b}\cdot\vec{a}+\vec{b}\cdot\vec{b}$$
$$= (\vec{a})^2+2(\vec{a}\cdot\vec{b})+(\vec{b})^2$$

(v) $$(\vec{a}-\vec{b})^2 = (\vec{a}-\vec{b})\cdot(\vec{a}-\vec{b}) = \vec{a}\cdot\vec{a}-\vec{a}\cdot\vec{b}-\vec{b}\cdot\vec{a}+\vec{b}\cdot\vec{b}$$
$$= (\vec{a})^2-2(\vec{a}\cdot\vec{b})+(\vec{b})^2$$

(vi) $$(\vec{a}+\vec{b})\cdot(\vec{a}-\vec{b}) = \vec{a}\cdot\vec{a}+\vec{a}\cdot(-\vec{b})+\vec{b}\cdot\vec{a}+\vec{b}\cdot(-\vec{b})$$
$$= \vec{a}\cdot\vec{a}-\vec{a}\cdot\vec{b}+\vec{b}\cdot\vec{a}-\vec{b}\cdot\vec{b} = (\vec{a})^2-(\vec{b})^2$$

24.32 IMPORTANT RESULTS OF DOT PRODUCT

1. *Magnitude of the scalar product of two parallel like vectors is equal to product of their magnitude.*

Proof. Let $\vec{a}$ and $\vec{b}$ be two vectors and $|\vec{a}| = a$ and $|\vec{b}| = b$.

$\vec{a}$ and $\vec{b}$ are like and parallel vectors, so angle between $\vec{a}$ and $\vec{b}$ is θ.

Then $$\vec{a}\cdot\vec{b} = ab\cos\theta$$
$$\Rightarrow \quad \vec{a}\cdot\vec{b} = ab\cos\theta = ab\cos 0° = ab\cdot 1 = ab$$
$$\Rightarrow \quad \vec{a}\cdot\vec{b} = ab$$

2. *The scalar product of two parallel vectors of opposite direction is negative to the product of their magnitude.*

Proof. *Let $\vec{a}$ and $\vec{b}$ be two parallel vectors of opposite direction, then angle between $\vec{a}$ and $\vec{b}$ is θ = 180°.*

$$\therefore \quad \vec{a}\cdot\vec{b} = ab\cos\theta = ab\cos 180° = ab(-1) = -ab$$

3. *The scalar product of two mutually perpendicular vectors is zero.*

Proof. Let $\vec{a}$ and $\vec{b}$ be two perpendicular vectors then angle between $\vec{a}$ and $\vec{b}$ is θ = 90°.

$$\therefore \quad \vec{a}\cdot\vec{b} = ab\cos\theta = ab\cos 90° = ab\cdot 0 = 0$$

4. *The square of any vector is equal to the square of its magnitude.*

Proof. Let $\vec{a}$ and $\vec{b}$ be two equal vectors.

$$\Rightarrow \quad \vec{a} = \vec{b}$$

⇒ $\vec{a}$ and $\vec{b}$ are like and parallel vectors.

∴ The angle between $\vec{a}$ and $\vec{b}$ is θ = 0°

$\Rightarrow$ $\quad \vec{a}\cdot\vec{b} = \vec{a}\cdot\vec{a} = a\cdot a\cos\theta = a\cdot a\cos 0° = a\cdot a = a^2 = |\vec{a}|^2 \ (\because a = |\vec{a}|)$

$\Rightarrow$ $\quad \vec{a}\cdot\vec{a} = |\vec{a}|^2$

24.33 CONDITION OF TWO VECTORS BEING PARALLEL

Let $\vec{a}$ and $\vec{b}$ be two vectors such that

$$\vec{a} = a_1\hat{i} + a_2\hat{j} + a_3\hat{k}$$

and

$$\vec{b} = b_1\hat{i} + b_2\hat{j} + b_3\hat{k}$$

We know that $\vec{a}$ and $\vec{b}$ are parallel $\Leftrightarrow \vec{a} = t\vec{b}$, where t is a scalar

$\Rightarrow$ $\quad a_1\hat{i} + a_2\hat{j} + a_3\hat{k} = t(b_1\hat{i} + b_2\hat{j} + b_3\hat{k})$

Comparing the coefficients of $\hat{i}$, $\hat{j}$ and $\hat{k}$ on both sides, we get

$$a_1 = tb_1,\ a_2 = tb_2,\ a_3 = tb_3$$

$\Rightarrow$ $$\boldsymbol{\frac{a_1}{b_1} = \frac{a_2}{b_2} = \frac{a_3}{b_3}}$$

which is the required condition of parallelism.

24.34 CONDITION OF TWO VECTORS BEING PERPENDICULAR

Let $\vec{a}$ and $\vec{b}$ be two vectors such that $\vec{a} = a_1\hat{i} + a_2\hat{j} + a_3\hat{k}$ and $\vec{b} = b_1\hat{i} + b_2\hat{j} + b_3\hat{k}$

Then, $\quad \vec{a}\cdot\vec{b} = a_1b_1 + a_2b_2 + a_3b_3$

Vectors $\vec{a}$ and $\vec{b}$ will be perpendicular if and only if $\vec{a}\cdot\vec{b} = 0$

$\Leftrightarrow$ $\quad \boldsymbol{a_1b_1 + a_2b_2 + a_3b_3 = 0}$

24.35 SCALAR PRODUCT OF UNIT VECTORS $\hat{i}, \hat{j}, \hat{k}$

Let *OX*, *OY* and *OZ* be three rectangular co-ordinate axes and their corresponding unit vectors are $\hat{i}$, $\hat{j}$ and $\hat{k}$.

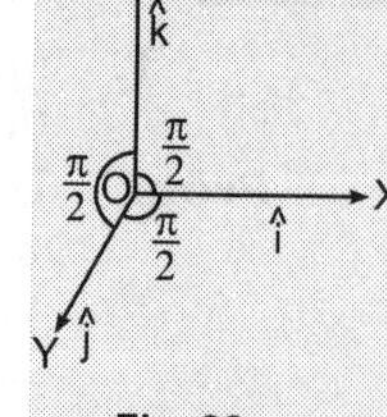

Fig. 22

Clearly $\quad |\hat{i}| = |\hat{j}| = |\hat{k}| = 1$

We know that angle between two unit vectors is $\frac{\pi}{2}$.

$\therefore$ $\quad \hat{i}\cdot\hat{j} = |\hat{i}|\cdot|\hat{j}|\cdot\cos\frac{\pi}{2} = 1\cdot 1\cdot 0 = 0$

Similarly $\quad \hat{j}\cdot\hat{k} = 0$ and $\hat{k}\cdot\hat{i} = 0$

Now $\quad \hat{i}\cdot\hat{i} = \hat{i}^2 = |\hat{i}|^2 = (1)^2 = 1$

Similarly $\quad \hat{j}\cdot\hat{j} = 1, \hat{k}\cdot\hat{k} = 1$

24.36 SOME IMPORTANT RESULTS

(1) Let $\quad \vec{a} = a_1\hat{i} + a_2\hat{j} + a_3\hat{k}$ and $\vec{b} = b_1\hat{i} + b_2\hat{j} + b_3\hat{k}$

Then
$$\vec{a}\cdot\vec{b} = (a_1\hat{i} + a_2\hat{j} + a_3\hat{k})\cdot(b_1\hat{i} + b_2\hat{j} + b_3\hat{k})$$
$$= a_1b_1\hat{i}\cdot\hat{i} + a_1b_2\hat{i}\cdot\hat{j} + a_1b_3\hat{i}\cdot\hat{k} + a_2b_1\hat{j}\cdot\hat{i} + a_2b_2\hat{j}\cdot\hat{j} + a_2b_3\hat{j}\cdot\hat{k}$$
$$+ a_3b_1\hat{k}\cdot\hat{i} + a_3b_2\hat{k}\cdot\hat{j} + a_3b_3\hat{k}\cdot\hat{k} \quad \text{...(i)}$$

We know that

$$\left.\begin{aligned} \hat{i}\cdot\hat{i} = \hat{j}\cdot\hat{j} = \hat{k}\cdot\hat{k} = 1 \\ \text{and} \quad \hat{i}\cdot\hat{j} = \hat{j}\cdot\hat{k} = \hat{k}\cdot\hat{i} = 0 \end{aligned}\right\} \quad \text{...(ii)}$$

Using (ii) in (i), we get

$$\vec{a}\cdot\vec{b} = a_1b_1(1) + a_1b_2(0) + a_1b_3(0) + a_2b_1(0) + a_2b_2(1) + a_2b_3(0) + a_3b_1(0) + a_3b_2(0) + a_3b_3(1)$$

$$= a_1b_1 + a_2b_2 + a_3b_3$$

$$\Rightarrow \quad \vec{a}\cdot\vec{b} = a_1b_1 + a_2b_2 + a_3b_3$$

which is the scalar products of the vectors $\vec{a}$ and $\vec{b}$ in terms rectangular components.

(2) From above result (1)

$$\vec{a}\cdot\vec{b} = a_1b_1 + a_2b_2 + a_3b_3 \quad \text{...(i)}$$

We know that

$$|\vec{a}| = \sqrt{a_1^2 + a_2^2 + a_3^2}$$

and

$$|\vec{b}| = \sqrt{b_1^2 + b_2^2 + b_2^3} \quad \text{...(ii)}$$

Now $\vec{a}\cdot\vec{b} = |\vec{a}|\cdot|\vec{b}|\cos\theta,$

$$\Rightarrow \quad \cos\theta = \frac{\vec{a}\cdot\vec{b}}{|\vec{a}|\cdot|\vec{b}|}$$

$$= \frac{a_1b_1 + a_2b_2 + a_3b_3}{\sqrt{a_1^2 + a_2^2 + a_3^2}\cdot\sqrt{b_1^2 + b_2^2 + b_3^2}} \quad \text{[From eqn. (i) and (ii)]}$$

$$\Rightarrow \quad \theta = \cos^{-1}\left[\frac{a_1b_1 + a_2b_2 + a_3b_3}{\sqrt{a_1^2 + a_2^2 + a_3^2}\cdot\sqrt{b_1^2 + b_2^2 + b_3^2}}\right]$$

which is the required angle between $\vec{a}$ and $\vec{b}$.

Solved Examples

1. *Prove that vectors in the following pairs are perpendicular to each other.*
$\hat{i} + 4\hat{j} + 3\hat{k}$ and $4\hat{i} + 2\hat{j} - 4\hat{k}$

SOLUTION. Scalar product of vectors

$= (\hat{i} + 4\hat{j} + 3\hat{k})\cdot(4\hat{i} + 2\hat{j} - 4\hat{k})$

$= 4(\hat{i}\cdot\hat{i}) + 8(\hat{j}\cdot\hat{j}) - 12(\hat{k}\cdot\hat{k})$

$= 4(1) + 8(1) - 12(1) = 0$

$(\hat{i}\cdot\hat{j} = 0, \hat{j}\cdot\hat{k} = 0, \hat{k}\cdot\hat{i} = 0)$

$\Rightarrow$ Both vectors are perpendicular.

2. *If $\vec{a} = \hat{i} + 2\hat{j} + 3\hat{k}, \vec{b} = 2\hat{i} - 3\hat{j} + \hat{k}$, find the value of $\vec{a}\cdot\vec{b}$.*

SOLUTION. We have

$\vec{a}\cdot\vec{b} = (\hat{i} + 2\hat{j} + 3\hat{k})\cdot(2\hat{i} - 3\hat{j} + \hat{k})$

$= 2(\hat{i}\cdot\hat{i}) - 6(\hat{j}\cdot\hat{j}) + 3(\hat{k}\cdot\hat{k})$

$= 2(1) - 6(1) + 3(1)$

$= 2 - 6 + 3 = -1$

3. *If $\vec{a} = 2\hat{i} - 6\hat{j} - 3\hat{k}, \vec{b} = 4\hat{i} + 3\hat{j} - \hat{k}$, find the value of $\vec{a}\cdot\vec{b}$.*

SOLUTION. We have

$\vec{a}\cdot\vec{b} = (2\hat{i} - 6\hat{j} - 3\hat{k})\cdot(4\hat{i} + 3\hat{j} - \hat{k})$

$= 8(\hat{i}\cdot\hat{i}) - 18(\hat{j}\cdot\hat{j}) + 3(\hat{k}\cdot\hat{k})$

$= 8(1) - 18(1) + 3(1)$

$= 8 - 18 + 3 = -7$

4. *Find the cosine of the angle between the vectors $2\hat{i} + 2\hat{j} - \hat{k}$ and $6\hat{i} - 3\hat{j} + 2\hat{k}$.*

SOLUTION. Let $\vec{a} = 2\hat{i} + 2\hat{j} - \hat{k}$ and $\vec{b} = 6\hat{i} - 3\hat{j} + 2\hat{k}$

$\vec{a}\cdot\vec{b} = (2\hat{i} + 2\hat{j} - \hat{k})\cdot(6\hat{i} - 3\hat{j} + 2\hat{k})$

$= 2\cdot6 + 2\cdot(-3) + (-1)\cdot2$

$= 12 - 6 - 2 = 4$

$|\vec{a}| = \sqrt{[(2)^2 + (2)^2 + (-1)^2]}$

$= \sqrt{4 + 4 + 1} = \sqrt{9} = 3$

$|\vec{b}| = \sqrt{[(6)^2 + (-3)^2 + (2)^2]}$

$= \sqrt{36 + 9 + 4} = \sqrt{49} = 7$

$\cos\theta = \frac{\vec{a}\cdot\vec{b}}{|\vec{a}|\cdot|\vec{b}|} = \frac{4}{3\cdot7} = \frac{4}{21}$

5. *Find the scalar product of the following vectors $4\hat{i}-4\hat{j}-\hat{k}$ and $\hat{i}+2\hat{j}+3\hat{k}$.*

SOLUTION. Let $\vec{a}=4\hat{i}-4\hat{j}-\hat{k}$ and $\vec{b}=\hat{i}+2\hat{j}+3\hat{k}$

Then, $\vec{a}\cdot\vec{b}=(4\hat{i}-4\hat{j}-\hat{k})\cdot(\hat{i}+2\hat{j}+3\hat{k})$

$$= 4(\hat{i}\cdot\hat{i})-8(\hat{j}\cdot\hat{j})-3(\hat{k}\cdot\hat{k})$$
$$= 4(1)-8(1)-3(1)$$
$$= 4-8-3=-7$$

6. *Find the angle between the vectors $2\hat{i}$ and $3\hat{i}-4\hat{j}$.*

SOLUTION. Let $\vec{a}=2\hat{i}$ and $\vec{b}=3\hat{i}-4\hat{j}$

Then, $\vec{a}\cdot\vec{b}=(2\hat{i})\cdot(3\hat{i}-4\hat{j})$

$$= 6(\hat{i}\cdot\hat{i})+0(\hat{j}\cdot\hat{j})+0(\hat{k}\cdot\hat{k})$$
$$= 6\cdot1+0\cdot1+0\cdot1=6$$

$$|\vec{a}|=|2\hat{i}|=\sqrt{[(2)^2+(0)^2+(0)^2]}$$
$$= \sqrt{4}=2$$

and $|\vec{b}|=|3\hat{i}-4\hat{j}|$

$$= \sqrt{[(3)^2+(-4)^2+(0)^2]}$$
$$= \sqrt{25}=5$$

Now, $\cos\theta=\dfrac{\vec{a}\cdot\vec{b}}{|\vec{a}|\cdot|\vec{b}|}=\dfrac{6}{2\times5}=\dfrac{6}{10}=\dfrac{3}{5}$

$\Rightarrow\ \theta=\cos^{-1}\left(\dfrac{3}{5}\right)$

7. *If $\vec{a}=2\hat{i}+\hat{j}+3\hat{k}$ and $\vec{b}=3\hat{i}-2\hat{j}+\hat{k}$ two vectors. Show that angle between them is 60°.*

SOLUTION. We have

$$\vec{a}\cdot\vec{b}=(2\hat{i}+\hat{j}+3\hat{k})\cdot(3\hat{i}-2\hat{j}+\hat{k})$$
$$= 6(\hat{i}\cdot\hat{i})-2(\hat{j}\cdot\hat{j})+3(\hat{k}\cdot\hat{k})$$
$$= 6-2+3=7$$

$$|\vec{a}|=|2\hat{i}+\hat{j}+3\hat{k}|$$
$$= \sqrt{[(2)^2+(1)^2+(3)^2]}=\sqrt{14}$$

and $|\vec{b}|=|3\hat{i}-2\hat{j}+\hat{k}|$

$$= \sqrt{[(3)^2+(-2)^2+(1)^2]}=\sqrt{14}$$

Now, $\cos\theta=\dfrac{\vec{a}\cdot\vec{b}}{|\vec{a}|\cdot|\vec{b}|}=\dfrac{7}{\sqrt{14}\times\sqrt{14}}$

$$= \frac{7}{14}=\frac{1}{2}$$

$\Rightarrow\ \theta=\cos^{-1}\left(\dfrac{1}{2}\right)\Rightarrow\ \theta=60°$

8. *Find the magnitude and angle between the vectors $3\hat{i}-2\hat{j}+\hat{k}$ and $2\hat{i}+3\hat{j}$.*

SOLUTION. Let $\vec{a}=3\hat{i}-2\hat{j}+\hat{k}$ and $\vec{b}=2\hat{i}+3\hat{j}$

Now, $|\vec{a}|=|3\hat{i}-2\hat{j}+\hat{k}|$

$$= \sqrt{[(3)^2+(-2)^2+(1)^2]}$$
$$= \sqrt{14}$$

and $|\vec{b}|=|2\hat{i}+3\hat{j}+0\hat{k}|$

$$= \sqrt{(2)^2+(3)^2}=\sqrt{13}$$

Also $\vec{a}\cdot\vec{b}=(3\hat{i}-2\hat{j}+\hat{k})\cdot(2\hat{i}+3\hat{j}+0\hat{k})$

$$= 6(\hat{i}\cdot\hat{i})-6(\hat{j}\cdot\hat{j})+0(\hat{k}\cdot\hat{k})$$
$$= 6-6+0=0$$

$\Rightarrow$ Both vectors are perpendicular to each other.

$\therefore\ \theta=90°$

9. *Find the angle between $2\hat{i}+2\hat{j}-\hat{k}$ and XY plane.*

SOLUTION. Let $\vec{a}=2\hat{i}+2\hat{j}-\hat{k}$ and $\vec{b}=\hat{k}$.

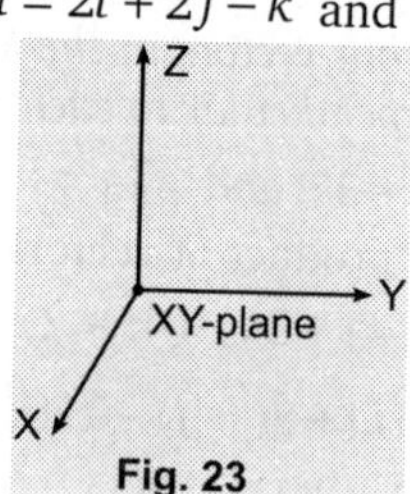

Fig. 23

Now, $|\vec{a}|=|2\hat{i}+2\hat{j}-\hat{k}|$

$$= \sqrt{[(2)^2+(2)^2+(-1)^2]}$$
$$= \sqrt{4+4+1}=\sqrt{9}=3$$

and $|\vec{b}|=|\hat{k}|=\sqrt{(1)^2}=1$

$$\vec{a}\cdot\vec{b}=(2\hat{i}+2\hat{j}-\hat{k})\cdot(\hat{k})$$
$$= 0+0-1(\hat{k}\cdot\hat{k})=0-1=-1$$

Now $\cos\theta=\dfrac{\vec{a}\cdot\vec{b}}{|\vec{a}|\cdot|\vec{b}|}=\dfrac{-1}{3\times1}=-\dfrac{1}{3}$

$\Rightarrow \theta = \cos^{-1}\left(-\frac{1}{3}\right)$

$\therefore$ The angle between $\vec{a}$ and XY-plane

$= 90° - \theta$

$= 90° - \cos^{-1}\left(-\frac{1}{3}\right)$

10. *Find the projection of the vector $\vec{A} = 4\hat{i} + 4\hat{j} - 10\hat{k}$ in the direction of $\vec{B} = \hat{i} - 2\hat{j} + 2\hat{k}$.*

SOLUTION. Projection of vector $\vec{A}$ in the direction of $\vec{B} = \frac{\vec{A}\cdot\vec{B}}{|\vec{B}|}$

$\vec{A}\cdot\vec{B} = (4\hat{i} + 4\hat{j} - 10\hat{k})\cdot(\hat{i} - 2\hat{j} + 2\hat{k})$

$= 4(\hat{i}\cdot\hat{i}) - 8(\hat{j}\cdot\hat{j}) - 20(\hat{k}\cdot\hat{k})$

$= 4 - 8 - 20 = -24$

$|\vec{B}| = \sqrt{\{(1)^2 + (-2)^2 + (2)^2\}} = \sqrt{9} = 3$

Hence, required projection

$= \frac{-24}{3} = -8 = 8$

11. *If $\vec{a} = 2\hat{i} - 3\hat{j} + 4\hat{k}$ and $\vec{b} = 2\hat{j} + 4\hat{k}$ then find the resolved part of $\vec{a}$ in the direction of $\vec{b}$.*

SOLUTION. $\vec{a}\cdot\vec{b} = 0 - 6(\hat{j}\cdot\hat{j}) + 16(\hat{k}\cdot\hat{k})$

$= -6\cdot1 + 16\cdot1 = 10$

$|\vec{b}| = \sqrt{(2)^2 + (4)^2}$

$= \sqrt{4 + 16} = \sqrt{20} = 2\sqrt{5}$

Projection of $\vec{a}$ in the direction of $\vec{b}$

$= \frac{\vec{a}\cdot\vec{b}}{|\vec{b}|} = \frac{10}{2\sqrt{5}} = \sqrt{5}$

$\therefore$ Resolved part

$= \sqrt{5}\left(\frac{\vec{b}}{|\vec{b}|}\right) = \sqrt{5}\left(\frac{2\hat{j} + 4\hat{k}}{2\sqrt{5}}\right)$

$= \hat{j} + 2\hat{k}$

Exercise-24.2

1. Find the scalar product of the following vectors:
   (i) $3\hat{i} + 8\hat{j} - 2\hat{k}$ and $5\hat{i} + \hat{j} + 2\hat{k}$
   (ii) $3\hat{i} + 4\hat{j}$ and $5\hat{j} - 10\hat{k}$
   (iii) $\hat{i} + \hat{j} - \hat{k}$ and $\hat{i} - \hat{j} + \hat{k}$ (NCERT)
2. Prove that the following vectors are perpendicular to each other :
   (i) $4\hat{i} + \hat{j} + 3\hat{k}$ and $2\hat{i} + 4\hat{j} - 4\hat{k}$
   (ii) $2\hat{i} - \hat{j} + \hat{k}$ and $-\hat{i} + 3\hat{j} + 5\hat{k}$
   (iii) $\hat{i} + 4\hat{j} + 3\hat{k}$ and $4\hat{i} + 2\hat{j} - 4\hat{k}$
   (iv) $4\hat{i} - \hat{j} + \hat{k}$ and $-\hat{i} + 3\hat{j} + 7\hat{k}$
3. Find the cosine of the angle between the vectors.
   (i) $\hat{i} + 2\hat{j} - \hat{k}$ and $-\hat{i} + \hat{j} - 2\hat{k}$
   (ii) $2\hat{i} + \hat{j} - 2\hat{k}$ and $3\hat{i} - 4\hat{j}$
4. If $\vec{a} = \hat{i} + 4\hat{j} + 3\hat{k}, \vec{b} = 4\hat{i} + 2\hat{j} + \lambda\hat{k}$, for what value of λ, $\vec{a}$ and $\vec{b}$ are perpendicular to each other?
5. If $\vec{a} = 15\hat{i} - \lambda\hat{j} + 30\hat{k}$ and $\vec{b} = 16\hat{i} + 12\hat{j} - 2\hat{k}$, for what value of λ, $\vec{a}$ and $\vec{b}$ are perpendicular to each other?
6. For what value of x, the vectors $x\hat{i} - 2x\hat{j} + 3\hat{k}$ and $-\hat{i} + \hat{j} + \hat{k}$ are mutually perpendicular?
7. Prove that the vectors $2\hat{i} - \hat{j} + \hat{k}, \hat{i} - 3\hat{j} - 5\hat{k}$, $3\hat{i} - 4\hat{j} - 4\hat{k}$ are the sides of a right angled triangle.
8. If $|\vec{a} + \vec{b}| = |\vec{a}|$, prove that vector $2\vec{a} + \vec{b}$ is perpendicular to $\vec{b}$.
9. The scalar product of the vector $\vec{r}$ with $3\hat{i} - 5\hat{k}, 2\hat{i} + 7\hat{j}, \hat{i} + \hat{j} + \hat{k}$ given by -1, 6 and 5 respectively. Find the value of $\vec{r}$.
10. Prove that the triangle whose vertices are $\hat{i} + 2\hat{j} + 3\hat{k}, 2\hat{i} + 3\hat{j} + \hat{k}, 3\hat{i} + \hat{j} + 2\hat{k}$ is an equilateral triangle.

Hint to Selected Problems

3. (i) use $\cos\theta = \frac{\vec{a}\cdot\vec{b}}{|\vec{a}|\cdot|\vec{b}|}$

4. $\vec{a}\cdot\vec{b} = 0$

$\Rightarrow (\hat{i} + 4\hat{j} + 3\hat{k})\cdot(4\hat{i} + 2\hat{j} + \lambda\hat{k}) = 0$

$\Rightarrow \quad 4 + 8 + 3\lambda = 0$

$\Rightarrow \quad \lambda = -4$

6. For perpendicularity show that $\vec{a}\cdot\vec{b} = 0$

8. $|\vec{a}+\vec{b}| = |\vec{a}|$

$\Rightarrow (\vec{a}+\vec{b})\cdot(\vec{a}+\vec{b}) = \vec{a}\cdot\vec{a}$

$\Rightarrow a^2 + b^2 + 2\vec{a}\cdot\vec{b} = a^2$

$\Rightarrow \quad b^2 + 2\vec{a}\cdot\vec{b} = 0$

For perpendicularity of $(2\vec{a}+\vec{b})$ and $\vec{b}$

$(2\vec{a}+\vec{b})\cdot\vec{b} = 2\vec{a}\cdot\vec{b} + b^2 = 0$

ANSWERS

1. (i) 19 (ii) 20 (iii) –1 **3.** (i) $\frac{1}{2}$ (ii) $\frac{2}{15}$ **4.** – 4 **5.** 15 **6.** 1
9. $3\hat{i} + 2\hat{k}$

24.37 APPLICATION OF SCALAR PRODUCT

We know that if a force F displaced a body to a distance d.
then work done by the force $\vec{F}\cdot\vec{d} = Fd\cos\theta$

$\Rightarrow$ The work done by the force is the scalar product of the force and displacement.

Solved Examples

1. *Prove that in an isosceles triangle, the median of the base is perpendicular to it.*

SOLUTION. **Given:** In an isosceles triangle ABC where $AB = AC$ and D be the mid point of base BC.

To prove: $AD \perp BC$

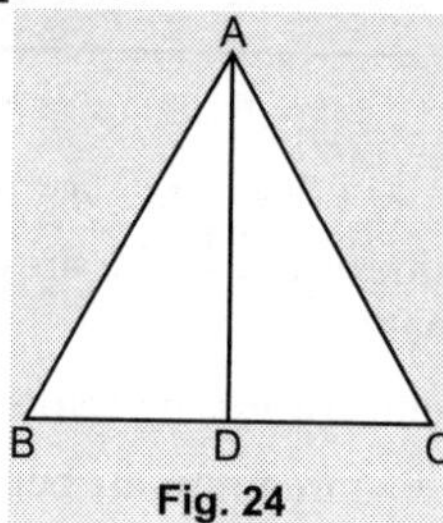

Fig. 24

Let $|\vec{b}| = AB$ and $|\vec{c}| = AC$

$\therefore \quad \overrightarrow{AD} = \frac{\vec{b}+\vec{c}}{2}$

and $\overrightarrow{BC} = \overrightarrow{BA} + \overrightarrow{AC} = \overrightarrow{AC} - \overrightarrow{AB} = \vec{c} - \vec{b}$

Now $\overrightarrow{AD}\cdot\overrightarrow{BC} = \frac{1}{2}(\vec{b}+\vec{c})\cdot(\vec{c}-\vec{b})$

$= \frac{1}{2}(\vec{c}+\vec{b})(\vec{c}-\vec{b})$

$= \frac{1}{2}[(\vec{c})^2 - (\vec{b})^2]$

$= \frac{1}{2}[(\overrightarrow{AC})^2 - (\overrightarrow{AB})^2]$

$= \frac{1}{2}[(\overrightarrow{AB})^2 - (\overrightarrow{AB})^2]$

$(\overrightarrow{AB} = \overrightarrow{AC})$

$\Rightarrow \overrightarrow{AD}$ and $\overrightarrow{BC}$ are perpendicular to each other.

2. *Prove that the parallelogram with equal diagonal is a rectangle.*

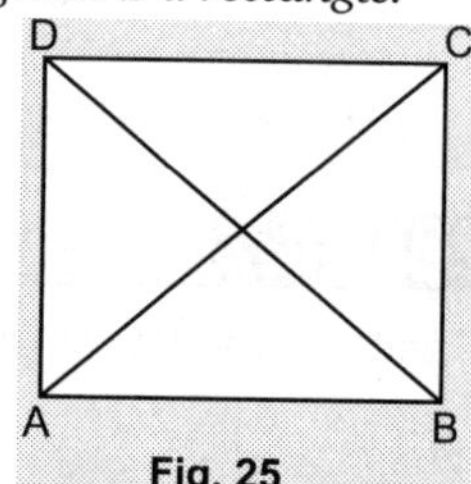

Fig. 25

SOLUTION. Let $ABCD$ be a parallelogram

and $\overrightarrow{AB} = \vec{b}, \overrightarrow{AD} = \vec{d}$

$\therefore \quad |\vec{b}| = AB$

and $\quad |\vec{d}| = AD$

$\therefore \quad \overrightarrow{AC} = \overrightarrow{AB} + \overrightarrow{BC} = \vec{b} + \vec{d}$

and $\quad \overrightarrow{BD} = \overrightarrow{BC} + \overrightarrow{CD} = \overrightarrow{BC} - \overrightarrow{DC}$

$= \vec{d} - \vec{b}$

diagonal AC = diagonal BD

$\Rightarrow \quad \overrightarrow{AC} = \overrightarrow{BD}$

$\Rightarrow \quad (\overrightarrow{AC})^2 = (\overrightarrow{BD})^2$

$\Rightarrow \quad (\vec{b}+\vec{d})^2 = (\vec{d}-\vec{b})^2$

$\Rightarrow \quad (\vec{b})^2 + 2(\vec{b}\cdot\vec{d}) + (\vec{d})^2$

$= (\vec{d})^2 - 2(\vec{d}\cdot\vec{b}) + (\vec{b})^2$

$\Rightarrow \quad 2(\vec{b}\cdot\vec{d}) = -2(\vec{d}\cdot\vec{b})$

$\Rightarrow \quad 2(\vec{b}\cdot\vec{d}) = -2(\vec{b}\cdot\vec{d})$

$\Rightarrow \quad 4(\vec{b}\cdot\vec{d}) = 0$

$\Rightarrow \quad (\vec{b}\cdot\vec{d}) = 0$

$\Rightarrow \quad \overrightarrow{AB} \cdot \overrightarrow{AD} = 0$

AB and AD are perpendicular to each other.

Hence parallelogram ABCD is a rectangle.

3. *Prove that the mid point of the hypotenuse of a right angled triangle is equidistant from its vertices.*

SOLUTION. Let in ΔABC, D be the mid point of BC

$$BD = DC \text{ or } \overrightarrow{BD} = \overrightarrow{DC}$$

Now $\quad \overrightarrow{AB} = \overrightarrow{AD} + \overrightarrow{DB}$

and $\quad \overrightarrow{AC} = \overrightarrow{AD} + \overrightarrow{DC} = \overrightarrow{AD} + \overrightarrow{BD}$

$\quad = \overrightarrow{AD} - \overrightarrow{DB}$

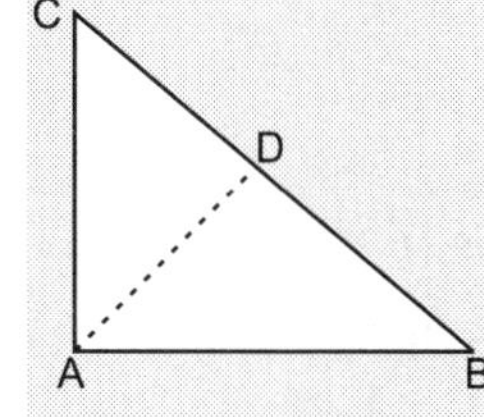

Fig. 26

But sides AB and AC are mutually perpendicular.

$$\overrightarrow{AB} \cdot \overrightarrow{AC} = 0$$

$\Rightarrow (\overrightarrow{AD} + \overrightarrow{DB}) \cdot (\overrightarrow{AD} - \overrightarrow{DB}) = 0$

$\Rightarrow \quad (\overrightarrow{AD})^2 - (\overrightarrow{DB})^2 = 0$

$\Rightarrow \quad AD^2 - DB^2 = 0$

$\Rightarrow \quad AD^2 = DB^2$

$\Rightarrow \quad AD = DB$

$\Rightarrow \quad DA = DB$

But $\quad DB = DC$

$\therefore \quad DA = DB = DC$

4. *A particle $\vec{D} = 2\hat{i} + \hat{j} - \hat{k}$ is displaced by the force $\vec{F} = 3\hat{i} + \hat{j} + 6\hat{k}$, find the work done.*

SOLUTION. We know that

work = force · displacement

$= (3\hat{i} + \hat{j} + 6\hat{k}) \cdot (2\hat{i} + \hat{j} - \hat{k})$

$= 6(\hat{i} \cdot \hat{i}) + (\hat{j} \cdot \hat{j}) - 6(\hat{k} \cdot \hat{k})$

$= 6(1) + (1) - 6(1) = 1$unit.

5. *Two forces $4\hat{i} + 3\hat{j}$ and $3\hat{i} + 2\hat{j}$ are applied on the particle then particle is displaced from $\hat{i} + 2\hat{j}$ to $5\hat{i} + 4\hat{j}$. Find total work done.*

SOLUTION. Let $\vec{F_1} = 4\hat{i} + 3\hat{j}$ and $\vec{F_2} = 3\hat{i} + 2\hat{j}$

Resultant force $\vec{F} = \vec{F_1} + \vec{F_2}$

$= (4\hat{i} + 3\hat{j}) + (3\hat{i} + 2\hat{j})$

$= 7\hat{i} + 5\hat{j}$

Let particle be displaced from A to B by the force $\vec{F}$.

$\overrightarrow{OA} = \hat{i} + 2\hat{j}$ and $\overrightarrow{OB} = 5\hat{i} + 4\hat{j}$

$\therefore \overrightarrow{AB} = \overrightarrow{OB} - \overrightarrow{OA} = (5\hat{i} + 4\hat{j}) - (\hat{i} + 2\hat{j})$

$= 4\hat{i} + 2\hat{j}$

Here total work done $= \vec{F} \cdot \overrightarrow{AB}$

$= (7\hat{i} + 5\hat{j}) \cdot (4\hat{i} + 2\hat{j})$

$= 28(\hat{i} \cdot \hat{i}) + 10(\hat{j} \cdot \hat{j})$

$= 28 + 10 = 38$ units.

24.38 VECTOR PRODUCT OR CROSS PRODUCT

Let $\vec{a}$ and $\vec{b}$ be two vectors then vector product of $\vec{a}$ and $\vec{b}$ is given by $ab\sin\theta$. It is denoted by $\vec{a} \times \vec{b}$ and read as $\vec{a}$ cross $\vec{b}$.

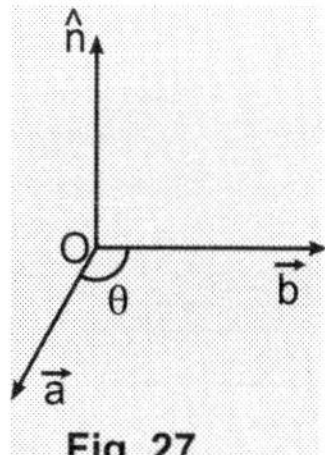

Fig. 27

- Vector product is also known as 'outer multiplication'.
- Vector product of two parallel vectors is always zero. $(\theta = 0 \Rightarrow \sin 0 = 0)$
- If $\vec{a} \times \vec{b} = 0$ then $\vec{a}$ and $\vec{b}$ will be parallel.
- The vector product of any vector with itself is always zero.
- If n be the unit normal vector along $\vec{a} \times \vec{b}$ then

$\therefore \quad \vec{a} \times \vec{b} = (|\vec{a}| \cdot |\vec{b}| \sin\theta)n = (ab\sin\theta)n \qquad |\vec{a}| = a, |\vec{b}| = b, 0 \le \theta \le \pi$

24.39 GEOMETRICAL INTERPRETATION OF THE VECTOR PRODUCT

Let $\vec{a}$ and $\vec{b}$ be two non-zero, non parallel vectors and θ be the angle between them.

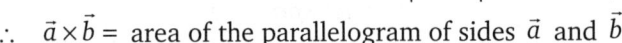

and $\qquad \overrightarrow{OA} = \vec{a}$, *i.e.*, $|\vec{a}| = OA = a$

$\qquad \overrightarrow{OB} = \vec{b}$, *i.e.*, $|\vec{b}| = OB = b$

$\Rightarrow \qquad |\vec{a}\times\vec{b}| = ab\sin\theta$

Fig. 28

From figure, $\qquad$ area of $OACB = 2(\text{area of } \Delta\, OAB)$

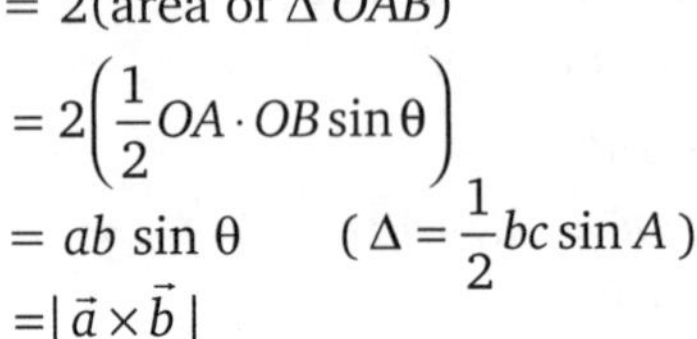

$$= 2\left(\frac{1}{2} OA \cdot OB \sin\theta\right)$$

$$= ab \sin\theta \qquad \left(\Delta = \frac{1}{2} bc \sin A\right)$$

$$= |\vec{a}\times\vec{b}|$$

$\therefore \quad \vec{a}\times\vec{b} =$ area of the parallelogram of sides $\vec{a}$ and $\vec{b}$

INTERPRETATION

(i) Area of the parallelogram with adjacent sides $\vec{a}$ and $\vec{b}$ is $|\vec{a}\times\vec{b}|$.

(ii) The vector area of a parallelogram with adjacent sides $\vec{a}$ and $\vec{b}$ is $\vec{a}\times\vec{b}$.

(iii) Area of a triangle whose two adjacent sides are $\vec{a}$ and $\vec{b}$ is $\frac{1}{2}|\vec{a}\times\vec{b}|$.

(iv) Vector area of a triangle whose two adjacent sides are $\vec{a}$ and $\vec{b}$ is $\frac{1}{2}(\vec{a}\times\vec{b})$.

24.40 PROPERTIES OF VECTOR PRODUCT

PROPERTY 1. *Vector multiplication is not commutative.*

PROOF. By definition of vector multiplication.

$$\vec{a}\times\vec{b} = ab\sin\theta\hat{n}$$

If the unit vector $\hat{n}$ is perpendicular to the vectors $\vec{a}$ and $\vec{b}$ moving in anticlockwise direction when we rotate it from $\vec{a}$ to $\vec{b}$.

If we rotate it from $\vec{b}$ to $\vec{a}$, then its direction will be opposite.

$\Rightarrow \quad$ Direction of $\vec{a}\times\vec{b}$ will be the opposite to the direction of $\vec{b}\times\vec{a}$.

i.e., $\qquad (\vec{a}\times\vec{b}) = -(\vec{b}\times\vec{a})$

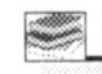

- Magnitude of $\vec{b}\times\vec{a}$ is also $ab \sin\theta$.

PROPERTY 2. *The vector product of two parallel vectors is always zero.*

PROOF. Let $\vec{a}$ and $\vec{b}$ be two parallel vectors.

$\therefore$ The angle between $\vec{a}$ and $\vec{b}$ $= 0°$ or $180°$

$\Rightarrow \qquad \sin 0° = \sin 180° = 0$

$\therefore \qquad \vec{a}\times\vec{b} = ab\sin\theta\hat{n} = ab\cdot 0 = 0$

- From above it is clear that $\vec{a}\times\vec{a} = 0$ *i.e.*, the vector product of two same vectors is zero.

PROPERTY 3. *Vector product is not associative.*

PROOF. Let $\vec{a}, \vec{b}$ and $\vec{c}$ be three vectors. Let $\vec{b} = \vec{c}$ then $\vec{b}\times\vec{c} = 0$

To prove: $\vec{a}\times(\vec{b}\times\vec{c})\neq(\vec{a}\times\vec{b})\times\vec{c}$

$$\text{LHS} = \vec{a}\times(\vec{b}\times\vec{c}) = a\times 0 = 0$$

$$\text{RHS} = (\vec{a}\times\vec{b})\times\vec{c}\neq 0$$

$\Rightarrow$ Vector product is not associative.

PROPERTY 4. *Vector product is associative w.r.t. a scalar.*

PROOF. Let $\vec{a}$ and $\vec{b}$ be two vectors and m, n be two scalars.

We have to prove that

$$(m\vec{a})\times(n\vec{b}) = mn(\vec{a}\times\vec{b}) = n\vec{a}\times m\vec{b}$$

Clearly the unit vector $\hat{n}$, perpendicular to $\vec{a}$ and $\vec{b}$ will also be perpendicular to $m\vec{a}$ and $n\vec{b}$.

$$(m\vec{a}\times n\vec{b}) = (ma)(nb)\sin\theta\hat{n} = mnab\sin\theta\hat{n}$$

$$= mn(\vec{a}\times\vec{b}) \qquad ...(i)$$

and $$n\vec{a}\times m\vec{b} = nmab\sin\theta\hat{n} = mnab\sin\theta\hat{n}$$

$$= mn(\vec{a}\times\vec{b}) \qquad ...(ii)$$

From (i) and (ii)

$$(m\vec{a})\times(n\vec{b}) = mn(\vec{a}\times\vec{b}) = (n\vec{a})\times(m\vec{a})$$

PROPERTY 5. *Vector product is distributive over the vector addition.*

PROOF. Let $\vec{a},\vec{b}$ and $\vec{c}$ be three vectors.

To prove that $\vec{a}\times(\vec{b}+\vec{c}) = \vec{a}\times\vec{b}+\vec{a}\times\vec{c}$

Case I: ***If vector are coplanar***

Clearly ΔABC and $\Delta A'B'C'$ are congruence.

Hence, sum of the area of parallelogram $ABB'A'$ and $BCC'B'$ is equal to the area of $ACC'A'$.

Here vector area of $ABB'A' = \vec{a}\times\vec{b}$

vector area of $BCC'B' = \vec{a}\times\vec{c}$

and vector area of $ACC'A' = \vec{a}\times(\vec{b}+\vec{c})$

Hence $\vec{a}\times(\vec{b}+\vec{c}) = \vec{a}\times\vec{b}+\vec{a}\times\vec{c}$

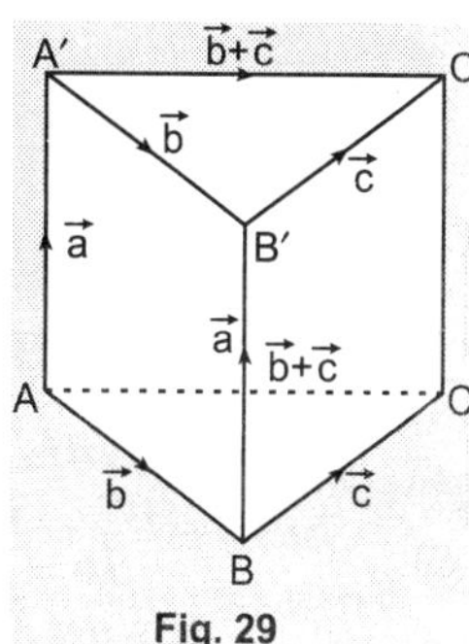

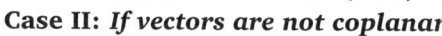

Fig. 29

Case II: ***If vectors are not coplanar.***

Consider a prism whose parallel sides are in the direction of $\vec{a}$.

Here vector area which is along the outward drawn normal is represented by $=\frac{1}{2}\vec{c}\times\vec{b}$ and $\frac{1}{2}\vec{b}\times\vec{c}$.

Clearly both are equal in magnitude but opposite in direction. Similarly the vector area of other faces will be represented by $\vec{b}\times\vec{a},\vec{c}\times\vec{a},\vec{a}\times(\vec{b}+\vec{c})$. We know that the vector area of any closed polyhedral (Here it is prism) is zero.

Therefore, $\vec{a}\times(\vec{b}+\vec{c})+\vec{b}\times\vec{a}+\vec{c}\times\vec{a} = 0$

$\Rightarrow$ $$\vec{a}\times(\vec{b}+\vec{c}) = -(\vec{b}\times\vec{a})-\vec{c}\times\vec{a} = \vec{a}\times\vec{b}+\vec{a}\times\vec{c}$$

Hence $$\vec{a}\times(\vec{b}+\vec{c}) = \vec{a}\times b+\vec{a}\times\vec{c}$$

- $(\vec{a}+\vec{b})\times(\vec{c}+\vec{d}) = \vec{a}\times\vec{c}+\vec{b}\times\vec{c}+\vec{a}\times d+\vec{b}\times\vec{d}$

24.41 VECTOR PRODUCT OF UNIT VECTORS $\hat{i}, \hat{j}$ AND $\hat{k}$

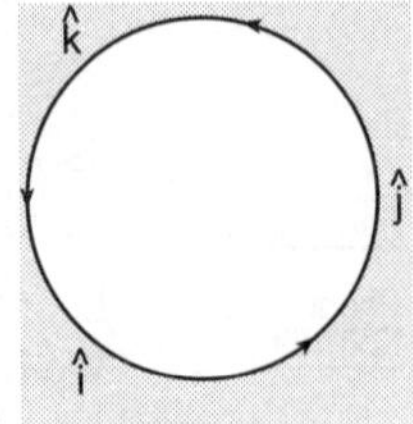

Fig. 30

Let $\hat{i}, \hat{j}$ and $\hat{k}$ be three unit vectors. Then by definition

$$\hat{i}\times\hat{i}=0;\quad \hat{i}\times\hat{j}=\hat{k};\quad \hat{j}\times\hat{i}=-\hat{k}$$
$$\hat{j}\times\hat{j}=0;\quad \hat{j}\times\hat{k}=\hat{i};\quad \hat{k}\times\hat{j}=-\hat{i}$$
$$\hat{k}\times\hat{k}=0;\quad \hat{k}\times\hat{i}=j;\quad \hat{i}\times\hat{k}=-\hat{j}$$

24.42 VECTOR PRODUCT IN TERMS OF UNIT VECTORS

Let $\vec{a}$ and $\vec{b}$ be two vectors such that

$$\vec{a}=a_1\hat{i}+a_2\hat{j}+a_3\hat{k}$$

and $$\vec{b}=b_1\hat{i}+b_2\hat{j}+b_3\hat{k}$$

Then $$\vec{a}\times\vec{b}=(a_1\hat{i}+a_2\hat{j}+a_3\hat{k})\times(b_1\hat{i}+b_2\hat{j}+b_3\hat{k})$$
$$=a_1b_1\hat{i}\times\hat{i}+a_1b_2\hat{i}\times\hat{j}+a_1b_3\hat{i}\times\hat{k}+a_2b_1\hat{j}\times\hat{i}+a_2b_2\hat{j}\times\hat{j}+a_2b_3\hat{j}\times\hat{k}$$
$$+a_3b_1\hat{k}\times\hat{i}+a_3b_2\hat{k}\times\hat{j}+a_3b_3\hat{k}\times\hat{k} \quad ...(i)$$

Using $\hat{i}\times\hat{i}=\hat{j}\times\hat{j}=\hat{k}\times\hat{k}=0$ and $\hat{i}\times\hat{j}=\hat{k}, \hat{j}\times\hat{k}=\hat{i}$ ... and $\hat{j}\times\hat{i}=-\hat{k}$ ... in eqn. (i), we get

$$\vec{a}\times\vec{b}=(a_2b_3-a_3b_2)\hat{i}+(a_3b_1-a_1b_3)\hat{j}+(a_1b_2-a_2b_1)\hat{k}$$

This result can also be written in the form of determinant as

$$\vec{a}\times\vec{b}=\begin{vmatrix}\hat{i} & \hat{j} & \hat{k}\\ a_1 & a_2 & a_3\\ b_1 & b_2 & b_3\end{vmatrix}$$

24.43 ANGLE BETWEEN TWO VECTORS

Let $\vec{a}=a_1\hat{i}+a_2\hat{j}+a_3\hat{k}$ and $\vec{b}=b_1\hat{i}+b_2\hat{j}+b_3\hat{k}$ be two vectors

Then clearly $|\vec{a}|=\sqrt{a_1^2+a_2^2+a_3^2}$

and $|\vec{b}|=\sqrt{b_1^2+b_2^2+b_3^2}$

We know that $\vec{a}\times\vec{b}=|\vec{a}|\cdot|\vec{b}|\sin\theta\hat{n}$ ...(i)

and $$\vec{a}\times\vec{b}=\begin{vmatrix}\hat{i} & \hat{j} & \hat{k}\\ a_1 & a_2 & a_3\\ b_1 & b_2 & b_3\end{vmatrix}=(a_2b_3-a_3b_2)\hat{i}+(a_3b_1-a_1b_3)\hat{j}+(a_1b_2-a_2b_1)\hat{k} \quad ...(ii)$$

From eqn. (i) and (ii)

$$|\vec{a}|\cdot|\vec{b}|\sin\theta\hat{n}=(a_2b_3-a_3b_2)\hat{i}+(a_3b_1-a_1b_3)\hat{j}+(a_1b_2-a_2b_1)\hat{k}$$

Squaring both the sides, we get

$$|\vec{a}|^2|\vec{b}|^2\sin^2\theta=(a_2b_3-a_3b_2)^2+(a_3b_1-a_1b_3)^2+(a_1b_2-a_2b_1)^2$$

$$\therefore \quad \sin^2\theta=\frac{(a_2b_3-a_3b_2)^2+(a_3b_1-a_1b_3)^2+(a_1b_2-a_2b_1)^2}{(a_1^2+a_2^2+a_3^2)(b_1^2+b_2^2+b_3^2)}$$

or $$\sin\theta=\frac{|\vec{a}\times\vec{b}|}{|\vec{a}|\cdot|\vec{b}|}=\frac{\text{magnitude of }(\vec{a}\times\vec{b})}{(\text{magnitude of }\vec{a})(\text{magnitude of }\vec{b})}$$

Solved Examples

1. *If $\vec{a} = \hat{i} + 2\hat{j} + 3\hat{k}, \vec{b} = 2\hat{i} - 3\hat{j} + \hat{k}$, write the value of $\vec{a} \times \vec{b}$ in determinant form.*

SOLUTION. We have $\vec{a} \times \vec{b} = \begin{vmatrix} \hat{i} & \hat{j} & \hat{k} \\ 1 & 2 & 3 \\ 2 & -3 & 1 \end{vmatrix}$

2. *If $\vec{a} = 3\hat{i} + 2\hat{j} + 2\hat{k}$ and $\vec{b} = 2\hat{i} + 4\hat{j} + 3\hat{k}$ then find the $(\vec{a} \times \vec{b})$ and $|\vec{a} \times \vec{b}|$.*

SOLUTION. $\vec{a} \times \vec{b} = \begin{vmatrix} \hat{i} & \hat{j} & \hat{k} \\ 3 & 2 & 2 \\ 2 & 4 & 3 \end{vmatrix}$

$$= \hat{i}(6-8) - \hat{j}(9-4) + \hat{k}(12-4)$$

$$= -2\hat{i} - 5\hat{j} + 8\hat{k}$$

$$|\vec{a} \times \vec{b}| = \sqrt{(-2)^2 + (-5)^2 + (8)^2}$$

$$= \sqrt{4 + 25 + 64} = \sqrt{93}$$

3. *Find the unit vector perpendicular to vectors $\hat{i} + \hat{j} + \hat{k}$ and $2\hat{i} + 3\hat{j} - \hat{k}$.*

SOLUTION. Let vector $\vec{a} = \hat{i} + \hat{j} + \hat{k}$ and $\vec{b} = 2\hat{i} + 3\hat{j} - \hat{k}$. Vector perpendicular to both vector $\vec{a}$ and $\vec{b}$ is given by

$$\vec{a} \times \vec{b} = \begin{vmatrix} \hat{i} & \hat{j} & \hat{k} \\ 1 & 1 & 1 \\ 2 & 3 & -1 \end{vmatrix}$$

$$= (-1-3)\hat{i} - (-1-2)\hat{j} + (3-2)\hat{k}$$

$$= -4\hat{i} + 3\hat{j} + \hat{k}$$

Required unit vector

$$= \frac{-4\hat{i} + 3\hat{j} + \hat{k}}{\sqrt{(-4)^2 + 3^2 + 1^2}} = \frac{-4\hat{i} + 3\hat{j} + \hat{k}}{\sqrt{26}}$$

4. *If $\vec{a} = 2\hat{i} + 5\hat{j} + 3\hat{k}, \vec{b} = 3\hat{i} + 3\hat{j} + 6\hat{k}$ and $\vec{c} = 2\hat{i} + 7\hat{j} + 4\hat{k}$, find the value of $(\vec{a} - \vec{b}) \times (\vec{c} - \vec{a})$ and $|(\vec{a} - \vec{b}) \times (\vec{c} - \vec{a})|$.*

SOLUTION. We have

$$\vec{a} - \vec{b} = (2\hat{i} + 5\hat{j} + 3\hat{k}) - (3\hat{i} + 3\hat{j} + 6\hat{k})$$

$$= -\hat{i} + 2\hat{j} - 3\hat{k}$$

and $\vec{c} - \vec{a} = (2\hat{i} + 7\hat{j} + 4\hat{k}) - (2\hat{i} + 5\hat{j} + 3\hat{k})$

$$= 0\hat{i} + 2\hat{j} + \hat{k}$$

$\therefore (\vec{a} - \vec{b}) \times (\vec{c} - \vec{a})$

$$= (-\hat{i} + 2\hat{j} - 3\hat{k}) \times (0\hat{i} + 2\hat{j} + \hat{k})$$

$$= \begin{vmatrix} \hat{i} & \hat{j} & \hat{k} \\ -1 & 2 & -3 \\ 0 & 2 & 1 \end{vmatrix}$$

$$= \hat{i}(2+6) - \hat{j}(-1+0) + \hat{k}(-2-0)$$

$$= 8\hat{i} + \hat{j} - 2\hat{k}$$

and $|(\vec{a} - \vec{b}) \times (\vec{c} - \vec{a})|$

$$= \sqrt{[8^2 + 1^2 + (-2)^2]}$$

$$= \sqrt{(64 + 1 + 4)} = \sqrt{69}$$

5. *Show that the sine of the angle between the vectors $\hat{i} + 3\hat{j} + 2\hat{k}$ and $2\hat{i} - 4\hat{j} + \hat{k}$ is $\sqrt{\frac{115}{147}}$.*

SOLUTION. Let $\vec{a} = \hat{i} + 3\hat{j} + 2\hat{k}$ and $\vec{b} = 2\hat{i} - 4\hat{j} + \hat{k}$

$$\vec{a} \times \vec{b} = \begin{vmatrix} \hat{i} & \hat{j} & \hat{k} \\ 1 & 3 & 2 \\ 2 & -4 & 1 \end{vmatrix}$$

$$= \hat{i}(3+8) - \hat{j}(1-4) + \hat{k}(-4-6)$$

$$= 11\hat{i} + 3\hat{j} - 10\hat{k}$$

$$\therefore |\vec{a} \times \vec{b}| = \sqrt{\{(11)^2 + (3)^2 + (-10)^2\}}$$

$$= \sqrt{230}$$

and $|\vec{a}| = \sqrt{(1^2 + 3^2 + 2^2)}$

$$= \sqrt{1 + 9 + 4} = \sqrt{14}$$

$$|\vec{b}| = \sqrt{[(2)^2 + (-4)^2 + 1^2]}$$

$$= \sqrt{4 + 16 + 1} = \sqrt{21}$$

Also $\sin\theta = \dfrac{|\vec{a} \times \vec{b}|}{|\vec{a}||\vec{b}|}$

$$= \frac{\sqrt{230}}{\sqrt{14} \times \sqrt{21}} = \frac{\sqrt{2} \times \sqrt{115}}{\sqrt{2} \times \sqrt{7} \times \sqrt{21}}$$

$$= \frac{\sqrt{115}}{\sqrt{147}} = \sqrt{\left(\frac{115}{147}\right)}$$

6. *If $\vec{a}\times\vec{b}=\vec{c}\times\vec{d}$ and $\vec{a}\times\vec{c}=\vec{b}\times\vec{d}$ then prove that $\vec{a}-\vec{d}$ and $\vec{b}-\vec{c}$ are parallel.*

SOLUTION. $\vec{a}-\vec{d}$ and $\vec{b}-\vec{c}$ will be parallel if $(\vec{a}-\vec{d})\times(\vec{b}-\vec{c})=0$.

Now, $(\vec{a}-\vec{d})\times(\vec{b}-\vec{c})$

$=\vec{a}\times(\vec{b}-\vec{c})-\vec{d}\times(\vec{b}-\vec{c})$

$=(\vec{a}\times\vec{b})-(\vec{a}\times\vec{c})-(\vec{d}\times\vec{b})+(\vec{d}\times\vec{c})$

$=(\vec{a}\times\vec{b})-(\vec{a}\times\vec{c})+(\vec{b}\times\vec{d})-(\vec{c}\times\vec{d})=0$

7. *If $\vec{a},\vec{b},\vec{c}$ be three vectors such that $\vec{a}+\vec{b}+\vec{c}=0$, prove that:*

$$\vec{a}\times\vec{b}=\vec{b}\times\vec{c}=\vec{c}\times\vec{a}$$

SOLUTION. We have $\vec{a}\times\vec{b}$

$=[-(\vec{b}+\vec{c})\times\vec{b}]=\vec{b}\times(\vec{b}+\vec{c})$

$[\because \vec{a}=-(\vec{b}+\vec{c})]$

$=(\vec{b}\times\vec{b})+(\vec{b}\times\vec{c})$

$=0+(\vec{b}\times\vec{c})=\vec{b}\times\vec{c}$ ...(i)

$\vec{c}\times\vec{a}=-\vec{a}\times\vec{c}=-[-(\vec{b}+\vec{c})\times\vec{c}]$

$=(\vec{b}+\vec{c})\times\vec{c}=-\vec{c}\times(\vec{b}+\vec{c})$

$=-[(\vec{c}\times\vec{b})+(\vec{c}\times\vec{c})]$

$=-[\vec{c}\times\vec{b}]-0=\vec{b}\times\vec{c}$ ...(ii)

From eqn. (i) and (ii)

$$\vec{a}\times\vec{b}=\vec{b}\times\vec{c}=\vec{c}\times\vec{a}$$

8. *For two vectors $\vec{a}$ and $\vec{b}$, prove the following :*

(*i*) $|\vec{a}\times\vec{b}|=a^2b^2-(\vec{a}\cdot\vec{b})^2$

(*ii*) $|\vec{a}\times\vec{b}|^2=\begin{vmatrix}\vec{a}\cdot\vec{a} & \vec{a}\cdot\vec{b}\\ \vec{a}\cdot\vec{b} & \vec{b}\cdot\vec{b}\end{vmatrix}$

SOLUTION. (i) We have

$|\vec{a}\times\vec{b}|=(\vec{a}\times\vec{b})$

$=(|\vec{a}|\cdot|\vec{b}|\cdot\sin\theta)^2$

$=|\vec{a}|^2\cdot|\vec{b}|^2\cdot\sin^2\theta$

$=a^2b^2\sin^2\theta=a^2b^2(1-\cos^2\theta)$

$=a^2b^2-a^2b^2\cos^2\theta$

$=a^2b^2-(ab\cos\theta)^2$

$=a^2b^2-(|\vec{a}|\cdot|\vec{b}|\cdot\cos\theta)^2$

$=a^2b^2-(\vec{a}\cdot\vec{b})^2$

(ii) We have

$|\vec{a}\times\vec{b}|^2=a^2b^2-(\vec{a}\cdot\vec{b})^2$

$=|\vec{a}|^2|\vec{b}|^2-(\vec{a}\cdot\vec{b})^2$

$=(\vec{a}\cdot\vec{a})(\vec{b}\cdot\vec{b})-(\vec{a}\cdot\vec{b})(\vec{a}\cdot\vec{b})$

$=\begin{vmatrix}\vec{a}\cdot\vec{a} & \vec{a}\cdot\vec{b}\\ \vec{a}\cdot\vec{b} & \vec{b}\cdot\vec{b}\end{vmatrix}$

9. *If $\vec{a}\cdot\vec{b}=0$ and $\vec{a}\times\vec{b}=0$, prove that $\vec{a}=0$ or $\vec{b}=0$.*

SOLUTION. Let $\vec{a}\cdot\vec{b}=0$ and $\vec{a}\times\vec{b}=0$

To prove either $\vec{a}=0$ or $\vec{b}=0$

$(\vec{a}\cdot\vec{b})=0 \Rightarrow (\vec{a}=0 \text{ or } \vec{b}=0 \text{ or } \vec{a}\perp\vec{b})$

$(\vec{a}\times\vec{b})=0 \Rightarrow (\vec{a}=0 \text{ or } \vec{b}=0 \text{ or } \vec{a}\,||\,\vec{b})$

$\vec{a}\perp\vec{b}$ and $\vec{a}\,||\,\vec{b}$ which is not possible at one time.

Therefore, $\vec{a}=0$ or $\vec{b}=0$.

10. *Find the value of λ and μ for which:*

$$(2\hat{i}+6\hat{j}+27\hat{k})\times(\hat{i}+\lambda\hat{j}+\mu\hat{k})=0$$

SOLUTION. Let $\vec{a}=2\hat{i}+6\hat{j}+27\hat{k}$ and $\vec{b}=\hat{i}+\lambda\hat{j}+\mu\hat{k}$

$$\therefore\quad \vec{a}\times\vec{b}=\begin{vmatrix}\hat{i} & \hat{j} & \hat{k}\\ 2 & 6 & 27\\ 1 & \lambda & \mu\end{vmatrix}$$

$=(6\mu-27\lambda)\hat{i}-(2\mu-27)\hat{j}+(2\lambda-6)\hat{k}$

Now $\vec{a}\times\vec{b}=0$

$\Leftrightarrow (6\mu-27\lambda)\hat{i}-(2\mu-27)\hat{j}+(2\lambda-6)k=0$

$\Leftrightarrow \quad 2\lambda-6=0, 2\mu-27=0$

$\Leftrightarrow \quad \lambda=3$ and $\mu=\dfrac{27}{2}$

11. *For three vectors $\vec{a},\vec{b}$ and $\vec{c}$, prove that*

$$\vec{a}\times(\vec{b}+\vec{c})+\vec{b}\times(\vec{c}+\vec{a})+\vec{c}\times(\vec{a}+\vec{b})=0$$

SOLUTION. We have LHS

$=\vec{a}\times(\vec{b}+\vec{c})+\vec{b}\times(\vec{c}+\vec{a})+\vec{c}\times(\vec{a}+\vec{b})$

$=(\vec{a}\times\vec{b})+(\vec{a}\times\vec{c})+(\vec{b}\times\vec{c})+(\vec{b}\times\vec{a})+(\vec{c}\times\vec{a})+(\vec{c}\times\vec{b})$

$=(\vec{a}\times\vec{b})+(\vec{a}\times\vec{c})+(\vec{b}\times\vec{c})-(\vec{a}\times\vec{b})-(\vec{a}\times\vec{c})-(\vec{b}\times\vec{c})$

$=0=$ RHS

12. *For three vectors $\vec{a}, \vec{b}$ and $\vec{c}$, prove that*

$$(\vec{a}-\vec{b})\times(\vec{a}+\vec{b}) = 2(\vec{a}\times\vec{b}).$$

SOLUTION. LHS $= (\vec{a}-\vec{b})\times(\vec{a}+\vec{b})$

$$= \vec{a}\times\vec{a}+\vec{a}\times\vec{b}-\vec{b}\times\vec{a}-\vec{b}\times\vec{b}$$
$$= \vec{a}\times\vec{b}-\vec{b}\times\vec{a} \quad (\vec{a}\times\vec{a}=\vec{b}\times\vec{b}=0)$$
$$=(\vec{a}\times\vec{b})-[-(\vec{a}\times\vec{b})]=(\vec{a}\times\vec{b})+(\vec{a}\times\vec{b})$$
$$= 2(\vec{a}\times\vec{b}) = \text{RHS}$$

13. *If $\vec{a}\times\vec{b}=\vec{a}\times\vec{c}$, prove that difference vector of $\vec{b}$ and $\vec{c}$ is parallel to the vector $\vec{a}$.*

SOLUTION. Given $\quad \vec{a}\times\vec{b}=\vec{a}\times\vec{c}$

$\Rightarrow (\vec{a}\times\vec{b})-(\vec{a}\times\vec{c})=0$

$\Rightarrow \quad \vec{a}\times(\vec{b}-\vec{c})=0$

$\Rightarrow (\vec{b}-\vec{c})$ is parallel to $\vec{a}$.

14. *If $\vec{a}\cdot\vec{b}=\vec{a}\cdot\vec{c}, \vec{a}\times\vec{b}=\vec{a}\times\vec{c}, \vec{a}\neq 0$, prove that $\vec{b}=\vec{c}$.*

SOLUTION. Given $\vec{a}\cdot\vec{b}=\vec{a}\cdot\vec{c}$ and $\vec{a}\neq 0$

$\Rightarrow \quad \vec{a}\cdot b-\vec{a}\cdot\vec{c}=0$ and $\vec{a}\neq 0$

$\Rightarrow \quad \vec{a}\cdot(\vec{b}-\vec{c})=0$ and $\vec{a}\neq\vec{0}$

$\Rightarrow \quad \vec{b}-\vec{c}=0$ or $\vec{a}\perp(\vec{b}-\vec{c})$

$\Rightarrow \quad \vec{b}=\vec{c}$ or $\vec{a}\perp(\vec{b}-\vec{c})$

It is also given that $\vec{a}\times b=\vec{a}\times\vec{c}$ and $\vec{a}\neq 0$

$\Rightarrow (\vec{a}\times\vec{b})-(\vec{a}\times\vec{c})=\vec{0}$ and $\vec{a}\neq\vec{0}$

$\Rightarrow \vec{a}\times(\vec{b}-\vec{c})=0$ and $\vec{a}\neq\vec{0}$

$\Rightarrow \quad \vec{b}-\vec{c}=0$ or $\vec{a}\,||\,(\vec{b}-\vec{c})$

$\Rightarrow \quad \vec{b}=\vec{c}$ or $\vec{a}\,||\,(\vec{b}-\vec{c})$

Hence it is clear that $\vec{b}=\vec{c}$

15. *For any two vectors $\vec{a}$ and $\vec{b}$, solve the following equation $\vec{r}\times\vec{b}=\vec{a}\times\vec{b}$ has the solution $\vec{r}=\vec{a}+t\vec{b}$.*

SOLUTION. Given equation $\vec{r}\times\vec{b}=\vec{a}\times\vec{b}$

$\Rightarrow \quad (\vec{r}-\vec{a})\times\vec{b}=0$

$\Rightarrow (\vec{r}-\vec{a})$ and $\vec{b}$ are parallel to each other.

$\therefore \quad \vec{r}-\vec{a}=t\vec{b}$

$\Rightarrow \vec{r}=\vec{a}+t\vec{b}$, where t is a scalar.

which is the required solution of the given equation.

16. *If $\vec{a}\times\vec{b}=\vec{b}\times\vec{c}\neq 0$, then prove that $\vec{a}+\vec{c}=t\vec{b}$ where t is a scalar.*

SOLUTION. Given: $\quad \vec{a}\times\vec{b}=\vec{b}\times\vec{c}$

$\Rightarrow \quad \vec{a}\times\vec{b}-\vec{b}\times\vec{c}=0$

$\Rightarrow (\vec{a}\times\vec{b})+(\vec{c}\times\vec{b})=0$

$\Rightarrow \quad (\vec{a}+\vec{c})\times\vec{b}=0$

$\Rightarrow (\vec{a}+\vec{c})$ and $\vec{b}$ are parallel.

$\therefore \quad (\vec{a}+\vec{c})=t\vec{b}$ where t is a scalar.

Exercise-24.3

1. Find the vector product of the following vectors:
   (i) $\vec{a}=3\hat{i}-\hat{j}+2\hat{k}, \vec{b}=\hat{i}+\hat{j}-4\hat{k}$
   (ii) $\vec{a}=2\hat{i}+\hat{j}+7\hat{k}, \vec{b}=3\hat{i}+\hat{j}-\hat{k}$
   (iii) $\vec{a}=\hat{i}+2\hat{j}-3\hat{k}, \vec{b}=3\hat{i}+2\hat{j}-\hat{k}$
   (iv) $\vec{a}=3\hat{i}-2\hat{j}+\hat{k}, \vec{b}=\hat{i}+4\hat{j}-2\hat{k}$
   (v) $\vec{a}=2\hat{i}-3\hat{j}-\hat{k}, \vec{b}=\hat{i}+4\hat{j}-2\hat{k}$
2. If $\vec{a}=\hat{i}+2\hat{j}-2\hat{k}$ and $\vec{b}=2\hat{i}+4\hat{j}+3\hat{k}$, find the value of $\vec{b}\times\vec{a}$.
3. Find the unit vector perpendicular to $2\hat{i}-\hat{j}+\hat{k}$ and $3\hat{i}+4\hat{j}-\hat{k}$. Also find the sine of angle between them.
4. Find $\vec{a}=\hat{i}+\hat{j}-2\hat{k}$ and $\vec{b}=2\hat{i}-\hat{j}+\hat{k}$, find a vector which is perpendicular to the plane of $\vec{a}$ and $\vec{b}$ and whose magnitude is 7.
5. Prove by vector method that
   (i) $\sin(\alpha-\beta) = \sin\alpha\cos\beta-\cos\alpha\sin\beta$
   (ii) $\cos(\alpha+\beta) = \cos\alpha\cos\beta-\sin\alpha\sin\beta$
6. If $\vec{a}=a_1\hat{i}+a_2\hat{j}+a_3\hat{k}$ and $\vec{b}=b_1\hat{i}+b_2\hat{j}+b_3\hat{k}$ be two non-zero parallel vectors, find the relation between $a_1, b_1; a_2, b_2$ and a_3, b_3.
7. If $\vec{a}=2\hat{i}-3\hat{j}-\hat{k}$ and $\vec{b}=\hat{i}+4\hat{j}-2\hat{k}$, find the value of $(\vec{a}+\vec{b})\times(\vec{a}-\vec{b})$.
8. If $\vec{a}=2\hat{i}-\hat{j}+\hat{k}$ and $\vec{b}=3\hat{i}+4\hat{j}-\hat{k}$, prove that $\vec{a}\times\vec{b}$ is a vector perpendicular to both $\vec{a}$ and $\vec{b}$.
9. Prove that the sine of the angle between $3\hat{i}+\hat{j}+2\hat{k}$ and $2\hat{i}-2\hat{j}+4\hat{k}$ is $\frac{2}{\sqrt{7}}$.

10. Prove that the sine of the angle between $2\hat{i}+3\hat{j}+6\hat{k}$ and $4\hat{i}-4\hat{j}-7\hat{k}$ is $\sqrt{\frac{1853}{63}}$.

11. Prove that the following:

$$(\vec{a}+\vec{b})\times\vec{c}=\vec{a}\times\vec{c}+\vec{b}\times\vec{c}$$

12. For the vectors $\vec{a}=\hat{i}+4\hat{j}+2\hat{k},\ \vec{b}=3\hat{i}-2\hat{j}+7\hat{k}$ and $\vec{c}=2\hat{i}-\hat{j}+4\hat{k}$, find a vector $\vec{d}$ which is perpendicular to $\vec{a}$ and $\vec{b}$ both.

Hint to Selected Problems

3. $\vec{a}\times\vec{b}=\begin{vmatrix}\hat{i} & \hat{j} & \hat{k}\\ 2 & -1 & 1\\ 3 & 4 & -1\end{vmatrix}=-3\hat{i}+5\hat{j}+11\hat{k}$

$\Rightarrow |\vec{a}\times\vec{b}|=\sqrt{9+25+121}=\sqrt{155}$

Now $n=\dfrac{\vec{a}\times\vec{b}}{|\vec{a}\times\vec{b}|}=\dfrac{-3\hat{i}+5\hat{j}+11\hat{k}}{\sqrt{155}}$

Now use $\sin\theta=\dfrac{|\vec{a}\times\vec{b}|}{|\vec{a}|\times|\vec{b}|}$

7. $\vec{a}+\vec{b}=3\hat{i}+\hat{j}-3\hat{k}$ and $\vec{a}-\vec{b}=\hat{i}-7\hat{j}+\hat{k}$

Now find the value of

$(\vec{a}+\vec{b})\times(\vec{a}-\vec{b})=\begin{vmatrix}\hat{i} & \hat{j} & \hat{k}\\ 3 & 1 & -3\\ 1 & -7 & 1\end{vmatrix}$

9. Use $\sin\theta=\dfrac{|\vec{a}\times\vec{b}|}{|\vec{a}|\cdot|\vec{b}|}$

11. $\vec{r}=(\vec{a}+\vec{b})\times\vec{c}-\vec{a}\times\vec{c}-\vec{b}\times\vec{c}$

Now $\vec{r}\cdot\vec{d}=[(\vec{a}+\vec{b})\times\vec{c}-\vec{a}\times\vec{c}-\vec{b}\times\vec{c}]\cdot\vec{d}$

$=[(\vec{a}+\vec{b})\times\vec{c}]\cdot\vec{d}-(\vec{a}\times\vec{c})\cdot\vec{d}-(\vec{b}\times\vec{c})\cdot\vec{d}$

$=(\vec{a}+\vec{b})\cdot(\vec{c}\times\vec{d})-\vec{a}\cdot(\vec{c}\times\vec{d})-\vec{b}.(\vec{c}\times\vec{d})$

$=\vec{a}\cdot(\vec{c}\times\vec{d})+\vec{b}\cdot(\vec{c}\times\vec{d})-\vec{a}(\vec{c}\times\vec{d})-\vec{b}\cdot(\vec{c}\times\vec{d})$

$=0$

$\vec{r}\cdot\vec{d}=0 \Rightarrow$ either $\vec{r}=0$ or $\vec{d}=0$

But $\vec{d}\neq 0 \therefore \vec{r}=0$

$\Rightarrow (\vec{a}+\vec{b})\times\vec{c}=\vec{a}\times\vec{c}+\vec{b}\times\vec{c}$

ANSWERS

1. (i) $2\hat{i}+14\hat{j}+4\hat{k}$ (ii) $-8\hat{i}+23\hat{j}-\hat{k}$ (iii) $4\hat{i}-8\hat{j}-4\hat{k}$ (iv) $-3\hat{i}+2\hat{j}+13\hat{k}$ (v) $10\hat{i}+3\hat{j}+11\hat{k}$ **2.** $-14\hat{i}+7\hat{j}$ **3.** $\dfrac{-3\hat{i}+5\hat{j}+11\hat{k}}{\sqrt{155}}, \dfrac{\sqrt{155}}{\sqrt{6}\sqrt{26}}$ **4.** $\dfrac{7}{\sqrt{59}}(\hat{i}-7\hat{j}-3\hat{k})$

6. $\dfrac{a_1}{b_1}=\dfrac{a_2}{b_2}=\dfrac{a_3}{b_3}$ **7.** $-20\hat{i}-6\hat{j}-22\hat{k}$ **12.** $32\hat{i}-\hat{j}-14\hat{k}$

24.44 APPLICATION OF VECTOR PRODUCT IN GEOMETRY

Use the following results of geometry whenever required:

(1) Two vectors $\vec{a}$ and $\vec{b}$ will be collinear (parallel) if and only if $\vec{a}\times\vec{b}=0$.

(2) Three points *A*, *B*, *C* will be collinear if and only if

$\overrightarrow{AB}\parallel\overrightarrow{AC}$ or $\overrightarrow{AB}\parallel\overrightarrow{BC}$ or $\overrightarrow{AC}\parallel\overrightarrow{BC}$ or $\overrightarrow{AB}\times\overrightarrow{AC}=0$ or $\overrightarrow{AB}\times\overrightarrow{BC}=0$ or $\overrightarrow{AC}\times\overrightarrow{BC}=0$

(3) Three points whose position vectors are given by $\vec{a},\vec{b}$ and $\vec{c}$ will be collinear if and only if $\vec{a}\times\vec{b}+\vec{b}+\vec{c}+\vec{c}\times\vec{a}=0$.

(4) Area of the parallelogram whose adjacent sides are $\vec{a}$ and $\vec{b}=|\vec{a}\times\vec{b}|$.

(5) Area of the parallelogram whose diagonals are $\vec{a}$ and $\vec{b}=\frac{1}{2}|\vec{a}\times\vec{b}|$.

(6) The area of the triangle whose two sides are $\vec{a}$ and $\vec{b}=\frac{1}{2}|\vec{a}\times\vec{b}|$.

(7) Three points *A*, *B* and *C* will be collinear if and only if area of $\Delta ABC=0$ or if and only if $\overrightarrow{AB}\times\overrightarrow{AC}=0$.

24.45 APPLICATION OF VECTOR PRODUCT IN MECHANICS

Vector moment of a force $\vec{F}$ about a point O is $\vec{r}\times\vec{F}$, where $\vec{r}$ is the position vector of any point on the line, also the magnitude of the moment $=|\vec{r}\times\vec{F}|$

Solved Examples

1. *Find the area of the parallelogram whose adjacent sides are $3\hat{i}+4\hat{j}$ and $\hat{i}+\hat{j}+\hat{k}$.*

SOLUTION. Let $\vec{a}=3\hat{i}+4\hat{j}, \vec{b}=\hat{i}+\hat{j}+\hat{k}$

$$\vec{a}\times\vec{b}=(3\hat{i}+4\hat{j}+0\hat{k})\times(\hat{i}+\hat{j}+\hat{k})$$

$$=\begin{vmatrix}\hat{i} & \hat{j} & \hat{k}\\ 3 & 4 & 0\\ 1 & 1 & 1\end{vmatrix}$$

$$=\hat{i}(4-0)-\hat{j}(3-0)+\hat{k}(3-4)$$

$$=4\hat{i}-3\hat{j}-\hat{k}$$

$\therefore$ Required area $=|\vec{a}\times\vec{b}|$

$$|\vec{a}\times\vec{b}|=|4\hat{i}-3\hat{j}-\hat{k}|$$

$$=\sqrt{\{(4)^2+(-3)^2+(-1)^2\}}$$

$$=\sqrt{26}\text{ sq. units.}$$

2. *Find the area of parallelogram whose diagonals are given by $\vec{a}=3\hat{i}+\hat{j}-2\hat{k}$ and $\vec{b}=\hat{i}-3\hat{j}+4\hat{k}$.*

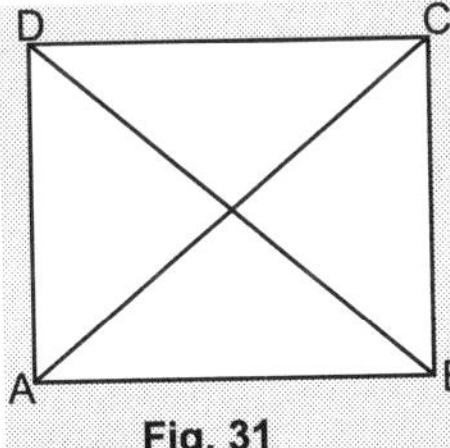

Fig. 31

SOLUTION. Let $\overline{AC}=\vec{a}=3\hat{i}+\hat{j}-2\hat{k}$ and $\overline{BD}=\vec{b}=\hat{i}-3\hat{j}+4\hat{k}$

So, $\frac{1}{2}(\vec{a}\times\vec{b})$

$$=\frac{1}{2}\{(3\hat{i}+\hat{j}-2\hat{k})\times(\hat{i}-3\hat{j}+4\hat{k})\}$$

$$=\frac{1}{2}\begin{vmatrix}\hat{i} & \hat{j} & \hat{k}\\ 3 & 1 & -2\\ 1 & -3 & 4\end{vmatrix}$$

$$=\frac{1}{2}[\hat{i}(4-6)-\hat{j}(12+2)+\hat{k}(-9-1)]$$

$$=\frac{1}{2}[-2\hat{i}-14\hat{j}-10\hat{k}]=-\hat{i}-7\hat{j}-5\hat{k}$$

Hence, area of the parallelogram $ABCD$

$$=\sqrt{[(-1)^2+(-7)^2+(-5)^2]}$$

$$=\sqrt{1+49+25}$$

$$=\sqrt{75}=5\sqrt{3}\text{ square units.}$$

3. *In the adjoining figure $\overrightarrow{OA}=3\hat{i}+2\hat{j}-\hat{k}$ and $\overrightarrow{OB}=\hat{i}+3\hat{j}+\hat{k}$. Find the area of ΔOAB.*

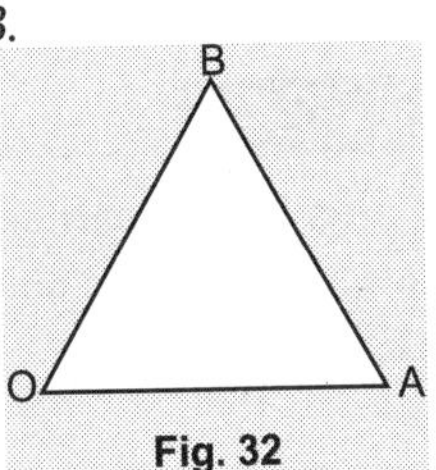

Fig. 32

SOLUTION. We have $\overrightarrow{OA}\times\overrightarrow{OB}=\begin{vmatrix}\hat{i} & \hat{j} & \hat{k}\\ 3 & 2 & -1\\ 1 & 3 & 1\end{vmatrix}$

$$=\hat{i}(2+3)-\hat{j}(3+1)+\hat{k}(9-2)$$

$$=5\hat{i}-4\hat{j}+7\hat{k}$$

Area of ΔOAB

$$=\frac{1}{2}|5\hat{i}-4\hat{j}+7\hat{k}|$$

$$=\frac{1}{2}\sqrt{[(5)^2+(-4)^2+(7)^2]}$$

$$=\frac{1}{2}\sqrt{(25+16+49)}$$

$$=\frac{1}{2}\sqrt{90}=\frac{1}{2}(3\sqrt{10})$$

$$=\frac{3}{2}\sqrt{10}\text{ square units.}$$

4. *Find the area of the triangle ABC of the vertices A(1, 2, 3), B(2, 3, 1) and C(3, 1, 2). Also find the angles of the triangle.*

SOLUTION. Let O be the origin then

$\overrightarrow{OA} = \hat{i} + 2\hat{j} + 3\hat{k}, \overrightarrow{OB} = 2\hat{i} + 3\hat{j} + \hat{k},$

$\overrightarrow{OC} = 3\hat{i} + \hat{j} + 2\hat{k}$

$\therefore\ \overrightarrow{AB} = \overrightarrow{OB} - \overrightarrow{OA}$

$= (2\hat{i} + 3\hat{j} + \hat{k}) - (\hat{i} + 2\hat{j} + 3\hat{k})$

$= \hat{i} + \hat{j} - 2\hat{k}$

and $\overrightarrow{AC} = \overrightarrow{OC} - \overrightarrow{OA}$

$= (3\hat{i} + \hat{j} + 2\hat{k}) - (\hat{i} + 2\hat{j} + 3\hat{k})$

$= 2\hat{i} - \hat{j} - \hat{k}$

$$\overrightarrow{AB} \times \overrightarrow{AC} = \begin{vmatrix} \hat{i} & \hat{j} & \hat{k} \\ 1 & 1 & -2 \\ 2 & -1 & -1 \end{vmatrix}$$

$= \hat{i}(-1-2) - \hat{j}(-1+4) + \hat{k}(-1-2)$

$= -3\hat{i} - 3\hat{j} - 3\hat{k}$

Area of $\Delta ABC = \frac{1}{2} |\overrightarrow{AB} \times \overrightarrow{AC}|$

$= \frac{1}{2}\sqrt{[(-3)^2 + (-3)^2 + (-3)^2]}$

$= \frac{1}{2}\sqrt{27} = \frac{3}{2}\sqrt{3}$ square unit

Now $\overrightarrow{BC} = \overrightarrow{OC} - \overrightarrow{OB} = \hat{i} - 2\hat{j} + \hat{k}$

$|\overrightarrow{AB}| = \sqrt{1+1+4} = \sqrt{6}$

$|\overrightarrow{AC}| = \sqrt{4+1+1} = \sqrt{6}$

$|\overrightarrow{BC}| = \sqrt{1+4+1} = \sqrt{6}$

Hence, each angle of the triangle $= 60° = \frac{\pi}{3}$.

Exercise-24.4

1. Prove that area of the parallelogram whose diagonals are $2\hat{i} + 4\hat{j} - 5\hat{k}$ and $\hat{i} + 2\hat{j} + 3\hat{k}$ is given by $\frac{11}{2}\sqrt{5}$ square unit.
2. Prove by vector method the two parallelogram on the same base between two parallel lines are equal in area.
3. Prove that area of the triangle with concurrent edges $\vec{a} = 3\hat{i} + 4\hat{j}$ and $\vec{b} = -5\hat{i} + 7\hat{j}$ is $20\frac{1}{2}$ square unit.
4. Prove that the point $2\hat{i} + 3\hat{j} + 4\hat{k}, \hat{i} - 3\hat{j} + 5\hat{k}$ and $-9\hat{j} + 6\hat{k}$ are collinear.
5. Prove that the area of the parallelogram whose adjacent sides are $3\hat{i} + 2\hat{j} - \hat{k}$ and $\hat{i} + 2\hat{j} + 3\hat{k}$ is $6\sqrt{5}$ square unit.
6. If the vectors $\hat{i} + 2\hat{j} + 3\hat{k}$ and $3\hat{i} - 2\hat{j} + \hat{k}$ represent two sides of a triangle. Prove that area of the triangle will be $4\sqrt{3}$ square unit.
7. Prove by vector method that moment of any force $\vec{F}$ about any point O does not depend on its line of force.
8. Three forces $\vec{P}_1 = \hat{i} - \hat{j} + \hat{k}, \vec{P}_2 = -\hat{i} + 2\hat{j} - \hat{k}$ and $\vec{P}_3 = \hat{i} - \hat{k}$ act on a particle A to displace it to B. Find total workdone when position vectors of A and B are respectively given by $4\hat{i} - 3\hat{j} - 2\hat{k}$ and $6\hat{i} + \hat{j} - 3\hat{k}$. Also find the moment of force $\vec{P}_1$ about (1, 0, 1).
9. The resultant force of two forces $\vec{F}_1 = 4\hat{i} + 3\hat{j} + 2\hat{k}$ and $\vec{F}_2 = 3\hat{i} + 2\hat{j} + \hat{k}$ act on a particle at (2, 3, 1). It displace this particle from (2, 3, 1) to (3, 4, 2). Prove that the workdone by the resultant force is 15 units.

Hint to Selected Problems

1. $$\vec{a} \times \vec{b} = \begin{vmatrix} \hat{i} & \hat{j} & \hat{k} \\ 2 & 4 & -5 \\ 1 & 2 & 3 \end{vmatrix} = 22\hat{i} - 11\hat{j}$$

$\therefore$ Required area $= \frac{1}{2}|\vec{a} \times \vec{b}|$

9. $\vec{F} = \vec{F}_1 + \vec{F}_2 = (4\hat{i} + 3\hat{j} + 2\hat{k}) + (3\hat{i} + 2\hat{j} + \hat{k})$

$= 7\hat{i} + 5\hat{j} + 3\hat{k}$

$\vec{d} = (3\hat{i} + 4\hat{j} + 2\hat{k}) - (2\hat{i} + 3\hat{j} + \hat{k}) = \hat{i} + \hat{j} + \hat{k}$

Total work done

$\vec{F} \cdot \vec{d} = (7\hat{i} + 5\hat{j} + 3\hat{k}) \cdot (\hat{i} + \hat{j} + \hat{k})$

ANSWERS

8. 7 unit, $\hat{i}-\hat{k}$

More Solved Examples

1. *If θ be the angle between the unit vectors a and b, prove that* $\sin\frac{\theta}{2}=\frac{1}{2}|\hat{a}-\hat{b}|$.

SOLUTION. Since, $|\hat{a}|=1$ and $|\hat{b}|=1$

$\therefore \quad \hat{a}\cdot\hat{b}=(1)(1)\cos\theta=\cos\theta \quad \ldots\text{(i)}$

$$|\hat{a}-\hat{b}|^2=(\hat{a}-\hat{b})^2$$
$$=(\hat{a})^2+(\hat{b})^2-2(\hat{a}\cdot\hat{b})$$
$$=|\hat{a}|^2+|\hat{b}|^2-2\cos\theta \text{ [From eqn. (i)]}$$
$$=1+1-2\cos\theta=2-2\left(1-2\sin^2\frac{\theta}{2}\right)$$
$$=4\sin^2\frac{\theta}{2}$$
$$\therefore\ 2\sin\frac{\theta}{2}=|\hat{a}-\hat{b}|$$
$$\Rightarrow \sin\frac{\theta}{2}=\frac{1}{2}|\hat{a}-\hat{b}|$$

2. *Find the cosine of the angle between x-axis and* $\hat{i}+\hat{j}+\hat{k}$.

SOLUTION. Let $\vec{a}=\hat{i}$ and $\vec{b}=\hat{i}+\hat{j}+\hat{k}$

$$\vec{a}\cdot\vec{b}=\hat{i}\cdot(\hat{i}+\hat{j}+\hat{k})=\hat{i}\cdot\hat{i}=1$$
$$|\vec{a}|=\sqrt{(1)^2}=1,$$
$$|\vec{b}|=\sqrt{(1)^2+(1)^2+(1)^2}=\sqrt{3}$$

Hence $\cos\theta=\dfrac{\vec{a}\cdot\vec{b}}{|\vec{a}|\cdot|\vec{b}|}=\dfrac{1}{1\cdot\sqrt{3}}=\dfrac{1}{\sqrt{3}}$

$$\therefore \qquad \theta=\cos^{-1}\left(\frac{1}{\sqrt{3}}\right)$$

3. *Find the projection of the vector* $(\hat{i}+3\hat{j}+7\hat{k})$ *on the vector* $(2\hat{i}-3\hat{j}+6\hat{k})$.

SOLUTION. Assume that

$\vec{a}=(\hat{i}+3\hat{j}+7\hat{k})$ and $\vec{b}=(2\hat{i}-3\hat{j}+6\hat{k})$

Now, projection of $\vec{a}$ on $\vec{b}=\dfrac{(\vec{a}\cdot\vec{b})}{|\vec{b}|}$

$$=\frac{(\hat{i}+3\hat{j}+7\hat{k})\cdot(2\hat{i}-3\hat{j}+6\hat{k})}{\sqrt{4+9+36}}$$
$$=\frac{2-9+42}{\sqrt{49}}=\frac{35}{7}=5$$

4. *Write the projection of* $(\vec{b}+\vec{c})$ *on* $\vec{a}$, *where* $\vec{a}=(2\hat{i}-2\hat{j}+\hat{k}),\vec{b}=(\hat{i}+2\hat{j}-2\hat{k})$ *and* $\vec{c}=(2\hat{i}-\hat{j}+4\hat{k})$.

SOLUTION. Consider $(\vec{b}+\vec{c})$

$$=(\hat{i}+2\hat{j}-2\hat{k})+(2\hat{i}-\hat{j}+4\hat{k})$$
$$=(1+2)\hat{i}+(2-1)\hat{j}+(-2+4)\hat{k}$$
$$=(3\hat{i}+\hat{j}+2\hat{k})$$

Now, projection of $(\vec{b}+\vec{c})$ on $\vec{a}$

$$=\frac{(\vec{b}+\vec{c})\cdot\vec{a}}{|\vec{a}|}$$
$$=\frac{(3\hat{i}+\hat{j}+2\hat{k})\cdot(2\hat{i}-2\hat{j}+\hat{k})}{\sqrt{2^2+(-2)^2+1^2}}$$
$$=\frac{6-2+2}{\sqrt{9}}=\frac{6}{3}=2$$

5. *Dot products of a vector with the vectors* $(\hat{i}-\hat{j}+\hat{k}),(2\hat{i}+\hat{j}-3\hat{k})$ *and* $(\hat{i}+\hat{j}+\hat{k})$ *are respectively 4, 0 and 2. Find the vector.*

SOLUTION. Assume that required vector is $(x\hat{i}+y\hat{j}+z\hat{k})$, then we have

$$(x\hat{i}+y\hat{j}+z\hat{k})\cdot(\hat{i}-\hat{j}+\hat{k})=4$$
$$\Rightarrow \qquad x-y+z=4 \qquad \ldots\text{(i)}$$
$$(x\hat{i}+y\hat{j}+z\hat{k})\cdot(2\hat{i}+\hat{j}-3\hat{k})=0$$
$$\Rightarrow \qquad 2x+y-3z=0 \qquad \ldots\text{(ii)}$$
$$(x\hat{i}+y\hat{j}+z\hat{k})\cdot(\hat{i}+\hat{j}+\hat{k})=2$$

$\Rightarrow \quad x + y + z = 2 \quad \ldots\text{(iii)}$

Adding eqn. (i) and (ii), we get

$$3x - 2z = 4 \quad \ldots\text{(iv)}$$

Adding eqn. (i) and (iii), we get

$$2x + 2z = 6 \quad \ldots\text{(v)}$$

From eqn. (iv) and (v), we get $x = 2$ and $z = 1$

Subtracting eqn. (i) from (iii), we get $y = -1$

Hence, $x = 2, y = -1, z = 1$

Thus, the required vector is $(2\hat{i} - \hat{j} + \hat{k})$.

6. *The scalar product of the vector $(\hat{i} + \hat{j} + \hat{k})$ with the unit vector along the sum of the vectors $(2\hat{i} + 4\hat{j} - 5\hat{k})$ and $(\lambda\hat{i} + 2\hat{j} + 3\hat{k})$ is equal to 1. Find the value of λ.*

SOLUTION. Consider $\vec{a} = (\hat{i} + \hat{j} + \hat{k})$, $\vec{b} = (2\hat{i} + 4\hat{j} - 5\hat{k})$ and $\vec{c} = (\lambda\hat{i} + 2\hat{j} + 3\hat{k})$, then

$$(\vec{b} + \vec{c}) = (2\hat{i} + 4\hat{j} - 5\hat{k}) + (\lambda\hat{i} + 2\hat{j} + 3\hat{k})$$

$$= (2 + \lambda)\hat{i} + 6\hat{j} - 2\hat{k}$$

Now, unit vector along $(\vec{b} + \vec{c})$

$$= \frac{(\vec{b} + \vec{c})}{|\vec{b} + \vec{c}|} = \frac{(2+\lambda)\hat{i} + 6\hat{j} - 2\hat{k}}{\sqrt{(2+\lambda)^2 + (6)^2 + (-2)^2}}$$

$$= \frac{(2+\lambda)\hat{i} + 6\hat{j} - 2\hat{k}}{\sqrt{\lambda^2 + 4\lambda + 44}}$$

It is given that $\dfrac{(\vec{b} + \vec{c})}{|\vec{b} + \vec{c}|} \cdot \vec{a} = 1$

$$\Rightarrow \frac{(2+\lambda)\hat{i} + 6\hat{j} - 2\hat{k}}{\sqrt{\lambda^2 + 4\lambda + 44}} \cdot (\hat{i} + \hat{j} + \hat{k}) = 1$$

$$\Rightarrow [(2+\lambda)\hat{i} + 6\hat{j} - 2\hat{k}] \cdot (\hat{i} + \hat{j} + \hat{k}) = \sqrt{\lambda^2 + 4\lambda + 44}$$

$$\Rightarrow (2+\lambda) + 6 - 2 = \sqrt{\lambda^2 + 4\lambda + 44}$$

$$\Rightarrow \quad 6 + \lambda = \sqrt{\lambda^2 + 4\lambda + 44}$$

$$\Rightarrow \lambda^2 + 4\lambda + 44 = (6 + \lambda)^2$$

$$\Rightarrow \lambda^2 + 4\lambda + 44 = 36 + \lambda^2 + 12\lambda$$

$$\Rightarrow \quad 8\lambda = 8$$

$$\Rightarrow \quad \lambda = 1$$

7. *Find λ when the projection of $\vec{a} = \lambda\hat{i} + \hat{j} + 4\hat{k}$ on $\vec{b} = (2\hat{i} + 6\hat{j} + 3\hat{k})$ is 4 units.*

SOLUTION. It is given that $\vec{a} = \lambda\hat{i} + \hat{j} + 4\hat{k}$ and $\vec{b} = (2\hat{i} + 6\hat{j} + 3\hat{k})$ and projection of $\vec{a}$ on $\vec{b}$ = 4 units.

Now, projection of $\vec{a}$ on $\vec{b} = \dfrac{(\vec{a} \cdot \vec{b})}{|\vec{b}|}$

$$\Rightarrow 4 = \frac{(\lambda\hat{i} + \hat{j} + 4\hat{k}) \cdot (2\hat{i} + 6\hat{j} + 3\hat{k})}{\sqrt{2^2 + 6^2 + 3^2}}$$

$$\Rightarrow 4 = \frac{(2\lambda + 6 + 12)}{\sqrt{4 + 36 + 9}}$$

$$\Rightarrow 4 = \frac{2\lambda + 18}{\sqrt{49}}$$

$$\Rightarrow 4 = \frac{2(\lambda + 9)}{7}$$

$$\Rightarrow 2(\lambda + 9) = 28$$

$$\Rightarrow \lambda + 9 = 14$$

$$\Rightarrow \lambda = 14 - 9 = 5$$

8. *Let $\vec{a} = \hat{i} + 4\hat{j} + 2\hat{k}, \vec{b} = 3\hat{i} - 2\hat{j} + 7\hat{k}$ and $\vec{c} = 2\hat{i} - \hat{j} + 4\hat{k}$. Find vector $\vec{p}$ which is perpendicular to both $\vec{a}$ and $\vec{b}$ and $\vec{p} \cdot \vec{c} = 18$.*

SOLUTION. Assume that $\vec{p} = (x\hat{i} + y\hat{j} + z\hat{k})$ and it is given that $\vec{p} \perp \vec{a}, \vec{p} \perp \vec{b}$ and $\vec{p} \cdot \vec{c} = 18$

$$\Rightarrow \vec{p} \cdot \vec{a} = 0, \vec{p} \cdot \vec{b} = 0 \text{ and } \vec{p} \cdot \vec{c} = 18$$

Now, $(x\hat{i} + y\hat{j} + z\hat{k}) \cdot (\hat{i} + 4\hat{j} + 2\hat{k}) = 0$

$$\Rightarrow \quad x + 4y + 2z = 0 \quad \ldots\text{(i)}$$

$$(x\hat{i} + y\hat{j} + z\hat{k}) \cdot (3\hat{i} - 2\hat{j} + 7\hat{k}) = 0$$

$\Rightarrow \quad 3x - 2y + 7z = 0 \quad \ldots(ii)$

$(x\hat{i} + y\hat{j} + z\hat{k})\cdot(2\hat{i} - \hat{j} + 4\hat{k}) = 0$

$\Rightarrow \quad 2x - y + 4z = 18 \quad \ldots(iii)$

From eqn. (i) and (ii)

$$\frac{x}{(28+4)} = \frac{y}{(6-7)} = \frac{z}{(-2-12)} = \lambda \text{ (say)}$$

$\Rightarrow x = 32\lambda,\ y = -\lambda$ and $z = -14\lambda$

Putting these values in eqn. (iii), we get

$64\lambda + \lambda - 56\lambda = 18 \Rightarrow 9\lambda = 18$

$\Rightarrow \quad \lambda = 2$

$x = 64,\ y = -2,\ z = -28$

Hence, the required vector

$$= 64\hat{i} - 2\hat{j} - 28\hat{k}$$

9. *If $\vec{a}$ and $\vec{b}$ are two unit vectors such that $\vec{a}+\vec{b}$ is also a unit vector, then find the angle between $\vec{a}$ and $\vec{b}$.*

SOLUTION. It is given that $\vec{a}$ and $\vec{b}$ are unit vectors, then we have $|\vec{a}| = 1$ and $|\vec{b}| = 1$.

and also $(\vec{a}+\vec{b})$ is a unit vector, then

$$|\vec{a}+\vec{b}|^2 = 1$$

$\Rightarrow \quad (\vec{a}+\vec{b})\cdot(\vec{a}+\vec{b}) = 1$

$\Rightarrow \vec{a}\cdot\vec{a} + \vec{a}\cdot\vec{b} + \vec{b}\cdot\vec{a} + \vec{b}\cdot\vec{b} = 1$

$\Rightarrow |\vec{a}|^2 + 2(\vec{a}\cdot\vec{b}) + |\vec{b}|^2 = 1,$

where $\vec{b}\cdot\vec{a} = \vec{a}\cdot\vec{b}$

$\Rightarrow \quad 2(\vec{a}\cdot\vec{b}) = -1$

$\Rightarrow \quad \vec{a}\cdot\vec{b} = -\frac{1}{2}$

$\Rightarrow \quad |\vec{a}|\cdot|\vec{b}|\cos\theta = -\frac{1}{2}$

(where θ is the angle between unit vectors $\vec{a}$ and $\vec{b}$)

$\Rightarrow \quad \cos\theta = -\frac{1}{2}$

$\Rightarrow \quad \theta = \frac{2\pi}{3}$

10. *If the vectors $\vec{a}$ and $\vec{b}$ are such that $|\vec{a}| = 3, |\vec{b}| = \frac{2}{3}$ and $\vec{a}\times\vec{b}$ is a unit vector then find the angle between $\vec{a}$ and $\vec{b}$.*

SOLUTION. Assume that θ be the angle between $\vec{a}$ and $\vec{b}$.

Then, we have

$$|\vec{a}\times\vec{b}| = 1$$

$\Rightarrow \quad |\vec{a}||\vec{b}|\sin\theta = 1$

$\Rightarrow \quad \left(3\times\frac{2}{3}\right)\sin\theta = 1$

$\Rightarrow \quad \sin\theta = \frac{1}{2}$

$\Rightarrow \quad \theta = 30°$

11. *Find λ and μ if $(\hat{i}+3\hat{j}+9\hat{k})\times(3\hat{i}-\lambda\hat{j}+\mu\hat{k}) = \vec{0}$.*

SOLUTION. Given, $(\hat{i}+3\hat{j}+9\hat{k})\times(3\hat{i}-\lambda\hat{j}+\mu\hat{k}) = \vec{0}$

i.e., $\begin{vmatrix} \hat{i} & \hat{j} & \hat{k} \\ 1 & 3 & 9 \\ 3 & -\lambda & \mu \end{vmatrix} = 0$

$\hat{i}(3\mu + 9\lambda) - \hat{j}(\mu - 27) + \hat{k}(-\lambda - 9)$

$= 0\hat{i} + 0\hat{j} + 0\hat{k}$

On comparing the coefficients of $\hat{i}, \hat{j}$ and $\hat{k}$, we get

$3\mu + 9\lambda = 0,\ -\mu + 27 = 0$

and $\quad -\lambda - 9 = 0$

Also, the value of μ and λ satisfy the equation $3\mu + 9\lambda = 0$

Hence, $\mu = 27$ and $\lambda = -9$.

Exercise-24.5

1. Show that the angle between $\vec{a} = 2\hat{i} + \hat{j} + 3\hat{k}$ and $\vec{b} = 3\hat{i} - 2\hat{j} + \hat{k}$ is 60°.
2. If $\vec{a} = \hat{i} + \hat{j} + \hat{k}$ and $\vec{b} = \hat{i} - \hat{j} + \hat{k}$, find the value of $\vec{a} \cdot \vec{b}$.
3. If $|\hat{a} + \hat{b}| = |\hat{a} - \hat{b}|$, show that $\hat{a}$ and $\hat{b}$ are mutually perpendicular.
4. Find the angle between the vectors $2\hat{i} + 3\hat{j} + 4\hat{k}$ and $2\hat{i} + 4\hat{j} - 4\hat{k}$.
5. If the position vectors of the point *A, B, C, D* are respectively given by $2\hat{i} + 4\hat{k}, 5\hat{i} + 3\sqrt{3}\hat{j} + 4\hat{k}, -2\sqrt{3}\hat{i} + \hat{k}, 6\hat{j} + \hat{k}$. Prove that *AB* and *CD* are parallel.
6. Prove that the triangle whose vertices are $2\hat{i} + 4\hat{j} - \hat{k}, 4\hat{i} + 5\hat{j} + \hat{k}$ and $3\hat{i} + 6\hat{j} - 3\hat{k}$ is an right angled isosceles triangle.
7. Prove that diagonals of a rhombus are mutually perpendicular.
8. Prove by vector method that in Δ*ABC*, the internal edge of $\angle A$ divide *BC* in the ratio of *AB* : *AC*.
9. Find the area of the triangle whose vertices are (1, 1, 2), (2, 3, 5) and (1, 5, 5). (NCERT)
10. Prove that three vectors given by $\vec{\alpha} = \hat{i} + 2\hat{j} + \hat{k}$, $\vec{\beta} = \hat{i} + \hat{j} - 3\hat{k}, \vec{\gamma} = 7\hat{i} - 4\hat{j} + \hat{k}$ are mutually perpendicular.
11. If $\vec{a} \times \vec{b} = \vec{c} \times \vec{d}$ and $\vec{a} \times \vec{c} = \vec{b} \times \vec{d}$, show that $\vec{a} - \vec{d}, \vec{b} - \vec{c}$ are parallel if $\vec{a} \neq \vec{d}, \vec{b} \neq \vec{c}$.
12. If $\vec{a}, \vec{b}, \vec{c}$ are the vertices of a triangle *ABC* show that area of Δ *ABC*
$$= \frac{1}{2}[\vec{b} \times \vec{c} + \vec{c} \times \vec{a} + \vec{a} \times \vec{b}]$$
Also, show that $\vec{a}, \vec{b}, \vec{c}$ will be collinear if $\vec{b} \times \vec{c} + \vec{c} \times \vec{a} + \vec{a} \times \vec{b} = 0$.
13. If *D, E, F* on the mid points of the side of Δ*ABC*, prove that $\Delta DEF = \frac{1}{4} \Delta ABC$.
14. Find the moment of the force $\vec{F} = 5\hat{i} + 10\hat{j} + 16\hat{k}$ acted on $2\hat{i} - 7\hat{j} + 10\hat{k}$ about the points $-5\hat{i} + 6\hat{j} - 10\hat{k}$.
15. A force of 6 unit acted on the line $\overrightarrow{AB}$ joining the points *A*(2, 1, 0) and *B*(3, –1, 2). Find the moment of force about the origin.
16. In Δ *ABC*, prove by vector method that $\frac{\sin A}{a} = \frac{\sin B}{b} = \frac{\sin C}{c}$

Hint to Selected Problems

1. Use $\cos\theta = \frac{\vec{a} \cdot \vec{b}}{|\vec{a}| \cdot |\vec{b}|}$

3. $|\vec{a} + \vec{b}| = |\vec{a} - \vec{b}| \Rightarrow |\vec{a} + \vec{b}|^2 = |\vec{a} - \vec{b}|^2$

$\Rightarrow (\vec{a} + \vec{b}) \cdot (\vec{a} + \vec{b}) = (\vec{a} - \vec{b}) \cdot (\vec{a} - \vec{b})$

Now simplify to get $\vec{a} \cdot \vec{b} = 0$

5. $\overrightarrow{AB} = (5\hat{i} + 3\sqrt{3}\hat{j} + 4\hat{k}) - (2\hat{i} - 4\hat{k})$

$= 3\hat{i} + 3\sqrt{3}\hat{j}$

$\overrightarrow{CD} = (6\hat{j} + \hat{k}) - (-2\sqrt{3}\hat{i} + \hat{k}) = 2\sqrt{3}\hat{i} + 6\hat{j}$

Now prove that $\overrightarrow{AB} \times \overrightarrow{CD} = 0$

9. Let $A = (1,1,2), B = (2,3,5)$ and $C = (1, 5, 5)$

$\overrightarrow{AB} = (2\hat{i} + 3\hat{j} + 5\hat{k}) - (\hat{i} + \hat{j} + 2\hat{k})$

$= \hat{i} + 2\hat{j} + 3\hat{k}$

$\overrightarrow{AC} = (\hat{i} + 5\hat{j} + 5\hat{k}) - (\hat{i} + \hat{j} + 2\hat{k})$

$= 4\hat{j} + 3\hat{k}$

Now, Area of $\Delta ABC = \frac{1}{2}|\overrightarrow{AB} \times \overrightarrow{AC}|$

11. Prove that $(\vec{a} - \vec{d}) \times (\vec{b} - \vec{c}) = 0$

ANSWERS

2. –1 **4.** $\theta = 90°$ **9.** $\frac{1}{2}\sqrt{61}$ square unit **14.** $-408\hat{i} - 12\hat{j} + 135\hat{k}$ **15.** $4\hat{i} - 8\hat{j} - 10\hat{k}$

24.46 SCALAR TRIPLE PRODUCT

Let $\vec{a},\vec{b},\vec{c}$ be three vectors, then $\vec{a}\cdot(\vec{b}\times\vec{c})$ is called scalar triple product and $\vec{a}\times(\vec{b}\times\vec{c})$ is called vector triple product.

- The scalar triple product $\vec{a}\cdot(\vec{b}\times\vec{c})$ in which three vectors make an ordered triads can be represented by $[\underline{a},\underline{b},\underline{c}]$ or $[\vec{a},\vec{b},\vec{c}]$.

24.47 SCALAR TRIPLE PRODUCT IN TERMS OF THE COMPONENTS OF THE VECTORS

Let $\quad \vec{a}=a_1\hat{i}+a_2\hat{j}+a_3\hat{k}$

$\vec{b}=b_1\hat{i}+b_2\hat{j}+b_3\hat{k}$

and $\quad \vec{c}=c_1\hat{i}+c_2\hat{j}+c_3\hat{k}$

Then $\quad \vec{b}\times\vec{c}=(b_1\hat{i}+b_2\hat{j}+b_3\hat{k})\times(c_1\hat{i}+c_2\hat{j}+c_3\hat{k})$

$=(b_2c_3-b_3c_2)i+(b_3c_1-b_1c_3)\hat{j}+(b_1c_2-b_2c_1)\hat{k}$

Therefore, $\quad \vec{a}\cdot(\vec{b}\times\vec{c})=(a_1\hat{i}+a_2\hat{j}+a_3\hat{k})\cdot[(b_2c_3-b_3c_2)\hat{i}+(b_3c_1-b_1c_3)\hat{j}+(b_1c_2-b_2c_1)\hat{k}]$

$=a_1(b_2c_3-b_3c_2)+a_2(b_3c_1-b_1c_3)+a_3(b_1c_2-b_2c_1)$

i.e., $\quad \vec{a}\cdot(\vec{b}\times\vec{c})=\begin{vmatrix}a_1 & a_2 & a_3\\ b_1 & b_2 & b_3\\ c_1 & c_2 & c_3\end{vmatrix}$

24.48 GEOMETRICAL INTERPRETATION OF SCALAR TRIPLE PRODUCT

Statement: *If the three concurrent edges of a parallelopiped be represented by $\vec{a},\vec{b}$ and $\vec{c}$ respectively. Then scalar triple product of $\vec{a},\vec{b}$ and $\vec{c}$ represent the volume of the parallelopiped.*

Verification: Let $\overrightarrow{OA}=\vec{a},\overrightarrow{OB}=\vec{b}$ and $\overrightarrow{OC}=\vec{c}$ be three non-zero vectors. We know that $\vec{a}\times\vec{b}$ is a vector quantity whose direction is that of the unit vector $\hat{n}$.

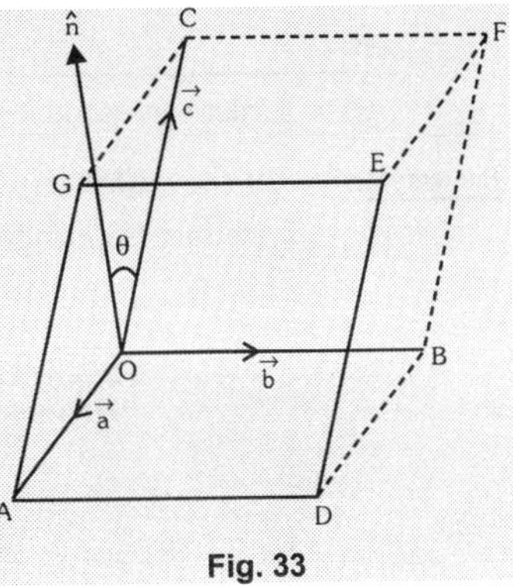

Fig. 33

Let angle between $(\vec{a}\times\vec{b})$ and $\vec{c}$ be θ. Then scalar triple product of vectors $\vec{a},\vec{b}$ and $\vec{c}$ is represented by $(\vec{a}\times\vec{b})\cdot\vec{c}$ or $[\vec{a}\vec{b}\vec{c}]$.

Now $\quad [\vec{a}\vec{b}\vec{c}]=(\vec{a}\times\vec{b})\cdot\vec{c}=|\vec{a}\times\vec{b}|\,|\vec{c}|\cos\theta \quad$ ...(i)

∴ Volume of the parallelopiped

= Area of the parallelogram *OADB* × height of the parallelopiped

$=(|\vec{a}\times\vec{b}|)\times(OC\cos\theta)=|\vec{a}\times\vec{b}|\,|\vec{c}|\cos\theta \quad$ ...(ii)

From eqns. (i) and (ii), we conclude that $[\vec{a}\vec{b}\vec{c}]=$ Volume of the parallelopiped

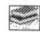

- If θ is an acute angle, then value of $[\vec{a},\vec{b},\vec{c}]$ is positive.
- If θ is an obtuse angle, then the value of $[\vec{a},\vec{b},\vec{c}]$ is negative.

24.49 PROPERTIES OF A SCALAR TRIPLE PRODUCT

PROPERTY 1. *In the scalar triple product the positions of the dot and cross can be interchanged without changing the value of the product provided the cyclic order of the vectors is maintained.*

PROOF. By definition of scalar triple product, we have

$$(\vec{a}\times\vec{b})\cdot\vec{c} = [(a_2b_3 - a_3b_2)\hat{i} + (a_3b_1 - a_1b_3)\hat{j} + (a_1b_2 - a_2b_1)\hat{k}]\cdot(c_1\hat{i} + c_2\hat{j} + c_3\hat{k})$$

$$= (a_2b_3 - a_3b_2)c_1 + (a_3b_1 - a_1b_3)c_2 + (a_1b_2 - a_2b_1)c_3$$

$$= \begin{vmatrix} c_1 & c_2 & c_3 \\ a_1 & a_2 & a_3 \\ b_1 & b_2 & b_3 \end{vmatrix} = -\begin{vmatrix} a_1 & a_2 & a_3 \\ c_1 & c_2 & c_3 \\ b_1 & b_2 & b_3 \end{vmatrix} \quad \text{(On interchanging } R_1 \text{ and } R_2\text{)}$$

$$= (-1)^2\begin{vmatrix} a_1 & a_2 & a_3 \\ b_1 & b_2 & b_3 \\ c_1 & c_2 & c_3 \end{vmatrix} \quad \text{(On interchanging } R_2 \text{ and } R_3\text{)}$$

$$= \begin{vmatrix} a_1 & a_2 & a_3 \\ b_1 & b_2 & b_3 \\ c_1 & c_2 & c_3 \end{vmatrix} = \vec{a}\cdot(\vec{b}\times\vec{c})$$

i.e., $(\vec{a}\times\vec{b})\cdot\vec{c} = \vec{a}\cdot(\vec{b}\times\vec{c})$

⇒ There is no change by interchanging the dot and cross sign.

- Scalar triple product can be written as $[\vec{a}\vec{b}\vec{c}]$ due to the above result.

PROPERTY 2. *In the scalar triple product for every change in cyclic order of the vectors, the value of the product is changed in sign though, not in magnitude.*

PROOF. Let $\vec{a},\vec{b},\vec{c}$ be three vectors, then

$$[\vec{a}\vec{b}\vec{c}] = (\vec{a}\times\vec{b})\cdot\vec{c} = -(\vec{b}\times\vec{a})\cdot\vec{c} \quad (\because \vec{a}\times\vec{b} = -\vec{b}\times\vec{a})$$

$$= -[\vec{b}\vec{a}\vec{c}] = -[\vec{b}\cdot(\vec{a}\times\vec{c})] = (-1)^2[\vec{b}\cdot(\vec{c}\times\vec{a})] \quad (\because \vec{a}\times\vec{c} = -\vec{c}\times\vec{a})$$

$$= [\vec{b}\vec{c}\vec{a}]$$

and
$$[\vec{a}\vec{b}\vec{c}] = \vec{a}\cdot(\vec{b}\times\vec{c}) = -\vec{a}\cdot(\vec{c}\times\vec{b}) = -[\vec{a}\vec{c}\vec{b}]$$

$$= -[(\vec{a}\times\vec{c})\cdot\vec{b}] = (-1)^2[(\vec{c}\times\vec{a})\cdot\vec{b}] = [\vec{c}\vec{a}\vec{b}]$$

Hence, it is clear that

$$[\vec{a}\vec{b}\vec{c}] = [\vec{b}\vec{c}\vec{a}] = [\vec{c}\vec{a}\vec{b}]$$

and
$$[\vec{a}\vec{b}\vec{c}] = -[\vec{b}\vec{a}\vec{c}] = -[\vec{a}\vec{c}\vec{b}]$$

PROPERTY 3. *If any two vectors of $\vec{a},\vec{b},\vec{c}$ are equal then their scalar triple product is zero.*

PROOF. We know that $[\vec{a}\vec{b}\vec{c}] = \begin{vmatrix} a_1 & a_2 & a_3 \\ b_1 & b_2 & b_3 \\ c_1 & c_2 & c_3 \end{vmatrix}$

If $\vec{a} = \vec{b}$, then

$$[\vec{a}\vec{a}\vec{c}] = \begin{vmatrix} a_1 & a_2 & a_3 \\ a_1 & a_2 & a_3 \\ c_1 & c_2 & c_3 \end{vmatrix} = 0 \quad \text{(Two columns of the determinant are equal)}$$

Similarly, we may prove that

$$[\vec{a}\vec{b}\vec{a}] = [\vec{a}\vec{b}\vec{b}] = 0$$

PROPERTY 4. *The scalar triple product of unit vectors is* 1.

i.e., $[\hat{i}\hat{j}\hat{k}] = [\hat{j}\hat{k}\hat{i}] = [\hat{k}\hat{i}\hat{j}] = 1$

PROPERTY 5. *If any two vectors are parallel then their scalar triple product is* 0.

24.50 CONDITION FOR THREE NON-PARALLEL, NON-ZERO VECTORS TO BE COPLANAR

THEOREM. *The necessary and sufficient condition for non-parallel and non-zero vectors $\vec{a}, \vec{b}$ and $\vec{c}$ are coplanar is $[\vec{a}, \vec{b}, \vec{c}] = 0$.*

PROOF. We know that if three vectors $\vec{a}, \vec{b}, \vec{c}$ are coplanar then volume of the parallelopiped whose three concurrent edges are represented by $\vec{a}, \vec{b}, \vec{c}$ is zero. Hence we can say that the condition that the three non-parallel and non-zero vectors may be coplanar is that their scalar triple product is zero, *i.e.*,$[\vec{a}\vec{b}\vec{c}] = 0$.

Conversely, if $[\vec{a}\vec{b}\vec{c}] = 0$ then $\vec{a} \cdot (\vec{b} \times \vec{c}) = 0$, *i.e.*, $\vec{a}$ is perpendicular to $(\vec{b} \times \vec{c})$ but by definition of cross product $(\vec{b} \times \vec{c})$ is perpendicular to both $\vec{b}$ and $\vec{c}$. Thus, $\vec{a}$ must lie in the plane of $\vec{b}$ and $\vec{c}$. Hence, $\vec{a}, \vec{b}$ and $\vec{c}$ are coplanar.

24.51 VECTOR TRIPLE PRODUCT

Let $\vec{a}, \vec{b}$ and $\vec{c}$ be three vectors, then vectors $[\vec{a} \times (\vec{b} \times \vec{c})]$ and $[(\vec{a} \times \vec{b}) \times \vec{c}]$ are called the vector triple product of vectors $\vec{a}, \vec{b}$ and $\vec{c}$.

Solved Examples

1. *If* $\vec{a} = \hat{i} - \hat{j} - 6\hat{k}, \vec{b} = \hat{i} - \hat{j} + 4\hat{k}$ *and* $\vec{c} = 2\hat{i} - 5\hat{j} + 3\hat{k}$, *find the value of* $[\vec{a}\vec{b}\vec{c}]$.

SOLUTION. By definition of scalar triple product, we have

$$[\vec{a}\vec{b}\vec{c}] = \begin{vmatrix} 1 & -1 & -6 \\ 1 & -1 & 4 \\ 2 & -5 & 3 \end{vmatrix}$$

$$= \begin{vmatrix} 0 & 0 & -10 \\ 1 & -1 & 4 \\ 2 & -5 & 3 \end{vmatrix} \quad (R_1 \to R_1 - R_2)$$

$= 30$

2. *If* $\vec{a} = \hat{i} + \hat{j} - \hat{k}, \vec{b} = 2\hat{i} + \hat{j} + 2\hat{k}$ *and* $\vec{c} = 3\hat{i} + \hat{j} + 3\hat{k}$, *find the value of* $(\vec{a} \times \vec{b}) \cdot \vec{c}$.

SOLUTION. By definition of scalar triple product

$$(\vec{a}\times\vec{b})\cdot\vec{c} = \begin{vmatrix} 1 & 1 & -1 \\ 2 & 1 & 2 \\ 3 & 1 & 3 \end{vmatrix}$$

$= 1(3-2) - 1(6-6) - 1(2-3)$
$= 1 - 0 + 1 = 2$

3. *If $\vec{a},\vec{b},\vec{c}$ be three vectors, prove that*

$$[\vec{a}+\vec{b}\;\vec{b}+\vec{c}\;\vec{c}+\vec{a}] = 2[\vec{a}\vec{b}\vec{c}]$$

SOLUTION. L.H.S.

$= [\vec{a}+\vec{b}\;\vec{b}+\vec{c}\;\vec{c}+\vec{a}]$

$= (\vec{a}+\vec{b})\cdot[(\vec{b}+\vec{c})\times(\vec{c}\times\vec{a})]$

$= (\vec{a}+\vec{b})\cdot[\vec{b}\times\vec{c}+\vec{b}\times\vec{a}+\vec{c}\times\vec{c}+\vec{c}\times\vec{a}]$

$= (\vec{a}+\vec{b})\cdot[\vec{b}\times\vec{c}-\vec{a}\times\vec{b}+0+\vec{c}\times\vec{a}]$

$(\because\; \vec{a}\times\vec{b} = -\vec{b}\times\vec{a}$ and $\vec{c}\times\vec{c} = 0)$

$= (\vec{a}+\vec{b})\cdot[\vec{b}\times\vec{c}-\vec{a}\times\vec{b}+\vec{c}\times\vec{a}]$

$= \vec{a}\cdot(\vec{b}\times\vec{c}) - \vec{a}\cdot(\vec{a}\times\vec{b}) + \vec{a}\cdot(\vec{c}\times\vec{a})$
$\quad + \vec{b}\cdot(\vec{b}\times\vec{c}) - \vec{b}\cdot(\vec{a}\times\vec{b}) + \vec{b}\cdot(\vec{c}\times\vec{a})$

$= [\vec{a}\vec{b}\vec{c}] - [\vec{a}\vec{a}\vec{b}] + [\vec{a}\vec{c}\vec{a}] + [\vec{b}\vec{b}\vec{c}]$
$\quad - [\vec{b}\vec{a}\vec{b}] + [\vec{b}\vec{c}\vec{a}]$

$= [\vec{a}\vec{b}\vec{c}] - 0 + 0 + 0 - 0 + [\vec{b}\vec{c}\vec{a}]$

$[\because\; [\vec{a}\vec{a}\vec{b}] = [\vec{a}\vec{c}\vec{a}] = [\vec{b}\vec{b}\vec{c}]$
$= [\vec{b}\vec{a}\vec{b}] = 0\,]$

$= [\vec{a}\vec{b}\vec{c}] + [\vec{b}\vec{c}\vec{a}] = [\vec{a}\vec{b}\vec{c}] + [\vec{a}\vec{b}\vec{c}]$

$= 2[\vec{a}\vec{b}\vec{c}] =$ R.H.S.

4. *Prove that the vectors $\hat{i}-2\hat{j}+3\hat{k}$, $-2\hat{i}+3\hat{j}-4\hat{k}$ and $\hat{i}-3\hat{j}+5\hat{k}$ are coplanar.*

SOLUTION. Let, $\vec{a} = \hat{i}-2\hat{j}+3\hat{k}$

$\vec{b} = -2\hat{i}+3\hat{j}-4\hat{k}$

and $\vec{c} = \hat{i}-3\hat{j}+5\hat{k}$

For three vectors to be coplanar, we have $[\vec{a}\vec{b}\vec{c}] = 0$

Therefore,

$$[\vec{a}\vec{b}\vec{c}] = \begin{vmatrix} 1 & -2 & 3 \\ -2 & 3 & -4 \\ 1 & -3 & 5 \end{vmatrix}$$

$= 1(15-12) - (-2)(-10+4) + 3(6-3)$

$= 3 + 2(-6) + 3(3) = 3 - 12 + 9 = 0$

$\Rightarrow [\vec{a}\vec{b}\vec{c}] = 0$

Hence, $\vec{a},\vec{b},\vec{c}$ are coplanar.

5. *Prove that the four points A, B, C, D represented by $(4,5,1), (0,-1,-1)$, $(3,9,4)$ and $(-4,4,4)$ are coplanar.*

SOLUTION. Let O be the origin, then

$\overrightarrow{OA} = 4\hat{i}-5\hat{j}+\hat{k}$

$\overrightarrow{OB} = 0\hat{i}-\hat{j}-\hat{k}$

$\overrightarrow{OC} = 3\hat{i}+9\hat{j}+4\hat{k}$

$\overrightarrow{OD} = -4\hat{i}+4\hat{j}+4\hat{k}$

Now, $\overrightarrow{AB} = \overrightarrow{OB} - \overrightarrow{OA}$

$= (0\hat{i}-\hat{j}-\hat{k}) - (4\hat{i}+5\hat{j}+\hat{k})$

$= -4\hat{i}-6\hat{j}-2\hat{k} = \vec{u}$ (say)

$\overrightarrow{AC} = \overrightarrow{OC} - \overrightarrow{OA}$

$= (3\hat{i}+9\hat{j}+4\hat{k}) - (4\hat{i}+5\hat{j}+\hat{k})$

$= -\hat{i}+4\hat{j}+3\hat{k} = \vec{v}$ (say)

$\overrightarrow{AD} = \overrightarrow{OD} - \overrightarrow{OA}$

$= (-4\hat{i}+4\hat{j}+4\hat{k}) - (4\hat{i}+5\hat{j}+\hat{k})$

$= -8\hat{i}-\hat{j}+3\hat{k} = \vec{w}$ (say)

The four points A, B, C, D will be coplanar if the vector $\overrightarrow{AB}, \overrightarrow{AC}$ and $\overrightarrow{AD}$, *i.e.*, $\vec{u},\vec{v}$ and $\vec{w}$ are coplanar.

$\therefore \qquad [\vec{u}\vec{v}\vec{w}] = 0$

$$\text{Now, } [\vec{u}\vec{v}\vec{w}] = \begin{vmatrix} -4 & -6 & -2 \\ -1 & 4 & 3 \\ -8 & -1 & 3 \end{vmatrix}$$

$= -4(12+3) + 6(-3+24) - 2(1+32)$

$= -60 + 126 - 66 = 0$

$\Rightarrow$ *A*, *B*, *C* and *D* are coplanar.

6. *Prove the following*

$\hat{i}\times(\vec{a}\times\hat{i})+\hat{j}\times(\vec{a}\times\hat{j})+\hat{k}\times(\vec{a}\times\hat{k})=2\vec{a}$

SOLUTION. We know that

$\vec{a}\times(\vec{b}\times\vec{c})=(\vec{a}\cdot\vec{c})\vec{b}-(\vec{a}\cdot\vec{b})\vec{c}$

$\therefore\ \hat{i}\times(\vec{a}\times\hat{i})=(\hat{i}\cdot\hat{i})\vec{a}-(\hat{i}\cdot\vec{a})\hat{i}$

$=\vec{a}-(\hat{i}\cdot\vec{a})\hat{i} \quad (\because \hat{i}\cdot\hat{i}=1)$ ...(i)

Similarly, $\hat{j}\times(\vec{a}\times\hat{j})=\vec{a}-(\hat{j}\cdot\vec{a})\hat{j}$ ...(ii)

and $\hat{k}\times(\vec{a}\times\hat{k})=\vec{a}-(\hat{k}\cdot\vec{a})\hat{k}$ ...(iii)

On adding eqns. (i), (ii) and (iii), we get

$\hat{i}\times(\vec{a}\times\hat{i})+\hat{j}\times(\vec{a}\times\hat{j})+\hat{k}\times(\vec{a}\times\hat{k})$

$=3\vec{a}-[(\hat{i}\cdot\vec{a})\hat{i}+(\hat{j}\cdot\vec{a})\hat{j}+(\hat{k}\cdot\vec{a})\hat{k}]$ ...(iv)

Let $\vec{a}=l\hat{i}+m\hat{j}+n\hat{k}$ ...(v)

then $\hat{i}\cdot\vec{a}=\hat{i}\cdot[l\hat{i}+m\hat{j}+n\hat{k}]$

$=l(\hat{i}\cdot\hat{i})+m(\hat{i}\cdot\hat{j})+n(\hat{i}\cdot\hat{k})$

$=l\cdot 1+m\cdot 0+n\cdot 0=l$

Similarly, $\hat{j}\cdot\vec{a}=m$ and $\hat{k}\cdot\vec{a}=n$

$\therefore$ from (v)

$\vec{a}=(\hat{i}\cdot\vec{a})\hat{i}+(\hat{j}\cdot\vec{a})\hat{j}+(\hat{k}\cdot\vec{a})\hat{k}$ ...(vi)

Using (vi) in (iv), we get

$\hat{i}\times(\vec{a}\times\hat{i})+\hat{j}\times(\vec{a}\times\hat{j})+\hat{k}\times(\vec{a}\times\hat{k})$

$=3\vec{a}-\vec{a}=2\vec{a}$

Exercise-24.6

1. Find the value of $\vec{c}\cdot(\vec{a}\times\vec{b})$ if $\vec{a}=5\hat{i}-4\hat{j}+\hat{k}$, $\vec{b}=-4\hat{i}+3\hat{j}-2\hat{k}, \vec{c}=\hat{i}-2\hat{j}-7\hat{k}$.
2. Prove that the points (1, 0, 0), (0, 1, 0), (0, 0, 1) and (1, 1, –1) are coplanar.
3. Prove that $[\hat{i}\,\hat{j}\,\hat{k}]=1$.
4. Find the value of $(2\hat{i}-3\hat{j})\cdot\{(\hat{i}+\hat{j}-\hat{k})\times(3\hat{i}-\hat{k})\}$
5. Find the value of $[\vec{a}\,\vec{b}\,\vec{c}]$ if
   (i) $\vec{a}=2\hat{i}+\hat{j}-3\hat{k}, \vec{b}=-\hat{i}+\hat{j}+2\hat{k}, \vec{c}=4\hat{i}+3\hat{k}$
   (ii) $\vec{a}=3\hat{i}-2\hat{j}+2\hat{k}, \vec{b}=6\hat{i}+4\hat{j}-2\hat{k}, \vec{c}=-3\hat{i}-2\hat{j}-4\hat{k}$
   (iii) $\vec{a}=\hat{i}+\hat{j}+\hat{k}, \vec{b}=\hat{i}-\hat{j}+\hat{k}, \vec{c}=\hat{i}+2\hat{j}-\hat{k}$
6. Find the value of $\vec{a}$ if the vectors $2\hat{i}-\hat{j}+\hat{k}$, $\hat{i}+2\hat{j}-3\hat{k}$ and $3\hat{i}+a\hat{j}+2\hat{k}$ are coplanar?
7. Find the value of λ if the vectors $2\hat{i}-\hat{j}+\hat{k}$, $\hat{i}+2\hat{j}-3\hat{k}$ and $3\hat{i}-\lambda\hat{j}+2\hat{k}$ are coplanar?
8. If $\vec{a},\vec{b},\vec{c}$ are mutually perpendicular vectors, prove that $[a\,b\,c]^2=a^2b^2c^2$
9. Prove that four points represented by $6\hat{i}-4\hat{j}+10\hat{k}$, $5\hat{i}-3\hat{j}+10\hat{k}, 4\hat{i}-6\hat{j}+10\hat{k}$, $2\hat{j}+10\hat{k}$ are coplanar.
10. If four points A, B, C, D represented by $3\hat{i}-2\hat{j}-\hat{k}$, $2\hat{i}+3\hat{j}-4\hat{k}$, $-\hat{i}+\hat{j}+2\hat{k}$, $4\hat{i}+5\hat{j}+\lambda\hat{k}$ are coplanar, find the value of λ.

Hint to Selected Problems

1. $\vec{a}\times\vec{b}=\begin{vmatrix}\hat{i} & \hat{j} & \hat{k}\\ 5 & -4 & 1\\ -4 & 3 & -2\end{vmatrix}=5\hat{i}+6\hat{j}-\hat{k}$

Now $\vec{c}\cdot(\vec{a}\times\vec{b})=(\hat{i}-2\hat{j}-7\hat{k})\cdot(5\hat{i}+6\hat{j}-\hat{k})$

$=1\cdot 5+(-2)6+(-7)(-1)$

3. $[\hat{i}\,\hat{j}\,\hat{k}]=\hat{i}\cdot[\hat{j}\times\hat{k}]=\hat{i}\cdot\hat{i}=1$

5. Use $[\vec{a}\,\vec{b}\,\vec{c}]=\begin{vmatrix}a_1 & a_2 & a_3\\ b_1 & b_2 & b_3\\ c_1 & c_2 & c_3\end{vmatrix}$

6. The condition of coplanarity of three vectors is given by

First vector = A(second vector) + B(third vector)

$\Rightarrow (2\hat{i}-\hat{j}+\hat{k})=A(\hat{i}+2\hat{j}-3\hat{k}) + B(3\hat{i}+a\hat{j}+5\hat{k})$

Now comparing the coefficient of $\hat{i}, \hat{j}$ and $\hat{k}$ on both the sides.

7. Same as question (6)

$\Rightarrow (2\hat{i} - \hat{j} + \hat{k}) = A(\hat{i} + 2\hat{j} - 3\hat{k})$

$$+ B(3\hat{i} - \lambda\hat{j} + 2\hat{k})$$

Now, comparing the coefficient of $\hat{i}, \hat{j}$ and $\hat{k}$ on both the sides.

9. For scalar values 1, λ, μ and ν

We can write

$(6\hat{i} - 4\hat{j} + 10\hat{k})\cdot 1 + \lambda(5\hat{i} - 3\hat{j} + 10\hat{k})$

$$+ \mu(4\hat{i} - 6\hat{j} + 10\hat{k}) + \nu(2\hat{j} + 10\hat{k}) = 0\hat{i} + 0\hat{j} + 0\hat{k}$$

Now, comparing the coefficients of $\hat{i}, \hat{j}$ and $\hat{k}$ on both the sides.

ANSWERS

1. 0 **4.** 4 **5.** (i) 29 (ii) –120 (iii) 4 **6.** – 4 **7.** $\frac{13}{7}$ **10.** $\lambda = -\frac{146}{17}$

❑❑❑❑❑❑

Chapter

25 Vector Calculus

25.1 SCALAR FUNCTION

Since we know that the quantity which is associated with the magnitude but not associated with direction is known as scalar quantity. Therefore every real number is a scalar quantity.

Let D be a subset of a set of real numbers. Then a function f defined over the subset D such that for all $t \in D$, $f(t)$ is obtained as a scalar quantity, is called a scalar function.

25.2 VECTOR FUNCTION

If the scalar fucntion $f(t)$ for all $t \in D$ is associated with some direction then this function is called a vector function and is therefore, denoted by $\vec{f}\,(t)$ or $\vec{f}$.

Let $f_1(t)$, $f_2(t)$, $f_3(t)$ be three components of a vector function $\vec{f}\,(t)$, then this function can be uniquely expressed as a linear combination of these three fixed non-coplanar vectors $f_1(t)\hat{i}, f_2(t)\hat{j}, f_3(t)\hat{k}$.

$$\therefore \qquad \vec{f}(t) = f_1(t)\hat{i} + f_2(t)\hat{j} + f_3(t)\hat{k}$$

where $\hat{i}, \hat{j}, \hat{k}$ are three mutually perpendicular non-coplanar unit vectors.

25.3 SCALAR AND VECTOR FIELDS

Scalar fields. A scalar point function f defined over some region R such that to each point $P(x, y, z)$ in space, there corresponds a unique scalar $f(P)$, is called a scalar field. For example

$$f(x, y, z) = x^2 + y^2 + z^2 - 3xyz.$$

Vector fields. A vector point function f defined over a region R such that to each point $P(x, y, z)$ there exists a unique vector $\vec{f}\,(P)$, is called vector field. For example

$$\vec{f}(x, y, z) = x^2y\hat{i} + x^3z\hat{j} - y^3z\hat{k}.$$

25.4 LIMIT AND CONTINUITY OF A VECTOR FUNCTION

Limit. A vector function $f(t)$ is said to have the limit l as t tends to t_0, for given $\varepsilon > 0$ there exists a positive number δ such that

$$\left|\vec{f}(t) - l\right| < \varepsilon \text{ whenever } 0 < |t - t_0| < \delta \text{ i.e., } \lim_{t \to t_0} \vec{f}(t) = l.$$

Continuity. A vector function $\vec{f}\,(t)$ is said to be continuous at t_0, if for given $\varepsilon > 0$ there must exists a positive number δ such that

$$\left|\vec{f}(t) - \vec{f}(t_0)\right| < \varepsilon \text{ whenever } |t - t_0| < \delta, \text{provided } \vec{f}\,(t_0) \text{ is defined.}$$

- A vector function $\vec{f}\,(t)$ is said to be continuous for every value of t in the domain over which $\mathbf{f}(t)$ is defined.

25.5 SOME RESULTS RELATED TO THE LIMIT AND CONTINUITY OF A VECTOR FUNCTION

1. The necessary and sufficient condition for a vcector function $\vec{f}$ (t) to be continuous at t_0 is that $\lim_{t \to t_0} \vec{f}(t) = \vec{f}(t_0)$.

2. If $\vec{f}(t) = f_1(t)\hat{i} + f_2(t)\hat{j} + f_3(t)\hat{k}$, then $\vec{f}(t)$ is continuous iff $f_1(t), f_2(t), f_3(t)$ are continuous.

3. If $\vec{f}(t) = f_1(t)\hat{i} + f_2(t)\hat{j} + f_3(t)\hat{k}$ and $\vec{l} = l_1\hat{i} + l_2\hat{j} + l_3\hat{k}$, then $\lim_{t \to t_0} \vec{f}(t) = \vec{l}$ iff $\lim_{t \to t_0} f_1(t) = l_1$, $\lim_{t \to t_0} f_2(t) = l_2$ and $\lim_{t \to t_0} f_3(t) = l_3$.

4. If $\vec{f}$ (t) and $\vec{g}$ (t) are vector functions of scalar variable t and $\phi(t)$ is a scalar function, then

(i) $\lim_{t \to t_0} [\vec{f}(t) \pm \vec{g}(t)] = \lim_{t \to t_0} \vec{f}(t) \pm \lim_{t \to t_0} \vec{g}(t)$

(ii) $\lim_{t \to t_0} [\vec{f}(t).\vec{g}(t)] = \left[\lim_{t \to t_0} \vec{f}(t)\right].\left[\lim_{t \to t_0} \vec{g}(t)\right]$

(iii) $\lim_{t \to t_0} [\vec{f}(t) \times \vec{g}(t)] = \left[\lim_{t \to t_0} \vec{f}(t)\right] \times \left[\lim_{t \to t_0} \vec{g}(t)\right]$

(iv) $\lim_{t \to t_0} \left|\vec{f}(t)\right| = \left|\lim_{t \to t_0} \vec{f}(t)\right|$

(v) $\lim_{t \to t_0} [\phi(t)\vec{f}(t)] = \left[\lim_{t \to t_0} \phi(t)\right]\left[\lim_{t \to t_0} \vec{f}(t)\right]$.

25.6 DIFFERENTIATION OF A VECTOR FUNCTION WITH RESPECT TO A SCALAR

Definition (1) *Let $\vec{f}$ (t) be a vector function of scalar variable t. The function $\vec{f}$ (t) is differentiable with respect to t if* $\lim_{\delta t \to 0} \frac{\vec{f}(t+\delta t) - \vec{f}(t)}{\delta t}$ *exists.*

and it is denoted by $\frac{d\vec{f}(t)}{dt}$.

Definition (2). *If $\frac{d\vec{f}(t)}{dt}$ exists, then $\vec{f}$ (t) is differentiable and $\frac{d\vec{f}(t)}{dt}$ is also a vector function of variable t. If $\frac{d\vec{f}(t)}{dt}$ is differentiable, then $\frac{d^2\vec{f}(t)}{dt^2}$ is called second derivative of $\vec{f}$ (t). Similarly we can find third, fourth, etc. derivaties of $\vec{f}$ (t).*

- If $\vec{r} = \vec{f}(t)$, then $\frac{d\vec{r}}{dt}, \frac{d^2\vec{r}}{dt^2}$, etc. are the first, second etc. derivaties of $r = \vec{f}$ (t) and also denoted by $\dot{\mathbf{r}}, \ddot{\mathbf{r}}$ respectively etc.

25.7 DIFFERENTIATION FORMULAE FOR THE VECTOR FUNCTION

Let $\vec{a}, \vec{b}, \vec{c}$ be differentiable vector function of a scalar variable f and ϕ be a differentiable scalar function of t, then

(i) $\frac{d}{dt}(\vec{a} \pm \vec{b}) = \frac{d\vec{a}}{dt} \pm \frac{d\vec{b}}{dt}$

(ii) $\frac{d}{dt}(\vec{a}.\vec{b}) = \vec{a}.\frac{d\vec{b}}{dt} + \frac{d\vec{a}}{dt}.\vec{b}$

(iii) $\frac{d}{dt}(\vec{a} \times \vec{b}) = \vec{a} \times \frac{d\vec{b}}{dt} + \frac{d\vec{a}}{dt} \times \vec{b}$

(iv) $\frac{d}{dt}(\phi\vec{a}) = \phi\frac{d\vec{a}}{dt} + \frac{d\phi}{dt}\vec{a}$

(v) $\frac{d}{dt}[\vec{a}\,\vec{b}\,\vec{c}] = \left[\frac{d\vec{a}}{dt}\vec{b}\,\vec{c}\right] + \left[\vec{a}\frac{d\vec{b}}{dt}\vec{c}\right] + \left[\vec{a}\,\vec{b}\frac{d\vec{c}}{dt}\right]$

(vi) $\frac{d}{dt}\{\vec{a}\times(\vec{b}\times\vec{c})\} = \frac{d\vec{a}}{dt}\times(\vec{b}\times\vec{c}) + \vec{a}\times\left[\frac{d\vec{b}}{dt}\times\vec{c}\right] + \vec{a}\times\left[\vec{b}\times\frac{d\vec{c}}{dt}\right].$

25.8 DERIVATIVE OF A CONSTANT VECTOR

Definition. *A vector is said to be constant vector if its magnitude as well as direction are fixed.*

Let $\vec{r}$ be a constant vector, then $\vec{r} = \vec{c}$ (a constant vector) ...(1)

$\therefore$ $\vec{r} + \delta\vec{r} = \vec{c}$. ...(2)

Subtract (1) from (2), we get $\delta\vec{r} = 0$.

Divide by δt and taking the limit as $\delta t \to 0$, we get $\lim_{\delta t\to 0}\frac{\delta\vec{r}}{\delta t} = 0$ or $\frac{d\vec{r}}{dt} = 0$.

Hence the derivative of a constant vector is a zero vector.

25.9 DERIVATIVE OF A VECTOR FUNCTION IN TERMS OF ITS COMPONENTS

Let $P(x, y, z)$ be any point in space and its position vector with respect to the origin O be $\vec{r}$ and let x, y, z be the function of scalar variable t, then we have

$$\vec{r} = x\hat{i} + y\hat{j} + z\hat{k} \quad ...(1)$$

where $\hat{i}, \hat{j}, \hat{k}$ are constant vectors.

$$\therefore \quad \vec{r} + \delta\vec{r} = (x+\delta x)\hat{i} + (y+\delta y)\hat{j} + (z+\delta z)\hat{k} \quad ...(2)$$

Subtract (1) from (2), we get

$$\delta\vec{r} = \delta x\hat{i} + \delta y\hat{j} + \delta z\hat{k}$$

Now divide this equation by δt and taking the limit as $\delta t \to 0$, we have

$$\lim_{\delta t\to 0}\frac{\delta\vec{r}}{\delta t} = \lim_{\delta t\to 0}\left(\frac{\delta x}{\delta t}\hat{i} + \frac{\delta y}{\delta t}\hat{j} + \frac{\delta z}{\delta t}\hat{k}\right)$$

$$\frac{d\vec{r}}{dt} = \left(\lim_{\delta t\to 0}\frac{\delta x}{\delta t}\right)\hat{i} + \left(\lim_{\delta t\to 0}\frac{\delta y}{\delta t}\right)\hat{j} + \left(\lim_{\delta t\to 0}\frac{\delta z}{\delta t}\right)\hat{k}$$

$$\therefore \quad \frac{d\vec{r}}{dt} = \frac{dx}{dt}\hat{i} + \frac{dy}{dt}\hat{j} + \frac{dz}{dt}\hat{k}.$$

Similarly, we can find $\frac{d^2\vec{r}}{dt^2}, \frac{d^3\vec{r}}{dt^3}$, etc.

25.10 DERIVATIVE OF A VECTOR FUNCTION OF FUNCTION

Let $\vec{r}$ be a function of a scalar variable u, and u is also a scalar function of scalar variable t.

$\therefore$ $\vec{r} = \vec{f}(u)$ ...(1)

and $u = g(t)$ ...(2)

$\therefore$ $\vec{r} + \delta\vec{r} = \vec{f}(u + \delta u)$ ...(3)

and $u + \delta u = g(t + \delta t)$ ...(4)

Subtract (1) from (3), we get

$$\delta\vec{r} = \vec{f}(u+\delta u) - \vec{f}(u) \quad ...(5)$$

and subtract (2) from (4), we get

$$\delta u = g(t+\delta t) - g(t) \quad ...(6)$$

Now divide (5) by δt, we have

$$\frac{\delta\vec{r}}{\delta t} = \frac{\vec{f}(u+\delta u) - \vec{f}(u)}{\delta t} = \frac{\vec{f}(u+\delta u) - \vec{f}(u)}{\delta u}\cdot\frac{\delta u}{\delta t}$$

$$\frac{\delta\vec{r}}{\delta t} = \frac{\vec{f}(u+\delta u) - \vec{f}(u)}{\delta u} \cdot \frac{g(t+\delta t) - g(t)}{\delta t}$$ [Using (6)]

Taking the limit $\delta t \to 0$, when $\delta t \to 0$, $\delta \vec{r} \to 0$ and $\delta u \to 0$, we get

$$\lim_{\delta t \to 0} \frac{\delta\vec{r}}{\delta t} = \lim_{\delta u \to 0} \frac{\vec{f}(u+\delta u) - \vec{f}(u)}{\delta u} \cdot \lim_{\delta t \to 0} \frac{g(t+\delta t) - g(t)}{\delta t}$$

$$\frac{d\vec{r}}{dt} = \frac{d\vec{f}}{du}\frac{dg}{dt} \quad \text{or} \quad \frac{d\vec{r}}{dt} = \frac{d\vec{r}}{du}\frac{du}{dt}$$ $[\because \vec{r} = \vec{f}(u), u = g(t)]$

THEOREM 1. *The vector $\vec{a}(t)$ has a constant magnitude if and only if $\vec{a}.\frac{d\vec{a}}{dt} = 0$.*

PROOF. Let us suppose $\vec{a}(t)$ has a constant magnitude. Therefore, $|\vec{a}(t)| = a(\text{constant})$

or $\vec{a} \cdot \vec{a} = a^2(\text{constant})$

$$\therefore \quad \frac{d}{dt}(\vec{a}\cdot\vec{a}) = \vec{a}\cdot\frac{d\vec{a}}{dt} + \frac{d\vec{a}}{dt}\cdot\vec{a} = 2\vec{a}\cdot\frac{da}{dt}$$ $(\because \vec{a}\cdot\vec{b} = \vec{b}\cdot\vec{a})$

Since $\vec{a}\cdot\vec{a} = a^2$

$$\frac{d}{dt}(\vec{a}\cdot\vec{a}) = \frac{d}{dt}(a^2) = 0.$$

$$\therefore \quad 2\vec{a}\cdot\frac{d\vec{a}}{dt} = 0 \quad \text{or} \quad \vec{a}\cdot\frac{d\vec{a}}{dt} = 0$$

Conversely, suppose $\vec{a}\cdot\frac{d\vec{a}}{dt} = 0$, then we get

$$\frac{d}{dt}(\vec{a}\cdot\vec{a}) = \vec{a}\cdot\frac{d\vec{a}}{dt} + \frac{d\vec{a}}{dt}\cdot\vec{a} = 2\vec{a}\cdot\frac{d\vec{a}}{dt}$$ $|\vec{a}.\vec{b} = \vec{b}.\vec{a}|$

$$\frac{d}{dt}(\vec{a}.\vec{a}) = 0 \quad \text{or} \quad \vec{a}.\vec{a} = \text{constant}$$

or $|\vec{a}|^2 = \text{constant}$ or $|\vec{a}| = \text{constant}$

THEOREM 2. *The vector function $\vec{a}(t)$ is constant vector if and only if $\frac{d\vec{a}}{dt} = 0$.*

PROOF. Let us suppose first $\vec{a}(t)$ is a constant vector such that $\vec{a}(t) = \vec{c}$ where c is a constant vector, then

$$\vec{a}(t+\delta t) = \vec{c}$$

$$\therefore \vec{a}(t+\delta t) - \vec{a}(t) = \vec{c} - \vec{c} = \vec{0}.$$

Divide by δt and taking the limit as $\delta t \to 0$, we get

$$\lim_{\delta t \to 0} \frac{\vec{a}(t+\delta t) - \vec{a}(t)}{\delta t} = \vec{0}. \Rightarrow \quad \frac{d\vec{a}}{dt} = \vec{0}.$$

Conversely, suppose $\frac{d\vec{a}}{dt} = \vec{0}$.

Let $\vec{a}(t) = a_1(t)\hat{i} + a_2(t)\hat{j} + a_3(t)\hat{k}$

$$\therefore \quad \frac{d\vec{a}}{dt} = \frac{da_1(t)}{dt}\hat{i} + \frac{da_2(t)}{dt}\hat{j} + \frac{da_3(t)}{dt}\hat{k}$$

$$\therefore \quad \frac{da_1(t)}{dt}\hat{i} + \frac{da_2(t)}{dt}\hat{j} + \frac{da_3(t)}{dt}\hat{k} = \vec{0}$$ $\left(\because \frac{d\vec{a}}{dt} = 0\right)$

This implies $$\frac{da_1}{dt} = 0, \frac{da_2}{dt} = 0, \frac{da_3}{dt} = 0.$$

Therefore, a_1, a_2, a_3 are all constants.

Hence $\vec{a}(t) = a_1\hat{i} + a_2\hat{j} + a_3\hat{k}$ is a constant vector.

THEOREM 3. *If the vector $\vec{a}$ has a constant magnitude $\vec{a}$, then $\vec{a}$ and $\frac{d\vec{a}}{dt}$ are perpendicular, provided $\left|\frac{d\vec{a}}{dt}\right| \neq 0$.*

PROOF. Since, we have that $|\vec{a}| = a$ (constant), then

$$\vec{a} \cdot \vec{a} = |\vec{a}|^2 = a^2 \text{ (constant)}$$

$$\therefore \quad \frac{d}{dt}(\vec{a} \cdot \vec{a}) = \vec{a} \cdot \frac{d\vec{a}}{dt} + \frac{d\vec{a}}{dt} \cdot \vec{a} = 2\vec{a} \cdot \frac{d\vec{a}}{dt}$$

and $$\frac{d}{dt}(\vec{a} \cdot \vec{a}) = \frac{d}{dt}(a^2) = 0$$

$$\therefore \quad 2\vec{a} \cdot \frac{d\vec{a}}{dt} = 0 \quad \text{or} \quad \vec{a} \cdot \frac{d\vec{a}}{dt} = 0.$$

This implies that vector $\vec{a}$ is perpendicular to $\frac{d\vec{a}}{dt}$, provided $\left|\frac{d\vec{a}}{dt}\right| \neq 0$.

THEOREM 4. *If a vector $\vec{a}$ is a differentiable vector function of t, then $\frac{d}{dt}\left(\vec{a} \times \frac{d\vec{a}}{dt}\right) = \vec{a} \times \frac{d^2\vec{a}}{dt^2}$.*

PROOF. Since, we have $$\frac{d}{dt}\left(\vec{a} \times \vec{b}\right) = \vec{a} \times \frac{d\vec{b}}{dt} + \frac{d\vec{a}}{dt} \times \vec{b}.$$

$$\therefore \quad \frac{d}{dt}\left(\vec{a} \times \frac{d\vec{a}}{dt}\right) = \vec{a} \times \frac{d}{dt}\left(\frac{d\vec{a}}{dt}\right) + \frac{d\vec{a}}{dt} \times \frac{d\vec{a}}{dt} = \vec{a} \times \frac{d^2\vec{a}}{dt^2} + \frac{d\vec{a}}{dt} \times \frac{d\vec{a}}{dt} = \vec{a} \times \frac{d^2\vec{a}}{dt^2}$$

$\left(\because \frac{d\vec{a}}{dt} \times \frac{d\vec{a}}{dt} = 0\right.$ *i.e.*, cross product of two same vector is zero.$\left.\right)$

THEOREM 5. *The vector $\vec{a}(t)$ has a constant direction if and only if $\vec{a} \times \frac{d\vec{a}}{dt} = \vec{0}$.*

PROOF. Suppose $\vec{a}(t)$ has a constant direction. Let $\hat{a}$ be the unit vector along $\vec{a}$ (t) and $|\vec{a}(t)| = a$, then

$$\vec{a}(t) = a\hat{a}.$$

$$\therefore \quad \frac{d\vec{a}}{dt} = \frac{d}{dt}(a\hat{a})$$

$$\frac{d\vec{a}}{dt} = \frac{da}{dt}\hat{a} + a\frac{d\hat{a}}{dt}$$

$$\therefore \quad \vec{a} \times \frac{d\vec{a}}{dt} = \vec{a} \times \left(\frac{da}{dt}\hat{a} + a\frac{d\hat{a}}{dt}\right) = \frac{da}{dt}\vec{a} \times \hat{a} + a\vec{a} \times \frac{d\hat{a}}{dt}$$

or $$\vec{a} \times \frac{d\vec{a}}{dt} = a\left(\vec{a} \times \frac{d\hat{a}}{dt}\right). \qquad \left(\because \vec{a} \times \hat{a} = \vec{a} \times \frac{\vec{a}}{a} = 0\right) \quad \ldots(1)$$

Since, $\vec{a}$ has a constant direction, then $\hat{a}$ is a constant vector, and thus we have $\frac{d\hat{a}}{dt} = \vec{0}$.

$$\therefore \qquad \vec{a} \times \frac{d\vec{a}}{dt} = a(\vec{a} \times \vec{0}) = \vec{0}.$$

Conversely, suppose $\vec{a} \times \frac{d\vec{a}}{dt} = 0$, then from (1)

$$a\left(\vec{a} \times \frac{d\hat{a}}{dt}\right) = 0 \quad \text{or} \quad \vec{a} \times \frac{d\hat{a}}{dt} = 0 \quad \text{or} \quad \hat{a} \times \frac{d\hat{a}}{dt} = 0 \qquad \ldots(2)$$

$[\because \vec{a} = a\hat{a}]$

Since $\hat{a}$ has a constant magnitude, then by theorem (1)

$$\hat{a} \times \frac{d\hat{a}}{dt} = 0 \,. \qquad \ldots(3)$$

From (2) and (3), we get $\frac{d\hat{a}}{dt} = \vec{0}$.

This implies $\hat{a}$ is a constant vector hence $\vec{a}$ has a constant directions.

25.11 CURVES IN THREE DIMENSIONAL SPACE

Let $f(x, y, z) = 0$ and $\phi(x, y, z) = 0$ be two surfaces, then a curve in three dimensional space is obtained by the intersection of the surfaces $f(x, y, z) = 0$ and $\phi(x, y, z) = 0$. Therefore, the equation is of the form

$$x = f_1(t), y = f_2(t), z = f_3(t) \qquad \ldots(1)$$

and it also represents a curve in three dimensional space. Where t takes the value between a and b, *i.e.* $a \le t \le b$. Let (x, y, z) be any point on the curve (1) and let **r** be its position vector, then we have

$$\vec{r} = x\hat{i} + y\hat{j} + z\hat{k} \qquad \text{and} \qquad \vec{f}(t) = f_1(t)\hat{i} + f_2(t)\hat{j} + f_3(t)\hat{k}.$$

$\therefore$ From (1), we have

$$x\hat{i} + y\hat{j} + z\hat{k} = f_1(t)\hat{i} + f_2(t)\hat{j} + f_3(t)\hat{k} \qquad \text{or} \qquad \vec{r} = \vec{f}(t). \qquad \ldots(2)$$

Thus equation (2) represents a curve in three dimensional space.

25.11.1 GEOMETRICAL INTERPRETATION OF $\frac{d\vec{r}}{dt}$

Let $\vec{r} = \vec{f}(t)$ be a curve in three dimensional space and let P and Q be two neighbouring points on this curve and $\vec{r}$ and $\vec{r} + \delta\vec{r}$ be the position vectors of P and Q respectively as shown in fig. 1.

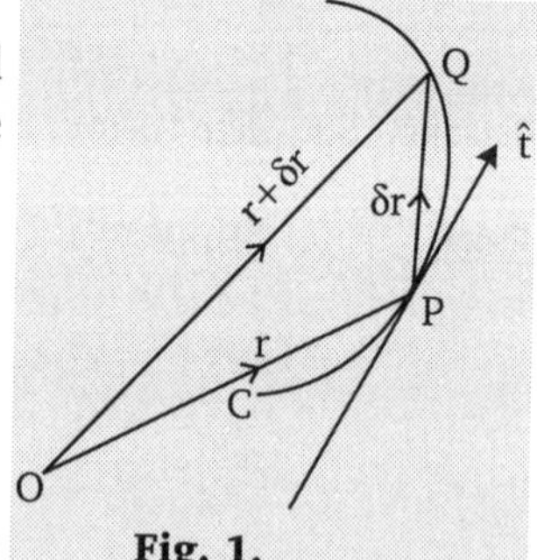

Fig. 1.

$$\therefore \quad \vec{r} = \overrightarrow{OP} = \vec{f}(t) \qquad \text{and} \qquad \overrightarrow{OQ} = \vec{r} + \delta\vec{r} = \vec{f}(t + \delta t)$$

$$\therefore \quad \overrightarrow{PQ} = \overrightarrow{OQ} - \overrightarrow{OP} = \vec{r} + \delta\vec{r} - \vec{r} = \delta\vec{r}.$$

Thus $\frac{\delta\vec{r}}{\delta t}$ is a vector parallel to the vector $\overrightarrow{PQ}$ (which is a chord).

As $\delta t \to 0$ *i.e.*, $Q \to P$, then the chord PQ tending to a line at P to the curve. This line is known as tangent.

$$\therefore \qquad \lim_{\delta t \to 0} \frac{\delta\vec{r}}{\delta t} = \frac{d\vec{r}}{dt}.$$

Hence, $\frac{d\vec{r}}{dt}$ is a vector which is parallel to the line (tangent) at P to the curve $\vec{r} = \vec{f}(t)$.

25.12 VELOCITY AND ACCELERATION VECTORS (GBTU–2010)

Let a particle be moving along the curve $\vec{r} = \vec{f}(t)$. At any instant t the moving particle is at P whose position vector is $\vec{r}$. In time interval δt the moving particle reached to the point Q whose position vector is $\vec{r} + \delta\vec{r}$.

$\therefore$ $\delta\vec{r}$ is the displacement of the moving particle in the time interval δt.

Thus $\frac{\delta\vec{r}}{\delta t}$ gives an average velocity of the particle during the interval δt. If the vector $\vec{v}$ represents the velocity vector at P, then

$$\vec{v} = \lim_{\delta t\to 0}\frac{\delta\vec{r}}{\delta t} = \frac{d\vec{r}}{dt}.$$

Since $\frac{d\vec{r}}{dt}$ is a vector along the tangent at P to the curve. Hence, the vector $\vec{v}$ of the particle always along the tangent.

Further, if $\delta\vec{v}$ is the change in velocity during the time interval δt, then $\frac{\delta\vec{v}}{\delta t}$ represents a vector which gives an average acceleration of the particle. Let $\vec{a}$ be the acceleration vector of the particle, then we have

$$\vec{a} = \lim_{\delta t\to 0}\frac{\delta\vec{v}}{\delta t} = \frac{d\vec{v}}{dt}.$$

Since $\vec{v} = \frac{d\vec{r}}{dt}$ therefore $\vec{a} = \frac{d}{dt}\left(\frac{d\vec{r}}{dt}\right) = \frac{d^2\vec{r}}{dt^2}$.

Hence $\vec{a} = \frac{d\vec{v}}{dt} = \frac{d^2\vec{r}}{dt^2}$.

- The equation $\vec{r} = (a\cos t)\hat{i} + (b\sin t)\hat{j} + 0.\hat{k}$ represents the equation of an ellipse.
- The equation $\vec{r} = (a\sec t)\hat{i} + (b\tan t)\hat{j} + 0.\hat{k}$ represents the equation of hyperbola.
- The equation $\vec{r} = (at^2)\hat{i} + (2at)\hat{j} + 0.\hat{k}$ represents the equation of a parabola.

Solved Examples

1. *If* $\vec{r} = (2\sin t)\hat{i} + (3\cos t)\hat{j} + t\hat{k}$, *find*

(i) $\frac{d\vec{r}}{dt}$ (ii) $\left|\frac{d\vec{r}}{dt}\right|$

(iii) $\frac{d^2\vec{r}}{dt^2}$ (iv) $\left|\frac{d^2\vec{r}}{dt^2}\right|$

SOLUTION. Since we know that $\hat{i}, \hat{j}, \hat{k}$ are constant vectors, so $\frac{d\hat{i}}{dt} = \vec{0}, \frac{d\hat{j}}{dt} = \vec{0}$ and $\frac{d\hat{k}}{dt} = \vec{0}$.

(i) $\vec{r} = (2\sin t)\hat{i} + (3\cos t)\hat{j} + t\hat{k}$,

$\therefore$ $\frac{d\vec{r}}{dt} = (2\cos t)\hat{i} - (3\sin t)\hat{j} + \hat{k}$

(ii) $\left|\frac{d\vec{r}}{dt}\right| = \sqrt{4\cos^2 t + 9\sin^2 t + 1}$

$= \sqrt{5(1+\sin^2 t)}.$

(iii) $\frac{d^2\vec{r}}{dt^2} = \frac{d}{dt}\left(\frac{d\vec{r}}{dt}\right)$

$= \frac{d}{dt}(2\cos t\hat{i} - 3\sin t\hat{j} + \hat{k})$

$= -2\sin t\hat{i} - 3\cos t\hat{j}.$

(iv) $\left|\frac{d^2\vec{r}}{dt^2}\right| = \sqrt{(4\sin^2 t + 9\cos^2 t)}$

$= \sqrt{(4 + 5\cos^2 t)}\,.$

2. *If $\hat{r}$ be a unit vector in the direction of $\vec{r}$, prove that*

$$\hat{r}\times\frac{d\hat{r}}{dt} = \frac{1}{r^2}\vec{r}\times\frac{dr}{dt}, \textit{where } |\vec{r}| = r.$$

SOLUTION. Since $\hat{r}$ is a unit vector along the vector r, so we have

$$\vec{r} = r\hat{r} \qquad ...(1)$$

$\because \quad |\vec{r}| = r.$

Differentiating w.r.t. t of both sides, we get

$$\frac{d\vec{r}}{dt} = \frac{d}{dt}(r\hat{r})$$

$$\therefore \quad \frac{d\vec{r}}{dt} = r\frac{d\hat{r}}{dt} + \frac{dr}{dt}\hat{r} \quad \ldots(2)$$

$$\text{Now } \vec{r} \times \frac{d\vec{r}}{dt} = \vec{r} \times \left(r\frac{d\hat{r}}{dt} + \frac{dr}{dt}\hat{r} \right)$$

$$= r\vec{r} \times \frac{d\hat{r}}{dt} + \frac{dr}{dt}\vec{r} \times \hat{r}$$

$$= r(r\hat{r}) \times \frac{d\hat{r}}{dt} + \frac{dr}{dt}r\hat{r} \times \hat{r}$$

$(\because \vec{r} = r\hat{r})$

$$= r^2\hat{r} \times \frac{d\hat{r}}{dt} + 0$$

($\because$ Cross product of same vector is zero, *i.e.*, $\hat{r} \times \hat{r} = \vec{0}$)

$$= r^2\hat{r} \times \frac{d\hat{r}}{dt}$$

$$\therefore \quad \hat{r} \times \frac{d\hat{r}}{dt} = \frac{1}{r^2}\vec{r} \times \frac{d\vec{r}}{dt}$$

3. *If* $\vec{r} = \vec{a} \sin \omega t + \vec{b} \cos \omega t + \frac{\vec{c}t}{\omega^2} \sin \omega t$, *prove that*

$$\frac{d^2\vec{r}}{dt^2} + \omega^2\vec{r} = \frac{2\vec{c}}{\omega}\cos \omega t,$$

where $\vec{a}, \vec{b}, \vec{c}$, *are constant vectors and* ω *is a constant scalar.*

Solution. Since $\vec{a}, \vec{b}, \vec{c}$, are constant vectors so

$$\frac{d\vec{a}}{dt} = 0, \frac{d\vec{b}}{dt} = 0 \text{ and } \frac{d\vec{c}}{dt} = 0.$$

and

$$\vec{r} = \vec{a}\sin \omega t + \vec{b}\cos \omega t + \frac{\vec{c}t}{\omega^2}\sin \omega t \quad \ldots(1)$$

$$\therefore \quad \frac{d\vec{r}}{dt} = \omega\vec{a}\cos \omega t - \omega\vec{b}\sin \omega t + \frac{\vec{c}}{\omega^2}\sin \omega t + \frac{\vec{c}t}{\omega}\cos \omega t$$

$$\text{and} \quad \frac{d^2\vec{r}}{dt^2} = \frac{d}{dt}\left(\frac{d\vec{r}}{dt}\right)$$

$$= -\omega^2\vec{a}\sin \omega t - \omega^2\vec{b}\cos \omega t + \frac{\vec{c}}{\omega}\cos \omega t + \frac{\vec{c}}{\omega}\cos \omega t - \vec{c}t\sin \omega t$$

$$= -\omega^2\left(\vec{a}\sin \omega t + \vec{b}\cos \omega t + \frac{\vec{c}t}{\omega^2}\sin \omega t\right) + \frac{2\vec{c}}{\omega}\cos \omega t$$

$$= -\omega^2\vec{r} + \frac{2\vec{c}}{\omega}\cos \omega t$$

$$\therefore \quad \frac{d^2\vec{r}}{dt^2} + \omega^2\vec{r} = \frac{2\vec{c}}{\omega}\cos \omega t.$$

4. *If* $\vec{r} = (\cos nt)\hat{i} + (\sin nt)\hat{j}$, *where n is a constant and t varies, show that*

$$\vec{r} \times \frac{d\vec{r}}{dt} = n\hat{k}.$$

Solution. Since $\hat{i}$ and $\hat{j}$ are constant vectors so

$$\frac{d\hat{i}}{dt} = \vec{0}, \frac{d\hat{j}}{dt} = \vec{0} \text{ and}$$

$$\vec{r} = (\cos nt)\hat{i} + (\sin nt)\hat{j} \quad \ldots(1)$$

Differentiating (1) w.r.t. 't', we get

$$\frac{d\vec{r}}{dt} = -n(\sin nt)\hat{i} + n(\cos nt)\hat{j} \quad \ldots(2)$$

Now

$$\vec{r} \times \frac{d\vec{r}}{dt} = \vec{r} \times [-n(\sin nt)\hat{i} + n(\cos nt)\hat{j}]$$

$$= [(\cos nt)\hat{i} + (\sin nt)\hat{j}] \times [-n(\sin nt)\hat{i} + n(\cos nt)\hat{j}]$$

[From (1)]

$$= (n\cos^2 nt)\hat{i} \times \hat{j} - n(\sin^2 nt)\hat{j} \times \hat{i}$$

$$= n(\cos^2 nt)\hat{k} + n(\sin^2 nt)\hat{k}$$

$[\because \hat{j} \times \hat{i} = -\hat{k} \text{ and } \hat{i} \times \hat{j} = \hat{k}]$

$$= (\cos^2 nt + \sin^2 nt)n\hat{k} = n\hat{k}$$

$(\because \cos^2 nt + \sin^2 nt = 1)$

$$\text{Hence,} \quad \vec{r} \times \frac{d\vec{r}}{dt} = n\hat{k}.$$

5. *If* $\frac{d\vec{a}}{dt} = \vec{c} \times \vec{a}, \frac{d\vec{b}}{dt} = \vec{c} \times \vec{b}$ *show that*

$$\frac{d}{dt}(\vec{a} \times \vec{b}) = \vec{c} \times (\vec{a} \times \vec{b}).$$

Solution. Since we know that

$$\frac{d}{dt}(\vec{a} \times \vec{b}) = \vec{a} \times \frac{d\vec{b}}{dt} + \frac{d\vec{a}}{dt} \times \vec{b}$$

$$= \vec{a}\times(\vec{c}\times\vec{b})+(\vec{c}\times\vec{a})\times\vec{b}$$
$$\left(\because \frac{d\vec{a}}{dt}=\vec{c}\times\vec{a}, \frac{d\vec{b}}{dt}=\vec{c}\times\vec{b}\right)$$
$$= [(\vec{a}\cdot\vec{b})\vec{c}-(\vec{a}\cdot\vec{c})\vec{b}] - [(\vec{b}\cdot\vec{a})\vec{c}-(\vec{b}\cdot\vec{c})\vec{a}]$$
$$= (\vec{a}\cdot\vec{b})\vec{c}-(\vec{a}\cdot\vec{c})\vec{b}-(\vec{a}\cdot\vec{b})\vec{c}+(\vec{b}\cdot\vec{c})\vec{a}$$
$$(\because \vec{a}\cdot\vec{b}=\vec{b}\cdot\vec{a})$$
$$= (\vec{b}\cdot\vec{c})\vec{a}-(\vec{a}\cdot\vec{c})\vec{b}$$
$$= (\vec{c}\cdot\vec{b})\vec{a}-(\vec{c}\cdot\vec{a})\vec{b}$$
($\because$ dot products is commutative.)
$$= \vec{c}\times(\vec{a}\times\vec{b}).$$
$$\therefore \frac{d}{dt}(\vec{a}\times\vec{b})=\vec{c}\times(\vec{a}\times\vec{b}).$$

6. *If $\vec{r}$ is a vector function of a scalar variable t, $|\vec{r}| = r$ and $\vec{a}$, $\vec{b}$ are constant vectors, then differentiate the following with respect to t :*

(i) $\vec{r}^2+\frac{1}{\vec{r}^2}$ (ii) $r^n\vec{r}$

(iii) $(a\vec{r}+r\vec{b})^2$.

SOLUTION. Since $\vec{a}$, $\vec{b}$ are constant vectors, so $\frac{d\vec{a}}{dt}=0, \frac{d\vec{b}}{dt}=0$ and $|\vec{a}|=a$ and $|\vec{r}|=r$.

(i) Let $\vec{R}=\vec{r}^2+\frac{1}{\vec{r}^2}$

$$\therefore \frac{d\vec{R}}{dt}=\frac{d}{dt}\left(\vec{r}^2+\frac{1}{\vec{r}^2}\right)$$
$$=\frac{d}{dt}(\vec{r}^2)+\frac{d}{dt}\left(\frac{1}{\vec{r}^2}\right)$$
$$=\frac{d}{dt}(\vec{r}.\vec{r})+\frac{d}{dt}\left(\frac{1}{\vec{r}.\vec{r}}\right)$$
$$=\frac{d}{dt}(r^2)+\frac{d}{dt}\left(\frac{1}{r^2}\right)$$
$$=2r\frac{dr}{dt}-\frac{2}{r^3}\frac{dr}{dt}$$

(ii) Let $\vec{R}=r^n\vec{r}$.

$$\frac{d\vec{R}}{dt}=\frac{d}{dt}(r^n\vec{r})=r^n\frac{d\vec{r}}{dt}+\frac{d(r^n)}{dt}\vec{r}$$
$$=r^n\frac{d\vec{r}}{dt}+nr^{n-1}\frac{d\vec{r}}{dt}\vec{r}.$$

(iii) Let $\vec{R}=(a\vec{r}+r\vec{b})^2$.

$$\therefore \frac{d\vec{R}}{dt}=\frac{d}{dt}(a\vec{r}+r\vec{b})^2$$
$$=2(a\vec{r}+r\vec{b}).\frac{d}{dt}(a\vec{r}+r\vec{b})$$
$$=2(a\vec{r}+r\vec{b}).\left(a\frac{d\vec{r}}{dt}+\frac{da}{dt}\vec{r}+r\frac{d\vec{b}}{dt}+\frac{dr}{dt}\vec{b}\right)$$
$$=2(a\vec{r}+r\vec{b}).\left(a\frac{d\vec{r}}{dt}+\frac{dr}{dt}\vec{b}\right)$$
$$\left(\because \frac{d\vec{a}}{dt}=0, \frac{d\vec{b}}{dt}=0\right)$$

7. *A particle moves along the curve $x = t^3 + 1$, $y = t^2$, $z = 2t + 5$, where t is the time. Find the components of its velocity and acceleration at $t = 1$ in the direction $\hat{i}+\hat{j}+3\hat{k}$.*

SOLUTION. Let $\vec{r}$ be the position vector of a moving particle at any time t at the point (x, y, z) on the curve, then

$\vec{r} = x\hat{i} + y\hat{j} + z\hat{k}$.

$$\vec{r}=(t^3+1)\hat{i}+t^2\hat{j}+(2t+5)\hat{k} \quad \text{...(1)}$$

where $\hat{i},\hat{j},\hat{k}$ are constant vector.

$$\therefore \frac{d\vec{r}}{dt}=3t^2\hat{i}+2t\hat{j}+2\hat{k} \quad \text{...(2)}$$

At t = 1

$$\frac{d\vec{r}}{dt}=3\hat{i}+2\hat{j}+2\hat{k}$$

It is a velocity vector whose components are 3, 2, 2.

Again from (2)

$$\frac{d^2\vec{r}}{dt^2}=6t\hat{i}+2\hat{j}.$$

At t = 1

$$\frac{d^2\vec{r}}{dt^2}=6\hat{i}+2\hat{j}.$$

This is the acceleration vector whose components are 6, 2, 0.

Now we have to find the components of velocity in the direction of $\hat{i}+\hat{j}+3\hat{k}$.

$\therefore$ Unit vector along the direction of $\hat{i}+\hat{j}+3\hat{k}$

$$= \frac{\hat{i} + \hat{j} + 3\hat{k}}{\sqrt{11}}.$$

Thus the component of velocity in the direction of $\hat{i} + \hat{j} + 3\hat{k}$ is

$$= (3\hat{i} + 2\hat{j} + 2\hat{k}) \cdot \frac{\hat{i} + \hat{j} + 3\hat{k}}{\sqrt{11}}$$

$$= \frac{3+2+6}{\sqrt{11}} = \frac{11}{\sqrt{11}} = \sqrt{11} \text{ units}$$

and the component of acceleration in the direction of $\hat{i} + \hat{j} + 3\hat{k}$ is

$$= (6\hat{i} + 2\hat{j}) \cdot \frac{\hat{i} + \hat{j} + 3\hat{k}}{\sqrt{11}}$$

$$= \frac{6+2}{\sqrt{11}} = \frac{8}{\sqrt{11}} \text{ units.}$$

8. *Show that*

$$\frac{d^2}{dt^2}\left(\vec{r} \times \frac{d\vec{r}}{dt}\right) = \frac{d\vec{r}}{dt} \times \frac{d^2\vec{r}}{dt^2} + \vec{r} \times \frac{d^3\vec{r}}{dt^3}.$$

SOLUTION.

$$\frac{d}{dt}\left(\vec{r} \times \frac{d\vec{r}}{dt}\right) = \frac{d\vec{r}}{dt} \times \frac{d\vec{r}}{dt} + \vec{r} \times \frac{d^2\vec{r}}{dt^2}$$

$$= \vec{r} \times \frac{d^2\vec{r}}{dt^2} \quad \left[\because \frac{d\vec{r}}{dt} \times \frac{d\vec{r}}{dt} = \vec{0}\right]$$

$$\therefore \frac{d^2}{dt^2}\left(\vec{r} \times \frac{d\vec{r}}{dt}\right) = \frac{d}{dt}\left(\vec{r} \times \frac{d^2\vec{r}}{dt^2}\right)$$

$$= \frac{d\vec{r}}{dt} \times \frac{d^2\vec{r}}{dt^2} + \vec{r} \times \frac{d^3\vec{r}}{dt^3}$$

9. *Show that the radial and transverse acceleration of a particle moving in a plane are* $\frac{d^2\vec{r}}{dt^2} - \vec{r}\left(\frac{d\theta}{dt}\right)^2$ *and* $2\frac{d\vec{r}}{dt} \cdot \frac{d\theta}{dt} + \vec{r}\frac{d^2\theta}{dt^2}$ *respectively.* (KURUKSHETRA–2006, RAJASTHAN–2005, 2006)

SOLUTION. Let $\hat{e}_r$ and $\hat{e}_\theta$ be two unit vectors along and perpendicular to radius vector OP where $\hat{i}$ and $\hat{j}$ be two mutually perpendicular unit vectors in the plane.

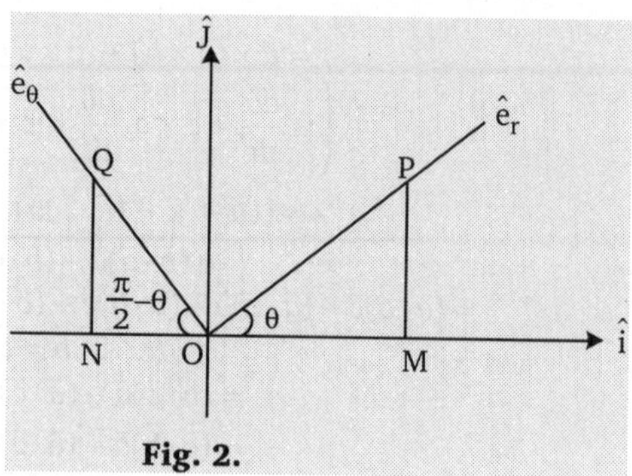

Fig. 2.

Then $\hat{e}_r = \overrightarrow{OP} = \overrightarrow{OM} + \overrightarrow{MP}$

$$= \cos\theta\hat{i} + \sin\theta\hat{j} \qquad \ldots(1)$$

and $\hat{e}_\theta = \cos\left(\frac{\pi}{2} + \theta\right)\hat{i} + \sin\left(\frac{\pi}{2} + \theta\right)\hat{j}$

$$= -\sin\theta\hat{i} + \cos\theta\hat{j} \qquad \ldots(2)$$

Also $\vec{r} = r\hat{e}_r = r\cos\theta\hat{i} + r\sin\theta\hat{j} \qquad \ldots(3)$

$$\frac{d\hat{e}_r}{dt} = (-\sin\theta\hat{i} + \cos\theta\hat{j})\frac{d\theta}{dt}$$

$$= \hat{e}_\theta \frac{d\theta}{dt} = \dot{\theta}\hat{e}_\theta \qquad \ldots(4)$$

$$\frac{d\hat{e}_\theta}{dt} = (-\cos\theta\hat{i} - \sin\theta\hat{j})\frac{d\theta}{dt}$$

$$= -\hat{e}_r \frac{d\theta}{dt} = -\dot{\theta}\hat{e}_r \qquad \ldots(5)$$

Now, $\frac{dr}{dt} = \frac{d}{dt}(\vec{r}\cos\theta\hat{i} + \vec{r}\sin\theta\hat{j})$

$$= \left(\frac{d\vec{r}}{dt}\cos\theta - \vec{r}\sin\theta\frac{d\theta}{dt}\right)\hat{i} + \left(\frac{d\vec{r}}{dt}\sin\theta + \vec{r}\cos\theta\frac{d\theta}{dt}\right)\hat{j}$$

$$= \frac{d\vec{r}}{dt}\left(\cos\theta\hat{i} + \sin\theta\hat{j}\right) + \vec{r}\frac{d\theta}{dt}\left(-\sin\theta\hat{i} + \cos\theta\hat{j}\right)$$

$$= \dot{\vec{r}}\,\hat{e}_r + \vec{r}\,\dot{\theta}\,\hat{e}_\theta$$

$\therefore$ Acceleration

$$\frac{d^2\vec{r}}{dt^2} = \ddot{\vec{r}}\,\hat{e}_r + \dot{\vec{r}}\frac{d\hat{e}_r}{dt} + \dot{\vec{r}}\,\dot{\theta}\,\hat{e}_\theta + \vec{r}\,\ddot{\theta}\,\hat{e}_\theta + \vec{r}\,\dot{\theta}\frac{d\hat{e}_\theta}{dt}$$

$$= \ddot{\vec{r}}\,\hat{e}_r + 2\dot{\vec{r}}\,\dot{\theta}\,\hat{e}_\theta + \vec{r}\,\ddot{\theta}\,\hat{e}_\theta - \vec{r}\,\dot{\theta}^2\,\hat{e}_r$$

$$= (\ddot{\vec{r}} - \vec{r}\,\dot{\theta}^2)\hat{e}_r + (2\dot{\vec{r}}\,\dot{\theta} + \vec{r}\,\ddot{\theta})\hat{e}_\theta$$

$$= \left[\frac{d^2\vec{r}}{dt^2} - \vec{r}\left(\frac{d\theta}{dt}\right)^2\right]\hat{e}_r + \frac{1}{\vec{r}}\frac{d}{dt}\left(\vec{r}^2\frac{d\theta}{dt}\right)\hat{e}_\theta$$

Hence, Radial acceleration

$$= \text{Acceleration along } \hat{e}_r = \frac{d^2\vec{r}}{dt^2} - \vec{r}\left(\frac{d\theta}{dt}\right)^2.$$

Transverse acceleration

$$= \text{Acceleration along } \hat{e}_\theta = \frac{1}{\vec{r}}\frac{d}{dt}\left(\vec{r}^2\frac{d\theta}{dt}\right) = 2\frac{d\vec{r}}{dt}\cdot\frac{d\theta}{dt} + \vec{r}\,\frac{d^2\theta}{dt^2}.$$

Exercise-25.1

1. If $\vec{r} = (t+1)\hat{i} + (t^2+t+1)\hat{j} + (t^3+t^2+t+1)\hat{k}$, find $\frac{d\vec{r}}{dt}, \frac{d^2\vec{r}}{dt^2}$.

2. If $\vec{a}, \vec{b}$ are constant vectors, ω is a constant, and **r** is a vector function of the scalar variable t given by $\vec{r}$ = cos $\omega t\ \vec{a}$ + sin $\omega t\ \vec{b}$. Show that

   (i) $\frac{d^2\vec{r}}{dt^2} + \omega^2\vec{r} = \vec{0}$

   (ii) $\vec{r} \times \frac{d\vec{r}}{dt} = \omega\vec{a} \times \vec{b}$ (UPTU-2007, BHOPAL-2007)

3. (i) If $\vec{r}$ is a unit vector, then show that
   $$\left|\vec{r} \times \frac{d\vec{r}}{dt}\right| = \left|\frac{d\vec{r}}{dt}\right|.$$

   (ii) If $\vec{r} \times d\vec{r} = \vec{0}$, show that $\hat{r}$ = constant.

4. If $\vec{r}$ is the position vector of a moving point and r is the modulus of $\vec{r}$, show that
   $$\vec{r}.\frac{d\vec{r}}{dt} = r\frac{dr}{dt}.$$

5. If $\vec{r}$ is a vector function of a scalar variable t and $\vec{a}$ is a constant vector, differentiate the following with respect to t :

   (i) $\vec{r} \times \vec{a}$ (ii) $\vec{r} \times \frac{d\vec{r}}{dt}$

   (iii) $\frac{\vec{r} \times \vec{a}}{\vec{r}.\vec{a}}$ (iv) $r^3\vec{r} + \vec{a} \times \frac{d\vec{r}}{dt}$

6. (i) If $\vec{r} = \sin t\hat{i} + \cos t\hat{j} + t\hat{k}$, find
   $$\left|\frac{d\vec{r}}{dt} \times \frac{d^2\vec{r}}{dt^2}\right|, \left|\frac{d^2\vec{r}}{dt^2}\right|.$$

   (ii) If $\vec{r} = a\cos t\hat{i} + a\sin t\hat{j} + at\tan\alpha\hat{k}$, find
   $$\left|\frac{d\vec{r}}{dt} \times \frac{d^2\vec{r}}{dt^2}\right| \text{ and } \frac{d\vec{r}}{dt}\cdot\left(\frac{d^2\vec{r}}{dt^2} \times \frac{d^3\vec{r}}{dt^3}\right).$$

7. If $\vec{r} = r^3\hat{i} + \left(2t^3 - \frac{1}{5t^2}\right)\hat{j}$, show that $\vec{r} \times \frac{d\vec{r}}{dt} = \hat{k}$.

8. Show that if $\vec{a}, \vec{b}, \vec{c}$ are constant vectors, then $\vec{r} = \vec{a}t^2 + \vec{b}t + \vec{c}$ is the path of a particle moving with constant acceleration.

9. If $\vec{r} = e^{nt}\vec{a} + e^{-nt}\vec{b}$, where $\vec{a}$, $\vec{b}$ are constant vectors, show that
   $$\frac{d^2\vec{r}}{dt^2} - n^2\vec{r} = \vec{0}.$$

10. Show that $\vec{r} = \vec{a}e^{nt} + \vec{b}e^{nt}$ is the solution of the differential equation
    $$\frac{d^2\vec{r}}{dt^2} - (m+n)\frac{d\vec{r}}{dt} + mn\vec{r} = 0.$$
    Hence solve the equation $\frac{d^2\vec{r}}{dt^2} - \frac{d\vec{r}}{dt} - 2\vec{r} = 0.$
    where $\vec{r} = \hat{i}$ and $\frac{d\vec{r}}{dt} = \hat{j}$ at t = 0.

11. If $\vec{a} = 5t^2\hat{i} + t\hat{j} - t^3\hat{k}$ and $\vec{b} = \sin t\hat{i} - \cos t\hat{j}$, then find

    (i) $\frac{d}{dt}(\vec{a}.\vec{b})$ (ii) $\frac{d}{dt}(\vec{a} \times \vec{b})$

    (iii) $\frac{d}{dt}(\vec{a}.\vec{a})$

12. A particle moves along the curve x = 4 cos$t$, y = 4 sin t, z = 6t. Find the velocity and acceleration at time t = 0 and $t = \frac{\pi}{2}$.

13. A particle moves along the curve $x = e^{-t}$, y = 2 cos 3t, z = 2 sin 3t. Find the velocity and acceleration at any time t and their magnitudes at t = 0. (PTU–2003, VTU–2003)

14. Find the unit tangent vector to any point on the curve $x = a$ cos t, $y = a$ sin t, $z = bt$.

15. A particle P is moving on a circle of radius r with constant angular velocity $\omega = \dfrac{d\theta}{dt}$ show that the acceleration is $-\omega^2 \vec{r}$.

16. The position vector of a moving particle at a time t is $\vec{r} = 3\cos t\hat{i} + 3\sin t\hat{j} + 4t\hat{k}$. Find the tangent and normal components of its acceleration at $t = 1$. (MARATHWADA–2008)

Hint to the Selected Problems

1. $\vec{r} = (t+1)\hat{i} + (t^2+t+1)\hat{j} + (t^3+t^2+t+1)\hat{k}$

$\therefore \quad \dfrac{d\vec{r}}{dt} = \hat{i} + (2t+1)\hat{j} + (3t^2+2t+1)\hat{k}$

$\dfrac{d^2\vec{r}}{dt^2} = 2\hat{j} + (6t+2)\hat{k}$.

2. $\vec{r} = (\cos\omega t)\vec{a} + (\sin\omega t)\vec{b}$

$\dfrac{d\vec{r}}{dt} = -\omega\sin\omega t\vec{a} + \omega\cos\omega t\vec{b}$

$\dfrac{d^2\vec{r}}{dt^2} = -\omega^2[\cos\omega t\vec{a} + \sin\omega t\vec{b}] = -\omega^2\vec{r}$

$\therefore \quad \dfrac{d^2\vec{r}}{dt^2} + \omega^2\vec{r} = \vec{0}$.

Similarly $\vec{r} \times \dfrac{d\vec{r}}{dt} = (\cos\omega t\vec{a} + \sin\omega t\vec{b})$

$\times(-\omega\sin\omega t\vec{a} + \omega\cos\omega t\vec{b})$

$= \omega\vec{a}\times\vec{b}$.

3. (i) Since $\vec{r}$ is a unit vector, then

$|\vec{r}| = 1 \quad \Rightarrow \quad \vec{r}.\vec{r} = 1$

$\Rightarrow \quad \dfrac{d}{dt}(\vec{r}.\vec{r}) = 0 \quad \Rightarrow \quad \vec{r}.\dfrac{d\vec{r}}{dt} = 0$

$\Rightarrow \quad \vec{r}$ is perpendicular to $\dfrac{d\vec{r}}{dt}$

$\therefore \quad \left|\vec{r}\times\dfrac{d\vec{r}}{dt}\right| = |\vec{r}|\left|\dfrac{d\vec{r}}{dt}\right|\sin\dfrac{\pi}{2} = \left|\dfrac{d\vec{r}}{dt}\right|$.

(ii) $\vec{r} = r\hat{r} \quad \Rightarrow \quad d\vec{r} = d(r\hat{r}) = rd\hat{r} + \hat{r}dr$

$\therefore \quad \vec{r}\times d\vec{r} = r\hat{r}\times(rd\hat{r} + \hat{r}dr) = r^2\hat{r} + d\hat{r}$

$\Rightarrow \quad \vec{0} = r^2\hat{r} + d\hat{r} \quad \Rightarrow \quad \hat{r}\times d\hat{r} = \vec{0}$

$\therefore \quad \vec{r}\times d\vec{r} = 0 \quad$ and $\quad \hat{r}\times d\hat{r} = 0$

$\Rightarrow \quad \hat{r}$ = constant.

4. Since $\quad \vec{r} = r\hat{r} \quad \Rightarrow \dfrac{d\vec{r}}{dt} = \dfrac{d}{dr}(r\hat{r}) = \dfrac{rd\hat{r}}{dt} + \hat{r}\dfrac{dr}{dt}$

$\therefore \quad \vec{r}.\dfrac{d\vec{r}}{dt} = \vec{r}.\left(r\dfrac{d\hat{r}}{dt} + \hat{r}\dfrac{dr}{dt}\right) = r\vec{r}.\dfrac{d\hat{r}}{dt} + \vec{r}.\hat{r}\dfrac{dr}{dt}$

$= r^2\hat{r}.\dfrac{d\hat{r}}{dt} + r(r\hat{r})\dfrac{dr}{dt} = 0 + r\dfrac{dr}{dt}$

$[\because \hat{r}.\hat{r} = 1]$

$= r\dfrac{dr}{dt}$.

6. (i) $\quad \vec{r} = \sin t\hat{i} + \cos t\hat{j} + t\hat{k}$

$\therefore \quad \dfrac{d\vec{r}}{dt} = \cos t\hat{i} - \sin t\hat{j} + \hat{k}$

$\dfrac{d^2\vec{r}}{dt^2} = -\sin t\hat{i} - \cos t\hat{j}$

$\therefore \quad \dfrac{d\vec{r}}{dt}\times\dfrac{d^2\vec{r}}{dt^2} = |\cos t\hat{i} - \sin t\hat{j} - \hat{k}| = \sqrt{2}$.

11. (i) $\quad \vec{a} = 5t^2\hat{i} + t\hat{j} - t^3\hat{k}$ and $\vec{b} = \sin t\hat{i} - \cos t\hat{j}$

$\vec{a}.\vec{b} = 5t^2\sin t - t\cos t$

$\therefore \quad \dfrac{d}{dt}(\vec{a}.\vec{b}) = \dfrac{d}{dt}(5t^2\sin t - t\cos t)$

$= 10t\sin t + 5t^2\cos t - \cos t + t\sin t$

$= 5t^2\cos t + 11t\sin t - \cos t$

Similarly, we can find $\dfrac{d}{dt}(\vec{a}\times\vec{b})$ and $\dfrac{d}{dt}(\vec{a}\cdot\vec{b})$

13. $\quad x = e^{-t}, y = 2\cos 3t, z = 2\sin 3t$

$\therefore \quad \vec{r} = e^{-t}\hat{i} + 2\cos 3t\hat{j} + 2\sin 3t\hat{k}$

so $\quad \dfrac{d\vec{r}}{dt} = -e^{-t}\hat{i} - 6\sin 3t\hat{j} + 6\cos 3t\hat{k}$

and $\quad \dfrac{d^2\vec{r}}{dt^2} = e^{-t}\hat{i} - 18\cos 3t\hat{j} - 18\sin 3t\hat{k}$

Velocity $= \mathrm{v} = \left(\dfrac{d\vec{r}}{dt}\right)_{\text{at } t=0} = -\hat{i} + 6\hat{k}$

$\therefore \quad |\mathrm{v}| = \sqrt{1+36} = \sqrt{37}$

and $\quad$ acceleration $= \left(\dfrac{d^2\vec{r}}{dt^2}\right)_{\text{at } t=0} = \hat{i} - 18\hat{j}$

$\therefore \quad \left|\dfrac{d^2\vec{r}}{dt^2}\right| = \sqrt{1+324} = \sqrt{325}$.

15. Let i and j be the two unit vectors perpendicular to the radii of the circle.

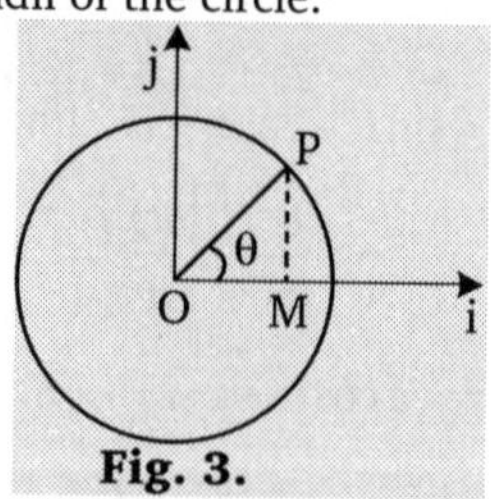

Fig. 3.

If P be any point on the circle such that OP makes an angle θ with the direction of i, then the position vector of P is given by

$$\vec{r} = \overrightarrow{OP} = \overrightarrow{OM} + \overrightarrow{MP} = (r\cos\theta)i + (r\sin\theta)j$$

where r is the radius of circle and hence constant and further $\frac{d\vec{r}}{dt}, \frac{d^2\vec{r}}{dt^2} = -\omega^2\vec{r}$.

ANSWERS

1. $\frac{d\vec{r}}{dt} = \hat{i} + (2t+1)\hat{j} + (3t^2+2t+1)\hat{k}$, $\frac{d^2\vec{r}}{dt^2} = 2\hat{j} + (6t+2)\hat{k}$ **5.** (i) $\frac{d\vec{r}}{dt} \times \vec{a}$ (ii) $\vec{r} \times \frac{d^2\vec{r}}{dt^2}$

(iii) $\frac{\frac{d\vec{r}}{dt} \times \vec{a}}{\vec{r}.\vec{a}} - \frac{\frac{d\vec{r}}{dt}.\vec{a}}{(\vec{r}.\vec{a})^2}(\vec{r} \times \vec{a})$ (iv) $3r^2\frac{dr}{dt}\vec{r} + r^3\frac{d\vec{r}}{dt} + \vec{a} \times \frac{d^2\vec{r}}{dt^2}$

6. (i) $\sqrt{2}, 1$ (ii) $a^2 \sec\alpha$, $a^3 \tan\alpha$ **10.** $\vec{r} = \frac{1}{3}(e^{2t} + 2e^{-t})\hat{i} + \frac{1}{3}(e^{2t} - e^{-t})\hat{j}$

11. (i) $(5t^2-1)\cos t + 11t\sin t$ (ii) $(t^3\sin t - 3t^2\cos t)\hat{i} - (t^3\cos t + 3t^2\sin t)\hat{j} + (5t^2\sin t - 11t\cos t - \sin t)\hat{k}$

(iii) $100t^3 + 2t + 6t^5$ **12.** $\vec{v} = 4\hat{j} + 6\hat{k}, \vec{a} = -4\hat{i}$ and $\vec{v} = -4\hat{i} + 6\hat{k}, \vec{a} = -4\hat{j}$

13. $|\vec{v}| = \sqrt{37}, \vec{a} = \sqrt{(325)}$ **14.** $\frac{1}{\sqrt{(a^2+b^2)}}[-a\sin t\hat{i} + a\cos\hat{j} + b\hat{k}]$ **16.** 0, 3

25.13 INTEGRATION OF A VECTOR FUNCTION

Let $\vec{F}(t)$ be a differentiable vector function and let $\vec{f}(t)$ be its differential coefficient, then

$$\frac{d}{dt}(\vec{F}(t)) = \vec{f}(t). \quad ...(1)$$

Therefore the integral of $\vec{f}(t)$ is $\vec{F}(t)$. Consequently we can say that integration is the reverse process of differentiation.

$$\therefore \quad \int \vec{f}(t)dt = \vec{F}(t). \quad ...(2)$$

This is an indefinite integral and the function $\vec{f}(t)$ which is being integrated is known as integrand.

Moreover, let $\vec{c}$ be a constant vector which is independent of t, then (1) can also be written as

$$\frac{d}{dt}[\vec{F}(t) + \vec{c}] = \vec{f}(t) \quad ...(3)$$

$$\therefore \quad \int \vec{f}(t)dt = \vec{F}(t) + \vec{c}. \quad ...(4)$$

This constant vector $\vec{c}$ is called constant of integration, since this vector $\vec{c}$ is taken to be arbitrary so the integral given by (4) is therefore known as indefinite integral.

If $\vec{f}(t)$ is defined over the closed interval $[a, b]$, then the integral given in (5)

$$\int_a^b \vec{f}(t)dt = [\vec{F}(t) + \vec{c}]_a^b = \vec{F}(b) - \vec{F}(a) \quad ...(5)$$

is called the definite integral and a and b are called limits of integration.

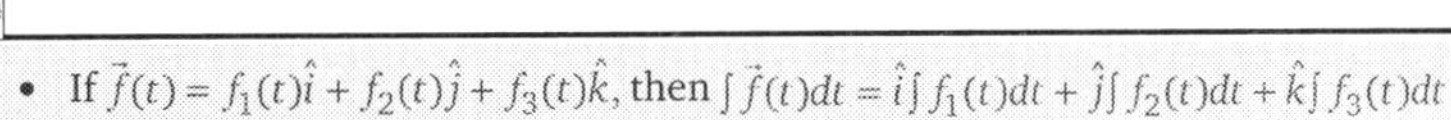

- If $\vec{f}(t) = f_1(t)\hat{i} + f_2(t)\hat{j} + f_3(t)\hat{k}$, then $\int \vec{f}(t)dt = \hat{i}\int f_1(t)dt + \hat{j}\int f_2(t)dt + \hat{k}\int f_3(t)dt$.

25.13.1 SOME IMPORTANT RESULTS

1. Since $\frac{d}{dt}(\vec{a}.\vec{b}) = \vec{a}.\frac{d\vec{b}}{dt} + \frac{d\vec{a}}{dt}.\vec{b}$, therefore g$\int\left(\vec{a}.\frac{d\vec{b}}{dt} + \frac{d\vec{a}}{dt}.\vec{b}\right)dt = \vec{a}.\vec{b} + \vec{c}$ where, $\vec{c}$ is a constant of integration.

2. $\frac{d}{dt}(\vec{a}\times\vec{b}) = \vec{a}\times\frac{d\vec{b}}{dt}+\frac{d\vec{a}}{dt}\times\vec{b}$, so $\int\left(\vec{a}\times\frac{d\vec{b}}{dt}+\frac{d\vec{a}}{dt}\times\vec{b}\right)dt = (\vec{a}\times\vec{b})+\vec{c}$, where, $\vec{c}$ is a constant vector.

3. Since $\vec{a}.\vec{a} = \vec{a}^2 \Rightarrow \frac{d}{dt}(\vec{a}.\vec{a}) = \vec{a}.\frac{d\vec{a}}{dt}+\frac{d\vec{a}}{dt}.\vec{a} = 2\vec{a}.\frac{d\vec{a}}{dt}$

$\therefore$ $\int\left(2\vec{a}.\frac{d\vec{a}}{dt}\right)dt = (\vec{a}.\vec{a})+c$ or $\int\left(2\vec{a}.\frac{d\vec{a}}{dt}\right)dt = \vec{a}^2+c$. Here, c is a scalar quantity.

4. Since

$$\frac{d}{dt}\left(\vec{a}\times\frac{d\vec{a}}{dt}\right) = \vec{a}\times\frac{d^2\vec{a}}{dt^2}+\frac{d\vec{a}}{dt}\times\frac{d\vec{a}}{dt} = \vec{a}\times\frac{d^2\vec{a}}{dt^2} \qquad \left(\because \frac{d\vec{a}}{dt}\times\frac{d\vec{a}}{dt} = 0\right)$$

$$\therefore \int\left(\vec{a}\times\frac{d^2\vec{a}}{dt^2}\right)dt = \left(\vec{a}\times\frac{d\vec{a}}{dt}\right)+\vec{c}$$

Here, $\vec{c}$ is a constant vectror of integration.

5. Since

$$\frac{d}{dt}\left(\vec{a}\times\frac{d\vec{b}}{dt}\right) = \vec{a}\times\frac{d^2\vec{b}}{dt^2}+\frac{d\vec{a}}{dt}\times\frac{d\vec{b}}{dt}$$

If $\vec{a}$ is a constant vector, then $\frac{d\vec{a}}{dt} = 0$ and $\frac{d}{dt}\left(\vec{a}\times\frac{d\vec{b}}{dt}\right) = \vec{a}\times\frac{d^2\vec{b}}{dt^2}$

$\therefore$ $\int\left(\vec{a}\times\frac{d^2\vec{b}}{dt^2}\right)dt = \left(\vec{a}\times\frac{d\vec{b}}{dt}\right)+\vec{c}$. Here, $\vec{c}$ is a constant vector of integration.

6. If **a** is a constant vector, we have that

$$\frac{d}{dt}(\vec{a}\times\vec{b}) = \vec{a}\times\frac{d\vec{b}}{dt} \qquad \left(\because \frac{d\vec{a}}{dt} = 0\right)$$

$\therefore$ $\int\left(\vec{a}\times\frac{d\vec{b}}{dt}\right)dt = (\vec{a}\times\vec{b})+\vec{c}$. Here, $\vec{c}$ is a constant vector which is constant of integration.

7. If c is constant scalar and $\vec{a}$ is a vector function of t, then $\int c\vec{a}dt = c\int\vec{a}dt$.

Solved Examples

1. *Interpret the relations*

$$\vec{r}.\frac{d\vec{r}}{ds} = 0 \quad \text{and} \quad \vec{r}\times\frac{d\vec{r}}{ds} = 0$$

SOLUTION. For $\vec{r}.\frac{d\vec{r}}{ds} = 0 \quad \Rightarrow \quad 2\vec{r}.\frac{d\vec{r}}{ds} = 0$

Integrating w.r.t. s we get

$$\int\left(2\vec{r}.\frac{d\vec{r}}{ds}\right)ds = \int 0ds$$

or $\vec{r}^{\,2} = a$ (constant)

$\Rightarrow$ $\vec{r}$ has constant magnitude.

Thus $\vec{r}$ describe a circle.

Again, for $\vec{r}\times\frac{d\vec{r}}{ds} = 0$

$\Rightarrow$ $\vec{r}$ and $\frac{d\vec{r}}{ds}$ are parallel.

Also $\frac{d\vec{r}}{ds}$ is a unit vector along tangent.

$\therefore$ $\vec{r}$ has constant direction that the tangent at every point is along **r**. Thus $\vec{r}$ describes a straight line.

2. *If*
$\vec{f}(t)=(t+1)\hat{i}+(t^2+t+1)\hat{j}+(t^3+t^2+t+1)\hat{k}$
find $\int_0^1 \vec{f}(t)dt$.

SOLUTION. Since

$$\vec{f}(t)=(t+1)\hat{i}+(t^2+t+1)\hat{j}+(t^3+t^2+t+1)\hat{k}$$

then $\int_0^1 \vec{f}(t)dt$

$$=\int_0^1[(t+1)\hat{i}+(t^2+t+1)\hat{j}+(t^3+t^2+t+1)\hat{k}]dt$$

$$=\hat{i}\int_0^1(t+1)dt+\hat{j}\int_0^1(t^2+t+1)dt+\hat{k}\int_0^1(t^3+t^2+t+1)dt$$

$$=\hat{i}\left(\frac{t^2}{2}+t\right)_0^1+\hat{j}\left(\frac{t^3}{3}+\frac{t^2}{2}+t\right)_0^1+\hat{k}\left(\frac{t^4}{4}+\frac{t^3}{3}+\frac{t^2}{2}+t\right)_0^1$$

$$=\frac{3}{2}\hat{i}+\frac{11}{6}\hat{j}+\frac{25}{12}\hat{k}.$$

3. *If* $\vec{r}=5t^2\hat{i}+t\hat{j}-t^3\hat{k}$, *then prove that*

$$\int_1^2\left(\vec{r}\times\frac{d^2\vec{r}}{dt^2}\right)dt=-14\hat{i}+75\hat{j}-15\hat{k}.$$

SOLUTION. Since $\vec{r}=5t^2\hat{i}+t\hat{j}-t^3\hat{k}$, then

$$\frac{d\vec{r}}{dt}=10t\hat{i}+\hat{j}-3t^2\hat{k}$$

again $\dfrac{d^2\vec{r}}{dt^2}=10\hat{i}-6t\hat{k}$.

$$\therefore\ \vec{r}\times\frac{d^2\vec{r}}{dt^2}=(5t^2\hat{i}+t\hat{j}-t^3\hat{k})\times(10\hat{i}-6t\hat{k})$$

$$=-30t^3\hat{i}\times\hat{k}+10t\hat{j}\times\hat{i}-6t^2\hat{j}\times\hat{k}-10t^3\hat{k}\times\hat{i}$$

$$=30t^3\hat{j}-10t\hat{k}-6t^2\hat{i}-10t^3\hat{j}$$

$$=-6t^2\hat{i}+20t^3\hat{j}-10t\hat{k}.$$

Now

$$\int_1^2\left(\vec{r}\times\frac{d^2\vec{r}}{dt^2}\right)=\int_1^2(-6t^2\hat{i}+20t^3\hat{j}-10t\hat{k})dt$$

$$=\left[-2t^3\hat{i}+5t^4\hat{j}-5t^2\hat{k}\right]_1^2$$

$$=-14\hat{i}+75\hat{j}-15\hat{k}.$$

4. *Find the value of* $\vec{r}$ *satisfying the equation*

$$\frac{d^2\vec{r}}{dt^2}=6t\hat{i}-24t^2\hat{j}+4\sin t\hat{k}$$

given that $\vec{r}=2\hat{i}+\hat{j}$ *and* $\dfrac{d\vec{r}}{dt}=0$ *at* $t=0$.

SOLUTION. We know that $\dfrac{d^2\vec{r}}{dt^2}=\dfrac{d}{dt}\left(\dfrac{d\vec{r}}{dt}\right)$. so

$$\frac{d\vec{r}}{dt}=\int\left(\frac{d^2\vec{r}}{dt^2}\right)dt+\vec{c}$$

(where $\vec{c}$ is constant vector taken to be as constant of integration.)

$$\frac{d\vec{r}}{dt}=\int(6t\hat{i}-24t^2\hat{j}+4\sin t\hat{k})dt+\vec{c}$$

$$\frac{d\vec{r}}{dt}=3t^2\hat{i}-8t^3\hat{j}-4\cos t\hat{k}+\vec{c}\quad\ldots(1)$$

Initially at $t=0$,

$$\frac{d\vec{r}}{dt}=0\Rightarrow\ 0=-4\hat{k}+\vec{c}$$

$$\therefore\quad \vec{c}=4\hat{k}\quad\ldots(2)$$

Form (1) and (2), we get

$$\frac{d\vec{r}}{dt}=3t^2\hat{i}-8t^3\hat{j}-4\cos t\hat{k}+4\hat{k}$$

Again integrating, we get

$$\vec{r}=\int(3t^2\hat{i}-8t^3\hat{j}-4\cos t\hat{k}+4\hat{k})+\vec{d}$$

Here, $\vec{d}$ is constant vector of integration.

$$\therefore\ \vec{r}=(t^3\hat{i}-2t^4\hat{j}-4\sin t\hat{k}+4t\hat{k})+\vec{d}\quad\ldots(3)$$

Again initially, at $t=0, \vec{r}=2\hat{i}+\hat{j}$.

$$\therefore\quad 2\hat{i}+\hat{j}=\vec{d}\quad\ldots(4)$$

Thus, form (3) and (4), we get the required result

$$\vec{r}=t^3\hat{i}-2t^4\hat{j}+4(t-\sin t)\hat{k}+2\hat{i}+\hat{j}$$

or $\vec{r}=(t^3+2)\hat{i}+(1-2t^4)\hat{j}+4(t-\sin t)\hat{k}$

Exercise-25.2

1. If $\vec{f}(t)=(t-t^2)\hat{i}+2t^3\hat{j}-3\hat{k}$, find

   (i) $\int \vec{f}(t)dt$ (ii) $\int_1^2 \vec{f}(t)dt$

2. Integrate $\vec{a}\times\frac{d^2\vec{r}}{dt^2}=\vec{b}$, where $\vec{a}$ and $\vec{b}$ are constant vectors.

3. Find the value of $\vec{r}$ satisfying the equation $\frac{d^2\vec{r}}{dt^2}=t\vec{a}+\vec{b}$ where $\vec{a}$ and $\vec{b}$ are constant vectors.

4. Given that $\vec{r}(t)=\begin{cases}2\hat{i}-\hat{j}+2\hat{k} & , t=2\\ 4\hat{i}-2\hat{j}+3\hat{k} & , t=3\end{cases}$

   Show that $\int_2^3\left(\vec{r}.\frac{d\vec{r}}{dt}\right)dt=10$.

5. Find $\int_0^1\left(e^t\hat{i}+e^{-2t}\hat{j}+t\hat{k}\right)dt$

6. If $\vec{r}=t\hat{i}-t^2\hat{j}+(t-1)\hat{k}$ and $\vec{s}=2t^2\hat{i}+6t\hat{k}$, evaluate (i) $\int_0^2\vec{r}.\vec{s}dt$ (ii) $\int_0^2\vec{r}\times\vec{s}dt$.

7. Solve the equation $\frac{d^2\vec{r}}{dt^2}=\vec{a}$ where $\vec{a}$ is a constant vector given that $\vec{r}=0$ and $\frac{d\vec{r}}{dt}=0$ when $t=0$.

8. If $\vec{f}(t)=t\hat{i}+(t^2-2t)\hat{j}+(3t^2+3t^3)\hat{k}$, find $\int_0^1\vec{f}(t)dt$.

9. If $\vec{a}=t\hat{i}-3\hat{j}+2t\hat{k},\vec{b}=\hat{i}-2\hat{j}+2\hat{k}$ and $\vec{c}=3\hat{i}+t\hat{j}-\hat{k}$, then evaluate $\int_1^2\vec{a}\cdot(\vec{b}\times\vec{c})dt$.

10. The acceleration of a particle at any time $t\geq 0$ is given by $\vec{a}=\frac{d\vec{v}}{dt}=12\cos 2t\hat{i}-8\sin 2t\hat{j}+16t\hat{k}$ if the velocity $\vec{v}$ and displacement $\vec{r}$, are zero at $t=0$, find $\vec{v}$ and $\vec{r}$ at any time t.

11. The acceleration of a particle at any time t is given by $\vec{a}=\frac{d\vec{v}}{dt}=e^t\hat{i}+e^{2t}\hat{j}+\hat{k}$, find v if $\vec{v}=\hat{i}+\hat{j}$ at $t=0$.

12. Find the value of $\vec{r}$ satisfying the equation $\frac{d^2\vec{r}}{dt^2}=\vec{a}$, where $\vec{a}$ is a constant vector. Also it is given that when $t=0$, $\vec{r}=0$ and $\frac{d\vec{r}}{dt}=\vec{u}$.

13. If $\vec{A}=\hat{i}+u^2\hat{j}-2u\hat{k}$ and $\vec{B}=e^u\hat{i}-u\hat{j}-\hat{k}$, find $\int(\vec{A}\times\vec{B})du$.

Hint to Selected Problems

1. $\vec{f}(t)=(t-t^2)\hat{i}+2t^3\hat{j}-3\hat{k}$

$$\therefore \int\vec{f}(t)dt=\int[(t-t^2)\hat{i}+2t^3\hat{j}-3\hat{k}]dt=\left(\frac{t^2}{2}-\frac{t^3}{3}\right)\hat{i}+\frac{t^4}{2}\hat{j}-3t\hat{k}$$

and $\int_1^2\vec{f}(t)dt=\left[\left(\frac{t^2}{2}-\frac{t^3}{3}\right)\hat{i}+\frac{t^4}{2}\hat{j}-3t\hat{k}\right]_1^2$

$$=\frac{-5}{6}\hat{i}+\frac{15}{2}\hat{j}-3\hat{k}$$

4. $\vec{r}(t)=\begin{cases}2\hat{i}-\hat{j}+2\hat{k} & , t=2\\ 4\hat{i}-2\hat{j}+3\hat{k} & , t=3\end{cases}$

Since $\int\left(\vec{r}.\frac{d\vec{r}}{dt}\right)dt=\frac{1}{2}\int\frac{d}{dt}(\vec{r}.\vec{r})dt=\frac{1}{2}(\vec{r}.\vec{r})$

$$\therefore \int_2^3\left(\vec{r}.\frac{d\vec{r}}{dt}\right)dt=\frac{1}{2}[\vec{r}(t).\vec{r}(t)]_2^3$$

$$=\frac{1}{2}[\vec{r}(3).\vec{r}(3)-\vec{r}(2).\vec{r}(2)]$$

$$=\frac{1}{2}[(4\hat{i}-2\hat{j}+3\hat{k}).(4\hat{i}-2\hat{j}+3\hat{k})-(2\hat{i}-\hat{j}+2\hat{k}).(2\hat{i}-\hat{j}+2\hat{k})]$$

$$=\frac{1}{2}[(16+4+9)-(4+1+4)]$$

$$=\frac{1}{2}[29-9]=\frac{1}{2}(20)=10.$$

9. $\vec{a}=t\hat{i}-3\hat{j}+2t\hat{k},\vec{b}=\hat{i}-2\hat{j}+2\hat{k},\vec{c}=3\hat{i}+t\hat{j}-\hat{k}$,

then $\vec{a}.(\vec{b}\times\vec{c})=\begin{vmatrix}t & -3 & 2t\\ 1 & -2 & 2\\ 3 & t & -1\end{vmatrix}$

$$=t(2-2t)+3(-1-6)+2t(t+6)$$

$$=2t-2t^2-21=2t^2+12t=14t-21$$

$$\therefore \int_1^2\vec{a}.(\vec{b}\times\vec{c})dt=\int_1^2(14t-21)dt=\left[7t^2-21t\right]_1^2$$

$$=(28-42)-(7-21)=0.$$

ANSWERS

1. (i) $\left(\frac{t^2}{2}-\frac{t^3}{3}\right)\hat{i}+\frac{t^4}{2}\hat{j}-3t\hat{k}+\vec{c}$ (ii) $-\frac{5}{6}\hat{i}+\frac{15}{2}\hat{j}-3\hat{k}$ **2.** $\vec{a}\times\vec{r}=\frac{1}{2}t^2\vec{b}+t\vec{c}+\vec{d}$

3. $\vec{r}=\frac{1}{6}t^3\vec{a}+\frac{1}{2}t^2\vec{b}+t\vec{c}+\vec{d}$ **5.** $(e-1)\hat{i}-\frac{1}{2}(e^{-2}-1)\hat{j}+\frac{1}{2}\hat{k}$ **6.** (i) 12 (ii) $-24\hat{i}-\frac{40}{3}\hat{j}+\frac{64}{5}\hat{k}$

7. $\vec{r}=\frac{1}{2}t^2\vec{a}$ **8.** $\frac{1}{2}\hat{i}-\frac{2}{3}\hat{j}+\frac{7}{4}\hat{k}$ **9.** 0 **10.** $\vec{v}=6\sin 2t\hat{i}+(4\cos 2t-4)\hat{j}+8t^2\hat{k}$

$\vec{r}=(3-3\cos 2t)\hat{i}+(2\sin 2t-4t)\hat{j}+\frac{8}{3}t^3\hat{k}$

11. $\vec{v}=e^t\hat{i}+\frac{1}{2}(e^{2t}+1)\hat{j}+t\hat{k}$ **12.** $\vec{r}=\frac{1}{2}t^2\vec{a}+t\vec{u}$

13. $-\frac{u^3}{3}\hat{i}-\hat{j}\left(-u+2ue^u-2e^u\right)+\hat{k}\left(-\frac{u^2}{2}-u^2e^u+2ue^u+2e^u\right)$.

25.14 PARTIAL DERIVATIVE OF VECTORS

Let $\vec{r} = \vec{f}(x, y, z)$ be a vector function of three scalar variables x, y, z. The first order partial derivative of $\vec{r}$ with respect to x is given by

$$\frac{\partial\vec{r}}{\partial x}=\lim_{\delta x\to 0}\frac{\vec{f}(x+\delta x,y,z)-\vec{f}(x,y,z)}{\delta x}, \text{ if this limit exists.}$$

Similarly we can find first order partial derivatives of $\vec{r}$ with respect to y and z respectively and are denoted by $\frac{\partial\vec{r}}{\partial y},\frac{\partial\vec{r}}{\partial z}$.

During the differentiation if y and z are treating as constant, then $\frac{\partial\vec{r}}{\partial x}$ is regarded as ordinary derivative. Likewise we can find higher order partial derivatives.

25.15 VECTOR DIFFERENTIAL OPERATOR

The vector differential operator is defined by the formula $\nabla=\frac{\partial}{\partial x}\hat{i}+\frac{\partial}{\partial y}\hat{j}+\frac{\partial}{\partial z}\hat{k}$.

Obviously, ∇ is a vector quantity. This vector ∇ is read as **nabla** or **del**.

25.16 GRADIENT OF A SCALAR FIELD

Let $f(x, y, z)$ be a scalar point function which is defined over some region R in space and also differentiable at each point (x, y, z) in R, then the gradient of $f(x, y, z)$ is defined as

$$\text{grad } f=\frac{\partial f}{\partial x}\hat{i}+\frac{\partial f}{\partial y}\hat{j}+\frac{\partial f}{\partial z}\hat{k} \text{ or grad } f=\left(\frac{\partial}{\partial x}\hat{i}+\frac{\partial}{\partial y}\hat{j}+\frac{\partial}{\partial z}\hat{k}\right)f=\nabla f$$

Thus gradient of f can also be written in terms of vector differential operator(∇). Since ∇ is a vector quantity, thus ∇f is a vector whose components are $\frac{\partial f}{\partial x},\frac{\partial f}{\partial y},\frac{\partial f}{\partial z}$. Hence, gradient of a scalar field is a vector field.

25.17 SOME FORMULAE RELATED TO GRADIENT

1. If f and g are two scalar point functions, then grad $(f + g)$ = grad f + grad g

or $\nabla(f+g)=\nabla f+\nabla g.$

PROOF. Since we know that

$$\nabla f = \frac{\partial f}{\partial x}\hat{i} + \frac{\partial f}{\partial y}\hat{j} + \frac{\partial f}{\partial z}\hat{k}$$

$$\therefore \quad \nabla(f+g) = \frac{\partial}{\partial x}(f+g)\hat{i} + \frac{\partial}{\partial y}(f+g)\hat{j} + \frac{\partial}{\partial z}(f+g)\hat{k}$$

$$= \frac{\partial f}{\partial x}\hat{i} + \frac{\partial g}{\partial x}\hat{i} + \frac{\partial f}{\partial y}\hat{j} + \frac{\partial g}{\partial y}\hat{j} + \frac{\partial f}{\partial z}\hat{k} + \frac{\partial g}{\partial z}\hat{k}$$

$$= \left(\frac{\partial f}{\partial x}\hat{i} + \frac{\partial f}{\partial y}\hat{j} + \frac{\partial f}{\partial z}\hat{k}\right) + \left(\frac{\partial g}{\partial x}\hat{i} + \frac{\partial g}{\partial y}\hat{j} + \frac{\partial g}{\partial z}\hat{k}\right) = \nabla f + \nabla g.$$

Hence, $\nabla(f+g) = \nabla f + \nabla g$.

2. *If f and g are two scalar point functions, then* $\nabla(fg) = f\nabla g + g\nabla f$.

or $$\text{grad } (fg) = f(\text{grad } g) + g(\text{grad } f).$$

PROOF. Since we know that $\nabla f = \frac{\partial f}{\partial x}\hat{i} + \frac{\partial f}{\partial y}\hat{j} + \frac{\partial f}{\partial z}\hat{k}$

$$\therefore \quad \nabla(fg) = \frac{\partial}{\partial x}(fg)\hat{i} + \frac{\partial}{\partial y}(fg)\hat{j} + \frac{\partial}{\partial z}(fg)\hat{k}$$

$$= \left(f\frac{\partial g}{\partial x} + g\frac{\partial f}{\partial x}\right)\hat{i} + \left(f\frac{\partial g}{\partial y} + g\frac{\partial f}{\partial y}\right)\hat{j} + \left(f\frac{\partial g}{\partial z} + g\frac{\partial f}{\partial z}\right)\hat{k}$$

$$= f\left(\frac{\partial g}{\partial x}\hat{i} + \frac{\partial g}{\partial y}\hat{j} + \frac{\partial g}{\partial z}\hat{k}\right) + g\left(\frac{\partial f}{\partial x}\hat{i} + \frac{\partial f}{\partial y}\hat{j} + \frac{\partial f}{\partial z}\hat{k}\right) = f\nabla g + g\nabla f.$$

Hence, $\nabla(fg) = f\nabla g + g\nabla f$.

3. *If f and g are scalar point functions and $g \neq 0$ for all point in the region R, then* $\nabla\left(\frac{f}{g}\right) = \frac{g\nabla f - f\nabla g}{g^2}$.

PROOF. Since $\nabla f = \frac{\partial f}{\partial x}\hat{i} + \frac{\partial f}{\partial y}\hat{j} + \frac{\partial f}{\partial z}\hat{k}$

$$\therefore \quad \nabla\left(\frac{f}{g}\right) = \frac{\partial}{\partial x}\left(\frac{f}{g}\right)\hat{i} + \frac{\partial}{\partial y}\left(\frac{f}{g}\right)\hat{j} + \frac{\partial}{\partial z}\left(\frac{f}{g}\right)\hat{k}$$

$$= \frac{1}{g^2}\left(g\frac{\partial f}{\partial x} - f\frac{\partial g}{\partial x}\right)\hat{i} + \frac{1}{g^2}\left(g\frac{\partial f}{\partial y} - f\frac{\partial g}{\partial y}\right)\hat{j} + \frac{1}{g^2}\left(g\frac{\partial f}{\partial z} - f\frac{\partial g}{\partial z}\right)\hat{k}$$

$$= \frac{1}{g^2}\left[g\left(\frac{\partial f}{\partial x}\hat{i} + \frac{\partial f}{\partial y}\hat{j} + \frac{\partial f}{\partial z}\hat{k}\right) - f\left(\frac{\partial g}{\partial x}\hat{i} + \frac{\partial g}{\partial y}\hat{j} + \frac{\partial g}{\partial z}\hat{k}\right)\right] = \frac{1}{g^2}[g\nabla f - f\nabla g]$$

$$= \frac{g(\nabla f) - f(\nabla g)}{g^2}.$$

Hence, $\nabla\left(\frac{f}{g}\right) = \frac{g\nabla f - f\nabla g}{g^2}$.

4. *If f is a scalar point function, then f is constant if and only if* $\nabla f = \vec{0}$.

PROOF. Suppose f is constant, then

$$\frac{\partial f}{\partial x} = 0, \frac{\partial f}{\partial y} = 0, \frac{\partial f}{\partial z} = 0 \qquad (\because f(x, y, z) = c)$$

$$\therefore \quad \nabla f = \frac{\partial f}{\partial x}\hat{i} + \frac{\partial f}{\partial y}\hat{j} + \frac{\partial f}{\partial z}\hat{k} = 0\hat{i} + 0\hat{j} + 0\hat{k} = \vec{0}.$$

Conversely, suppose $\nabla f = \vec{0}$. Then we have $\nabla f = \frac{\partial f}{\partial x}\hat{i} + \frac{\partial f}{\partial y}\hat{j} + \frac{\partial f}{\partial z}\hat{k} = \vec{0}$. So,

$$\frac{\partial f}{\partial x} = 0, \frac{\partial f}{\partial y} = 0, \frac{\partial f}{\partial z} = 0.$$

Hence, $f(x, y, z) = c$ (constant)

- $\nabla(f - g) = \nabla f - \nabla g$
- $\nabla(cf) = c\nabla f$, where c is a constant.
- $\nabla\left(\frac{1}{f}\right) = -\frac{\nabla f}{f^2}$, where $f \neq 0 \ \forall \ (x, y, z) \in \mathbf{R}$.

25.18 DIRECTIONAL DERIVATIVES

Let us consider a scalar field given by a scalar point function $f(P) = f(x, y, z)$ where P is any point in space whose co-ordinates are (x, y, z). Since we know that the first order partial derivatives of f are the rates of change of f in the direction of co-ordinate axes. Now we shall have to discuss the rate of change of f in any direction, this leads the notion of a directional derivative.

Let us choose a point P in space and a direction at P, given by a unit vector $\hat{a}$. Let C be the ray from P in the direction of $\hat{a}$ and let Q be any point on this ray C such that PQ is as shown in fig. 4.

Then the limit

$$\frac{\partial f}{\partial s} = \lim_{s \to 0} \frac{f(Q) - f(P)}{s}, \text{ where } s = PQ$$

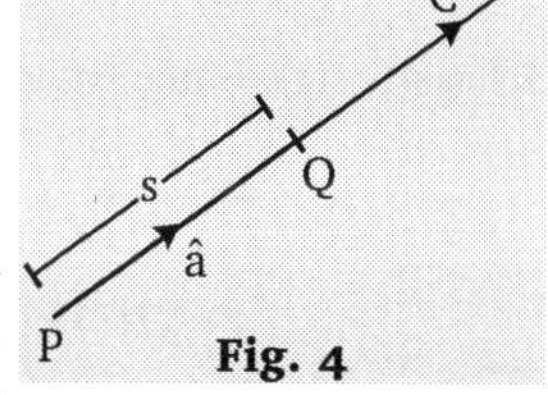

Fig. 4

if exists is called the directional derivative of f at P in the direction of $\hat{a}$. In fact there are infinitely many directional derivatives of f at P, each corresponding to a certain direction. But if a cartesian co-ordinates system is given, then we may represent any such derivative in terms of the first order partial derivatives of f at P. If the position vector P is $\vec{p}$, then the ray C can be written as

$$\vec{r}(s) = x(s)\hat{i} + y(s)\hat{j} + z(s)\hat{k} \qquad \ldots(1)$$

$$= \vec{p} + s\hat{a} \, (s \geq 0)$$

and $\frac{\partial f}{\partial s}$ is the derivative of the function $f[x(s), y(s), z(s)]$ with respect to the arc length s of C. Hence, assuming that f has continuous partial derivative of first order, we have

$$\frac{\partial f}{\partial s} = \frac{\partial f}{\partial x}\frac{dx}{ds} + \frac{\partial f}{\partial y}\frac{dy}{ds} + \frac{\partial f}{\partial z}\frac{dz}{ds} \qquad \ldots(2)$$

Form (1)

$$\frac{d\vec{r}}{ds} = \frac{dx}{ds}\hat{i} + \frac{dy}{ds}\hat{j} + \frac{dz}{ds}\hat{k} = \hat{a} \qquad \ldots(3)$$

Since we have

$$\text{grad} f = \frac{\partial f}{\partial x}\hat{i} + \frac{\partial f}{\partial y}\hat{j} + \frac{\partial f}{\partial z}\hat{k}. \quad \ldots(4)$$

Thus, equation (2) becomes

$$\frac{\partial f}{\partial s} = \left(\frac{\partial f}{\partial x}\hat{i} + \frac{\partial f}{\partial y}\hat{j} + \frac{\partial f}{\partial z}\hat{k}\right).\left(\frac{dx}{ds}\hat{i} + \frac{dy}{ds}\hat{j} + \frac{dz}{ds}\hat{k}\right)$$

$$= (\text{grad} f).\hat{a} \quad \text{[From (3) and (4)]}$$

or

$$\frac{\partial f}{\partial s} = \hat{a} \cdot \text{grad } f = \hat{a} \cdot \nabla f.$$

Hence, the directional derivative $\frac{\partial f}{\partial s}$ is given as $\hat{a} \cdot \nabla f$.

- If $\hat{a} = \hat{i}$, then $\frac{\partial f}{\partial s} = \hat{i}.\nabla f = \hat{i}.\left(\frac{\partial f}{\partial x}\hat{i} + \frac{\partial f}{\partial y}\hat{j} + \frac{\partial f}{\partial z}\hat{k}\right) = \frac{\partial f}{\partial x}$. Similarly, if $\hat{a} = \hat{j}, \hat{k}$, then $\frac{\partial f}{\partial s} = \frac{\partial f}{\partial y}, \frac{\partial f}{\partial s} = \frac{\partial f}{\partial z}$.
- Maximum value of the directional derivative is $|\text{grad} f|$.

Solved Examples

1. *If $r = |\vec{r}|$ where $\vec{r} = x\hat{i} + y\hat{j} + z\hat{k}$, prove that*

(i) $\nabla f(r) = f'(r)\nabla r$

(ii) $\nabla r = \frac{\vec{r}}{r}$ (GBTU–2011)

(iii) $\nabla f(r) \times \vec{r} = 0$

(iv) $\nabla r^n = nr^{n-2}\vec{r}$.

(v) $\nabla r^{-3} = -3r^{-5}\vec{r}$.

SOLUTION. (i) Since we know that

$$\nabla f = \frac{\partial f}{\partial x}\hat{i} + \frac{\partial f}{\partial y}\hat{j} + \frac{\partial f}{\partial z}\hat{k} \quad \ldots(1)$$

$$\therefore \nabla f(r) = \frac{\partial}{\partial x}(f(r))\hat{i} + \frac{\partial}{\partial y}(f(r))\hat{j} + \frac{\partial}{\partial z}(f(r))\hat{k}$$

or $$\nabla f(r) = f'(r)\frac{\partial r}{\partial x}\hat{i} + f'(r)\frac{\partial r}{\partial y}\hat{j} + f'(r)\frac{\partial r}{\partial z}\hat{k}$$

$$\nabla f(r) = f'(r)\left[\frac{\partial r}{\partial x}\hat{i} + \frac{\partial r}{\partial y}\hat{j} + \frac{\partial r}{\partial z}\hat{k}\right]$$

$$\nabla f(r) = f'(r)\nabla r. \text{ [Using (i)]}$$

(ii) We have $\nabla r = \frac{\partial r}{\partial x}\hat{i} + \frac{\partial r}{\partial y}\hat{j} + \frac{\partial r}{\partial z}\hat{k}$

Since $\vec{r} = x\hat{i} + y\hat{j} + z\hat{k}$

$$\therefore |\vec{r}|^2 = x^2 + y^2 + z^2$$

or $r^2 = x^2 + y^2 + z^2$ $(\because |\vec{r}| = r)$

$$\therefore \frac{\partial r}{\partial x} = \frac{x}{r}, \frac{\partial r}{\partial y} = \frac{y}{r}, \frac{\partial r}{\partial z} = \frac{z}{r}$$

$$\therefore \nabla r = \frac{x}{r}\hat{i} + \frac{y}{r}\hat{j} + \frac{z}{r}\hat{k}$$

$$= \frac{1}{r}(x\hat{i} + y\hat{j} + z\hat{k})$$

or $$\nabla r = \frac{\vec{r}}{r}.$$

(iii) $\nabla f(r) = f'(r)\nabla r$ [From (i)]

$$= f'(r)\frac{\vec{r}}{r} \quad \text{[From (ii)]}$$

Now $\nabla f(r) \times \vec{r} = \frac{f'(r)}{r}\vec{r} \times \vec{r} = \vec{0}$

$(\because \vec{r} \times \vec{r} = \vec{0})$

(iv) Since

$$\nabla f(r) = f'(r)\nabla r \quad \text{(From (i))}$$

Let $f(r) = r^n$.

$$\therefore \nabla r^n = nr^{n-1}\nabla r = nr^{n-1}\left(\frac{\vec{r}}{r}\right)$$

$$\left(\because \nabla r = \frac{\vec{r}}{r}\right)$$

$$= nr^{n-2}\vec{r}$$

or $\nabla r^n = nr^{n-2}\vec{r}$.

(v) From part (iv), $\nabla r^n = nr^{n-2}\vec{r}$

$$\Rightarrow \nabla r^{-3} = -3r^{-3-2}\vec{r} = -3r^{-5}\vec{r}.$$

2. *If $f(x, y, z) = 3x^2y - y^3z^2$, find grad f and $|\text{grad } f|$ at $(1, -2, -1)$.*

SOLUTION. Since we know that

$$\text{grad } f = \nabla f = \frac{\partial f}{\partial x}\hat{i} + \frac{\partial f}{\partial y}\hat{j} + \frac{\partial f}{\partial z}\hat{k}$$

$$= \frac{\partial}{\partial x}(3x^2y - y^3z^2)\hat{i} + \frac{\partial}{\partial y}(3x^2y - y^3z^2)\hat{j} + \frac{\partial}{\partial z}(3x^2y - y^3z^2)\hat{k}$$

$$= 6xy\hat{i} + (3x^2 - 3y^2z^2)\hat{j} + (-2y^3z)\hat{k}$$

At $(1, -2, -1)$

$$\text{grad } f = -12\hat{i} - 9\hat{j} - 16\hat{k}$$

and $|\text{grad } f| = \sqrt{144 + 81 + 256} = \sqrt{481}$.

3. *If $\phi(x, y, z) = xy^2z$ and $\vec{f}(x, y, z) = xz\hat{i} - xy\hat{j} + yz\hat{k}$, show that $\frac{\partial^3}{\partial x^2 \partial z}(\phi\vec{f})$ at $(2, -1, 1)$ is $4\hat{i} + 2\hat{j}$.*

(BHOPAL–2008)

SOLUTION. We have $\phi\vec{f} = x^2y^2z^2\hat{i} - x^2y^3z\hat{j} + xy^3z^2\hat{k}$.

$$\therefore \frac{\partial}{\partial z}(\phi\vec{f}) = 2x^2y^2z\hat{i} - x^2y^3\hat{j} + 2xy^3z\hat{k}$$

$$\frac{\partial^2}{\partial x \partial z}(\phi\vec{f}) = 4xy^2z\hat{i} - 2xy^3\hat{j} + 2y^3z\hat{k}$$

$$\frac{\partial^3}{\partial x^2 \partial z}(\phi\vec{f}) = 4y^2z\hat{i} - 2y^3\hat{j}$$

At $(2, -1, 1)$

$$\frac{\partial^3(\phi\vec{f})}{\partial x^2 \partial z} = 4(-1)^2(1)\hat{i} - 2(-1)^3\hat{j}$$

$$= 4\hat{i} + 2\hat{j}.$$

4. *Find $\nabla\phi$ and $|\nabla\phi|$ when*

$$\phi = (x^2 + y^2 + z^2)e^{-(x^2+y^2+z^2)^{1/2}}.$$

SOLUTION. Let $r^2 = x^2 + y^2 + z^2$, then ϕ can be written as

$$\phi = r^2e^{-r} \qquad \ldots(1)$$

$$\text{Now } \nabla\phi = \frac{\partial\phi}{\partial x}\hat{i} + \frac{\partial\phi}{\partial y}\hat{j} + \frac{\partial\phi}{\partial z}\hat{k} \qquad \ldots(2)$$

By (1),

$$\frac{\partial\phi}{\partial x} = \frac{\partial\phi}{\partial r}\frac{\partial r}{\partial x} = (2re^{-r} - r^2e^{-r})\frac{\partial r}{\partial x}.$$

Again by $r^2 = x^2 + y^2 + z^2$,

$$2r\frac{\partial r}{\partial x} = 2x \Rightarrow \frac{\partial r}{\partial x} = \frac{x}{r}.$$

$$\therefore \quad \frac{\partial\phi}{\partial x} = r(2 - r)e^{-r}\frac{x}{r} = (2 - r)e^{-r}x$$

Similarly, $\frac{\partial\phi}{\partial y} = (2 - r)e^{-r}y$

and $\frac{\partial\phi}{\partial z} = (2 - r)e^{-r}z$

$\therefore$ By (2), we have

$$\nabla\phi = (2 - r)e^{-r}(x\hat{i} + y\hat{j} + z\hat{k})$$

$$= (2 - r)e^{-r}\vec{r}.$$

Also, $|\nabla\phi| = |(2 - r)e^{-r}\vec{r}| = (2 - r)e^{-r}|\vec{r}|$

$$= (2 - r)e^{-r}r = (2 - r)re^{-r}$$

5. *Prove that*

(i) $\nabla(\vec{r}.\vec{a}) = \vec{a}$ (UPTU–2008)

(ii) $\nabla[\vec{r}\ \vec{a}\ \vec{b}] = \vec{a} \times \vec{b}$.

where $\vec{a}$ and $\vec{b}$ are constant vectors.

SOLUTION. Suppose $\vec{a} = a_1\hat{i} + a_2\hat{j} + a_3\hat{k}$

and $\vec{r} = x\hat{i} + y\hat{j} + z\hat{k}, \vec{b} = b_1\hat{i} + b_2\hat{j} + b_3\hat{k}$,

then $\quad \vec{r}.\vec{a} = xa_1 + a_2y + a_3z$

$$\text{and } \vec{r}.(\vec{a} \times \vec{b}) = \begin{vmatrix} x & y & z \\ a_1 & a_2 & a_3 \\ b_1 & b_2 & b_3 \end{vmatrix}$$

$$= x(a_2b_3 - a_3b_2) + y(a_3b_1 - a_1b_3) + z(a_1b_2 - a_2b_1)$$

(i) $\nabla(\vec{r}.\vec{a}) = \nabla(xa_1 + a_2y + a_3z)$

$$= a_1\nabla(x) + a_2\nabla(y) + a_3\nabla(z)$$
$$= a_1\hat{i} + a_2\hat{j} + a_3\hat{k}$$
$$(\because \nabla(x) = \hat{i}, \nabla(y) = \hat{j}, \nabla(z) = \hat{k})$$
$$= a$$

(ii) $\nabla[\vec{r}\ \vec{a}\ \vec{b}] = \nabla(\vec{r}.(\vec{a}\times\vec{b}))$

$$= \nabla[x(a_2b_3 - a_3b_2) + y(a_3b_1 - a_1b_3) + z(a_1b_2 - a_2b_1)]$$
$$= \nabla[x(a_2b_3 - a_3b_2)] + \nabla[y(a_3b_1 - a_1b_3)] + \nabla[z(a_1b_2 - a_2b_1)]$$
$$= (a_2b_3 - a_3b_2)\nabla(x) + (a_3b_1 - a_1b_3)\nabla(y) + (a_1b_2 - a_2b_1)\nabla(z)$$
$$= (a_2b_3 - a_3b_2)\hat{i} + (a_3b_1 - a_1b_3)\hat{j} + (a_1b_2 - a_2b_1)\hat{k}$$
$$= \begin{vmatrix} \hat{i} & \hat{j} & \hat{k} \\ a_1 & a_2 & a_3 \\ b_1 & b_2 & b_3 \end{vmatrix} = \vec{a}\times\vec{b}$$

$\therefore \quad \nabla[\vec{r}\ \vec{a}\ \vec{b}] = \vec{a}\times\vec{b}$.

6. *If* $\phi = (3r^2 - 4r^{1/2} + 6r^{-1/3})$, *show that* $\nabla\phi = 2(3 - r^{-3/2} - r^{-7/3})\vec{r}$.

SOLUTION. Let $\vec{r} = x\hat{i} + y\hat{j} + z\hat{k}$

then $|\vec{r}| = r = \sqrt{(x^2 + y^2 + z^2)}$.

Now $\nabla\phi = \dfrac{\partial\phi}{\partial x}\hat{i} + \dfrac{\partial\phi}{\partial y}\hat{j} + \dfrac{\partial\phi}{\partial z}\hat{k}$

$$= \frac{\partial\phi}{\partial r}\frac{\partial r}{\partial x}\hat{i} + \frac{\partial\phi}{\partial r}\frac{\partial r}{\partial y}\hat{j} + \frac{\partial\phi}{\partial r}\frac{\partial r}{\partial z}\hat{k}$$

$$\nabla\phi = \frac{\partial\phi}{\partial r}\left(\frac{\partial r}{\partial x}\hat{i} + \frac{\partial r}{\partial y}\hat{j} + \frac{\partial r}{\partial z}\hat{k}\right) \quad \ldots(1)$$

$$\left.\begin{aligned} &\text{Since} \quad \phi = 3r^2 - 4r^{1/2} + 6r^{-1/3} \\ &\therefore \quad \frac{\partial\phi}{\partial r} = (6r - 2r^{-1/2} - 2r^{-4/3}) \\ &\text{and} \quad r^2 = x^2 + y^2 + z^2 \\ &\therefore \quad \frac{\partial r}{\partial x} = \frac{x}{r}, \frac{\partial r}{\partial y} = \frac{y}{r}, \frac{\partial r}{\partial z} = \frac{z}{r} \end{aligned}\right\} \quad \ldots(2)$$

Using (2), equation (1) becomes

$$\therefore \quad \nabla\phi = (6r - 2r^{-1/2} - 2r^{-4/3})\frac{1}{r}(x\hat{i} + y\hat{j} + z\hat{k})$$
$$= 2(3 - r^{-3/2} - r^{-7/3})\,\vec{r}.$$

7. *Find the directional derivative of* $f(x, y, z) = x^2yz + 4xz^2$ *at the point* $(1, -2, -1)$ *in the direction of the vector* $2\hat{i} - \hat{j} - 2\hat{k}$.

(UPTU–2006, JNTU–2006, VTU–2007, ROHTAK–2006)

SOLUTION. Let $\vec{a} = 2\hat{i} - \hat{j} - 2\hat{k}$, then

$$\hat{a} = \frac{\vec{a}}{|\vec{a}|} = \frac{2\hat{i} - \hat{j} - 2\hat{k}}{\sqrt{4+1+4}} = \frac{1}{3}(2\hat{i} - \hat{j} - 2\hat{k}).$$

Since $f(x, y, z) = x^2yz + 4xz^2$

$$\therefore \quad \frac{\partial f}{\partial x} = 2xyz + 4z^2$$
$$\frac{\partial f}{\partial y} = x^2z, \frac{\partial f}{\partial z} = x^2y + 8xz$$
$$\therefore \quad \nabla f = \frac{\partial f}{\partial x}\hat{i} + \frac{\partial f}{\partial y}\hat{j} + \frac{\partial f}{\partial z}\hat{k}$$
$$= (2xyz + 4z^2)\hat{i} + x^2z\hat{j} + (x^2y + 8xz)\hat{k}$$

At $(1, -2, -1)$ $\nabla f = 8\hat{i} - \hat{j} - 10\hat{k}$.

Now directional derivative of f at $(1, -2, -1)$ in the direction of $2\hat{i} - \hat{j} - 2\hat{k}$ is

$$\nabla f\cdot\hat{a} = (8\hat{i} - \hat{j} - 10\hat{k}).\left(\frac{1}{3}(2\hat{i} - \hat{j} - 2\hat{k})\right)$$
$$= \frac{1}{3}(16 + 1 + 20) = \frac{37}{3}.$$

8. *Find the directional derivative of* $\phi = (x^2 + y^2 + z^2)^{-\frac{1}{2}}$ *at the point* $(3, 1, 2)$ *in the direction of the vector* $yz\hat{i} + zx\hat{j} + xy\hat{k}$.

SOLUTION. We have $\quad \phi = (x^2 + y^2 + z^2)^{-\frac{1}{2}}$

Therefore,

$$\text{grad}\,\phi = \hat{i}\frac{\partial\phi}{\partial x} + \hat{j}\frac{\partial\phi}{\partial y} + \hat{k}\frac{\partial\phi}{\partial z}$$

$$= \hat{i}\left(-\frac{1}{2}(x^2+y^2+z^2)^{-3/2}.2x\right) + \hat{j}\left(-\frac{1}{2}(x^2+y^2+z^2)^{-3/2}.2y\right) + \hat{k}\left(-\frac{1}{2}(x^2+y^2+z^2)^{-3/2}.2z\right)$$

$$= -\frac{(x\hat{i}+y\hat{j}+z\hat{k})}{(x^2+y^2+z^2)^{3/2}}$$

$$= -\frac{3\hat{i}+\hat{j}+2\hat{k}}{14\sqrt{14}} \text{ at } (3, 1, 2).$$

Let $\hat{a}$ be the unit vector in the given direction then

$$\hat{a} = \frac{yz\hat{i}+zx\hat{j}+xy\hat{k}}{\sqrt{y^2z^2+z^2x^2+x^2y^2}}$$

$$= \frac{2\hat{i}+6\hat{j}+3\hat{k}}{7} \text{ at } (3, 1, 2).$$

Hence $\qquad \dfrac{d\phi}{ds} = \hat{a}.\text{grad } \phi$

$$= \frac{2\hat{i}+6\hat{j}+3\hat{k}}{7}\left(-\frac{3\hat{i}+\hat{j}+2\hat{k}}{14\sqrt{14}}\right)$$

$$= -\frac{2(3)+6\cdot 1+3\cdot 2}{7\cdot 14\cdot\sqrt{14}} = -\frac{9}{49\sqrt{14}}$$

9. *Find the directional derivative of* $\phi = 5x^2y - 5y^2z + \frac{5}{2}z^2x$ *at the point* $P(1, 1, 1)$ *in the direction of the line* $\frac{x-1}{2} = \frac{y-3}{2} = \frac{z}{1}$.

SOLUTION. We have $\qquad \phi = 5x^2y - 5y^2z + \frac{5}{2}z^2x$

$$\therefore \text{grad } \phi = \hat{i}\frac{\partial\phi}{\partial x} + \hat{j}\frac{\partial\phi}{\partial y} + \hat{k}\frac{\partial\phi}{\partial z}$$

$$= (10xy + \frac{5}{2}z^2)\hat{i} + (5x^2 - 10yz)\hat{j} + (-5y^2 + 5zx)\hat{k}$$

$$= \frac{25}{2}\hat{i} - 5\hat{j} \text{ at the point } (1, 1, 1)$$

$\therefore$ Required direction derivative

$$= \left(\frac{25}{2}\hat{i} - 5\hat{j}\right).\left(\frac{2}{3}\hat{i} - \frac{2}{3}\hat{j} + \frac{1}{3}\hat{k}\right)$$

$$= \frac{25}{3} + \frac{10}{3} = \frac{35}{3}.$$

Exercise-25.3

1. If $\phi(x, y, z) = x^2y + y^2x + z^2$, find $\nabla\phi$ at the point (1, 1, 1).
2. If $\vec{f}(x, y, z) = x^2yz\hat{i} - 2xz^3\hat{j} + xz^2\hat{k}$, $\phi(x, y, z) = 2z\hat{i} + y\hat{j} - x^2\hat{k}$, find the value of $\frac{\partial^2}{\partial x\partial y}(\vec{f}\times\phi)$ at (1, 0, –2).
3. If $|\vec{r}| = r$ where $\vec{r} = x\hat{i} + y\hat{j} + z\hat{k}$, prove that
   (i) $\nabla\left(\frac{1}{r}\right) = -\frac{\vec{r}}{r^3}$ (ii) $\nabla \log r = \frac{\vec{r}}{r^2}$
4. Prove that $f(r)\nabla r = \nabla\int f(r)dr$.
5. (i) Interpret the symbol $\vec{a}.\nabla$. (ii) Prove that $(\vec{a}.\nabla)\phi = \vec{a}.\nabla\phi$.
   (iii) Prove that $(\vec{a}.\nabla)\vec{r} = \vec{a}$.
6. Find the grad f, where f is given by $f(x, y, z) = x^3 - y^3 + xz^2$, at the point (1, –1, 2).
7. If $u = x + y + z$, $v = x^2 + y^2 + z^2$, $w = yz + zx + xy$, prove that (grad u) . [(grad v) × (grad w)] = 0. (UKTU–2010, UPTU–2002)
8. f and p are two scalar point functions such that f is a function of p, show that $\nabla f = \frac{df}{dp}\nabla p$.
9. If
   $$\vec{F} = \left(y\frac{\partial f}{\partial z} - z\frac{\partial f}{\partial y}\right)\hat{i} + \left(z\frac{\partial f}{\partial x} - x\frac{\partial f}{\partial z}\right)\hat{j} + \left(x\frac{\partial f}{\partial y} - y\frac{\partial f}{\partial x}\right)\hat{k}.$$
   Prove that
   (i) $\vec{F} = \vec{r}\times\nabla f$ (ii) $\vec{F}\cdot\vec{r} = 0$
   (iii) $\vec{F}\,.\,\nabla f = 0$
10. Prove that the directional derivative of a scalar field f at a point $P(x, y, z)$ in the direction of a unit vector $\hat{a}$ is given by
    $$\frac{\partial f}{\partial s} = \nabla f.\hat{a}$$
11. Find the directional derivative of the function
    $$f(x, y, z) = x^2 - y^2 + 2z^2.$$
    at the point $P(1, 2, 3)$ in the direction of the line PQ where Q is the point (5, 0, 4).
12. In what direction from the point (1, 1, –1) is the directional derivative of $f = x^2 - 2y^2 + 4z^2$ a maximum? Also find the value of this maximum directional derivative.

13. Find the directional derivative of the function $f = xy + yz + zx$ in the direction of the vector $2\hat{i}+3\hat{j}+6\hat{k}$ at the point (3, 1, 2).

14. Find the greatest value of the derivative of the function $f = 2x^2 - y - z^4$ at the point (2, –1, 1).

15. Find the directional derivative $\partial f/\partial s$ of $f(x, y, z) = 2x^2 + 3y^2 + z^2$ at the point $P(2, 1, 3)$ in the direction of the vector $\vec{a} = \hat{i} - 2\hat{k}$.

16. Find the directional derivative of $f = x^2 + y^2 + z^2$ at (1, 2, 3) in the direction of the line

$$\frac{x}{3} = \frac{y}{4} = \frac{z}{5}.$$

17. Find the directional derivative of the function $f(x, y, z) = 4e^{x + 5y - 13z}$ at the point (1, 2, 3) in the direction towards the point (–3, 5, 7).

18. In what direction from (3, 1, –2) is the directional derivative of $\phi = x^2y^2z^4$ maximum and what is its magnitude. (ROHTAK–2003)

19. Show that grad $(e^{r^2}) = 2e^{r^2} \cdot \vec{r}$.

20. Show that grad $f(r) \times \vec{r} = 0$.

21. Show that the directional derivative of $\frac{1}{r}$ in the direction of $\vec{r}$ where $\vec{r} = x\hat{i} + y\hat{j} + z\hat{k}$ is $-\frac{1}{r^2}$.

22. Show that the directional derivative of $\frac{1}{r^2}$ in the direction of $\vec{r}$ where $\vec{r} = x\hat{i} + y\hat{j} + z\hat{k}$ is $-\frac{2}{r^3}$.

Hint to Selected Problems

1. $\phi(x,y,z) = x^2y + y^2x + z^2$

$$\therefore\ \nabla\phi = \frac{\partial\phi}{\partial x}\hat{i} + \frac{\partial\phi}{\partial y}\hat{j} + \frac{\partial\phi}{\partial z}\hat{k}$$

$$= (2xy + y^2)\hat{i} + (x^2 + 2xy)\hat{j} + 2z\hat{k}$$

$$\therefore\ [\nabla\phi]_{(1,1,1)} = 3\hat{i} + 3\hat{j} + 2\hat{k}\,.$$

3. (ii) Since $\nabla f(r) = f(r)\nabla r = f'(r)\frac{\vec{r}}{r}$.

$$\therefore\ \nabla \log r = \frac{d}{dt}(\log r)\frac{\vec{r}}{r} = \frac{1}{r}\frac{\vec{r}}{r} = \frac{\vec{r}}{r^2}.$$

(iv) $\vec{r} = x\hat{i} + y\hat{j} + z\hat{k}$ $\therefore$ $d\vec{r} = dx\hat{i} + dy\hat{j} + dz\hat{k}$.

$$\therefore\ \nabla\phi . d\vec{r} = \left(\frac{\partial\phi}{\partial x}\hat{i} + \frac{\partial\phi}{\partial y}\hat{j} + \frac{\partial\phi}{\partial z}\hat{k}\right).(dx\hat{i} + dy\hat{j} + dz\hat{k})$$

$$= \frac{\partial\phi}{\partial x}dx + \frac{\partial\phi}{\partial y}dy + \frac{\partial\phi}{\partial z}dz = d\phi.$$

5. Let $\vec{a} = a_1\hat{i} + a_2\hat{j} + a_3\hat{k}, \vec{r} = x\hat{i} + y\hat{j} + z\hat{k}$.

$$\therefore\ \vec{a}\cdot\nabla = a_1\frac{\partial}{\partial x} + a_2\frac{\partial}{\partial y} + a_3\frac{\partial}{\partial z}$$

Now
$$(\vec{a}\cdot\nabla)\vec{r} = a_1\frac{\partial\vec{r}}{\partial x} + a_2\frac{\partial\vec{r}}{\partial y} + a_3\frac{\partial\vec{r}}{\partial z}$$

$$= a_1\hat{i} + a_2\hat{j} + a_3\hat{k} = \vec{a}$$

7. $u = x + y + z, v = x^2 + y^2 + z^2, w = yz + zx + xy$

$$\text{grad} v = \frac{\partial v}{\partial x}\hat{i} + \frac{\partial v}{\partial y}\hat{j} + \frac{\partial v}{\partial z}\hat{k} = 2x\hat{i} + 2y\hat{j} + 2z\hat{k}$$

$$\text{grad } w = \frac{\partial w}{\partial x}\hat{i} + \frac{\partial w}{\partial y}\hat{j} + \frac{\partial w}{\partial z}\hat{k}$$

$$= (z+y)\hat{i} + (z+x)\hat{j} + (y+x)\hat{k}$$

$$(\text{grad } v)\times(\text{grad } w) = \begin{vmatrix} \hat{i} & \hat{j} & \hat{k} \\ 2x & 2y & 2z \\ z+y & z+x & y+x \end{vmatrix}$$

$$= \hat{i}(2y^2 + 2xy - 2z^2 - 2zx) + \hat{j}(2z^2 + 2yz - 2xy - 2x^2) + \hat{k}(2xz + 2x^2 - 2yz - 2y^2)$$

$$\text{grad } u = \frac{\partial u}{\partial x}\hat{i} + \frac{\partial u}{\partial y}\hat{j} + \frac{\partial u}{\partial z}\hat{k} = \hat{i} + \hat{j} + \hat{k}$$

$\therefore$ (grad u)$\cdot$[(grad v) $\times$ (grad w)]

$$= (2y^2 + 2xy - 2z^2 - 2zx) + (2z^2 + 2yz - 2xy - 2x^2) + (2xz + 2x^2 - 2yz - 2y^2) = 0.$$

8. Since $f = f(p)$

$$\therefore\ \nabla f = \nabla(f(p))$$

$$= \frac{\partial}{\partial x}(f(p))\hat{i} + \frac{\partial}{\partial y}(f(p))\hat{j} + \frac{\partial}{\partial z}(f(p))\hat{k}$$

$$= \frac{df}{dp}\frac{\partial p}{\partial x}\hat{i} + \frac{df}{dp}\frac{\partial p}{\partial y}\hat{j} + \frac{df}{dp}\frac{\partial p}{\partial z}\hat{k}$$

$$= \frac{df}{dp}\left(\frac{\partial p}{\partial x}\hat{i} + \frac{\partial p}{\partial y}\hat{j} + \frac{\partial p}{\partial z}\hat{k}\right) = \frac{df}{dp}\nabla p.$$

11. $f(x,y,z) = x^2 - y^2 + 2z^2$

$$\therefore\ \frac{\partial f}{\partial x} = 2x, \frac{\partial f}{\partial y} = -2y, \frac{\partial f}{\partial z} = 4z.$$

$$\therefore\ \nabla f = \frac{\partial f}{\partial x}\hat{i} + \frac{\partial f}{\partial y}\hat{j} + \frac{\partial f}{\partial z}\hat{k} = 2x\hat{i} - 2y\hat{j} + 4z\hat{k}$$

at $P(1, 2, 3)$ $\nabla f = 2\hat{i} - 4\hat{j} + 12\hat{k}$

Now $\overrightarrow{PQ} = 4\hat{i} - 2\hat{j} + \hat{k}$

$\therefore$ directional derivative along $\overrightarrow{PQ}$ is

$$(\nabla f).\frac{\overrightarrow{PQ}}{|\overrightarrow{PQ}|} = \frac{(8+8+12)}{\sqrt{16+4+1}}$$

$$= \frac{28}{\sqrt{21}} = \frac{28\sqrt{21}}{21} = \frac{4}{3}\sqrt{21}.$$

12. Same as **11**.

13. Same as **11**.

14. Same as **11**.

15. Same as **11**.

ANSWERS

1. $3\hat{i}+3\hat{j}+2\hat{k}$ **2.** $-4\hat{i}-8\hat{j}$ **6.** $7\hat{i}-3\hat{j}+4\hat{k}$ **11.** $\frac{4}{3}\sqrt{21}$

12. $2\hat{i}-4\hat{j}-8\hat{k}, 2\sqrt{(21)}$ **13.** $45/7$ **14.** 9 **15.** $-4/\sqrt{5}$ **16.** $\frac{52}{\sqrt{50}}$

17. $-4\sqrt{41}e^{-28}$ **18.** $96(\hat{i}+3\hat{j}-3\hat{k}), 96\sqrt{19}$

25.19 LEVEL SURFACES

Let us consider a scalar function $f(x, y, z)$ and suppose that for each constant c the equation

$$f(x, y, z) = c = \text{constant}$$

represents a surface in space (in three dimensional space). Then assuming c takes all values, we obtain a family of surfaces, which are known as level surfaces.

SOME RESULTS

(1) Let $f(x, y, z)$ be a scalar point function over some region R, then show that through any point on R there passes one and only one, level surface of f.

(2) grad $(f) = \nabla f$ is a normal vector to the surface $f(x, y, z) = c$, where c is a constant.

25.20 TANGENT AND NORMAL TO THE LEVEL SURFACE

(i) Tangent Plane. Let $f(x, y, z) = c$ be the equation of a level surfaces and let $P(x, y, z)$ be any point on this surface whose position vector be $\vec{r}$.

$$\therefore \quad \vec{r} = x\hat{i} + y\hat{j} + z\hat{k}. \quad \ldots(1)$$

Since ∇f is perpendicular to the tangent plane at $P(x, y, z)$. Let Q be any variable point on the surface tangent plane to the whose co-ordinates are (X, Y, Z) and whose position vector is $\vec{R}$.

$$\therefore \quad \overrightarrow{PQ} = \vec{R} - \vec{r} = (X-x)\hat{i} + (Y-y)\hat{j} + (Z-z)\hat{k}.$$

Since $\overrightarrow{PQ}$ is along the tangent plane at P, then ∇f is perpendicular to $\overrightarrow{PQ}$.

$$\therefore \quad \nabla f.\overrightarrow{PQ} = 0$$

$$\left(\frac{\partial f}{\partial x}\hat{i} + \frac{\partial f}{\partial y}\hat{j} + \frac{\partial f}{\partial z}\hat{k}\right)((X-x)\hat{i} + (Y-y)\hat{j} + (Z-z)\hat{k}) = 0$$

or
$$(X-x)\frac{\partial f}{\partial x} + (Y-y)\frac{\partial f}{\partial y} + (Z-z)\frac{\partial f}{\partial z} = 0$$

This is the equation of a tangent plane at $P(x, y, z)$ to the level surface $f(x, y, z) = c$.

(ii) Normal. In this case the point Q is taken on the normal to the surface $f(x, y, z) = c$. So that the direction ratios of the line PQ are $X - x, Y - y, Z - z$

or
$$\overrightarrow{PQ} = (X-x)\hat{i} + (Y-y)\hat{j} + (Z-z)\hat{k}$$

Thus the vector $\overrightarrow{PQ}$ is now parallel to the ∇f.

$$\therefore \quad \nabla f \times \overrightarrow{PQ} = \vec{0}$$

or $\left(\frac{\partial f}{\partial x}\hat{i}+\frac{\partial f}{\partial y}\hat{j}+\frac{\partial f}{\partial z}\hat{k}\right)\times((X-x)\hat{i}+(Y-y)\hat{j}+(Z-z)\hat{k})=\vec{0}$

$$\left[\frac{\partial f}{\partial y}(Z-z)-\frac{\partial f}{\partial z}(Y-y)\right]\hat{i}+\left[\frac{\partial f}{\partial z}(X-x)-\frac{\partial f}{\partial x}(Z-z)\right]\hat{j}+\left[\frac{\partial f}{\partial x}(Y-y)-\frac{\partial f}{\partial y}(X-x)\right]\hat{k}=\vec{0}$$

or $$\frac{\partial f}{\partial y}(Z-z)-\frac{\partial f}{\partial z}(Y-y)=0$$

$\frac{\partial f}{\partial z}(X-x)-\frac{\partial f}{\partial x}(Z-z)=0$ and $\frac{\partial f}{\partial x}(Y-y)-\frac{\partial f}{\partial y}(X-x)=0$.

From these three equations we obtain the equation to the normal which is as follows :

$$\frac{X-x}{\frac{\partial f}{\partial x}}=\frac{Y-y}{\frac{\partial f}{\partial y}}=\frac{Z-z}{\frac{\partial f}{\partial z}}.$$

- If $f(x, y, z) = c$, then $\frac{\partial f}{\partial x},\frac{\partial f}{\partial y},\frac{\partial f}{\partial z}$ are the direction ratios of the normal to the surface.

Solved Examples

1. *Find a unit normal vector to the level surface $x^2y + 2xz = 4$ at the point (2, –2, 3).*

SOLUTION. Let $f(x,y,z) \equiv x^2y+2xz-4=0$.

$$\therefore \quad \frac{\partial f}{\partial x}=2xy+2z, \frac{\partial f}{\partial y}=x^2, \frac{\partial f}{\partial z}=2x.$$

$$\therefore \quad \nabla f=\frac{\partial f}{\partial x}\hat{i}+\frac{\partial f}{\partial y}\hat{j}+\frac{\partial f}{\partial z}\hat{k}$$

$$=(2xy+2z)\hat{i}+x^2\hat{j}+2\,x\hat{k}$$

At (2, –2, 3), $\nabla f=-2\hat{i}+4\hat{j}+4\hat{k}$.

The unit normal vector is given by

$$\frac{\nabla f}{|\nabla f|}=\frac{-2\hat{i}+4\hat{j}+4\hat{k}}{\sqrt{(4+16+16)}}=\frac{-\hat{i}+2\hat{j}+2\hat{k}}{3}.$$

2. *Find the unit normal to the surface $x^4-3xyz+z^2+1=0$ at the point (1, 1, 1).*

SOLUTION. Suppose $f(x, y, z)=x^4-3xyz+z^2+1=0$, then

$$\frac{\partial f}{\partial x}=4x^3-3yz, \frac{\partial f}{\partial y}=-3xz,$$

$$\frac{\partial f}{\partial z}=-3xy+2z.$$

$$\therefore \quad \nabla f=\frac{\partial f}{\partial x}\hat{i}+\frac{\partial f}{\partial y}\hat{j}+\frac{\partial f}{\partial z}\hat{k}$$

or $$\nabla f=(4x^3-3yz)\hat{i}-3xz\hat{j}+(2z-3xy)\hat{k}$$

At (1, 1, 1), $\nabla f=\hat{i}-3\hat{j}-\hat{k}$.

The unit normal vector is given by

$$\frac{\nabla f}{|\nabla f|}=\frac{\hat{i}-3\hat{j}-\hat{k}}{\sqrt{(1+9+1)}}=\frac{1}{\sqrt{11}}(\hat{i}-3\hat{j}-\hat{k}).$$

3. *Find a unit vector normal to the surface $xy^3z^2=0$ at the point (–1, –1, 2).*

(UPTU–2008, MUMBAI–2008)

SOLUTION. We have $\phi = xy^3z^2$

$$\therefore \quad \text{grad}\,\phi=\hat{i}\frac{\partial \phi}{\partial x}+\hat{j}\frac{\partial \phi}{\partial y}+\hat{k}\frac{\partial \phi}{\partial z}$$

$$=\hat{i}\frac{\partial}{\partial x}(xy^3z^2)+\hat{j}\frac{\partial}{\partial y}(xy^3z^2)+\hat{k}\frac{\partial}{\partial z}(xy^3z^2)$$

$$=\hat{i}(y^3z^2)+\hat{j}(3xy^2z^2)+\hat{k}(2xy^3z)$$

$=-4\hat{i}-12\hat{j}+4\hat{k}$ at the point (–1, –1, 2)

Hence, required unit normal vector to the surface is

$$=\frac{-4\hat{i}-12\hat{j}+4\hat{k}}{\sqrt{(-4)^2+(-12)^2+4^2}}$$

$$=-\frac{1}{\sqrt{11}}(\hat{i}+3\hat{j}-\hat{k}).$$

4. *Find the equation of the tangent plane to the surface $yz - zx + xy + 5 = 0$ at the point (1, –1, 2).*

SOLUTION. Let $f = yz - zx + xy + 5 = 0$, then

$$\frac{\partial f}{\partial x} = -z + y, \frac{\partial f}{\partial y} = z + x, \frac{\partial f}{\partial z} = y - x.$$

$$\therefore \quad \nabla f = \frac{\partial f}{\partial x}\hat{i} + \frac{\partial f}{\partial y}\hat{j} + \frac{\partial f}{\partial z}\hat{k}.$$

$$= (y - z)\hat{i} + (z + x)\hat{j} + (y - x)\hat{k}.$$

At (1, –1, 2), $\nabla f = -3\hat{i} + 3\hat{j} - 2\hat{k}$.

Let $Q(X, Y, Z)$ be any point on the tangent plane to the surface and P is given as (1, –1, 2)

$\therefore \overrightarrow{PQ} = (X-1)\hat{i} + (Y+1)\hat{j} + (Z-2)\hat{k}$.

For the equation of the tangent at (1, –1, 2), we have

$$\nabla f . \overrightarrow{PQ} = 0$$

$$\Rightarrow (X-1)(-3) + (Y+1)(3) + (Z-2)(-2) = 0$$

$$-3X + 3Y - 2Z + 3 + 3 + 4 = 0$$

or $$3X - 3Y + 2Z = 10$$

or $$3x - 3y + 2z = 10$$

5. *Find the angle between the surface $x^2 + y^2 + z^2 = 9$ and $z = x^2 + y^2 - 3$ at the point (2, –1, 2).*

(VTU–2010, KOTTAYAM–2005)

SOLUTION. Let the given surfaces be

$$f_1(x, y, z) \equiv x^2 + y^2 + z^2 = 9$$

as $f_1(x, y, z) = c_1$ ...(1)

$$f_2(x, y, z) \equiv x^2 + y^2 - z = 3$$

as $f_2(x, y, z) = c_2$ ...(2)

Normal vector to surface (1) is

$$\hat{n}_1 = \text{grad } f_1$$

$$= \left(\hat{i}\frac{\partial}{\partial x} + \hat{j}\frac{\partial}{\partial y} + \hat{k}\frac{\partial}{\partial z}\right)(x^2 + y^2 + z^2)$$

$$= 2x\hat{i} + 2y\hat{j} + 2z\hat{k}$$

At point (2, –1, 2),

$$\hat{n}_1 = 2.2\hat{i} + 2(-1)\hat{j} + 2.2\hat{k}$$

$$= 4\hat{i} - 2\hat{j} + 4\hat{k}.$$

Normal vector to surface (2) is

$$\hat{n}_2 = \text{grad } f_2$$

$$= \left(\hat{i}\frac{\partial}{\partial x} + \hat{j}\frac{\partial}{\partial y} + \hat{k}\frac{\partial}{\partial z}\right)(x^2 + y^2 - z)$$

$$= 2x\hat{i} + 2y\hat{j} - \hat{k}.$$

At point (2, –1, 2),

$$\hat{n}_2 = 2.2\hat{i} + 2(-1)\hat{j} - \hat{k} = 4\hat{i} - 2\hat{j} - \hat{k}.$$

Now let θ be the angle between surfaces (1) and (2), then the angle between their normals $\hat{n}_1$ and $\hat{n}_2$ is also θ.

$$\therefore \quad \cos\theta = \frac{\hat{n}_1.\hat{n}_2}{|\hat{n}_1||\hat{n}_2|}$$

$$= \frac{4.4 + (-2)(-2) + 4(-1)}{\sqrt{(4)^2 + (-2)^2 + (4)^2}\sqrt{(4)^2 + (-2)^2 + (-1)^2}}$$

$$= \frac{16 + 4 - 4}{\sqrt{36}\sqrt{21}} = \frac{16}{6\sqrt{21}} = \frac{8}{3\sqrt{21}}$$

$$\therefore \quad \theta = \cos^{-1}\left(\frac{8}{3\sqrt{21}}\right).$$

Exercise-25.4

1. Find the unit vector normal to the surfce $x^2 - y^2 + z = 2$ at the point (1, –1, 2).
2. Find the vector normal to the surface $z = x^2 + y^2$ at the point (–1, –2, 5).
3. Find the unit normal to the surface $x^2 + y - z = 4$ at the point (2, 0, 0).
4. Find the equation of the tangent plane and normal to the surface $xyz = 4$ at the point (1, 2, 2).
5. Find the equation of the tangent plane and normal to the surface $x^2 + y^2 + z^2 = 25$ at the point (4, 0, 3).
6. Find the equation of the tangent plane and normal to the surface $z = x^2 + y^2$ at the point (2, –1, 5).
7. If $\hat{n}$ be a unit vector normal to the level surface $f(x, y, z) = c$ at a point $P(x, y, z)$ and n be the distance of P from some fixed point A in the direction of $\hat{n}$ so that δn represents element of normal at P in the direction of $\hat{n}$, then grad $f = \frac{df}{dn}\hat{n}$.

8. Prove that grad f is a vector in the direction of which the maximum value of the directional derivative of f.

9. Find the angle between the normals to the surface $xy = z^2$ at the points (4, 1, 2) and (3, 3, –3). (UKTU–2012)

Hint to Selected Problems

1. $f \equiv x^2 - y^2 + z - 2 = 0.$

$\therefore \quad \nabla f = \frac{\partial f}{\partial x}\hat{i} + \frac{\partial f}{\partial y}\hat{j} + \frac{\partial f}{\partial z}\hat{k} = 2x\hat{i} - 2y\hat{j} + \hat{k}$

At (1, –1, 2)

$\nabla f = 2\hat{i} + 2\hat{j} + \hat{k}$

$\therefore$ Unit normal to the surface f

$= \frac{\nabla f}{|\nabla f|} = \frac{2\hat{i} + 2\hat{j} + \hat{k}}{3}.$

4. $f(x, y, z) \equiv xyz - 4$

$\therefore \quad \frac{\partial f}{\partial x} = yz, \frac{\partial f}{\partial y} = xz, \frac{\partial f}{\partial z} = xy$

$\therefore$ at (1, 2, 2) $\nabla f = 4\hat{i} + 2\hat{j} + 2\hat{k}$.

The equation of the tangent plane at (1, 2, 2) is

$[(x-1)\hat{i} + (y-2)\hat{j} + (z-2)\hat{k}].(4\hat{i} + 2\hat{j} + 2\hat{k}) = 0$

or $4(x-1) + 2(y-2) + 2(z-2) = 0$

or $4x + 2y + 2z - 12 = 0$

or $2x + y + z - 6 = 0$

and the equation of the normal at (1, 2, 2) is

$\frac{x-1}{4} = \frac{y-2}{2} = \frac{z-2}{2}$

or $\frac{x-1}{2} = \frac{y-2}{1} = \frac{z-2}{1}$

6. Same as (4).

ANSWERS

1. $\frac{1}{3}(2\hat{i} + 2\hat{j} + \hat{k})$ **2.** $2\hat{i} + 4\hat{j} + \hat{k}$ **3.** $\frac{1}{3\sqrt{2}}(4\hat{i} + \hat{j} - \hat{k})$

4. $2x + y + z = 6; \frac{x-1}{2} = \frac{y-2}{1} = \frac{z-2}{1}$ **5.** $4x + 3z = 25; \frac{x-4}{4} = \frac{y}{0} = \frac{z-3}{3}$

6. $4x - 2y - z = 5; \frac{x-2}{4} = \frac{y+1}{-2} = \frac{z-5}{-1}$ **9.** $\cos^{-1}\left(\frac{1}{\sqrt{22}}\right)$

25.21 DIVERGENCE OF A VECTOR FIELD

Let $\vec{V}$ (x, y, z) be a differentiable vector function, where x, y, z are cartesian co-ordinates in space and let V_1, V_2, V_3 be the components of $\vec{V}$, then the function

$$\operatorname{div} \vec{V} = \frac{\partial V_1}{\partial x} + \frac{\partial V_2}{\partial y} + \frac{\partial V_3}{\partial z} \qquad \ldots(1)$$

is called the divergence of $\vec{V}$.

Since we have that the differential operator $\nabla \equiv \frac{\partial}{\partial x}\hat{i} + \frac{\partial}{\partial y}\hat{j} + \frac{\partial}{\partial z}\hat{k}$ and the vector $\vec{V} = \vec{V}_1\hat{i} + \vec{V}_2\hat{j} + \vec{V}_3\hat{k}$.

Then
$$\nabla.\vec{V} = \frac{\partial V_1}{\partial x} + \frac{\partial V_2}{\partial y} + \frac{\partial V_3}{\partial z} \qquad \ldots(2)$$

From equation (1) and (2), we get

$$\operatorname{div} \vec{V} = \nabla.\vec{V}$$

Hence, divergence of a vector function $\vec{V}$ can also be written as $\nabla.\vec{V}$. Consequently divergence of a vector function is scalar because dot product of ∇ and $\vec{V}$ gives a scalar quantity.

- Though dot product is cummulative but ∇ being operator which operates right side function only, we have $\nabla.\vec{f} \neq \vec{f}.\nabla$.
- If div $\vec{V} = 0$, then the vector $\vec{V}$ is called solenoidal vector.
- If the vector $\vec{V}$ is a velocity vector of a fluid and if div $\vec{V} = 0$, then the fluid is incompressible.
- $\operatorname{div} \vec{V} = \nabla.\vec{V} = \Sigma\hat{i}.\frac{\partial \vec{V}}{\partial x}$.

25.22 CURL OF A VECTOR FIELD

(UPTU–2006, 07,08; GBTU–2012)

Let $\vec{V}$ (x, y, z) be a vector function of x, y, z where (x, y, z) are right handed cartesian co-ordinates in space and let

$$\vec{V}(x,y,z) = V_1(x,y,z)\hat{i} + V_2(x,y,z)\hat{j} + V_3(x,y,z)\hat{k}$$

be a differentiable vector function. Then the function

$$\text{curl } \vec{V} = \nabla \times \vec{V} = \begin{vmatrix} \hat{i} & \hat{j} & \hat{k} \\ \dfrac{\partial}{\partial x} & \dfrac{\partial}{\partial y} & \dfrac{\partial}{\partial z} \\ V_1 & V_2 & V_3 \end{vmatrix} = \left(\frac{\partial V_3}{\partial y} - \frac{\partial V_2}{\partial z}\right)\hat{i} + \left(\frac{\partial V_1}{\partial z} - \frac{\partial V_3}{\partial x}\right)\hat{j} + \left(\frac{\partial V_2}{\partial x} - \frac{\partial V_1}{\partial y}\right)\hat{k}$$

is called the curl of the vector function V or the curl of the vector field definded by Curl $\vec{V}$ is a vector quantity.

- If curl $\vec{V} = 0$, then the vector $\vec{V}$ is called irrotational.
- $\text{Curl } \vec{V} = \nabla \times \vec{V} = \Sigma \hat{i} \times \dfrac{\partial \vec{V}}{\partial x}$.
- Curl $\vec{V}$ is perpendicular to $\vec{V}$.
- In the case of a rigid body rotation, the curl of the velocity field has the direction of the axis of rotation and its magnitude equals twice the angular speed of the rotation.

25.23 LAPLACIAN OPERATOR

If the function $f(x, y, z)$ is a twice differentiable scalar function, then we have

$$\text{grad } f = \frac{\partial f}{\partial x}\hat{i} + \frac{\partial f}{\partial y}\hat{j} + \frac{\partial f}{\partial z}\hat{k}$$

Since grad f is a vector function, then

$$\text{div (grad } f) = \left(\frac{\partial}{\partial x}\hat{i} + \frac{\partial}{\partial y}\hat{j} + \frac{\partial}{\partial z}\hat{k}\right) \cdot \left(\frac{\partial f}{\partial x}\hat{i} + \frac{\partial f}{\partial y}\hat{j} + \frac{\partial f}{\partial z}\hat{k}\right)$$

$$= \frac{\partial^2 f}{\partial x^2} + \frac{\partial^2 f}{\partial y^2} + \frac{\partial^2 f}{\partial z^2} = \left(\frac{\partial^2}{\partial x^2} + \frac{\partial^2}{\partial y^2} + \frac{\partial^2}{\partial z^2}\right) f$$

$$\therefore \quad \text{div (grad } f) = \nabla^2 f. \qquad \ldots(1)$$

Thus, R.H.S. of (1) is the Laplacian of f. Consequently the Laplacian is defined as

$$\nabla^2 = \left(\frac{\partial^2}{\partial x^2} + \frac{\partial^2}{\partial y^2} + \frac{\partial^2}{\partial z^2}\right).$$

Hence, ∇^2 is a Laplacian operator.

- The equation $\nabla^2 f = 0$ is called Laplace's equation.
- If $\vec{f}$ is a scalar point function, then $\nabla^2 \vec{f}$ is a scalar quantity.
- If $\vec{f}$ is a vector point function, then $\nabla^2 \vec{f}$ is a vector quantity.
- If a function f satisfies the Laplace's equation then f is called harmonic function.
- Stoke's states that $\oint_C \vec{A}.d\vec{r} = \iint_S (\text{curl } \vec{A}).\hat{n}\, dS$. This theorem will discuss later on.

Solved Examples

1. *Prove that the followings:*
(i) *div* $\vec{r} = 3$ (ii) *curl* $\vec{r} = \vec{0}$

where $\vec{r} = x\hat{i} + y\hat{j} + z\hat{k}$.

SOLUTION. (i) Since div $\vec{r} = \nabla \times \vec{r}$

$$= \left(\frac{\partial}{\partial x}\hat{i} + \frac{\partial}{\partial y}\hat{j} + \frac{\partial}{\partial z}\hat{k}\right).(x\hat{i} + y\hat{j} + z\hat{k})$$

$$= \frac{\partial x}{\partial x} + \frac{\partial y}{\partial y} + \frac{\partial z}{\partial z} = 1 + 1 + 1 = 3.$$

(ii) Curl $\vec{r} = \nabla \times \vec{r}$

$$= \begin{vmatrix} \hat{i} & \hat{j} & \hat{k} \\ \frac{\partial}{\partial x} & \frac{\partial}{\partial y} & \frac{\partial}{\partial z} \\ x & y & z \end{vmatrix}$$

$$= \hat{i}\left(\frac{\partial z}{\partial y} - \frac{\partial y}{\partial z}\right) + \hat{j}\left(\frac{\partial x}{\partial z} - \frac{\partial z}{\partial x}\right) + \hat{k}\left(\frac{\partial y}{\partial x} - \frac{\partial x}{\partial y}\right)$$

$$= \hat{i}(0-0) + \hat{j}(0-0) + \hat{k}(0-0) = \vec{0}.$$

2. *If* $\vec{a}$ *is a constant vector, find*
(i) *div* $(\vec{r} \times \vec{a})$ (ii) *curl* $(\vec{r} \times \vec{a})$

where $\vec{r} = x\hat{i} + y\hat{j} + z\hat{k}$.

SOLUTION. Let $\vec{a} = a_1\hat{i} + a_2\hat{j} + a_3\hat{k}$ be a constant vector, then

$$\vec{r} \times \vec{a} = \begin{vmatrix} \hat{i} & \hat{j} & \hat{k} \\ x & y & z \\ a_1 & a_2 & a_3 \end{vmatrix}$$

$$= \hat{i}(ya_3 - za_2) + \hat{j}(za_1 - xa_3) + \hat{k}(xa_2 - ya_1)$$

(i) div$(\vec{r} \times \vec{a}) = \nabla.(\vec{r} \times \vec{a})$

$$= \frac{\partial}{\partial x}(ya_3 - za_2) + \frac{\partial}{\partial y}(za_1 - xa_3) + \frac{\partial}{\partial z}(xa_2 - ya_1)$$

$$= 0 + 0 + 0 = 0$$

(ii) curl $(\vec{r} \times \vec{a}) = \nabla \times (\vec{r} \times \vec{a})$

$$= \begin{vmatrix} \hat{i} & \hat{j} & \hat{k} \\ \frac{\partial}{\partial x} & \frac{\partial}{\partial y} & \frac{\partial}{\partial z} \\ (ya_3 - za_2) & (za_1 - xa_3) & (xa_2 - ya_1) \end{vmatrix}$$

$$= \hat{i}\left[\frac{\partial}{\partial y}(xa_2 - ya_1) - \frac{\partial}{\partial z}(za_1 - xa_3)\right] + \hat{j}\left[\frac{\partial}{\partial z}(ya_3 - za_2) - \frac{\partial}{\partial x}(xa_2 - ya_1)\right] + \hat{k}\left[\frac{\partial}{\partial x}(za_1 - xa_3) - \frac{\partial}{\partial y}(ya_3 - za_2)\right]$$

$$= \hat{i}[-a_1 - a_1] + \hat{j}[-a_2 - a_2] + \hat{k}[-a_3 - a_3]$$

$$= -2(a_1\hat{i} + a_2\hat{j} + a_3\hat{k}) = -2\vec{a}$$

Similarly, we can show that

$$\frac{1}{2}\text{curl } (\vec{a} \times \vec{r}) = \vec{a}.$$

3. *If* $\vec{V}$ *is differentiable vector function and* f *is a scalar point function, then show that*
(i) *div* $(f\vec{V}) = f$ *div* $\vec{V} + \vec{V}.(\text{grad} f)$
(ii) *curl* $(f\vec{V}) = (\nabla f) \times \vec{V} + f(\nabla \times \vec{V})$

SOLUTION. (i) Since we know that

$$\text{div } (f\vec{V}) = \nabla.(f\vec{V})$$

$$= \left(\hat{i}\frac{\partial}{\partial x} + \hat{j}\frac{\partial}{\partial y} + \hat{k}\frac{\partial}{\partial z}\right).(f\vec{V})$$

$$= \hat{i}\cdot\frac{\partial}{\partial x}(f\vec{V}) + \hat{j}\cdot\frac{\partial}{\partial y}(f\vec{V}) + \hat{k}\cdot\frac{\partial}{\partial z}(f\vec{V})$$

$$= \hat{i}\cdot\left(\frac{\partial f}{\partial x}\vec{V} + f\frac{\partial \vec{V}}{\partial x}\right) + \hat{j}\cdot\left(\frac{\partial f}{\partial y}\vec{V} + f\frac{\partial \vec{V}}{\partial y}\right) + \hat{k}\cdot\left(\frac{\partial f}{\partial z}\vec{V} + f\frac{\partial \vec{V}}{\partial z}\right)$$

$$= \left[\hat{i}\cdot\left(\frac{\partial f}{\partial x}\vec{V}\right) + \hat{j}\cdot\left(\frac{\partial f}{\partial y}\vec{V}\right) + \hat{k}\cdot\left(\frac{\partial f}{\partial z}\vec{V}\right)\right] + \left[\hat{i}\cdot\left(f\frac{\partial \vec{V}}{\partial x}\right) + \hat{j}\cdot\left(f\frac{\partial \vec{V}}{\partial y}\right) + \hat{k}\cdot\left(\frac{\partial \vec{V}}{\partial z}f\right)\right]$$

$$= \left[\left(\frac{\partial f}{\partial x}\hat{i}\right)\cdot\vec{V} + \left(\frac{\partial f}{\partial y}\hat{j}\right)\cdot\vec{V} + \left(\frac{\partial f}{\partial z}\hat{k}\right)\cdot\vec{V}\right] + \left[f\left(\hat{i}\cdot\frac{\partial \vec{V}}{\partial x}\right) + f\left(\hat{j}\cdot\frac{\partial \vec{V}}{\partial y}\right) + f\left(\hat{k}\cdot\frac{\partial \vec{V}}{\partial z}\right)\right]$$

$$= \left[\left(\frac{\partial f}{\partial x}\cdot\hat{i} + \frac{\partial f}{\partial z}\cdot\hat{k} + \frac{\partial f}{\partial y}\cdot\hat{j}\right)\vec{V}\right] + \left[f\left(\hat{i}\cdot\frac{\partial \vec{V}}{\partial x} + \hat{j}\cdot\frac{\partial \vec{V}}{\partial y} + \hat{k}\cdot\frac{\partial \vec{V}}{\partial z}\right)\right]$$

$$= (\nabla f).\vec{V} + f(\nabla.\vec{V})$$

$$\therefore\ \text{div}(f\vec{V}) = f(\text{div}\vec{V}) + \vec{V}\cdot(\text{grad } f)$$

(ii) $\text{Curl}(f\vec{V}) = \nabla\times(f\vec{V})$

$$= \left(\hat{i}\frac{\partial}{\partial x} + \hat{j}\frac{\partial}{\partial y} + \hat{k}\frac{\partial}{\partial z}\right)\times(f\vec{V})$$

$$= \left(\hat{i}\frac{\partial}{\partial x}\right)\times(f\vec{V}) + \left(\hat{j}\frac{\partial}{\partial y}\right)\times(f\vec{V}) + \left(\hat{k}\frac{\partial}{\partial z}\right)\times(f\vec{V})$$

$$= \hat{i}\times\frac{\partial}{\partial x}(f\vec{V}) + \hat{j}\times\frac{\partial}{\partial y}(f\vec{V}) + \hat{k}\times\frac{\partial}{\partial z}(f\vec{V})$$

$$= \hat{i}\times\left(\frac{\partial f}{\partial x}\vec{V} + f\frac{\partial \vec{V}}{\partial x}\right) + \hat{j}\times\left(\frac{\partial f}{\partial y}\vec{V} + f\frac{\partial \vec{V}}{\partial y}\right) + \hat{k}\times\left(\frac{\partial f}{\partial z}\vec{V} + f\frac{\partial \vec{V}}{\partial z}\right)$$

$$= \left[\left(\frac{\partial f}{\partial x}\hat{i}\right)\times\vec{V} + \left(\frac{\partial f}{\partial y}\hat{j}\right)\times\vec{V} + \left(\frac{\partial f}{\partial z}\hat{k}\right)\times\vec{V}\right] + \left[f\left(\hat{i}\times\frac{\partial \vec{V}}{\partial x}\right) + f\left(\hat{j}\times\frac{\partial \vec{V}}{\partial y}\right) + f\left(\hat{k}\times\frac{\partial \vec{V}}{\partial z}\right)\right]$$

$$= \left(\frac{\partial f}{\partial x}\hat{i} + \frac{\partial f}{\partial y}\hat{j} + \frac{\partial f}{\partial z}\hat{k}\right)\times\vec{V} + f\left(\hat{i}\times\frac{\partial \vec{V}}{\partial x} + \hat{j}\times\frac{\partial \vec{V}}{\partial y} + \hat{k}\times\frac{\partial \vec{V}}{\partial z}\right)$$

$$= (\nabla f)\times\vec{V} + f(\nabla\times\vec{V})\cdot$$

$$\therefore\ \text{curl}(f\vec{V}) = (\nabla f)\times\vec{V} + f(\nabla\times\vec{V})\cdot$$

4. *Find the divergence of the following vector functions :*

(*i*) $\vec{f} = x^2\hat{i} + y^2\hat{j} - z\hat{k}$

(*ii*) $\vec{f} = xyz(\hat{i} + \hat{j} + \hat{k})$

(*iii*) $\vec{f} = yz^2\hat{i} - zx^2\hat{k}$

SOLUTION. (i) We have $\text{div}\,\vec{f} = \nabla.\vec{f}$

$$= \left(\hat{i}\frac{\partial}{\partial x} + \hat{j}\frac{\partial}{\partial y} + \hat{k}\frac{\partial}{\partial z}\right).(x^2\hat{i} + y^2\hat{j} - z\hat{k})$$

$$= \frac{\partial}{\partial x}(x^2) + \frac{\partial}{\partial y}(y^2) + \frac{\partial}{\partial z}(-z)$$

$$= 2x + 2y - 1$$

(ii) $\vec{f} = xyz(\hat{i} + \hat{j} + \hat{k})$

$\therefore\ \text{div}\,\vec{f} = \nabla.\vec{f}$

$$= \left(\hat{i}\frac{\partial}{\partial x} + \hat{j}\frac{\partial}{\partial y} + \hat{k}\frac{\partial}{\partial z}\right)\cdot xyz.(\hat{i} + \hat{j} + \hat{k})$$

$$= \frac{\partial}{\partial x}(xyz) + \frac{\partial}{\partial y}(xyz) + \frac{\partial}{\partial z}(xyz)$$

$$= yz + zx + xy$$

(iii) $\vec{f} = yz^2\hat{i} - zx^2\hat{k}$

$\therefore\ \text{div}\,\vec{f} = \nabla.\vec{f}$

$$= \left(\hat{i}\frac{\partial}{\partial x} + \hat{j}\frac{\partial}{\partial y} + \hat{k}\frac{\partial}{\partial z}\right).(yz^2\hat{i} - zx^2\hat{k})$$

$$= \frac{\partial}{\partial x}(yz^2) - \frac{\partial}{\partial z}(zx^2)$$

$$= 0 - x^2 = -x^2.$$

5. *Find curl* $\vec{f}$ *if*

(*i*) $\vec{f} = z^2\hat{i} + x^2\hat{j} + y^2\hat{k}$

(*ii*) $\vec{f} = xz\hat{i} - yz\hat{j}$

SOLUTION. (i) $\vec{f} = z^2\hat{i} + x^2\hat{j} + y^2\hat{k}$

We have curl $\vec{f} = \nabla\times\vec{f}$

$$= \begin{vmatrix} \hat{i} & \hat{j} & \hat{k} \\ \dfrac{\partial}{\partial x} & \dfrac{\partial}{\partial y} & \dfrac{\partial}{\partial z} \\ z^2 & x^2 & y^2 \end{vmatrix}$$

$$= \hat{i}\left(\frac{\partial}{\partial y}(y)^2 - \frac{\partial}{\partial z}(x)^2\right) + \hat{j}\left(\frac{\partial}{\partial z}(z)^2 - \frac{\partial}{\partial x}(y)^2\right) + \hat{k}\left(\frac{\partial}{\partial x}(x)^2 - \frac{\partial}{\partial y}(z)^2\right)$$

$$= 2y\hat{i} + 2z\hat{j} + 2x\hat{k} = 2(y\hat{i} + z\hat{j} + x\hat{k}).$$

(ii) $\vec{f} = xz\hat{i} - yz\hat{j}$

$\therefore$ curl $\vec{f} = \nabla \times \vec{f}$

$$= \begin{vmatrix} \hat{i} & \hat{j} & \hat{k} \\ \frac{\partial}{\partial x} & \frac{\partial}{\partial y} & \frac{\partial}{\partial z} \\ xz & -yz & 0 \end{vmatrix}$$

$$= \hat{i}\left(\frac{\partial}{\partial z}(yz)\right) + \hat{j}\left(\frac{\partial}{\partial z}(xz)\right) + \hat{k}\left(-\frac{\partial}{\partial x}(yz) - \frac{\partial}{\partial y}(xz)\right)$$

$$= y\hat{i} + x\hat{j} + \hat{k}(0-0) = y\hat{i} + x\hat{j}.$$

6. *Prove that*

div $(\vec{a}\times\vec{b}) = \vec{b}\cdot curl\,\vec{a} - \vec{a}\,.\,curl\,\vec{b}$

or $\nabla\cdot(\vec{a}\times\vec{b}) = \vec{b}\cdot(\nabla\times\vec{a}) - \vec{a}\cdot(\nabla\times\vec{b})$

SOLUTION. We have div $(\vec{a}\times\vec{b}) = \nabla\cdot(\vec{a}\times\vec{b})$

$$= \left(\hat{i}\frac{\partial}{\partial x} + \hat{j}\frac{\partial}{\partial y} + \hat{k}\frac{\partial}{\partial z}\right).(\vec{a}\times\vec{b})$$

$$= \left(\hat{i}\frac{\partial}{\partial x}\right).(\vec{a}\times\vec{b}) + \left(\hat{j}\frac{\partial}{\partial y}\right).(\vec{a}\times\vec{b}) + \left(\hat{k}\frac{\partial}{\partial z}\right).(\vec{a}\times\vec{b})$$

$$= \hat{i}.\frac{\partial}{\partial x}(\vec{a}\times\vec{b}) + \hat{j}.\frac{\partial}{\partial y}(\vec{a}\times\vec{b}) + \hat{k}.\frac{\partial}{\partial z}(\vec{a}\times\vec{b})$$

$$= \hat{i}.\left(\frac{\partial\vec{a}}{\partial x}\times\vec{b} + \vec{a}\times\frac{\partial\vec{b}}{\partial x}\right) + \hat{j}.\left(\frac{\partial\vec{a}}{\partial y}\times\vec{b} + \vec{a}\times\frac{\partial\vec{b}}{\partial y}\right) + \hat{k}.\left(\frac{\partial\vec{a}}{\partial z}\times\vec{b} + \vec{a}\times\frac{\partial\vec{b}}{\partial z}\right)$$

$$= \hat{i}.\left(\frac{\partial\vec{a}}{\partial x}\times\vec{b}\right) + \hat{i}.\left(\vec{a}\times\frac{\partial\vec{b}}{\partial x}\right) + \hat{j}.\left(\frac{\partial\vec{a}}{\partial y}\times\vec{b}\right) + \hat{j}.\left(\vec{a}\times\frac{\partial\vec{b}}{\partial y}\right) + \hat{k}.\left(\frac{\partial\vec{a}}{\partial z}\times\vec{b}\right) + \hat{k}.\left(\vec{a}\times\frac{\partial\vec{b}}{\partial z}\right)$$

$$= \left[\hat{i}.\left(\frac{\partial\vec{a}}{\partial x}\times\vec{b}\right) + \hat{j}.\left(\frac{\partial\vec{a}}{\partial y}\times\vec{b}\right) + \hat{k}.\left(\frac{\partial\vec{a}}{\partial z}\times\vec{b}\right)\right] + \left[\hat{i}.\left(\vec{a}\times\frac{\partial\vec{b}}{\partial x}\right) + \hat{j}.\left(\vec{a}\times\frac{\partial\vec{b}}{\partial y}\right) + \hat{k}.\left(\vec{a}\times\frac{\partial\vec{b}}{\partial z}\right)\right]$$

Using $\vec{a}.(\vec{b}\times\vec{c}) = \vec{a}\times(\vec{b}.\vec{c})$

and $\vec{a}.(\vec{b}\times\vec{c}) = -\vec{a}.(\vec{c}\times\vec{b})$

$$= \left[\left(\hat{i}\times\frac{\partial\vec{a}}{\partial x}\right).\vec{b} + \left(\hat{j}\times\frac{\partial\vec{a}}{\partial y}\right).\vec{b} + \left(\hat{k}\times\frac{\partial\vec{a}}{\partial z}\right).\vec{b}\right] - \left[\hat{i}.\left(\frac{\partial\vec{b}}{\partial x}\times\vec{a}\right) + \hat{j}.\left(\frac{\partial\vec{b}}{\partial y}\times\vec{a}\right) + \hat{k}.\left(\frac{\partial\vec{b}}{\partial z}\times\vec{a}\right)\right]$$

$$= \left(\hat{i}\times\frac{\partial\vec{a}}{\partial x} + \hat{j}\times\frac{\partial\vec{a}}{\partial y} + \hat{k}\times\frac{\partial\vec{a}}{\partial z}\right).\vec{b} - \left(\hat{i}\times\frac{\partial\vec{b}}{\partial x} + \hat{j}\times\frac{\partial\vec{b}}{\partial y} + \hat{k}\times\frac{\partial\vec{b}}{\partial z}\right).\vec{a}$$

$$= (\nabla\times\vec{a}).\vec{b} - (\nabla\times\vec{b}).\vec{a}$$

$$\therefore \nabla\cdot(\vec{a}\times\vec{b}) = \vec{b}\cdot(\nabla\times\vec{a}) - \vec{a}\cdot(\nabla\times\vec{b}) \qquad (\because \vec{a}.\vec{b} = \vec{b}.\vec{a})$$

7. *Prove that*

curl $(\vec{a}\times\vec{b}) = \vec{b}\cdot\nabla)\ \vec{a} - \vec{b}$ *div* $\vec{a}$

$-((\vec{a}\cdot\nabla)\vec{b} + \vec{a}$ *div* $\vec{b}$

SOLUTION. We have curl $(\vec{a}\times\vec{b}) = \nabla\times(\vec{a}\times\vec{b})$

$$= \left(\hat{i}\frac{\partial}{\partial x} + \hat{j}\frac{\partial}{\partial y} + \hat{k}\frac{\partial}{\partial z}\right)\times(\vec{a}\times\vec{b})$$

$$= \hat{i}\times\frac{\partial}{\partial x}(\vec{a}\times\vec{b}) + \hat{j}\times\frac{\partial}{\partial y}(\vec{a}\times\vec{b}) + \hat{k}\times\frac{\partial}{\partial z}(\vec{a}\times\vec{b})$$

$$= \hat{i}\times\left(\frac{\partial\vec{a}}{\partial x}\times\vec{b} + \vec{a}\times\frac{\partial\vec{b}}{\partial x}\right) + \hat{j}\times\left(\frac{\partial\vec{a}}{\partial y}\times\vec{b} + \vec{a}\times\frac{\partial\vec{b}}{\partial y}\right) + \hat{k}\times\left(\frac{\partial\vec{a}}{\partial z}\times\vec{b} + \vec{a}\times\frac{\partial\vec{b}}{\partial z}\right)$$

$$= \hat{i} \times \left(\frac{\partial \vec{a}}{\partial x} \times \vec{b} \right) + \hat{i} \times \left(\vec{a} \times \frac{\partial \vec{b}}{\partial x} \right)$$

$$+ \hat{j} \times \left(\frac{\partial \vec{a}}{\partial y} \times \vec{b} \right) + \hat{j} \times \left(\vec{a} \times \frac{\partial \vec{b}}{\partial y} \right)$$

$$+ \hat{k} \times \left(\frac{\partial \vec{a}}{\partial z} \times \vec{b} \right) + \hat{k} \times \left(\vec{a} \times \frac{\partial \vec{b}}{\partial z} \right)$$

$$= \left[\hat{i} \times \left(\frac{\partial \vec{a}}{\partial x} \times \vec{b} \right) + \hat{j} \times \left(\frac{\partial \vec{a}}{\partial y} \times \vec{b} \right) + \right.$$

$$\left. + \hat{k} \times \left(\frac{\partial \vec{a}}{\partial z} \times \vec{b} \right) \right] + \left[\hat{i} \times \left(\vec{a} \times \frac{\partial \vec{b}}{\partial x} \right) \right.$$

$$\left. + \hat{j} \times \left(\vec{a} \times \frac{\partial \vec{b}}{\partial y} \right) + \hat{k} \times \left(\vec{a} \times \frac{\partial \vec{b}}{\partial z} \right) \right]$$

$$= \left[(\hat{i} \cdot \vec{b}) \frac{\partial \vec{a}}{\partial x} - \left(\hat{i} \cdot \frac{\partial \vec{a}}{\partial x} \right) \vec{b} + (\hat{j} \cdot \vec{b}) \frac{\partial \vec{a}}{\partial y} \right.$$

$$\left. - \left(\hat{j} \cdot \frac{\partial \vec{a}}{\partial y} \right) \vec{b} + (\hat{k} \cdot \vec{b}) \frac{\partial \vec{a}}{\partial z} - \left(\hat{k} \cdot \frac{\partial \vec{a}}{\partial z} \right) \vec{b} \right]$$

$$- \left[(\hat{i} \cdot \vec{a}) \frac{\partial \vec{b}}{\partial x} - \left(\hat{i} \cdot \frac{\partial \vec{b}}{\partial x} \right) \vec{a} + (\hat{j} \cdot \vec{a}) \frac{\partial \vec{b}}{\partial y} \right.$$

$$\left. - \left(\hat{j} \cdot \frac{\partial \vec{b}}{\partial y} \right) \vec{a} + (\hat{k} \cdot \vec{a}) \frac{\partial \vec{b}}{\partial z} - \left(\hat{k} \cdot \frac{\partial \vec{b}}{\partial z} \right) \vec{a} \right]$$

Using $\vec{a} \cdot \vec{b} = \vec{b} \cdot \vec{a}$, we get

$$= \left[\left(\vec{b} \cdot \hat{i} \frac{\partial \vec{a}}{\partial x} + \vec{b} \cdot \hat{j} \frac{\partial \vec{a}}{\partial y} + \vec{b} \cdot \hat{k} \frac{\partial \vec{a}}{\partial z} \right) \right.$$

$$\left. - \left(\hat{i} \cdot \frac{\partial \vec{a}}{\partial x} + \hat{j} \cdot \frac{\partial \vec{a}}{\partial y} + \hat{k} \cdot \frac{\partial \vec{a}}{\partial z} \right) \vec{b} \right]$$

$$- \left[\left(\vec{a} \cdot \hat{i} \frac{\partial \vec{b}}{\partial x} + \vec{a} \cdot \hat{j} \frac{\partial \vec{b}}{\partial y} + \vec{a} \cdot \hat{k} \frac{\partial \vec{b}}{\partial z} \right) \right.$$

$$\left. - \left(\hat{i} \cdot \frac{\partial \vec{b}}{\partial x} + \hat{j} \cdot \frac{\partial \vec{b}}{\partial y} + \hat{k} \cdot \frac{\partial \vec{b}}{\partial z} \right) \vec{a} \right]$$

$$= \left[\left(\vec{b} \cdot \hat{i} \frac{\partial}{\partial x} + \vec{b} \cdot \hat{j} \frac{\partial}{\partial y} + \vec{b} \cdot \hat{k} \frac{\partial}{\partial z} \right) \vec{a} - (\nabla \cdot a) \vec{b} \right]$$

$$- \left[\left(\vec{a} \cdot \hat{i} \frac{\partial}{\partial x} + \vec{a} \cdot \hat{j} \frac{\partial}{\partial y} + \vec{a} \cdot \hat{k} \frac{\partial}{\partial z} \right) \vec{b} - (\nabla \cdot b) \vec{a} \right]$$

$$= (\vec{b} \cdot \nabla) \vec{a} - (\nabla \cdot \vec{a}) \vec{b} - (\vec{a} \cdot \nabla) \vec{b} + (\nabla \cdot \vec{b}) \vec{a}$$

Hence, curl $(\vec{a} \times \vec{b}) = (\vec{b} \cdot \nabla)\vec{a} - \vec{b}$ div $\vec{a}$ $- (\vec{a} \cdot \nabla)\vec{b} + \vec{a}$ div $\vec{b}$.

Similar Problem

(1) Prove that grad $(\vec{a} \cdot \vec{b}) = (\vec{b} \cdot \nabla)\vec{a} + (\vec{a} \cdot \nabla)\vec{b} + \vec{b} \times$ curl $\vec{a} + \vec{a} \times$ curl $\vec{b}$.

8. *Prove that the curl of the gradient of f(scalar function) is zero, i.e.* $\nabla \times (\nabla f) = \vec{0}$

or

If $f = r^n$, *then* $\nabla \times (\nabla r^n) = 0$

SOLUTION. Since we have

$$\nabla f = \frac{\partial f}{\partial x} \hat{i} + \frac{\partial f}{\partial y} \hat{j} + \frac{\partial f}{\partial z} \hat{k}$$

$$\therefore \nabla \times (\nabla f) = \begin{vmatrix} \hat{i} & \hat{j} & \hat{k} \\ \frac{\partial}{\partial x} & \frac{\partial}{\partial y} & \frac{\partial}{\partial z} \\ \frac{\partial f}{\partial x} & \frac{\partial f}{\partial y} & \frac{\partial f}{\partial z} \end{vmatrix}$$

$$= \hat{i} \left[\frac{\partial^2 f}{\partial y \partial z} - \frac{\partial^2 f}{\partial z \partial y} \right] + \hat{j} \left[\frac{\partial^2 f}{\partial z \partial x} - \frac{\partial^2 f}{\partial x \partial z} \right]$$

$$+ \hat{k} \left[\frac{\partial^2 f}{\partial x \partial y} - \frac{\partial^2 f}{\partial y \partial x} \right]$$

Since $\frac{\partial^2 f}{\partial y \partial z} = \frac{\partial^2 f}{\partial z \partial y}$ etc.

$$\therefore \nabla \times (\nabla f) = 0\hat{i} + 0\hat{j} + 0\hat{k} = \vec{0}$$

9. *Prove that the div(curl* $\vec{V}$ *) = 0.*

i.e. $\nabla \cdot (\nabla \times \vec{V}) = 0$.

SOLUTION. Since we have

$$\nabla \times V = \begin{vmatrix} \hat{i} & \hat{j} & \hat{k} \\ \frac{\partial}{\partial x} & \frac{\partial}{\partial y} & \frac{\partial}{\partial z} \\ V_1 & V_2 & V_3 \end{vmatrix}$$

where $\vec{V} = V_1\hat{i} + V_2\hat{j} + V_3\hat{k}$ (say).

$$\therefore \nabla \times \vec{V} = \hat{i} \left(\frac{\partial V_3}{\partial y} - \frac{\partial V_2}{\partial z} \right) + \hat{j} \left(\frac{\partial V_1}{\partial z} - \frac{\partial V_3}{\partial x} \right)$$

$$+ \hat{k} \left(\frac{\partial V_2}{\partial x} - \frac{\partial V_1}{\partial y} \right)$$

Now $\nabla \cdot (\nabla \times \vec{V})$

$$= \frac{\partial}{\partial x}\left(\frac{\partial V_3}{\partial y} - \frac{\partial V_2}{\partial z}\right) + \frac{\partial}{\partial y}\left(\frac{\partial V_1}{\partial z} - \frac{\partial V_3}{\partial x}\right) + \frac{\partial}{\partial z}\left(\frac{\partial V_2}{\partial x} - \frac{\partial V_1}{\partial y}\right)$$

$$= \frac{\partial^2 V_3}{\partial x \partial y} - \frac{\partial^2 V_2}{\partial x \partial z} + \frac{\partial^2 V_1}{\partial y \partial z} - \frac{\partial^2 V_3}{\partial y \partial x} + \frac{\partial^2 V_2}{\partial z \partial x} - \frac{\partial^2 V_1}{\partial z \partial y}$$

Since $\frac{\partial^2 V_1}{\partial y \partial z} = \frac{\partial^2 V_1}{\partial z \partial y}$ etc.

$\therefore \nabla \cdot (\nabla \times \vec{V}) = 0.$

10. $\nabla^2 f(r) = f''(r) + \frac{2}{r} f'(r)$

(BHOPAL–2008, SVTU–2008, VTU–2006)

SOLUTION. Since we have

$$\nabla^2 f(r) = \nabla \cdot (\nabla f(r)) = \nabla \cdot (f'(r) \nabla r) \quad (\because \nabla f(r) = f'(r)\nabla r)$$

$$= \nabla \cdot \left(f'(r)\frac{\vec{r}}{r}\right) \quad \left(\because \nabla r = \frac{\vec{r}}{r}\right)$$

$$= \nabla \cdot \left(\frac{f'(r)}{r}\vec{r}\right) = \frac{f'(r)}{r}\nabla . \vec{r} + \vec{r} . \nabla\left\{\frac{f'(r)}{r}\right\}$$

$$[\because \nabla f(\vec{V}) = f \nabla \cdot \vec{V} + \vec{V} \cdot (\nabla f)]$$

$$= \frac{3}{r} f'(r) + \vec{r} . \left\{\frac{f'(r)}{r}\right\}' \nabla r$$

$$= \frac{3}{r} f'(r) + \vec{r} . \left\{\frac{r f''(r) - f'(r)}{r^2}\right\} \frac{\vec{r}}{r}$$

$$= \frac{3}{r} f'(r) + \frac{r f''(r) - f'(r)}{r^2} \frac{\vec{r} \cdot \vec{r}}{r}$$

$$= \frac{3}{r} f'(r) + \frac{r f''(r) - f'(r)}{r^2} \frac{r^2}{r}$$

$$= \frac{3}{r} f'(r) + \frac{r f''(r) - f'(r)}{r}$$

$$= f''(r) + \frac{2}{r} f'(r)$$

Hence, $\nabla^2 f(r) = f''(r) + \frac{2}{r} f'(r)$.

11. *Solve* $\nabla^2 f(r) = 0$.

SOLUTION. We have

$$\nabla^2 f(r) = f''(r) + \frac{2}{r} f'(r)$$

Since $\nabla^2 f(r) = 0$ given

$$\therefore f''(r) + \frac{2}{r} f'(r) = 0$$

or $$\frac{f''(r)}{f'(r)} = -\frac{2}{r}$$

Integrating w.r.t. 'r', we get

$$\log f'(r) = -2 \log r + \log c_1$$

where c_1 is a constant of integration.

$$\therefore \quad f'(r) = \frac{c_1}{r^2}.$$

Again integrating w.r.t. 'r', we get

$$f(r) = -\frac{c_1}{r} + c_2$$

where c_1 and c_2 are constant of integration.

12. *Prove that* $\nabla^2 \left(\frac{1}{r}\right) = 0.$ (PTU–2003)

SOLUTION. Since we have

$$\nabla^2 \left(\frac{1}{r}\right) = \nabla \cdot \left(\nabla\left(\frac{1}{r}\right)\right) = \nabla \cdot \left(-\frac{1}{r^2}\nabla r\right)$$

$$[\because \text{grad} f(r) = f'(r) \text{ grad } r]$$

$$= \nabla \cdot \left(-\frac{1}{r^3}\vec{r}\right) \quad \left[\because \nabla r = \frac{\vec{r}}{r}\right]$$

$$= \left(-\frac{1}{r^3}\right)\nabla \cdot \vec{r} + \vec{r} \cdot \text{grad}\left(-\frac{1}{r^3}\right)$$

$$= -\frac{3}{r^3} + \vec{r} \cdot \left(\frac{3}{r^4}\text{grad } r\right)$$

$$= -\frac{3}{r^3} + \vec{r} \cdot \left(\frac{3}{r^4}\frac{\vec{r}}{r}\right)$$

$$= -\frac{3}{r^3} + \frac{3}{r^5}\vec{r} \cdot \vec{r} = -\frac{3}{r^3} + \frac{3}{r^5} r^2 \quad (\because \vec{r} . \vec{r} = r^2)$$

$$= -\frac{3}{r^3} + \frac{3}{r^3} = 0.$$

$$\therefore \nabla^2 \left(\frac{1}{r}\right) = 0.$$

13. *Prove that*

(*i*) $\nabla \times (\nabla \times a) = \nabla(\nabla . \vec{a}) - \nabla^2 \vec{a}$.

(*ii*) $\vec{a} \times (\nabla \times \vec{r}) = \nabla(\vec{a} . \vec{r}) - (\vec{a} . \nabla)\vec{r}$.

where $\vec{a} = x\hat{i} + y\hat{j} + z\hat{k}$ (UPTU–2008)

SOLUTION. (i) Let $\vec{a} = a_1\hat{i} + a_2\hat{j} + a_3\hat{k}$. Then

$$\nabla \times \vec{a} = \begin{vmatrix} \hat{i} & \hat{j} & \hat{k} \\ \frac{\partial}{\partial x} & \frac{\partial}{\partial y} & \frac{\partial}{\partial z} \\ a_1 & a_2 & a_3 \end{vmatrix}$$

$$= \left(\frac{\partial a_3}{\partial y} - \frac{\partial a_2}{\partial z}\right)\hat{i} + \left(\frac{\partial a_1}{\partial z} - \frac{\partial a_3}{\partial x}\right)\hat{j} + \left(\frac{\partial a_2}{\partial x} - \frac{\partial a_1}{\partial y}\right)\hat{k}$$

$\therefore\ \nabla\times(\nabla\times\vec{a})$

$$= \begin{vmatrix} \hat{i} & \hat{j} & \hat{k} \\ \frac{\partial}{\partial x} & \frac{\partial}{\partial y} & \frac{\partial}{\partial z} \\ \frac{\partial a_3}{\partial y} - \frac{\partial a_2}{\partial z} & \frac{\partial a_1}{\partial z} - \frac{\partial a_3}{\partial x} & \frac{\partial a_2}{\partial x} - \frac{\partial a_1}{\partial y} \end{vmatrix}$$

$$= \Sigma\left[\left\{\frac{\partial}{\partial y}\left(\frac{\partial a_2}{\partial x} - \frac{\partial a_1}{\partial y}\right) - \frac{\partial}{\partial z}\left(\frac{\partial a_1}{\partial z} - \frac{\partial a_3}{\partial x}\right)\right\}\hat{i}\right]$$

$$= \Sigma\left[\left\{\left(\frac{\partial^2 a_2}{\partial x \partial y} + \frac{\partial^2 a_3}{\partial x \partial z}\right) - \left(\frac{\partial^2 a_1}{\partial y^2} - \frac{\partial^2 a_1}{\partial z^2}\right)\right\}\hat{i}\right]$$

$$= \Sigma\left[\left\{\frac{\partial}{\partial x}\left(\frac{\partial a_1}{\partial x} + \frac{\partial a_2}{\partial y} + \frac{\partial a_3}{\partial z}\right) - \left(\frac{\partial^2 a_1}{\partial x^2} + \frac{\partial^2 a_1}{\partial y^2} + \frac{\partial^2 a_1}{\partial z^2}\right)\right\}\hat{i}\right]$$

$$= \Sigma\left[\left\{\frac{\partial}{\partial x}(\nabla\cdot\vec{a}) - (\nabla^2 \cdot a_1)\right\}\hat{i}\right]$$

$$= \left(\Sigma\hat{i}\frac{\partial}{\partial x}\right)(\nabla\cdot\vec{a}) - \nabla^2(\Sigma a_1\hat{i})$$

$$= \nabla(\nabla\cdot\vec{a}) - \nabla^2\vec{a}.$$

(ii) LHS $= \vec{a}\times(\nabla\times\vec{r}) = \vec{a}\times\vec{0} = 0$ $\quad [\because \text{curl } \vec{r} = 0]$

RHS $= \nabla(\vec{a}\cdot\vec{r}) - (\vec{a}\cdot\nabla)\vec{r}$

$$= \nabla(a_1x + a_2y + a_3z) - \left(a_1\frac{\partial}{\partial x} + a_2\frac{\partial}{\partial y} + a_3\frac{\partial}{\partial z}\right)\vec{r}$$

$$= \hat{i}(a_1) + \hat{j}(a_2) + \hat{k}(a_3) - (a_1\hat{i} + a_2\hat{j} + a_3\hat{k})$$

$$= \vec{0} = \text{LHS}$$

14. *If f and g are two scalar point functions, show that*

(i) *div* $(f\nabla g) = f\nabla^2 g + \nabla f\cdot\nabla g$

(ii) *div* $(f\nabla g)$ – *div* $(g\nabla f) = f\nabla^2 g - g\nabla^2 f$

SOLUTION. (i) Since $\nabla g = \frac{\partial g}{\partial x}\hat{i} + \frac{\partial g}{\partial y}\hat{j} + \frac{\partial g}{\partial z}\hat{k}$

$$\therefore\ f\nabla g = f\frac{\partial g}{\partial x}\hat{i} + f\frac{\partial g}{\partial y}\hat{j} + f\frac{\partial g}{\partial z}\hat{k}$$

and

$$\text{div}(f\nabla g) = \frac{\partial}{\partial x}\left(f\frac{\partial g}{\partial x}\right) + \frac{\partial}{\partial y}\left(f\frac{\partial g}{\partial y}\right) + \frac{\partial}{\partial z}\left(f\frac{\partial g}{\partial z}\right)$$

$$= f\frac{\partial^2 g}{\partial x^2} + \frac{\partial f}{\partial x}\frac{\partial g}{\partial x} + f\frac{\partial^2 g}{\partial y^2} + \frac{\partial f}{\partial y}\frac{\partial g}{\partial y} + f\frac{\partial^2 g}{\partial z^2} + \frac{\partial f}{\partial z}\frac{\partial g}{\partial z}$$

$$= f\left(\frac{\partial^2 g}{\partial x^2} + \frac{\partial^2 g}{\partial y^2} + \frac{\partial^2 g}{\partial z^2}\right) + \frac{\partial f}{\partial x}\frac{\partial g}{\partial x} + \frac{\partial f}{\partial y}\frac{\partial g}{\partial y} + \frac{\partial f}{\partial z}\frac{\partial g}{\partial z}$$

$$= f\nabla^2 g + \left(\frac{\partial f}{\partial x}\hat{i} + \frac{\partial f}{\partial y}\hat{j} + \frac{\partial f}{\partial z}\hat{k}\right)\cdot\left(\frac{\partial g}{\partial x}\hat{i} + \frac{\partial g}{\partial y}\hat{j} + \frac{\partial g}{\partial z}\hat{k}\right)$$

$$= f\nabla^2 g + (\nabla f)\cdot(\nabla g)$$

Hence, div $(f\nabla g) = f\nabla^2 g + (\nabla f)\cdot(\nabla g)$ ...(1)

(ii) Similarly, we may get

div $(g\nabla f) = g\nabla^2 f + (\nabla g).(\nabla f)$ ...(2)

Form (1) and (2), we get

div $(f\nabla g)$ – div $(g\nabla f) = f\nabla^2 g - g\nabla^2 f$

15. *Prove that div grad* $(r^n) = n(n+1)r^{n-2}$.

(BHOPAL–2008, JNTU–2006, SVTU–2006)

SOLUTION. Since we have

$$\text{grad}\,(r^n) = (nr^{n-1}\,\text{grad}\,r)$$
$$[\because \text{grad}\,f(r) = f'(r)(\nabla r)]$$
$$= nr^{n-1}\frac{\vec{r}}{r} \quad \left[\because \text{grad}\,r = \frac{\vec{r}}{r}\right]$$
$$= nr^{n-2}\vec{r}$$

Now

$$\text{div grad}\,(r^n) = \text{div}(nr^{n-2}\vec{r})$$
$$= n\,\text{div}(r^{n-2}\vec{r})$$
$$= n[r^{n-2}\nabla\cdot\vec{r} + \vec{r}\cdot\text{grad}\,(r^{n-2})]$$
$$= n[3r^{n-2} + \vec{r}\cdot((n-2)r^{n-3}\text{grad}\,r)] \quad (\because \nabla\cdot\vec{r} = 3)$$
$$= n\left[3r^{n-2} + \vec{r}\cdot\left((n-2)r^{n-3}\frac{\vec{r}}{r}\right)\right]$$
$$= n[3r^{n-2} + (n-2)r^{n-4}\vec{r}\cdot\vec{r}]$$
$$= n[3r^{n-2} + (n-2)r^{n-4}r^2] \quad [\because \vec{r}\cdot\vec{r} = r^2]$$
$$= n(n+1)r^{n-2}$$

$\therefore$ div grad $r^n = n(n+1)r^{n-2}$.

16. *If* $\vec{u} = y\hat{i} + z\hat{j} + x\hat{k}, \vec{v} = xy\hat{i} + yz\hat{j} + zx\hat{k}$, *find*

(i) *curl* $(\vec{u}\times\vec{v})$ (ii) $\vec{u}\times$ *curl* $\vec{v}$

(iii) $\vec{v}\times$ *curl* $\vec{u}$ (iv) *div* $(\vec{u}\times\vec{v})$

SOLUTION. (i) Since

$$\vec{u} = y\hat{i} + z\hat{j} + x\hat{k}, \vec{v} = xy\hat{i} + yz\hat{j} + zx\hat{k}.$$

$$\therefore \vec{u}\times\vec{v} = \begin{vmatrix} \hat{i} & \hat{j} & \hat{k} \\ y & z & x \\ xy & yz & zx \end{vmatrix}$$
$$= \hat{i}(z^2x - xyz) + \hat{j}(x^2y - xyz) + \hat{k}(y^2z - xyz).$$

Then curl $(\vec{u}\times\vec{v})$

$$= \begin{vmatrix} \hat{i} & \hat{j} & \hat{k} \\ \frac{\partial}{\partial x} & \frac{\partial}{\partial y} & \frac{\partial}{\partial z} \\ (z^2x - xyz) & (x^2y - xyz) & (y^2z - xyz) \end{vmatrix}$$

$$= \hat{i}\left[\frac{\partial}{\partial y}(y^2z - xyz) - \frac{\partial}{\partial z}(x^2y - xyz)\right] + \hat{j}\left[\frac{\partial}{\partial z}(z^2x - xyz) - \frac{\partial}{\partial x}(y^2z - xyz)\right] + \hat{k}\left[\frac{\partial}{\partial x}(x^2y - xyz) - \frac{\partial}{\partial y}(z^2x - xyz)\right]$$

$$= \hat{i}[(2yz - xz) - (-xy)] + \hat{j}[2zx - xy + yz] + \hat{k}[2xy - yz + xz]$$

$$= (2yz - xz + xy)\hat{i} + \hat{j}(2zx - xy + yz) + \hat{k}(2xy - yz + xz).$$

(ii) $$\text{curl}\,\vec{v} = \begin{vmatrix} \hat{i} & \hat{j} & \hat{k} \\ \frac{\partial}{\partial x} & \frac{\partial}{\partial y} & \frac{\partial}{\partial z} \\ xy & yz & zx \end{vmatrix}$$

$$= \hat{i}\left[\frac{\partial}{\partial y}(zx) - \frac{\partial}{\partial z}(yz)\right] + \hat{j}\left[\frac{\partial}{\partial z}(xy) - \frac{\partial}{\partial x}(zx)\right] + \hat{k}\left[\frac{\partial}{\partial x}(yz) - \frac{\partial}{\partial y}(xy)\right]$$

$$= -y\hat{i} - z\hat{j} - x\hat{k}$$
$$= -(y\hat{i} + z\hat{j} + x\hat{k}) = -\vec{u}$$

$\therefore$ $\vec{u}\times\text{curl}\,\vec{v} = \vec{u}\times -\vec{u} = -(\vec{u}\times\vec{u}) = 0$

(iii) $$\text{curl}\,\vec{u} = \begin{vmatrix} \hat{i} & \hat{j} & \hat{k} \\ \frac{\partial}{\partial x} & \frac{\partial}{\partial y} & \frac{\partial}{\partial z} \\ y & z & x \end{vmatrix}$$

$$= \hat{i}(-1) + \hat{j}(-1) + \hat{k}(-1)$$
$$= -(\hat{i} + \hat{j} + \hat{k})$$

$\therefore$ $\vec{v}\times\text{curl}\,\vec{u}$

$$= (xy\hat{i} + yz\hat{j} + zx\hat{k})\times\{-(\hat{i} + \hat{j} + \hat{k})\}$$
$$= -[xy\hat{k} - xy\hat{j} - yz\hat{k} + yz\hat{i} + zx\hat{j} - zx\hat{i}]$$
$$= \hat{i}(zx - yz) + \hat{j}(xy - zx) + (yz - xy)\hat{k}.$$

(iv) $\vec{u}\times\vec{v}$

$= (z^2x - xyz)\hat{i} + (x^2y - xyz)\hat{j} + (y^2z - xyz)\hat{k}.$

$\therefore$ div $(\vec{u}\times\vec{v})$

$$= \frac{\partial}{\partial x}(z^2x - xyz) + \frac{\partial}{\partial y}(x^2y - xyz) + \frac{\partial}{\partial z}(y^2z - xyz).$$

$= z^2 - yz + x^2 - xz + y^2 - xy$

$= x^2 + y^2 + z^2 - xy - yz - zx.$

17. *If f and g are two scalar point functions, show that div(g $\nabla f \times f \nabla g$) = 0.*

SOLUTION. Since we have

div $(\vec{a}\times\vec{b}) = \vec{b}\cdot$ curl $\vec{a} - \vec{a}$ curl $\vec{b}$

Let $\vec{a} = g\,\nabla f$ and $\vec{b} = f\,\nabla g$

$\therefore$ div$(g\,\nabla f \times f\,\nabla g)$

$= f\,\nabla g\cdot$curl $(g\,\nabla f) - g\,\nabla f\cdot$curl$(f\,\nabla g)$

$= f\,\nabla g.g$ curl grad $f - g\,\nabla f\cdot f$ curl grad g

$= 0 - 0.$

($\because$ curl grad $f = \vec{0}$, curl grad $g = \vec{0}$)

Hence, div$(g\,\nabla f \times f\,\nabla g) = 0.$

18. *Prove that $r^n\vec{r}$ is an irrotational vector for any value of n but is solenodial if n + 3 = 0.* (GBTU–2010, VTU–2006, UPTU–2006, PTU–2005, 06, KOTTAYAM–2005)

SOLUTION. Since we know that if $\vec{a}$ is irrotational, then $\nabla\times\vec{a} = 0$

$\therefore\ \nabla\times(r^n\vec{r}) = (\text{grad } r^n)\times\vec{r} + r^n \text{ curl } \vec{r}$

$= (nr^{n-1}\text{ grad } r)\times\vec{r} + \vec{0}$ [$\because$ curl $\vec{r} = 0$]

$$= \left(nr^{n-1}\frac{\vec{r}}{r}\right)\times\vec{r} \qquad \left[\because \text{grad } r = \frac{\vec{r}}{r}\right]$$

$= nr^{n-2}\,\vec{r}\times\vec{r} = \vec{0}$

[$\because$ Vector product of two same vectors is zero.]

Hence $r^n\vec{r}$ is irrotational for any value of n.

Further since if $\vec{a}$ is solenoidal, then $\nabla.\vec{a} = 0$

$\therefore\ \nabla\cdot(r^n\vec{r}) = (\text{grad } r^n).\vec{r} + r^n\,\nabla.\vec{r}$

$= (nr^{n-1}\text{ grad}\vec{r}).\vec{r} + 3r^n$ [$\because \nabla.\vec{r} = 3$]

$$= \left(nr^{n-1}\frac{\vec{r}}{r}\right).\vec{r} + 3r^n \qquad \left[\because \text{grad } r = \frac{\vec{r}}{r}\right]$$

$= nr^{n-2}\,\vec{r}.\vec{r} + 3r^n$

$= nr^{n-2}r^2 + 3r^n \qquad [\because \vec{r}.\vec{r} = r^2]$

$= nr^n + 3r^n = r^n(n+3).$

If $n + 3 = 0$, then $\nabla.(r^n\vec{r}) = 0$, and hence $r^n\vec{r}$ is solenoidal.

19. *If $\vec{a}$ and $\vec{b}$ are irrotational, prove that $\vec{a}\times\vec{b}$ is solenoidal.*

(GBTU–2010, MADRAS–2003, VTU–2001)

SOLUTION. Since $\vec{a}$ and $\vec{b}$ are irrotational, then

$\nabla\times\vec{a} = 0, \nabla\times\vec{b} = 0.$

Now we have to prove that $\vec{a}\times\vec{b}$ is solenoidal.

$\therefore\ \nabla\cdot(\vec{a}\times\vec{b}) = \vec{b}\cdot\text{curl }\vec{a} - \vec{a}\cdot\text{curl }\vec{b}$

$= \vec{b}\cdot(\nabla\times\vec{a}) - \vec{a}\cdot(\nabla\times\vec{b})$

$= 0 - 0 = 0.\quad [\because \nabla\times\vec{a} = 0, \nabla\times\vec{b} = 0]$

Thus, $\nabla.(\vec{a}\times\vec{b}) = 0.$

Hence $(\vec{a}\times\vec{b})$ is solenoidal.

20. *Show that the vector field $\vec{F} = \dfrac{\vec{r}}{r^3}$ is irrotaitonal as well as solenoidal. Find the scalar potential.* (UPTU–2006)

SOLUTION. We know that

curl $(u.\vec{a}) = u$ curl $\vec{a}$ + (grad $u)\times\vec{a}$

Therefore,

$$\text{curl}\left(\frac{1}{r^3}\cdot\vec{r}\right) = \frac{1}{r^3}\text{curl}\,\vec{r} + \left(\text{grad}\frac{1}{r^3}\right)\times\vec{r}$$

$$= \frac{1}{r^3}\,\vec{0} + \left(-\frac{3}{r^4}\hat{r}\right)\times\vec{r}$$

$$= \vec{0} - \frac{3}{r^5}(\vec{r}\times\vec{r}) = \vec{0} - \vec{0} = \vec{0}$$

$\Rightarrow \qquad \vec{F}$ is irrotational.

Also, we know that for the vector field $\vec{F}$ to be solenoidal, div $\vec{F} = 0$

We know that

div $(u\vec{a}) = u$ div $\vec{a} + \vec{a}$.grad u

$$\therefore\ \text{div}\left(\frac{\vec{r}}{r^3}\right) = \frac{1}{r^3}\text{div}\,\vec{r} + \vec{r}.\text{grad}\left(\frac{1}{r^3}\right)$$

$$= \frac{3}{r^3} + r\left(-\frac{3}{r^4}\frac{\vec{r}}{r}\right) \qquad (\because \text{div } \vec{r} = 3)$$

$$= \frac{3}{r^3} - \frac{3}{r^5}r^2 = \frac{3}{r^3} - \frac{3}{r^3} = 0$$

$\Rightarrow$ $\vec{F}$ is solenoidal.

Now, let $\vec{F} = \nabla\phi$, where ϕ is scalar potential.

$\therefore$ $\vec{F}.d\vec{r} = \nabla\phi.d\vec{r}$

$\vec{F}.d\vec{r} = d\phi$

$$\therefore d\phi = \frac{x\hat{i} + y\hat{j} + z\hat{k}}{(x^2+y^2+z^2)^{3/2}}(dx\hat{i} + dy\hat{j} + dz\hat{k})$$

$$= \frac{xdx + ydy + zdz}{(x^2+y^2+z^2)^{3/2}}$$

$$= d[-(x^2+y^2+z^2)^{-1/2}]$$

$$\Rightarrow \quad \phi = -\frac{1}{\sqrt{x^2+y^2+z^2}} + c.$$

$$\therefore \quad \phi = -\frac{1}{r} + c.$$

Exercise-25.5

1. If $\vec{f} = x^2y\hat{i} - 2xz\hat{j} + 2yz\hat{k}$, find
   (i) div $\vec{f}$ (ii) curl $\vec{f}$
   (iii) curl curl $\vec{f}$
2. If $\vec{f} = xy^2\hat{i} + 2x^2yz\hat{j} - 3yz^2\hat{k}$, then at the point (1, –1, 1) find
   (i) div $\vec{f}$ (ii) curl $\vec{f}$
3. If $\vec{f} = \text{grad}(x^3 + y^3 + z^3 - 3xyz)$, find
   (i) div $\vec{f}$ (ii) curl $\vec{f}$
4. (i) Determine the constant λ so that the vector $\vec{f} = (x+3y)\hat{i} + (y-2z)\hat{j} + (x+\lambda z)\hat{k}$ is solenoidal.
   (ii) Find the constants a, b, c so that the vector
   $$\vec{f} = (x+2y+az)\hat{i} + (bx-3y-z)\hat{j} + (4x+cy+2z)\hat{k}$$
   is irrotational, *i.e.* curl $\vec{f} = \vec{0}$.
5. Show that the vector
   $$\vec{f} = (\sin y + z)\hat{i} + (x\cos y - z)\hat{j} + (x-y)\hat{k}$$
   is irrotational.
6. Show that $\nabla^2\left(\frac{x}{r^2}\right) = -\frac{2x}{r^4}$.
7. If $\vec{v} = (x\hat{i} + y\hat{j} + z\hat{k})/(x^2+y^2+z^2)^{3/2}$, find
   (i) $\nabla\cdot\vec{v}$ (ii) $\nabla\times\vec{v}$
8. If $\vec{v} = (x+y+1)\hat{i} + \hat{j} + (-x-y)\hat{k}$, prove that
   $$\vec{v}\cdot(\nabla\times\vec{v}) = 0$$
9. If
   $$\vec{v} = (y^2+z^2-x^2)\hat{i} + (z^2+x^2-y^2)\hat{j} + (x^2+y^2-z^2)\hat{k},$$
   find (i) div $\vec{v}$ (ii) curl $\vec{v}$
10. Prove that
    (i) div $(\vec{a} + \vec{b})$ = div $\vec{a}$ + div $\vec{b}$
    (ii) curl $(\vec{a} + \vec{b})$ = curl $\vec{a}$ + curl $\vec{b}$
11. Prove that div $\nabla\phi = \nabla^2\phi$, *i.e.* $\nabla\cdot\nabla\phi = \nabla^2\phi$, where ϕ is a scalar point function.
12. If $\vec{f} = x^2y\hat{i} + xz\hat{j} + 2yz\hat{k}$, prove that div curl $\vec{f} = 0$.
13. Prove that div $\hat{r} = 2/r$, where $\hat{r}$ is a unit vector.
14. Prove that the vector $f(r)\,\vec{r}$ is irrotational.
15. Prove that :
    (i) $\nabla^2(fg) = f\nabla^2g + 2\nabla f\cdot\nabla g + g\nabla^2 f$
    (ii) div $(\nabla f \times \nabla g) = 0$
    where f and g are two scalar point function.
16. Prove that : $\nabla\cdot\left\{r\nabla\left(\frac{1}{r^3}\right)\right\} = \frac{3}{r^4}$.
17. If $\vec{a}$ is a constant vector, prove that
    (i) div $\{r^n(\vec{a} \times \vec{r})\} = 0$
    (ii) curl $\left(\frac{\vec{a}\times\vec{r}}{r^3}\right) = -\frac{\vec{a}}{r^3} + \frac{3\vec{r}}{r^5}(\vec{a}\cdot\vec{r})$
18. If $\vec{f} = f_1\hat{i} + f_2\hat{j} + f_3\hat{k}$, show that
    (i) $\nabla\cdot\vec{f} = \nabla f_1\cdot\hat{i} + \nabla f_2\cdot\hat{j} + \nabla f_3\cdot\hat{k}$
    (ii) $\nabla\times\vec{f} = \nabla f_1\times\hat{i} + \nabla f_2\times\hat{j} + \nabla f_3\times\hat{k}$
19. Prove that :
    (i) $\vec{a}.\nabla\left(\frac{1}{r}\right) = -\frac{\vec{a}.\vec{r}}{r^3}$
    (ii) $\vec{b}\cdot\nabla\left[\vec{a}\cdot\nabla\left(\frac{1}{r}\right)\right] = -\frac{\vec{a}\cdot\vec{b}}{r^3} + \frac{3(\vec{a}\cdot\vec{r})(\vec{b}\cdot\vec{r})}{r^5}$
20. Prove that div $\left\{\frac{f(r)}{r}\vec{r}\right\} = \frac{1}{r^2}\frac{d}{dr}r^2f(r)$.
21. Prove that curl $(g\nabla f) = \nabla g\times\nabla f = -$ curl $(f\nabla g)$.
22. Prove that curl $(\vec{a}\times r)r^n = (n+2)r^n\vec{a} - nr^{n-2}(\vec{r}\cdot\vec{a})\vec{r}$.
23. If $\hat{a}$ is a constant unit vector, prove that
    $$\hat{a}\cdot\{\nabla(\vec{v}\cdot\hat{a}) - \nabla\times(\vec{v}\times\hat{a})\} = \text{div }\vec{v}$$
24. Prove that $\nabla^2\left[\nabla\cdot\left(\frac{\vec{r}}{r^2}\right)\right] = 2r^{-4}$.

25. Prove that $\frac{1}{2}\nabla\vec{a}^2 = (\vec{a}\cdot\nabla)\vec{a} + \vec{a}\times \text{curl}\,\vec{a}$

26. Prove that curl grad $r^n = \vec{0}$.

27. If $\vec{a}$ and $\vec{b}$ are constant vectors, prove that $\nabla[(\vec{a}\cdot\vec{b})\vec{r}] = \vec{a}\cdot\vec{b}$.

28. If $\vec{a}$ is a constant vector, prove that

(i) $\nabla(\vec{a}\cdot\vec{u}) = (\vec{a}\cdot\nabla)\vec{u} + \vec{a}\times \text{curl}\,\vec{u}$

(ii) $\nabla\cdot(\vec{a}\times\vec{u}) = -\vec{a}\cdot \text{curl}\,\vec{u}$

(iii) $\nabla\times(\vec{a}\times\vec{u}) = \vec{a}\ \text{div}\,\vec{u} - (\vec{a}\cdot\nabla)\vec{u}$

29. If $\vec{u} = \left(\frac{1}{r}\right)\vec{r}$, then prove that

(i) $\nabla\times\vec{u} = 0$

(ii) $\text{grad}(\text{div}\,\vec{u}) = -\left(\frac{2}{r^3}\right)\vec{r}$.

30. Prove that

(i) $\text{div}(\vec{a}\times\vec{r}) = \vec{r}\cdot \text{curl}\,\vec{a}$

(ii) $\text{div}(\vec{r}\times\vec{a}) = 0$

(iii) $\text{curl}(\vec{r}\times a) = -2a$

31. If $\vec{V} = \dfrac{x\hat{i}+y\hat{j}+z\hat{k}}{\sqrt{x^2+y^2+z^2}}$, show that

$$\nabla\vec{V} = \frac{2}{\sqrt{x^2+y^2+z^2}} \text{ and } \nabla\times\vec{V} = 0.$$

32. Show that

$$\vec{A} = (6xy+z^3)\hat{i} + (3x^2-z)\hat{j} + (3xz^2-y)\hat{k}$$

is irrotational. (UKTU–2011)

33. Show that the fluid motion given by

$$\vec{V} = (y\sin z + \sin x)\hat{i} + (x\sin z + 2yz)\hat{j} + (xy\cos z + y^2)\hat{k}$$

is irrotational.

Hint to Selected Problems

1. $\vec{f} = x^2y\hat{i} - 2xz\hat{j} + 2yz\hat{k}$

(i) $\nabla\cdot\vec{f} = \frac{\partial}{\partial x}(x^2y)\hat{i} + \frac{\partial}{\partial y}(-2xz)\hat{j} + \frac{\partial}{\partial z}(2yz)\hat{k}$

$= 2xy + 0 + 2y = 2y(x+1)$.

3. $\vec{f} = \text{grad}(x^3+y^3+z^3-3xyz)$

Let $\phi = x^3+y^3+z^3-3xyz$.

$\therefore\ \vec{f} = \nabla\phi$.

(i) $\nabla\cdot\vec{f} = \nabla.(\nabla\phi) = \nabla^2\phi = \frac{\partial^2\phi}{\partial x^2} + \frac{\partial^2\phi}{\partial y^2} + \frac{\partial^2\phi}{\partial z^2}$

$= 6x + 6y + 6z = 6(x+y+z)$.

(ii) $\nabla\times(\nabla\phi) = 0$.

4. (ii) $\vec{f} = (x+2y+az)\hat{i} + (bx-3y-z)\hat{j} + (4x+cy+2z)\hat{k}$

$$\nabla\times\mathbf{f} = \begin{vmatrix} \hat{i} & \hat{j} & \hat{k} \\ \frac{\partial}{\partial x} & \frac{\partial}{\partial y} & \frac{\partial}{\partial z} \\ x+2y+az & bx-3y-z & 4x+cy+2z \end{vmatrix}$$

$= (c+1)\hat{i} + (a-4)\hat{j} + (b-2)\hat{k}$

For irrotaional, we have $\nabla\times\vec{f} = 0$.

$\therefore\quad c = -1,\ a = 4,\ b = 2$.

8. $\vec{v} = (x+y+1)\hat{i} + \hat{j} + (-x-y)\hat{k}$, then

$$\nabla\times\vec{v} = \begin{vmatrix} \hat{i} & \hat{j} & \hat{k} \\ \frac{\partial}{\partial x} & \frac{\partial}{\partial y} & \frac{\partial}{\partial z} \\ (x+y+1) & 1 & (-x-y) \end{vmatrix}$$

$= \hat{i}[-1-0] - \hat{j}[-1-0] + \hat{k}[0-1] = -\hat{i} + \hat{j} - \hat{k}$

$\therefore\ \vec{v}.\nabla\times\vec{v} = -(x+y+1) + 1 + x + y = 0$.

11. $\text{div}(\nabla\phi) = \nabla.(\nabla\phi) = \nabla.\left[\frac{\partial\phi}{\partial x}\hat{i} + \frac{\partial\phi}{\partial y}\hat{j} + \frac{\partial\phi}{\partial z}\hat{k}\right]$

$= \frac{\partial}{\partial x}\left(\frac{\partial\phi}{\partial x}\right) + \frac{\partial}{\partial y}\left(\frac{\partial\phi}{\partial y}\right) + \frac{\partial}{\partial z}\left(\frac{\partial\phi}{\partial z}\right)$

$= \frac{\partial^2\phi}{\partial x^2} + \frac{\partial^2\phi}{\partial y^2} + \frac{\partial^2\phi}{\partial z^2} = \nabla^2\phi$.

16. Since $\nabla f(r) = f'(r).\nabla r = f'(r)\left(\frac{\vec{r}}{r}\right)$.

$\therefore\quad \nabla\left(\frac{1}{r^3}\right) = -\frac{3}{r^5}\vec{r}$.

$\therefore\quad \nabla\left\{r\nabla\left(\frac{1}{r^3}\right)\right\} = \nabla\cdot\left(-\frac{3}{r^4}\vec{r}\right)$

$= \left(-\frac{3}{r^4}\right)\nabla\cdot\vec{r} + \vec{r}\nabla\left(-\frac{3}{r^4}\right)$

$= -\frac{9}{r^4} + \vec{r}\cdot\left(\frac{12}{r^6}\vec{r}\right) = -\frac{9}{r^4} + \frac{12}{r^6}(\vec{r}\cdot\vec{r})$.

$= -\frac{9}{r^4} + \frac{12}{r^6}(r^2) = -\frac{9}{r^4} + \frac{12}{r^4} = \frac{3}{r^4}$.

17. (ii) $\text{curl}\left\{\frac{\vec{a}\times\vec{r}}{r^3}\right\}$

$= \nabla\left(\frac{1}{r^3}\right)\times(\vec{a}\times\vec{r}) + \frac{1}{r^3}\nabla\times(\vec{a}\times\vec{r})$

$$= -\frac{3}{r^3}\left(\frac{\vec{r}}{r}\right)\times(\vec{a}\times\vec{r}) + \frac{1}{r^3}(0-0-\vec{a}+3\vec{a})$$

$$= -\frac{3}{r^5}[(\vec{r}\cdot\vec{r})\vec{a} - (\vec{r}\cdot\vec{a})\vec{r}] + \frac{2\vec{a}}{r^3}$$

$$= -\frac{3\vec{a}}{r^3} + \frac{3\vec{r}}{r^5}(\vec{r}\cdot\vec{a}) + \frac{2\vec{a}}{r^3} = -\frac{\vec{a}}{r^3} + \frac{3\vec{r}}{r^5}(\vec{r}\cdot\vec{a})$$

19. (i) $\vec{a}\cdot\nabla\left(\frac{1}{r}\right) = \vec{a}\cdot\left[-\frac{1}{r^2}\frac{\vec{r}}{r}\right] = \frac{\vec{a}\cdot\vec{r}}{r^3}$

(ii) $\vec{b}\cdot\nabla\left[\vec{a}\cdot\nabla\left(\frac{1}{r}\right)\right] = \vec{b}\cdot\nabla\left[-\frac{\vec{a}.\vec{r}}{r^3}\right]$

$$= \vec{b}\cdot\left[-\frac{\vec{a}}{r^3} + \frac{3(\vec{a}\cdot\vec{r})}{r^5}\vec{r}\right] = -\frac{\vec{a}\cdot\vec{b}}{r^3} + \frac{3(\vec{a}\cdot\vec{r})(\vec{b}\cdot\vec{r})}{r^5}$$

24. $\nabla\cdot\left(\frac{\vec{r}}{r^2}\right) = \nabla\left(\frac{1}{r^2}\right)\cdot\vec{r} + \frac{1}{r^2}(\nabla\cdot\vec{r})$

$$= -\frac{2}{r^3}\left(\frac{\vec{r}}{r}\right)\cdot\vec{r} + \frac{3}{r^2} = -\frac{2}{r^2} + \frac{3}{r^2} = \frac{1}{r^2}$$

$$\therefore\ \nabla^2\left[\nabla\cdot\left(\frac{\vec{r}}{r^2}\right)\right] = \nabla^2\cdot\left(\frac{1}{r^2}\right) = \nabla\left(\nabla\left(\frac{1}{r^2}\right)\right)$$

$$= \nabla\cdot\left[-\frac{2\vec{r}}{r^4}\right]$$

$$= \nabla\left(-\frac{2}{r^4}\right)\cdot\vec{r} + \left(-\frac{2}{r^4}\right)\nabla\cdot\vec{r}$$

$$= \frac{8}{r^4} - \frac{6}{r^4} = \frac{2}{r^4} = 2r^{-4}.$$

ANSWERS

1. (i) $2y(x+1)$ (ii) $(2x+2z)\hat{i} - (x^2+2z)\hat{k}$ (iii) $(2x+2)\hat{j}$

2. (i) div $\vec{f} = 9$ (ii) curl $\vec{f} = -\hat{i} - 2\hat{k}$

3. (i) div $\vec{f} = 6(x+y+z)$ (ii) curl $\vec{f} = 0$

4. (i) $\lambda = -2$ (ii) $a = 4, b = 2\ c = -1$

7. (i) $\frac{3}{2}\cdot\frac{1}{(x^2+y^2+z^2)^{3/2}}$ (ii) $\vec{0}$

9. (i) $-2x - 2y - 2z$ (ii) $2(y-z)\hat{i} + 2(z-x)\hat{j} + 2(x-y)\hat{k}$

□□□□□□

Chapter

26 Geometry

26.1 INTRODUCTION

Coordinate Geometry is the branch of mathematics in which two numbers are used to represent the position of a point with respect to two mutually perpendicular number lines called coordinate axes.

The French mathematician and philosopher Rene Descaotes first published his book La Geometric in 1637 in which he used algebra in the study of geometry. This he did by representing points in the plane by ordered pairs of real number called cartesian coordinates and representing lines and curves by algebraic equations.

26.1.1 Coordinate Axes

The adjoining figure 1 shows two number lines XOX' and YOY' intersecting each other at their zeros.

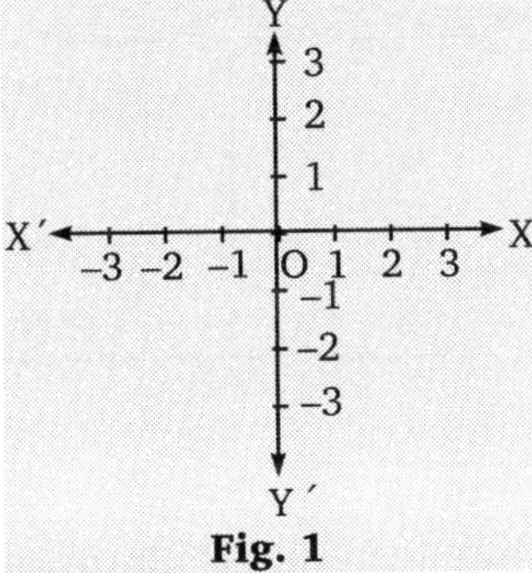

Fig. 1

XOX' and YOY' are called coordinate axes out of which XOX' is called the x-axis, YOY' is called y-axis and their point of intersection is called the origin.

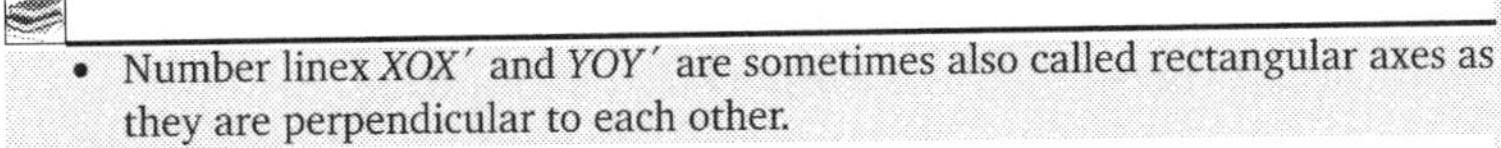

- Number linex XOX' and YOY' are sometimes also called rectangular axes as they are perpendicular to each other.

26.1.2 Convention of Signs

The distance measured along OX and OY are taken as positive and those along OX' and OY' are taken as negative as shown in figure 1.

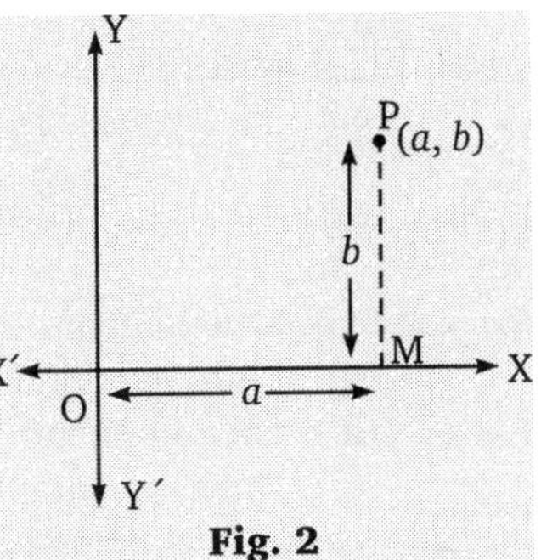

Fig. 2

26.1.3 Coordinate of a point in a plane

Let P be a point in a plane. Let the distance of P from the y-axis $= a$ units.

And, the distance of P from the x-axis = b units. Then we say that the coordinate of P are (a, b). a is called the x-coordinate or abscissa of P and b is called the y-coordinate or ordinate of P.

- (x, y) and (y, x) do not represent the same point unless $x = y$.
  e.g. (5, 4) and (4, 5) represent two different points.
- In stating the co-ordinates of a point the abscissa proceeds the ordinate. The two are separated by a comma and enclosed in a bracket. Thus a point, whose abscissa is x and whose ordinate is y designated by the notation (x, y), *i.e.*, (abscissa, ordinate)
- Since at origin the value of x-coordinate is 0 and the value of y-coordinate is also 0, therefore, the coordinate of origin = (0, 0).
- Since for every point on x-axis, its distance from x-axis is 0, *i.e.*, ordinate is 0. Therefore, the coordinate of a point on x-axis are taken as $(x, 0)$.
- For every point on y-axis its distance from y-axis is 0, *i.e.*, abscissa is 0, therefore, the coordinate of a point on y-axis are taken as $(0, y)$.

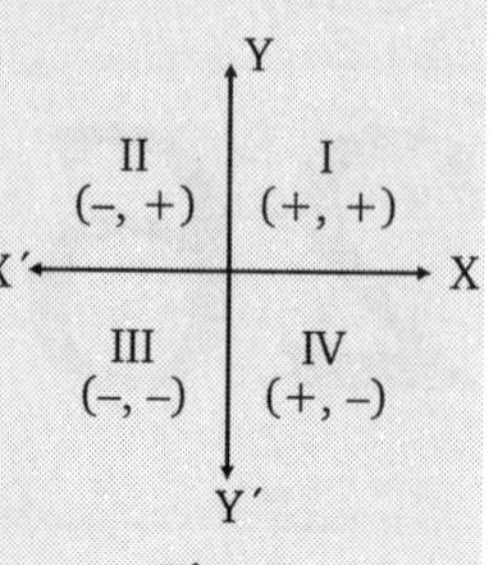

Fig. 3

26.1.4 QUADRANTS

Let $X'OX$ and YOY' be the coordinate axes.

These axes divide the plane of the paper into four regions, called Quadrants. The Regions XOY, YOX', $X'OY'$ and $Y'OX$ are respectively known as first, second, third and fourth quadrants.

Using the convention of sings, we have the sings of the coordinates in various quadrant given below.

Region	Quadrant	Nature of x and y	Signs of coordinate
XOY	I	$x > 0, y > 0$	(+ , +)
YOX'	II	$x < 0, y > 0$	(– , +)
$X'OY'$	III	$x < 0, y < 0$	(– , –)
$Y'OX$	IV	$x > 0, y < 0$	(+ , –)

Solved Examples

1. *In which quadrant will the point lie if*

(*i*) *the ordinate is 3 and the abscissa is – 4 ?*

(*ii*) *the abscissa is – 5 and the ordinate is – 3 ?*

(*iii*) *the ordinate is 4 and the abscissa is 5 ?*

(*iv*) *the ordinate is –4 and the abscissa is 8?*

SOLUTION. (i) Second quadrant

(ii) Third quadrant

(iii) First quadrant

(v) Fourth quadrant.

2. *In which quadrant do the given point lie?*

(*i*) (4 , –2) (*ii*) (– 3 , 7)

(*iii*) (– 1, –2) (*iv*) (3, 6).

SOLUTION. (i) Fourth quadrant

(ii) Second quadrant

(iii) Third quadrant

(iv) First quadrant

3. *On which axes do the given points lie?*

(*i*) (7, 0) (*ii*) (0, –3)

(*iii*) (0, 6) (*iv*) (–5, 0)

SOLUTION. (i) In (7, 0), we have the ordinate = 0.

$\therefore$ (7, 0) lies on the x-axis.

(ii) In (0, – 3) we have the abscissa = 0.

$\therefore$ (0, – 3) lies on the y-axis.

(iii) In (0, 6) we have the abscissa = 0.
$\therefore$ (0, 6) lies on the y-axis.

(iv) In (–5, 0) we have the ordinate = 0.
$\therefore$ (– 5, 0) lies on the x-axis.

4. *Plot the points (– 3, 0), (2 ,3), (– 4, 3) and (3,– 5) in a rectangular coordinate system.*

SOLUTION. See the adjoining Figure 4.

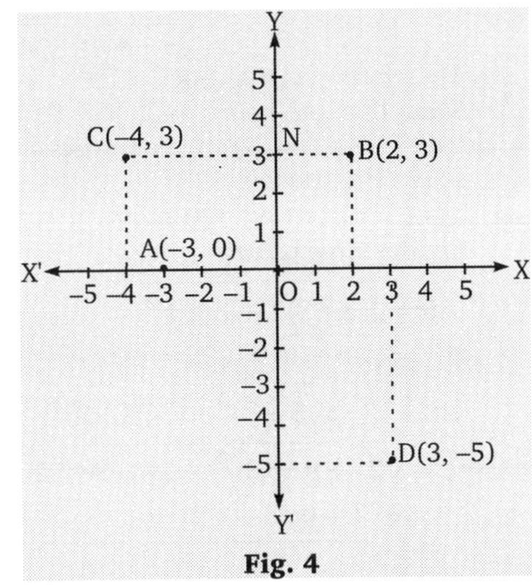

Fig. 4

26.2 DISTANCE BETWEEN TWO POINTS

The distance between two points $A(x_1, y_1)$ and $B(x_2, y_2)$ is given by the formula

$$AB = \sqrt{(x_2 - x_1)^2 + (y_2 - y_1)^2}$$

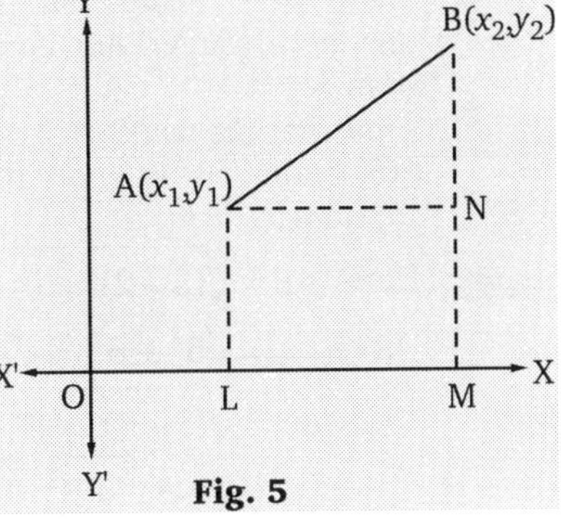

Fig. 5

PROOF. Let $A(x_1, y_1)$ and $B(x_2, y_2)$ be the given points.
Let $X'OX$ and YOY' be the coordinate axes.
Draw $AL \perp OX$, $BM \perp OX$ and $AN \perp BM$. Then

$$OL = x_1, OM = x_2, AL = y_1 \text{ and } BM = y_2$$

$$AN = LM = OM - OL = (x_2 - x_1)$$

$$BN = BM - NM = BM - AL = (y_2 - y_1) \quad [\because NM = AL]$$

Now, ΔANB is a right-angled, so by Pythagoras theorem, we have

$$AB^2 = AN^2 + BN^2 = (x_2 - x_1)^2 + (y_2 - y_1)^2$$

$$AB = \sqrt{(x_2 - x_1)^2 + (y_2 - y_1)^2}$$

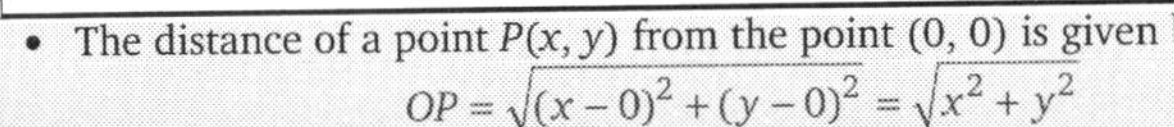

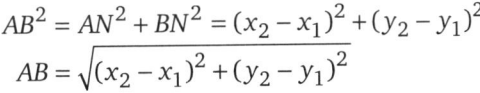

- The distance of a point $P(x, y)$ from the point (0, 0) is given by
$$OP = \sqrt{(x-0)^2 + (y-0)^2} = \sqrt{x^2 + y^2}$$

WORKING PROCEDURE

In order to prove that a figure is a :

STEP 1. Square, prove that four sides are equal and the diagonals are also equal.

STEP 2. Rhombus, prove that the four sides are equal.

STEP 3. Rectangle, prove that opposite sides are equal and the diagonals are also equal.

STEP 4. Parallelogram, prove that the opposite sides are equal.

Solved Examples

1. *Find the distance between the points (3, 4) and (6, –3).*

SOLUTION. The given points are $A(3, 4)$ and $B(6, –3)$.

Here $x_1 = 3, y_1 = 4$ and $x_2 = 6, y_2 = -3$.

$$AB = \sqrt{(x_2 - x_1)^2 + (y_2 - y_1)^2}$$

$$= \sqrt{(6-3)^2 + (-3-4)^2}$$

$$= \sqrt{9+49} = \sqrt{58}$$

Therefore $AB = \sqrt{58}$

2. *Show that the points (–3, –3), (3, 3) and $C(-3\sqrt{3}, 3\sqrt{3})$ are the vertices of an equilateral triangle.*

SOLUTION. $A(-3, -3)$, $B(3, 3)$ and $C(-3\sqrt{3}, 3\sqrt{3})$ are the three points.

$$AB = \sqrt{(3+3)^2 + (3+3)^2}$$
$$= \sqrt{36+36} = \sqrt{72} = 6\sqrt{2}$$
$$AC = \sqrt{(-3\sqrt{3}+3)^2 + (3\sqrt{3}+3)^2}$$
$$= \sqrt{27+9-18\sqrt{3}+27+9+18\sqrt{3}}$$
$$= \sqrt{72} = 6\sqrt{2}$$
$$BC = \sqrt{(-3\sqrt{3}-3)^2 + (3\sqrt{3}-3)^2}$$
$$= \sqrt{72} = 6\sqrt{2}$$

Then $AB = BC = AC$.

Therefore, triangle ABC is an equilateral triangle.

3. *Show that the points $A(2, -2)$, $B(8, 4)$, $C(5, 7)$ and $D(-1, 1)$ are the vertices of a rectangle.* [UPTU–2007]

SOLUTION. Here, $AB = \sqrt{(8-2)^2 + (4+2)^2}$

$$= \sqrt{6^2 + 6^2} = \sqrt{72}$$
$$BC = \sqrt{(5-8)^2 + (7-4)^2}$$
$$= \sqrt{(-3)^2 + 3^2} = \sqrt{18}$$
$$CD = \sqrt{(-1-5)^2 + (1-7)^2}$$
$$= \sqrt{(-6)^2 + (-6)^2} = \sqrt{72}$$
$$DA = \sqrt{(2+1)^2 + (-2-1)^2}$$
$$= \sqrt{3^2 + (-3)^2} = \sqrt{18}$$
$$AC = \sqrt{(5-2)^2 + (7+2)^2}$$
$$= \sqrt{3^2 + 9^2} = \sqrt{90}$$
$$BD = \sqrt{(-1-8)^2 + (1-4)^2}$$
$$= \sqrt{(-9)^2 + (-3)^2} = \sqrt{90}$$

Thus, the opposite sides of the quadrilateral $ABCD$ are equal and its diagonals are also equal. Hence, it is a rectangle.

4. *Find the value of a if the distance between the points (3, a) and (4, 1) is $\sqrt{10}$.* [UPTU–2003]

SOLUTION. The required distance is given by

$$\sqrt{(4-3)^2 + (1-a)^2} = \sqrt{10}$$
$$\Rightarrow \quad 1 + (1-a)^2 = 10$$
$$\Rightarrow \quad (1-a)^2 = 9$$
$$\Rightarrow \quad 1-a = \pm 3$$
$$\Rightarrow \quad a = 1 \pm 3 = -2, 4$$

5. *Find the value of x, if the distance between the points (x, –1) and (3, 2) is 5.*

SOLUTION. Let $P(x, -1)$ and $Q(3, 2)$ be the given points, then :

$$PQ = 5 \quad \text{[Given]}$$
$$\Rightarrow \quad \sqrt{(x-3)^2 + (-1-2)^2} = 5$$
$$\Rightarrow \quad (x-3)^2 + 9 = 5^2$$
$$\Rightarrow \quad (x^2 - 6x + 18) = 25$$
$$\Rightarrow \quad x^2 - 6x - 7 = 0$$
$$\Rightarrow \quad (x-7)(x+1) = 0$$
$$\Rightarrow \quad x = 7 \text{ or } x = -1$$

6. *Find the point on the y-axis which is equidistant from the points (3, 4) and (6, 7).*

SOLUTION. Given points are $A(3, 4)$ and $B(6, 7)$. Required point P is on the y-axis. Its abscissa = 0.

Suppose its ordinate = y.

Then coordinate of P are $(0, y)$.

Now $PA = PB$

$$\Rightarrow \quad \sqrt{(0-3)^2 + (y-4)^2} = \sqrt{(0-6)^2 + (y-7)^2}$$
$$\Rightarrow \quad 9 + y^2 - 8y + 16 = 36 + y^2 - 14y + 49$$
$$\Rightarrow \quad -8y + 14y = 36 + 49 - 9 - 16$$
$$\Rightarrow \quad 6y = 60$$
$$\Rightarrow \quad y = 10$$

Therefore, the required point is (0, 10).

7. *If the point (x, y) is equidistant from the points (a + b, b – a) and (a – b, a + b) prove that bx = ay.*

SOLUTION. Let $P(x, y)$, $Q(a + b, b - a)$ and $R(a - b, a + b)$ be the given points.

Then $PQ = PR$ (given)

$$\Rightarrow \sqrt{[x-(a+b)]^2+[y-(b-a)]^2}$$
$$= \sqrt{[x-(a-b)]^2+[y-(b+a)]^2}$$
$$\Rightarrow [x-(a+b)]^2+[y-(b-a)]^2$$
$$= [x-(a-b)]^2+[y-(b+a)]^2$$
$$\Rightarrow x^2-2x(a+b)+(a+b)^2$$
$$+y^2-2y(b-a)+(b-a)^2$$
$$= x^2+(a-b)^2-2x(a-b)$$

$$\Rightarrow -2x(a+b)-2y(b-a)$$
$$= -2x(a-b)-2y(a+b)$$
$$\Rightarrow ax+bx+by-ay$$
$$= ax-bx+ay+by$$
$$\Rightarrow \quad 2bx = 2ay$$
$$\Rightarrow \quad bx = ay$$

26.3 COLLINEAR POINTS

Three points A, B, C are said to be collinear if they lie on the same straight line.

WORKING PROCEDURE : TEST FOR COLLINEARITY OF THREE POINTS

- In order to show that three given points A, B, C are collinear. We find distances AB, BC and AC. If the sum of any two of these distance is equal to the third distance then the given points are collinear.

Solved Examples

1. *Using distance formula, show that the points (–3, 2), (1, –2) and (9, –10) are collinear.*

SOLUTION. $A(-3, 2)$, $B(1, -2)$ and $C(9, -10)$ are the given points.

Now, $AB = \sqrt{(1+3)^2+(-2-2)^2}$
$= \sqrt{16+16} = 4\sqrt{2}$ units

$BC = \sqrt{(9-1)^2+(-10+2)^2}$
$= \sqrt{64+64} = 8\sqrt{2}$ units

$AC = \sqrt{(9+3)^2+(-10-2)^2}$
$= \sqrt{144+144} = 12\sqrt{2}$ units

$\Rightarrow AB+BC=4\sqrt{2}+8\sqrt{2}=12\sqrt{2}=AC$.

Therefore, the three points are collinear.

2. *Show that the points (1, 1), (–2, 7) and (3, –3) are collinear.*

SOLUTION. Let $A(1, 1)$, $B(-2, 7)$ and $C(3, -3)$ be the given points.

Then we have

$AB = \sqrt{(-2-1)^2+(7-1)^2}$
$= \sqrt{9+36} = 3\sqrt{5}$

$BC = \sqrt{(3+2)^2+(-3-7)^2}$
$= \sqrt{25+100} = 5\sqrt{5}$

and $AC = \sqrt{(3-1)^2+(-3-1)^2}$
$= \sqrt{4+16} = 2\sqrt{5}$

Clearly $BC = AB + AC$.

Hence, A, B and C are collinear.

Exercise-26.1

1. Find the distance between the points :
   (i) $A(7, 13)$, $B(10, 9)$
   (ii) $P(-4, 7)$ and $Q(1, -5)$
2. Find the distance of the point $P(6, -6)$ from the origin.
3. Find the value or values of k for which the distance between the point $A(k, -5)$ and $B(2, 7)$ is 13 units.
4. Prove that the points $A(-3, 0)$, $B(1, -3)$ and $C(4, 1)$ are the vertices of an isosceles right angled triangle. Find the area of this triangle.
5. Prove that the points $A(a, a)$, $B(-a, -a)$, $C(-\sqrt{3a}, \sqrt{3a})$ are the vertices of an equilateral triangle. Calculate the area of this rectangle.
6. Prove that the points $A(1, -3)$, $B(13, 9)$, $C(10, 12)$, $D(-2, 0)$ taken in order are the angular points of a rectangle. Find the area of the rectangle.
7. Prove that the points $A(1, 1)$, $B(-2, 7)$ and $C(3, -3)$ are collinear.

8. If $P(2, -1)$, $Q(3, 4)$, $R(-2, 3)$ and $S(-3, -1)$ be four points in a plane. Show that $PQRS$ is a rhombus but not a square. Find the area of the rhombus.

Hint to the Selected Problems

5. Let $A(a, -a)$, $B(-a, -a)$ and $C(-\sqrt{3}a, \sqrt{3}a)$

$AB = 2\sqrt{2}\,a$ units, $BC = 2\sqrt{2}\,a$ units

$AC = 2\sqrt{2}$ a units, $AB = BC = AC = 2\sqrt{2}a$

Area of $\Delta ABC = \frac{\sqrt{3}}{4}(\text{side})^2 = \frac{\sqrt{3}}{4}\times(2\sqrt{2}a)^2$

$= (2\sqrt{3}a^2)$ sq. units.

6. $AB = 12\sqrt{2}$ units, $BC = 3\sqrt{2}$ units,

$DC = 12\sqrt{2}$ units, $AD = 3\sqrt{2}$ units

$AB = DC$ & $BC = AD, AC = 3\sqrt{34}$ units

$BD = 3\sqrt{34}$ units, $AC = BD$

Hence, $ABCD$ is a rectangle.

ANSWERS

1. (i) 5 units (ii) 13 units **2.** $6\sqrt{2}$ units **3.** $k = -3$ or $k = 7$

4. 12.5 sq units **5.** $(2\sqrt{3}a^2)$ sq units **8.** 24 sq units

26.4 SECTION FORMULA

The coordinates of the point $P(x, y)$ which divides the line segment joining $A(x_1, y_1)$ and $B(x_2, y_2)$ internally in the ratio $m : n$ are given by

$$x = \frac{mx_2 + nx_1}{m+n}, y = \frac{my_2 + ny_1}{m+n}$$

PROOF. Let $X'OX$ and YOY' be the coordinate axes.

Let $A(x_1, y_1)$ and $B(x_2, y_2)$ be the end points of the given line segments AB.

If $P(x, y)$ is the point which divides AB in the ratio $m : n$.

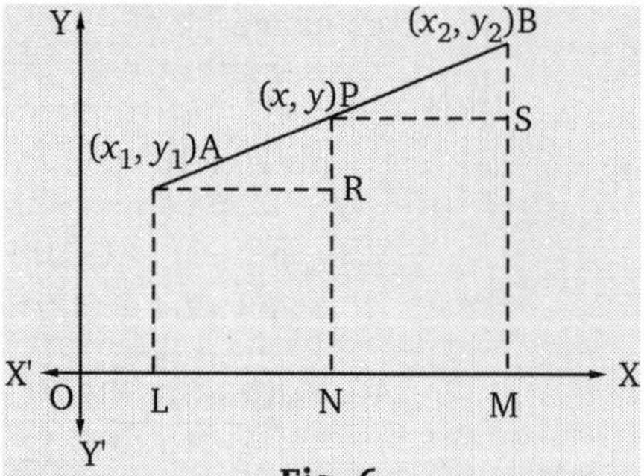

Then $$\frac{AP}{PB} = \frac{m}{n}$$

Draw

$$AL \perp OX; BM \perp OX; PN \perp OX$$
$$AR \perp PN; PS \perp BM$$

Fig. 6

Now $AR = LN = ON - OL = (x - x_1)$

$PS = NM = OM - ON = (x_2 - x)$

$PR = PN - RN = PN - AL = (y - y_1)$

$BS = BM - SM = BM - PN = y_2 - y$

Clearly, ΔARP and ΔPSB are similar and therefore, their sides are proportional.

$$\frac{AP}{PB} = \frac{AR}{PS} = \frac{PR}{BS}$$

$$\Rightarrow \quad \frac{m}{n} = \frac{x - x_1}{x_2 - x} = \frac{y - y_1}{y_2 - y}$$

$$\Rightarrow \quad \frac{m}{n} = \frac{x - x_1}{x_2 - x} \quad \text{and} \quad \frac{m}{n} = \frac{y - y_1}{y_2 - y}$$

$$\Rightarrow \quad mx_2 - mx = nx - nx_1 \text{ and } my_2 - my = ny - ny_1$$

$$\Rightarrow \quad (m+n)x = mx_2 + nx_1 \text{ and } (m+n)y = my_2 + ny_1$$

$$x = \frac{mx_2 + nx_1}{m+n}, y = \frac{my_2 + ny_1}{m+n}$$

Hence, the coordinate of P are $\left(\frac{mx_2 + nx_1}{m+n}, \frac{my_2 + ny_1}{m+n}\right)$

26.5 MID POINT FORMULA

The coordinates of the midpoint M on a line segment AB with end points $A(x_1, y_1)$ and $B(x_2, y_2)$ are $\left(\frac{x_1 + x_2}{2}, \frac{y_1 + y_2}{2}\right)$.

- The coordinate of the point P, which divides the line-segment joining $A(x_1, y_1)$ and $B(x_2, y_2)$ internally, in the ratio $k : 1$ are given by $\left(\frac{kx_2 + x_1}{k+1}, \frac{ky_2 + y_1}{k+1}\right)$.
- The coordinate of the point which divides the line segment joining the points (x_1, y_1) and (x_2, y_2) externally in the ratio $m : n$ are given by $x = \frac{mx_2 - nx_1}{m-n}, y = \frac{my_2 - ny_1}{m-n}$.

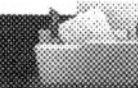

Solved Examples

1. *Find the coordinates of the point which divides the line segment joining the points (6, 3) and (–4, 5) in the ratio 3:2 (i) internally and (ii) externally.*

SOLUTION. Let $P(x, y)$ be the required point.

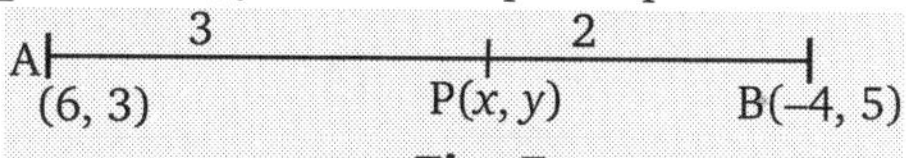

A (6, 3) —3— P(x, y) —2— B(–4, 5)

Fig. 7

(i) For internal division, we have

$$x = \frac{3 \times -4 + 2 \times 6}{3+2}$$

and $$y = \frac{3 \times 5 + 2 \times 3}{3+2}$$

$x = 0$ and $y = \frac{21}{5}$

So the coordinates of P are $\left(0, \frac{21}{5}\right)$.

(ii) For external division, we have

A (6, 3) — B(–4, 5) — P(x, y)

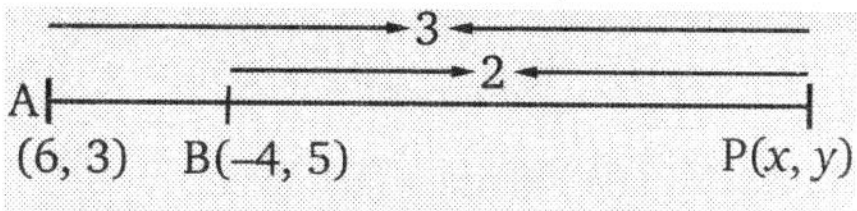

Fig. 8

$$x = \frac{3 \times -4 - 2 \times 6}{3-2}$$

and $$y = \frac{3 \times 5 - 2 \times 3}{3-2}$$

$x = -24$ and $y = 9$.

So, the coordinates of point are (–24, 9).

2. *In what ratio does the point (–2, 3) divide the line segment joining the points (–3, 5) and (4, –9).*

SOLUTION. Let the required ratio be $k : 1$

Compairing x-coordinate

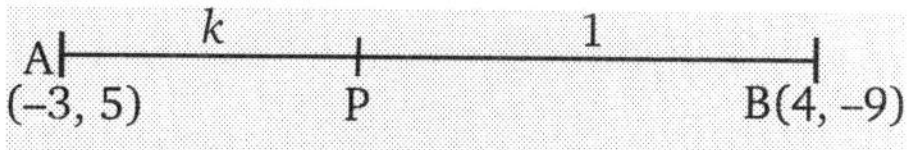

A (–3, 5) —k— P —1— B(4, –9)

Fig. 9

$$\frac{k \times 4 + 1 \times (-3)}{k+1} = -2$$

$$\Rightarrow \quad \frac{4k-3}{k+1} = -2 \Rightarrow 4k - 3 = -2k - 2$$

$$\Rightarrow \quad 6k = 1 \Rightarrow k = 1/6$$

Compairing y-coordinate

$$\frac{k \times (-9) + (1) \times 5}{k+1} = 3$$

$\Rightarrow \quad \dfrac{9k+5}{k+1} = 3 \Rightarrow -9k + 5 = 3k + 3$

$\Rightarrow \quad 12k = 2 \Rightarrow \quad k = 1/6$

Hence, the required ratio is 1 : 6.

3. *In what ratio does the y-axis divide the line segment joining the point (–4, 5) and (3, –7)?*

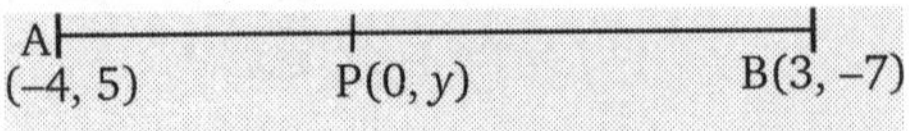

A (–4, 5) P(0, y) B(3, –7)

Fig.10

SOLUTION. The line segment joining the points $A(-4, 5)$ and $B(3, -7)$ is divided by the y-axis at the point $P(0, y)$ in the ratio $k : 1$.

Compairing x-coordinate, we have

$$\frac{k \times 3 + 1 \times (-4)}{k+1} = 0$$

$\Rightarrow \quad 3k - 4 = 0$

$\Rightarrow \quad 3k = 4 \quad \Rightarrow k = 4/3.$

Therefore, the required ratio is 4 : 3.

4. *Find the ratio in which the line $3x + y - 9 = 0$ divides the line segment joining $A(1, 3)$ and $B(2, 7)$.*

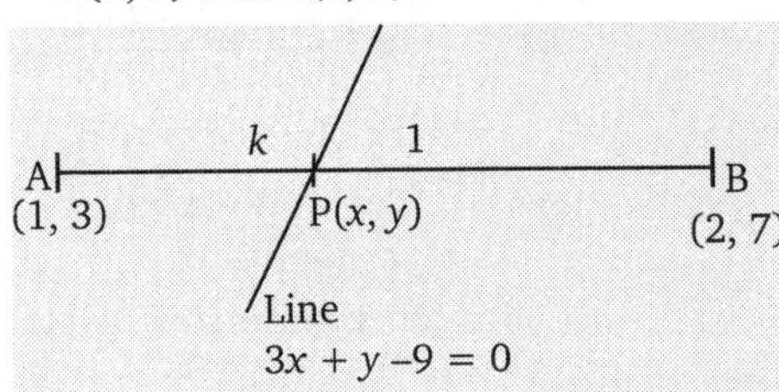

Fig. 11

SOLUTION. The equation of the given line is

$$3x + y - 9 = 0 \qquad \ldots(1)$$

meets the line segment joining $A(1, 3)$ and $B(2, 7)$ at the point $P(x, y)$ and divides the segment internally in the ratio $k : 1$.

By section formula :

$$x = \frac{2k+1}{k+1}, y = \frac{7k+3}{k+1}$$

i.e., Coordinate of P are

$$\left(\frac{2k+1}{k+1}, \frac{7k+3}{k+1}\right)$$

The point P lies on the line whose equation is given by (1)

Therefore, $3\left(\dfrac{2k+1}{k+1}\right) + \left(\dfrac{7k+3}{k+1}\right) - 9 = 0.$

$\Rightarrow \quad 6k + 3 + 7k + 3 - 9k - 9 = 0$

$\Rightarrow \quad 4k - 3 = 0$

$\Rightarrow \quad k = 3/4$

Hence, the required ratio is 3 : 4.

5. *Find the coordinates of point which divides the line joining the point (1, 2) and (–3, 4) in the ratio 2 : 3 internally.* [RGPV–2005]

SOLUTION. Let $A(1, 2)$ and $B(-3, 4)$ be the given points.

Point P divides A and B in the ratio 2 : 3

$\Rightarrow \quad PA : PB = 2:3$

$\therefore$ Coordinates of P are

$$\left(\frac{2 \times -3 + 3 \times 1}{2+3}, \frac{2 \times 4 + 3 \times 2}{2+3}\right)$$

i.e., $\left(\dfrac{-6+3}{5}, \dfrac{8+6}{5}\right)$, *i.e.*, $\left(\dfrac{-3}{5}, \dfrac{14}{5}\right)$.

6. *If A(–1, –3), B(1, –1) and C(5, 1) are the vertices of a triangle ABC, find the length of median through A.*

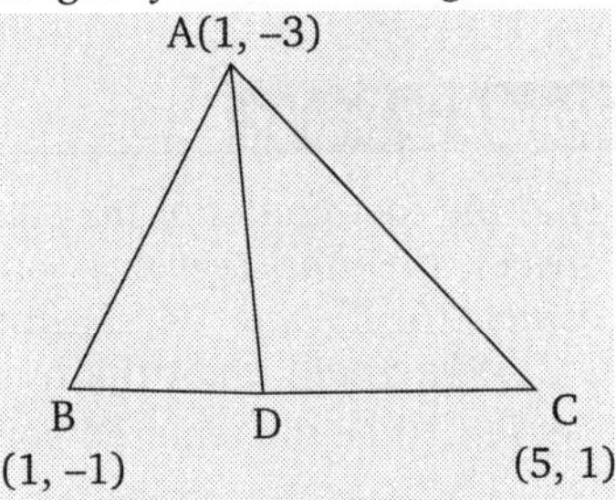

Fig. 12

SOLUTION. Let D be the middle point of BC.

Then AD is the median through A and

D is the point $\left(\dfrac{1+5}{2}, \dfrac{-1+1}{2}\right)$, *i.e.*, (3, 0)

Therefore,

$$AD = \sqrt{\{3-(-1)\}^2 + \{0+3\}^2}$$

$$= \sqrt{4^2 + (3)^2} = 5.$$

7. *A quadrilateral has the vertices at the points (–4, 2), (2, 6), (8, 5) and (9, –7). Show that the mid-points of the sides of this quadrilateral are the vertices of a parallelogram.*

SOLUTION. Let $ABCD$ be the given quadrilateral with vertices $A(-4, 2)$, $B(2, 6)$, $C(8, 5)$ and $D(9, -7)$. Let E, F, G and H be the mid-points of the sides AB, BC, CD and DA respectively.

Then the coordinates of E are $\left(\frac{-4+2}{2}, \frac{2+6}{2}\right)$, *i.e.*, $(-1, 4)$.

The coordinates of F are $\left(\frac{2+8}{2}, \frac{6+5}{2}\right)$, *i.e.*, $\left(5, \frac{11}{2}\right)$.

The coordinates of G are $\left(\frac{8+9}{2}, \frac{5-7}{2}\right)$, *i.e.*, $\left(\frac{17}{2}, -1\right)$.

and the coordinates of H are $\left(\frac{-4+9}{2}, \frac{2-7}{2}\right)$, *i.e.*, $\left(\frac{5}{2}, \frac{-5}{2}\right)$.

Now, the coordinates of the mid-point of EG are $\left(\frac{-1+\frac{17}{2}}{2}, \frac{4-1}{2}\right)$, *i.e.*, $\left(\frac{15}{4}, \frac{3}{2}\right)$.

and the coordinate of the mid-point of FH are $\left(\frac{5+\frac{5}{2}}{2}, \frac{\frac{11}{2}-\frac{5}{2}}{2}\right)$, *i.e.*, $\left(\frac{15}{4}, \frac{3}{2}\right)$

Thus, we see that the diagonals EG and FH of the quadrilateral $EFGH$ bisect each other. Hence, $EFGH$ is a parallelogram.

8. *Three consecutive vertices of a parallelogram are $A(1, 2)$, $B(1, 0)$ and $C(4, 0)$. Find the fourth vertex D.*

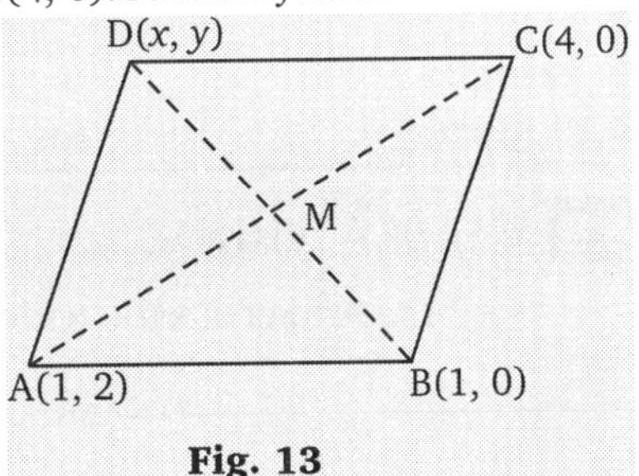

Fig. 13

SOLUTION. Let the coordinates of the vertex D be (x, y). Diagonals AC and BD of the parallelogram $ABCD$ bisect each other at M, *i.e.*, M is mid-point of AC as well as of BD.

Mid-point of

$$AC = \left(\frac{1+4}{2}, \frac{2+0}{2}\right) = \left(\frac{5}{2}, 1\right) \quad \ldots(1)$$

$$\text{Mid-point of } BD = \left(\frac{x+1}{2}, \frac{y+0}{2}\right) \quad \ldots(2)$$

Eq. (1) and (2) have same coordinates of the point M.

Then $\frac{x+1}{2} = \frac{5}{2}$ and $\frac{y}{2} = 1$

$\Rightarrow x = 4$ and $y = 2$. Therefore, the coordinates of D are $(4, 2)$.

Exercise-26.2

1. Find the coordinates of the point which divides the line segment joining the points $A(4, -3)$ and $B(9, 7)$ in the ratio $3 : 2$.
2. Find the coordinates of the mid-point of the line segment joining the points $A(-5, 4)$ and $B(7, -8)$.
3. Find the ratio in which the point $P(m, 6)$ divides the joining $A(-4, 3)$ and $B(2, 8)$. Also, find the value of m.
4. In what ratio does point $P(2, -5)$ divide the line segment joining $A(-3, 5)$ and $(4, -9)$.
5. In what ratio is the line segment joining the point $A(6, 3)$ and $B(-2, -5)$ divide by the x-axis.
   Also, find the coordinates of the point of intersection of AB and the x-axis.
6. Find the ratio in which the y-axis divides the line segment joining the points $A(-4, 10)$ and $B(7, -1)$.
   Also, find the coordinates of their point of intersection.
7. The coordinates of one end point of diameter AB of a circle are $A(4, -1)$ and the coordinates of the centre of the circle are $C(1, -3)$. Find the coordinates of B.
8. The three vertices of a parallelogram $ABCD$, taken in order are $A(1, -2)$, $B(3, 6)$ and $C(5, 10)$. Find the coordinates of the fourth vertex D.
9. Find the lengths of the medians of a ΔABC whose vertices are $A(7, -3)$, $B(5, 3)$ and $C(3, -1)$.

10. Let $D(3, -2)$, $E(-3, 1)$ and $F(4, -3)$ be the mid-points of the sides BC, CA and AB respectively of ΔABC. Then, find the coordinates of the vertices A, B and C.

ANSWERS

1. (7, 3), (3, 5)	**2.** (1, –2)	**3.** $m = \frac{-2}{5}$	**4.** 5 : 2
5. (3, 0)	**6.** 4 : 7, (0, 6)	**7.** (2, –5)	**8.** (3, 2)
9. 5, 5, $\sqrt{10}$	**10.** $A(-2, 0)$, $B(10, -6)$, $C(-4, 2)$		

26.6 AREA OF A TRIANGLE

The Area of a ΔABC with vertices $A(x_1, y_1)$, $B(x_2, y_2)$ and $C(x_3, y_3)$ is given by

$$\text{area}\,(\Delta ABC) = \left|\frac{1}{2}[x_1(y_2 - y_3) + x_2(y_3 - y_1) + x_3(y_1 - y_2)]\right|$$

PROOF. Let $A(x_1, y_1)$, $B(x_2, y_2)$ and $C(x_3, y_3)$ be the vertices of the given ΔABC. Draw AL, BM and CN perpendicular to the x-axis.

Then $ML = (x_1 - x_2)$, $LN = (x_3 - x_1)$ and $MN = (x_3 - x_2)$

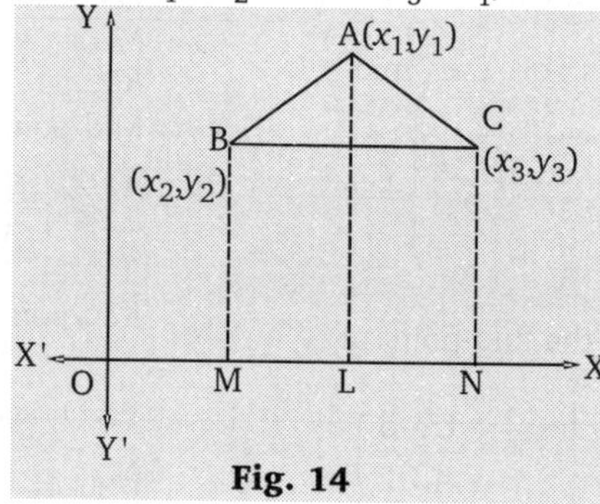

Fig. 14

Area of ΔABC

$$= \text{area (trap. } BMLA) + \text{area (trap. } ALNC) - \text{area (trap. } BMNC)$$

$$= \left[\frac{1}{2}(AL + BM) \times ML\right] + \left[\frac{1}{2}(AL + CN) \times LN\right] - \left[\frac{1}{2}(BM + CN) \times MN\right]$$

$$= \frac{1}{2}(y_1 + y_2)(x_1 - x_2) + \frac{1}{2}(y_1 + y_3)(x_3 - x_1) - \frac{1}{2}(y_2 + y_3)(x_3 - x_2)$$

$$= \frac{1}{2}[x_1(y_1 + y_2 - y_1 - y_3) + x_2(y_2 + y_3 - y_1 - y_2) + x_3(y_1 + y_3 - y_2 - y_3)]$$

$$= \frac{1}{2}[x_1(y_2 - y_3) + x_2(y_3 - y_1) + x_3(y_1 - y_2)]$$

Since, the area is never negative. Therefore,

$$\text{area}\,(\Delta ABC) = \frac{1}{2}[x_1(y_2 - y_3) + x_2(y_3 - y_1) + x_3(y_1 - y_2)]$$

- The area of a triangle is always taken as positive real quantity. Some times the result from the area formula given negative value in that case we reject the negative sign.
- The three points (x_1, y_1), (x_2, y_2) and (x_3, y_3) are collinear, *i.e.*, in a line if $x_1(y_2 - y_3) + x_2(y_3 - y_1) + x_3(y_1 - y_2) = 0$ because in this situation the area of the triangle reduces to zero.

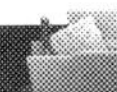

Solved Examples

1. *Find the area of the triangle whose vertices are (4, 3), (5, 4) and (11, 2).*

SOLUTION. Let $A(4, 3)$, $B(5, 4)$ and $C(11, 2)$ be the three vertices of the given triangle.

$$x_1 = 4, x_2 = 5, x_3 = 11$$
$$y_1 = 3, y_2 = 4, y_3 = 2$$

Area of ΔABC

$$= \frac{1}{2}[x_1(y_2 - y_3) + x_2(y_3 - y_1) + x_3(y_1 - y_2)]$$

$$= \frac{1}{2}[4(4-2) + 5(2-3) + 11(3-4)]$$

$$= \frac{1}{2}[8 - 5 - 11] = -4$$

Rejecting negative sign, we have the area of the given triangle equal to 4 square units.

2. *Find the area of a triangle formed by the lines: $y = 2x$, $y = x$ and $y = 3x + 4$.*

SOLUTION. Let the equations of the sides AB, BC and CA of ΔABC be $y - x = 0$, $y - 2x = 0$ and $y - 3x - 4 = 0$ respectively.

Solving these equations in pairs, the coordinates of A, B and C are (–2, –2), (0, 0) and (– 4, – 8) respectively.

Area of ΔABC

$$= \frac{1}{2}[x_1(y_2 - y_3) + x_2(y_3 - y_1) + x_3(y_1 - y_2)]$$

$$= \frac{1}{2}[(-2)(0+8) + 0.(-8+2) + (-4)(-2-0)]$$

$$= \frac{1}{2}[-16+8] = \frac{1}{2}[-8] = 4 \text{ sq. units,}$$

neglecting the negative sign.

3. *Four points $A(6, 3)$, $B(-3, 5)$, $C(4, -2)$ and $D(x, 3x)$ are given in such a way that $\frac{\Delta DBC}{\Delta ABC} = \frac{1}{2}$, find x.*

SOLUTION.

$$\frac{\text{Area of } \Delta DBC}{\text{Area of } \Delta ABC} = \frac{\frac{1}{2}[x(5+2) - 3(-2-3x) + 4(3x-5)]}{\frac{1}{2}[6(5+2) - 3(-2-3) + 4(3-5)]}$$

$$\frac{1}{2} = \frac{7x + 6 + 9x + 12x - 20}{42 + 15 - 8}$$

$$\frac{1}{2} = \frac{28x - 14}{49}$$

$$\Rightarrow \frac{1}{2} = \frac{4x-2}{7}$$

$$\Rightarrow \frac{7}{2} = 4x - 2$$

$$\Rightarrow x = \frac{11}{8}$$

4. *Find the value of k so that the point $A(-2, 3)$, $B(3, -1)$ and $C(5, k)$ be collinear.*

SOLUTION. We have $x_1 = -2, x_2 = 3, x_3 = 5$
$y_1 = 3, y_2 = -1, y_3 = k.$

Area of ΔABC

$$= \frac{1}{2}[x_1(y_2 - y_3) + x_2(y_3 - y_1) + x_3(y_1 - y_2)]$$

$$= \frac{1}{2}[-2(-1-k) + 3(k-3) + 5(3+1)]$$

$$= \frac{1}{2}[2 + 2k + 3k - 9 + 20] = \frac{1}{2}[5k + 13]$$

Now, the three points are collinear if the area of $\Delta ABC = 0$

i.e., $\frac{1}{2}(5k+13) = 0$

$$5k + 13 = 0$$
$$k = -13/5.$$

5. *For what value of k the points $(k, 2-2k)$, $(-k+1, 2k)$ and $(-4-k, 6-2k)$ are collinear.*

SOLUTION. Let the three points be $A(x_1, y_1) = (k, 2-2k)$, $B(x_2, y_2) = (-k+1, 2k)$ and $C(x_3, y_3) = (-4-k, 6-2k)$.

If the given points are collinear, then

$$x_1(y_2 - y_3) + x_2(y_3 - y_1) + x_3(y_1 - y_2) = 0$$

$$\Rightarrow k(2k - 6 + 2k) + (-k+1)(6 - 2k - 2 + 2k) + (-4-k)(2 - 2k - 2k) = 0$$

$$\Rightarrow k(4k-6) - 4(k-1) + (4+k)(4k-2) = 0$$

$$\Rightarrow 4k^2 - 6k - 4k + 4 + 4k^2 + 14k - 8 = 0$$

$$\Rightarrow 8k^2 + 4k - 4 = 0$$

$$\Rightarrow 2k^2 + k - 1 = 0$$

$$\Rightarrow (2k-1)(k+1) = 0$$

$$\Rightarrow k = 1/2 \text{ or } k = -1.$$

Hence, the given points are collinear for $k = 1/2$ or $k = -1$.

6. *Prove that the points (a, b + c), (b, c + a), (c, a + b) are collinear.*

Solution. Here $x_1 = a, y_1 = b + c, y_2 = c + a, x_3 = c, y_3 = a + b, x_2 = b$

Now area of the triangle formed by the given points

$$= \frac{1}{2}[(x_1y_2 + x_2y_3 + x_3y_1) - (y_1x_2 + y_2x_3 + y_3x_1)]$$

$$= \frac{1}{2}[\{a(c+a) + b(a+b) + c(b+c)\} - \{(b+c)b + (c+a)c + (a+b)a\}]$$

$$= \frac{1}{2}[ac + a^2 + ab + b^2 + bc + c^2 - b^2 - bc - c^2 - ac - a^2 - ab] = 0$$

Hence, the given points are collinear.

7. *Find the area of the quadrilateral ABCD whose vertices are respectively A(1, 1), B(7, –3), C(12, 2) and D(7, 21).*

Solution. Area of quadrilateral *ABCD*

$= |\text{Area of } (\Delta ABC)| + |\text{Area of } \Delta ACD|$

Now Area of ΔABC

$$= \frac{1}{2}|1\times(-3-2) + 7(2-1) + 12\times(1+3)|$$

$$= \frac{1}{2}|-5+7+48|$$

$= 25$ sq units

Area of ΔACD

$$= \frac{1}{2}|1\times(2-21)+12(21-1)+7(1-2)|$$

$$= \frac{1}{2}|-19+240-7| = 107 \text{ sq. units.}$$

∴ Area of quadrilateral $ABCD = 25 + 107 = 132$ sq. units.

8. *If the vertices of a triangle have integral coordinates prove that the triangle cannot be equilateral.*

Solution. Let $A(x_1, y_1)$, $B(x_2, y_2)$ and $C(x_3, y_3)$ be the vertices of triangle *ABC*, then the area of ΔABC is given by

$$\Delta = \frac{1}{2}[x_1(y_2 - y_3) + x_2(y_3 - y_1) + x_3(y_1 - y_2)]$$

= A rational number

If possible let the triangle *ABC* be an equilateral triangle, then its area is given by

$$\Delta = \frac{\sqrt{3}}{4}(\text{side})^2 = \frac{\sqrt{3}}{4}(AB)^2$$

$$= \frac{\sqrt{3}}{4} \times \text{a positive number}$$

= an irrational number

This is a contradiction to the fact that the area is a rational number. Hence, the triangle cannot be equilateral.

9. *The co-ordinates of vertices B and C of triangle are (1, – 2), (2, 3) lies on the line 2x + y – 2 = 0. The area of the triangle is 8 units. Then find the vertices coordinates of A.* [RGPV–2001]

Solution. Given points are $B(1, -2)$, $C(2, 3)$ and $A(x, y)$ lie on the line $2x + y - 2 = 0$

The coordinate of *A* are $(x, 2 - 2x)$

Area of ΔABC

$$= \frac{1}{2}[x_1(y_2 - y_3) + x_2(y_3 - y_1) + x_3(y_1 - y_2)]$$

$$\pm 8 = \frac{1}{2}[x(-2-3) + 1(3-(2-2x) + 2(2-2x+2)]$$

$$\pm 16 = [-5x + 1 + 2x + 8 - 4x]$$

$$\pm 16 = -7x + 9$$

$16 - 9 = -7x$ (taking positive sign)

$7 = -7x$

$x = -1$ put $x = -1$ in $y = 2 - 2x$ and get $y = 2 + 2 = 4$.

∴ Coordinate of *A* are $(-1, 4)$.

Taking negative sign $-16 = -7x + 9$

$$-16 - 9 = -7x \Rightarrow \quad x = \frac{25}{7}$$

Put $x = 25/7$ in $y = 2 - 2x$

We get $y = 2 - 2\times\frac{25}{7} = \frac{14-50}{7} = -\frac{36}{7}$

∴ Coordinate of *A* are $\left(\frac{25}{7}, -\frac{36}{7}\right)$ or $(-1, 4)$.

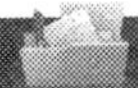

Exercise-26.3

1. Find the area of the triangle whose vertices are $A(2, 7)$, $B(3, -1)$ and $C(-5, 6)$.
2. Find the value of k for which the area formed by the triangle with vertices $A(k, 2k)$, $B(-2, 6)$, $C(3, 1)$ is 5 square units.
3. Show that the points $A(-1, 1)$, $B(5, 7)$ and $C(8, 10)$ are collinear.
4. For what value of k the points $A(1, 5)$, $B(k, 1)$ and $C(4, 11)$ are collinear ?
5. If the vertices of a triangle are $A(1, k)$, $B(4, -3)$ and $C(-9, 7)$ and its area is 15 sq. units, then find the value of k.

ANSWERS

1. 28.5 sq. units **2.** $k = 2, k = 2/3$ **4.** $k = -1$ **5.** $k = -3$ or $k = \frac{21}{13}$

26.7 LOCUS AND EQUATION TO A LOCUS

26.7.1 Locus

The curve described by a point which moves under given condition or conditions is called its locus.

For example :

Suppose C is a point in the plane of the paper and P is a variable point in the plane of the paper such that its distance from C is always equal to r(say). Obviously all the positions of the moving point P lie on the circumference of a circle whose radius is r. The circumference of this circle is therefore the Locus of the point P when it moves under the condition that its distance from point C is always equal to constant r.

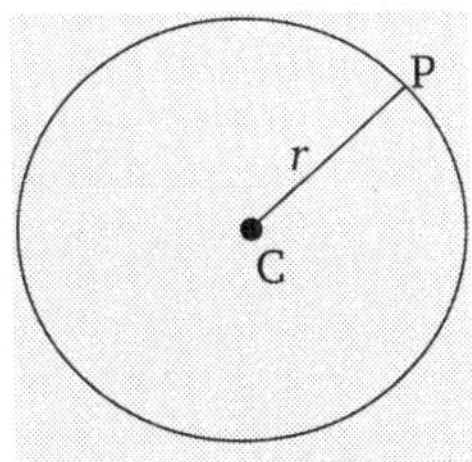

Fig. 15

26.7.2 Equation of the Locus of a Point

The equation of the locus of a point is the relation which is satisfied by the coordinates of every point on the locus of the point.

Working Procedure

Step 1. Assume the coordinates of the point say (h, k) whose locus is to be found.

Step 2. Write the given condition in mathematical form involving h, k.

Step 3. Eliminate the variables, if any.

Step 4. Replace h by x and k by y in the result obtained in step-3. The equation so obtained is the locus of the point which moves under some stated conditions.

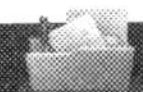

Solved Examples

1. *Find the locus of a point P such that the sum of the squares of abscissa and ordinate is equal to the product of abscissa and ordinate.*

Solution. Let $P(h, k)$ be any point on the locus.

$\therefore$ h is abscissa and k is ordinate of P.

By the given geometrical condition, we get

$$h^2 + k^2 = hk$$

Hence, locus of (h, k) is $x^2 + y^2 = xy$.

2. *Find the equation to the locus of a point equidistant from the points A(1, 3) and B(–2, 1).*

Solution. Let $P(h, k)$ be any point on the locus.

Then $PA = PB$ (given)

$\Rightarrow$ $PA^2 = PB^2$

$\Rightarrow (h-1)^2 + (k-3)^2 = (h+2)^2 + (k-1)^2$

$\Rightarrow$ $6h + 4k = 5$

Hence, locus (h, k) is $6x + 4y = 5$.

3. *A point moves so that the sum of its distances from (ae, 0) and (–ae, 0) is 2a, prove that the equation to its locus is*

$$\frac{x^2}{a^2} + \frac{y^2}{b^2} = 1 \text{ where } b^2 = a^2(1 - e^2).$$

SOLUTION. Let $P(h, k)$ be the moving point such that the sum of its distance from $A(ae, 0)$ and $B(-ae, 0)$ is $2a$.

Then $PA + PB = 2a$

$$\Rightarrow \sqrt{(h-ae)^2+(k-0)^2} + \sqrt{(h+ae)^2+(k-0)^2} = 2a$$

$$\Rightarrow \sqrt{(h-ae)^2+k^2} = 2a - \sqrt{(h+ae)^2+k^2}$$

$$\Rightarrow (h-ae)^2+k^2 = 4a^2+(h+ae)^2 + k^2 - 4a\sqrt{(h+ae)^2+k^2}$$

(squaring both sides)

$$\Rightarrow -4aeh - 4a^2 = -4a\sqrt{(h+ae)^2+k^2}$$

$$\Rightarrow (eh+a) = \sqrt{(h+ae)^2+k^2}$$

$$\Rightarrow (eh+a)^2 = (h+ae)^2 + k^2$$

$$\Rightarrow e^2h^2 + a^2 + 2aeh = h^2 + a^2e^2 + 2aeh + k^2$$

$$\Rightarrow h^2(1-e^2) + k^2 = a^2(1-e^2)$$

$$\Rightarrow \frac{h^2}{a^2} + \frac{k^2}{a^2(1-e^2)} = 1$$

Hence, locus of (h, k) is given by

$$\frac{h^2}{a^2} + \frac{k^2}{a^2(1-e^2)} = 1$$

or $\frac{x^2}{a^2} + \frac{y^2}{b^2} = 1$, where $b^2 = a^2(1-e^2)$

4. *A rod of length l slides with its ends on two perpendicular lines, find the locus of its mid-point.*

SOLUTION. Let the two perpendicular lines be the coordinate axes. Let AB be a rod of length l. Let the coordinate of A and B be $(a, 0)$ and $(0, b)$ respectively. As the rod slides, the values of a and b change. So a and b are two variables.

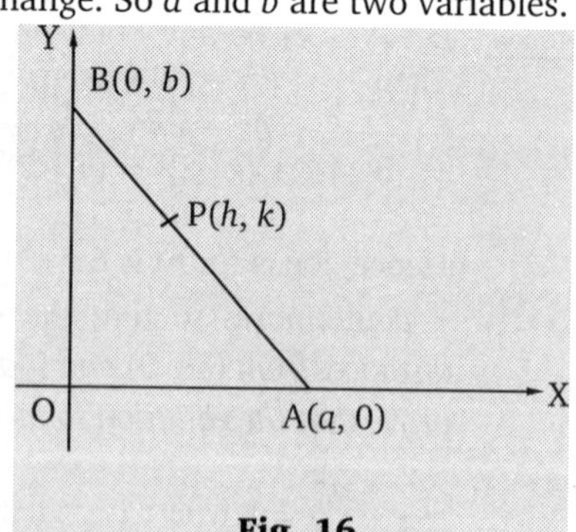

Fig. 16

Let $P(h, k)$ be the mid point of the rod AB in one of the indefinite position it attains. Then

$$h = \frac{a+0}{2} \text{ and } k = \frac{0+b}{2} \Rightarrow h = \frac{a}{2} \text{ and } k = \frac{b}{2} \quad \ldots(1)$$

From ΔOAB, we have

$$AB^2 = OA^2 + OB^2$$
$$= a^2 + b^2 = l^2$$

$$\Rightarrow (2h)^2 + (2k)^2 = l^2 \quad \text{(From (1))}$$

$$\Rightarrow 4h^2 + 4k^2 = l^2$$

Hence, the locus of (h, k) is $4x^2 + 4y^2 = l^2$.

5. *If O is the origin and Q is a variable point on $x^2 = 4y$. Find the locus of the mid-point of OQ.*

SOLUTION. Let the coordinates of Q be (a, b) and let $P(h, k)$ be the mid-point of OQ. Then

$$h = \frac{a+0}{2} = \frac{a}{2} \text{ and } k = \frac{0+b}{2} = \frac{b}{2}$$

$$\Rightarrow a = 2h \text{ and } b = 2k. \quad \ldots(1)$$

Here a and b are two variables which are to be eliminated. Since (a, b) lies on $x^2 = 4y$

Therefore, $a^2 = 4b$

$$\Rightarrow (2h)^2 = 4(2k)$$

$$\Rightarrow h^2 = 2k \quad \text{[using (1)]}$$

Hence, the locus of (h, k) is $x^2 = 2y$.

6. *A point moves so that its distance from (3, 0) is twice the distance from (–3, 0). Find the equation of the locus.*

SOLUTION. Let A represent the point $(3, 0)$, B the point $(-3, 0)$. Further, point $(-3, 0)$ and $P(h, k)$ be the moving point.

According to the question:

$$PA = 2PB$$

or $(PA)^2 = 4(PB)^2$

$$[(h-3)^2 + (k-0)^2] = 4[(h+3)^2 + (k-0)^2]$$

$$\Rightarrow h^2 + 9 - 6h + k^2 = 4h^2 + 36 + 24h + 4k^2$$

$$\Rightarrow 3h^2 + 3k^2 + 30h + 27 = 0$$

Hence, the required locus is $3x^2 + 3y^2 + 30x + 27 = 0$.

7. *Find the locus of a point such that the line segments having end points (2, 0) and (–2, 0) subtend a right angle at that point.*

SOLUTION. Let $A(2, 0)$ and $B(-2, 0)$ be the given points and $P(h, k)$ be the variable point.

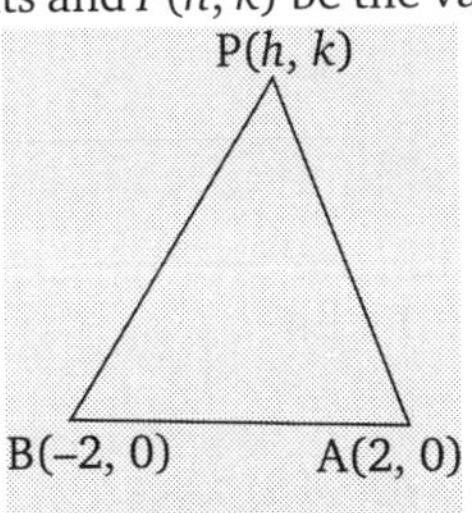

Fig. 17

According to the question

$$\angle APB = 90°$$

$\therefore$ *i.e.*, ΔAPB is a right angle.

$$AB^2 = PA^2 + PB^2$$

$$[2 - (-2)]^2 + [0 - 0]$$
$$= [(2 - h)^2 + (0 - k)^2] + [(-2 - h)^2 + (0 - k)^2]$$

$$16 = (2 - h)^2 + k^2 + (-2 - h)^2 + k^2$$

$$16 = 4 + h^2 - 4h + 2k^2 + 4 + h^2 + 4h$$

$$16 = 2h^2 + 2k^2 + 8$$

$$h^2 + k^2 = 4.$$

Hence, the required locus is $x^2 + y^2 = 4$.

8. *Find the equation to the locus of a point which moves so that the sum of its distance from (3, 0) and (–3, 0) is less then 9.*

SOLUTION. Let $A(3, 0)$ and $B(-3, 0)$ be the two given points and (h, k) be the coordinates of the moving point P whose locus is to be found. According to the question

$$PA + PB < 9$$

or $\sqrt{(h-3)^2+k^2}+\sqrt{(h+3)^2+k^2}<9$

$$\sqrt{(h-3)^2+k^2}<\left\{9-\sqrt{(h+3)^2+k^2}\right\}$$

Squaring both sides, we get

$$(h-3)^2+k^2<81-18\sqrt{(h+3)^2+k^2}+(h+3)^2+k^2$$

$$-12h-81<-18\sqrt{(h+3)^2+k^2}$$

or $4h+27>6\sqrt{(h+3)^2+k^2}$

Again squaring both the sides, we get

$$16h^2+729+216h>36[h^2+9+6h+k^2]$$

$$20h^2 + 36k^2 < 405$$

The required locus of the point (h, k) is $20x^2 + 36y^2 < 405$.

Exercise-26.4

1. Find the equation to the locus of a point equidistant from the points $A(1, 3)$ and $B(-2, 1)$.
2. If $A = (2, -2)$, B is a point on the locus $y^2 = 4x$. Find the equation of the locus of a point which divides AB internally in the ratio 1:2.
3. $A = (-3, 0)$ and $B(3, 0)$ are two given points. Find the equation of the locus of point P such that $PA + PB = 10$.
4. If B is $(4, -3)$, $C(0, 2)$ and point A lies on the locus $y = 1 + x$. Then find the equation of locus of centroid of triangle ABC.
5. Find the equation of the circle having segment AB as a diameter where $A(-1, 4)$ and $B(3, -2)$.
6. Find the equation of the locus of a point such that the sum of the squares of its distance from (5, –3) and (2, –2) is 20.
7. Let $A = (0, 5)$ and $B(0, -5)$. Find the equation of the locus of point P such that $PA - PB = 4$.
8. $A(1, 2)$ and $B(4, -5)$ are two vertices of ΔABC. Find the locus of the third vertex C if the centroid lie on the locus $2x + 3y = 11$.

ANSWERS

1. $6x + 4y = 5$ **2.** $9y^2 - 12x + 24y + 32 = 0$ **3.** $\frac{x^2}{25}+\frac{y^2}{16}=1$

4. $9x^2 - 24x - 3y + 16 = 0$ **5.** $x^2 + y^2 - 2x - 2y - 11 = 0$

6. $2x^2 + 2y^2 - 14x + 8y + 19 = 0$ **7.** $\frac{-x^2}{21}+\frac{y^2}{4}=1$ **8.** $2x + 3y = 32$

26.8 THE STRAIGHT LINES

A straight line is the locus of all those points which are collinear with two given points. Since, we know that one and only one line can be drawn from any two given points. So straight line is a curve such that every point on the line segment joining any two points on it lies on it.

- Every first degree equation in x, y represents a straight line.
- The x-axis and all lines parallel to it are called horizontal lines.
- The y-axis and all lines parallel to it are called vertical lines.

26.9 SLOPE OR GRADIENT OF A LINE

Geometrically, tangent of the angle that a line makes with the positive direction of the x-axis in anticlockwise sense is called the slope or gradient of the line.

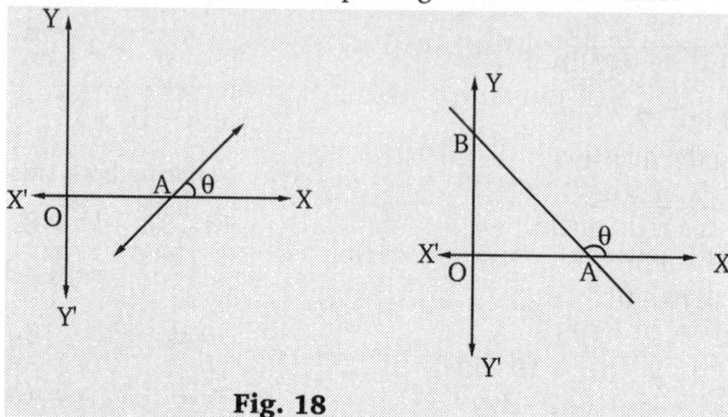

Fig. 18

The slope of a line is generally denoted by m. Thus $m = \tan\theta$.

- Slope of any line parallel to x-axis is zero.
- Slope of any line parallel to y-axis, *i.e.*, perpendicular to x-axis is infinite. Thus, not defined.
- Slope of the general equation of line $ax + by + c = 0$ is
$$m = -\frac{a}{b} = -\frac{\text{coefficient of } x}{\text{coefficient of } y}.$$
- Slope of a line equally inclined with axes is 1 or –1 as it makes 45° or 135° angle with x-axis.
- The angle of inclination of a line with the positive direction of x-axis in anticlockwise sense always lies between 0° and 180°.
- When $m < 0$, $\tan\theta < 0$, *i.e.*, $\theta > 90°$. Therefore, the angle of inclination is obtuse.
- When $m = 0$, $\tan\theta = 0$, *i.e.*, $\theta = 0°$. Therefore, the line is parallel to x-axis.
- When $m > 0$, $\tan\theta > 0$, *i.e.*, $\theta < 90°$. Therefore, the angle of inclination is acute.

26.10 SLOPE OF A LINE THROUGH TWO POINTS

Let L be the line through two fixed points $A(x_1, y_1)$ and $B(x_2, y_2)$ respectively. Let us draw perpendicular from A on x and y axis respectively so as to meet at $M(x_1, 0)$ and $P(0, y_1)$. Also through B perpendiculars on x and y axes meet at $N(x_2, 0)$ and $Q(0, y_2)$.

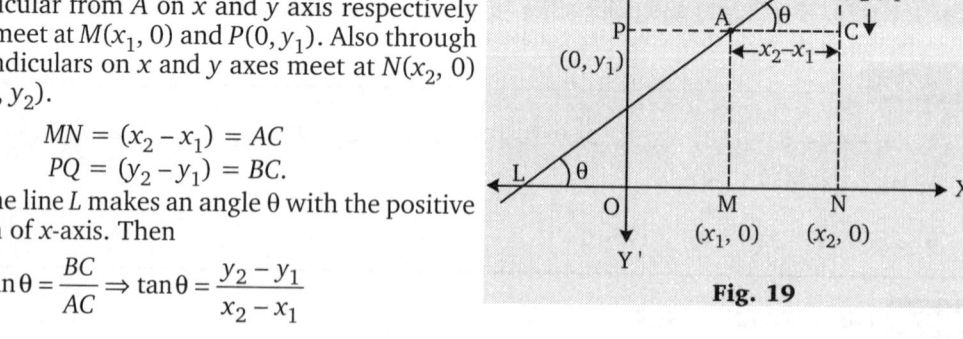

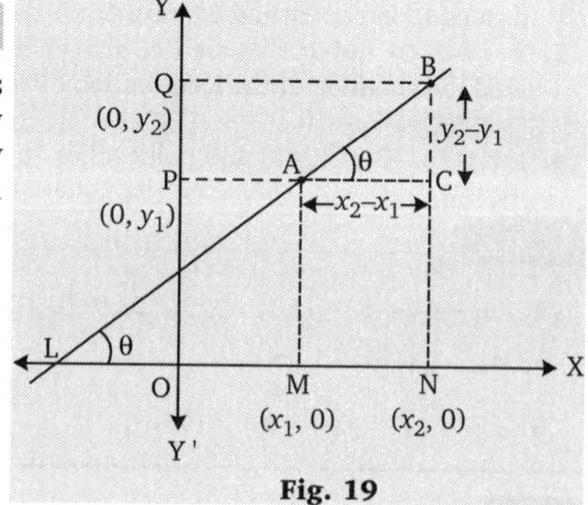

Fig. 19

Now $MN = (x_2 - x_1) = AC$

and $PQ = (y_2 - y_1) = BC$.

Let the line L makes an angle θ with the positive direction of x-axis. Then

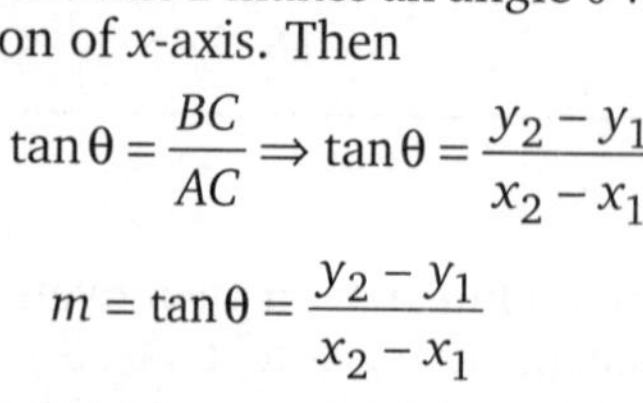

$$\tan\theta = \frac{BC}{AC} \Rightarrow \tan\theta = \frac{y_2 - y_1}{x_2 - x_1}$$

$$m = \tan\theta = \frac{y_2 - y_1}{x_2 - x_1}$$

Which is the required slope of the line joining the points $A(x_1, y_1)$ and $B(x_2, y_2)$.

- Let $A(x, y)$ and $O = (0, 0) = B$. Then slope of line $AB = \frac{y-0}{x-0} = \frac{y}{x}$ = slope of OA.

26.10.1 CONDITION OF PARALLELISM OF LINES

It two lines of slopes m_1 and m_2 are parallel, then angle θ made by them with positive direction of x-axis are equal.

So $$m_1 = m_2$$

26.10.2 CONDITION FOR PERPENDICULARITY OF TWO LINES

If m_1 and m_2 are the slopes of two mutually perpendicular lines

then $$m_1 = -\frac{1}{m_2} \text{ or } m_1 m_2 = -1$$

Solved Examples

1. *Find the slope of a line which makes an angle of 30° with the positive direction of x-axis.*

SOLUTION. Let m be the slope of the line.

Then $m = \tan\theta = \tan 30° = \frac{1}{\sqrt{3}}$.

2. *Find the slope of the line joining A(3, 4) and B(6, 8).*

SOLUTION. Slope of line $AB = \frac{y_2 - y_1}{x_2 - x_1} = \frac{8-4}{6-3} = \frac{4}{3}$.

3. *Determine x so that the line passing through (3, 4) and (x, 5) makes 135° angle with the positive direction of x-axis.*

SOLUTION. Since the line passing through (3, 4) and $(x, 5)$ makes an angle of 135° with x-axis. Therefore, its slope is tan 135° = –1.

But slope of the line is also equal to

$$\frac{5-4}{x-3}$$

$$\therefore\ -1 = \frac{5-4}{x-3} \Rightarrow -x + 3 = 1 \Rightarrow x = 2.$$

4. *Show that the points A(2, 3), B(4, 5) and C(3, 2) are the vertices of a right angled triangle.*

SOLUTION. The given points are $A(2, 4)$, $B(4, 5)$ and $C(3, 2)$.

Slope of line $AB = \frac{5-3}{4-2} = \frac{2}{2} = 1$

Slope of line $BC = \frac{2-5}{3-4} = \frac{-3}{-1} = 3$

and slope of line $AC = \frac{2-3}{3-2} = -1$

∴ (Slope of line AB)×(Slope of line AC) $= 1 \times (-1) = -1$

⇒ line AB is perpendicular to line AC.

∴ ABC is a triangle right angled at A.

5. *Find k, if the points (–1, 3), (8, k) and (2, 1) are collinear.*

SOLUTION. The points (–1, 3), (8, k) and (2, 1) are collinear then slope of AB = slope of AC.

$$\text{Slope of } AB = \frac{k-3}{8-(-1)} = \frac{k-3}{9}$$

$$\text{and Slope of } AC = \frac{1-3}{2-(-1)} = \frac{-2}{3}$$

$$\therefore\ \frac{k-3}{9} = \frac{-2}{3} \Rightarrow 3(k-3) = -18$$

$$\Rightarrow\ 3k - 9 = -18$$
$$k = -3$$

6. *Find angle made by the lines x cos 30° + y sin 30° + sin 120° = 0 with the positive direction of x-axis.*

SOLUTION. The equation of the given line is

$$x \cos 30° + y \sin 30° + \sin 120° = 0 \quad \text{...(1)}$$

$$y = \frac{-\cos 30° x}{\sin 30°} \frac{-\sin 120°}{\sin 30°}$$

$$y = -\cot 30° x - \frac{\sqrt{3}/2}{1/2}$$

⇒ $y = \tan 120° x - \sqrt{3}$, which is the slope intercept form. Hence, the angle made by the given line with the positive direction of x-axis is 120°.

7. *Reduce $4x + 3y - 9 = 0$ to the normal form and find the distance (perpendicular distance p) from origin.*

SOLUTION. We have $4x + 3y - 9 = 0$ or $4x + 3y = 9$

Dividing both sides by $\sqrt{(4)^2 + (3)^2} = 5$,

we get $\frac{4}{5}x + \frac{3}{5}y = \frac{9}{5}$, which is the normal form.

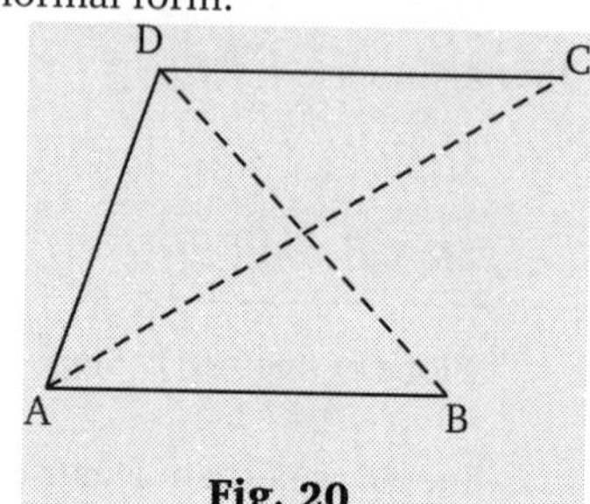

Fig. 20

Hence, the length of perpendicular from the origin to the line is $p = \frac{9}{5}$.

8. *Prove that the points (–1, 0), (3, 1), (2, 2) and (–2, 1) are the vertices of a parallelogram.*

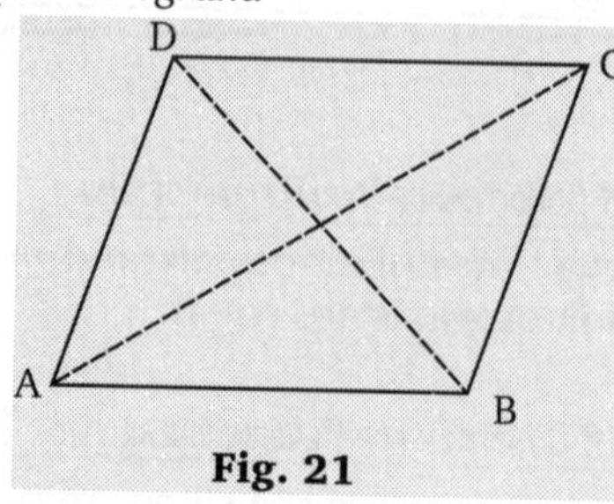

Fig. 21

SOLUTION. Let $A(-1, 0)$, $B(3, 1)$, $C(2, 2)$ and $D(-2, 1)$ be the vertices of the parallelogram, $ABCD$ taken in order. The mid-points of diagonals AC and BD are

$$AC = \left(\frac{-1+2}{2}, \frac{0+2}{2}\right) = \left(\frac{1}{2}, 1\right)$$

and $BD = \left(\frac{3-2}{2}, \frac{1+1}{2}\right) = \left(\frac{1}{2}, 1\right)$.

Since, the mid-points of AC and BD are same. Also, slope of $AB \times$ slope of $AD \neq -1$. and slope of $AC \times$ slope of $BD \neq -1$. Hence, $ABCD$ is a parallelogram.

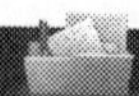

Exercise-26.5

1. Find the slope of a line whose inclination to the positive direction of x-axis in anticlockwise sense is :
   (i) 60°   (ii) 0°
   (iii) 150°   (iv) 120°
2. Find the slope of the line passing through (2, 3) and (1, 4).
3. Show that the points (1, 3), (2, 5) and (4, 9) are collinear.
4. Let $A(6, 4)$ and $B(2, 12)$ be two given points. Find the slope of a line perpendicular to AB.
5. Determine x so that 2 is the slope of the line through (2, 5) and (x, 3).
6. Without using Pythagoras theorem, show that the points (1, 2), (4, 5) and (6, 3) represent the vertices of a right angle triangle.
7. Show that the points $P(-4, -5)$, $Q(-2, 2)$, $R(5, 4)$ and $S(3, -3)$ are the vertices of a rhombus.
8. Show that the following points represent a rectangle (0, 0), (0, 5), (6, 5), (6, 0).
9. Show that the following points represent a square (3, 2), (0, 5), (–3, 2), (0 – 1).
10. Prove that the lines.
    (i) $x + 3y + 4 = 0$ and $2x + 6y - 7 = 0$ are parallel.
    (ii) $2x + 3y + 3 = 0$ and $3x - 2y + 5 = 0$ are perpendicular.

Hint to Selected Problems

6. Let $A(1, 2)$, $B(4, 5)$ and $C(6, 3)$ be the vertices of the given triangle.

Slope of $AB = \frac{5-2}{4-1} = \frac{3}{3} = 1 = m_1$(say)

Similarly, Slope of $BC = -1 = m_2$(say)

and Slope of $AC = \frac{1}{5} = m_3$(say)

$m_1 \times m_2 = 1 \times -1 = -1 \Rightarrow AB \perp BC$

7. $m_1 = \frac{7}{2}$, $m_2 = \frac{7}{2}$, $m_3 = \frac{2}{7}$ and $m_4 = \frac{2}{7}$

$PQ \parallel RS$ and $QR \parallel PS$

So $PQRS$ is a parallelogram.

Also (slope of PR) × (slope of SQ)

$$= \frac{4+5}{5+4} \times \frac{-3-2}{3-(-2)} = \frac{9}{9} \times \frac{-5}{5} = -1$$

$\Rightarrow$ The diagonals PR and QS are perpendicular.

ANSWERS

1. (i) $\sqrt{3}$ (ii) 0 (iii) $-\frac{1}{\sqrt{3}}$ (iv) $-\sqrt{3}$

2. 7 4. $\frac{1}{2}$ 5. $x = 1$

26.11 EQUATION OF LINES IN STANDARD FORM

26.11.1 Slope or Tangent Form

Find the equation of a line whose y-intercept 'c' and slope 'm' are given.

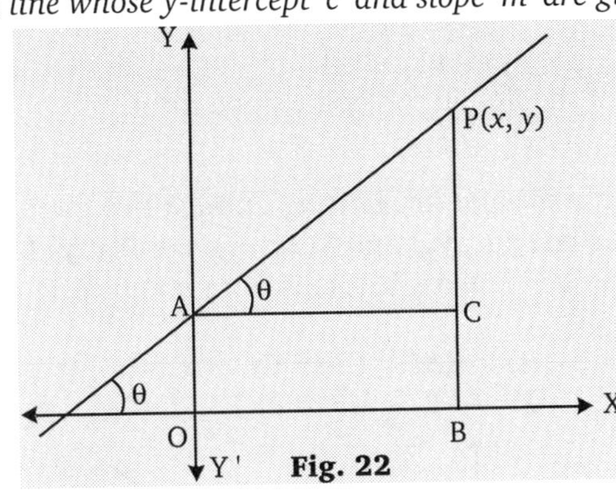

Fig. 22

Let the given line meet y-axis in A and let $P(x, y)$ be any point on it. As the y-intercept of the line is c.

$\therefore$ Coordinates of A are $(0, c)$.

Draw PB $\perp$ to x-axis and $AC \perp PB$.

Then $\tan\theta = \frac{PC}{AC} = \frac{PB - BC}{OB}$

$\Rightarrow$ $\tan\theta = \frac{BP - OA}{OB}$ $\Rightarrow$ $m = \frac{y - c}{x}$

$\Rightarrow$ $y = mx + c$

which is called the slope intercept form of the equation of a straight line.

- If c becomes zero, the equation $y = mx + c$ reduces to $y = mx$ which is the equation of a line passing through the origin.
- If $m = 0, c \neq 0$, then equation $y = mx + c$ reduces to $y = c$ which is the equation of a line parallel to x-axis at a distance c from it.
- If $m = 0, c = 0$, then the equation becomes $y = 0$ which represents the x-axis.

26.11.2 Point-Slope Form

To find the equation of a line passing through the given point (x_1, y_1) and having slope m:

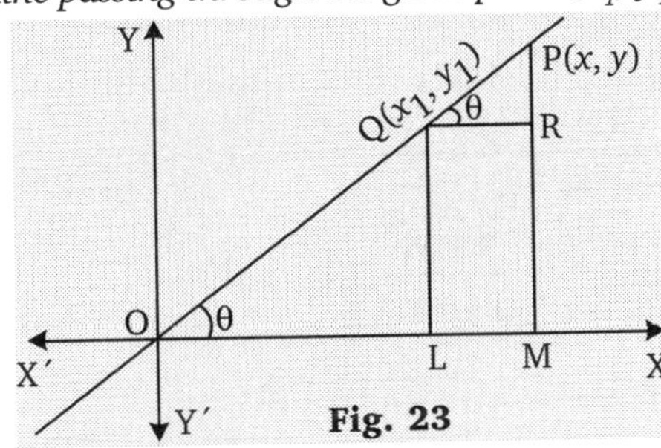

Fig. 23

Let the given point (x_1, y_1) be represented by Q. Let $P(x, y)$ be any point on the line. Draw PM and QL perpendicular to x-axis from points P and Q and $QR \perp MP$. Then

$$PR = MP - MR = MP - QL = y - y_1$$

and $$QR = LM = OM - OL = x - x_1$$

Then $$\tan\theta = \frac{PR}{QR} = \frac{y - y_1}{x - x_1}$$

$$m = \frac{y - y_1}{x - x_1}$$

$$y - y_1 = m(x - x_1)$$

which is the equation of the line in the point-slope form.

26.11.3 Two Points Form

To find the equation of the straight line passing through two given points:

Let the two given points be $Q(x_1, y_1)$ and $R(x_2, y_2)$. Let $P(x, y)$ be any point on the line. Draw RL, QM and PN perpendiculars to x-axis from points R, Q and P respectively.

Let $RS \perp QM$ and $QT \perp PN$.

Then $$RS = LM = OM - OL = x_1 - x_2$$

$$QS = MQ - MS = MQ - RL = y_1 - y_2$$

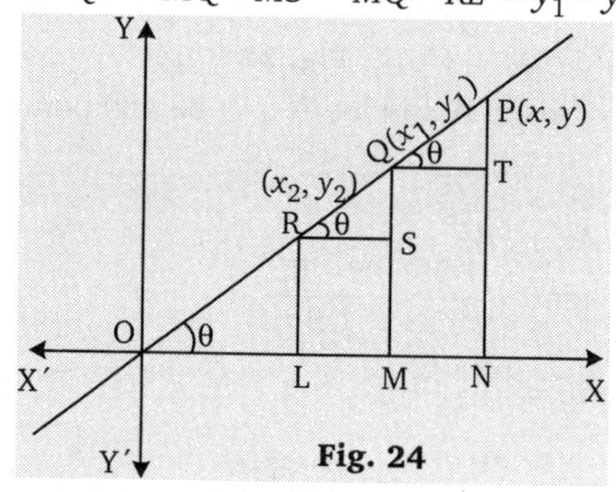

Fig. 24

$$QT = MN = ON - OM = x - x_1$$

$$PT = NP - NT = NP - MQ = y - y_1$$

In $\Delta RQS, \tan\theta = \dfrac{QS}{RS} = \dfrac{y_1 - y_2}{x_1 - x_2}$ ...(1)

In $\Delta QTP, \tan\theta = \dfrac{PT}{QT} = \dfrac{y - y_1}{x - x_1}$ ...(2)

From (1) and (2), we get

$$\frac{y_1 - y_2}{x_1 - x_2} = \frac{y - y_1}{x - x_1}$$

$$\frac{x - x_1}{x_1 - x_2} = \frac{y - y_1}{y_1 - y_2}$$

$$\frac{x - x_1}{x_2 - x_1} = \frac{y - y_1}{y_2 - y_1}$$

$$y - y_1 = \frac{y_2 - y_1}{x_2 - x_1}(x - x_1)$$

which is the required equation of line in two point form.

26.11.4 Intercept Form

To find the equation of the line which cuts off intercepts a and b on x-axis and y-axis respectively.

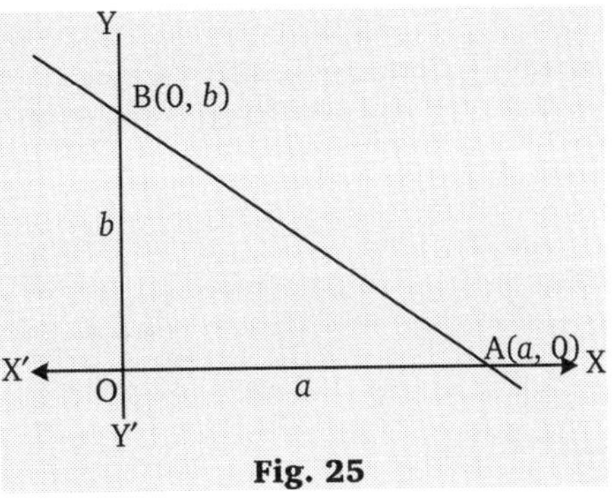

Fig. 25

Let the line meet x-axis at point A and y-axis is at point B. As the respective intercepts are a and b. So $OA = a$ and $OB = b$.

Coordinates of A and B are $(a, 0)$ and $(0, b)$ respectively.

Using two point form, the equation of line is

$$\frac{x-a}{0-a} = \frac{y-0}{b-0}$$

$$\frac{-x}{a} + 1 = \frac{y}{b}$$

$$\frac{x}{a} + \frac{y}{b} = 1.$$

Which is the equation of the line in the intercept form.

26.11.5 Normal or Perpendicular Form

To find the equation of a line in terms of the perpendicular segment p, from the origin to the lines and the angle a which the perpendicular segment makes with the x-axis.

Let l be the given line meeting x-axis and y-axis at the points A and B respectively. Let $OC \perp l$ and $\angle AOC = \alpha$, $OC = p$.

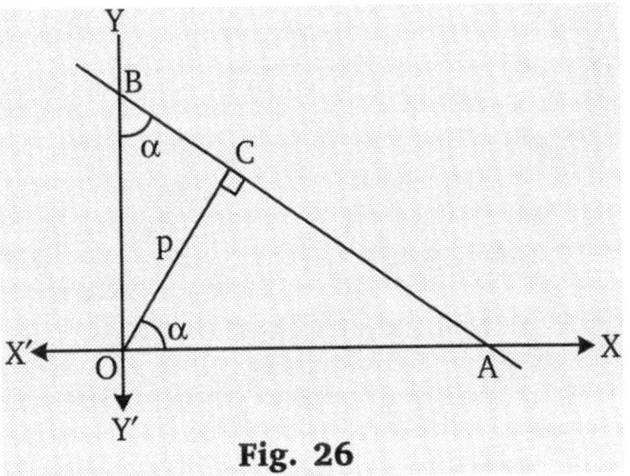

Fig. 26

Now $$\frac{OA}{OC} = \sec\alpha$$

$$\frac{OA}{p} = \sec\alpha$$

$$OA = p \sec\alpha$$

Again $$\frac{OB}{OC} = \operatorname{cosec}\alpha$$

$$\frac{OB}{p} = \operatorname{cosec}\alpha$$

$$OB = p \operatorname{cosec}\alpha$$

Using the intercept form of the equation of the line, the equation of the given line is

$$\frac{x}{OA} + \frac{y}{OB} = 1$$

$$\frac{x}{p\sec\alpha} + \frac{y}{p\operatorname{cosec}\alpha} = 1$$

or $x\cos\alpha + y\sin\alpha = p$

which is the required equation of the line.

26.11.6 Parametric Form

To find the equation of a straight line in the parametric form:

$$\frac{x-x_1}{\cos\theta} = \frac{y-y_1}{\sin\theta} = r, \text{ where } r \text{ is the parameter.}$$

Let the given line passes through the point $A(x_1, y_1)$ and be inclined at an angle θ with the positive direction of x-axis.

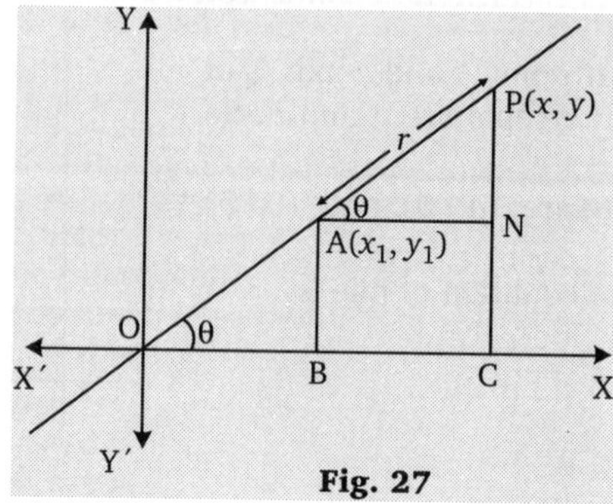

Fig. 27

Let $P(x, y)$ be any point and $AP = r$.

Draw AB and PC perpendiculars to x-axis from A and P respectively and $AN \perp PC$.

Now $$AN = BC = OC - OB = x - x_1$$

$$PN = PC - CN = PC - AB = y - y_1$$

Also $$AP = r.$$

In right angle triangle ΔANP.

$$\cos\theta = \frac{AN}{AP} = \frac{x - x_1}{r}$$

i.e., $$\frac{x - x_1}{\cos\theta} = r \quad \ldots(1)$$

and $$\sin\theta = \frac{PN}{AP} = \frac{y - y_1}{r}$$

$\Rightarrow$ $$\frac{y - y_1}{\sin\theta} = r \quad \ldots(2)$$

From (1) and (2), we get $\dfrac{x - x_1}{\cos\theta} = \dfrac{y - y_1}{\sin\theta} = r$

Which is the equation of the line in the parametric form.

- Parametric form of equation of a line is also known as symmetrical form of equation.
- From $\dfrac{x - x_1}{\cos\theta} = \dfrac{y - y_1}{\sin\theta} = r$, we have $x = x_1 + r\cos\theta$, $y = y_1 + r\sin\theta$, thus the coordinates of any point at a distance r from (x_1, y_1) are $(x_1 + r\cos\theta, y_1 + r\sin\theta)$.

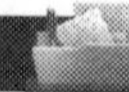

Solved Examples

1. *Find the equation of a line which cuts off an intercept –2 on the axis of y and makes an angle of 45° with the positive direction of x-axis.*

SOLUTION. Here, $c = -2$, and $m = \tan 45° = 1$.

Substituting these values in $y = mx + c$, we get $y = x - 2$ which is required equation of the line.

2. *Find the equation of a line through* (4, 3) *with slope* 2.

SOLUTION. Equation of line passing through (x_1, y_1) and with slope m is

$$y - y_1 = m(x - x_1)$$

$\therefore$ The required equation of the line is

$$y - 3 = 2(x - 4)$$

$$\Rightarrow \quad 2x - y - 5 = 0.$$

3. *Find the equation of a line which passes through the point (–2, 3) and makes an angle of 30° with the positive direction of x-axis.*

SOLUTION. Here $\theta = 30^\circ$

$$\Rightarrow \quad m = \tan\theta = \tan 30^\circ = \frac{1}{\sqrt{3}}$$

The point on the line is (–2, 3).

Using point slope form, the equation of line is

$$y - 3 = \frac{1}{\sqrt{3}}(x+2)$$

$$\Rightarrow \quad \sqrt{3}y - 3\sqrt{3} = x + 2$$

$$\Rightarrow x - \sqrt{3}y + (3\sqrt{3}+2) = 0.$$

4. *Find the equation of the straight line passing through the points (–3, 4) and (1, –3).* [RGPV–2004]

SOLUTION. Equation of the straight line passing through (x_1, y_1) and (x_2, y_2) is given by

$$y - y_1 = \frac{y_2 - y_1}{x_2 - x_1}(x - x_1) \quad \ldots(1)$$

Now, we have $x_1 = -3, y_1 = 4$

$x_2 = 1, y_2 = -3$

Putting these values in equation (1) we have

$$y - 4 = \frac{-3-4}{1+3}(x+3)$$

$$\Rightarrow \quad 4(y-4) = -7x - 21$$

$$\Rightarrow \quad 4y - 16 = -7x - 21$$

$$\Rightarrow \quad 7x + 4y + 5 = 0.$$

5. *Find the equation of the line which passes through the point (3, 4) and the sum of its intercept on the axes is 14.* [UPTU(B.PHARMA)–2008]

SOLUTION. Let the intercept made by the line on x-axis be a.

Then intercept on y-axis $= 14 - a$.

$\therefore$ Equation of the line is given by

$$\frac{x}{a} + \frac{y}{14-a} = 1 \quad \ldots(1)$$

As the point (3, 4) lies on it, we have

$$\frac{3}{a} + \frac{4}{14-a} = 1$$

$$3(14-a) + 4a = 14a - a^2$$

$$\Rightarrow 42 - 3a + 4a = 14a - a^2$$

$$\Rightarrow a^2 - 13a + 42 = 0$$

$$\Rightarrow (a-7)(a-6) = 0$$

$$a = 7, 6.$$

Putting these values of a in (1), we get equation of the lines

$$\frac{x}{7} + \frac{y}{7} = 1 \text{ or } x + y = 7$$

$$\text{and } \frac{x}{6} + \frac{y}{8} = 1 \text{ or } 4x + 3y = 24$$

6. *Find the ratio in which the line segment joining the points (2, 3) and (4, 5) is divided by the line joining the points (6, 8) and (–3, –2).*

SOLUTION. The equation of the line joining the points (6, 8) and (–3, –2) is

$$\frac{y-8}{-2-8} = \frac{x-6}{-3-6} \text{ (Two points form).}$$

$$\Rightarrow \quad \frac{y-8}{-10} = \frac{x-6}{-9}$$

or $\quad 9y - 72 = 10x - 60$

$$10x - 9y + 12 = 0 \quad \ldots(1)$$

Let this line divide the join of (2, 3) and (4, 5) at the point P in the ratio of $k : 1$.

Then the coordinates of P are

$$\left(\frac{4k+2}{k+1}, \frac{5k+3}{k+1}\right)$$

Now, the point P on the line (1)

Therefore,

$$10 \times \frac{4k+2}{k+1} - 9 \times \frac{5k+3}{k+1} + 12 = 0$$

$$40k + 20 - 45k - 27 + 12k + 12 = 0$$

$$7k = -5$$

$$k = -5/7.$$

Since, the value of k is negative, the line is divided externally.

Hence, the required ratio is 5 : 7 externally.

7. *Find the equation of a line passing through the point (3, –2) and perpendicular to the line x – 3y + 5 = 0.* [UPTU–2006]

SOLUTION. Slope of the given line $x - 3y + 5 = 0$ is

$$m_1 = \frac{1}{3}$$

As the line is perpendicular to line passing through (3, –2).

$$m_1 \times m_2 = -1.$$

$$\Rightarrow \quad \frac{1}{3} \times m_2 = -1$$

$$\Rightarrow \quad m_2 = -3.$$

And required equation is

$$(y + 2) = -3(x - 3)$$
$$\Rightarrow \quad y + 2 = -3x + 9$$
$$\Rightarrow \quad 3x + y - 7 = 0$$

8. *Find the equation of the straight line which passes through (1, 2) and is perpendicular to the line $4x - 3y = 8$.*

SOLUTION. The equation of any straight line perpendicular to the line $4x - 3y - 8 = 0$ is

$$3x + 4y + \lambda = 0 \quad ...(1)$$

If the line (1) passes through the point (1, 2) then

$$3 + 8 + \lambda = 0$$
$$\lambda = -11.$$

Putting $\lambda = -11$ in (1) the required equation of the line is

$$3x + 4y - 11 = 0$$

9. *Find the equation of perpendicular bisector of the line segment joining the points A(2, 3) and B(6, –5).*

SOLUTION. Slope $= \dfrac{-5-3}{6-2} = \dfrac{-8}{4} = -2.$

$\therefore$ Slope of a line perpendicular to the line $AB = \dfrac{1}{2}$. $\quad [\because m_1 m_2 = -1]$

The coordinates of the middle point M of AB are

$$\left(\frac{2+6}{2}, \frac{3+(-5)}{2}\right), i.e., (4, -1).$$

Hence, the equation of the perpendicular bisector of AB, *i.e.*, the equation of the line passing through m and perpendicular to AB is

$$y + 1 = \frac{1}{2}(x - 4)$$
$$\Rightarrow \quad x - 2y = 6.$$

10. *Find the equation of the straight line passing through the point ($a \cos^3\theta$, $a \sin^3\theta$) and perpendicular to the line $x \sec\theta + y \operatorname{cosec}\theta = a$.*

SOLUTION. The slope of the given line $x \sec\theta + y \operatorname{cosec}\theta = a$ is

$$\frac{-\sec\theta}{\operatorname{cosec}\theta}, i.e., \frac{-\sin\theta}{\cos\theta}$$

$\therefore$ The slope of a line perpendicular to the given line $= \dfrac{\cos\theta}{\sin\theta}$

Now, the equation of the straight line which passes through the point ($a \cos^3\theta$, $a \sin^3\theta$) and whose slope is $\dfrac{\cos\theta}{\sin\theta}$, is

$$y - a\sin^3\theta = \frac{\cos\theta}{\sin\theta}(x - a\cos^3\theta)$$

$\Rightarrow x \cos\theta - y \sin\theta = a(\cos^4\theta - \sin^4\theta)$

or $x \cos\theta - y \sin\theta$

$= a(\cos^2\theta + \sin^2\theta)(\cos^2\theta - \sin^2\theta)$

Hence, $x \cos\theta - y \sin\theta = a \cos 2\theta$.

11. *Find the equation of the straight line, the portion of which intercepted between the axes is divided by the point (–2, 6) in the ratio 3 : 2.* [UPTU(B.PHARMA)–2007]

SOLUTION. Let the equation of the straight line be

$$\frac{x}{a} + \frac{y}{b} = 1 \quad ...(1)$$

The line (1) meet x-axis at the point $A(a, 0)$ and y-axis at the point $B(0, b)$. Then the point (–2, 6) divides the line AB in the ratio 3 : 2.

By section formula, we have

$$(-2, 6) \equiv \left(\frac{2a + 3\times 0}{2+3}, \frac{2\times 0 + 3\times b}{2+3}\right)$$

$$\Rightarrow \quad -2 = \frac{2a}{5} \text{ and } 6 = \frac{3b}{5}$$

or $\quad a = -5, b = 10.$

Putting the value of a and b in (1), the required equation of the line is

$$\frac{x}{-5} + \frac{y}{10} = 1$$

or $\quad y - 2x = 10$

12. *A straight line, drawn through the point A(2, 1) makes an angle $\frac{\pi}{4}$ with positive x-axis and intersects line $x + 2y + 1 = 0$ at point B. Find the length AB.* [UPTU(B.PHARMA)–2003]

SOLUTION. The equation of any line passing through the given point $A(2, 1)$ and making an angle $\dfrac{\pi}{4}$ with x-axis is

$$\frac{x-2}{\cos 45^\circ} = \frac{y-1}{\sin 45^\circ} = r(\text{say}) \quad ...(1)$$

where r represents the distance of any point B on this line from the given point $A(2, 1)$. The coordinates (x, y) of any point B on the line (1) are

$$(2+r\cos 45°, 1+r\sin 45°),$$

i.e., $\left(2+r.\frac{1}{\sqrt{2}}, 1+r.\frac{1}{\sqrt{2}}\right)$

If the point B lies on the line $x + 2y + 1 = 0$, then

$$\left(2+r.\frac{1}{\sqrt{2}}\right)+2\left(1+r.\frac{1}{\sqrt{2}}\right)+1=0$$

$$\left(5+r.\frac{3}{\sqrt{2}}\right)=0 \text{ or } r=-\frac{5}{3}\sqrt{2}$$

Hence, the length $AB=-\frac{5\sqrt{2}}{3}$

13. *Find the equation of the straight line which divides the line joining the point (2, 3) and (–5, 8) in the ratio 3 : 4 and is also perpendicular to it.*

[UPTU(B.PHARMA)–2006]

SOLUTION. The equation of the line joining the points (2, 3) and (–5, 8) is

$$y-3=\frac{8-3}{-5-2}(x-2)$$

or $\quad y-3=\frac{5}{-7}(x-2)$

$\Rightarrow -7y + 21 = 5x - 10$

$\Rightarrow \quad 5x + 7y = 31 \qquad \ldots(1)$

The slope of line (1) is $\frac{-5}{7}$ and so the slope of the line perpendicular to it will be $\frac{7}{5}$. The coordinates (h, k) of the point dividing line (1) in the ratio 3 : 4 are given by

$$h=\frac{3\times(-5)+4\times 2}{3+4}$$

and $\quad k=\frac{3\times 8+4\times 3}{3+4}$

i.e., $h = -1$ and $k=\frac{36}{7}$

Hence, the equation of the line passing through (h, k) and having slope $\frac{7}{5}$ is

$$y-k=\frac{7}{5}(x-h)$$

$\Rightarrow \quad y-\frac{36}{7}=\frac{7}{5}(x-(-1))$

or $\quad 49x - 35y + 229 = 0.$

14. *Find the equation of a line at a distance of 3 units from the origin such that the perpendicular from the origin to the line makes an angle $\tan^{-1}\left(\frac{3}{4}\right)$ with the positive direction of x-axis.*

[UPTU(B.PHARMA)–2006]

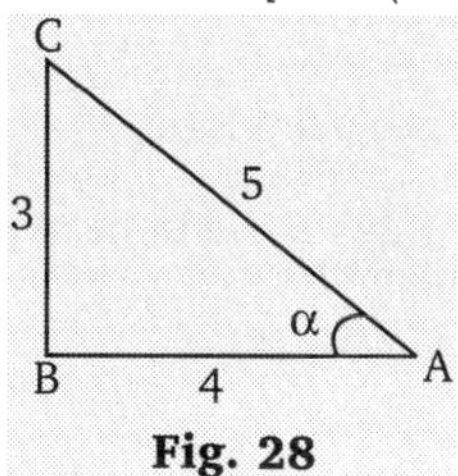

Fig. 28

SOLUTION. We have $p = 3$ and $\alpha=\tan^{-1}\frac{3}{4}$

$\Rightarrow \qquad \tan\alpha=\frac{3}{4}$

$\Rightarrow \qquad \cos\alpha=\frac{4}{5}$ and $\sin\alpha=\frac{3}{5}$

Hence, the equation of the line in normal form is

$$x\cos\alpha + y\sin\alpha = p$$

or $\quad x\times\frac{4}{5}+y\times\frac{3}{5}=3$

$\Rightarrow \qquad 4x + 3y = 15$

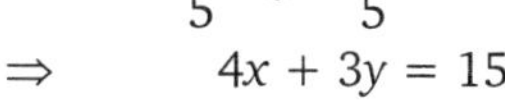

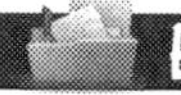

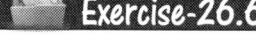

Exercise-26.6

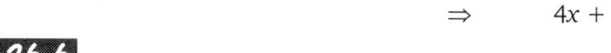

1. The x-intercept of a line is double to its y-intercept. If it passes through (2, 3), find its equation.
2. A line makes equal intercept on the coordinate axes and passes through (1, 3). Find its equation.
3. Find the equation of the line passing through the points (2, 3) and (–1, –4).
4. If length and inclination of the perpendicular from the origin on the line is 4 and 135° respectively. Find the equation of the line.
5. If $A(0, 2)$, $B(4, 1)$, $C(1, 3)$ are the vertices of a ΔABC, find the equation of (i) side AB (ii) median CF and (iii) attitude on side BC.

6. Find the equation of the line which passes through the point (–3, 8) and the sum of its intercept on the axes is 7.
7. Find the equation of the line through (2, 3) so that the segment of the line intercepted between the axes is bisected at this point.
8. The length of the perpendicular from the origin to a line is 6 and the line makes an angle of 30° with the positive direction of *y*-axis. Find the equation of the line.
9. Find the equation of the line through the point (2, 3) and making an angle of 45° with the *x*-axis. Also determine the length of intercept on it between *A* and the line $x + y + 1 = 0$.

Hint to Selected Problems

5. Given A = (0, 2), B(4, 1) and C(1, 3)

(i) Equation of *AB* is

$$\frac{y-2}{2-1}=\frac{x-0}{0-4}$$

$\Rightarrow \quad x + 4y = 8.$

$\therefore x + 4y = 8$ is the eq^n. of side *AB*.

(ii) Median *CF* :

$$F = \text{the mid of } AB = \left(\frac{0+4}{2},\frac{2+1}{2}\right)$$

$$F = \left(2,\frac{3}{2}\right) \text{ and } C = (1, 3)$$

Using two point form $\dfrac{y-y_1}{y_1-y_2}=\dfrac{x-x_1}{x_1-x_2}$

$\Rightarrow 3x + 2y - 9 = 0$ is the required equation of median *CF*.

(iii) Altitude $AD \perp BC$

Slope of $BC = \dfrac{3-1}{1-4} = -\dfrac{2}{3}$

Slope of $AD = \dfrac{3}{2} (\because AD \perp BC)$

Equation of *AD* is $y - y_1 = m(x - x_1)$

$$y-2=\frac{3}{2}(x-0)$$

$\Rightarrow 3x - 2y + 4 = 0.$

9.

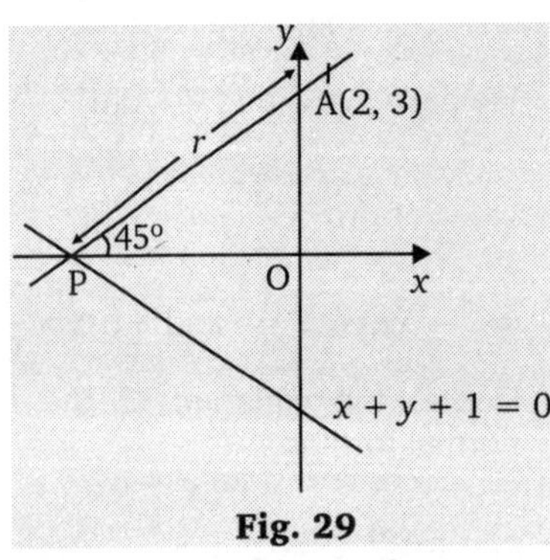

Fig. 29

The equation of a line through *A* and making an angle of 45° with the *x*-axis is

$$\frac{x-2}{\cos 45^\circ}=\frac{y-3}{\sin 45^\circ}$$

$$\Rightarrow \quad \frac{x-2}{\frac{1}{\sqrt{2}}}=\frac{y-3}{\frac{1}{\sqrt{2}}}$$

$\Rightarrow x - y + 1 = 0.$

Suppose the line meets the line $x + y + 1 = 0$ at *P* such that $AP = r$.

Then the coordinates of *P* are given by

$$\frac{x-2}{\cos 45^\circ}=\frac{y-3}{\sin 45^\circ}=r$$

$$\Rightarrow \quad x=2+\frac{r}{\sqrt{2}},\ y=3+\frac{r}{\sqrt{2}}$$

Thus, the coordinate of *P* are

$$\left(2+\frac{r}{\sqrt{2}},3+\frac{r}{\sqrt{2}}\right)$$

Since *P* lies on $x + y + 1 = 0$

$$\therefore\ 2+\frac{r}{\sqrt{2}}+3+\frac{r}{\sqrt{2}}+1=0$$

$$r=-3\sqrt{2}$$

$\Rightarrow$ length of $AP = |r| = 3\sqrt{2}$

Thus, the length of intercept $= 3\sqrt{2}$

ANSWERS

1. $x + 2y + 4 = 0$ **2.** $x + y + 4 = 0$ **3.** $7x - 3y + 2 = 0$ **4.** $x - y - 4\sqrt{2} = 0$

5. (i) $x + 4y = 8$ (ii) $3x + 2y - 9 = 0$ (iii) $3x - 2y + 4 = 0$ **6.** $4x + 3y = 12$

7. $3x + 2y - 12 = 0$ **8.** $\sqrt{3}x + y - 12 = 0$ **9.** $x - y + 1 = 0, 3\sqrt{2}$

26.12 TRANSFORMATION OF GENERAL EQUATION IN DIFFERENT STANDARD FORMS

The general equation of a straight line is $ax + by + c = 0$ which can be transformed to various standard forms as discussed below :

(1) *Transformation of $ax + by + c = 0$ in the slope intercept form ($y = mx + c$)*

We have $ax + by + c = 0 \Rightarrow by = -ax - c \Rightarrow \quad y = \left(-\frac{a}{b}\right)x + \left(-\frac{c}{b}\right)$

This is of the form $y = mx + c$, where $m = -\frac{a}{b}$ and $c = -\frac{c}{b}$

Thus, for the straight line $ax + by + c = 0$

$$m = \text{slope} = -\frac{a}{b} = -\frac{\text{coefficient of } x}{\text{coefficient of } y}$$

and $$y\text{-intercept} = -\frac{c}{b} = -\frac{\text{constant term}}{\text{coeff. of } y}$$

- To determine the slope of a line by the formula $m = -\frac{\text{coefficient of } x}{\text{coefficient of } y}$ we must transfer all terms in the equation on one side. Transformation of $Ax + By + C = 0$ intercept form $\left(\frac{x}{a} + \frac{y}{b} = 1\right)$:

We have $Ax + By + C = 0 \quad \Rightarrow \quad Ax + By = -C$

$$\Rightarrow \quad \frac{Ax}{-C} + \frac{By}{-C} = 1$$

$$\Rightarrow \quad \frac{x}{\left(-\frac{C}{A}\right)} + \frac{y}{\left(-\frac{C}{B}\right)} = 1.$$

This is of the form $\frac{x}{a} + \frac{y}{b} = 1$. Thus, for the straight line $Ax + By + C = 0$.

Intercept on x-axis $= \frac{-C}{A} = \frac{-\text{constant term}}{\text{coefficient of } x}$

Intercept on y-axis $= \frac{-C}{B} = \frac{-\text{constant term}}{\text{coefficient of } y}$

(2) *Transformation of $Ax + By + C = 0$ in normal form ($x\cos\alpha + y\sin\alpha = p$)*

We have $\quad Ax + By + C = 0 \quad \ldots(1)$

Let $\quad x\cos\alpha + y\sin\alpha - p = 0 \quad \ldots(2)$

be the normal form of $Ax + By + C = 0$. Then (1) and (2) represent the same straight line

$$\frac{A}{\cos\alpha} = \frac{B}{\sin\alpha} = \frac{C}{-p}$$

$$\Rightarrow \quad \cos\alpha = \frac{-Ap}{C} \text{ and } \sin\alpha = \frac{-Bp}{C} \quad \ldots(3)$$

$$\Rightarrow \cos^2\alpha + \sin^2\alpha = \frac{A^2p^2}{C^2} + \frac{B^2p^2}{C^2}$$

$$\Rightarrow \quad 1 = \frac{p^2}{C^2}(A^2 + B^2)$$

$$\Rightarrow \qquad p = \pm\frac{C}{\sqrt{A^2+B^2}}$$

But, p denotes the length of the perpendicular from the origin to the line and is always positive.

$$\therefore \qquad p = \frac{C}{\sqrt{A^2+B^2}}$$

Putting the value of p in (3) we get

$$\cos\alpha = \frac{-A}{\sqrt{A^2+B^2}}, \ \sin\alpha = \frac{-B}{\sqrt{A^2+B^2}}$$

So, the equation (2) takes the form

$$\frac{-A}{\sqrt{A^2+B^2}}x - \frac{B}{\sqrt{A^2+B^2}}y - \frac{C}{\sqrt{A^2+B^2}} = 0.$$

This is the required normal form of the line $Ax + By + C = 0$.

Solved Examples

1. *Reduce $3x - 4y + 5 = 0$ to slope form and find its intercept on y-axis.*

SOLUTION. The given equation $3x - 4y + 5 = 0$ can be written as

$$4y = 3x + 5$$

$$\Rightarrow \qquad y = \frac{3}{4}x + \frac{5}{4}$$

$$\text{Intercept on } y\text{-axis} = \frac{5}{4}$$

2. *Reduce the lines $3x - 4y + 4 = 0$ and $4x - 3y + 12 = 0$ to the normal form and hence determine which line is nearer to the origin.*

SOLUTION. We have $3x - 4y + 4 = 0$

$$\Rightarrow \qquad -3x + 4y = 4$$

$$\Rightarrow \qquad -\frac{3x}{\sqrt{(-3)^2+4^2}} + \frac{4y}{\sqrt{(-3)^2+4^2}} = \frac{4}{\sqrt{(-3)^2+4^2}}$$

$$\Rightarrow \qquad -\frac{3}{5}x + \frac{4}{5}y = \frac{4}{5}$$

This is the normal form of $3x - 4y + 4 = 0$ and the length of the perpendicular from the origin to it is given by

$$p_1 = \frac{4}{5}$$

Now $\quad 4x - 3y + 12 = 0$

$$-4x + 3y = 12$$

$$\Rightarrow \qquad \frac{-4x}{\sqrt{(-4)+3^2}} + \frac{3y}{\sqrt{(-4)^2+(3)^2}} = \frac{12}{\sqrt{(-4)+3^2}}$$

$$\Rightarrow \qquad -\frac{4}{5}x + \frac{3}{5}y = \frac{12}{5}$$

This is the normal form of $4x - 3y + 12 = 0$ and the length of the perpendicular from origin to it is given by $p_2 = \frac{12}{5}$.

Clearly $p_2 > p_1$ therefore, line $3x - 4y + 4 = 0$ is nearer to the origin.

26.13 POINT OF INTERSECTION OF TWO LINES

Let two lines be

$$A_1x + B_1y + C_1 = 0 \qquad \ldots(1)$$

$$A_2x + B_2y + C_2 = 0 \qquad \ldots(2)$$

Let (x_1, y_1) be the point of intersection of these two lines.

Then $\quad A_1x_1 + B_1y_1 + C_1 = 0 \qquad \ldots(3)$

and $\quad A_2x_1 + B_2y_1 + C_2 = 0$ ...(4)

From (3) and (4), we have

$$\frac{x_1}{B_1C_2 - B_2C_1} = \frac{y_1}{C_1A_2 - C_2A_1} = \frac{1}{A_1B_2 - A_2B_1}$$

$$\Rightarrow \quad x_1 = \frac{B_1C_2 - B_2C_1}{A_1B_2 - A_2B_1} \text{ and } y_1 = \frac{C_1A_2 - C_2A_1}{A_1B_2 - A_2B_1}$$

Hence, the coordinates of the point of intersection of the two lines (1) and (2) are

$$\left(\frac{B_1C_2 - B_2C_1}{A_1B_2 - A_2B_1}, \frac{C_1A_2 - C_2A_1}{A_1B_2 - A_2B_1}\right)$$

- To find the coordinates of the point of intersection of two non-parallel lines, we solve the given equations simultaneously and the values of x and y so obtained determine the coordinates of the point of intersection.
- The coordinates of the point of intersection determined above do not exist if

  $A_1B_2 - A_2B_1 = 0$, *i.e.*, if $\quad \frac{A_1}{A_2} = \frac{B_1}{B_2} \neq \frac{C_1}{C_2}$

- If $\frac{A_1}{A_2} = \frac{B_1}{B_2} = \frac{C_1}{C_2}$, then the lines are coincident.
- If there is only one point which satisfied both equation the system of equations is called consistent.

  In that case $\frac{A_1}{A_2} \neq \frac{B_1}{B_2} \neq \frac{C_1}{C_2}$.

26.14 CONDITION OF CONCURRENCY OF THREE GIVEN LINES

Let the equation of the three lines be

$$a_1x + b_1y + c_1 = 0 \quad \text{...(1)}$$

$$a_2x + b_2y + c_2 = 0 \quad \text{...(2)}$$

$$a_3x + b_3y + c_3 = 0 \quad \text{...(3)}$$

For given lines to be concurrent, no two of these lines can be parallel or coincident, *i.e.*,

$$\frac{a_1}{b_1} \neq \frac{a_2}{b_2} \neq \frac{a_3}{b_3} \quad \text{...(4)}$$

and the point of intersection of any two lines must lie on the third line.

Now, the point of intersection of (1) and (2) can be obtained as below:

$$\frac{x}{b_1c_2 - b_2c_1} = \frac{y}{c_1a_2 - a_1c_2} = \frac{1}{a_1b_2 - a_2b_1}$$

$$x = \frac{b_1c_2 - b_2c_1}{a_1b_2 - a_2b_1}$$

$$y = \frac{c_1a_2 - a_1c_2}{a_1b_2 - a_2b_1}$$

Now, the point $\left(\frac{b_1c_2 - b_2c_1}{a_1b_2 - a_2b_1}, \frac{c_1a_2 - a_1c_2}{a_1b_2 - a_2b_1}\right)$ lies on (3) because the lines are concurrent

$$a_3\left(\frac{b_1c_2 - b_2c_1}{a_1b_2 - a_2b_1}\right) + b_3\left(\frac{c_1a_2 - a_1c_2}{a_1b_2 - a_2b_1}\right) + c_3 = 0.$$

$\Rightarrow a_3(b_1c_2 - b_2c_1) + b_3(c_1a_2 - a_1c_2) + c_3(a_1b_2 - a_2b_1) = 0.$

$\Rightarrow a_1(b_2c_3 - b_3c_2) + b_1(c_2a_3 - a_2c_3) + c_1(a_2b_3 - a_3b_2) = 0.$ ...(5)

Thus, for the given three lines to be concurrent, the condition (4) and (5) must hold.

Solved Examples

1. *Find the coordinates of the point of intersection of the lines $2x - y + 3 = 0$ and $x + 2y - 4 = 0$.*

SOLUTION. Solving simultaneously the equation $2x - y + 3 = 0$ and $x + 2y - 4 = 0$, we obtain

$$\frac{x}{4-6} = \frac{y}{3+8} = \frac{1}{4+1}$$

$$\Rightarrow \frac{x}{-2} = \frac{y}{11} = \frac{1}{5} \Rightarrow x = \frac{-2}{5}, y = \frac{11}{5}.$$

Hence, $(-2/5, 11/5)$ is the required point of intersection.

2. *Show that lines $x - y - 6 = 0$, $4x - 3y - 20 = 0$ and $6x + 5y + 8 = 0$ are concurrent. Also, find their common point of intersection.*

SOLUTION. The given lines are

$x - y - 6 = 0$ ...(1)

$4x - 3y - 20 = 0$ ...(2)

$6x + 5y + 8 = 0$ ...(3)

Solving (1) and (2) by cross multiplication, we get

$$\frac{x}{20-18} = \frac{y}{-24+20} = \frac{1}{-3+4}$$

$$x = 2, y = -4$$

Thus, the two lines intersect at the point $(2, -4)$. Putting $x = 2, y = -4$ in (3), we get

$$6 \times 2 + 5 \times (-4) + 8 = 0$$

So $(2, -4)$ lies on (3).

Hence, the given lines are concurrent and their common point of intersection is $(2, -4)$.

3. *Find the value of k, so that the lines $x - 2y + 1 = 0$; $2x - 5y + 3 = 0$ and $5x - 4y + k = 0$ are concurrent.*

SOLUTION. The equation of the lines are :

$x - 2y + 1 = 0$ ...(1)

$2x - 5y + 3 = 0$ ...(2)

$5x - 4y + k = 0$ ...(3)

Solving (1) and (2) by cross multiplication method, we get

$$\frac{x}{-6+5} = \frac{y}{2-3} = \frac{1}{-5+4}$$

$$\Rightarrow \quad \frac{x}{-1} = \frac{y}{-1} = \frac{1}{-1}$$

$$\Rightarrow \quad x = 1, y = 1$$

$\therefore$ The point of intersection of (1) and (2) is $(1, 1)$.

This point will lie on (3) if $5 - 4 + k = 0$ or $k = -1$.

Thus, for concurrency of (1), (2) and (3), $k = -1$.

26.15 ANGLE BETWEEN TWO INTERSECTING LINES

THEOREM 1. *The angle θ between the line $y = m_1x + c_1$ and $y = m_2x + c_2$ is given by* $\tan\theta = \frac{m_1 - m_2}{1 + m_1m_2}$.

PROOF. Let l_1 and l_2 be two lines $y = m_1x + c_1$ and $y = m_2x + c_2$ respectively. Let l_1 intersect l_2 at P making an angle θ between them. Let l_1 and l_2 meet x-axis at R and Q respectively and l_1 and l_2 making an angle α and β respectively, with the positive direction of x-axis.

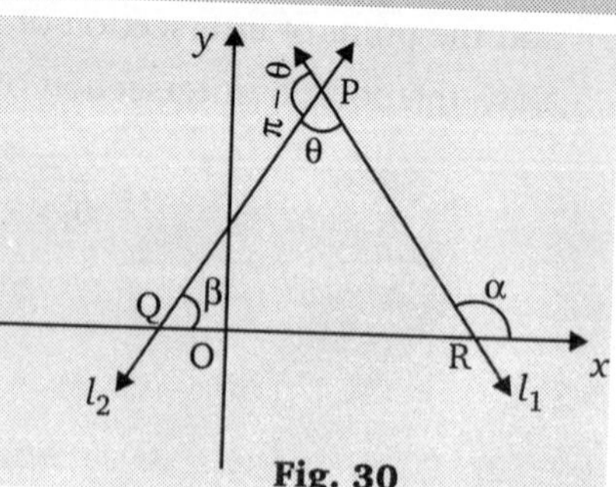

Fig. 30

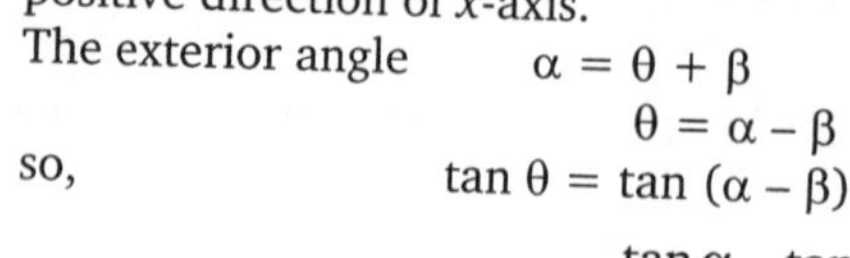

The exterior angle $\alpha = \theta + \beta$

$$\theta = \alpha - \beta$$

so, $\tan\theta = \tan(\alpha - \beta)$

$$\Rightarrow \quad \tan\theta = \frac{\tan\alpha - \tan\beta}{1 + \tan\alpha\tan\beta}$$

or $$\tan\theta = \frac{m_1 - m_2}{1 + m_1 m_2}$$

$\Rightarrow$ $$\theta = \tan^{-1}\frac{m_1 - m_2}{1 + m_1 m_2}$$

- The value of tan θ can be both positive and negative because between two lines there are two distinct angles. If this value is +ve, then the angle between the lines is acute and if it is –ve the angle is obtuse.

THEOREM 2. *The angle θ between the lines $a_1x + b_1y + c_1 = 0$ and $a_2x + b_2y + c_2 = 0$ is given by*

$$\tan\theta = \left|\frac{a_2b_1 - a_1b_2}{a_1a_2 + b_1b_2}\right|.$$

PROOF. Let m_1 and m_2 be the slopes of the lines $a_1x + b_1y + c_1 = 0$ and $a_2x + b_2y + c_2 = 0$. Then

$$m_1 = \frac{-a_1}{b_1} \text{ and } m_2 = \frac{-a_2}{b_2}$$

Now $$\tan\theta = \left|\frac{m_1 - m_2}{1 + m_1 m_2}\right|$$

$\Rightarrow$ $$\tan\theta = \left|\frac{-\frac{a_1}{b_1} + \frac{a_2}{b_2}}{1 + \left(-\frac{a_1}{b_1}\right)\left(-\frac{a_2}{b_2}\right)}\right|$$

$\Rightarrow$ $$\tan\theta = \left|\frac{a_2b_1 - a_1b_2}{a_1a_2 + b_1b_2}\right|$$

Hence $$\theta = \tan^{-1}\left|\frac{a_2b_1 - a_1b_2}{a_1a_2 + b_1b_2}\right|.$$

26.15.1 CONDITION OF PERPENDICULARITY

Two lines are perpendicular, if the angle between them is a right angle, *i.e.*, $\alpha = 90^\circ$

$$\tan\alpha = \tan 90^\circ = \infty$$

$\Rightarrow$ $$\frac{m_1 - m_2}{1 + m_1 m_2} = \infty$$

$\Rightarrow$ $$1 + m_1m_2 = 0$$

$\Rightarrow$ $$m_1m_2 = -1$$

Hence, two lines are perpendicular if the product of their slopes is –1.

26.15.2 CONDITION OF PARALLELISM

Two lines are parallel, if the angle between them is either 0 or π, *i.e.*, $\alpha = 0$ or π

$\therefore$ $$\tan\alpha = \tan 0 \text{ or } \tan\pi = 0$$

$\Rightarrow$ $$\frac{m_1 - m_2}{1 + m_1 m_2} = 0$$

$\Rightarrow$ $$m_1 - m_2 = 0$$

$\Rightarrow$ $$m_1 = m_2$$

Solved Examples

1. *Find the acute angle between the line $9x + 3y - 5 = 0$ and $2x + 4y + 3 = 0$.*

SOLUTION. We have $9x + 3y - 5 = 0$ ...(1)

$2x + 4y + 3 = 0$ ...(2)

Slope of (1) ⇒ $m_1 = -\frac{9}{3} = -3$

Slope of (2) ⇒ $m_2 = -\frac{2}{4} = -\frac{1}{2}$

The acute angle between the lines is given by

$$\tan\theta = \left|\frac{m_1 - m_2}{1 + m_1 m_2}\right|$$

$$\tan\theta = \left|\frac{-3 + 1/2}{1 + 3/2}\right|$$

$$\Rightarrow \quad \tan\theta = \left|\frac{-5}{5}\right| \quad \Rightarrow \quad \tan\theta = 1$$

$$\Rightarrow \quad \theta = 45^\circ.$$

2. *If A(–2, 1), B(2, 3) and C(–2, –4) are three points, find the angle between BA and BC.*

SOLUTION. Let m_1 and m_2 be the slope of BA and BC respectively. Then

$$m_1 = \frac{3-1}{2-(-2)} = \frac{2}{4} = \frac{1}{2}$$

and $m_2 = \frac{-4-3}{-2-2} = \frac{7}{4}$

Let θ be the angle between BA and BC. Then

$$\tan\theta = \left|\frac{m_1 - m_2}{1 + m_1 m_2}\right|$$

$$\Rightarrow \quad \left|\frac{7/4 - (1/2)}{1 + 7/4(1/2)}\right| = \left|\frac{10/8}{15/8}\right| = \pm\frac{2}{3}$$

$$\Rightarrow \quad \theta = \tan^{-1}\left(\frac{2}{3}\right).$$

3. *The angle between two lines is 45°. If the slope of one of them is 1/4. Find the slope of other.*

SOLUTION. Here, $\theta = 45^\circ$, $m_1 = 1/4$. Let the slope of the required line be m.

Now $\tan\theta = \left|\frac{m_1 - m}{1 + m_1 m}\right|$

$$\Rightarrow \quad \tan 45^\circ = \frac{|m_1 - m|}{1 + m_1 m}$$

$$\Rightarrow \quad 1 = \frac{|1/4 - m|}{1 + m/4}$$

$$\Rightarrow \quad 1 + \frac{m}{4} = \pm\left(\frac{1}{4} - m\right)$$

For +ve sign $1 + \frac{m}{4} = \frac{1}{4} - m$

$$\Rightarrow \quad \frac{5}{4}m = \frac{-3}{4} \quad \Rightarrow \quad m = \frac{-3}{5}$$

For –ve sign $1 + \frac{m}{4} = -\frac{1}{4} + m$

$$\Rightarrow \quad \frac{5}{4} = \frac{3}{4}m \quad \Rightarrow \quad m = \frac{5}{3}$$

The possible slope of the lines are

$$\frac{5}{3}, \frac{-3}{5}.$$

4. *Find the angle between the lines:*

$x - y\sqrt{3} - 5 = 0$ *and* $\sqrt{3}x + y - 7 = 0$

[UPTU–2001]

SOLUTION. The given two lines are:

$x - y\sqrt{3} - 5 = 0$ ...(1)

and $\sqrt{3}x + y - 7 = 0$ ...(2)

Here m_1 = Slope of the line (1)

$$= -\frac{1}{-\sqrt{3}} = \frac{1}{\sqrt{3}}$$

m_2 = Slope of the line (2)

$$= \frac{-\sqrt{3}}{1} = -\sqrt{3}$$

Clearly, $m_1 \times m_2 = -1$.

Hence, the two lines are at right angles.

5. *The line joining (–5, 7) and (0, –2) is perpendicular to the line joining (1, 3) and (4, x). Then find x.* [UPTU–2003]

SOLUTION. Here m_1 = Slope of the line joining the points (–5, 7) and (0, –2).

$$= \frac{-2-7}{0-(-5)} = \frac{-9}{5}.$$

and m_2 = Slope of the line joining the points (1, 3) and (4, x).

$$= \frac{x-3}{4-1} = \frac{x-3}{3}.$$

If the given two lines are perpendicular, then $m_1 m_2 = -1$

$$\Rightarrow \left(-\frac{9}{5}\right)\left(\frac{x-3}{3}\right) = -1$$

$$\Rightarrow -9(x-3) = -15$$

$$\Rightarrow x = 14/3.$$

26.15.3 Distance of a Point from a Line

Let $ax + by + c = 0$ be any equation of the line and $P(x_1, y_1)$ be any point in space, then the perpendicular distance d of the point p from the line is

$$d = \left|\frac{ax_1 + by_1 + c}{\sqrt{a^2 + b^2}}\right|$$

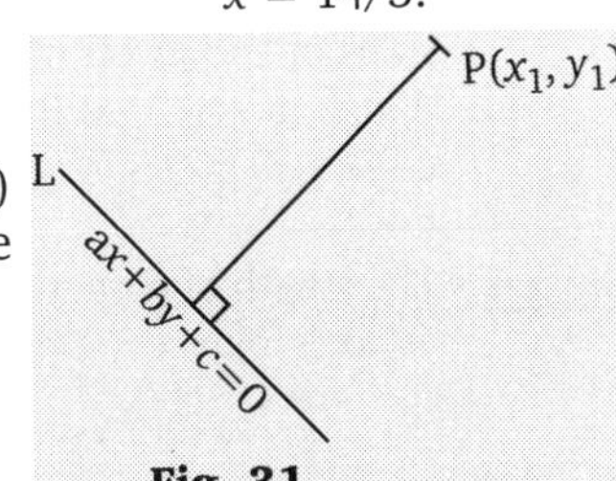

Fig. 31

26.15.4 Distance between Two Parallel Lines

Let $ax + by + c_1 = 0$ and $ax + by + c_2 = 0$ be two equation of parallel lines, then the distance between the two lines is given by

$$d = \left|\frac{c_2 - c_1}{\sqrt{a^2 + b^2}}\right|$$

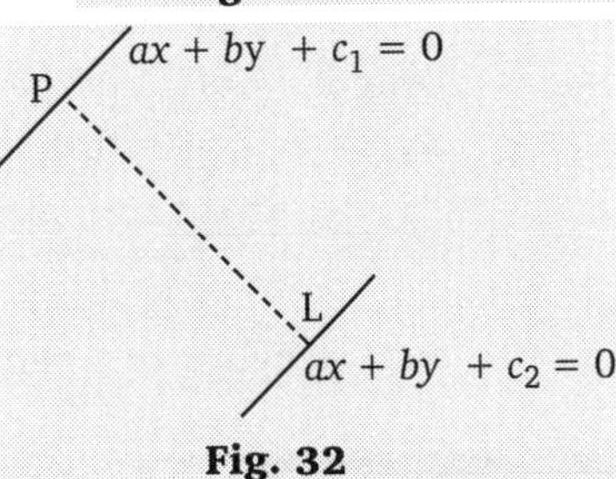

Fig. 32

Solved Examples

1. *Find the length of the perpendicular drawn from the point (–2, 3) on the line $12x - 5y + 1 = 0$.*

Solution. We know that the length of the perpendicular segment from point (x_1, y_1) on $ax + by + c = 0$ is

$$\left|\frac{ax_1 + by_1 + c}{\sqrt{a^2 + b^2}}\right|$$

$\therefore$ Here $a = 12, b = -5, c = 1, x_1 = -2, y_1 = 3$

$\therefore$ Length of the required perpendicular segment

$$= \left|\frac{12 \times (-2) + (-5) \times 3 + 1}{\sqrt{(12)^2 + (-5)^2}}\right|$$

$$= \left|\frac{-24 - 15 + 1}{13}\right| = \left|\frac{-38}{13}\right| = \frac{38}{13}.$$

2. *Find the distance between the parallel lines $2x - 3y + 9 = 0$ and $4x - 6y + 1 = 0$.*

Solution. As the given lines are parallel, they have same distance between them through out. So, we shall find the distance of any point on the first line from the second line. And (0, 3) is a point on the line $2x - 3y + 9 = 0$.

Perpendicular distance of the point (0, 3) from $4x - 6y + 1 = 0$ is

$$\left|\frac{4 \times 0 - 6 \times 3 + 1}{\sqrt{4^2 + (-6)^2}}\right| = \left|\frac{-17}{\sqrt{52}}\right| = \frac{17}{2\sqrt{13}}$$

Hence, the distance between the given lines is $\frac{17}{2\sqrt{13}}$.

3. *Are the points (2, –4) and (0, 5) on the same or opposite sides of the line $2x - 5y + 6 = 0$?*

Solution. Perpendicular distance of (2, – 4) from the given line is

$$P_1 = \frac{2 \times 2 - 5(-4) + 6}{\sqrt{4 + 25}}$$

$$= \frac{4 + 20 + 6}{\sqrt{29}} = \frac{30}{\sqrt{29}}. \qquad ...(1)$$

Perpendicular distance of (0, 5) from the given line is

$$P_2 = \frac{2 \times 0 - 5 \times 5 + 6}{\sqrt{4 + 25}} = \frac{-25 + 6}{\sqrt{29}}$$

$$= \frac{-19}{\sqrt{29}}. \qquad ...(2)$$

Since (1) and (2) are of opposite signs, therefore, the point are on opposite sides of the given line.

4. *Which of the lines $2x - y + 3 = 0$ and $x - 4y - 7 = 0$ is farther from the origin?* [RGPV–2001]

SOLUTION. The length of perpendicular from (x_1, y_1) on $ax + by + c = 0$ is

$$= \left|\frac{ax_1 + by_1 + c}{\sqrt{a^2 + b^2}}\right|$$

Length of perpendicular of $2x - y + 3 = 0$ from origin

$$p_1 = \left|\frac{2 \times 0 - 0 + 3}{\sqrt{4+1}}\right| = \frac{3}{\sqrt{5}}.$$

and length of perpendicular of $x - 4y - 7 = 0$ from origin

$$p_2 = \left|\frac{0 - 4 \times 0 - 7}{\sqrt{1+16}}\right| = \frac{7}{\sqrt{17}}.$$

as $p_1 > p_2$

$\therefore$ $2x - y + 3 = 0$ is farther from origin.

5. *Find the distance between the two parallel straight lines $y = mx + c$ and $y = mx + d$.* [RGPV–2002]

SOLUTION. Putting $y = 0$ in $y = mx + c$, we get $x = -c/m$. Thus $\left(-\frac{c}{m}, 0\right)$ is a point on the line $y = mx + c$. Length of perpendicular from $\left(-\frac{c}{m}, 0\right)$ to $y = mx + d$ is given by

$$p = \left|\frac{m \times -\frac{c}{m} - 0 + d}{\sqrt{m^2 + 1}}\right| = \left|\frac{d - c}{\sqrt{m^2 + 1}}\right|$$

Exercise-26.7

1. Find the length of the perpendicular from the origin on the line $4x - 3y = 7$.
2. Find the distance of the point $(3, -2)$ from the line $7x - 5y - 29 = 0$. Determine whether the point lies on the origin side of the line.
3. For what value of k will the point $(3, k)$ lie on the origin side of the line $2x + 3y + 6 = 0$.
4. Find the foot of the perpendicular drawn from the point $(-2, -1)$ on to the line $3x + 2y - 5 = 0$.
5. Show that the point $(1, 2)$ is equidistant from the lines $5x - 2y - 9 = 0$ and $5x - 2y + 7 = 0$.
6. Find the distance between the pair of parallel lines $2x - 3y + 4 = 0$ and $4x - 6y - 5 = 0$.
7. If a and b are the intercepts of a line on the x and y axis respectively and P be its perpendicular distance from the origin then show that $\frac{1}{p^2} = \frac{1}{a^2} + \frac{1}{b^2}$.

Hint to Selected Problems

4. Let $P(-2, -1) = (x_1, y_1)$ and $M = (h, k)$ be the foot of the perpendicular on to $3x + 2y - 5 = 0$. Now (h, k) are given by

$$\frac{h - x_1}{a} = \frac{k - y_1}{b} = -\frac{(ax_1 + by_1 + c)}{a^2 + b^2}$$

$$\Rightarrow \frac{h+2}{3} = \frac{k+1}{2} = \frac{-(-6-2-5)}{9+4}$$

$$\Rightarrow \frac{h+2}{3} = \frac{k+1}{2} = 1$$

$\Rightarrow$ $h + 2 = 3, k + 1 = 2$

$\Rightarrow$ $h = 1, k = 1$

$\therefore$ The foot of perpendicular $(1, 1)$.

7. $\frac{x}{a} + \frac{y}{b} = 1 = bx + ay = ab$

$\Rightarrow bx + ay - ab = 0 \qquad ...(1)$

$$p = \left|\frac{-ab}{\sqrt{a^2 + b^2}}\right| = p^2 = \frac{a^2 \times b^2}{a^2 + b^2}$$

$$\Rightarrow \frac{1}{p^2} = \frac{a^2 + b^2}{a^2 \times b^2} = \frac{1}{a^2} + \frac{1}{b^2}.$$

ANSWERS

1. 7/5 **2.** $\frac{2}{\sqrt{74}}$, origin lie on the opposite side of the line **3.** $k < 4$ **4.** (1, 1) **6.** $\frac{\sqrt{13}}{2}$

□□□□□□

Chapter

27 Fourier Series

27.1 INTRODUCTION

In this chapter, we shall study a special type of functional series extensively studied by Joseph Fourier. Joseph Fourier represented expansions in trigonometrical series in connection with boundary value problem in conduction of heat. Although such expansions had been studied earlier, these series bear the name 'Fourier series'because of the major contributions of Fourier in this field.

27.2 PERIODIC FUNCTIONS

A function $f(x)$ which satisfies the relation $f(x + T) = f(x)$for all real x and some fixed T is called a periodic function. The smallest positive number T, for which this relation holds, is called the period of $f(x)$.

If T is the period of $f(x)$. Then

$$f(x) = f(x + T) = f(x + 2T) = \ldots = f(x + nT) = \ldots$$

Also, $$f(x) = f(x - T) = f(x - 2T) = \ldots = f(x - nT) = \ldots$$

$\therefore$ $$f(x) = f(x \pm nT), \text{ where } n \text{ is a positive integer.}$$

For example: Consider the function $f(x) = \sin x$. We have

$$\sin x = \sin (x + 2\pi) = \sin (x + 4\pi) = \ldots.$$

Here, $f(x) = \sin x$ is a periodic function with period 2π. This function is also called sinusoidal periodic function.

We have studied about the Macluarian's theorem which is used to expand a function provided the function's derivative are continuous. Now, the need arise to expand functions which have discontinuities in their derivatives. By Fourier series, we can expand both types of functions under certain conditions as an infinite series of sine and cosine of x and it's integral multiple of a function $f(x)$ is defined in the interval $c < x < c + 2\pi$.

Then, Fourier series of $f(x)$ is given by

$$f(x) = \frac{a_0}{2} + \sum_{n=1}^{\infty} a_n \cos nx + \sum_{n=1}^{\infty} b_n \sin nx \quad \ldots(1)$$

where a_0, a_n and b_n are called Fourier coefficient of $f(x)$ and their values are given as :

$$a_0 = \frac{1}{\pi} \int_c^{c+2\pi} f(x)dx \quad \ldots(2)$$

$$a_n = \frac{1}{\pi} \int_c^{c+2\pi} f(x)\cos nx\, dx \quad \ldots(3)$$

$$b_n = \frac{1}{\pi} \int_c^{c+2\pi} f(x)\sin nx\, dx \quad \ldots(4)$$

The series (1) with coefficients a_0, a_n and b_n given by (2), (3) and (4) respectively is called the Fourier series of $f(x)$ and the coefficients a_0, a_n and b_n are called the Fourier coefficients corresponding to $f(x)$.

(i) When $c = 0$, the interval becomes $0 < x < 2\pi$ and formula for a_0, a_n, b_n is obtained by putting $c = 0$.

(ii) When $c = -\pi$, then interval becomes $-\pi < x < \pi$. In this interval, the formula for a_0, a_n and b_n becomes as under :

(a) When $f(x)$ is an odd function, then

$$a_0 = \frac{1}{\pi}\int_{-\pi}^{\pi} f(x)dx = 0$$

$$a_n = \frac{1}{\pi}\int_{-\pi}^{\pi} f(x)\cos nx\,dx = 0 \quad \text{[By property of definite integral]}$$

$$b_n = \frac{1}{\pi}\int_{-\pi}^{\pi} f(x)\sin nx\,dx = \frac{2}{\pi}\int_{0}^{\pi} f(x)\sin x dx$$

Hence, if function $f(x)$ is odd, its Fourier expansion contains only sine series,

i.e., $$f(x) = \sum_{n=1}^{\infty} b_n \sin nx, \text{where } b_n = \frac{2}{\pi}\int_0^{\pi} f(x)\sin nx\,dx.$$

(b) When $f(x)$ is even function, then formula for a_0, a_n and b_n are given by

$$a_0 = \frac{1}{\pi}\int_{-\pi}^{\pi} f(x)dx = \frac{2}{\pi}\int_0^{\pi} f(x)dx$$

$$a_n = \frac{1}{\pi}\int_{-\pi}^{\pi} f(x)\cos nx\,dx = \frac{2}{\pi}\int_0^{\pi} f(x)\cos nx\,dx$$

and $$b_n = \frac{1}{\pi}\int_{-\pi}^{\pi} f(x)\sin nx\,dx = 0 \quad [\because f(x) \sin nx \text{ is odd.}]$$

Hence, if a periodic function $f(x)$ is even, its Fourier expansion contains only cosine terms,

i.e., $f(x) = \frac{a_0}{2} + \sum_{n=1}^{\infty}\int_0^{\pi} f(x)dx$, where

$$a_0 = \frac{2}{\pi}\int_0^{\pi} f(x)dx \text{ and } a_n = \frac{2}{\pi}\int_0^{\pi} f(x).\cos nx\,dx$$

27.3 SOME IMPORTANT RESULTS

The following results are useful in the Fourier series :

(i) $\sin n\pi = 0, \cos n\pi = (-1)^n, \cos\left(n+\frac{1}{2}\right)\pi = 0$, where $n \in \mathbf{Z}$.

(ii) $\int uv = uv_1 - u'v_2 + u''v_3 - u'''v_4 + \ldots$, where $u' = \frac{du}{dx}, u'' = \frac{d^2u}{dx^2}, \ldots$ $v_1 = \int v dx, v_2 = \int v_1 dx, \ldots$

(iii) $\int_0^{2\pi} \sin nx\,dx = 0$ (iv) $\int_0^{2\pi} \cos nx\,dx = 0$

(v) $\int_0^{2\pi} \sin^2 nx\,dx = \pi$ (vi) $\int_0^{2\pi} \cos^2 nx\,dx = \pi$

(vii) $\int_0^{2\pi} \sin nx.\sin mx\, dx = 0$ (viii) $\int_0^{2\pi} \cos nx.\cos mx\, dx = 0$

(ix) $\int_0^{2\pi} \sin nx.\cos mx\, dx = 0$ (x) $\int_0^{2\pi} \sin mx.\cos nx\, dx = 0$

(xi) $\int e^{ax} \sin bx\, dx = \dfrac{e^{ax}}{a^2+b^2}(a \sin bx - b \cos bx) + c$

(xii) $\int e^{ax} \cos bx\, dx = \dfrac{e^{ax}}{a^2+b^2}(a \cos bx + b \sin bx) + c$

27.4 DETERMINATION OF FOURIER COEFFICIENTS: EULER'S FORMULAE

The fourier series is given by

$$f(x) = \frac{a_0}{2} + a_1 \cos x + a_2 \cos 2x + \dots + a_n \cos nx$$
$$+ b_1 \sin x + \dots + b_2 \sin 2x + \dots + b_n \sin nx + \dots$$

or $$f(x) = \frac{a_0}{2} + \sum_{n=1}^{\infty} a_n \cos nx + \sum_{n=1}^{\infty} b_n \sin nx. \quad \text{...(i)}$$

To find a_0 : Integrating both sides of equation (1) from $x = c+0, x = c+2\pi$

$$\int_c^{c+2\pi} f(x)dx = \frac{a_0}{2}\int_c^{c+2\pi} dx + \int_c^{c+2\pi}\left(\sum_{n=1}^{\infty} a_n \cos nx\right)dx + \int_c^{c+2\pi}\left(\sum_{n=1}^{\infty} b_n \sin nx\right)dx$$

$$= \frac{a_0}{2}(c + 2\pi - c) + 0 + 0 = a_0\pi$$

$$\Rightarrow \quad a_0 = \frac{1}{\pi}\int_c^{c+2\pi} f(x)dx.$$

To find a_n : Multipling each side of equation (1) by cos nx and integrate w.r.t. x., between the limit c to $c+2\pi$.

$$\int_c^{c+2\pi} f(x)\cos nx\, dx = \frac{a_0}{2}\int_c^{c+2\pi} \cos nx\, dx + \int_c^{c+2\pi}\left(\sum_{n=1}^{\infty} a_n \cos nx\right)\cos nx\, dx + \int_c^{c+2\pi}\left(\sum_{n=1}^{\infty} b_n \sin nx\right)\cos nx\, dx$$

$$= 0 + a_n\pi + 0 = a_n\pi$$

$$\Rightarrow \quad a_n = \frac{1}{\pi}\int_c^{c+2\pi} f(x)\cos nx\, dx.$$

To find b_n : Multiplying each side of equation (1) by sin nx and integrate w.r.t. x between the limit c to $c + 2\pi$.

$$\int_c^{c+2\pi} f(x)\sin nx\, dx = \frac{a_0}{2}\int_c^{c+2\pi} \sin nx dx + \int_c^{c+2\pi}\left(\sum_{n=1}^{\infty} a_n \cos nx\right)\sin nx\, dx + \int_c^{c+2\pi}\left(\sum_{n=1}^{\infty} b_n \sin nx\right)\sin nx\, dx$$

$$= 0 + 0 + b_n\pi = b_n\pi$$

$$\Rightarrow \quad b_n = \frac{1}{\pi}\int_c^{c+2\pi} f(x)\sin nx\, dx$$

These values of a_0, a_n and b_n are called Euler's formulae.

27.5 DIRICHLET'S CONDITIONS

Any function $f(x)$ can be expressed as a Fourier series
$\frac{a_0}{2} + \sum_{n=1}^{\infty} a_n \cos nx + \sum_{n=1}^{\infty} b_n \sin nx$, where a_0, a_n and b_n are constants.

(i) $f(x)$ is finite and single valued in the interval $c < x < c + 2\pi$.
(ii) $f(x)$ is periodic with period 2π
(iii) $f(x)$ and $f'(x)$ are piecewise continuous in the interval $c < x < c + 2\pi$.

The Fourier series with its coefficients converge to

(a) $f(x)$ if x is a point of continuity.
(b) $\frac{f(x+0)+f(x-0)}{2}$, if x is a point of discontinuity.

- The conditions (i), (ii) and (iii) imposed on $f(x)$ are sufficient but not necessary. *i.e.*, if the conditions are satisfied, the convergence is guranteed. However, if they are not satisfied the series may or may not converge.

Solved Examples

1. *Expand the function $f(x) = x \sin x$ as a Fourier series in interval $-\pi \le x \le \pi$. Deduce that*

$$\frac{1}{1.3} - \frac{1}{3.5} + \frac{1}{5.7} - \frac{1}{7.9} + \ldots = \frac{\pi - 2}{4}$$

SOLUTION. Since $x \sin x$ is an even function of x, so $b_n = 0$, then Fourier series is given by

$$f(x) = x \sin x = \frac{a_0}{2} + \sum_{n=1}^{\infty} a_n \cos nx,$$

where $a_0 = \frac{2}{\pi}\int_0^{\pi} x \sin x dx$

$$= \frac{2}{\pi}[-x\cos x + \sin x]_0^{\pi}$$

$$= \frac{2}{\pi}(-\pi \cos \pi) = 2$$

$$a_n = \frac{2}{\pi}\int_0^{\pi} x \sin x \cos nx \, dx$$

$$= \frac{1}{\pi}\int_0^{\pi} x.2\cos nx \sin x \, dx$$

$$= \frac{1}{\pi}\int_0^{\pi} x\{\sin(n+1)x - \sin(n-1)x\}dx$$

$$= \frac{1}{\pi}\left[x\left\{\frac{-\cos(n+1)x}{n+1} + \frac{\cos(n+1)x}{n-1}\right\} -1\left\{\frac{-\sin(n+1)x}{(n+1)^2} + \frac{\sin(n-1)x}{(n+1)^2}\right\}\right]_0^{\pi}$$

$$= \frac{1}{\pi}\left[\pi\left\{\frac{-\cos(n+1)\pi}{n+1} + \frac{\cos(n-1)\pi}{n-1}\right\}\right]$$

$$= \frac{\cos(n-1)\pi}{n-1} - \frac{\cos(n+1)\pi}{n+1}; n \ne 1$$

$$= \begin{cases} \frac{1}{n-1} - \frac{1}{n+1} = \frac{2}{n^2-1} & \text{if } n \text{ is odd } n \ne 1 \\ \frac{-1}{n-1} + \frac{1}{n+1} = \frac{-2}{n^2-1} & \text{if } n \text{ is even} \end{cases}$$

When $n=1$, then

$$a_1 = \frac{2}{\pi}\int_0^{\pi} x \sin x \cos x dx$$

$$= \frac{1}{\pi}\int_0^{\pi} x \sin 2x dx$$

$$= \frac{1}{\pi}\left[x\left(\frac{-\cos 2x}{2}\right) - \left(\frac{-\sin 2x}{4}\right)\right]_0^{\pi}$$

$$= \frac{1}{\pi}\left[\frac{-\pi\cos 2\pi}{2}\right] = -\frac{1}{2}$$

$$\therefore \; x \sin x = 1 - \frac{1}{2}\cos x - 2\left[\frac{\cos 2x}{2^2-1} - \frac{\cos 3x}{3^2-1} + \frac{\cos 4x}{4^2-1} - \frac{\cos 5x}{5^2-1} + \ldots\right]$$

Putting $x = \frac{\pi}{2}$, we get

$$\frac{\pi}{2} = 1 - 2\left(\frac{-1}{2^2-1} + \frac{1}{4^2-1} - \frac{1}{6^2-1} + \ldots\right)$$

$$\Rightarrow \frac{\pi}{2} - 1 = 2\left(\frac{1}{3} - \frac{1}{15} + \frac{1}{35} - \ldots\right)$$

$$\Rightarrow \frac{\pi - 2}{4} = \left(\frac{1}{1.3} - \frac{1}{3.5} + \frac{1}{5.7} - \ldots.\right).$$

2. *Find the Fourier series to represent e^{ax} in interval $-\pi < x < \pi$.*

SOLUTION. Let $f(x) = e^{ax}$

$$= \frac{a_0}{2} + \sum_{n=1}^{\infty} a_n \cos nx + \sum_{n=1}^{\infty} b_n \sin nx$$

$$a_0 = \frac{1}{\pi}\int_{-\pi}^{\pi} f(x)\,dx = \frac{1}{\pi}\int_{-\pi}^{\pi} e^{ax}\,dx$$

$$= \frac{1}{\pi}\left[\frac{e^{ax}}{a}\right]_{-\pi}^{\pi}$$

$$= \frac{1}{a\pi}(e^{a\pi} - e^{-a\pi}) = \frac{2\sinh a\pi}{\pi a}$$

$$a_n = \frac{1}{\pi}\int_{-\pi}^{\pi} f(x)\cos nx\,dx$$

$$= \frac{1}{\pi}\int_{-\pi}^{\pi} e^{ax}\cos nx\,dx$$

$$= \left[\frac{e^{ax}}{\pi(a^2+n^2)} a\cos nx + a\sin nx\right]_{-\pi}^{\pi}$$

$$= \frac{a\cos n\pi(e^{a\pi} - e^{-a\pi})}{\pi(a^2+n^2)}$$

$$= \frac{2a(-1)^n \sinh a\pi}{\pi(a^2+n^2)}$$

Similarly, we can set

$$b_n = \frac{2n(-1)^n \sinh a\pi}{\pi(a^2+n^2)}$$

$$\therefore\ e^{ax} = \frac{\sinh a\pi}{a\pi} + \sum_{n=1}^{\infty}\frac{2a(-1)^n \sinh a\pi}{\pi(a^2+n^2)}\cos nx + \sum_{n-1}^{\infty}\frac{2n(-1)^n \sinh a\pi}{\pi(a^2+n^2)}\sin n\pi$$

$$= \frac{2\sinh a\pi}{\pi}\left[\frac{1}{2a} - a\left(\frac{\cos x}{a^2+1^2} - \frac{\cos 2x}{a^2+2^2} + \frac{\cos 3x}{a^2+3^2} - \ldots\right) - \left(\frac{\sin x}{a^2+1^2} - \frac{2\sin 2x}{a^2+2^2} + \frac{3\sin 3x}{a^2+3^2} - \ldots\right)\right]$$

3. *Obtain the Fourier series for the function $f(x) = x^2, -\pi < x < \pi$. Sketch the graph f function f(x). Hence, show that*

(i) $\frac{1}{1^2} + \frac{1}{2^2} + \frac{1}{3^2} + \frac{1}{4^2} + \ldots = \sum_{n=1}^{\infty}\frac{1}{n^2} = \frac{\pi^2}{6}$

(ii) $\frac{1}{1^2} - \frac{1}{2^2} + \frac{1}{3^2} - \frac{1}{4^2} + \ldots = \frac{\pi^2}{12}$

(iii) $\frac{1}{1^2} + \frac{1}{3^2} + \frac{1}{5^2} + \ldots = \sum_{n=1}^{\infty}\frac{1}{(2n-1)^2} = \frac{\pi^2}{8}$

SOLUTION. $f(x) = x^2$ is an even function, therefore $b_n = 0$

Now $f(x) = x^2 = \frac{a_0}{2} + \sum_{n=1}^{\infty} a_n \cos nx.$

Then $a_0 = \frac{2}{\pi}\int_0^{\pi} f(x)\,dx = \frac{2}{\pi}\int_0^{\pi} x^2\,dx$

$$= \frac{2}{\pi}\left[\frac{x^3}{3}\right]_0^{\pi} = \frac{2}{3}\pi^2$$

$$a_n = \frac{2}{\pi}\int_0^{\pi} f(x)\cos nx\,dx = \frac{2}{\pi}\int_0^{\pi} x^2\cos nx\,dx$$

$$= \frac{2}{\pi}\left[x^2\left(\frac{\sin nx}{n}\right) - 2x\left(\frac{-\cos nx}{n^2}\right) + 2\left(\frac{-\sin nx}{n^2}\right)\right]_0^{\pi}$$

$$= \frac{2}{\pi}\left[2\pi\frac{\cos n\pi}{n^2}\right] = 4\frac{(-1)^n}{n^2}$$

$$\therefore\ x^2 = \frac{\pi^2}{3} - 4\left(\frac{\cos x}{1^2} - \frac{\cos 2x}{2^2} + \frac{\cos 3x}{3^2} - \frac{\cos 4x}{4^2} + \ldots\right)$$

$$x^2 = \frac{\pi^2}{3} + 4\sum_{n=1}^{\infty}\frac{(-1)^n}{n^2}\cos nx \quad \ldots (1)$$

Put $x=\pi$ in (1), we get

$$\pi^2 = \frac{\pi^2}{3} - 4\left(-\frac{1}{1^2} - \frac{1}{2^2} - \frac{1}{3^2} - \frac{1}{4^2} - \ldots\right)$$

$$\Rightarrow \frac{2\pi^2}{3} = -4\left(-\frac{1}{1^2} - \frac{1}{2^2} - \frac{1}{3^2} - \frac{1}{4^2} - \ldots\right)$$

$$\therefore \frac{1}{1^2}+\frac{1}{2^2}+\frac{1}{3^2}+\frac{1}{4^2}...=\frac{\pi^2}{6} \quad ...(2)$$

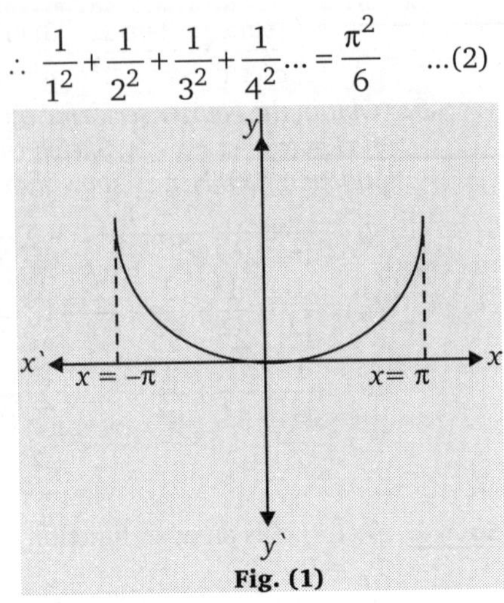

Fig. (1)

Put $x = 0$ in (1), we get

$$0=\frac{\pi^2}{3}-4\left(-\frac{1}{1^2}-\frac{1}{2^2}-\frac{1}{3^2}-\frac{1}{4^2}-...\right)$$

$$\therefore \frac{1}{1^2}-\frac{1}{2^2}-\frac{1}{3^2}-\frac{1}{4^2}-...=\frac{\pi^2}{12} \quad ...(3)$$

Adding (2) and (3), we get

$$\frac{\pi^2}{4}=2\left(\frac{1}{1^2}+\frac{1}{3^2}+\frac{1}{5^2}+...\right)$$

$$\therefore \frac{1}{1^2}+\frac{1}{3^2}+\frac{1}{5^2}+...=\frac{\pi^2}{8}.$$

4. *Obtain the Fouries series for $f(x) = e^{-x}$ in the interval $0 < x < 2\pi$.*

SOLUTION. Let $f(x) = e^{-x}$. The Fourier series of $f(x)$ can be written as

$$f(x)=e^{-x}=\frac{a_0}{2}+\sum_{n=1}^{\infty} a_n \cos nx + \sum_{n=1}^{\infty} b_n \sin nx$$

Then, $$a_0=\frac{1}{\pi}\int_0^{2\pi} f(x)dx=\frac{1}{\pi}\int_0^{2\pi} e^{-x}dx$$

$$=\frac{1}{\pi}.\left[-e^{-x}\right]_0^{2\pi}=\frac{1-e^{-2\pi}}{\pi}$$

$$a_n=\frac{1}{\pi}\int_0^{2\pi} f(x)\cos nx\,dx$$

$$=\frac{1}{\pi}\int_0^{2\pi} e^{-x}\cos nx\,dx$$

$$=\frac{1}{\pi(1+n^2)}[e^{-x}(-\cos nx+n\sin nx)]_0^{2\pi}$$

$$=\frac{1-e^{-2\pi}}{\pi(1+n^2)}$$

$$b_n=\frac{1}{\pi}\int_0^{2\pi} f(x)\sin nx\,dx$$

$$=\frac{1}{\pi}\int_0^{2\pi} e^{-x}\sin nx\,dx$$

$$=\left[\frac{e^{-x}}{\pi(1+n^2)}-\sin nx-n\cos nx\right]_0^{2\pi}$$

$$=\frac{1-e^{-2\pi}}{\pi}.\frac{n}{1+n^2}$$

$$\therefore e^{-x}=\frac{1-e^{-2\pi}}{\pi}\left[\frac{1}{2}+\left(\frac{1}{2}\cos x+\frac{1}{5}\cos 2x+\frac{1}{10}\cos 3x+...\right)\right]$$

$$+\left(\frac{1}{2}\sin x+\frac{2}{5}\sin 2x+\frac{3}{10}\sin 3x+...\right)$$

$$=\frac{1-e^{-2\pi}}{2\pi}+\frac{1-e^{-2\pi}}{\pi}\sum_{n=1}^{\infty}\frac{\cos nx}{1+n^2}+\frac{1-e^{-2\pi}}{\pi}\sum_{n=1}^{\infty}\frac{n\sin nx}{1+n^2}$$

5. *Find the Fourier series of the function defined as*

$$f(x)=\begin{cases} x+\pi & ; \quad 0\le x\le \pi \\ -x-\pi & ; \quad -\pi\le x\le 0\end{cases}$$ *and*

$f(x + 2\pi) = f(x)$

SOLUTION. Let $$f(x)=\frac{a_0}{2}+\sum_{n=1}^{\infty} a_n \cos nx + \sum_{n=1}^{\infty} b_n \sin nx$$

Then, $$a_0=\frac{1}{\pi}\int_{-\pi}^{\pi} f(x)dx$$

$$=\frac{1}{\pi}\int_{-\pi}^{0} f(x)dx+\frac{1}{\pi}\int_0^{\pi} f(x)dx$$

$$=\frac{1}{\pi}\int_{-\pi}^{0}(-x-\pi)dx+\frac{1}{\pi}\int_0^{\pi}(x+\pi)dx$$

$$= \frac{1}{\pi}\left[\left(-\frac{x^2}{2} - \pi x\right)_{-\pi}^{0} + \left(\frac{x^2}{2} + \pi x\right)_{0}^{\pi}\right]$$

$$= \frac{1}{\pi}\left\{\left(\frac{\pi^2}{2} - \pi^2\right) + \left(\frac{\pi^2}{2} + \pi^2\right)\right\} = \pi$$

$$a_n = \frac{1}{\pi}\int_{-\pi}^{\pi} f(x)\cos nx\, dx$$

$$= \frac{1}{\pi}\int_{-\pi}^{0} f(x).\cos nx\, dx + \frac{1}{\pi}\int_{0}^{\pi} f(x).\cos nx\, dx$$

$$= \frac{1}{\pi}\int_{-\pi}^{0} (-x-\pi)\cos nx\, dx + \frac{1}{\pi}\int_{0}^{\pi} (x+\pi)\cos nx\, dx$$

$$= \frac{1}{\pi}\left[(-x-\pi)\frac{\sin nx}{n} - (-1)\left\{-\frac{\cos nx}{n^2}\right\}\right]_{-\pi}^{0} + \frac{1}{\pi}\left[(x+\pi)\frac{\sin nx}{n} - (-1)\left\{-\frac{\cos nx}{n^2}\right\}\right]_{0}^{\pi}$$

$$= \frac{1}{\pi}\left[-\frac{1}{n^2} + \frac{(-1)^n}{n^2}\right] + \frac{1}{\pi}\left[\frac{(-1)^n}{n^2} - \frac{1}{n^2}\right]$$

$$= \frac{2}{n^2\pi}[(-1)^n - 1]$$

$$= \begin{cases} -\dfrac{4}{n^2\pi} & ; \text{ if } n \text{ is odd} \\ 0 & ; \text{ if } n \text{ is even} \end{cases}$$

Also, $b_n = \frac{1}{\pi}\int_{-\pi}^{\pi} f(x)\sin nx\, dx$

$$= \frac{1}{\pi}\left\{\int_{-\pi}^{0} f(x).\sin nx\, dx + \int_{0}^{\pi} f(x).\sin nx\, dx\right\}$$

$$= \frac{1}{\pi}\left\{\int_{-\pi}^{0} (-x-\pi)\sin nx\, dx + \int_{0}^{\pi} (x+\pi)\sin nx\, dx\right\}$$

$$= \frac{1}{\pi}\left[(-x-\pi)\left(-\frac{\cos nx}{n}\right) - (-1)\left\{-\frac{\sin nx}{n^2}\right\}\right]_{-\pi}^{0} + \frac{1}{\pi}\left[(x+\pi)\left(-\frac{\cos nx}{n}\right) - (-1)\left\{-\frac{\sin nx}{n^2}\right\}\right]_{0}^{\pi}$$

$$= \frac{1}{\pi}\left[\frac{\pi}{n}\right] + \frac{1}{\pi}\left[\frac{-2\pi}{n}(-1)^n + \frac{\pi}{n}\right]$$

$$= \frac{1}{n}[1 - 2(-1)^n + 1] = \frac{2}{n}[1 - (-1)^n]$$

$$= \begin{cases} \dfrac{4}{n} & , \text{ if } n \text{ is odd} \\ 0 & , \text{ if } n \text{ is even} \end{cases}$$

The required Fourier series is given by

$$f(x) = \frac{a_0}{2} + a_1\cos x + a_2\cos 2x + \dots + b_1\sin x + b_2\sin 2x + \dots$$

$$= \frac{\pi}{2} - \frac{4}{\pi}\left(\frac{\cos x}{1^2} + \frac{\cos 3x}{3^2} + \dots\right) + 4\left(\frac{\sin x}{1} + \frac{\sin 3x}{3} + \dots\right)$$

6. *Find the Fourier series for the function $f(x) = x + x^2$, $-\pi < x < \pi$. Hence, show that*

(*i*) $\frac{\pi^2}{6} = 1 + \frac{1}{2^2} + \frac{1}{3^2} + \frac{1}{4^2} + \dots$

(*ii*) $\frac{\pi^2}{12} = \frac{1}{1^2} - \frac{1}{2^2} + \frac{1}{3^2} - \frac{1}{4^2} + \dots$

SOLUTION. Let the Fourier series be

$$x + x^2 = \frac{a_0}{2} + \sum_{n=1}^{\infty} a_n\cos nx + \sum_{n=1}^{\infty} b_n\sin nx \quad \dots(1)$$

Here, $a_0 = \frac{1}{\pi}\int_{-\pi}^{\pi} (x + x^2)dx$

$$= \frac{1}{\pi}\left[\int_{-\pi}^{\pi} x\,dx + \int_{-\pi}^{\pi} x^2\,dx\right]$$

$$= \frac{2}{\pi}\int_0^{\pi} x^2 dx = \frac{2}{3}\pi^2$$

$$a_n = \frac{1}{\pi}\int_{-\pi}^{\pi} (x + x^2)\cos nx\,dx$$

$$= \frac{1}{\pi}\left[\int_{-\pi}^{\pi} x\cos nx\,dx + \int_{-\pi}^{\pi} x^2 \cos nx\,dx\right]$$

$$= \frac{2}{\pi}\int_0^{\pi} x^2 \cos nx\,dx$$

$$= \frac{2}{\pi}\left[\left(x^2\frac{\sin nx}{n}\right)_0^{\pi} - \int_0^{\pi} 2x.\frac{\sin nx}{n}dx\right]$$

$$= -\frac{4}{n\pi}\int_0^{\pi} x\sin nx\,dx$$

$$= -\frac{4}{n\pi}\left[\left\{x\left(-\frac{\cos nx}{n}\right)\right\}_0^{\pi} - \int_0^{\pi} 1.\left(-\frac{\cos nx}{n}\right)dx\right]$$

$$= -\frac{4}{n\pi}\left(-\frac{\pi}{n}\cos n\pi\right) = \frac{4}{n^2}\cos n\pi$$

$$= \frac{4}{n^2}(-1)^n$$

$$b_n = \frac{1}{\pi}\int_{-\pi}^{\pi} (x + x^2)\sin nx dx$$

$$= \frac{2}{\pi}\int_0^{\pi} x\sin nx\,dx + \frac{2}{\pi}\int_0^{\pi} x^2 \sin nx\,dx$$

$$\left[\because \int_0^{\pi} x^2 \sin nx\,dx = 0\right]$$

$$= \frac{2}{\pi}\left(-\frac{\pi}{n}\cos n\pi\right) = -\frac{2}{n}(-1)^n.$$

From (1),

$$x + x^2 = \frac{\pi^2}{3} + 4\sum_{n=1}^{\infty}\frac{(-1)^n}{n^2}\cos nx - 2\sum_{n=1}^{\infty}\frac{(-1)^n}{n}\sin nx$$

$$f(x) = \frac{\pi^2}{3} + 4\left[-\frac{1}{1^2}\cos x + \frac{1}{2^2}\cos 2x - \frac{1}{3^2}\cos 3x + \ldots\right] - 2\left[-\frac{1}{1}\sin x + \frac{1}{2}\sin 2x - \frac{1}{3}\sin 3x + \ldots\right]. \quad \ldots(2)$$

We observe that the series on the R.H.S. given by equation (2), always represents $x + x^2$ for all values of x except the end points $-\pi$ or π.

At the point of discontinuity

$$f(-\pi) = \frac{1}{2}(\text{L.H.L.} + \text{R.H.L.})$$

$$= \frac{1}{2}[f(-\pi - 0) + f(-\pi + 0)]$$

$$= \frac{1}{2}[f(\pi - 0) + f(-\pi + 0)]$$

$$= \frac{1}{2}[\pi + \pi^2 + (-\pi) + (-\pi)^2] = \pi^2.$$

Putting $x = -\pi$ in equation (2), we get

$$\pi^2 = \frac{\pi^2}{3} + 4\left[\frac{1}{1^2} + \frac{1}{2^2} + \frac{1}{3^2} + \frac{1}{4^2} + \ldots\right]$$

$$\frac{\pi^2}{6} = 1 + \frac{1}{2^2} + \frac{1}{3^2} + \frac{1}{4^2} + \ldots \quad \ldots(3)$$

Again, putting $x = 0$ in equaton (2), we get

$$0 = \frac{\pi^2}{3} + 4\left[-\frac{1}{1^2} + \frac{1}{2^2} - \frac{1}{3^2} + \frac{1}{4^2} - \ldots\right]$$

$$\frac{\pi^2}{12} = \frac{1}{1^2} - \frac{1}{2^2} + \frac{1}{3^2} - \frac{1}{4^2}\ldots$$

7. *Express $f(x) = |x|$, $-\pi < x < \pi$, as Fourier series. Hence, show that*

$$\frac{1}{1^2} + \frac{1}{3^2} + \frac{1}{5^2} + \ldots = \frac{\pi^2}{8}.$$

SOLUTION. Here, $f(-x) = |-x| = |x| = f(x)$

$\therefore f(x)$ is an even function and hence $b_n = 0$.

$$\text{Let, } f(x) = |x| = \frac{a_0}{2} + \sum_{n=1}^{\infty} a_n \cos nx$$

$$\text{Then, } a_0 = \frac{2}{\pi}\int_0^{\pi} f(x)dx = \frac{2}{\pi}\int_0^{\pi} |x|\,dx$$

$$= \frac{2}{\pi}\int_0^{\pi} x\,dx = \frac{2}{\pi}\left[\frac{x^2}{2}\right]_0^{\pi} = \pi$$

$$a_n = \frac{2}{\pi}\int_0^{\pi} f(x)\cos nx\,dx$$

$$= \frac{2}{\pi}\int_0^{\pi} |x|.\cos nx dx = \frac{2}{\pi}\int_0^{\pi} x\cos nx dx$$

$$= \frac{2}{\pi}\left[x\left(\frac{\sin nx}{n}\right) - 1\left(-\frac{\cos nx}{n^2}\right)\right]_0^{\pi}$$

$$= \frac{2}{\pi}\left[\frac{\cos nx}{n^2} - \frac{1}{n^2}\right]$$

$$= \frac{2}{\pi n^2}[(-1)^n - 1]$$

$$= \begin{cases} 0 & , \text{ if } n \text{ is even} \\ -\dfrac{4}{\pi n^2} & , \text{ if } n \text{ is odd} \end{cases}$$

Hence,

$$|x| = \frac{\pi}{2} - \frac{4}{\pi}\left(\cos x + \frac{\cos 3x}{3^2} + \frac{\cos 5x}{5^2} + \ldots\right) \quad \ldots(1)$$

Deduction. Putting $x = 0$, in the equation (1), we get

$$\frac{1}{1^2} + \frac{1}{3^2} + \frac{1}{5^2} + \ldots = \frac{\pi^2}{8}$$

Exercise-27.1

1. Express $f(x) = \frac{1}{2}(\pi - x)$ in a Fourier series in the interval $0 < x < 2\pi$.
2. Find the Fourier series to represent the function $f(x) = |\sin x|, -\pi < x < \pi$.
3. Obtain the Fourier series to represent $f(x) = \frac{1}{4}(\pi - x)^2, 0 < x < 2\pi$. Hence, obtain the following relation:

   (i) $\frac{1}{1^2} + \frac{1}{2^2} + \frac{1}{3^2} + \frac{1}{4^2} + \ldots = \frac{\pi^2}{6}$

   (ii) $\frac{1}{1^2} - \frac{1}{2^2} + \frac{1}{3^2} - \frac{1}{4^2} + \ldots = \frac{\pi^2}{12}$

   (iii) $\frac{1}{1^2} + \frac{1}{3^2} + \frac{1}{5^2} + \ldots = \frac{\pi^2}{8}$
4. Expand in a Fourier series the function $f(x) = x$ in the interval $0 < x < 2\pi$, sketch its graph from $x = -4\pi$ to $x = 4\pi$.
5. Show that for $-\pi < x < \pi$

   $\sin ax =$
   $$\frac{2\sin a\pi}{\pi}\left(\frac{\sin x}{1^2 - a^2} - \frac{2\sin 2x}{2^2 - a^2} + \frac{3\sin 3x}{3^2 - a^2} - \ldots\right)$$
6. Obtain a Fourier expansion for $\sqrt{1 - \cos x}$ in the interval $-\pi < x < \pi$.
7. Obtain a Fourier series to represent e^{-ax} from $x = -\pi$ to $x = \pi$. Hence derive series for $\frac{\pi}{\sinh \pi}$.
8. Find the Fourier series to represent the periodic function:
   $$f(x) = \begin{cases} x & , -\pi/2 < x < \pi/2 \\ \pi - x & , \pi/2 < x < 3\pi/2 \end{cases}$$
9. Find a series of sines and cosines to multiples of x which will represent $\frac{\pi}{\sinh \pi}e^x$ in the interval $-\pi < x < \pi$.
10. Prove that
    $$x^2 = \frac{\pi^2}{3} + 4\sum_{n=1}^{\infty}(-1)^n \frac{\cos nx}{n^2}, -\pi < x < \pi.$$
11. Prove that in the interval
    $$x\cos x = -\frac{1}{2}\sin x + 2\sum_{n=2}^{\infty}\frac{n(-1)^n}{n^2 - 1}\sin nx$$
12. If $f(x) = \cos \omega x, -\pi < x < \pi$, where ω is a fraction as a fourier series, prove that
    $$\cot\theta = \frac{1}{\theta} + \frac{2\theta}{\theta^2 - \pi^2} + \frac{2\theta}{\theta^2 - 4\pi^2} + \ldots$$

Hint to the Selected Problems

4. $a_0 = \frac{1}{\pi}\int_0^{2\pi}\frac{1}{4}(\pi - x)^2 dx = \frac{1}{4\pi}\left[\frac{(\pi - x)^3}{-3}\right]_0^{2\pi}$

$$= -\frac{1}{12\pi}[-\pi^3 - \pi^3] = \frac{\pi^2}{6}$$

$$a_n = \frac{1}{\pi}\int_0^{2\pi} f(x)\cos nx\,dx$$

$$= \frac{1}{\pi}\int_0^{2\pi}\frac{1}{4}(\pi - x)^2\cos nx\,dx$$

$$= \frac{1}{4\pi}\left[(\pi - x)^2\frac{\sin nx}{n} - \{-2(\pi - x)\}\left(-\frac{\cos nx}{n^2}\right) + 2\left(\frac{-\sin nx}{n^3}\right)\right]_0^{2\pi}$$

$$b_n = \frac{1}{\pi}\int_0^{2\pi}\frac{1}{4}(\pi - x)^2\sin nx\,dx$$

$$= \frac{1}{4\pi}\left[(\pi - x)^2\left(-\frac{\cos nx}{n}\right) - \{-2(\pi - x)\}\left(-\frac{\sin nx}{n^2}\right) + 2\left(\frac{\cos nx}{n^3}\right)\right]_0^{2\pi}$$

$$= \frac{1}{4\pi}\left[\left(-\frac{\pi^2}{n} + \frac{2}{n^3}\right) - \left(-\frac{\pi^2}{n} + \frac{2}{n^3}\right)\right] = 0$$

$$\therefore\ f(x) = \frac{\pi^2}{12} + \sum_{n=1}^{\infty} \frac{\cos nx}{n^2}$$

$$= \frac{\pi^2}{1^2} + \frac{\cos x}{1^2} + \frac{\cos 2x}{2^2} + \frac{\cos 3x}{3^2} + \ldots \quad \ldots(1)$$

(i) Putting $x=0$ in equation (1), we get

$$\frac{\pi^2}{4} = \frac{\pi^2}{12} + \left(\frac{1}{1^2} + \frac{1}{2^2} + \frac{1}{3^2} + \frac{1}{4^2} + \ldots\right)$$

$$\frac{\pi^2}{6} = \frac{1}{1^2} + \frac{1}{2^2} + \frac{1}{3^2} + \frac{1}{4^2} + \ldots \quad \ldots(2)$$

(ii) Putting $x=\pi$ in equation (1), we get

$$0 = \frac{\pi^2}{12} + \left[\left(\frac{-1}{1^2}\right) + \frac{1}{2^2} + \left(-\frac{1}{3^2}\right) + \frac{1}{4^2} + \ldots\right]$$

$$\frac{\pi^2}{12} = \frac{1}{1^2} - \frac{1}{2^2} + \frac{1}{3^2} - \frac{1}{4^2} + \ldots \quad \ldots(3)$$

(iii) Adding equations (2) and (3), we get

$$\frac{\pi^2}{6} + \frac{\pi^2}{12} = 2\left(\frac{1}{1^2} + \frac{1}{3^2} + \frac{1}{5^2} + \ldots\right)$$

$$\frac{\pi^2}{4} = 2\left(\frac{1}{1^2} + \frac{1}{3^2} + \frac{1}{5^2} + \ldots\right) \quad \ldots(3)$$

$$\frac{\pi^2}{8} = \frac{1}{1^2} + \frac{1}{3^2} + \frac{1}{5^2} + \ldots$$

5. Here, $a_0 = 0$, $a_n = 0$

[$\because f(x)$ is an odd function]

$$b_n = \frac{2}{\pi}\int_0^{\pi} \sin ax \sin nx\, dx$$

$$= \frac{1}{\pi}\int_0^{\pi} [\cos(n-a)x - \cos(n+a)x]\, dx$$

$$= \frac{1}{\pi}\left[\frac{\sin(n-a)x}{(n-a)} - \frac{\sin(n+a)x}{n+a}\right]_0^{\pi}$$

$$= \frac{1}{\pi}\left[\frac{\sin(n-a)\pi}{n-a} - \frac{\sin(n+a)\pi}{n+a}\right]$$

$$= \frac{1}{\pi}\left[\frac{(-1)^n(-\sin a\pi)}{n-a} - \frac{(-1)^n \sin a\pi}{n+a}\right]$$

$$= \frac{(-1)^n \sin a\pi}{\pi}\left[\frac{1}{n-a} + \frac{1}{n+a}\right]$$

$$= (-1)^{n+1} \frac{2n \sin a\pi}{\pi(n^2 - a^2)}$$

$$\sin ax = \frac{2\sin a\pi}{\pi} \sum_{n=1}^{\infty} \frac{(-1)^{n+1} n}{n^2 - a^2} \sin nx$$

$$= \frac{2\sin a\pi}{\pi}\left[\frac{\sin x}{1^2 - a^2} - \frac{2\sin 2x}{2^2 - a^2} + \frac{3\sin 3x}{3^2 - a^2} - \ldots\right]$$

9. $f(n) = \frac{1}{2l}\int_{-l}^{l} f(x)dx$

$$+ \frac{1}{l}\sum_{n=1}^{\infty}\left[\cos\frac{n\pi x}{l} - \int_{-l}^{l} f(x).\cos\frac{n\pi x}{l}dx + \sin\frac{n\pi x}{l}\int_{-l}^{l} f(x)\sin\frac{n\pi x}{l}dx\right]$$

$$\frac{\pi}{2\sin n\pi}e^x = \frac{1}{2\pi}\int_{-\pi}^{\pi}\frac{\pi}{2\sin n\pi}e^x dx$$

$$+ \frac{1}{\pi}\sum_{n=1}^{\infty} \cos nx \int_{-\pi}^{\pi} \frac{\pi}{2\sin n\pi} e^x \cos nu\, du$$

$$+ \frac{1}{\pi}\sum_{n=1}^{\infty} \sin nx \int_{-\pi}^{\pi} \frac{\pi}{2\sin n\pi} e^x \sin nu\, du.$$

We have $\int_{-\pi}^{\pi} e^u du = \left[e^u\right]_{-\pi}^{\pi} = 2\sin n\pi$

$$\int_{-\pi}^{\pi} e^u \cos nu\, du$$

$$= \left[e^u \frac{\sin nu}{n}\right]_{-\pi}^{\pi} - \frac{1}{n}\int_{-\pi}^{\pi} e^u \sin nu\, du$$

$$= \frac{1}{n^2}\left[e^u \cos nu\right]_{-\pi}^{\pi} - \frac{1}{n^2}\int_{-\pi}^{\pi} e^u \cos nu\, du$$

$$\left(1 + \frac{1}{n^2}\right)\int_{-\pi}^{\pi} e^u \cos nu\, du = \frac{1}{n^2}(e^{\pi} - e^{-\pi})\cos n\pi$$

$$\int_{-\pi}^{\pi} e^u \cos nu\, du = \frac{2}{1+n^2}\sin n\pi \cos n\pi$$

$$\int_{-\pi}^{\pi} e^u \sin nu\, du$$

$$= \left[\frac{-e^u \cos nu}{n}\right]_{-\pi}^{\pi} + \frac{1}{n}\int_{-\pi}^{\pi} e^u \cos nu\, du$$

$$= -\frac{1}{n}(e^{\pi} - e^{\pi})\cos n\pi + \frac{1}{n}\left[\left\{\frac{e^u \sin nu}{n}\right\}_{-\pi}^{\pi} - \int_{-\pi}^{\pi} \frac{e^u \sin nu}{n} du\right]$$

$$\left(1 + \frac{1}{n^2}\right)\int_{-\pi}^{\pi} e^u \sin nu\, du = -\frac{1}{n}(e^{\pi} - e^{-\pi})\cos n\pi$$

$$\int_{-\pi}^{\pi} e^u \sin nu\, du = \frac{2}{1+n^2}\sin n\pi \cos n\pi$$

$$\frac{\pi}{2\sin n\pi}e^x = \frac{1}{2}+\sum_{n=1}^{\infty}\frac{\cos n\pi}{1+n^2}\cos nx - \sum_{n=1}^{\infty}\left\{\frac{n}{1+n^2}\cos n\pi \sin nx\right\}$$

$$= \frac{1}{2}-\left(\frac{1}{2}\cos x-\frac{1}{2}\cos 2x+\frac{1}{10}\cos 3x-\frac{1}{17}\cos 4x+\dots\right)+\left(\frac{1}{2}\sin x-\frac{2}{5}\sin 2x+\frac{3}{10}\sin 3x-\frac{4}{17}\sin 4x+\dots\right)$$

ANSWERS

1. $f(x)=\sum_{n=1}^{\infty}\frac{\sin nx}{n}$ **2.** $|\sin x|=\frac{2}{\pi}\cdot\frac{4}{\pi}\left(\frac{\cos 2x}{3}+\frac{\cos 4x}{15}+\dots+\frac{\cos 2nx}{4n^2-1}+\dots\right)$

3. $f(x)=\frac{\pi^2}{12}+\sum_{n=1}^{\infty}\frac{\cos nx}{n^2}=\frac{\pi^2}{12}+\frac{\cos x}{1^2}+\frac{\cos 2x}{2^2}+\frac{\cos 3x}{3^2}+\dots$ **4.** $f(x)=\pi-2\,.\sum_{n=1}^{\infty}\frac{\sin nx}{n}$

5. $\sin ax=\frac{2\sin a\pi}{\pi}\sum_{n=1}^{\infty}\frac{(-1)^{n+1}}{n^2-a^2}\sin nx$ **6.** $\sqrt{1-\cos x}=\frac{2\sqrt{2}}{\pi}-\frac{4\sqrt{2}}{\pi}\sum_{n=1}^{\infty}\frac{\cos nx}{4n^2-1}$

7. $e^{-ax}=2\frac{\sin h\, a\pi}{\pi}\left[\left(\frac{1}{2a}-\frac{a\cos x}{1^2+a^2}+\frac{a\cos 2x}{2^2+a^2}-\dots\right)-\left(\frac{\sin x}{1^2+a^2}-\frac{2\sin 2x}{2^2+a^2}+\frac{3\sin 3x}{3^2+a^2}\dots\right)\right]$

$$\frac{\pi}{\sinh\pi}=2\left[\frac{1}{2^2+1}-\frac{1}{3^2+1}+\frac{1}{4^2+1}-\dots\right]$$

8. $f(x)=\frac{4}{\pi}\left[\frac{\sin x}{1^2}-\frac{\sin 3x}{3^2}+\frac{\sin 5x}{5^2}-\dots\right]$

9. $\frac{\pi}{2\sin n\pi}e^x=\frac{1}{2}+\sum_{n=1}^{\infty}\frac{\cos n\pi}{1+n^2}\cos nx-\sum_{n=1}^{\infty}\left\{\frac{n}{1+n^2}\cos nx\sin n\pi\right\}$

$$=\frac{1}{2}-\left(\frac{1}{2}\cos x-\frac{1}{2}\cos 2x+\frac{1}{10}\cos 3x-\frac{1}{17}\cos 4x+\dots\right)$$

27.6 FOURIER SERIES FOR DISCONTINUOUS FUNCTIONS

At the point of discontinuity, the value of function for Fourier series is obtained by the average of left hand limit and right hand limit of function at the point of discontinuity.

Solved Examples

1. *Obtain Fourier series for the function* $f(x)=\begin{cases} x & ; \quad -\pi<x<0 \\ -x & ; \quad 0<x<\pi \end{cases}$ *and hence show that* $\frac{1}{1^2}+\frac{1}{3^2}+\frac{1}{5^2}+\dots=\frac{\pi^2}{8}$.

SOLUTION. We know that

$$f(x)=\frac{a_0}{2}+\sum_{n=1}^{\infty}a_n\cos nx+\sum_{n=1}^{\infty}b_n\sin nx \qquad \dots(1)$$

$$a_0=\frac{1}{\pi}\int_{-\pi}^{\pi}f(x)dx$$

$$=\frac{1}{\pi}\left[\int_{-\pi}^{0}x\,dx+\int_{0}^{\pi}-x\,dx\right]$$

$$=\frac{1}{\pi}\left[\left(\frac{x^2}{2}\right)_{-\pi}^{0}-\left(\frac{x^2}{2}\right)_{0}^{\pi}\right]$$

$$=\frac{1}{\pi}\left[0-\frac{\pi^2}{2}-\frac{\pi^2}{2}\right]=-\pi$$

$$a_n = \frac{1}{\pi}\int_{-\pi}^{\pi} f(x)\cos nx dx$$

$$= \frac{1}{\pi}\left[\int_{-\pi}^{0} x\cos nx dx + \int_0^{\pi} -x\cos nx dx\right]$$

$$= \frac{1}{\pi}\left[\left(\frac{x\sin nx}{n}\right)_{-\pi}^{0} - \int_{-\pi}^{0}\frac{\sin nx}{n}dx + \left(-x\frac{\sin nx}{n}\right)_0^{\pi} - \int_0^{\pi}(-1)\frac{\sin nx}{n}dx\right]$$

$$= \frac{1}{\pi}\left[\frac{1}{n^2}(\cos nx)_{-\pi}^{0} - \frac{1}{n^2}(\cos nx)_0^{\pi}\right]$$

$$= \frac{1}{\pi}\left[\left\{\frac{1-(-1)^n}{n^2}\right\} - \left\{\frac{(-1)^n - 1}{n^2}\right\}\right]$$

$$= \frac{1}{\pi}\left[\frac{2\{1-(-1)^n\}}{n^2}\right] = \frac{2}{\pi n^2}[1-(-1)^n]$$

$$= \begin{cases} 0 & ; \text{ if } n \text{ is even} \\ \dfrac{4}{\pi n^2} & ; \text{ if } n \text{ is odd} \end{cases}$$

$$b_n = \frac{1}{\pi}\int_{-\pi}^{\pi} f(x)\sin nx dx$$

$$= \frac{1}{\pi}\left[\int_{-\pi}^{0} x\sin nx dx + \int_0^{\pi} -x\sin nx\, d x\right]$$

$$= \frac{1}{\pi}\left[\left(x\frac{-\cos nx}{n}\right)_{-\pi}^{0} - \int_{-\pi}^{0}\frac{-\cos nx}{n}dx + \left(x\frac{\cos nx}{n}\right)_0^{\pi} - \int_0^{\pi}(-1)\frac{-\cos nx}{n}dx\right]$$

$$= \frac{1}{\pi}\left[\frac{-\pi}{n}(-1)^n + \frac{1}{n}(-1)^n\right] = 0$$

From (1),

$$f(x) = -\frac{\pi}{2} + \frac{4}{\pi}\left(\frac{\cos x}{1^2} + \frac{\cos 3x}{3^2} + \frac{\cos 5x}{5^2} + \ldots\right)$$

At the point of discontinuity

$$f(0) = \frac{1}{2}[f(0^-) + f(0^+)] = \frac{1}{2}[0-0] = 0$$

Putting, $x = 0$ in (2), we get

$$0 = -\frac{\pi}{2} + \frac{4}{\pi}\left(\frac{1}{1^2} + \frac{1}{3^2} + \frac{1}{5^2} + \ldots\right)$$

Hence, $\dfrac{1}{1^2} + \dfrac{1}{3^2} + \dfrac{1}{5^2} + \ldots = \dfrac{\pi^2}{8}$

2. *Obtain the Fourier series to represent f(x) given as follows*

$$f(x) = \begin{cases} x & ; \text{ for } 0 \le x \le \pi \\ 2\pi - x & ; \text{ for } \pi \le x \le 2\pi \end{cases}$$

SOLUTION. Let

$$f(x) = \frac{a_0}{2} + \sum_{n=1}^{\infty} a_n \cos nx + \sum_{n=1}^{\infty} b_n \sin nx, 0 \le x \le 2\pi \quad \ldots(1)$$

where $a_0 = \dfrac{1}{\pi}\int_0^{2\pi} f(x)dx$

$$= \frac{1}{\pi}\left[\int_0^{\pi} x\, dx + \int_{\pi}^{2\pi}(2\pi - x)dx\right]$$

$$= \frac{1}{\pi}\left[\left(\frac{x^2}{2}\right)_0^{\pi} + \left(2\pi x - \frac{x^2}{2}\right)_{\pi}^{2\pi}\right]$$

$$= \frac{1}{\pi}\left[\frac{\pi^2}{2} + 2\pi(2\pi - x) - \frac{1}{2}(4\pi^2 - \pi^2)\right]$$

$$= \frac{1}{\pi}(\pi^2) = \pi$$

$$a_n = \frac{1}{\pi}\int_0^{2\pi} f(x)\cos nx dx$$

$$= \frac{1}{\pi}\left[\int_0^{\pi} x\cos nx dx + \int_0^{2\pi}(2\pi - x)\cos nx dx\right]$$

$$= \frac{1}{\pi}\left[\left\{\frac{x\sin nx}{n} + \frac{\cos nx}{n^2}\right\}_0^{\pi} + \left\{(2\pi - x)\frac{\sin nx}{n} - \frac{\cos nx}{n^2}\right\}_{\pi}^{2\pi}\right]$$

$$= \frac{1}{\pi}\left[\left(\frac{\cos n\pi - 1}{n^2}\right) - \left(\frac{1-\cos n\pi}{n^2}\right)\right]$$

$$= \frac{2}{n^2\pi}[(-1)^n - 1]$$

$$= \begin{cases} 0 & , \text{ if } n \text{ is even} \\ -\dfrac{4}{n\pi^2} & , \text{ if } n \text{ is odd} \end{cases}$$

Again $b_n = \dfrac{1}{\pi}\int_0^{2\pi} f(x).\sin nx\, dx$

$$= \frac{1}{\pi}\left[\int_0^{\pi} x \sin nx\, dx + \int_{\pi}^{2\pi} (2\pi - x)\sin nx\, dx\right]$$

$$= \frac{1}{\pi}\left[\left\{-\frac{x\cos nx}{n} + \frac{\sin nx}{n^2}\right\}_0^{\pi} + \left\{-(2\pi - x)\frac{\cos nx}{n} - \frac{\sin nx}{n^2}\right\}_{\pi}^{2\pi}\right]$$

$$= \left[\frac{-\pi\cos n\pi}{n} + \frac{\pi\cos n\pi}{n}\right] = 0$$

Therefore,

$$f(x) = \frac{\pi}{2} - \frac{4}{\pi}\left[\cos x + \frac{\cos 3x}{3^2} + \frac{\cos 5x}{5^2} + \ldots\right],$$
$$0 \le x \le 2\pi$$

which is the required Fourier series for $f(x)$.

Exercise-27.2

1. Find the Fourier series for the following function:

$$f(x) = \begin{cases} x^2 &, \quad 0 \le x \le \pi \\ -x^2 &, \quad -\pi \le x \le 0 \end{cases}$$

2. Find the Fourier series to represent the function:

$$f(x) = \begin{cases} -k &, \quad \text{when } -\pi < x < 0 \\ k &, \quad \text{when } 0 < x < \pi \end{cases}$$

Also deduce that $\dfrac{\pi}{4} = 1 - \dfrac{1}{3} + \dfrac{1}{5} - \dfrac{1}{7} + \ldots$

3. Find the Fourier series for the function:

$$f(x) = \begin{cases} -1 &, \quad -\pi < x < -\pi/2 \\ 0 &, \quad -\pi/2 < x < \pi/2 \\ 1 &, \quad \pi/2 < x < \pi \end{cases}$$

4. Find the Fourier series expansion for $f(x)$ if

$$f(x) = f(x) = \begin{cases} -\pi &, \quad -\pi < x < 0 \\ x &, \quad 0 < x < \pi \end{cases}$$

Deduce that $\dfrac{1}{1^2} + \dfrac{1}{3^2} + \dfrac{1}{5^2} + \ldots = \dfrac{\pi^2}{8}$

5. Find the Fourier expansion of the function derived in one period by the relations:

$$f(x) = \begin{cases} 1 &, \quad 0 < x < \pi \\ 2 &, \quad \pi < x < 2\pi \end{cases}$$ and deduce that

$$\frac{\pi}{4} = 1 - \frac{1}{3} + \frac{1}{5} - \frac{1}{7} + \ldots$$

6. An alternating current after passing through a rectifier has the form

$$i = \begin{cases} I_0 \sin x & \text{for} \quad 0 \le x < \pi \\ 0 & \text{for} \quad \pi \le x \le 2\pi \end{cases}$$

where I_0 is the maximum current and the period is 2π. Express i as a Fourier series.

Hints to Selected Problems

3. $a_0 = \frac{1}{\pi}\int_{-\pi}^{-\frac{\pi}{2}}(-1)dx + \frac{1}{\pi}\int_{-\pi/2}^{\pi/2} 0dx + \frac{1}{\pi}\int_{\frac{\pi}{2}}^{\pi} 1dx = 0$

$$a_n = \frac{1}{\pi}\int_{-\pi}^{-\pi/2}(-1)\cos nxdx + \frac{1}{\pi}\int_{-\pi/2}^{\pi/2}(0)\cos nxdx + \frac{1}{\pi}\int_{\pi/2}^{\pi}(1)\cos nx\, dx = 0$$

$$b_n = \frac{1}{\pi}\int_{-\pi}^{\pi/2}(-1)\sin nxdx + \frac{1}{\pi}\int_{-\pi}^{\pi/2}(0)\sin nxdx + \frac{1}{\pi}\int_{\pi/2}^{\pi}(1)\sin nx\, dx = 0$$

$$= \frac{2}{n\pi}\left[\cos\frac{n\pi}{2} - \cos n\pi\right]$$

$$b_1 = \frac{2}{\pi}, b_2 = -\frac{2}{\pi}, b_3 = \frac{2}{3\pi}$$

$$f(x) = \frac{1}{\pi}\left[2\sin x - 2\sin 2x + \frac{2}{3}\sin 3x + \ldots\right]$$

ANSWERS

1. $f(x) = 2\left(\pi - \dfrac{4}{\pi}\right)\sin x - \pi\sin 2x + \dfrac{2}{3}\left(\pi - \dfrac{4}{9\pi}\right)\sin 3x - \dfrac{\pi}{2}\sin 4x + ..$

2. $f(x) = \dfrac{4k}{\pi}\left(\sin x + \dfrac{\sin 3x}{3} + \dfrac{\sin 5x}{5} + \ldots\right)$

3. $f(x) = \dfrac{2}{\pi}\left[\sin x - \sin 2x + \dfrac{\sin 3x}{3} + \ldots\right]$

4. $f(x) = \frac{\pi}{4} - \frac{2}{\pi}\left(\cos x + \frac{\cos 3x}{3^2} + \frac{\cos 5x}{5^2} + ...\right) + \left(3\sin x - \frac{\sin 2x}{2} + \sin 3x - \frac{\sin 4x}{4} + ...\right)$

5. $f(x) = \frac{3}{2} - \frac{2}{\pi}\left(\sin x + \frac{\sin 3x}{3} + \frac{\sin 5x}{5} + ...\right)$

6. $i = \frac{I_0}{\pi} + \frac{I_0}{2}\sin x - \frac{2I_0}{\pi}\left(\frac{\cos 2x}{2^2-1} + \frac{\cos 4x}{4^2-1} + \frac{\cos 6x}{6^2-1} + ...\right)$

27.7 CHANGE OF INTERVAL

In many problems, the interval of Fourier expansion is $2l$ and not 2π. In order to apply this theory, this interval must be transformed into an interval of length 2π.

Consider a periodic function $f(x)$ defined in the interval $C<x<C+2l$. To change the interval into one of lenght 2π, we put

$$\frac{x}{l} = \frac{z}{\pi} \text{ or } z = \frac{\pi x}{l} \text{ so that at } x = c, z = \frac{\pi c}{l} = d(\text{say})$$

When $x = C + 2l, z = \frac{\pi(C+2l)}{l} = \frac{\pi c}{l} + 2\pi = d + 2\pi$

Thus, the function $f(x)$ of period $2l$ in $(C, C+2l)$ is transformed to the function $f\left(\frac{lz}{\pi}\right) = F(z)$ say, or period in $(d, d+2\pi)$ and then function $F(z)$ can be expressed as a Fourier series

$$F(z) = \frac{a_0}{2} + \sum_{n=1}^{\infty} a_n \cos nz + \sum_{n=1}^{\infty} b_n \sin nz \qquad ... (1)$$

where, $a_0 = \frac{1}{\pi}\int_d^{d+2\pi} F(z)dz; a_n = \frac{1}{\pi}\int_d^{d+2\pi} F(z)\cos nz\, dz$

and $b_n = \frac{1}{\pi}\int_d^{d+2\pi} F(z)\sin nz\, dz$

Now, making the inverse substitution $z = \frac{\pi x}{l}, dz = \frac{\pi}{l}dx$, when $z= d, x = C$ and when $z = d + 2\pi, x = C + 2l$. The expression (1) becomes

$$F(z) = F\left(\frac{\pi x}{l}\right) = F(x) = \frac{a_0}{2} + \sum_{n=1}^{\infty} a_n \cos\frac{n\pi x}{l} + \sum_{n=1}^{\infty} b_n \sin\frac{n\pi x}{l} \qquad ... (2)$$

The coefficient a_0, a_n, b_n in (2) becomes

$$a_0 = \frac{1}{l}\int_C^{C+2l} f(x)dx,\ a_n = \frac{1}{l}\int_C^{C+2l} f(x)\cos\frac{n\pi x}{l}dx,$$

$$b_n = \frac{1}{l}\int_C^{C+2\pi} f(x)\sin\frac{n\pi x}{l}dx$$

- If $C = 0$, the interval become $0 < x < 2l$ and the a_0, a_n, b_n are given by
  $a_0 = \frac{1}{l}\int_0^{2l} f(x)dx, a_n = \frac{1}{l}\int_0^{2l} f(x)\cos\frac{n\pi x}{l}dx,\ b_n = \frac{1}{l}\int_0^{2l} f(x)\sin\frac{n\pi x}{l}dx$.
- If $C = -l$, the interval become $-l < x < l$ and a_0, a_n, b_n are given by
  $a_0 = \frac{1}{l}\int_{-l}^{l} f(x)dx, a_n = \frac{1}{l}\int_{-l}^{l} f(x)\cos\frac{n\pi x}{l}dx, b_n = \frac{1}{l}\int_{-l}^{l} f(x)\sin\frac{n\pi x}{l}dx.$

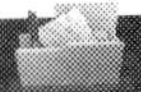

Solved Examples

1. *Find the Fourier series to represent $f(x) = x^2 - 2$ when $-2 \le x \le 2$.*

SOLUTION. Here, $b_n = 0$ because $f(x)$ is an even function

Let $f(x) = x^2 - 2 = \frac{a_0}{2} + \sum_{n=1}^{\infty} a_n \cos\frac{n\pi x}{2}$

$[\because 2l = 4 \Rightarrow l = 2]$

Then, $a_0 = \frac{2}{2}\int_0^2 (x^2 - 2)dx$

$$= \left[\frac{x^3}{3} - 2x\right]_0^2$$

$$= \frac{8}{3} - 4 = -\frac{4}{3}$$

and $a_n = \frac{2}{2}\int_0^2 (x^2 - x)\cos\frac{n\pi x}{2}dx$

$$= \left[(x^2-2)\frac{\sin n\pi x/2}{(n\pi/2)} - 2x\left(-\frac{\cos\frac{n\pi x}{2}}{(n^2\pi^2/4)} + 2\left(\frac{\sin\frac{n\pi x}{2}}{(n^3\pi^3/8)}\right)\right)\right]_0^2$$

$$= \frac{16\cos n\pi}{n^2\pi^2} = \frac{16(-1)^n}{n^2\pi^2}$$

$\therefore\ f(x) = (x^2 - 2)$

$$= -\frac{2}{3} + \frac{16}{\pi^2}\sum\frac{(-1)^n}{n^2}\cos\frac{n\pi x}{2}$$

$$= -\frac{2}{3} - \frac{16}{\pi^2}\left(\cos\frac{\pi x}{2} - \frac{1}{4}\cos\pi x + \frac{1}{9}\cos\frac{3\pi x}{2} - \ldots\right)$$

2. *Obtain the Fourier series for the function*

$$f(x) = \begin{cases} \pi x & ; \quad 0 \le x \le 1 \\ \pi(2-x) & ; \quad 1 \le x \le 2 \end{cases}$$

SOLUTION. Here, $2l = 2 \Rightarrow l = 1$.

Let $f(x) = \frac{a_0}{2} + \sum_{n=1}^{\infty} a_n \cos n\pi x + \sum_{n=1}^{\infty} b_n \sin n\pi x$

where $a_0 = \int_0^2 f(x)dx$

$$= \int_0^1 \pi x dx + \int_1^2 \pi(2-x)dx$$

$$= \pi\left[\frac{x^2}{2}\right]_0^1 + \pi\left[2x - \frac{x^2}{2}\right]_1^2$$

$$= \pi\left(\frac{1}{2}\right) + \pi\left[(4-2) - \left(2 - \frac{1}{2}\right)\right] = \pi$$

$a_n = \int_0^2 f(x)\cos n\pi x\, dx$

$$= \int_0^1 \pi x\cos n\pi x\, dx + \int_1^2 \pi(2-x)\cos n\pi x\, dx$$

$$= \left[\pi x\frac{\sin n\pi x}{n\pi} - \pi\left(-\frac{\cos n\pi x}{n^2\pi^2}\right)\right]_0^1 + \left[\pi(2-x)\frac{\sin n\pi x}{n\pi} - (-\pi)\left(-\frac{\cos n\pi x}{n^2\pi^2}\right)\right]_1^2$$

$$= \left(\frac{\cos n\pi}{n^2\pi} - \frac{1}{n^2\pi}\right) + \left[-\frac{\cos 2n\pi}{n^2\pi} + \frac{\cos n\pi}{n^2\pi}\right]$$

$$= \frac{2}{n^2\pi}(\cos n\pi - 1)$$

$$= \frac{2}{n^2\pi}[(-1)^n - 1]$$

$$= \begin{cases} 0 & ; \quad \text{if } n \text{ is even} \\ -\frac{4}{n^2\pi} & ; \quad \text{if } n \text{ is odd} \end{cases}$$

$b_n = \int_0^2 f(x)\sin n\pi x dx$

$$= \int_0^1 \pi x\sin n\pi x\, dx + \int_1^2 \pi(2-x)\sin n\pi x\, dx$$

$$= \left[\pi x\left(\frac{-\cos n\pi x}{n\pi}\right) - \pi\left(-\frac{\sin n\pi x}{n^2\pi^2}\right)\right]_0^1$$

$$+\left[-\pi(2-x)\frac{\cos n\pi x}{n\pi} - (-\pi)\left(-\frac{\sin n\pi x}{n^2\pi^2}\right)\right]_1^2$$

$$=\left[-\frac{\cos n\pi}{n}\right]+\left[\frac{\cos n\pi}{n}\right]=0$$

$$f(x)=\frac{\pi}{2}-\frac{4}{\pi}\left(\frac{\cos \pi x}{1^2}+\frac{\cos 3\pi x}{3^2}+\frac{\cos 5\pi x}{5^2}+\ldots\right)$$

3. *Find Fourier expansion for the function $f(x) = x - x^2$, $-1 < x < 1$.*

SOLUTION. Let $f(x)=\frac{a_0}{2}+\sum_{n=1}^{\infty} a_n \cos n\pi x + \sum_{n=1}^{\infty} b_n \sin n\pi x$

Then, $a_0 = \int_{-1}^{1}(x-x^2)dx$

$$=\int_{-1}^{1} x dx - \int_{-1}^{1} x^2 dx$$

$$=0-2\int_0^1 x^2 dx = -2\left[\frac{x^3}{3}\right]_0^1 = -\frac{2}{3}$$

$$a_n = \int_{-1}^{1}(x-x^2)\cos n\pi x\, dx$$

$$=\int_{-1}^{1} x\cos n\pi x\, dx - \int_{-1}^{1} x^2 \cos n\pi x\, dx$$

$$=0-2\int_0^1 x^2 \cos n\pi x\, dx$$

$$=-2\left[x^2\frac{\sin n\pi x}{n\pi}-2x\left(-\frac{\cos n\pi x}{n^2\pi^2}\right)+2\left(-\frac{\sin n\pi x}{n^3\pi^3}\right)\right]_0^1$$

$$=-2\left[\frac{2\cos n\pi}{n^2\pi^2}\right]=-\frac{4(-1)^n}{n^2\pi^2}$$

$$b_n=\int_{-1}^{1}(x-x^2)\sin n\pi x dx$$

$$=\int_{-1}^{1} x\sin n\pi x\, dx - 1\int_{-1}^{1} x^2 \sin n\pi x dx$$

$$=2\int_0^1 x\sin n\pi x\, dx - 0$$

$$=2\left[x\left(-\frac{\cos n\pi x}{n\pi}\right)-1\left(-\frac{\sin n\pi x}{n^2\pi^2}\right)\right]_0^1$$

$$=2\left[-\frac{\cos n\pi}{n\pi}\right]=-2\frac{(-1)^n}{n\pi}$$

$$\therefore\ x-x^2=-\frac{1}{3}+\frac{4}{\pi^2}\left(\frac{\cos\pi x}{1^2}-\frac{\cos 2\pi x}{2^2}+\frac{\cos 3\pi x}{3^2}-\ldots\right)+\frac{2}{\pi}\left(\frac{\sin \pi x}{1}-\frac{\sin 2\pi x}{2}+\frac{\sin 3\pi x}{3}-\ldots\right).$$

Exercise-27.3

1. Develop $f(x)$ in a Fourier series in the interval (0, 2) if $f(x)=\begin{cases} x, & 0<x<1 \\ 0, & 1<x<2 \end{cases}$
2. Given $f(x)=\begin{cases} 0, & 0<x<c \\ 1, & c<x<2c \end{cases}$ expand $f(x)$ in a Fourier series of period $2c$.
3. Expand $f(x)$ in Fourier series in the interval (–2, 2) when $f(x)=\begin{cases} 0, & -2<x<0 \\ 1, & 0<x<2 \end{cases}$.
4. Find a Fourier series for the function given by $f(t)=\begin{cases} t, & 0<t<1 \\ 1-t, & 1<t<2 \end{cases}$
5. Find a Fourier series corresponding to the function $f(x)$ defined in (–2, 2) as follows: $f(x)=\begin{cases} 2, & \text{if } -2\le x\le 0 \\ x, & \text{if } 0<x<2 \end{cases}$
6. Find a Fourier series for the function $f(x)=\begin{cases} 0, & \text{when } -2<x<-1 \\ k, & \text{when } -1<x<1 \\ 0, & \text{when } 1<x<2 \end{cases}$

Hints to Selected Problems

2. $a_0=\frac{1}{c}\int_0^{2c} f(x)dx=\frac{1}{c}\int_0^c 0.dx+\frac{1}{c}\int_c^{2c}1.dx$

$$=\frac{1}{c}[x]_c^{2c}=1$$

$$a_n=\frac{1}{c}\int_0^{2c} f(x)\cos\frac{n\pi x}{c}dx$$

$$=\frac{1}{c}\int_0^c 0.\cos\frac{n\pi x}{c}dx+\frac{1}{c}\int_c^{2c}1.\cos\frac{n\pi x}{c}dx$$

$$= \frac{1}{c}\left[\frac{c}{n\pi}\sin\frac{n\pi x}{c}\right]_c^{2c}$$

$$= \frac{1}{n\pi}[\sin 2n\pi - \sin n\pi] = 0$$

$$b_n = \frac{1}{c}\int_0^{2c} f(x).\sin\frac{n\pi x}{c}dx$$

$$= \frac{1}{c}\int_0^c 0.\sin\frac{n\pi x}{c}dx + \frac{1}{c}\int_c^{2c} 1.\sin\frac{n\pi x}{c}dx$$

$$= \frac{1}{c}\left[-\frac{c}{n\pi}\cos\frac{n\pi x}{c}\right]_c^{2c}$$

$$= -\frac{1}{n\pi}[\cos 2n\pi - \cos n\pi] = -\frac{1}{n\pi}[1-(-1)^n]$$

$$= \begin{cases} -\dfrac{2}{n\pi} & , \text{ when } n \text{ is odd} \\ 0 & , \text{ when } n \text{ is even} \end{cases}$$

Then, $f(x) = \frac{1}{2} - \frac{2}{\pi}\left(\frac{1}{1}\sin\frac{\pi x}{c} + \frac{1}{3}\sin\frac{3\pi x}{c} + \ldots\right)$

5. $a_0 = \frac{1}{l}\int_{-l}^{l} f(x)dx = \frac{1}{2}\left[\int_{-2}^{0} 2dx + \int_0^2 x\,dx\right]$

$$= \frac{1}{2}\left[(2x)_{-2}^{0} + \left(\frac{x^2}{2}\right)_0^2\right] = 3$$

$$a_n = \frac{1}{l}\int_{-l}^{l} f(x)\cos\left(\frac{n\pi x}{l}\right)dx$$

$$= \frac{1}{2}\left[\int_{-2}^{0} 2\cos\frac{n\pi x}{2}dx + \int_0^2 x\cos\frac{n\pi x}{2}dx\right]$$

$$= \frac{1}{2}\left[\frac{4}{n\pi}\left(\sin\frac{n\pi x}{2}\right)_{-2}^{0}\right.$$

$$\left. + \left(x\frac{2}{n\pi}\sin\frac{n\pi x}{2} + \frac{4}{n^2\pi^2}\cos\frac{n\pi x}{2}\right)_0^2\right]$$

$$= \frac{1}{2}\left[\frac{4}{n^2\pi^2}\cos n\pi - \frac{4}{n^2\pi^2}\right]$$

$$= \frac{2}{n^2\pi^2}[(-1)^n - 1]$$

$$= \begin{cases} -\dfrac{4}{n^2\pi^2} & , \text{ when } n \text{ is odd} \\ 0 & , \text{ when } n \text{ is even} \end{cases}$$

$$b_n = \frac{1}{l}\int_{-l}^{l} f(x)\sin\left(\frac{n\pi x}{l}\right)dx$$

$$= \frac{1}{2}\left[2\int_{-2}^{0}\sin\frac{n\pi x}{2}dx + \int_0^2 x\sin\frac{n\pi x}{2}dx\right]$$

$$= \frac{1}{2}\left[2\left(-\frac{2}{n\pi}\cos\frac{n\pi x}{2}\right)\right]_{-2}^{0}$$

$$+ \frac{1}{2}\left[x\left(-\frac{2}{n\pi}\cos\frac{n\pi x}{2}\right) + (1)\frac{4}{n^2\pi^2}\sin\frac{n\pi x}{2}\right]_0^2$$

$$= \frac{1}{2}\left[-\frac{4}{n\pi} + \frac{4}{n\pi}\cos n\pi\right]$$

$$+ \frac{1}{2}\left[-\frac{4}{n\pi}\cos n\pi + \frac{4}{n^2\pi^2}\sin n\pi\right]$$

$$= \frac{1}{2}\left[-\frac{4}{n\pi}\right] = -\frac{2}{n\pi}$$

$$f(x) = \frac{3}{2} - \frac{4}{\pi^2}\left\{\frac{1}{1^2}\cos\frac{\pi x}{2} + \frac{1}{3^2}\cos\frac{3\pi x}{2} + \ldots\right\}$$

$$-\frac{2}{\pi}\left\{\frac{1}{1}\sin\frac{\pi x}{2} + \frac{1}{2}\sin\frac{2\pi x}{2} + \frac{1}{3}\sin\frac{3\pi x}{3} + \ldots\right\}.$$

ANSWERS

1. $f(x) = \frac{1}{4} - \frac{2}{\pi^2}\left(\cos\pi x + \frac{\cos 3\pi x}{3^2} + \frac{\cos 5\pi x}{5^2} + \ldots\right) + \frac{1}{\pi}\left(\sin\pi x - \frac{\sin 2\pi x}{2} + \frac{\sin 3\pi x}{3} + \ldots\right)$

2. $f(x) = \frac{1}{2} - \frac{2}{\pi}\left\{\sin\frac{\pi x}{c} + \frac{1}{3}\sin\frac{3\pi x}{c} + \ldots\right\}$ **3.** $f(x) = \frac{1}{2} + \frac{2}{\pi^2}\left(\sin\frac{\pi x}{2} + \frac{1}{3}\sin\frac{3\pi x}{2} + \frac{1}{5}\sin\frac{5\pi x}{2} + \ldots\right)$

4. $f(t) = -\frac{4}{\pi^2}\left(\cos\pi t + \frac{\cos 3\pi t}{3^2} + \frac{\cos 5\pi t}{5^2} + \ldots\right) + \frac{2}{\pi}\left(\sin\pi t + \sin\frac{3\pi t}{3} + \ldots\right)$

5. $f(x) = \frac{3}{2} - \frac{4}{\pi^2}\left\{\frac{1}{1^2}\cos\frac{\pi x}{2} + \frac{1}{3^2}\cos\frac{3\pi x}{2} + \ldots\right\} - \frac{2}{\pi}\left\{\sin\frac{\pi x}{2} + \frac{1}{2}\sin\frac{2\pi x}{2} + \frac{1}{3}\sin\frac{3\pi x}{2} + \ldots\right\}$

6. $f(x) = \frac{k}{2} + \frac{2R}{\pi}\left(\cos\frac{\pi x}{2} - \frac{1}{3}\cos\frac{3\pi x}{2} + \frac{1}{5}\cos\frac{5\pi x}{5} - \ldots\right)$

27.8 HALF-RANGE SERIES

When we require to expand a function $f(x)$ in the range $(0, \pi)$ in a Fourier series of period 2π or more generally in the range $(0, l)$ in a Fourier series of period $2l$, a function $f(x)$ defined over the interval $0 < x < l$ is capable of two distinct half range series.

The half range cosine series is $f(x) = \dfrac{a_0}{2} + \sum\limits_{n=1}^{\infty} a_n \cos\dfrac{n\pi x}{l}$

where, $a_0 = \dfrac{2}{l}\int_0^l f(x).dx$, and $a_n = \dfrac{2}{l}\int_0^l f(x)\cos\dfrac{n\pi x}{l}dx$

The half range sine series is

$$f(x) = \sum_{n=1}^{\infty} b_n \sin\frac{n\pi x}{l}, \text{where } b_n = \frac{2}{l}\int_0^l f(x)\sin\frac{n\pi x}{l}dx$$

Solved Examples

1. *If* $f(x) = \begin{cases} x & ; \quad 0 < x < \pi/2 \\ \pi - x & ; \quad \pi/2 < x < \pi \end{cases}$

Show that

(*i*) $f(x) = \dfrac{4}{\pi}\left[\sin x - \dfrac{\sin 3x}{3^2} + \dfrac{\sin 5x}{5^2} - \dots\right]$

(*ii*) $f(x) = \dfrac{\pi}{4} - \dfrac{2}{\pi}\left[\dfrac{\cos 2x}{1^2} + \dfrac{\cos 6x}{3^2} + \dfrac{\cos 10x}{5^2} + \dots\right]$

SOLUTION. (i) Half range sine series, we have $l = \pi$ so

$$f(x) = \sum_{n=1}^{\infty} b_n \sin\frac{n\pi x}{\pi} = \sum_{n=1}^{\infty} b_n \sin nx$$

$$b_n = \frac{2}{\pi}\int_0^{\pi} f(x)\sin nx\,dx$$

$$= \frac{2}{\pi}\left[\int_0^{\pi/2} x\sin nx\,dx + \int_{\pi/2}^{\pi}(\pi - x)\sin nx\,dx\right]$$

$$= \frac{2}{\pi}\left[x\left(-\frac{\cos nx}{n}\right) - 1\left(-\frac{\sin nx}{n^2}\right)\right]_0^{\pi/2} + \frac{2}{\pi}\left[(\pi - x)\left(-\frac{\cos nx}{nx}\right) - (-1)\left(-\frac{\sin nx}{n^2}\right)\right]_0^{\pi}$$

$$= \frac{2}{\pi}\left[-\frac{\pi}{2n}\cos\frac{n\pi}{2} + \frac{1}{n^2}\sin\frac{n\pi}{2}\right] + \frac{2}{\pi}\left[\frac{\pi}{2n}\cos\frac{n\pi}{2} + \frac{1}{n^2}\sin\frac{n\pi}{2}\right]$$

$$= \frac{2}{\pi}\left[\frac{2}{n^2}\sin\frac{n\pi}{2}\right] = \frac{4}{\pi n^2}\sin\frac{n\pi}{2}$$

$$f(x) = \frac{4}{\pi}\left[\sin x - \frac{\sin 3x}{3^2} + \frac{\sin 5x}{5^2} - \dots\right]$$

(ii) Half range cosine series

Let $\quad f(x) = \dfrac{a_0}{2} + \sum\limits_{n=1}^{\infty} a_n \cos nx$

Then, $a_0 = \dfrac{2}{\pi}\int_0^{\pi} f(x)dx$

$$= \frac{2}{\pi}\left[\int_0^{\pi/2} x\,dx + \int_{\pi/2}^{\pi}(\pi - x)dx\right]$$

$$= \frac{2}{\pi}\left[\frac{x^2}{2}\right]_0^{\pi/2} + \left[\pi x - \frac{x^2}{2}\right]_{\pi/2}^{\pi}$$

$$= \frac{2}{\pi}\left[\frac{\pi^2}{8} + \left(\pi^2 - \frac{\pi^2}{2}\right) - \left(\frac{\pi^2}{2} - \frac{\pi^2}{8}\right)\right]$$

$$= \frac{2}{\pi}\left[\frac{\pi^2}{4}\right] = \frac{\pi}{2}$$

$$a_n = \frac{2}{\pi}\int_0^{\pi} f(x)\cos nx\,dx$$

$$= \frac{2}{\pi}\left[\int_0^{\pi/2} x\cos nx\,dx + \int_{\pi/2}^{\pi}(\pi - x)\cos nx\,dx\right]$$

$$= \frac{2}{\pi}\left[\frac{x\sin nx}{n} - 1\left(-\frac{\cos nx}{n^2}\right)\right]_0^{\pi/2} + \frac{2}{\pi}\left[(\pi - x)\frac{\sin nx}{n} - (-1)\left(-\frac{\cos nx}{n^2}\right)\right]_{\pi/2}^{\pi}$$

$$= \frac{2}{\pi}\left[\frac{\pi}{2n}\sin\frac{n\pi}{2} + \frac{1}{n^2}\cos\frac{n\pi}{2} - \frac{1}{n^2}\right] + \frac{2}{\pi}\left[-\frac{\cos n\pi}{n^2} - \frac{\pi}{2n}\sin\frac{n\pi}{2} + \frac{1}{n^2}\cos\frac{n\pi}{2}\right]$$

$$= \frac{2}{\pi}\left[\frac{2}{n^2}\cos\frac{n\pi}{2} - \frac{\cos n\pi}{n^2} - \frac{1}{n^2}\right]$$

$$= \frac{2}{\pi n^2}\left[2\cos\frac{n\pi}{2} - \cos n\pi - 1\right]$$

Put $n = 0, 1, 2, 3, \ldots$ in equation (1), we get

$a_1 = 0,$

$$a_2 = \frac{2}{\pi.2^2}(2\cos\pi - \cos 2\pi - 1) = \frac{-2}{1^2.\pi}$$

$a_3 = 0, a_4 = 0, a_5 = 0,$

$$a_6 = \frac{2}{6^2\pi}(2\cos 3\pi - \cos 6\pi - 1) = \frac{-2}{3^2\pi}$$

$a_7 = a_8 = a_9 = 0,$

$$a_{10} = \frac{2}{10^2.\pi}(2\cos 5\pi - \cos 10\pi - 1) = \frac{-2}{5^2\pi}$$

Hence, $$f(x) = \frac{\pi}{4} - \frac{2}{\pi}\left[\frac{\cos 2x}{1^2} + \frac{\cos 6x}{3^2} + \frac{\cos 10x}{5^2} + \ldots\right]$$

2. *Develop $\sin\frac{\pi x}{l}$ in half range cosine series in range $0 < x < l$.*

SOLUTION. Let $\sin\frac{\pi x}{l} = \frac{a_0}{2} + \sum_{n=1}^{\infty} a_n \cos\frac{n\pi x}{l}$

where,

$$a_0 = \frac{2}{l}\int_0^l \sin\frac{\pi x}{l}dx = \frac{2}{l}\left[-\frac{\cos(\pi x/l)}{\pi/l}\right]_0^l$$

$$= \frac{2}{\pi}[\cos\pi - 1] = \frac{4}{\pi}$$

and $$a_n = \frac{2}{l}\int_0^l \sin\frac{\pi x}{l}\cos\frac{n\pi x}{l}dx$$

$$= \frac{1}{l}\int_0^l\left[\sin(n+1)\frac{\pi x}{l} - \sin(n-1)\frac{\pi x}{l}\right]dx$$

$$= \frac{1}{l}\left[-\frac{\cos(n+1)\frac{\pi x}{l}}{(n+1)\pi/l} + \frac{\cos(n-1)\frac{\pi x}{l}}{(n-1)\pi/l}\right]_0^l$$

$$= \frac{1}{\pi}\left[-\frac{(-1)^{n+1}}{n+1} + \frac{(-1)^{n-1}}{n-1} + \frac{1}{n+1} - \frac{1}{n-1}\right]$$

(i) When n is odd

$$a_n = \frac{1}{\pi}\left[-\frac{1}{n+1} + \frac{1}{n-1} + \frac{1}{n+1} - \frac{1}{n-1}\right] = 0$$

(ii) When n is even

$$a_n = \frac{1}{\pi}\left[\frac{1}{n+1} - \frac{1}{n-1} + \frac{1}{n+1} - \frac{1}{n-1}\right]$$

$$= \frac{2}{\pi}\left[\frac{1}{n+1} - \frac{1}{n-1}\right]$$

$$= \frac{-4}{\pi(n+1)(n-1)}, n \neq 1$$

$$\therefore \sin\frac{\pi x}{l} = \frac{2}{\pi} - \frac{4}{\pi}\left[\frac{\cos\frac{2\pi x}{l}}{1.3} + \frac{\cos\frac{4\pi x}{l}}{3.5} + \frac{\cos\frac{6\pi x}{l}}{5.7} + \ldots\right]$$

3. *Obtain the half range sine series for function $f(x)=x^2$ in the interval $0<x<3$.*

SOLUTION. The Fouries half range sine series in the interval $(0, c)$ is given by

$$f(x) = \sum_{n=1}^{\infty} b_n \sin nx \qquad \ldots(1)$$

where, $b_n = \frac{2}{c}\int_0^c f(x)\sin\frac{n\pi x}{c}dx$

Here, $c = 3$ and $f(x) = x^2$

$$\therefore \quad b_n = \frac{2}{3}\int_0^3 x^2 \sin\frac{n\pi x}{3}dx$$

$$= \frac{2}{3}\left[x^2\left(\frac{-3}{n\pi}\right)\left(\cos\frac{n\pi x}{3}\right) + 2x\left(\frac{3}{n\pi}\right)\left(\frac{3}{n\pi}\right)\sin\frac{n\pi x}{3} - 2\left(\frac{3}{n\pi}\right)\left(\frac{3}{n\pi}\right)\left(\frac{3}{n\pi}\right)\cos\frac{n\pi x}{3}\right]_0^3$$

$$= \frac{2}{3}\left[\left\{-\frac{27}{n\pi}(-1)^n - \frac{54}{n^3\pi^3}(-1)^n\right\} + \frac{54}{n^3\pi^3}\right]$$

$$= \frac{2}{3}\left[\frac{54}{n^3\pi^3}\{1-(-1)^n\} - \frac{27}{n\pi}(-1)^n\right]$$

$$= \begin{cases} \frac{2}{3}\left(\frac{108}{n^3\pi^3} + \frac{27}{n\pi}\right) & , \text{ if } n \text{ is odd} \\ -\frac{18}{n\pi} & , \text{ if } n \text{ is even} \end{cases}$$

Hence, the required half range sine series is

$$f(x) = b_1 \sin x + b_2 \sin 2x + b_3 \sin 3x + ...$$

$$= \frac{2}{3}\left[\frac{108}{\pi^3}\left(\frac{\sin x}{1^3} + \frac{\sin 3x}{3^3} + \frac{\sin 5x}{5^3} + ...\right) + \frac{27}{\pi}\left(\frac{\sin x}{1} + \frac{\sin 3x}{3} + \frac{\sin 5x}{5} + ...\right) - \frac{18}{\pi}\left(\frac{\sin 2x}{2} + \frac{\sin 4x}{4} + ...\right)\right]$$

4. (i) *Express $f(x) = x$ as a half range sine series in $0 < x < 2$,*

(ii) *Express $f(x) = x$ as a half-range cosine series in $0 < x < 2$.*

SOLUTION. (i) The Fourier sine series For $F(x)$ in (0, 2) is $f(x) = \sum_{n=1}^{\infty} b_n \sin\frac{n\pi x}{2}$

where $b_n = \frac{2}{2}\int_0^2 f(x)\sin\frac{n\pi x}{2}dx$

$$= \int_0^2 x\sin\frac{n\pi x}{2}dx$$

$$= \left[-\frac{2x}{n\pi}\cos\frac{n\pi x}{2} + \frac{4}{n^2\pi^2}\sin\frac{n\pi x}{2}\right]_0^2$$

$$= \frac{-4(-1)^n}{n\pi}$$

$\Rightarrow b_1 = 4/\pi_1, b_2 = -4/2\pi,$

$b_3 = 4/3\pi, b_4 = -4/4\pi$, etc.

Required half range Fourier sine series

is $f(x) = \frac{4}{\pi}\left[\sin\frac{\pi x}{2} - \frac{1}{2}\sin\frac{2\pi x}{2} + \frac{1}{3}\sin\frac{3\pi x}{2} - \frac{1}{4}\sin\frac{4\pi x}{2} + ...\right]$

(ii) The Fourier cosine series for $f(x)$ in (0, 2) is

$$f(x) = \frac{a_0}{2} + \sum_{n=1}^{\infty} a_n \cos\frac{n\pi x}{2}$$

where $a_0 = \frac{2}{2}\int_0^2 f(x)dx = \int_0^2 x\,dx = 2$

and $a_n = \frac{2}{2}\int_0^2 f(x)\cos\frac{n\pi x}{2}dx$

$$= \int_0^2 x\cos\frac{n\pi x}{2}dx$$

$$= \left[\frac{2x}{n\pi}\sin\frac{n\pi x}{2} + \frac{4}{n^2\pi^2}\cos\frac{n\pi x}{2}\right]_0^2$$

$$= \frac{4}{n^2\pi^2}[(-1)^n - 1]$$

$\Rightarrow a_1 = -8/\pi^2, a_2 = 0, a_3 = -8/3^2\pi^2,$

$a_4 = 0, a_5 = -8/5^2\pi^2$, etc.

Required half range Fourier cosine series is given by

$$f(x) = 1 - \frac{8}{\pi^2}\left[\frac{\cos\pi\frac{x}{2}}{1^2} + \frac{\cos 3\pi\frac{x}{2}}{3^2} + \frac{\cos 5\pi\frac{x}{2}}{5^2} + ...\right].$$

5. *Obtain the half range sine series for e^x in $0 < x < 1$.*

SOLUTION. Let $e^x = \sum_{n=1}^{\infty} b_n \sin n\pi x \qquad [\because l = 1]$

Then,

$$b_n = 2\int_0^1 e^x \sin n\pi x\,dx$$

$$= 2\left[\frac{e^x}{1+(n\pi)^2}(\sin n\pi x - n\pi\cos n\pi x)\right]_0^1$$

$$= 2\left[\frac{e}{1+(n\pi)^2}(-n\pi\cos n\pi x) - \frac{1}{1+(n\pi)^2}(-n\pi)\right]$$

$$= \frac{2}{1+n^2\pi^2}[-en\pi(-1)^n + n\pi]$$

$$= \frac{2n\pi}{1+n^2\pi^2}[1-e(-1)^n]$$

Hence, $e^x = 2\pi\sum_{n=1}^{\infty}\frac{n[1-e(-1)^n]}{1+n^2\pi^2}$

$$= 2\pi\left[\frac{1+e}{1+\pi^2}\sin\pi x + \frac{2(1-e)}{1+4\pi^2}\sin 2\pi x + \frac{3(1+e)}{1+9\pi^2}\sin 3\pi x + ...\right]$$

6. *Expand*

$$f(x) = \begin{cases} \frac{1}{4} - x & ,\text{if } 0 < x < \frac{1}{2} \\ x - \frac{3}{4} & ,\text{if } \frac{1}{2} < x < 1 \end{cases}$$

as the Fourier series of sine terms.

SOLUTION. The Fourier sine series for $f(x)$ in (0, 1) is $f(x) = \sum_{n=1}^{\infty} b_n \sin n\pi x$

where, $b_n = \frac{2}{1}\int_0^1 f(x)\sin n\pi x\,dx$

$$= 2\left[\int_0^{1/2}\left(\frac{1}{4} - x\right)\sin n\pi x\,dx + \int_{1/2}^{1}\left(x - \frac{3}{4}\right)\sin n\pi x\,dx\right]$$

$$= 2\left|-\left(\frac{1}{4} - x\right)\frac{\cos n\pi x}{n\pi} - \frac{\sin n\pi x}{n\pi}\right|_0^{1/2} + 2\left|-\left(x - \frac{3}{4}\right)\frac{\cos n\pi x}{n\pi} + \frac{\sin n\pi x}{n^2\pi^2}\right|_{1/2}^{1}$$

$$= 2\left[\frac{1}{4n\pi}\cos\frac{n\pi}{2} + \frac{1}{4n\pi} - \frac{\sin n\pi/2}{n^2\pi^2}\right] + 2\left[-\frac{1}{4n\pi}\cos n\pi - \frac{1}{4n\pi}\cos\frac{n\pi}{2} - \frac{\sin n\pi/2}{n^2\pi^2}\right]$$

$$= \frac{1}{2n\pi}[1-(-1)^n] - \frac{4\sin n\pi/2}{n^2\pi^2}$$

$$\Rightarrow b_1 = \frac{1}{\pi} - \frac{4}{\pi^2}, b_2 = 0,$$

$$b_3 = \frac{1}{3\pi} + \frac{4}{3^2\pi^2},$$

$$b_4 = 0, b_5 = \frac{1}{5} - \frac{4}{5^2\pi^2}, b_6 = 0 \text{ etc.}$$

The required Fourier series is

$$f(x) = \left(\frac{1}{\pi} - \frac{4}{\pi^2}\right)\sin \pi x + \left(\frac{1}{3\pi} + \frac{4}{3^2\pi^2}\right)\sin 3\pi x + \left(\frac{1}{5\pi} - \frac{4}{5^2\pi^2}\right)\sin 5\pi x + \ldots.$$

27.9 PARSEVEL'S IDENTITY FOR FOURIER SERIES

Consider the Fourier series $\frac{a_0}{2} + \sum_{n=1}^{\infty}(a_n \cos nx + b_n \sin nx)$ *.If f(x) converges uniformly to f(x) at every point of the interval* $(0, 2\pi)$*, then*

$$\frac{1}{\pi}\int_0^{2\pi}\{f(x)\}^2 dx = \frac{a_0^2}{2} + \sum_{n=1}^{\infty}(a_n^2 + b_n^2)$$

Proof. Let the series $\frac{a_0}{2} + \sum_{n=1}^{\infty}(a_n \cos nx + b_n \sin nx)$ represent the Fourier series of $f(x)$. Also, let this series converges uniformly to $f(x)$ at every point of the interval $(0, 2\pi)$ so that

$$f(x) = \frac{a_0}{2} + \sum_{n=1}^{\infty}(a_n \cos nx + b_n \sin nx) \qquad \ldots(1)$$

and that term by term integration is possible.

To prove that $\frac{1}{\pi}\int_0^{2\pi}\{f(x)\}^2 dx = \frac{a_0^2}{2} + \sum(a_n^2 + b_n^2)$

We have $a_n = \frac{1}{\pi}\int_0^{2\pi} f(x).\cos nx\,dx \qquad (n = 0, 1, 2, 3, \ldots)$

$b_n = \frac{1}{\pi}\int_0^{2\pi} f(x).\sin nx\,dx \qquad (n = 0, 1, 2, 3 \ldots)$

Multiplying (1) by $f(x)$ and then integrating from $x=0$ to $x=2\pi$, we get

$$\int_0^{2\pi}\{f(x)\}^2 dx = \frac{a_0}{2} + \int_0^{2\pi} f(x)\,dx + \sum_{n=1}^{\infty}\left[a_n\int_0^{2\pi} f(x).\cos nx dx + b_n\int_0^{2\pi} f(x)\sin nx dx\right]$$

$$= \frac{a_0}{2}.\pi a_0 + \sum_{n=1}^{\infty} (\pi a_n^2 + \pi b_n^2)$$

Dividing by π, we get $\frac{1}{\pi}\int_0^{2\pi} \{f(x)\}^2 dx = \frac{a_0^2}{2} + \sum_{n=1}^{\infty} (a_n^2 + b_n^2)$.

Solved Examples

1. *Obtain the Fourier series expansion of $f(x) = x^2$ in $-\pi < x < \pi$ and prove that $\sum_{n=1}^{\infty} \frac{1}{n^4} = \frac{\pi^4}{90}$ by using Parsevel's theorem.*

SOLUTION. Since $f(x) = x^2$ is even function so $b_n = 0$

Let the Fourier series expansion of $f(x)$ is given by

$$f(x) = x^2 = \frac{a_0}{2} + \sum_{n=1}^{\infty} a_n \cos nx \quad ...(1)$$

where,

$$a_0 = \frac{2}{\pi}\int_0^{\pi} f(x)dx = \frac{2}{\pi}\int_0^{\pi} x^2 dx = \frac{2\pi^2}{3}$$

$$a_n = \frac{2}{\pi}\int_0^{\pi} f(x)\cos nx\, dx$$

$$= \frac{2}{\pi}\int_0^{\pi} x^2 \cos nx\, dx$$

$$\Rightarrow a_n = \frac{2}{\pi}\left[x^2 \frac{\sin nx}{n} + 2x.\frac{\cos nx}{n^2} - 2\frac{\sin nx}{n^2}\right]_0^{\pi}$$

$$= \frac{4(-1)^2}{n^2}$$

$\therefore$ (1) becomes,

$$x^2 = \frac{\pi^2}{3} + 4\sum_{n=1}^{\infty} \frac{(-1)^n \cos nx}{n^2} \quad ...(2)$$

which is the required Fourier expansion.

Now, by Parsevel's theorem, we have

$$\int_{-\pi}^{\pi} \{f(x)\}^2 dx = \pi\left[\frac{a_0^2}{2} + \sum_{n=1}^{\infty} (a_n^2 + b_n^2)\right]$$

Hence, $\int_{-\pi}^{\pi} x^4 dx = \pi\left[\frac{4\pi^4}{2.9} + \sum_{n=1}^{\infty} \frac{16}{n^4}\right]$

$$\Rightarrow \left(\frac{x^5}{5}\right)_{-\pi}^{\pi} = \frac{2\pi^5}{9} + \pi\sum_{n=1}^{\infty} \frac{16}{n^4}$$

or $$\frac{2\pi^5}{5} - \frac{2\pi^5}{9} = \pi\sum_{n=1}^{\infty} \frac{16}{n^4}$$

$$\Rightarrow \frac{\pi^4}{90} = \sum_{n=1}^{\infty} \frac{1}{n^4}.$$

2. *By using the sine series for $f(x) = 1$ in $0 < x < \pi$, show that*

$$\frac{\pi^2}{8} = 1 + \frac{1}{3^2} + \frac{1}{5^2} + \frac{1}{7^2} + ...$$

SOLUTION. The Fourier sine series for $f(x) = 1$ in $(0, \pi)$ is $f(x) = \Sigma\, b_n \sin nx$,

where, $b_n = \frac{2}{\pi}\int_0^{\pi} f(x)\sin nx\, dx$

$$= \frac{2}{\pi}\int_0^{\pi} (1).\sin nx dx = \frac{2}{\pi}\left(-\frac{\cos nx}{n}\right)_0^{\pi}$$

$$= -\frac{2}{n\pi}[\cos n\pi - 1] = -\frac{2}{n\pi}[(-1)^n - 1]$$

$$= \begin{cases} \frac{4}{n\pi} &, \text{ if } n \text{ is odd} \\ 0 &, \text{ if } n \text{ is even} \end{cases}$$

The Fourier sine series is

$$1 = \frac{4}{\pi}\sin x + \frac{4}{3\pi}\sin 3x + \frac{4}{5\pi}\sin 5x + \frac{4}{7\pi}\sin 7x + ...$$

By Parsevel's formula, we get

$$\int_0^{\pi} [f(x)]^2 dx = \frac{\pi}{2}[b_1^2 + b_2^2 + b_3^2 + b_4^2 + b_5^2 + ...]$$

$$\Rightarrow \int_0^{\pi} (1)^2 dx = \frac{\pi}{2}\left[\left(\frac{4}{\pi}\right)^2 + \left(\frac{4}{3\pi}\right)^2 + \left(\frac{4}{5\pi}\right)^2 + \left(\frac{4}{7\pi}\right)^2 + ...\right]$$

$$\Rightarrow [x]_0^{\pi} = \left(\frac{\pi}{2}\right)\left(\frac{16}{\pi^2}\right)\left[1 + \frac{1}{3^2} + \frac{1}{5^2} + \frac{1}{7^2} + ...\right]$$

$$\Rightarrow \pi = \frac{\pi}{2}\left(\frac{16}{\pi^2}\right)\left[1+\frac{1}{3^2}+\frac{1}{5^2}+\frac{1}{7^2}+\ldots\right]$$

Hence, $\frac{\pi^2}{8} = 1+\frac{1}{3^2}+\frac{1}{5^2}+\frac{1}{7^2}+\ldots.$

Exercise-27.4

1. Find the Fourier half range even expansion of the function $f(x)=(-x/l)+1, 0\le x\le l$.

2. Find a series of sines of multiples of x which will represent $f(x)$ in the interval $(0, \pi)$,

$$\text{where } f(x) = \begin{cases} \frac{1}{3}\pi & , \quad 0 < x < \frac{1}{3}\pi \\ 0 & , \quad \frac{1}{3}\pi < x < \frac{2}{3}\pi \\ -\frac{1}{3}\pi & , \quad \frac{2}{3} < x < \pi \end{cases}$$

Also, represent this function by a series of cosines of multiples of x as well. Draw graph of these series and find the sine and cosine series where $x = -\frac{1}{3}\pi, -\frac{2}{3}\pi, -\pi$

3. Find the half range cosine series for function $f(x) = (x-1)^2$ in the interval $0 < x < 1$. Hence show that

(i) $\frac{1}{1^2}+\frac{1}{2^2}+\frac{1}{3^2}+\frac{1}{4^2}+\ldots=\frac{\pi^2}{6}$,

(ii) $\frac{1}{1^2}-\frac{1}{2^2}+\frac{1}{3^2}-\frac{1}{4^2}+\ldots=\frac{\pi^2}{12}$,

(iii) $\frac{1}{1^2}+\frac{1}{3^2}+\frac{1}{5^2}+\frac{1}{7^2}+\ldots=\frac{\pi^2}{8}$.

4. If $f(x) = mx, \quad 0\le x\le \pi/2$
$\quad = m(\pi - x), \quad \pi/2 \le x \le \pi$

Then show that

$$f(x) = \frac{4m}{\pi}\left[\frac{\sin x}{1^2} - \frac{\sin 3\pi}{3^2} + \frac{\sin 5x}{5^2} - \ldots\right].$$

5. If $f(x) = \begin{cases} \frac{hx}{a} & , \quad 0 < x < a \\ \frac{h(l-x)}{l-a}, & a < x < l \end{cases}$

Prove that for all values of x between 0 and l

$$f(x) = \frac{2hl^2}{a(l-a)\pi^2}\left[\sin\frac{\pi a}{l}\sin\frac{\pi x}{l}\sin\frac{\pi x}{l} + \frac{1}{2^2}\sin\frac{2\pi a}{l}\sin\frac{2\pi x}{l}+\ldots\right].$$

6. Expand $\pi x - x^2$ is a half range sine series in the interval $(0, \pi)$ upto first three terms.

7. Obtain a half range cosine series for

$$f(x) = \begin{cases} kx & , \quad \text{for} \quad 0 \le x \le l/2 \\ k(l-x) & , \quad \text{for} \quad l/2 \le x \le l \end{cases}$$

Deduce the sum of the series $\frac{1}{1^2}+\frac{1}{3^2}+\frac{1}{5^2}+\ldots.$

8. Find the half range sine series for the function $f(t) = t - t^2$ in the interval $0 < t < 1$.

Hints to Selected Problems

1. $a_n = \frac{2}{l}\int_0^l f(x)\cos\frac{n\pi x}{l}dx$

$$= \frac{2}{l}\int_0^l \left(-\frac{x}{l}+1\right)\cos\frac{n\pi x}{l}dx$$

$$a_n = \frac{2}{l}\int_0^l f(x)\cos\frac{n\pi x}{l}dx$$

$$= \frac{2}{l}\int_0^l \left(-\frac{x}{l}+1\right)\cos\frac{n\pi x}{l}dx$$

$$= \frac{2}{l}\left[\left(-\frac{x}{l}+1\right)\left(\frac{l}{n\pi}\sin\frac{n\pi x}{l}\right) - \left(-\frac{1}{l}\right)\left(-\frac{l^2}{n^2\pi^2}\cos\frac{n\pi x}{l}\right)\right]_0^l$$

$$= \frac{2}{l}\left[0 - \frac{l}{n^2\pi^2}\cos n\pi + \frac{l}{n^2\pi^2}\right] = \frac{2}{n^2\pi^2}[1-(-1)^n]$$

$$= \begin{cases} \frac{4}{n^2\pi^2} & , \quad \text{when } n \text{ is odd} \\ 0 & , \quad \text{when } n \text{ is odd} \end{cases}$$

and $b_n = 0$

$$f(x) = \frac{1}{2} + \frac{4}{\pi^2}\left[\frac{1}{1^2}\cos\frac{\pi x}{l} + \frac{1}{3^2}\cos\frac{3\pi x}{l} + \frac{1}{5^2}\cos\frac{5\pi x}{l}+\ldots\right].$$

2. $b_n = \frac{2}{\pi}\int_0^\pi f(v)\sin nv dv$

$$= \frac{2}{\pi}\left[\int_0^{\pi/2}\frac{\pi}{3}\sin nv dv + \int_{\pi/3}^{2\pi/3} 0.\sin nv\,dv + \int_{2\pi/3}^{\pi} -\frac{\pi}{3}.\sin nv dv\right]$$

$$= \frac{2}{3}\left[-\frac{\cos nv}{n}\right]_0^{\pi/3} - \frac{2}{3}\left[-\frac{\cos nv}{n}\right]_{2\pi/3}^{\pi}$$

$$= \frac{2}{3n}\left[1 - \cos\frac{n\pi}{3} + \cos n\pi - \cos\frac{2n\pi}{3}\right]$$

$$= -\frac{8}{3n}\sin\frac{n\pi}{6}\sin\frac{n\pi}{3}.\cos\frac{n\pi}{2}$$

$$f(x) = -\frac{8}{3}\sum_{n=1}^{\infty}\frac{1}{n}\sin\frac{n\pi}{6}\sin\frac{n\pi}{3}\cos\frac{n\pi}{2}\sin nx$$

$$=\frac{1}{2}\left[\frac{1}{2}\sin 2x+\frac{1}{2}\sin 4x+\frac{1}{3}\sin 3x+\frac{1}{10}\sin 10x+...\right]$$

$$a_0=\frac{1}{\pi}\int_0^{\pi} f(v)dv$$

$$=\frac{1}{\pi}\int_0^{\pi/3}\frac{\pi}{3}dv+\int_{\pi/3}^{2\pi/3}0.dv+\int_{2\pi/3}^{\pi}-\frac{\pi}{3}dv=0$$

$$a_n=\frac{2}{\pi}\int_0^{\pi} f(v)\cos nv\,dv$$

$$=\frac{2}{\pi}\left[\int_0^{\pi/3}\frac{\pi}{3}.\cos nvdv+\int_{\pi/3}^{2\pi/3}0.dv+\int_{2\pi/3}^{\pi/3}-\frac{\pi}{3}.\cos nv\,dv\right]$$

$$=\frac{2}{3n}\left[\sin\frac{n\pi}{3}+\sin\frac{2n\pi}{3}\right]=\frac{4}{3n}\sin\frac{n\pi}{2}\cos\frac{n\pi}{6}$$

$$f(x)=\frac{4}{3}\sum_{n=1}^{\infty}\frac{1}{n}\cos\frac{n\pi}{6}\sin\frac{n\pi}{2}.\cos nx$$

$$=\frac{2}{\sqrt{3}}\left[\cos x-\frac{1}{5}\cos 5x+\frac{1}{7}\cos 7x-\frac{1}{11}\cos 11x+...\right]$$

6. $b_n=\frac{2}{\pi}\int_0^{\pi}(\pi x-x^2)\sin x\,dx$

$$=\frac{2}{\pi}\left[(\pi x-x^2)\left(-\frac{\cos nx}{n}\right)-(\pi-2x).\left(-\frac{\sin nx}{n^2}\right)+(-2)\left(\frac{\cos nx}{n^3}\right)\right]_0^{\pi}$$

$$=\frac{2}{\pi}\left[-\frac{2\cos n\pi}{n^3}+\frac{2}{n^3}\right]$$

$$=\frac{4}{\pi n^3}[1-(-1)^n]=0 \text{ or } \frac{8}{n\pi^3}$$

according as n is even or odd

$$\pi x-x^2=\frac{8}{\pi}\left(\sin x+\frac{\sin 3x}{3^3}+\frac{\sin 5x}{5^3}+...\right).$$

7. $a_0=\frac{2}{l}\int_0^l f(x)dx$

$$=\frac{2}{l}\left[\int_0^{l/2}kxdx+\int_{l/2}^{l}k(l-x)dx\right]=\frac{kl}{2}$$

$$a_n=\frac{2}{l}\left[\int_0^{l/2}k.x\cos\frac{n\pi x}{l}dx+\int_{l/2}^{l}k(l-x)\frac{\cos n\pi x}{l}dx\right]$$

$$=\frac{2kl}{n^2\pi^2}\left[2\cos\frac{n\pi}{2}-1-\cos n\pi\right]$$

When n is odd, $\cos\frac{n\pi}{2}=0$ and $\cos n\pi=-1$,

$\Rightarrow a_n=0\Rightarrow a_1=a_3=a_5=...=0$

When n is even,

$$a_2=\frac{2kl}{2^2\pi^2}[2\cos\pi-1-\cos 2\pi]=-\frac{8kl}{2^2\pi^2}$$

$$a_4=\frac{2kl}{4^2\pi^2}[2\cos 2\pi-1-\cos 4\pi]=0$$

$$a_6=\frac{2kl}{6^2\pi^2}[2\cos 3\pi-1-\cos 6\pi]$$

$$=\frac{2kl}{6^2\pi^2}(-2-1-1)=-\frac{8kl}{6^2\pi^2} \text{ and so on}$$

$$f(x)=\frac{kl}{4}-\frac{8kl}{\pi^2}\left[\frac{1}{2^2}\cos\frac{2\pi x}{l}+\frac{1}{6^2}\cos\frac{6\pi x}{l}+...\right] \quad ...(1)$$

Putting $x=1, f(x)=0$

From (1), we have $0=\frac{kl}{4}-\frac{8kl}{\pi^2}\left(\frac{1}{2^2}+\frac{1}{6^2}+...\right)$

$$\frac{1}{2^2}+\frac{1}{6^2}+...=\frac{\pi^2}{32}$$

$$\Rightarrow\ \frac{1}{2^2}\left(\frac{1}{1^2}+\frac{1}{3^2}+...\right)...=\frac{\pi^2}{32}.$$

Hence $\frac{1}{1^2}+\frac{1}{3^2}+...=\frac{\pi^2}{8}$

ANSWERS

1. $f(x)=\frac{1}{2}+\frac{4}{\pi^2}\left[\frac{1}{1^2}\cos\frac{\pi x}{l}+\frac{1}{3^2}\cos\frac{3\pi x}{l}+\frac{1}{5^2}\cos\frac{5\pi x}{l}+...\right]$

2. $f(x)=\frac{1}{2}\left[\frac{1}{2}\sin 2x+\frac{1}{2}\sin 4x+\frac{1}{8}\sin 8x+\frac{1}{10}\sin 10x...\right]$

and $f(x)=\frac{2}{\sqrt{3}}\left[\cos x-\frac{1}{5}\cos 5x+\frac{1}{7}\cos 7x-\frac{1}{11}\cos 11x+...\right]$

3. $\frac{1}{3}+\frac{4}{\pi^2}\left(\cos\pi x+\frac{\cos 2\pi x}{2^2}+\frac{\cos 3\pi x}{3^2}+...\right)$ **6.** $\pi x-x^2=\frac{8}{\pi}\left(\sin x+\frac{\sin 3x}{3^2}+\frac{\sin 5x}{5^3}+...\right)$

7. $\frac{2kl}{n^2\pi^2}\left[2\cos\frac{n\pi}{2}-1-\cos n\pi\right]$ **8.** $f(t)=\frac{a}{2}+\frac{2a}{\pi}\left[\sin x+\frac{1}{3}\sin 3x+\frac{1}{5}\sin 5x+\frac{1}{7}\sin 7x+...\right]$

□□□□□□

Index

A

C

D